MICROBIOLOGY SECOND EDITION

MICHAEL J. TAUSSIG
MA PhD
Principal Scientific Officer,
Department of Immunology,
Institute of Animal Physiology,
Babraham, Cambridge; and former
Fellow of Trinity College,
University of Cambridge

PADDINGTON COLLEGE LIBRARY
PADDINGTON GREEN
LONDON W2 1NB

D0248509

Blackwell Scientific Publications
OXFORD LONDON
EDINBURGH BOSTON MELBOURNE

© 1984 by Blackwell Scientific Publications
Editorial offices:
Osney Mead, Oxford, OX2 0EL
8 John Street, London, WC1N 2ES
9 Forrest Road, Edinburgh, EH1 2QH
52 Beacon Street, Boston, Massachusetts 02108, USA
99 Barry Street, Carlton, Victoria 3053, Australia

All rights reserved. No part of this publication may
be reproduced, stored in a retrieval system, or
transmitted, in any form or by any means,
electronic, mechanical, photocopying, recording or
otherwise without the prior permission of the
copyright owner

First published 1979
Reprinted 1980
Italian translation 1982
Second edition 1984

Set by Setrite Typesetters Ltd,
Hong Kong and
printed and bound in Great Britain
by Butler & Tanner Ltd
Frome, Somerset

DISTRIBUTORS

USA
    Blackwell Mosby Book Distributors
    11830 Westline Industrial Drive
    St Louis, Missouri 63141

Canada
    Blackwell Mosby Book Distributors
    120 Melford Drive, Scarborough
    Ontario, M1B 2X4

Australia
    Blackwell Scientific Book Distributors
    31 Advantage Road, Highett
    Victoria 3190

British Library
Cataloguing in Publication Data

Taussig, Michael J.
    Processes in pathology and microbiology. — 2nd ed.
    1. Pathology
    I. Title
    616.07   RB111

    ISBN 0-632-01206-4

PADDINGTON
COLLEGE LIBRARY.
Date   5.3.85.
Acc. No.   38377
Class No.   616.07

FOR HANNA, GURION AND
AURELL, AND
IN MEMORY OF
GEORGE, ALMA AND MOSHE

CONTENTS

PREFACE TO SECOND EDITION

Those familiar with *Processes in Pathology* will realise that this edition is almost twice as long as its predecessor, an increase largely explained by the expanded scope of the book, which now includes medical microbiology as well as general pathology. A shortcoming of the first edition was that it did not fully explore the events in infectious disease, concentrating on host responses (inflammation, immune response) to the exclusion of the other side of the host/pathogen relationship. I have tried to correct this imbalance by adding two new sections dealing with virology and bacteriology respectively, and some parasitology has also been incorporated into the 'immune response' section. The new Section 3 is a systematic account of medical virology, including viral structure and replication and a description of the major virus families infecting man. Section 4, also new, covers medical bacteriology, and here the emphasis is on factors determining pathogenicity. Thus, considerable space is devoted to the mechanisms of toxin action and to bacterial genetics, both areas where there have been many exciting recent advances, as well as prokaryotic structure in relation to pathogenicity. In describing bacterial genera of medical importance, I have tried to explain as far as possible how principles of pathogenicity operate in the human host. By bringing together medical microbiology and general pathology between the same covers, I hope the book now provides the student with a fairly comprehensive guide to disease processes.

The contents of the first edition have also been enlarged and brought up to date in several areas. In Section 1 (Inflammation) I have added a subsection on leucocyte chemotaxis, introduced the recent progress in the roles of prostaglandins and leukotrienes, and added accounts of C-reactive protein and amyloid. Progress in immunological research has continued apace since the book first appeared and among other revisions to Section 2 I have included the recent exciting discoveries in immunoglobulin genetics, monoclonal antibody (hybridoma) technology, the increased understanding of the functions of the major histocompatibility complex, and the role of leukotrienes in anaphylaxis. In the neoplasia section, some rewriting has been necessary to take account of recent research into the molecular biology of transformation; the carcinogenic properties of asbestos and hepatitis B virus, both subjects of much current interest, are also discussed more fully than before. The sections on the circulation and genetics of disease have also been revised within their existing frameworks.

I am greatly indebted to several colleagues and friends for reading parts of the new manuscript or providing photographs, and to others who have given most generously of their time, advice and photographic material. My chief advisor and critic has again been Dr Donald Kellaway (Department of Pathology, Cambridge), who has been an invaluable source of help on all matters pathological, as well as a kind and dear friend. He bore the brunt of reading the manuscript and for his countless hints and suggestions I will be eternally grateful. For Section 3, I am particularly thankful to Dr June Almeida (Wellcome Research Laboratories) for many superb electron micrographs; Professor Robert Horne (John Innes Institute) for making available photographs of his models of adenovirus and herpesvirus, as well as for electron micrographs and for reading part of the text; Dr Hugh Field (Department of Pathology, Cambridge) for occupying a Christmas holiday with reading the entire section and making many valuable suggestions; Dr David Secher (MRC Laboratory of Molecular Biology, Cambridge) for help with interferon; Dr Derek Wight (Department of Pathology, Cambridge) for advice on hepatitis viruses; Dr Brian Mahey (Department of Pathology, Cambridge) for bringing me up to date on influenza viruses, as well as other kind advice; Dr Margaret Periera (Central Public Health Laboratory, London), for information on nomenclature of influenza viruses; Dr Fred Brown (Animal Virus Research Institute, Pirbright) for electron micrographs of rabies virus; and not least to Dr Alfred Glücksmann (Babraham) for reading the text and making several useful suggestions. For Section 4, I am grateful to Dr Ed Munn (Babraham) for electron micrographs of flagella; Dr Peter Walker (Wellcome Research Laboratories) for the electron micrograph of enterobacteria; Dr Audrey Glauert (Strangeways Research Laboratory, Cambridge) for electron micrographs of platelets reacting with endotoxin and for discussion of other topics; Dr John Gordon (Babraham) for advice on the reaction of platelets with endotoxin; Dr Mike Smith (Babraham) for correcting me on the effects of cholera toxin on intestinal cells; Dr Ann Silver (Babraham) for help with neurotoxins; and Dr Derek Symons, for reading the passage on endotoxin. For the revisions to Section 1, I thank Dr Jeremy Pearson (Babraham) for electron micrographs of leucocyte emigration; Dr Mark Pepys (Royal Postgraduate Medical School, London) for correcting the text on C-reactive protein and amyloid; and Dr Basil Herbertson (Department of Pathology, Cambridge) for general comments. For Section 2, expert advice was sought from Dr David White (Department of Surgery, Cambridge) on cyclosporin A; Dr Richard Binns (Babraham) on lymphocyte recirculation and rosette formation; Professor Nevin Hughes-Jones (Babraham) on anti-Rh antibodies and complement activation; Dr Arnold Feinstein and Mr Neil Richardson (Babraham) on immunoglobulin structure (they also provided the photograph of the IgG model); and Mr Leslie Wright (Babraham) on monoclonal antibodies to progesterone. For Section 5, Dr Gordon was again most helpful on the subject of platelets, and the electron micrographs of cell junctions in Section 6 were very kindly provided by Dr Peter Wooding (Babraham). I would like to express particular appreciation to Dr Mary MacDonald (Department of Pathology, University of Edinburgh) for her extensive comments on the first edition, many of which have now been incorporated. I would also like to thank the various sources of published photographic material, as acknowledged in figure legends. My thanks also to Dr Bill Mason (Babraham) for initiating me into word processing, Mr Andrew Holliman (Babraham) for several helpful suggestions, and Mrs Joan Payne for occasional typing. Finally, my students, in recent years mostly from Newnham College and Corpus Christi College, have rarely hesitated to offer their critical appraisal of 'the book', as well as keeping me in tune with their scientific needs.

It is a pleasure to express my gratitude to Blackwell Scientific Publications Ltd., especially to Mr John Robson (Production Manager) and his assistant, Miss Caroline Hawes. In addition to their natural courtesy, they have also been efficiency personified. My thanks also to Mr Per Saugman for his sympathetic co-operation over several years.

Writing a textbook, although arduous, is instructive for the author, but seldom amusing for his family. Mine have tolerated the antisocial working hours with good grace and to them I offer my thanks, apologies, and the dedication of this book.

SECTION 1   INFLAMMATION

Introduction

Inflammation is the response of living tissue to injury. It is a fundamental pathological process, in Florey's words 'the backbone of pathology'. The term covers the progressive changes which occur when a tissue is damaged, but not destroyed, from the time of the original injury to final healing. Inflammation is thus a process not a state. The stimuli which give rise to inflammation may be physical, as in a cut or a burn, or chemical, after contact with noxious substances; they may be bacterial, as in infection by pathogenic micro-organisms, or immunological, in the conditions known as hypersensitivity. The basic events which follow these diverse stimuli, however, are generally similar. The end results of inflammation are often beneficial in that the inflammatory response leads, as far as possible, to the return of tissues to normal functioning after physical and chemical injury, and is a main line of defence against pathogenic microbes. A beneficial outcome is not always the case, however; inflammation can lead to fibrous scarring and, especially where hypersensitivity is involved, the inflammatory response can itself be a major cause of tissue damage.

Terminology

The occurrence of inflammation in a tissue or organ is indicated by the suffix *-itis*, as in appendicitis, meningitis, glomerulonephritis, and so forth. Inflammation is divided on the basis of duration into *acute* and *chronic*: acute inflammation lasts for hours or days, while chronic inflammation persists for weeks or months.

The stimuli which give rise to acute or chronic inflammation and the course of events in each are often sufficiently distinctive to justify describing the acute and chronic process separately.

ACUTE INFLAMMATION

Main features of acute inflammation

The major or 'cardinal' signs of acute inflammation have been recognised for literally thousands of years. Celsus (30 B.C.−A.D. 38) formulated them as *rubor* (redness), *tumor* (swelling), *calor* (heat) and *dolor* (pain). To these is generally added *functio laesa* (loss of function) traditionally ascribed to Galen (A.D. 130−200). The understanding of the biological changes underlying these signs had to wait for detailed microscopic observations, the pioneering description being that of Cohnheim (1882). The main features of acute inflammation which he described in the tongue or foot-web of the frog hold good for inflammation as it occurs in many different situations in the human body. They may be summarised as follows.

1   Dilatation of blood vessels in the injured area. As a result, flow of blood through the area is at first greatly increased, though with time the loss of fluid from the blood leads to progressive reduction in blood flow.

2 Increased permeability of vessel walls to protein. Blood vessel walls normally permit the free passage of water and low molecular weight solutes, but are only slightly permeable to plasma proteins. This permeability is increased during inflammation and leads to the accumulation of a protein-rich fluid termed the *inflammatory exudate*, in the extravascular space.

3 Emigration of white blood cells from the blood vessels into the exudate. Typically, leucocytes line up on the inner surface of the blood vessel, a process known as *pavementing* or *margination*, pass through the vessel wall between endothelial cells, and then migrate by amoeboid movement through the extravascular space towards the site of injury.

Thus acute inflammation is essentially a vascular phenomenon and all the changes which occur, including pavementing and emigration of leucocytes, are consequences of the primary vascular responses. The outward signs of inflammation can also be explained on this basis. Redness and heat are both due to increased blood flow through the inflamed area resulting from vasodilatation. Swelling is caused by the accumulation of exudate. Pain is the result of the increase in tissue tension and the action of chemical substances released during inflammation. Swelling, pain and cell death can lead to loss of function of the inflamed part.

The triple response

Clearly, vascular changes play a major role in acute inflammation. The triple response, described first by Lewis (1927), is often used as an example of the vascular changes in the skin to mild mechanical injury. It can readily be produced by a firm stroke with a ruler on the forearm or back. An immediate reddening or flush occurs at the site of injury; a zone of redness, known as a *flare*, then spreads outwards from the injured area; finally, a swelling or *weal* develops inside the injured area. The reaction reaches its peak within a few minutes of the injury being given. The triple response illustrates three of the cardinal signs — redness, heat and swelling. Briefly, the mechanism is as follows. As a result of the injury, various chemical substances, termed the *chemical mediators* of inflammation and including vasoactive amines and kinins (p. 28) are released locally. Their immediate effect is to cause vasodilatation at the site of the injury, producing the observed flush. The flare which follows, an area of surrounding vasodilatation, is of nervous origin and is due to an axon reflex which results from stimulation of local nerve endings in the skin by the chemical mediators. In acute inflammation in general, however, the nervous contribution is not considered vital, since the main features of inflammation can occur in denervated tissue. The weal is the result of local increased permeability of the blood vessels, again caused by chemical mediators, resulting in local accumulation of a fluid exudate.

The small blood vessels

The arterioles, capillaries and venules of the microcirculation are the blood vessels mainly involved in inflammation. The dilatation of local vessels is an essential early feature of acute inflammation. After very brief initial contraction, the arteriolar walls relax to increase blood flow. In the case of capillaries, which in their normal state often contain plasma but not red cells, the term dilatation really means the relaxation of precapillary sphincters to allow them to fill with blood. The basic structure of capillaries consists of a layer of endothelium surrounded by a basement membrane and pericapillary cells (Figure 1.1). An important feature of the vessel wall shown in Figure 1.1 is the intercellular junction between endothelial cells. These junctions are normally closed, but during inflammation they separate to produce gaps between the endothelial cells, which can be visualised by electron microscopy as shown in Figure 1.2. The gaps, which form under the influence of the chemical mediators of inflammation, are the physical basis of increased permeability of capillaries and venules during inflammation and permit the rapid movement of fluid from the blood into the tissue. Exudation of fluid and leucocyte emigration take place from capillaries and postcapillary venules.

Normal tissue fluid and exudate

It is important here to understand the mechanism of formation of normal tissue fluid. This was described by Starling as the result of a balance between the hydrostatic pressure at the arteriolar end of a tissue blood supply tending to force water out of the blood vessels, and the resulting increased osmotic pressure of the blood, due principally to the plasma proteins, which tends to draw water back into the vessels from the tissues at the venous end. This is illustrated in Figure 1.3a. It is important to note that under normal circumstances, the capillaries allow water, salts and solute

Figure 1.1 Cross-section of a capillary as seen in the electron microscope (at about ×20,000 magnification).

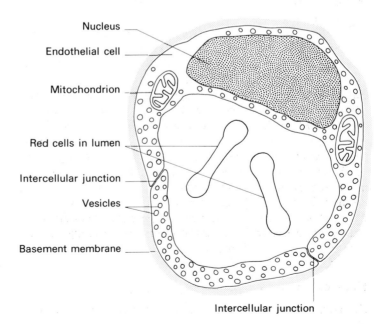

Nucleus

Endothelial cell

Mitochondrion

Red cells in lumen

Intercellular junction

Vesicles

Basement membrane

Intercellular junction

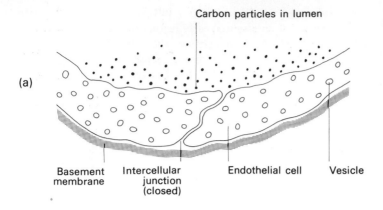

Carbon particles in lumen

(a)

Basement membrane | Intercellular junction (closed) | Endothelial cell | Vesicle

Figure 1.2 Wall of small blood vessel (a) in normal state, and (b) in inflammation. Carbon particles have been injected to demonstrate permeability change (as seen in electron micrographs, approximately ×30,000).

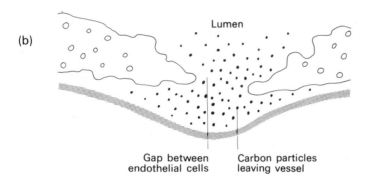

(b)

Lumen

Gap between endothelial cells | Carbon particles leaving vessel

up to molecular weight of about 10,000 to pass freely into the surrounding tissue; they are only very slightly permeable to plasma proteins, which have molecular weights considerably higher than 10,000. The accumulation of excess tissue fluid will result if the vessels become more permeable to proteins, since the difference in osmotic pressure between tissue fluid and blood will disappear and water will cease to return at the venous end (Figure 1.3b). The presence of excess fluid in tissues is known as *oedema*, of which inflammatory exudate is a particular example. (Other examples of oedema can be found in Section 5.) In addition to the increased permeability to protein via gaps in the endothelial wall, it can be shown that there is a local increase in the hydrostatic pressure inside the blood vessels in inflammation, which doubtless also contributes to exudate formation. The amount of protein in the exudate is variable. In mild inflammation, exudate tends to be watery with a low protein content, as exemplified by a blister. This is termed *serous* exudation. In more severe acute inflammation, a protein-rich *fibrinous* exudation takes place, with clotting of the exudate through formation of fibrin from fibrinogen it contains. Good examples occur in the alveoli of the lungs in lobar pneumonia and in the pericardium in fibrinous pericarditis. A third type of exudation, in which pus is formed, *suppurative* or *purulent* exudation, is described on page 26.

Figure 1.3 Exchange of fluid across walls of small blood vessels (a) under normal conditions, and (b) in acute inflammation.

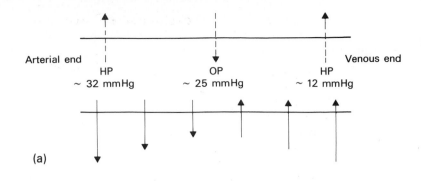

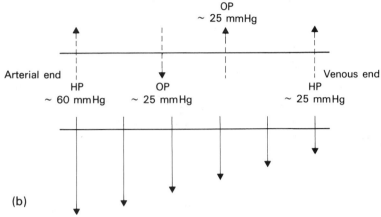

(b)

HP = Hydrostatic pressure of blood over that of extracellular fluid
OP = Osmotic pressure of plasma proteins
-- -→ Direction of pressure
——→ Net movement of fluid

Functions of exudate

The inflammatory exudate has several important functions, particularly in relation to infection by pathogenic bacteria. Bacteria often produce tissue-damaging toxins which will be diluted by the exudate. As noted above, the exudate frequently clots, with deposition of fibrin which creates a mechanical obstruction to the spread of bacteria. Other very important protein components of exudate are the gamma globulins which include the *antibodies* to neutralise toxins (antitoxins) and assist in the uptake of bacteria by phagocytic cells (opsonins, described further below). Finally, the exudate is continuously drained off by the lymphatic vessels, and antigens such as bacteria and their toxins are thereby carried to the lymph nodes where immune responses can be mounted.

Lymphatics

The draining of the exudate during acute inflammation and resolution takes place mainly through the lymphatic system. The lymphatic vessels form an extensive network in practically all the

7

tissues of the body. In the tissues themselves, the terminal lymphatics are blind-ending, thin-walled tubes with a wall of endothelium and basement membrane very similar to the blood vessels of the microcirculation. The colourless fluid they contain—lymph—drains from them into larger collecting lymphatics, eventually to still larger collecting channels and finally into the thoracic duct or the right lymph duct. These in turn discharge into veins at the root of the neck. Situated on the path from terminal lymphatics to the thoracic duct are the lymph nodes, about which more will be said in Section 2. Part of the function of the lymph nodes is to act as filters of the lymph, removing foreign proteins, particles, bacteria, etc., and initiating immune responses to them.

In normal tissues the function of lymphatics is to drain the extracellular fluid as it forms, eventually returning it and the small amount of protein it contains, to the blood. In acute inflammation, lymphatic drainage is greatly increased in volume and richer in protein. Despite their thin-walled structure, lymphatics do not collapse as the pressure of the inflammatory exudate on them increases; instead they are held open by fine fibres attached to the vessel wall, which stretch as the tissue fills with exudate. Protein enters lymphatics through gaps between adjacent endothelial cells, in much the same way as it leaves the blood vessels. Bacteria are often transported in the lymph to the local lymph nodes. Virulent organisms, such as *Streptococcus pyogenes*, may cause inflammation in the walls of lymphatic vessels, which can then be seen as thin red streaks in the skin extending from the focus of infection (*lymphangiitis*); acute inflammation in the lymph nodes also frequently occurs, resulting in painful swelling of the nodes (*lymphadenitis*). This latter process greatly increases the filtering capacity of the node by jamming the sinus channels with neutrophils and later with macrophages.

Migration of leucocytes into the exudate

In addition to proteins, the main component of inflammatory exudate is cellular, the most prominent cell types involved being the neutrophil polymorphonuclear leucocytes (neutrophils) and macrophages (derived from blood monocytes). The cellular component is most pronounced in bacterial infection, especially with pyogenic (pus-forming) organisms such as *Streptococcus pyogenes* and *Staphylococcus aureus*, and rather less in purely physical injury. We have seen that, as a result of initial vaso-dilatation, the blood flow through an area of inflammation is at first much increased. Typically, the cellular components of the blood are found centrally in the bloodstream (axial flow) while the plasma flows peripherally and adjacent to the vessel wall. With time, the loss of plasma through the endothelium, due to its increased permeability, causes a slowing of the blood flow, which in turn results in more contact between blood cells and the endothelium of the vessel. It is then observed that leucocytes adhere to the endothelium, the inner surface of which may eventually become lined with a layer of adherent leucocytes (pavementing of leucocytes) as shown in Figure 1.4a. Since this process is only observed during inflammation, it has been asumed in the past that a change in the endothelium renders it 'sticky' for leucocytes at this time. However, tissue culture studies show that neutrophils have a natural tendency to stick to normal endothelium (Figure 1.5a); thus to some extent at least, the adherence which occurs during inflammation is probably due simply to the increased opportunity for neutrophils to make contact with the

Figure 1.4 Emigration of leucocytes in inflammation, drawn after electron micrographs. (a) Margination (pavementing) of neutrophil polymorphonuclear leucocytes; (b) and (c) stages in emigration.

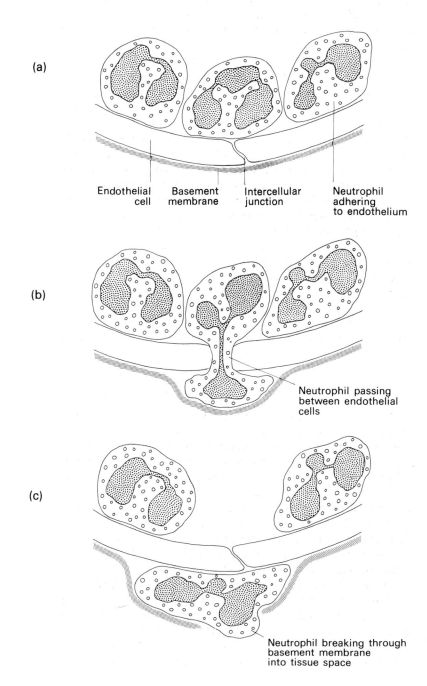

(a)

Endothelial cell Basement membrane Intercellular junction Neutrophil adhering to endothelium

(b)

Neutrophil passing between endothelial cells

(c)

Neutrophil breaking through basement membrane into tissue space

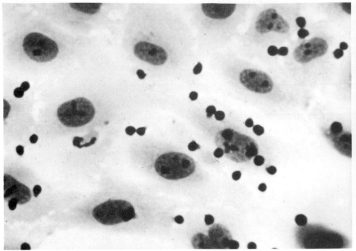

(a)

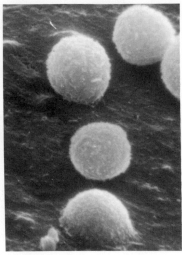

(b)

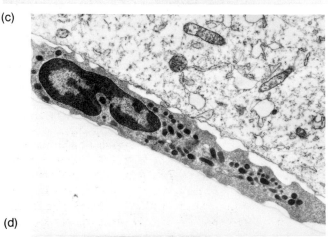

(c)

(d)

Figure 1.5 The interaction between neutrophils and endothelial cells as observed in culture.

(a) Adherence of blood neutrophils to a layer of cultured endothelial cells grown on the surface of a culture dish. The large grey ovals are nuclei of endothelial cells, with prominent nucleoli; the small dark circles are neutrophils adherent to the upper surface of the endothelial cell layer. On the left of the field is a neutrophil in which the multilobed nucleus is visible; this cell is underneath the endothelial layer, having migrated through an intercellular junction and become spread out in the process.

(b) Scanning electron microscopy of adherent neutrophils on the endothelial surface (×2,000).

(c) Emigration of a neutrophil between two endothelial cells as seen by transmission electron microscopy of a thin section (×8,000).

(d) A neutrophil, having completed its emigration, spread out underneath an endothelial cell (×8,000).

(Courtesy of Dr J.E. Beesley and Dr J.D. Pearson.)

vessel wall as blood flow slows. Nevertheless, adherence is increased during acute inflammation by chemical mediators such as leukotrienes (p. 35). Adherence is calcium-dependent and selective for certain cell types—neutrophils and monocytes adhere to endothelium whereas lymphocytes, which are not generally found in acute inflammatory exudates, do not. The adherent cells are rounded and at this stage easily mistaken for lymphocytes under the light microscope or scanning electron microscope (Figure 1.5a, b).

Having adhered, neutrophils and monocytes actively traverse the vessel wall, a process known as *emigration* (Figure 1.4b, c). It has been shown by electron microscopy that leucocytes pass between endothelial cells by thrusting a pseudopodium into the intercellular junction and then flowing through in amoeboid fashion (Figure 1.5c). Gaps are not required for leucocyte emigration. (Emigration of leucocytes is sometimes called 'diapedesis', which would seem a very appropriate description; however, the original meaning of diapedesis is the passive extrusion of *red cells* from the vessels under pressure during acute inflammation, e.g. in lobar pneumonia, the red cells being forced through the intercellular junctions in the wake of leucocytes.) Having penetrated the endothelium, the emigrating cell finds itself 'spread out' in the narrow space between the endothelium and the basement membrane (Figure 1.5a, d); it moves within this space until it is able to penetrate the basement membrane and continue its migration towards the site of the inflammatory stimulus.

Chemotaxis

The movement of leucocytes in the extravascular space is directional, towards the site of injury, and is the result of *chemotaxis*—the movement of cells along a gradient of concentration of an attractant. Various components of inflammation can be shown to attract neutrophils, including bacterial products, extracts of thermally injured skin, products of neutrophils and mast cells (*leukotrienes*, p. 35), and factors derived from the blood plasma, especially those of the *complement* system (p. 30). Chemotaxis is vital in bringing neutrophils and monocytes to the site of tissue damage, since without an attractive stimulus the distribution of leucocytes in the tissue would be random. Chemotaxis is studied in a Boyden chamber, in which a suspension of leucocytes is separated from the chemotactic substance by a micropore filter. To cross the filter, the cells must pass actively through its pores, which only happens under chemotactic attraction. The filter can then be removed and the number of cells passing through from the cell chamber to the opposite side of the filter are counted. In this way it can be shown that many bacteria release chemotactic products, which may be toxins or simply normal products of their metabolism. It would be an advantage for organisms to prevent chemotaxis, and some toxins such as streptococcal streptolysin have the ability to inhibit neutrophil chemotaxis. Their effectiveness *in vivo*, however, is not known.

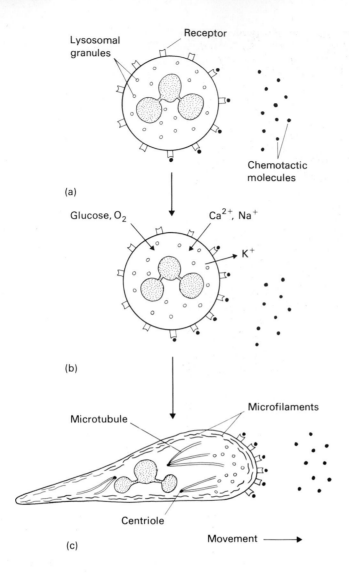

(a)

Lysosomal granules

Receptor

Chemotactic molecules

(b)

Glucose, O_2

Ca^{2+}, Na^+

K^+

(c)

Microtubule

Microfilaments

Centriole

Movement ⟶

Figure 1.6 Cellular events in neutrophil chemotaxis.
(a) Chemotactic molecules bind to receptors at the neutrophil surface.
(b) Ion fluxes, including entry of calcium, are triggered and metabolic processes activated.
(c) Change of cell shape occurs, with reorganisation of cytoskeletal contractile elements (microfilaments, microtubules) and surface receptors. Movement in the direction of the chemotactic attractant begins.
(d) Scanning electron microscopy of human blood monocytes migrating through pores of a polycarbonate filter in response to a chemotactic lymphokine. One cell has passed completely through a pore and is migrating diagonally across the field, while a second is in the process of emerging. ($\times 4000$). (From Snyderman and Goetzl, 1981.)*

Neutrophils migrate rapidly along a chemotactic gradient, whereas monocytes move rather slowly. This may account in part for the delay in appearance of monocytes in inflammatory exudates. Neutrophils contain a substance which attracts monocytes, which could also explain the sequential appearance of these cells in acute inflammation. Sensitised lymphocytes also produce monocyte chemotactic factors (lymphokines) which are important in cell-mediated immunity (p. 147). The absence of lymphocytes from acute inflammatory exudate reflects selectivity of chemotactic factors for different cell types.

Two general models have been proposed to account for the ability of a cell to move along a concentration gradient. One, called *temporal sensing*, explains chemotaxis of motile bacteria: the organisms evidently register changes in concentration at different times in their progress and adjust their mode of movement (directional swimming or random tumbling) accordingly

*Unless cited in full in the text, references will be found in the Further Reading lists at the end of each section.

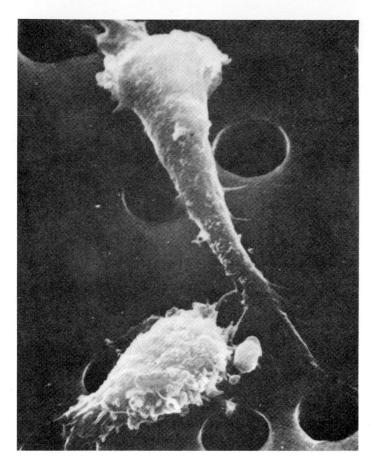

(d)

(see p. 405). In contrast, leucocytes, which crawl over surfaces rather than swim, are able to detect changing concentrations of substances along the length of the individual cell, so-called *spatial sensing*. An extremely finely-tuned mechanism must be involved, as it is estimated that neutrophils can respond to gradients of as little as 0.1% across the cell surface.

When a leucocyte encounters a chemotactic stimulus, changes rapidly occur in cell morphology, internal organisation and metabolism. The initiating event is the *binding* of the chemotactic agent at specific receptors on the plasma membrane (Figure 1.6a). This leads to alterations of membrane permeability, including a substantial net influx of calcium ions, and enhanced utilisation of glucose and oxygen (Figure 1.6b). Calcium seems to play a central role in the chemotactic response, both by activation of enzymes (adenylate cyclase, phospholipase, etc.) and by a direct involvement in cell motility itself. Shortly after the events at the membrane, neutrophils and monocytes change their shape from spherical to elongated and become orientated in the direction of the attractive stimulus; the cell now has a broad 'front' end or lamellipod and a long, thin, trailing 'tail' or uropod (Figure 1.6c, d). Membrane receptors are reorganised and cluster at the leading edge. The change in cell morphology is the result of a rearrange-

13

ment of actin microfilaments just beneath the membrane; thus, cytochalasin B, an agent which blocks this rearrangement, inhibits the shape change and chemotaxis. Microtubules are also rearranged. It is not altogether clear how the changes in membrane permeability are coupled to those in cell morphology. Cyclic nucleotides (cyclic AMP, cyclic GMP) may be involved: chemotactic substances do cause a rise in intracellular levels of cyclic nucleotides, though at concentrations much above those needed to stimulate chemotaxis. Methylation of intracellular proteins is also involved in leucocyte chemotaxis, and it is interesting to note that this is also part of bacterial chemotaxis (p. 406).

Leucocytes involved in acute inflammation

The morphology of the cells involved in acute inflammation is shown in Figure 1.7. The neutrophils are granulocytes which arise from specific precursors in the bone marrow; they are end

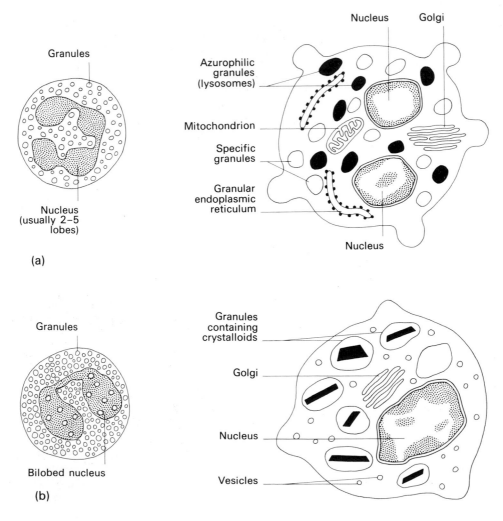

cells, incapable of further division. Their important morphological feature, besides the typical lobed nucleus, is the presence in the cytoplasm of two types of granule, the azurophilic *lysosomal granules* and the neutrophilic *specific granules*. The lysosomes contain degradative enzymes which play a major role in neutrophil function, including phosphatases, myeloperoxidase, nucleases, nucleotidase, lysozyme, cathepsin, β-glucuronidase, collagenase, elastase, kallikrein and plasminogen (precursor of plasmin or fibrinolysin). The more numerous specific granules contain lactoferrin and lysozyme. Because of their short life-span (3–4 days), neutrophils often tend to die at the site of inflammation and in so doing release their lysosomal enzymes, which then proceed to digest both the dead neutrophils themselves (autolysis) and dead tissue cells round about, as well as extravascular fibrin. The solubilisation of debris is the main role of neutrophils in sterile inflammation, such as mild thermal

Figure 1.7 *and on facing page.* Cells involved in acute inflammation. In each case the appearance in the light microscope is shown on the left and in electron microscope on the right.
(a) Neutrophil; (b) Eosinophil; (c) Monocyte; (d) Mast cell.

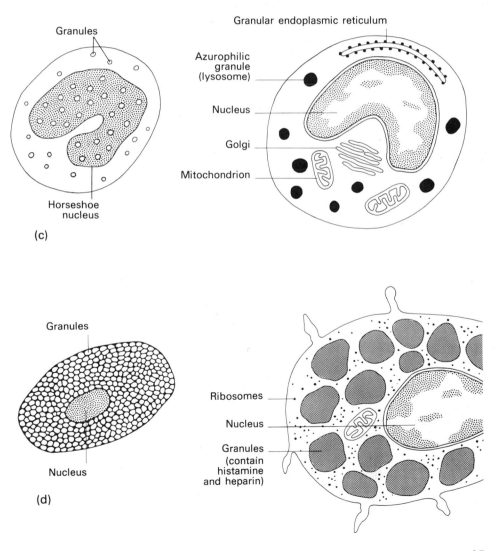

burns. The other major function of neutrophils is their ability to take up, kill and intracellularly digest pathogenic bacteria by the process known as *phagocytosis*. This is of paramount importance in infectious disease, where neutrophils are often the first line of defence against bacterial invaders. During infections, such as those due to pyogenic cocci, in which acute inflammation is prominent, the number of neutrophils in the blood is increased from the normal levels of $2.5-7.5 \times 10^6$ per ml to $10-20 \times 10^6$ per ml (*neutrophil leucocytosis*), the degree depending on the severity and duration of the infection. Sustained leucocytosis is due to an increased rate of production of neutrophils from the bone marrow. Neutrophils also contain, and release, a substance called *endogenous pyrogen*, which is partly responsible for the development of fever during acute inflammation. This is a lipoprotein, probably released during phagocytosis, which acts on the thermoregulatory centres of the brain. Fever during inflammation is probably of little advantage and rarely harmful.

Sometimes, eosinophil polymorphonuclear leucocytes (eosinophils) rather than neutrophils are found in areas of inflammation, particularly in helminth infections and in hypersensitivity reactions including hay fever and allergic asthma. In addition to other enzymes, eosinophil granules contain some which degrade certain mediators of inflammation such as histamine (see p. 156).

The other major cell type in acute inflammation is the macrophage. Macrophages are derived from blood monocytes, and apart from obvious morphology (Figure 1.7) they differ from polymorphs both in their longer life-span and their ability to divide in areas of inflammation. Whereas neutrophils dominate the early stages of acute inflammation, macrophages are usually the main cell type in the later stages. The transition from neutrophil to macrophage predominance occurs as soon as infecting micro-organisms have been brought under control and, for example, can be produced at will in experimental pneumococcal infection by termination with penicillin. Their ability to withstand the acid environment in inflammatory exudate also contributes to their survival. The main function of macrophages is again phagocytosis. Macrophages are able to take up and digest a somewhat wider range of substances than neutrophils—including effete (old) erythrocytes, debris and fragments of tissue-cells, and masses of fibrin—which gives them great importance in the later stages (resolution) of inflammation. Bacteria are also actively phagocytosed by macrophages. In this respect, however, neutrophils are probably more significant in acute bacterial infections, as evidenced by the susceptibility to such infection of patients with severe granulocytopenia (lack of granulocytes in the blood).

The role of platelets in acute inflammation is considered separately on p. 38.

Phagocytosis, opsonins and complement

The importance of phagocytosis in bacterial defence was the subject of great controversy at the turn of the century.

Metchnikoff (1882), from his observations of macrophages in starfish larvae, proposed that immunity to bacteria was by phagocytosis and destruction. The theory of 'cellular immunity' was vigorously opposed by the proponents of 'humoral immunity' — which was supported by the discovery of antibacterial substances in cell-free serum by Buchner (1890) and of antitoxin by Behring and Kitasato (1890). The opposing theories were reconciled by the discovery, by Neufeld and Rimpeau (1904), that the phagocytosis of pneumococci was enhanced by serum of animals injected with killed pneumococci. The active substances in serum were termed *opsonins* (Gk. opsonein — to prepare food for); they are now known to be antibodies against the bacterial surface.

The ability to resist phagocytosis is a key factor in the virulence of the pathogenic bacteria which live as *extracellular parasites* and cause acute infectious diseases — streptococci, pneumococci, staphylococci, etc. They are promptly destroyed once taken up by neutrophils and must perforce resist phagocytosis to survive. They do this by possessing an antiphagocytic *capsule* or other surface material, typical examples being the capsular polysaccharides of pneumococci, the M protein and capsular hyaluronic acid of *Streptococcus pyogenes*, and the capsular protein (polyglutamic acid) of *Bacillus anthracis*. The importance of the capsule can easily be demonstrated, for example, in pneumococci, where the smooth encapsulated strains are virulent whereas the rough non-encapsulated strains are not. Moreover, removal of the capsule from normally virulent smooth strains by enzymatic digestion renders them phagocytosable and avirulent. Extracellular pathogenic organisms often cause direct tissue damage by production of *exotoxins*, which can have a variety of harmful effects. Some exotoxins aid the survival of the pathogen by being toxic for leucocytes — *Staph. aureus* α-toxin and the streptolysins S and O secreted by *Strep. pyogenes* are examples of leucocidic toxins. Streptolysin O acts by causing disintegration of the neutrophil granules; this releases into the cell the degradative enzymes which are normally sequestered in lysosomes and the cell is rapidly killed in consequence. A summary of the 'tactics' used by different organisms to avoid phagocytosis is given in Table 1.1 and a more extensive description can be found in Section 4.

The extent to which neutrophils can phagocytose encapsulated bacteria in the absence of opsonins is dependent on the architecture of the infected tissues. If the leucocyte can trap the organism against tissue surfaces, in the interstices of fibrin clots, or between adjacent leucocytes in concentrated exudates, phagocytosis — here termed surface phagocytosis — will occur. This may well be vital in the early stages of acute bacterial disease and clearly will be more effective in close knit tissues than in body cavities. Where surface phagocytosis is not sufficient to prevent the onset of disease, opsonins are essential. Opsonins are antibodies directed specifically against the bacterial surface capsule or wall. They are secreted by cells in the lymphoid organs, the lymph nodes, spleen, etc. (see Section 2 for details of antibody structure and production). The antibody molecules possess at least two identical combining sites with which they can react with surface structures on the organism. (A structure with which an antibody combines is called an *antigen*, Section 2). The function of the opsonising antibodies is to bind to the bacterium and thereby promote phagocytosis; once coated by opsonin, the organisms are readily taken up and destroyed by neutrophils. The latter are equipped to recognise opsonised bacteria by means of receptors at their surface for the 'tail' part (Fc) of the bound antibody molecule. Hence antibody-coated bacteria will combine

Table 1.1 Mechanisms by which pathogenic bacteria avoid the action of phagocytes.

Micro-organism	Mechanism
Streptococci	Produce exotoxins (streptolysins) which kill leucocytes and inhibit chemotaxis. Possess antiphagocytic surface component (M protein).
Pneumococci, *Haemophilus influenzae*, *Klebsiella pneumoniae*	Possess antiphagocytic polysaccharide capsule.
Staphylococci	Produce exotoxins (α-toxin) which kill leucocytes. Wall component (protein A) interferes with opsonisation by binding to Fc region of antibody. Resist intracellular killing.
Bacillus anthracis	Antiphagocytic capsular component (poly-D-glutamic acid).
Escherichia coli	Resist phagocytosis and intracellular killing (K antigen).
Salmonella typhi	Resist phagocytosis and intracellular killing (Vi antigen).
Mycobacteria	Resist intracellular killing and enzymatic digestion (high lipid content of cell wall).

with the neutrophil surface at Fc receptor sites and phagocytosis follows. An interesting bacterial antiphagocytic mechanism is directed at inhibition of opsonisation. *Staphylococcus aureus* organisms possess and release a wall component called *protein A*, which, by binding specifically to the antibody Fc region, prevents the uptake of opsonised organisms by Fc receptors on the neutrophil membrane. Note that opsonins, like all antibodies, are highly specific, in that an opsonin made in response to pneumococcal capsular polysaccharide will not react with, say, streptococcal M protein or indeed with the walls of any other organisms. Thus, for each organism, a different range of specific opsonins must be synthesized by the immune system and this process takes a few days to reach a peak after infection (Section 2).

The coating of the bacterial surface can be accomplished by opsonins alone, but usually also involves the plasma protein system known as *complement*. Complement consists of a sequence of nine proteins, normally present in inactive forms in the blood, which are closely involved both in the immune system and inflammation (p. 30). In the case of phagocytosis, once opsonising antibodies have bound, complement components are activated by and become physically fixed in large amounts to and around the opsonins at the bacterial surface. This aids phagocytosis because neutrophils and macrophages carry *complement receptors*, by means of which they can combine with complement fixed on the organism; together with the Fc receptors, these further encourage efficient binding of the opsonised microbes to the phagocytes. The walls of Gram-negative bacteria, such as *Salmonella* and *E. coli*, can activate complement by a pathway which is antibody-independent (the alternative pathway, p. 31). Complement-assisted phagocytosis for these organisms then occurs in the absence of specific antibody production. Another important consequence of the fixation or activation of complement is the production of various *phlogistic* (inflammation-producing) factors, in particular factors which are chemotactic for neutrophils, and others which cause vasodilatation and increase vascular permeability (p. 31). The overall effect is thus to amplify the inflammatory process and attract neutrophils to the scene at precisely the time that bacteria can be phagocytosed by the presence of opsonins.

The importance of these events is dramatically illustrated by pneumococcal *lobar pneumonia*. In a typical untreated case, pneumococci multiply in the lung alveoli, stimulating an acute inflammatory outpouring of exudate and neutrophils which rapidly spreads through an entire lobe (p. 515). The patient is extremely ill for 6 or 7 days, but then a dramatic improvement and drop in fever occurs, termed the *crisis*. The crisis corresponds to the production of ample amounts of opsonising antibody to coat the organisms, which can then be phagocytosed by the hitherto virtually helpless neutrophils. The process of recovery is then well under way. The period of 6–7 days is the time needed for the patient's immune system to make an antibody response to the pneumococci, in particular against the capsular polysaccharide which prevents phagocytosis. It should be noted that this process is far from completely efficient, untreated lobar pneumonia having a mortality of up to 30%. It used to be treated with antipneumococcal serum and today antibiotics provide a more reliable means of destroying pneumococci than waiting for the immune system to intervene.

Killing of organisms by phagocytes

The process of phagocytosis itself begins with *ingestion* of the organism into the cytoplasm, where it is found enclosed in a membrane-bound vacuole known as a phagosome (Figure 1.8a). Note that the internal lining of the phagosome is the outer surface of the plasma membrane, which becomes inverted in forming the phagosome. Ingestion is accompanied by an increase in glycolysis. The ability to respire anaerobically is important to neutrophils, which are often required to phagocytose in hypoxic conditions, as in the interior of abscesses. There is also

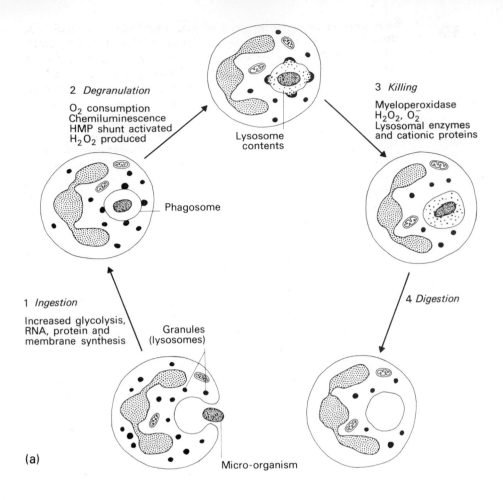

2 *Degranulation*

O$_2$ consumption
Chemiluminescence
HMP shunt activated
H$_2$O$_2$ produced

Lysosome
contents

3 *Killing*

Myeloperoxidase
H$_2$O$_2$, O$_2^-$
Lysosomal enzymes
and cationic proteins

Phagosome

1 *Ingestion*

Increased glycolysis,
RNA, protein and
membrane synthesis

Granules
(lysosomes)

4 *Digestion*

Micro-organism

(a)

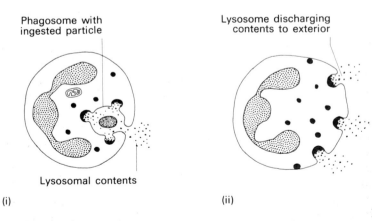

Phagosome with
ingested particle

Lysosome discharging
contents to exterior

Lysosomal contents

(i)

(ii)

(b)

Figure 1.8 (a) Stages in phagocytosis by neutrophils (after Cline). (b) Mechanisms of release of neutrophil lysosome contents: (i) regurgitation during feeding; (ii) reverse endocytosis (after Weissmann *et al*.).

increased synthesis of proteins and membrane phospholipids. The phagosome collides and fuses with neutrophil lysosomes, which contain the enzymes and other agents necessary for the killing and digestion of micro-organisms; there is visible degranulation of neutrophils. At this point, other important metabolic changes occur, known collectively as the *respiratory burst* and consisting of a sharp increase in oxygen consumption, stimulation of the hexose monophosphate (HMP) shunt, and production of reduced forms of oxygen, notably the superoxide anion O_2^-, the hydroxyl radical $OH^{\cdot}$ and hydrogen peroxide H_2O_2. The oxygen uptake is not related to mitochondrial respiration, being unaffected by mitochondrial inhibitors, but rather to the oxygen-dependent killing of micro-organisms within the phagosome, as described below.

The *killing* in neutrophils of bacteria and fungi is accomplished both by oxygen-dependent and independent mechanisms. The latter include the following lysosomal agents. (i) Cationic proteins of the lysosome bind to and damage bacterial walls. (ii) Enzymes such as lysozyme and elastase attack the peptidoglycan of the bacterial cell wall. Lysozyme, in collaboration with complement, may kill Gram-negative organisms. In general, however, lysosomal enzymes are probably more important as agents of digestion of dead organisms than in killing. (iii) Lactoferrin is an iron-binding protein with anti-microbial properties. (iv) The high acidity within the phagosome (pH 3.5–4.0) may have a bactericidal effect; it probably results from lactic acid production in glycolysis. Many lysosomal enzymes, such as acid hydrolases, have acid pH optima, which allow them to function in an acid environment.

The *oxygen-dependent killing* of micro-organisms is brought about by H_2O_2, free radicals such as O_2^- and $OH^{\cdot}$ and possibly by singlet oxygen $^1O_2$. Its importance has been underlined by the frequency and severity with which certain infectious diseases occur in patients with inherited deficiencies of the oxygen-dependent bactericidal systems, as in chronic granulomatous disease (below). The trapping of oxygen by the cell is carried out by an enzyme usually termed *NADPH oxidase* which, as Figure 1.9 shows, reduces oxygen to O_2^-, oxidising NADPH to $NADP^+$. The activation of this enzyme is a key step in the oxygen-dependent system as it (a) makes available $NADP^+$ for the HMP shunt, which therefore becomes stimulated, and (b) traps oxygen for bacterial killing. The oxidase is apparently present on the plasma membrane, and therefore on the inner lining of the phagosome, and is activated soon after contact of the membrane with a particulate stimulus, such as an organism being phagocytosed. As will be discussed further below, the inherited absence of NADPH oxidase in chronic granulomatous disease abolishes all the reactions of the respiratory burst. The superoxide anion O_2^- is a free radical produced by the one-electron reduction of molecular oxygen; it is very reactive and highly damaging to animal cells, as well as to micro-organisms. In the phagosome, it is converted by the enzyme *superoxide dismutase* into H_2O_2; this reaction is the main source of H_2O_2 for subsequent use in microbial killing.

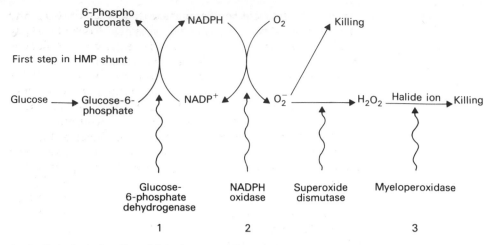

First step in HMP shunt

1, 2, 3 indicate location of inherited defects in killing:

1 Glucose-6-phosphate dehydrogenase deficiency
2 Chronic granulomatous disease
3 Myeloperoxidase deficiency

(a)

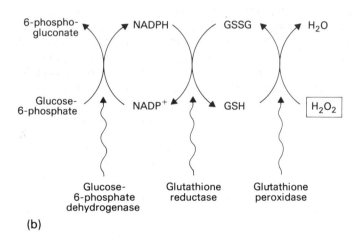

(b)

H$_2$O$_2$ is also toxic to cells and, if it leaks out of the phagosome into the cytoplasm, is destroyed by reaction with *glutathione peroxidase*; in this way the cell is protected from the toxic action of the highly potent substances it generates to kill bacteria. Figure 1.9b shows this detoxification reaction.

Hydrogen peroxide is probably the most important oxygen-derived killing agent in the phagosome. Its bactericidal effect involves a lysosomal enzyme, *myeloperoxidase*, and halide ions such as iodide I$^-$ or chloride Cl$^-$ (the 'H$_2$O$_2$-halide-myeloperoxidase' system). In the presence of H$_2$O$_2$ and halide, myeloperoxidase catalyses at least two mechanisms of bacterial killing. In one, halogenation of the bacterial wall occurs; iodine and chlorine are incorporated into the wall and it is postulated that this leads to death of the organism. The iodination of bacteria has become the basis of a widely used test of neutrophil function. In the second mechanism, myeloperoxidase and H$_2$O$_2$ damage the

Figure 1.9 (a) Pathway of oxygen-dependent killing of micro-organisms in neutrophils and its inherited deficiencies. (b) Pathway of detoxification of hydrogen peroxide in the neutrophil cytoplasm. GSH: reduced glutathione. GSSG: oxidised glutathione.

wall by converting amino acids in it into aldehydes; the latter may also have significant antimicrobial activity. While the H_2O_2-halide-myeloperoxidase system is considered to be the major one involved in killing, superoxide may be an additional microbicidal agent if present in large amount. The hydroxyl radical OH· is another highly reactive group with antibacterial properties; it may be formed by the interaction of O_2^- with H_2O_2 or alkyl peroxides. The decay of free radicals such as O_2^- and OH· to the ground state is probably responsible for the low intensity burst of light, or *chemiluminescence*, which accompanies phagocytosis and which can be sensitively detected in a liquid scintillation spectrometer. Another agent of possible importance is *singlet oxygen* ($^1O_2$), a form of molecular oxygen which differs from atmospheric (triplet) oxygen in the distribution of the electrons around the two oxygen nuclei. (The terms 'singlet' and 'triplet' refer to emission spectra of the two oxygen species.) $^1O_2$ oxidises double bonds and is capable of inflicting lethal damage on cells. It may also be a product of the reaction of O_2^- with H_2O_2. It seems likely that all these mechanisms will contribute to oxygen-dependent killing; indeed the neutrophil seems to be provided with a capacity to kill which is in considerable excess over its actual requirements.

There are significant differences between macrophages and neutrophils in the killing of organisms. Although macrophage lysosomes contain a variety of enzymes, including lysozyme, they lack the cationic proteins and lactoferrin found in neutrophils. Moreover, myeloperoxidase is not present in tissue macrophages or monocytes. However, there are indications that a hydrogen peroxide killing system is used by macrophages, perhaps in conjunction with catalase rather than myeloperoxidase. Thus, the characteristic burst of oxygen consumption, activation of the HMP shunt and hydrogen peroxide generation follow phagocytosis by macrophages as well as neutrophils. Nevertheless, normal macrophages are less effective in killing certain pathogens, such as the fungus *Candida albicans*, than neutrophils, which possess myeloperoxidase. The microbicidal activity of macrophages is greatly improved after contact with soluble lymphocyte products known as *lymphokines* (p. 61) and this is important in enabling them to deal with intracellular organisms such as the mycobacteria. After activation, macrophages enlarge and take on a ruffled appearance; they exhibit enhanced phagocytosis and HMP shunt activity and increased levels of lysosomal hydrolases. Activated macrophages are sometimes referred to as 'angry' macrophages (see pp. 60–61 for further discussion).

Once killed, most micro-organisms are *digested* and solubilised by lysosomal enzymes. For some organisms, however, destruction of the wall presents a problem to the phagocytes. The significance of the persistence of bacterial products lies in the prolonged stimulation of the immune system which they evoke. A good example of resistance to enzymatic attack is provided by the mycobacteria; the high lipid content of their walls makes them particularly insensitive to lysosomal degradation. For this reason the organisms are not only particularly resistant to killing by macrophages, but stimulate a tissue-damaging immunological reaction (hypersensitivity) which continues even after the organisms have been killed. Such reactions play an important role in tuberculosis and leprosy (p. 62).

Defects in phagocytosis

There are several inherited deficiencies in killing of micro-organisms by phagocytes, which lead to susceptibility to life-threatening bacterial and fungal infections. Most defects occur in the oxidative killing system. *Chronic granulomatous disease* is a childhood disease with X-linked inheritance (Section 7) in which there is susceptibility to infection by an unusual group of organisms including *Staphylococcus aureus* and *Staphylococcus epidermidis, Aerobacter aerogenes, Serratia marcescens* and *Aspergillus*. The infections are severe and slow to heal; healing is accompanied by characteristic granuloma formation (p. 59) in different organs. The disease is often fatal, though the prophylactic use of antibiotics is proving helpful. A defect is found in both neutrophils and macrophages and can be detected by the nitroblue tetrazolium dye reduction test and neutrophil microbicidal assays (below). After engulfing organisms normally, phagocytic cells of patients with chronic granulomatous disease fail to show the expected respiratory burst: there is no rise in oxygen consumption, increase in HMP shunt or production of O_2^- or H_2O_2. The metabolic basis is a deficiency of NADPH oxidase (Figure 1.9a), emphasizing the central importance of this enzyme to the reactions of the respiratory burst. However, the defective neutrophils continue to kill a range of bacteria, including streptococci and pneumococci, and children with chronic granulomatous disease rarely suffer from infections with these organisms. The reason for this selective susceptibility to certain infections lies in the way the organisms handle the H_2O_2 which they themselves produce. Many organisms produce H_2O_2 during metabolism; some also destroy this endogenous H_2O_2 via the enzyme catalase, while others lack catalase and excrete their H_2O_2 to the outside. Pneumococci and streptococci are of the catalase-negative class; they thus suicidally provide the neutrophil with a source of H_2O_2 which the phagocyte uses to kill the organism (note that myeloperoxidase functions normally in chronic granulomatous disease if the neutrophil is provided with H_2O_2). *Staph. aureus* and all the other organisms which give rise to chronic infections in this disease are catalase positive and destroy rather than excrete endogenously produced H_2O_2; they give the neutrophil nothing to work with and are therefore poorly killed.

Not surprisingly, severe deficiency of *glucose-6-phosphate dehydrogenase* (G6PD), one of the enzymes required to generate NADPH in the hexose monophosphate shunt, produces, in addition to haemolytic anaemia (see Section 7), manifestations similar to chronic granulomatous disease. All respiratory burst phenomena are absent due to the lack of NADPH. Note that, although it is not the only reaction in the HMP shunt to generate NADPH, the G6PD step is the first in the shunt sequence, so that G6PD deficiency essentially shuts down all NADPH production by this pathway. Very few patients with G6PD deficiency sufficient to lead to severe infections have been described to date. Another rare abnormality of the oxygen-dependent killing system is *myeloperoxidase deficiency*. However, in marked contrast to chronic granulomatous disease or severe G6PD deficiency, this does not usually lead to troublesome infections. The respiratory burst is normal and O_2^- and H_2O_2 are produced; in fact there is a greater than normal production of these active agents, as if to compensate for the lack of myeloperoxidase. Because of the multiplicity of possible pathways of oxygen-dependent killing, neutrophils lacking myeloperoxidase are able to destroy ingested bacteria, though the killing time is prolonged; destruction of micro-organisms is complete and protects the myeloperoxidase-deficient patient from the infections which characterise NADPH oxidase deficiency.

An unusual aberration occurs in the *Chédiak-Higashi syndrome*, an autosomal recessive condition (Section 7) in which there are a variety of recurrent bacterial infections, partial albinism, abnormalities of the central nervous system and a high incidence of lymphomas. A characteristic feature is the abnormally large size of the lysosomes of neutrophils and platelets. Lysosomal activities and hydrogen peroxide production appear normal and the lysosomes are peroxidase positive; yet there is an inability to kill many organisms, both catalase positive and negative. Leucocyte chemotaxis is also defective, apparently due to an inability to rearrange microfilaments in response to chemotactic stimuli. Infection and development of lymphoid neoplasms lead to an early death.

Tests widely used to measure the killing activity of neutrophils include the nitroblue tetrazolium dye or NBT test and the neutrophil microbicidal assay. The NBT test measures the ability of neutrophils to generate and use the reducing power of the HMP shunt (NBT is reduced by reaction with O_2^-). Neutrophils are encouraged to take up the NBT dye by incubation with the dye in the presence of latex particles; the latter are phagocytosed and the dye is taken up simultaneously. Initially a clear yellow, NBT turns deep blue on reduction in the neutrophil and the colour change can be observed microscopically or measured quantitatively by extraction in pyridine. Failure to change colour occurs consistently in chronic granulomatous disease and in some cases of G6PD deficiency. In the microbicidal assay, neutrophils are allowed to engulf a suspension of *Staphylococcus aureus* and the intracellular survival of the organisms is followed at various times by lysis of the neutrophils and plating out surviving bacteria. The iodination of ingested particles is also a useful test for myeloperoxidase-mediated killing.

Release of enzymes from neutrophils

Enzymes and other constituents of lysosomes can be released from the neutrophil to the outside, either as a result of death of the cell at the site of inflammation or as a side-effect of phagocytosis. While enzyme shedding serves a useful function, by digesting tissue debris and providing a source of mediators of inflammation (below), it can also lead to tissue damage, a fact of particular importance in certain hypersensitivity reactions mediated by antigen–antibody complexes (p. 160). The external release of lysosomal contents during phagocytosis, without death of the neutrophil, occurs in two ways. The first has been descriptively termed 'regurgitation during feeding', indicating the accidental leakage of enzymes from a phagosome with which lysosomes have fused, but which is still connected to the outside as a result of incomplete closure of the plasma membrane (Figure 1.8b). The second method, 'reverse endocytosis', follows the binding of antigen–antibody complexes to the neutrophil surface at Fc receptors. The disturbance of the cell membrane can cause lysosomes to fuse with the plasma membrane itself and discharge their contents to the outside (Figure 1.8b). Among the enzymes released are some which can damage connective tissue, such as elastase and collagenase. They are inhibited by serum α_1-antitrypsin, and the inherited deficiency of this inhibitor enables these enzymes to produce serious damage in the lung (p. 41).

A good example of acute inflammation following the release of lysosomal enzymes from killed neutrophils occurs in joints in the acute arthritic attacks of *gout*. Gout is the result of hyperuricaemia (Section 7, p. 847). Crystals of monosodium urate are deposited in and around joints and are taken up by neutrophils. The urate crystals are able to form hydrogen bonds with phospholipids of the phagosome membrane, and the disturbance which this causes disrupts the phagosome and releases its lysosomal contents into the cell cytoplasm. The neutrophil is rapidly killed as a result and the enzymes are shed into the joint, where they cause damage and initiate intense attacks of acute inflammation. Before they die, neutrophils which have engulfed monosodium urate crystals produce a chemotactic substance (crystal-induced chemotactic factor) which attracts more neutrophils, and this will further exacerbate the inflammatory response. Colchicine suppresses gouty arthritis by preventing the merger of lysosomal granules with the phagosome and interfering with neutrophil motility and phagocytosis (see p. 847 for further details of gout).

Suppuration and abscess formation

The ability to resist uptake or destruction by phagocytes is essential to the formation of pus, *suppuration*. Pyogenic (pus-forming) organisms, among which are many of the extracellular parasites already mentioned, include staphylococci, some streptococci, pneumococci, meningococci, gonococci, *Escherichia coli* and related bacilli. The process of suppuration can be observed in boils and pimples in the skin which are frequently caused by *Staph. aureus*. A localised, circumscribed collection of pus is termed an *abscess*. Pus itself consists of dead phagocytes, predominantly neutrophils, inflammatory exudate and tissue debris.

The main features of pyogenic organisms which result in suppuration are (a) their production of substances which can cause the massive emigration of neutrophils and then kill them, (b) their ability to avoid removal by phagocytosis, often by possessing an antiphagocytic capsule, or (c) their capacity to resist destruction within the phagocytic cell. We have seen that, given time, the host will produce opsonins and also antitoxins in response to the antigenic stimulus. Meanwhile, however, the accumulation of leucocytes and their death *in situ* give rise to pus, formed chiefly by autolysis of neutrophils by their own lysosomal enzymes released on cell death. The creamy nature and colour of pus and its viscosity are caused by its high concentration of 'pus cells' (neutrophils) and also in particular free nucleic acids; the green hue it sometimes acquires is due to myeloperoxidase. As this process continues in solid tissue, an abscess cavity forms, which eventually becomes walled off from the surrounding tissue by a process of repair (p. 43). The wall of young connective tissue (granulation tissue, p. 44), containing collagen fibres and new blood vessels, is termed the *pyogenic membrane*. Leucocytes continue to migrate into the abscess from blood vessels in the pyogenic membrane. An abscess may form in a body cavity by a somewhat different process in which part of the cavity is first walled off by a layer of fibrin deposited from fibrinous exudate onto several surfaces forming an *adhesion*. The abscess cavity then forms inside the fibrin walls, which gradually become vascularised and fibrous. An example of this process occurs in the peritoneal cavity in acute appendicitis and serves to localise infection in an 'appendix abscess' in cases where perforation of the appendix wall has occurred, adhesions forming between the omentum and adjacent intestine.

An abscess may be terminated by the influx of antibodies to neutralise toxins and opsonise bacteria. It is treated by surgical incision which relieves the pressure (and the throbbing pain) and drains the contents. Untreated, it expands along the line of least resistance, destroying more tissue until it points at a surface and ruptures. If rupture is to the outside, as at the surface of the skin, the infection is generally effectively ended. Rupture into a body cavity has the very serious result of discharging toxins and bacteria into hitherto uninfected tissues and even their dissemination by the bloodstream. This may occur with the appendix abscess, with the severe consequence of peritonitis, and is obviously to be avoided wherever possible. After discharge of an abscess, the cavity collapses, its walls come together under pressure of surrounding tissues and are bound first by fibrin and then fibrous connective tissue. A scar marks the site of the abscess.

Ulceration

When injury occurs to the surface of an organ or tissue, the epithelium and surface fabric may be destroyed, leaving an inflamed area of erosion called an *ulcer*. The classic examples are the peptic ulcers of the stomach and duodenum, which frequently become chronic. These form pits in the stomach or intestinal wall from 0.5 to 4 cm in diameter, with steep sides and a flat base. The floor of the ulcer consists of dead tissue and inflammatory exudate produced from the base and margins where the acute response is occurring and where there is an intense neutrophil infiltration. With chronic ulcers, a process of repair takes place in the deeper layers in the base with formation of fibrous tissue (p. 58 and Figure 1.19). The causes of the common ulcers in the gastro-intestinal tract are complex. Hyperacidity is certainly the important factor in duodenal ulcers, but is less significant in gastric ulcers. The pathogenesis of the latter is still mysterious.

Intracellular bacteria

In contrast with the rapid destruction of extracellular bacteria once inside phagocytic cells, there are a number of bacteria which are able to survive and grow inside normal macrophages after being phagocytosed. Important examples are *Mycobacterium tuberculosis* and *M. leprae*, the causative agents of tuberculosis and leprosy respectively, *Salmonella typhi* (typhoid fever) and *Brucella abortus* (brucellosis). Note (a) that (except for *M. leprae*) these organisms are not obligate intracellular parasites, but can grow equally well extracellularly, and (b) that they are only found inside cells because they have been phagocytosed by macrophages which cannot destroy them. The 'lepra cell' of some forms of leprosy, for example, is a macrophage packed with living, dividing *M. leprae* organisms inhabiting a cell which is unable to destroy them. However, in many cases the macrophage can in due course become activated and its ability to kill and digest engulfed organisms increased. It is the balance which is then set up between the persistence of the microbes and their breakdown products and the ability of the macrophage to remove them that results in the protracted course of chronic infectious disease which these organisms often cause. These events are discussed at greater length under chronic inflammation (pp. 59–63).

CHEMICAL MEDIATORS OF INFLAMMATION

We have seen that important vascular and cellular events follow on tissue injury, notably vasodilatation, increased permeability and leucocyte emigration. Clearly, there must exist a linking step between the occurrence of the injury and the stimulation of the vascular changes; that link is provided by the chemical mediators of inflammation. These are substances which are often widely distributed in a sequestered or inactive form throughout the body and are released or activated locally at the site of inflammation. The may act directly or indirectly on blood vessels, or be chemotactic for leucocytes. After release they tend to be rapidly inactivated locally, a feature which is important in the control of inflammation. Furthermore, many of these substances, especially the kinin and complement systems, are linked by a series of interactions which tend to amplify their effects in a manner well-described by the term *positive feedback*. Control is therefore an important aspect of inflammation, in the sense of limiting the reactions involved and preventing the spontaneous activation of phlogistic factors when they are not required. Certain pathological conditions result when this control breaks down.

HISTAMINE

This vasoactive amine is particularly important in the initiation and early stages of acute inflammation. It is very widely distributed in tissues, being found particularly in mast cells (tissue basophils, Figure 1.7d), which characteristically lie in the connective tissue close to blood vessels, and in blood basophils and platelets. Its main pharmacological actions are the contraction of extravascular smooth muscle, the dilatation of blood vessels, and the increase of vascular permeability by causing formation of gaps between endothelial cells. Inflammatory changes can often be shown to involve two main phases—an immediate, but passing increase in permeability is followed by a latent period of variable duration before the main phase of increased permeability and leucocyte migration (Figure 1.10). In such cases, the immediate effects are generally due to histamine release in the damaged tissue and can be abolished by antihistamines. Such drugs therefore often delay the development of acute inflammation without affecting the eventual outcome. Histamine is of particular importance in immediate-type hypersensitivities or allergies, such as hay-fever, allergic asthma, etc. (Section 2). When injected into the skin it produces a typical weal-and-flare reaction reminiscent of the triple response, in which it is also probably involved. Soon after its release from mast cells, histamine is inactivated by histaminase or acetylation. In rodents, another vasoactive amine, 5-hydroxytryptamine (5-HT, serotonin) is also released from mast cells and plays the same role as histamine.

KININS AND KININ-GENERATING ENZYMES

The *kinins* are biologically active polypeptides which are produced by the action of enzymes known as *kallikreins* on a kinin-precursor called kininogen (a plasma α_2-globulin). The best known and probably most significant, is *bradykinin*, a nonapeptide produced by the action of plasma kallikrein on kininogen; a closely related decapeptide known as kallidin is formed by urinary or glandular kallikrein. Another important kinin, C2-kinin, is produced from complement (below).

The name 'bradykinin' derives from the Greek, *bradys*—slow, and *kinein*—to move, because smooth muscle contracted slower in response to it than to histamine or acetylcholine. Bradykinin produces extravascular smooth muscle contraction, vasodilatation, increased permeability through 'gap' formation (it is the most active permeability factor known), pain, an axon reflex, and possibly margination and emigration of leucocytes. It is clearly important as a general mediator of the prolonged phase of inflammation (Fig. 1.10). The vasodilatory effects of bradykinin may be mediated via an action on vascular endothelium, leading to release of the prostaglandin called prostacyclin (PGI_2, p. 631).

The kallikrein enzymes are present in plasma as inactive precursors, *prekallikreins*, which are activated following tissue damage by a serum β-globulin known as *Hageman factor*, and more especially by fragments derived from Hageman factor (Figure 1.13). Kinins are broken down by kininases and their accumulation thus prevented.

COMPLEMENT

The complement system plays an important role in both inflammation and immunity. It has already been mentioned in connection with chemotaxis of leucocytes and opsonisation of encapsulated bacteria. The system consists of nine protein components which are present in inactive form in plasma. (Complement components are numbered from 1 to 9 and referred to as C1, C2, etc. Activated forms are indicated by a bar—C$\bar{1}$, etc.) Several complement components are enzymes which act on one another in sequence; the result is essentially an amplification mechanism, generating relatively large effects from limited stimuli, analogous to the enzyme cascade mechanism of the blood clotting system. The following complement components and fragments have important roles in acute inflammation (Figures 1.11, 1.12).

1 A kinin-like fragment generated from component C2, with properties of vasodilatation and increasing vascular permeability. *C2-kinin* is distinct from bradykinin and kallidin, and is important in the condition of hereditary angio-oedema (below).

2 C3, the component present in highest concentration in the blood. When fixed at the surface of a bacterium, as a result of the combination of an opsonising antibody and the bacterial wall, C3 promotes phagocytosis. Receptors for fixed C3 exist at the surface

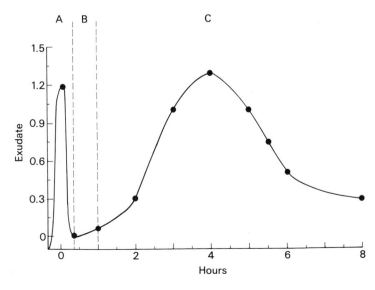

Figure 1.10 Diphasic permeability change in acute inflammation. Responses of this type can be produced experimentally in guinea-pig skin by thermal injury or acute bacterial infection.
A Immediate phase, mediated by histamine or 5-HT.
B Latent period.
C Delayed phase, mediated by kinins, prostaglandins and leukotrienes.

of phagocytic cells to aid the uptake of complement-coated micro-organisms.

3 During the activation of the complement sequence, small fragments are split off from components C3 and C5, and are termed C3a and C5a. These are *anaphylatoxins*, substances which cause the release of histamine from mast cells, which in turn results in vasodilatation and increased permeability. C5a is also a powerful chemotactic stimulus for neutrophils.

4 An activated complex of three complement components known as $\overline{C567}$ is produced and is chemotactic for neutrophils, though less significant in this respect than C5a.

5 When all the complement components have been fixed at a cell surface, damage to the membrane occurs. This is readily demonstrated with thin-walled cells such as red cells, where complement fixation leads to haemolysis. In the same way, complement, in conjunction with the enzymatic action of lysozyme, can be bactericidal for several Gram-negative bacteria; with Gram-positive organisms, however, complement probably has little direct damaging effect on the cell (p. 386).

The best known stimulus to the activation of complement is the formation of an antibody–antigen complex, a typical example of which in acute inflammation of bacterial origin is the combination of opsonins in the exudate with the bacterial capsule or cell wall. The sequence of events involved in complement activation in this way—known as the *classical* pathway—is shown in outline in Figure 1.11. Although this sequence of reactions is triggered by combination of antibody with antigen, only certain classes of antibody (see Section 2) can activate complement by the classical pathway. There is also an independent route of complement activation called the *alternative* pathway, which bypasses the early complement components (C1, C4, C2) and depends on

Figure 1.11 The 'classical' pathway of complement activation.

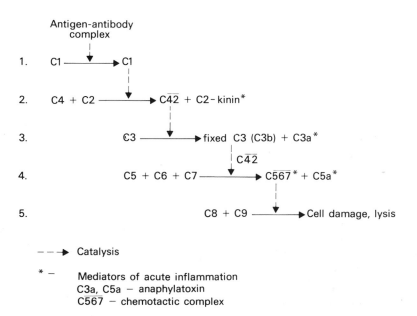

(After Lachmann)

31

other serum proteins (factor B, properdin and others) to generate an enzyme which activates C3. From the C3 stage, the sequence of events and in particular the production of phlogistic fragments, etc., are essentially the same in both the classical and alternative pathways. The alternative pathway can be triggered by certain polysaccharides and by the lipopolysaccharide (endotoxin) which forms part of the envelope of Gram-negative bacteria. The alternative pathway enables complement-assisted phagocytosis and inflammation to proceed before the influx of antibody. A more detailed account of the complement system can be found in Section 2.

There are other potentially important stimuli, besides antibody–antigen reactions, for the activation of complement during inflammation. Particularly significant are certain proteolytic enzymes which are released or activated in acute inflammation. *Plasmin* and *thrombin*, for example, both of which are activated during inflammation (below), can start the whole complement sequence by acting on C1, or may act directly on C3 to generate anaphylatoxin. Enzymes released from the lysosomes of dead neutrophils can also activate complement in the same way. Thus a self-prolonging cycle of leucocyte emigration can be set up: leucocytes enter an area of tissue damage and die *in situ*, releasing lysosomal enzymes, the latter in turn acting on complement to produce vasoactive and chemotactic products which further increase leucocyte emigration (Figure 1.12). The same type of enhancement sequence follows antibody-stimulated complement activation: opsonins in exudate combine with bacteria, fix complement and enhance phagocytosis, while at the same time complement factors are released which cause further exudation of plasma containing opsonins and leucocytes, and so the cycle is repeated (Figure 1.12).

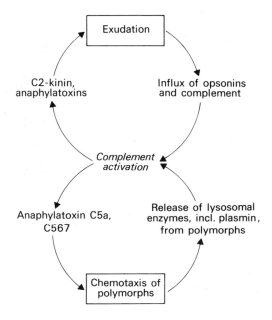

Figure 1.12 Role of complement products in acute inflammation.

Clearly the activation of complement and the consequent enhancement of acute inflammation will often have beneficial results, particularly in acute infectious disease. On the other hand, complement-induced inflammation under other circumstances has decidedly harmful effects and is an important cause of tissue damage in a variety of conditions. The main areas of damage are often in the kidneys, joints, heart and skin, and conditions where complement is involved include glomerulonephritis, rheumatoid arthritis, rheumatic fever, drug allergies and several others. The pathogenesis of these conditions is discussed at greater length in Section 2.

PLASMIN (FIBRINOLYSIN).

This is an important enzyme which normally exists in blood and phagocyte lysosomes as its inactive precursor, plasminogen. Plasmin is generated by activated Hageman factor following tissue damage (Figure 1.13), as well as by bacterial enzymes such as streptokinase and by tissue elements such as endothelium. It has the following activities:

1 Digestion of fibrin—important because of the large amounts of fibrin which can be laid down during inflammation (see Fibrinolysis, Section 5).

2 Action on activated Hageman factor to produce subunits of Hageman factor, which in their turn activate prekallikrein and thus lead to kinin formation (Figure 1.13).

3 Action on complement, already described, leading to generation of phlogistic and chemotactic factors. (The significance of this reaction *in vivo* has yet to be determined.)

Figure 1.13 Pathways for production of mediators of inflammation.

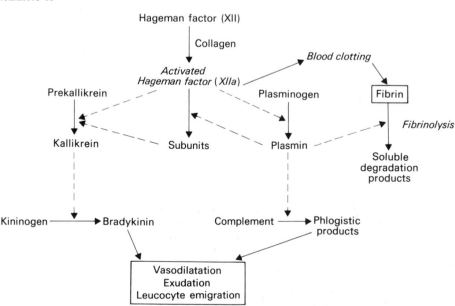

This has been referred to in various connections above and is potentially a central component of the inflammatory process. Hageman factor is a serum β-globulin, of molecular weight 110,000, originally described as the factor in blood which is activated by glass to cause intrinsic blood clotting (factor XII). It is known to be activated by other surfaces also, and particularly important in the present context are its activation by collagen and basement membrane. Besides causing blood coagulation, the main actions of Hageman factor are (a) the conversion of plasminogen to plasmin, and (b) the conversion of prekallikrein to kallikrein (Figure 1.13). Plasmin acts back on Hageman factor, producing subunits which are more potent activators of prekallikrein than Hageman factor itself. Since plasmin, and also kallikrein, activate complement to produce a variety of important phlogistic fragments already described above, and since kallikrein generates bradykinin from kininogen, the activation of Hageman factor is clearly a key event in inflammation. The result is the production of several important vasoactive and chemotactic substances to cause increased vascular permeability, formation of exudate and emigration of leucocytes. The central role of Hageman factor in these processes is shown in Figure 1.13. (An account of the functions of Hageman factor in blood clotting and fibrinolysis can be found in Section 5.)

PROSTAGLANDINS AND LEUKOTRIENES

The prostaglandins (PGs) are a family of molecules of universal distribution which mediate a variety of pharmacological effects in different tissues. They were discovered in the 1930's and the name was coined by von Euler, who believed them to be products of the prostate gland. They are 20-carbon fatty acids that contain a 5-carbon ring; the major classes are designated PGA, PGB, PGE and PGF, followed by a subscript (1,2,3) which denotes the number of double bonds outside the ring (Figure 1.14). Many tissues have the capacity to synthesize prostaglandins and generally do so when stimulated; tissue damage and inflammation are stimuli leading to prostaglandin production. Prostaglandins are not stored, but are synthesized when required. The precursor molecule is *arachidonic acid* and this is produced by the action of *phospholipase A_2* on phopholipids present in cell membranes. It is envisaged that neutrophil (lysosomal) phospholipase is activated during acute inflammation and this is the starting point for production of prostaglandins via arachidonic acid. The pathway of prostaglandin synthesis involves the action of an enzyme called *cyclo-oxygenase* (prostaglandin synthetase) which converts arachidonic acid into an intermediate cyclic endoperoxide; subsequent enzymatic steps then generate the range of prostaglandins (Figure 1.15a).

There is considerable evidence that prostaglandins such as PGE_1 and PGE_2 act as mediators and regulators of acute inflammation. They fulfil the essential criteria for mediators

Figure 1.14 Structures of some representative molecules derived from arachidonic acid.

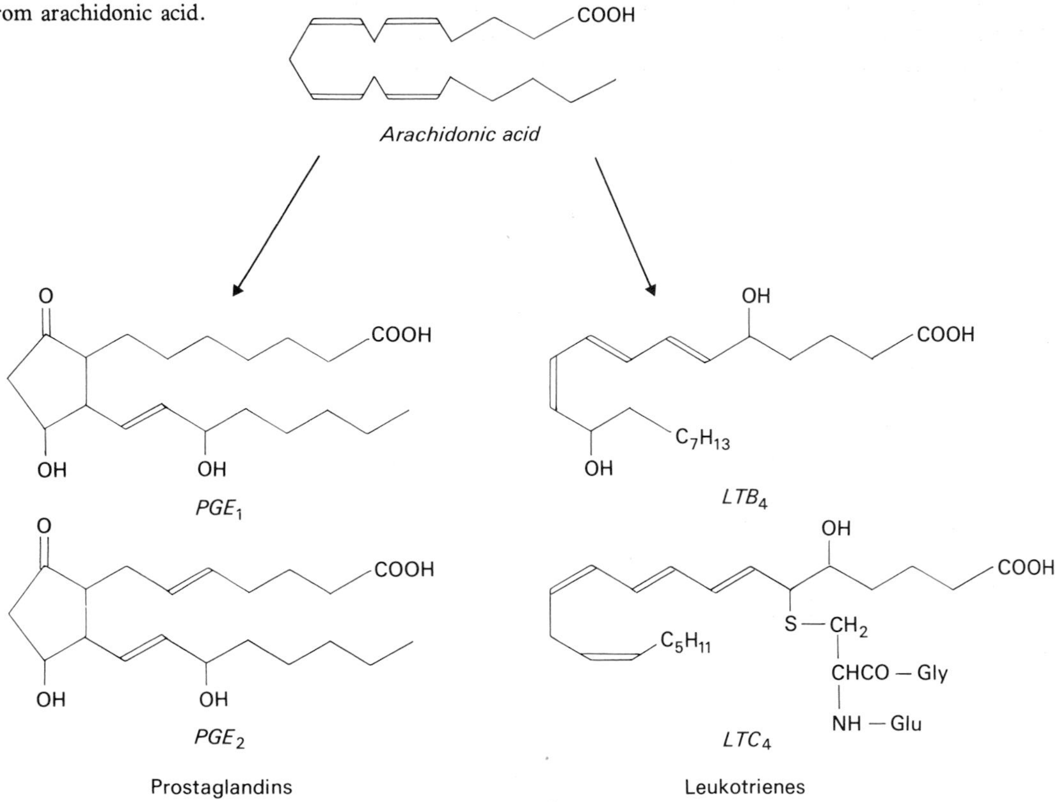

Arachidonic acid

PGE_1

PGE_2

Prostaglandins

LTB_4

LTC_4

Leukotrienes

recognised by Sir Henry Dale in 1929, namely the ability to produce the cardinal signs of inflammation, release during the course of an inflammatory response, and inhibition by known anti-inflammatory agents. PGE_1 and PGE_2 cause vasodilatation and increased permeability when injected into normal human skin, and seem to act directly on capillaries and venules rather than via release of agents such as histamine. It is also possible to demonstrate their production during experimental inflammation. Another important prostaglandin is the unstable molecule *prostacyclin* (PGI_2), which is produced by the endothelial cells of blood vessels. PGI_2 causes vasodilatation and increased permeability and may be one route of action of kinins; bradykinin, for example, stimulates release of PGI_2 from vascular endothelium.

Recently, a second pathway of arachidonic acid metabolism was discovered in which this molecule is acted on by an enzyme called *lipoxygenase* (Figure 1.15a). This pathway gives rise to a group of biologically active lipids called *leukotrienes* (LTs), so named because they were first found in neutrophils and their common structural feature is a conjugated triene. Leukotrienes are structurally distinct from prostaglandins, but are also unsaturated fatty acids (Figure 1.14). The major molecules in the group are designated LTA_4, LTB_4, LTC_4, LTD_4 and LTE_4.

35

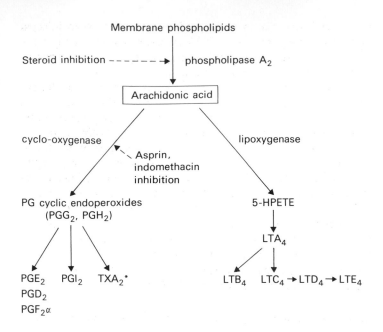

Figure 1.15 Products of arachidonic acid in inflammation. (a) Pathways of arachidonic acid metabolism. (*see Section 5 for thromboxanes). (b) Prostaglandins and leukotrienes in acute inflammation. (see also Table 1.2).

(a)

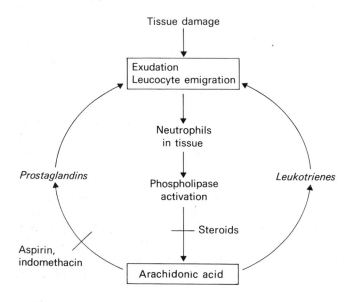

(b)

Leukotrienes are known to be produced by neutrophils and mast cells. An important role in inflammation is ascribed to LTB_4, which causes adherence of neutrophils to endothelium of post-capillary venules as well as being a powerful chemotactic agent for neutrophils; it is thus probably important in the migration of leucocytes to sites of inflammation. LTC_4 and LTD_4 are also potentially important inflammatory mediator molecules, since they cause dilatation and increased permeability of small blood vessels and give rise to a weal-and-flare reaction when injected into human skin (see also p. 156 for their role in anaphylaxis). Leukotrienes and prostaglandins may act synergistically during acute inflammation to enhance each other's effects.

Prostaglandins and leukotrienes seem to be responsible for the delayed, prolonged phase of acute inflammation (Figure 1.10). Thus, in skin burns for example, there are two discernable phases of vascular permeability, an immediate phase lasting about 10 minutes and a delayed phase which begins after 30 minutes and persists for several hours or days. In some model systems, such as acute inflammation induced in the paw of the rat by injection of carrageenin, three distinct phases of mediator action are demonstrable. The immediate reaction is due to release of histamine and serotonin from mast cells (only histamine in man); kinins mediate a second phase, while the third and more prolonged phase is caused by prostaglandins and leukotrienes. The involvement of the products of arachidonic acid metabolism in the inflammatory response is summarised in Figure 1.15b and Table 1.2.

Table 1.2 Role of prostaglandins and leukotrienes in inflammation.

Activity	Mediators
Vasodilatation	PGE_1, PGE_2, PGI_2; LTC_4, LTD_4
Increased permeability	PGE_2, PGI_2; LTC_4, LTD_4, LTE_4
Pain	PGE_2, PGI_2
Neutrophil migration (adherence, chemotaxis)	LTB_4

The anti-inflammatory actions of aspirin, indomethacin and steroids result from inhibition of the pathways of arachidonic acid metabolism (Figure 1.15a). Aspirin and indomethacin inhibit cyclo-oxygenase and thus block the formation of prostaglandins. Anti-inflammatory steroids, on the other hand, prevent the generation of arachidonic acid from phospholipids, evidently by inducing the synthesis of a protein which inhibits phospholipase A_2; thus steroids prevent the formation of prostaglandins *and* leukotrienes, which may account for some of their therapeutic effects not shared by aspirin-type agents. It is likely that, in time, new anti-inflammatory drugs will be developed which inhibit both the cyclo-oxygenase and lipoxygenase pathways; such agents might be as effective as steroids, but lack their undesirable side effects.

In addition to producing acute inflammation, however, PGE_1 and PGE_2 have also been found to inhibit inflammatory changes, preventing histamine release from mast cells and the shedding of lysosomal enzymes by neutrophils. The differential effects of prostaglandins are probably related to their concentration in the tissue; thus, lower concentrations of PGE_1 and PGE_2 stimulate inflammation, while an excess is inhibitory. The prostaglandins can therefore be regarded as regulators of inflammation, in that they can both mediate and suppress the response. At the cellular level, these opposing influences are the result of alteration in the levels of cyclic nucleotides cyclic AMP and cyclic GMP, as described below.

NEUTROPHILS AS A SOURCE OF MEDIATORS

The release of neutrophil lysosomal contents provides a source of several mediators of inflammation. (a) Lysosomal proteases, among them plasmin, generate complement fragments such as C3a and C5a by acting directly on C3 and C5. C5a stimulates further release of lysosomal contents by reverse endocytosis (p. 26) and attracts more neutrophils by chemotaxis. (b) Neutrophil lysosomes contain a kallikrein which generates bradykinin from kininogen. (c) Cationic proteins, which have been noted above for their antibacterial properties, cause degranulation of mast cells and release of histamine, etc. (d) Neutrophils are a source of phospholipase, required for prostaglandin production in the tissue, and they also synthesize prostaglandins and leukotrienes. Thus, neutrophils may have a central role in promoting and regulating the events of acute inflammation, including vessel wall permeability and their own influx into the site. A widely accepted view is that the action of enzymes shed from neutrophil lysosomes increases permeability by damaging endothelial cells or breaking down material in the junctions between them; the enzymes may also act on the basement membrane. Note that two of the molecules directly or indirectly generated by neutrophils, namely leukotriene LTB_4 and the complement fragment C5a, are powerful chemotactic agents for neutrophils, hence tending to perpetuate inflammation in the cyclical manner described on p. 32. Moreover, in the presence of neutrophils, these chemotactic products also induce increased vascular permeability. One suggestion is that the physical swelling of neutrophils trapped temporarily beneath endothelial junctions could cause gaps to form; swelling of neutrophils *in vitro* in response to C5a has been described.

PLATELETS AS A SOURCE OF MEDIATORS

Platelets are the smallest cellular elements in the blood, where they are found at a concentration of $2-4 \times 10^8$ per ml. They play a central role in blood clotting and haemostasis (arrest of bleeding) as well as in pathological changes in the circulation such as thrombosis and atherosclerosis. (Platelet physiology and function is described in Section 5). Platelet granules contain a variety of substances which can act as mediators of inflammation, and in addition platelets can synthesize prostaglandins. The platelet α granules are lysosomal, containing proteolytic enzymes and cationic substances which can increase vascular permeability. Other granules, called dense bodies, contain ADP and the vasoactive amine 5-hydroxytryptamine (5-HT, serotonin), which has activities similar to histamine and causes smooth muscle contraction and increased permeability. The release of active substances from platelets occurs after they have *adhered* to a foreign surface, as happens when collagen is revealed by vascular damage; granule contents are then shed to the outside in the *platelet release reaction*. ADP released from the dense bodies causes another characteristic reaction of platelets, namely *aggregation*, in which a mass of tightly packed platelets is formed. Further release of mediators occurs, so that aggregation becomes self-amplifying (Figure 1.16). The aggregation of platelets reveals on the platelet surface an important component of the blood clotting system, a phospholipid called *platelet factor 3*. We have noted that exudate frequently clots, due to conversion of plasma fibrinogen to fibrin. The clotting mechanism (detailed in Section 5) is initiated by the activation of Hageman factor on contact with collagen. Besides several other plasma clotting factors, the generation of the clotting enzyme *thrombin* requires platelet factor 3 (Figure 1.16). Thrombin itself also acts back on platelets to cause further aggregation, another example of 'positive feedback'.

Besides collagen, thrombin and ADP, there are two other stimuli to platelet activation during acute inflammation. Human platelets have an Fc receptor enabling them to bind to antigen–antibody complexes, which in inflammatory responses to bacterial infection are formed when, for example, opsonins combine with bacterial capsules or when antitoxins bind to toxins. Binding of platelets to such complexes via Fc receptors causes the release of platelet mediators. (In many species other than man, platelets also bind the fixed C3 component of complement). The other activating stimulus is a factor released from basophils and, significantly, from mast cells on degranulation. This is termed *platelet activating factor* or PAF. The release of 5-HT triggered by PAF could supplement the increased permeability caused by histamine (Figure 1.16). The importance of mediators derived from platelets, in relation to histamine and plasma

Figure 1.16 Role of platelets in inflammation.
* PAF—platelet activating factor.

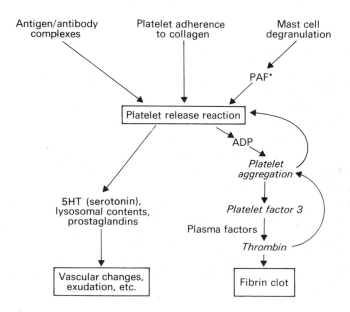

mediators, is difficult to estimate. 5-HT, as noted, has effects similar to those of histamine; however, it is more important as a mediator in rodents, which are particularly sensitive to its effects, than in man and other species. Platelet lysosomal enzymes will contribute to the generation of phlogistic molecules from plasma proteins such as complement. Finally, platelets may be a significant source of the prostaglandins PGE_1 and PGE_2, which, as noted above, are important in the production and control of inflammation. In summary, platelets can produce several mediators of potential importance in acute inflammation, as well as activating the blood clotting system which lays down fibrin.

LYMPHOKINES

Sensitised T lymphocytes (Section 2) produce a variety of biologically active proteins known as lymphokines. Their main effects are the accumulation and activation of macrophages, though some cause increased vascular permeability. They are of special importance in delayed hypersensitivity reactions and chronic inflammation, and are described on p. 61–62 and in Section 2.

Intracellular control of mediator release

Several of the mediators described are released from cellular stores, e.g. histamine from mast cells and basophils, platelet mediators, lysosomal contents from neutrophils, and so on. The stimuli which cause the release or secretion of mediators react with the surface of the cells, often via specific cell surface receptors. Inside the cell, the 'message' to release is conveyed by *cyclic nucleotides*, in particular by cyclic AMP and cyclic GMP. Release of mediators is accompanied by a *fall* in cyclic AMP levels and a *rise* in cyclic GMP; similarly, agents which raise the cyclic AMP level and lower cyclic GMP are inhibitory to the release of mediators. Examples of inhibitors which have been shown to increase intracellular cyclic AMP include PGE_1, which inhibits the release of histamine from mast cells; theophylline; and histamine itself which can suppress its own release in a negative-feedback loop. Adenylate cyclase, the enzyme which forms cyclic AMP from AMP, is present in the membrane of platelets and mast cells, and an effect on this enzyme is probably the common route for agents which react with the cell surface. However, it is probably the relative balance between cyclic AMP and cyclic GMP levels, acting in opposition to each other, which determines the outcome. It is interesting to note that other examples of secretion, such as of enzymes from salivary glands or hormones from the anterior pituitary gland, are controlled in the reverse manner, i.e. secretion is accompanied by a *rise* in cyclic AMP which acts as the intracellular trigger.

Control of inflammation

In view of the properties of self-amplification inherent in inflammation, the need for adequate control is particularly vital.

One method of control already mentioned is the rapid enzymatic destruction of active substances once they are formed. Another is the existence of natural inhibitors of mediators, including antagonists for histamine, kinins, anaphylatoxins, complement components, kallikrein, plasmin, etc. One such factor is C$\bar{1}$ inhibitor, which besides inhibiting activated C1, also inhibits activated Hageman factor and its fragments, as well as plasmin and kallikrein. A deficiency of C$\bar{1}$ inhibitor, therefore, has serious effects and is the basis of *hereditary angio-oedema*, an acute and painful condition characterised by local oedema in patches in the skin or in the respiratory or alimentary tract. The cause seems to be the uncontrolled production of C2-kinin, by the pathway shown in Figure 1.11, resulting in increased vascular permeability and hence oedema. Another hereditary deficiency affects serum anti-elastase, identical with serum α_1-antitrypsin, an inhibitor of the enzyme elastase which is released from leucocyte lysosomes. Lack of the inhibitor is associated with *emphysema*, the abnormal increase in the size of air spaces distal to the terminal bronchioles in the lung, due in this case to damage to the bronchiole wall. During bouts of pulmonary inflammation, elastase is released from leucocytes and, in the absence of its inhibitor, causes damage to elastic fibres in the bronchiole wall.

Carcinoid syndrome

This provides an unusual example of excessive production into the circulation of certain vasoactive inflammatory mediators, notably 5-hydroxytryptamine (5-HT), bradykinin and prostaglandins. The syndrome results from a malignant neoplasm (p. 691) of argentaffin cells, most commonly in the appendix, but sometimes elsewhere in the bowel and in the stomach or lung. The argentaffin cells form part of a diffuse collection of endocrine cells, chiefly of the gastrointestinal tract, the function of which is obscure. A characteristic clinical indication of a tumour of these cells is the 'carcinoid flush', a paroxysmal flushing of the skin of the face, neck and upper extremities, which may be spontaneous or precipitated by emotion or ingestion of food or alcohol. Other features of the syndrome are diarrhoea, fibrosis of the valves of the right side of the heart and occasionally asthma. The basis of these features lies in the production by the neoplastic cells of 5-HT and bradykinin. 5-HT is produced in large amount and the presence in the urine of its major metabolite, 5-hydroxyindole-acetic acid, forms a diagnostic test for the disease. The tumour tissue also contains kallikrein in high concentration, which is responsible for generation of bradykinin. The increased levels of prostaglandins present in the circulation may be released from the lungs in response to 5-HT stimulation. It seems that bradykinin is involved principally in the carcinoid flush itself, while 5-HT is the major factor in the diarrhoea. Valvular heart disease also seems to be an effect of 5-HT; the left side of the heart is protected by the metabolic destruction of 5-HT in the lungs. Carcinoids of the stomach produce histamine, which also leads to a characteristic flushing.

C-reactive protein

In many diseases involving acute inflammation, such as acute infections and rheumatological conditions, an increase in the concentration of certain serum proteins (other than specific antibodies) can be demonstrated, a phenomenon known as the *acute phase reaction*. One protein showing dramatic concentration changes is *C-reactive protein* (CRP), so called because it was discovered in the ability of sera of patients acutely ill with pneumonia to precipitate the C polysaccharide of pneumococci (p. 513). C-reactive protein is normally present in trace amounts in the blood, but within a few hours of acute injury or inflammation its plasma level may rise remarkably by more than a hundredfold, reaching peak concentrations of up to 300 μg/ml within 24–48 hours. At the end of the inflammatory response, its plasma level returns to normal. It is synthesized by hepatocytes and its increased production in inflammation may be triggered by PGE_1 or endogenous pyrogen (p. 16). In structure, C-reactive protein consists of five polypeptide subunits arranged in disc-like form (mol.wt 105,000). As well as C polysaccharide, it binds to other polysaccharides present in a wide range of bacteria, fungi and parasites, and to phospholipids (e.g. lecithin) and sphingo-lipids (e.g. sphingomyelin) which are major constituents of animal cell membranes. Its affinity is greatest for molecules containing *phosphoryl choline* and binding is calcium dependent.

An important property of human C-reactive protein is that, once bound to a target molecule, it activates *complement* by the classical pathway; indeed, it is as efficient in complement activation as IgG antibody, leading to release of active complement fragments and, if the target is on a cell surface, to cell lysis. Thus, like antibody, C-reactive protein acts as an opsonin and cytotoxic agent and initiates inflammation, suggesting that it may be a primitive, but wide-ranging, defensive protein. Injection of pneumococcal C polysaccharide into the skin of patients with a high serum level of C-reactive protein leads to a typical weal-and-flare reaction; however, the significance of C-reactive protein in acute inflammatory responses in general is unknown. Its main function is probably to assist in clearing from the blood potentially toxic materials, such as bacterial products or substances released from damaged tissue, during the course of infections or other diseases.

The presence of C-reactive protein in plasma is an indication of a tissue-damaging process, the rise in its level being especially sensitive and rapid in microbial infection. Thus, measurement of the C-reactive protein level is a useful diagnostic aid in acute infections where standard microbiological investigations are difficult, as in neonatal septicaemia and meningitis. It is also of value in assessment of inflammatory disorders, including rheumatoid arthritis, rheumatic fever, ankylosing spondylitis and Crohn's disease.

Another acute phase protein, serum amyloid A, is discussed on p. 66.

TERMINATION OF ACUTE INFLAMMATION: RESOLUTION, REPAIR AND REGENERATION

The most favourable end of acute inflammation is the complete return to normal structure and function of the inflamed part. This process is termed *resolution*. It can only occur, however, where tissue damage has been limited, as in mild physical or chemical injury or where an infecting organism has not caused large areas of destruction, and where parenchymatous cells are capable of *regeneration*. (Inflammation can occur without cell death). Furthermore, for resolution to occur, fibrin must be removed rapidly from the site of inflammation. When either extensive tissue damage has taken place, or where fibrin persists after inflammation, or when specialised parenchymal cells cannot regenerate, a process of *repair* takes place, the result of which is the replacement of the dead tissue and fibrin by fibrous collagen and formation of a scar. The extent of fibrous repair is variable, depending on the capacity of specialised tissue cells to regenerate. The term *healing* includes the processes of resolution, regeneration and repair.

Resolution

Resolution involves the complete removal of inflammatory exudate, fibrin, dead tissue cells and their breakdown products, the reversal of the vasodilatation and vascular permeability of inflammation, and the regeneration of tissue cells. The end result is the return of the area to normal. Most of the fluid and the degraded proteins of the exudate are removed by the lymphatics. The dominant cell type in the exudate in resolving inflammation is the macrophage, in contrast with the largely neutrophil composition of exudate throughout the earlier stages of acute inflammation. Macrophages engulf and destroy dead neutrophils, many of which die *in situ* as related above; they also take up any dead tissue cells and red cells present in the exudate, as well as digesting quantities of fibrin. Most of the fibrin, however, is solubilised extracellularly by plasma fibrinolysin (plasmin) or the same enzyme released from neutrophil lysosomes. A good illustration of resolution is provided by lobar pneumonia. As already noted, infection of the lung by pneumococci is followed eventually by filling of one or more lobes with exudate, deposition of fibrin and neutrophil infiltration. When the organisms have been killed off, either by the neutrophils after opsonisation or by chemotherapy, there is a change in the cellular exudate from predominantly neutrophil to macrophage infiltration, fibrin is digested and exudate is drained off. There is also considerable activity in the local lymph nodes, the sinuses of which are packed with macrophages containing dead neutrophils and cell fragments. Eventually, if resolution is complete, the air spaces can return to normal.

Repair

Where tissue damage is extensive or when fibrin is not rapidly cleared after acute inflammation, the process of healing is by repair rather than resolution. This involves the ingrowth from the surrounding connective tissue of an initially vascular tissue containing capillary loops, fibroblasts and leucocytes and known as *granulation tissue*. With time, the fibroblasts lay down collagen fibres and the capillaries disappear, leaving an avascular area of fibrosis or *scar*. Repair by granulation and fibrosis occurs in any part of the body where a deposit of clot, exudate or dead tissue occurs, and is given the general name of *organisation*. Fibrous repair is also an important feature of chronic inflammation (p. 57). The process of repair is exemplified by the healing of wounds, especially those of the skin, and since this typifies repair following acute inflammation it will be described in some detail.

Wound healing

A body wound is repaired by the formation of fibrous tissue. Much of our knowledge of the events involved comes from observations made with the rabbit ear chamber, formed by placing transparent plates on either side of a hole punched in a rabbit's ear so that the healing changes can be followed microscopically. The wound is first filled by a blood clot containing fibrin, trapped red cells and leucocytes; in the surrounding tissue there is an immediate phase of acute inflammation with exudation, further fibrin deposition and infiltration by neutrophils as already described. Inflammation is soon followed by healing, which begins at the margins of the wound where pre-existing tissue adjoins the clot. Macrophages play an important role, invading the clot and removing it by digesting red cells, fibrin and cellular debris. Degradation products of haemoglobin (haemosiderin, bilirubin) accumulate in the macrophage granules and give them a yellow colour. The clot is also digested by enzymes released from dead neutrophils, as well as plasmin. Macrophage invasion is followed by the growth into the wound of capillaries which originate from blood vessels at the periphery. The endothelium of the latter vessels migrates and divides, growing out at first as capillary sprouts or buds, solid protruberant cords composed of endothelial cells. The sprouts grow at a rate of between 0.1–0.6 mm per day and eventually develop a lumen into which blood flows. The young vessels extend into the area cleared by macrophages and join one another (anastomose) to form capillary loops through which the blood flow is established. Capillary loops are a characteristic feature of the growing edge of a healing wound. The newly formed vessels are fragile and more permeable, both to red cells and fluid, than mature vessels; red cells extruded from them are taken up and disposed of by macrophages. Neutrophils adhere to the margins of very young vessels, as in areas of inflammation, and emerge from them, especially at the growing edge, where they contribute to digestion of debris. While all the young vessels are initially capillaries, they soon differentiate into arterioles and venules, the former acquiring a smooth muscle coat and a vasomotor nerve supply. The ingrowth of lymphatics follows a similar course to that of capillaries, though it begins later and is more irregular.

At the same time as blood vessels grow into the wound, fibroblasts in the peripheral connective tissue are stimulated to divide and follow macrophages into the clot. They are responsible for the production of *collagen*, the essential material which heals wounds. Collagen is laid down in the area from which macrophages have partially cleared clot and debris and into which new blood vessels are growing and supplying nutrient. Collagen is evident about six days after the first appearance of fibroblasts, initially as thin reticulin fibres which soon mature into the thick collagen bundles of fibrous tissue. Fibroblasts also produce the mucopolysaccharides (glycosaminoglycans) of the ground substance. Most of the blood vessels are obliterated with time as the fibrous tissue thickens, so that a pale avascular scar is formed. An important feature of fibrous tissue is its tendency to contract (*cicatrisation or contracture*), which reduces the size of the wound but can also lead to potentially dangerous tissue distortion and obstruction of blood vessels. The shrinkage of the collagen fibres results in their orientation along tension lines across the wound.

Skin wounds

The processes which occur in surgical and accidental skin wounds in man are essentially those described above. It is usual to distinguish healing in which the sides of the wound are brought close together, e.g. by stitching, known as *healing by first intention*, from that in which the edges of the wound are allowed to gape, called *healing by second intention*. However, the process of repair is essentially similar in both and the differences are quantitative rather than qualitative.

Healing by first intention

This is the rule with surgical incisions and small, clean, accidental wounds, which are sutured so that there is the minimum of space between the sides. During the first 24 hours, the space is filled with clot and exudate and invaded by neutrophils and monocytes as a result of inflammatory changes. Epithelial cells migrate over the surface and into the wound and proliferate rapidly (see below). Epithelium also grows into the incision and down the suture tracks, but these epithelial ingrowths later disappear and the final scar is covered by normal epithelium. Mitoses in connective tissue are found at the end of the first day. By the third day, capillary sprouts can be seen. Reticulin fibres appear on the fourth or fifth day and rapidly mature into fibrous tissue. This is usually strong enough to take strain after 8–10 days when stitches are removed. An incision into the abdominal wall (a laparotomy wound) heals in about three weeks, though it may take several months for the repaired area to reach its maximal strength. The young scar tissue is initially vascular and appears red or, when cold, bluish; it becomes progressively less vascular and the scar develops into a fine white line.

Healing by second intention

This occurs with larger wounds where the margins are separated. An early event, not seen in healing by first intention, is the *contraction* of the wound, which can reduce its size very considerably and even close it altogether in fur-bearing animals. This is very helpful in minimising the area to be repaired and accelerating healing. It is less important in man; surface wounds on the back and abdomen may show useful contraction, but not on the front of the thorax or limbs. This wound contraction is not caused by collagen fibres and should be distinguished from shrinkage of scars. It is the result of a contractile property of fibroblasts themselves, which contain cytoplasmic fibrils of actomyosin. Other differences between healing by first and second intention are the result of the greater area which has to be covered in the latter. The degree of inflammation and the amount of debris to be cleared by macrophages are proportionately greater. Epithelialisation proceeds from the margins of the wound, first by cells from the lower layers of the epidermis sliding across the wounded surface (under the scab of dried clot). A few hours later, mitosis takes place in the epidermal cells of the skin around the cut edge and later in the spreading epithelium itself. Cells continue to divide and migrate across the surface until they meet at the middle of the wound; division and migration then both cease, an effect known as *contact inhibition*. In this phenomenon, cells of the same differentiated type recognise each other, adhere to each other and evidently interchange signals which inhibit mitosis and movement. Its basis is discussed at greater length in Section 6 (p. 710).

Meanwhile, granulation tissue forms from the base and sides of the wound. The base of the wound appears red and finely granular when viewed with a hand lens; it was this which originated the term 'granulation'. Each granule consists of a loop of new capillaries, with surrounding macrophages and fibroblasts; the granules are extremely delicate and bleed easily when touched. The granulation tissue increases in thickness until the wound is filled. In this way, fibrous tissue heals the area and a scar forms covered by a layer of epidermis. Maturation of the fibrous tissue takes several months and it remains pink (or blue when cold) much longer than in healing by first intention. Gradually, however, the vessels disappear and the scar is paler than the surrounding skin. In contrast with the neat scar of healing by first intention, the scar tissue of healing by second intention is large and distorted. Its tendency to shrink has already been noted.

Occasionally, a large, bulging scar is formed by excessive collagen production; such a raised area is called a *keloid*. The tendency to form keloids is seen mostly in Negroes, and from its occurrence in families appears to be inherited as a dominant trait (Section 7). In susceptible individuals, keloid formation is seen in both first and second intention healing.

Organisation

Wound healing provides an illustration of the general process of organisation, which occurs in any part of the body as a sequel to deposition of clot, fibrinous exudate or necrosis. The organisation of thrombi in blood vessels is described on p. 646; dead areas of tissues, such as infarcts, are also replaced by fibrous tissue (p. 649). Lobar pneumonia has been cited as an example of efficient resolution following inflammation; in some cases of lobar pneumonia, however, when removal of fibrin is for some reason insufficiently rapid, organisation occurs instead and results in fibrosis of part of the lung. Fibrinous exudate in the pleural, pericardial or abdominal cavities may be turned into fibrous tissue which binds the organs together by fibrous bands or *adhesions*. These tend to contract and their shrinkage can lead to distortion and functional disturbance of affected organs. In the peritoneal cavity, for example, obstruction of the intestinal tract or its blood supply may result. The contracture of fibrous tissue may have very serious effects in vital organs, such as the stenosis and distortion of the mitral and aortic valves of the heart following acute rheumatic fever, which can lead to regurgitation. On the other hand, newly formed fibrous tissue may stretch if subjected to tension. This can occur in the abdomen, where a laparotomy scar may stretch and allow abdominal contents to protrude (herniate) into a fibrous sac. Another instance occurs in the wall of the aorta in atherosclerotic or syphilitic arterial disease, where a local dilatation (aneurysm) may result following scarring of the media.

Factors affecting wound healing

Wound healing is influenced both by local and general factors. The former include the apposition of wound edges, infection, and the adequacy of the local blood supply; among general factors, deficiency of vitamin C and certain amino acids and the presence of a raised glucocorticoid level can retard wound healing.

Local factors

Apposition. The influence on healing in the skin of the proximity of the wound edges has been emphasised above. In the skin and other soft tissues where repair is by fibrous union, this is achieved by suturing, but exactness is not required in placing the edges of the wound together. In contrast, regeneration of bone demands a more precise apposition of the fragments to be healed and strict immobilisation of the broken ends during the healing process. Movement between the broken ends prevents new bone formation and leads instead to fibrous repair.

Infection. Bacterial infection of wounds occurs most frequently with pyogenic organisms (streptococci, staphylococci) from clothes, skin or the respiratory tract; occasionally contamination is by tetanus or gas gangrene organisms from the soil. Granulation tissue provides an important barrier against infection, and introduction of organisms into a wound is much less likely to cause serious infection if the wound has granulated. The effect of infection is to prolong the phase of inflammation, increasing exudation and leading to pus formation. If it is not too severe, healing proceeds, though much more slowly than normal and with the formation of a larger amount of scar tissue. Severe infections prevent healing altogether. Streptococcal and staphylococcal infection may result in secondary haemorrhage, which is most usual about a week after injury. In case of infection, suturing of the wound is delayed until the organisms have been cleared; even late suturing is beneficial as it enables healing to proceed more rapidly, prevents further infection and reduces the amount of scarring.

Blood supply. An adequate blood supply is required for efficient healing. This is probably the reason leg ulcers heal slowly in patients with varicose veins and why the severance of blood supply to fractures leads to necrosis rather than healing.

General factors

Scurvy. Deficiency of ascorbic acid (vitamin C) causes poor wound healing with inadequate formation of collagen, so that the edges of wounds do not knit together. Exudation, clotting and epithelialisation are unaffected, but in severe deficiency the wound edges separate after a few days and the wound 'breaks down'. Lack of ascorbic acid makes it impossible for fibroblasts to synthesize mature collagen, apparently because it is required for hydroxylation of proline residues in the collagen molecule. In scurvy, only the precursor form, protocollagen, is synthesized, which cannot form fibrous tissue.

Sulphur-containing amino acids. Wound healing can continue normally during starvation, provided there is sufficient methionine or cysteine available. Deficiency of these amino acids has effects similar to scurvy, i.e. inadequate collagen synthesis.

Glucocorticoids. Cortisone and related agents inhibit repair by preventing the formation of new blood vessels and the proliferation and migration of fibroblasts. This has been of great importance in ophthalmology. Local application of appropriate corticosteroids to a damaged cornea in man inhibits fibrous repair, while resolution and regeneration occur, thus avoiding adhesions and opacities due to scar formation without preventing satisfactory healing. In some other species, regeneration and fibrosis may be equally depressed.

Regeneration

The proliferation of connective tissue and blood vessels occurs in all organs in response to wounding or loss of tissue. However, in addition to the development of fibrous repair, a variable degree of regeneration also occurs. Regeneration consists of the proliferation of tissue cells and their differentiation into specialised tissue structures. The effect of healing processes on the structure and function of organs depends on the relative contributions of fibrous repair and regeneration.

Since regeneration depends to a large extent on the ability of differentiated cells to multiply, it is helpful to classify somatic cells according to the degree to which they have preserved this property. *Labile cells* continue to multiply throughout life and include those of the epidermis, the mucous membranes of the alimentary, respiratory and urinary tracts, the uterine endometrium and the bone marrow and lymph nodes. *Stable cells* do not normally multiply in the fully grown body, but retain the ability to divide throughout adult life should the need arise; cells of the liver, pancreas, thyroid, adrenal cortex and renal tubular epithelium are in this category, and regeneration can thus take place from cells which survive tissue injury. *Permanent cells*, such as neurones and skeletal muscle fibres, lose the ability to multiply about the time of birth; damage to the central nervous system, for example, never evokes mitosis of nerve cells. As applied to permanent cells, the term regeneration merely means replacement of part of the cell where this is possible without cell division, e.g. regrowth of an axon or dendrite or of part of a muscle fibre. Some examples of regeneration are discussed below.

SKIN

Healing in the skin has been discussed above. The skin has limited powers of regeneration; scar tissue is covered by epidermis, but specialised structures such as sweat and sebaceous glands and hair follicles are not regenerated.

MUCOUS MEMBRANES

The regeneration of structures of mucosal epithelia in the gastro-intestinal and respiratory tracts is far more efficient than in skin epithelium. In the gastro-intestinal tract, for example, the complicated glandular structures of the stomach and small intestine can all regenerate after injury. Note that the muscularis mucosae and underlying muscle are only repaired by fibrous tissue. In one important instance, the repair of gastric epithelium fails to take place, namely in the chronic peptic ulcer (p. 58). The ulcerated area is devoid of mucosa; granulation and fibrous repair tissue form at the base of the ulcer, but inflammation continues from the margins. Failure of epithelial healing may be due in part to stomach acidity, but since this does not normally inhibit healing of stomach mucosa, other factors, as yet unknown, must be involved.

ARTERIAL ENDOTHELIUM

The occurrence of endothelial damage in arteries and its repair is of considerable importance in the pathogenesis of arterial disease, especially atherosclerosis, and reference should be made to Section 5 for a full discussion of the events involved. In brief, denuded intima is first lined by deposition of platelets from the blood; the platelet layer subsequently dissolves as endothelial cells grow out from the edge to cover the area. Fibrous changes in the intima take place at the same time and in certain circumstances can give rise to pathological lesions (see p. 652). The regeneration of large areas of arterial endothelium is a slow process, taking many weeks, in marked contrast to the vigorous proliferation of endothelial cells in the capillaries of granulation tissue. Endothelial regeneration is also important following surgical replacement of segments of diseased arteries, such as the aorta, by vessels constructed from synthetic fibres. Grafts of Dacron tubing are used for this purpose and it is remarkable that not only endothelium and connective tissue, but a structural artery wall with intima and smooth muscle layers forms in the synthetic tube. Before grafting, the tube is dipped in blood which is allowed to clot. Once the tube is grafted onto the artery, granulation tissue grows into and organises the clot from the periarterial tissues and new endothelium lines the tube in a few weeks. Similar repair processes occur in veins, but denudation here is more likely to result in significant thrombosis than in arteries (see Section 5).

LIVER

The liver provides a remarkable example of complete and rapid regeneration. When portions of the liver are removed, either surgically or through disease, a vigorous proliferation of parenchymal cells proceeds, leading to an exact restoration of liver mass. Experimentally, up to 90% of the liver can be removed by partial hepatectomy and the remaining 10% will both maintain liver function and regenerate the original mass and normal liver structure (though not precisely the original shape). Repeated partial hepatectomy, at intervals of a few weeks, can be performed on the same liver and each time the liver regenerates anew. In experiments such as these, 1 g of the original liver was calculated to generate 18 g of liver tissue.

In the normal liver, as in all other organs, cellular proliferation exactly balances cell loss. Maintenance of the steady state requires only a low frequency of mitosis, and only one cell in several thousand is found in division at any time. Following partial hepatectomy, cellular changes in the remaining cells can be observed after as little as an hour and proliferation enters an early burst with a maximum at about 24 hours. Subsequent proliferation proceeds rather more slowly; in the rat, the original weight is restored in about two weeks following removal of 75% of the liver. In restoring liver mass after resection of this degree, nearly every liver parenchymal cell divides at least once. In contrast with the scattered mitoses which occur throughout the lobule in the normal liver, in regeneration proliferation is most marked, during the first 24 hours, at the periphery, moving in a wave to the centre of the lobule by about 42 hours. This transfer of mitotic activity is due to migration inwards of dividing cells from the periphery. The mechanisms whereby the dramatic stimulation of mitotic activity occurs are not understood; some possibilities are discussed below (p. 53).

In liver regeneration following partial hepatectomy, there is a normal balance between parenchyma and fibrous stroma, i.e. fibrous repair does not interfere with regeneration. However, in liver disease due to infection, intoxication or bile duct obstruction, fibrous repair may outweigh regeneration, leading to the condition of *cirrhosis* (or 'biliary cirrhosis' in the case of bile duct obstruction). The most familiar example is the cirrhosis of chronic alcoholism (portal cirrhosis). Sheets of fibrous tissue, a massive overgrowth of the periportal stroma, divide the liver up into irregular islands, replacing the normal lobular architecture. In addition to fibrosis, the characteristic feature of the cirrhotic liver is the active regeneration of the surviving liver tissue; numerous functional regenerating nodules are found among the fibrous tissue (nodular hyperplasia). Another prominent feature is the proliferation of bile ducts to connect with the regenerating nodules. Cirrhosis leads eventually to liver failure, portal hypertension and their complications.

MUSCLE

Skeletal muscle fibres, like neurones, are permanent cells which do not divide after birth; post-natal growth consists purely of addition of cytoplasmic mass with no increase in fibre number. Multiplication of nuclei in the syncytia is rarely seen after birth, and then only in the first few months. Regeneration is possible to a certain degree after injury, but is limited to a cytoplasmic response (i.e. regrowth of sarcoplasm); lost muscle mass can only be replaced by hypertrophy of surviving fibres.

After mechanical trauma, the sarcolemma is disrupted and sarcoplasm exposed; severely injured fibres die and are not replaced. In cells which have been less seriously damaged, the dead portion of the fibre disintegrates and the fragments are removed by phagocytosis by macrophages, followed by regrowth of the fibre from the truncated ends. Multinucleated sprouts or tongues of sarcoplasm extend into the damaged area; nuclei are acquired from the remaining intact portion of the fibre, apparently by redistribution rather than mitosis. If the connective tissue around the fibres (the endomysium) has been destroyed, regenerating fibres are orientated irregularly and the wound is largely replaced by fibrous tissue. On the other hand, when skeletal muscle is injured in continuity, e.g. by crushing, the outgrowing tongues of sarcolemma on either side of the wound unite in the correct alignment. In skeletal muscle which has been divided surgically, healing is generally by formation of fibrous tissue between the severed edges, with little loss of function, though here too the continuity of the muscle may be restored by regeneration. Similarly, after other forms of injury in which the connective tissue of the endomysial tube remains in place, regenerating fibres can reoccupy their former positions; this occurs after *Zenker's degeneration*, a toxic injury to muscles of the abdominal wall seen in patients with severe typhoid fever.

Cardiac muscle which has been killed by prolonged interruption of its blood supply, as in *myocardial infarction*, does not regenerate, but is replaced by a fibrous scar; this is an important consequence of coronary thrombosis (Section 5). However, if parts of individual fibres are damaged, with preservation of their surrounding connective tissue, a cytoplasmic form of regeneration is possible as for skeletal muscle; this occurs after diphtheria or coxsackievirus infection in young persons.

Smooth muscle cells retain some capacity to proliferate, as seen for example in the fibrous plaques of atherosclerosis (p. 652) and in young arterioles developing during wound healing. However, healing of smooth muscle after surgical incision in the bowel or uterus occurs by fibrous repair.

NERVOUS TISSUE

Nerve cells do not divide and consequently cannot be replaced if they die; nor is there any useful regeneration of axons in the CNS. However, if the nerve fibres in the peripheral system are injured so that the cell survives, the axons or dendrites can be regenerated. The process involved in peripheral axonal regeneration depends on whether injury is by pressure, sufficiently severe to destroy the axon at the point of application, or by severance. In both cases, the distal part of the fibre dies along its entire length, because it is separated from the nerve body, and must be regenerated to restore nerve function. Its myelin sheath also degenerates, being reduced to droplets which are phagocytosed by macrophages; the latter also take up remnants of dead axons. The degeneration of the axon and its myelin is called *Wallerian*, after the first description by Waller. Following injury by compression, however, the continuity of the endoneurial tubes, in which the axons are found, is not interrupted and new axoplasm from the surviving proximal side can push into the endoneurial tube that was formerly occupied by the axon from the same neuron. Axoplasm grows into the tube at a rate of about 2–3 mm per day and function is restored when it reaches the terminals of the fibre. Schwann cells produce a new myelin sheath. On the other hand, if the nerve has been severed, the cut ends must be brought into apposition for regeneration to occur; if they are not approximated, fibrous tissue is laid down between them and blocks re-innervation. Regeneration again follows Wallerian degeneration of the dead distal portion of the fibre and removal of debris by macrophages. The proximal stump also degenerates for a short distance near the cut. Schwann cells then proliferate, at first from the distal stump and later from the proximal stump, and grow into the gap to establish continuity between the cut ends. Next, axon sprouts grow out from the proximal stump into the network of Schwann cells; each axon sends out several branches and some are able to find the endoneurial channels remaining between Schwann cells in the degenerated distal stump (Figure 1.17). Those which are successful grow along the old pathway, becoming enfolded by Schwann cells which lay down a new myelin sheath. In this way motor function and sensation can eventually

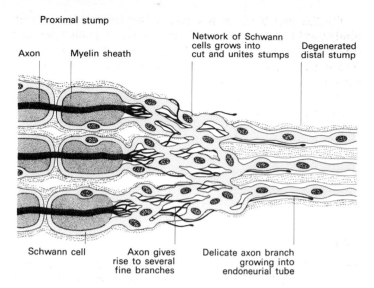

Figure 1.17 Regeneration of a severed nerve (after Ham (1979) *Histology*, 8th edn. Harper & Row).

Proximal stump

Axon Myelin sheath

Network of Schwann cells grows into cut and unites stumps

Degenerated distal stump

Schwann cell

Axon gives rise to several fine branches

Delicate axon branch growing into endoneurial tube

be restored. Essentially similar events seem to occur in the central nervous system, though functional recovery is generally poor.

Control of repair and regeneration

It is evident that during healing processes tissue cells are required to increase their rate of division, and indeed do so in striking fashion. In the regenerating liver, for example, nearly all parenchymal cells divide at least once in the seven days following large scale partial hepatectomy, which contrasts with the relative scarcity of mitosis in the normal liver; epithelial cells in the healing skin increase their mitotic activity up to fifteen times that of normal; and fibroblasts show intensive proliferation in areas undergoing repair. Moreover, when repair and regeneration are complete, the cells return to their previous lower level of mitosis and re-establish the normal state characteristic of the tissue, in which division occurs only to balance cell loss. It is important to know how the normal steady state is achieved, i.e. how tissue mass is regulated, in order to understand the changes which occur in regeneration and repair. Unfortunately our knowledge is at present incomplete, and experimental evidence on the relative importance of different mechanisms of growth control is inconclusive.

One method of growth regulation which can be observed to occur during epithelial regeneration is *contact inhibition*, the phenomenon in which direct contact between similar cells suppresses both division and motility. The cellular basis of contact inhibition is explained more fully in Section 6 in connection with its apparent breakdown in the growth of tumours. When normal cells make contact, they form junctions which permit the passage of low molecular weight substances between them (gap junctions, p. 714) and it is possible that a large number of cells in a tissue form an interconnecting network by means of such permeability junctions. This would enable intercellular signals, including signals to initiate or inhibit

53

division, to be transmitted rapidly throughout a tissue. It is particularly significant that tumour cells, which grow without heeding the normal tissue regulatory signals, can in some cases be shown to lack intercellular gap junctions. However, the role of cell contacts in the exquisite regulation of tissue mass is difficult to evaluate at present.

An alternative view is that cell growth in tissues is regulated locally by soluble mediators released by tissue cells themselves. The soluble regulators may either be stimulators or inhibitors of cell division. Much attention has been given in recent years to the latter, namely tissue-specific inhibitors of cell multiplication called *chalones*. A cybernetic theory of tissue regulation is proposed, in which chalones are feedback inhibitors, produced by differentiated tissue cells and acting to suppress mitosis in dividing cells (Figure 1.18a). The larger the differentiated cell mass, the more chalone inhibition is produced, until the steady state is established in which division only occurs to replace dead cells. According to the chalone theory, in regeneration or repair, cells enter mitosis because the level of chalone in the tissue falls due to cell loss in wounding. Thus, proliferation of epithelial and connective tissue cells in healing of skin wounds is attributed to the loss of differentiated, chalone-secreting cells consequent on the damage. Similarly, shedding of chalone-producing cells at an accelerated rate from the epidermis should stimulate proliferation of the basal layer, thus accounting for the epidermal thickening (hyperplasia) caused by excessive wear and tear on the skin.

Some experiments on the effects of wounding in the mouse ear seem to support the chalone model. The mouse ear is so thin that soluble regulators might be able to diffuse across its width, from one epidermal surface to the other. Thus, if an area of epidermis is stripped off, events on the opposite side might reveal a local decrease in inhibitor level in the wounded area or alternatively production of mitotic stimulators. The results of such experiments are in better agreement with the inhibitor rather than the stimulator concept, as mitotic activity on the other side of the ear occurred in an area opposite the centre of the wound rather than its edges, while proliferation on the wounded side was maximal at the margin (Figure 1.18b). Moreover, the increased mitotic activity on the other side of the ear is prevented by retransplantation of skin to the wounded surface. Other evidence for the existence of soluble inhibitors in the epidermis has come from experiments in which discs either of impermeable or permeable material were inserted between the regenerating edges of epithelium in wounded skin. If the disc was impermeable, e.g. cellophane, the two edges of epidermis grew around it on either side, ultimately linking to form a pocket; whereas if the disc was a permeable filter, epidermal edges grew up to the disc and then stopped (Figure 1.18b). The implication was that soluble regulatory substances were responsible for growth inhibition and were able to penetrate the filter. (Compare this with the concept of contact inhibition). However, *in vitro*, contact between cell layers is essential for inhibition of mitosis and movement.

Several years ago indications were found that regulators of

Figure 1.18 (a) The chalone theory as applied to control of epidermal growth (after Iversen (1969) in *Homeostatic regulators*, ed. Wolstenholme G. & Knight J., Churchill, p. 29).
(b) Chalone experiments.
I   The predicted patterns of mitosis in the mouse ear epidermis opposite an extended wound on the assumption in (i) that a stimulator substance is released from the edges of the wound, and in (ii) that an epidermal inhibitor (chalone) is reduced in concentration. The experimental result corresponded more closely with (ii) (after Bullough & Laurence (1960) *Proc. Roy. Soc. B.*, **151**, 517).
II   Behaviour of epidermis when regeneration was interrupted by (i) a disc of impermeable material or (ii) a permeable filter, inserted into the wound. In (i) the epidermis migrated around the disc, but in (ii) the epidermis stopped growing on either side of the implant, implying passage of a soluble inhibitor (indicated by dots) (after Mizuno & Fujii (1969) J. Fac. Sci. Univ. Tokyo, **11**, 475).

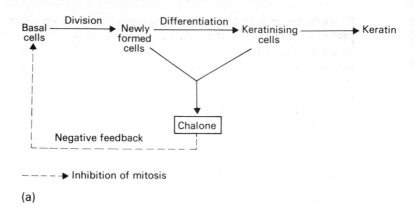

(a)

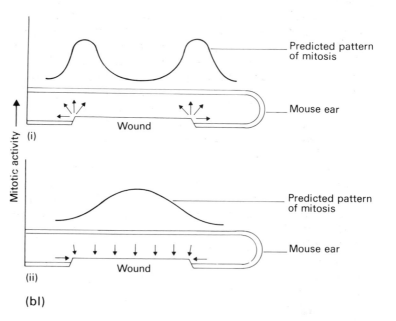

(bl)

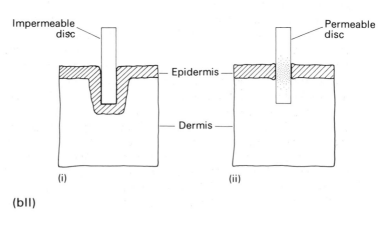

(bll)

regeneration were present in the bloodstream, in experiments in which two rats were connected together surgically so that they shared a common vascular system (parabiosis). When partial hepatectomy was performed on one rat, proliferation commenced in the livers of both animals. The effect on the normal liver was greatest when total hepatectomy was performed on the partner. Hence a signal seemed to have been transmitted in the bloodstream from the injured rat to the normal partner to commence division of liver cells. (The possibility that liver hypertrophy was stimulated by an increased work load on the remaining liver should be borne in mind as an alternative explanation.) Assuming that the signal was derived from the injured tissue itself, rather than a tissue-specific hormone produced elsewhere, it is more likely to have been a reduction in level of an inhibitor than release of a stimulator from damaged tissue, as evidenced by the effect of total liver removal. More recently, there have been several descriptions of a specific inhibitor obtained by homogenisation of liver; it also seems to be present in the circulation. (Note that cell regeneration in most tissues is assumed to reflect a *local* fall in chalone production rather than changes in circulating chalone levels.)

The study of chalones has proceeded to extraction of soluble inhibitors from tissues, e.g. 'epidermal chalones' have been obtained from skin extracts and show specificity for epidermal cells in culture. *In vitro*, chalones are not species specific in their action—an extract of pig skin will inhibit division in the mouse epidermis (but not mouse liver). Their precise mode of action is so far unknown, but it appears that they act mainly to arrest the cell cycle in the G_1 phase, which precedes DNA synthesis, though G_2 (post-synthetic) arrest can also occur (see p. 709). An action on the intracellular concentration of cyclic nucleotides (increase of cyclic AMP, fall in cyclic GMP) is a predictable intervening step. In this regard it is interesting that the inhibition of division in the epidermis by specific chalone requires the presence of a stress hormone, such as adrenaline, which is known to act by increasing activity of membrane adenylate cyclase and hence formation of cyclic AMP. The characterisation of chalones is as yet in its infancy and there has been little success in purification.

In contrast to the chalones, there may also exist soluble local stimulators of mitosis, which would be released on tissue injury. Such substances have been called 'wound hormones', 'trephones' and more recently 'antichalones'. For example, in the skin, if epidermis is separated from dermis and placed in culture, the activity of the normally dividing basal cells ceases and all the cells die; but if the separated epidermis is replaced on dermis, basal cell mitosis is restimulated and the tissue remains normal. Other connective tissue sources can substitute for dermis. The implication is that the dermis produces a nontissue-specific stimulator of mitosis, the effect of which is normally counterbalanced in the skin by the specific epidermal chalone. Proliferation on injury could occur through a shift in the normal balance, with reduced chalone inhibition. Obviously, the details of such mechanisms are vague at the moment, though in principle the idea that tissue size is regulated by antagonistic stimulatory/inhibitory mediators is attractive. Further progress depends on isolation and characterisation of the molecules involved. (See p. 719 for discussion of chalones in neoplasia.)

CHRONIC INFLAMMATION

As a matter of definition, the distinction between acute and chronic inflammation is made solely on the basis of duration—any inflammation lasting for weeks or months is termed chronic, regardless of its cause or histological characteristics. However, within this definition two types of chronic inflammation can be distinguished. In some cases, chronic merely supercedes acute inflammation where the latter is not resolved in the normal way. On the other hand, chronic inflammation is often a distinct process from the outset, with only a brief initial acute phase and with several features which can distinguish it from acute inflammation. An essential feature of all chronic inflammation is that processes of inflammation and repair occur simultaneously; this is an important difference from acute inflammation, where inflammatory and healing events are sequential.

Persistent suppuration

Persistent suppuration is the general example of chronic inflammation following on acute inflammation. This occurs where an abscess fails to heal after rupture or surgical drainage, but continues to suppurate, often because the fibrous wall of the abscess cavity has become so rigid that its collapse is prevented. Residual micro-organisms can then lead to renewal of inflammation. Examples of chronic abscesses occur in the pleural cavity in empyema, or when an abscess forms in bone as in osteomyelitis. The presence of a 'foreign body' in a wound—indigestible foreign material such as dirt or wood—also causes prolonged suppuration, perhaps by harbouring bacteria or having an inhibitory or toxic effect on neutrophils. The foreign body may even be an indigestible tissue fragment of host origin. In a boil or carbuncle of the skin, for example, a portion of dense collagen of the dermis may separate as a 'slough' and lie free in the pus, as a result of tissue necrosis caused by the staphylococcal toxins p. 525. The resistance of the collagen to digestion by lysosomal enzymes leads to the persistence of suppuration. Clearly, in these cases the events involved in the chronic inflammation are essentially the same as the acute inflammation of which it is a continuation.

The ultimate result of the repair which accompanies persistent, nonresolving, acute inflammation is fibrous scarring. A good example of this is found in the kidneys. If an acute bacterial infection is overcome quickly, resolution occurs; if it persists and becomes chronic, exudation is accompanied by formation of granulation tissue and eventually fibrous scarring (e.g. chronic pyelonephritis, p. 549). Scar formation in the kidney is obviously highly detrimental to its function, and chronic pyelonephritis is important as a cause both of renal failure and systemic hypertension.

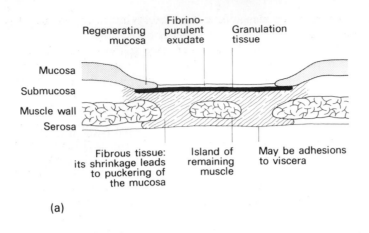

Regenerating mucosa | Fibrino-purulent exudate | Granulation tissue

Mucosa
Submucosa
Muscle wall
Serosa

Fibrous tissue: its shrinkage leads to puckering of the mucosa | Island of remaining muscle | May be adhesions to viscera

(a)

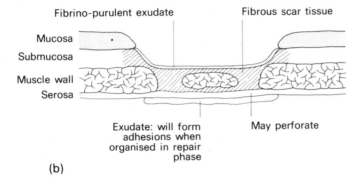

Fibrino-purulent exudate | Fibrous scar tissue

Mucosa
Submucosa
Muscle wall
Serosa

Exudate: will form adhesions when organised in repair phase | May perforate

(b)

Figure 1.19 Chronic peptic ulcer.
(a) Repair phase.
(b) Active phase.

Chronic ulceration

This is exemplified by the peptic ulcers of the stomach and duodenum when they fail to heal. The base of the ulcer becomes fibrous and, in addition to the neutrophil infiltration of the acute stage, there is an accumulation of lymphocytes, plasma cells and macrophages. At the same time, a typical acute inflammatory response may be present at the exposed base and margins of the ulcer, with suppurative exudation from the granulation tissue (Figure 1.19). Phases of repair alternate with active acute inflammation; during the latter, the granulation tissue may be destroyed, with possible perforation. Stomach muscle is destroyed in chronic ulceration and, since it cannot regenerate, is replaced by scar tissue. Contracture of the fibrous tissue can lead to pyloric stenosis or to narrowing of the lumen which is so extreme as to produce an 'hourglass' stomach. Occasionally, carcinoma of the stomach develops at the site of a chronic peptic ulcer.

Stimuli to chronic inflammation

We are now concerned with chronic inflammation when it occurs as a *distinct process* from the outset, with minimal acute inflammation. It follows many diverse stimuli, which are often mild in comparison with those leading to acute inflammation. Their common denominator is *persistence*. Chief examples are the following.

1 Prolonged chemical, particulate or physical irritation by inert materials. The presence of almost any inanimate, particulate, persistent foreign material in a tissue will provoke a chronic response termed a *foreign body reaction*. Good examples are provided by the chronic inflammatory conditions of the lungs in response to insoluble particles of silica and asbestos (silicosis, asbestosis), as well as the reactions in tissues to splinters of wood, suture materials, metal objects such as bullets, and so on.

2 Infection by certain micro-organisms, especially those which can persist in phagocytes as intracellular parasites but have low toxicity. Major infectious diseases involving chronic inflammation include tuberculosis, leprosy, syphilis and brucellosis. Hypersensitivity (Section 2) is an important part of the inflammatory process in these cases, due to persistence of microbial antigens.

3 Autoimmune reactions, that is immune responses directed against the individual's own tissues (Section 2), are important in several chronic inflammatory diseases, including rheumatoid arthritis, chronic thyroiditis and chronic hepatitis. Here too, hypersensitvity is involved in the inflammatory process, and the antigen is persistent.

4 In some cases, the aetiology is unknown, e.g. sarcoidosis, a disease resembling tuberculosis with lesions in lymph nodes and various internal organs.

Granulomas

In comparison with acute inflammation, chronic lesions are often characterised by dense cellular infiltration and proliferation rather than by a fluid exudate and are said to be proliferative or formative rather than exudative. A wide variety of cells may be present in chronic inflammation, including neutrophils, eosinophils, macrophages and the epithelioid and giant cells derived from them, lymphocytes, plasma cells and fibroblasts. In contrast with the neutrophils characteristic of much acute inflammation, macrophages and lymphocytes are frequently the dominant cell types in chronic inflammation. The accumulated mass of cells of different types—some engaged in phagocytosis or immune activity, others intent on healing by laying down collagen—which is typical of chronic inflammation is termed a *granuloma*.

The predominance in chronic inflammation of macrophages and lymphocytes is particularly the case in the classic example of a granuloma, namely the tubercle of tuberculosis (see Figure 1.20). Two cell types derived from macrophages are characteristic, *epithelioid cells* and *giant cells*. Epithelioid cells, named from their histological resemblance to certain types of epithelium, are differentiated macrophages, which have lost the ability to phagocytose, but can take up subcellular material by pinocytosis. Their function is removal of small irritant material, while larger matter is dealt with by the phagocytic macrophages. Besides their presence in the tubercle, they are also found in the granulomas of

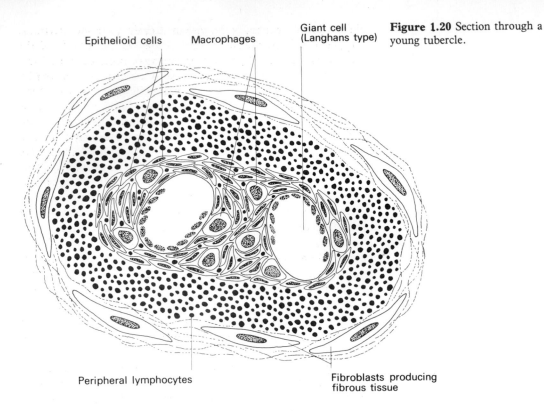

Epithelioid cells   Macrophages   Giant cell (Langhans type)

Figure 1.20 Section through a young tubercle.

Peripheral lymphocytes

Fibroblasts producing fibrous tissue

brucellosis, sarcoidosis and tuberculoid leprosy. Indigestible material which is too large for single macrophages to take up often causes macrophages to fuse and form giant cells. These are multinucleate, with the nuclei typically being arranged either in a ring around the periphery of the cell or clumped at one pole (Figure 1.20). As many as 200 nuclei may be present in a single giant cell. The peripheral ring, or 'horseshoe', arrangement of the nuclei is commonly found in the tubercle giant cells, which are called *Langhans giant cells*, while the alternative arrangement occurs in foreign body giant cells. The latter accumulate around indigestible foreign material such as talc, silica, wood splinters, glass fragments, etc. Both types of giant cell may be found in such responses. The function of giant cells is apparently to ingest foreign material by phagocytosis.

While macrophages are the chief phagocytic cells in chronic inflammation, they are often not immediately able to break down the very persistent organisms or materials which cause chronic inflammation. In order to improve their ability to take up and destroy such substances, *activation* of macrophages can take place and is accomplished by products of lymphocytes (below). Activated macrophages are more phagocytic, more metabolically active and have higher levels of lysosomal enzymes than normal macrophages (p. 23). Activation is important in enabling them to deal with organisms such as tubercle bacilli, which are very resistant to intracellular degradation.

The presence of lymphocytes in a granuloma such as the tubercle is an indication of an immunological contribution to its origin, which is generally the case in chronic bacterial infections. In these situations, the small lymphocytes can be considered the effector cells of chronic inflammation; they produce the soluble mediators of chronic inflammation, substances known as *lymphokines*, which can cause the accumulation of macrophages and their enhanced ability to kill ingested micro-organisms. As will be described in Section 2, these are the processes involved in cell-mediated immunity, immunity dependent on the activity of sensitised lymphocytes rather than humoral antibody. When they are present, the granuloma can be considered the site of a chronic cell-mediated immune response. The role of lymphocytes is particularly well illustrated by the polar forms of leprosy. In *lepromatous* leprosy, the granuloma consists of an accumulation of undifferentiated macrophages, known as 'lepra cells', packed with living organisms (*Mycobacterium leprae*) which they are unable to destroy; lymphocytes are absent. By contrast, in *tuberculoid* leprosy, where lymphocytes are present in the infiltrate, macrophages are activated and all organisms are killed off by them. Epithelioid cells are present. The difference between the two conditions is the absence of cell-mediated immunity to *M. leprae* in lepromatous leprosy, and its presence in the tuberculoid form p. 601.

The pleomorphic composition of a granuloma (i.e. presence of mixed cell types) is important as a practical guide in distinguishing unusual chronic inflammation from certain tumours of connective tissue origin. In the latter, in contrast, only one type of cell is expected to be present, even if varying in size and shape. One example where difficulties arise in drawing conclusions of this type from histology is Hodgkin's disease, where granulomas occur which show the pleomorphism usually associated with inflammation and contain lymphocytes, macrophages, and fibrous tissue. The Hodgkin's granulomas are, however, neoplastic in origin (reticulum cell tumours) in which the presence of granulocytes and other inflammatory cells is a secondary phenomenon.

Tubercle formation

The processes involved in formation of an immunologically-induced granuloma, such as the tubercle of tuberculosis, can be summarised as follows. Initial infection with *Mycobacterium tuberculosis* is followed by uptake of the organisms by local macrophages in which, at least at first, they continue to grow and divide; the macrophage at this stage is unable to destroy them. The infecting organism is antigenic and with time comes into contact with and stimulates a small number of the circulating lymphocyte population, which then respond by multiplication in the local lymph nodes (see Section 2 for details). A population of 'sensitised' lymphocytes, specifically able to recognise and respond to *M. tuberculosis*, is thus produced. On further contact with the organism at the site of infection, they now respond by the production of lymphokines, protein 'factors' with a variety of effects, principally on macrophages. Chief among them are macrophage *migration inhibition factor* (MIF), which causes the immobilisation of macrophages at the site of reaction, and *macrophage activation factor* (MAF), which induces their activation into cells which can kill and destroy their ingested micro-organisms, and their transformation into epithelioid cells. The activation of macrophages is nonspecific in that these cells have enhanced antibacterial activity against a variety of parasites (*Listeria, Brucella, Salmonella*), not merely against the inducing mycobacteria. Other lymphokines include lymph node permeability factor, so called because it was first extracted from lymph nodes, which increases local vascular permeability; factors chemotactic for macrophages and lymphocytes; and a blastogenic factor which induces mitosis in neighbouring lymphocytes. Although a state of specific cell-mediated immunity to *M. tuberculosis* now exists, the disease assumes a chronic nature. This is because of the persistence of viable organisms and the difficulty in degrading and digesting dead organisms, in spite of macrophage activation. A certain state of balance between bacterial survival and host immune response thus exists, and it is this which determines the outcome of the disease.

In tuberculosis, the patient is not only immune, in the sense of ability to destroy the organism, but is also *hypersensitive*—it is the very immune response itself, rather than the virulence of the organism, which leads to tissue damage. This hypersensitivity is readily demonstrable in anyone who has had tuberculosis or been immunised with BCG vaccine (attenuated bovine *M. tuberculosis*). Injection into the skin of tuberculin, a soluble protein product obtained by culture of *M. tuberculosis*, gives a typical delayed inflammatory response which reaches a peak after 24–48 hours. The inflammation is characterised by macrophage and lymphocyte infiltration—obviously reminiscent of the constitution of the tubercle—and is termed a *delayed hypersensitivity* response (discussed further in Section 2). If sufficiently violent, necrosis and ulceration can result. Essentially the same cellular processes underlie both delayed hypersensitivity and the formation of the tubercle, as well as much of the damage to the tissue which follows should the growth of the tubercle fail to be arrested (below). The interplay between hypersensitivity and immunity was first demonstrated by Robert Koch in a classic experiment which is generally known as the *Koch phenomenon*. Koch injected a guinea-pig subcutaneously with tubercle bacilli; after a period of apparent quiescence lasting 10–14 days, a nodule formed at the site of injection, which ulcerated and the ulcer enlarged until the animal died. At the same time, the regional lymph nodes became infected. While these events were in progress, Koch reinjected live tubercle bacilli at a separate site on the same animal and observed very different events. Here an inflammatory response developed after 1–2 days, the skin became thickened, darker and eventually necrotic, finally sloughing off. The skin lesion soon healed and there was no spread of infection to the local lymph nodes. Significantly, this reaction could be obtained with dead as well as living bacilli. The vigorous skin reaction developed as a result of *sensitisation* to the organism following the first infection;

besides the local death of the tissue (hypersensitivity) the reaction also eliminated the bacteria and prevented their spread to the lymph nodes (immunity). Thus hypersensitivity and immunity are part of a single process. Note that despite its demonstrable resistance to second infection, the animal nevertheless died because by the time immunity had developed, the first infection had already taken hold.

Fate of the tubercle

The tubercle may develop in several ways. If immunity to the bacilli is sufficiently great, as it often is in man, *healing* may occur by the laying down of fibrous tissue around and within the tubercle; a large tubercle may thus become encapsulated by fibrous tissue and the disease thereby arrested. At the same time as fibrous tissue is being formed, the cell mass within the tubercle begins to break down in a characteristic way: a necrotic centre forms which, because of its cheesy appearance, is called *caseous*. This process, known as *caseation*, occurs early in the development of the tubercle in man and is an important feature. If healing does not occur, or is only partial, cellular infiltration into the tubercle continues, which thus grows, becoming visible to the naked eye as a tiny body about 1 mm in diameter; dozens of these may be seen scattered throughout tuberculous tissue (miliary tubercles). Adjacent tubercles may then coalesce to form large lesions. As this process continues, healing often proceeds simultaneously, which we have noted to be a typical feature of chronic inflammation.

Areas of caseous necrosis usually contain only small numbers of bacilli. However, the caseous zone may in due course soften and *liquefy* due to enzymatic digestion, and the organisms then multiply rapidly in the liquefied material. As a result of liquefaction, the lesion resembles an abscess, and as there is none of the vasodilatation of acute inflammation, it is sometimes called a 'cold abscess'. Release of liquefied debris containing organisms into the bronchus is one of the chief methods of spread of tuberculosis through the lung, provoking an intense hypersensitivity reaction and leading to rapidly fatal tuberculous bronchopneumonia (galloping consumption). At the same time, discharge of the material in the sputum is the main source of infection with human tubercle bacilli; the latter, being obligate aerobes, grow more freely in an open tissue and multiply massively after release from the cold abscess. Instead of softening, areas of caseous necrosis may *calcify*, by deposition of calcium carbonate and calcium phosphate. This is another way in which the lesion is arrested. Calcified lesions, which are easily detected by X-rays, may still carry viable bacilli. (The pathological processes in tuberculosis are further discussed in Section 4, p. 596).

Foreign body response

There are many instances of chronic granulomatous inflammation where the immune system is not involved. Virtually any foreign insoluble particles, no matter how inert, can provoke chronic inflammatory responses, including wood, metals, plastic, carbon, silica, asbestos, and so on. In surgery, suture materials such as catgut provoke the accumulation of macrophages and giant cells, and talc (magnesium silicate), previously used as a powder on surgeons' gloves, also causes a typical foreign body response with eventual fibrosis. The characteristic cells of foreign body reactions are macrophages and giant cells, the latter formed by fusion of macrophages as a reaction to the particulate stimulus which is too large to be phagocytosed by a single cell. Extensive fibrosis accompanies the response. *Silicosis* and *asbestosis* are important examples of foreign body inflammation in the lung (*pneumoconioses*, diseases of the lung caused by inhalation of metallic or mineral particles) and are serious occupational hazards for workers exposed to these dusts. With silica, a direct toxic effect on macrophages occurs which parallels the formation of the foreign body granuloma. Silica particles which are small enough to be phagocytosed are taken up by macrophages and are present in phagosomes in the cytoplasm. Lysosomal enzymes are released into the phagosome in an attempt to digest the silica particle. Not only is this obviously fruitless, but silica forms hydrogen bonds with the inside of the phagosome membrane, causing the disruption of the phagosome and release of its enzymatic contents into the cytoplasm. This causes the death of the macrophage and additional damage to surrounding lung tissue. Enzymatic damage also stimulates the infiltration of more macrophages, in which the process is repeated, as well as the development of fibrous tissue. Fibrosing granulomatous foci thus develop in the lung. After progressing slowly for a number of years, silicosis leads ultimately to respiratory difficulties and eventual incapacity. Asbestosis, but not silicosis, predisposes to neoplasia of the lung (see Section 6, p. 700).

Fibrosis

We have noted that the simultaneous occurrence of processes of repair and inflammatory cellular infiltration is the most characteristic feature of chronic inflammation. Fibroblasts continually lay down fibrous tissue, whether in the walls of a chronic abscess, the base of a chronic ulcer, or around the tubercle or foreign body granuloma. The fibrosis of chronic inflammation is a consequence of tissue destruction and, except for tissue loss itself, is its most deleterious outcome, both because of the replacement of functioning tissue by collagen fibres and because of the effect on the organ of scar contracture. The following are a few instances of damage to vital organs by chronic inflammatory fibrosis. In chronic inflammation of the liver (chronic hepatitis, cirrhosis) the fibrous tissue prevents the regeneration of normal hepatic lobules and, by interfering with blood flow, leads to portal hypertension. In the stomach, chronic ulceration and fibrosis lead to pyloric stenosis. Kidney damage produced by chronic pyelonephritis is a cause both of renal failure and hypertension. Chronic inflammation of the joints as in rheumatoid arthritis can end in fibrous ankylosis and immobilisation. On the other hand, fibrous repair is also necessary and when it is depressed by steroids the consequences can be serious, e.g. perforation of peptic ulcers into the peritoneum and the growth and dissemination of tubercle bacilli.

Amyloidosis

Chronic inflammatory diseases, both of the granulomatous and suppurative types, may be complicated by extracellular deposition in various organs of protein material called *amyloid*. It occurs in longstanding tuberculosis, syphilis, leprosy, rheumatoid arthritis, chronic osteomyelitis and chronic pyelonephritis; in the West, rheumatoid arthritis is the commonest predisposing condition, while in countries such as India, tuberculosis is the major cause of amyloidosis. When it is a complication of an existing disease, as in these cases, the condition is called *secondary amyloidosis*; however, it may also occur where no pre-exisiting clinical state is recognised, and is then called *primary amyloidosis*. Until recently, amyloidosis was an untreatable and usually lethal disease, the pathogenesis of which was mysterious; today, there is a growing understanding of its origins, though the prognosis is still grave.

In secondary amyloidosis, deposits occur in the walls of small blood vessels (arterioles, venules) throughout the body and are most prominent in the liver, kidneys, spleen and adrenals. Amyloid is deposited in the walls of liver sinusoids, in the basement membrane of renal tubules and glomeruli, and either diffusely or as many scattered nodules in the spleen ('sago spleen'). The liver and spleen are enlarged in consequence (hepatosplenomegaly), but disturbance of organ function is most noticeable in the kidney, where increased permeability of the glomerular capillaries leads to severe proteinuria and generalised oedema (nephrotic syndrome) and eventually to renal failure. In primary amyloidosis, in contrast, the heart, tongue, alimentary tract and skin are the most affected sites, with death commonly due to heart failure.

Organs in which amyloid deposits are extensive often have a waxy appearance to the naked eye. Histologically, amyloid is a homogeneous, eosinophilic deposit; it is demonstrated by staining with *Congo red*, stained sections showing a green birefringence in polarised light which is highly characteristic. It is also strongly stained brown with iodine, a reaction which gave rise to its name (amyloid—'starch-like'), though it does not contain polysaccharide. Another characteristic property is metachromasia, i.e. staining a different colour from the dye itself, with toluidine blue and crystal violet.

The electron microscope shows that amyloid is deposited as an array of rigid, linear *fibrils* of indefinite length and 75–100 Å diameter, each fibril consisting of a pair of intertwining filaments (Figure 1.21). The fibrillar structure is responsible for Congo red binding and the green polarisation colour. When studied in more detail by X-ray crystallography, it became evident that the

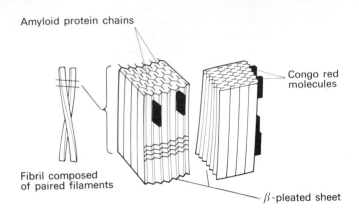

Amyloid protein chains

Congo red molecules

Fibril composed of paired filaments

β-pleated sheet

Figure 1.21 Structure of an amyloid fibril. (After Glenner, 1980.)

amyloid fibril is not helical in structure, as are collagen or keratin fibres, but has a *β-pleated sheet structure* which is unique among fibrous mammalian proteins (Figure 1.21). In this configuration, polypeptide chains are fully extended, not tightly coiled as in the α-helix, and are stabilised by hydrogen bonds between NH and CO groups in adjacent strands rather than within the same polypeptide chain. (The designation 'β' was applied to the pleated sheet simply because it was the second protein structure elucidated by Pauling and Corey, the first being the α-helix.) In nature, a good example of a β-pleated sheet is found in silk fibroin, but among native fibrous proteins of vertebrate tissues it is most unusual. However, this conformation can arise when common serum proteins are partially digested by proteolytic enzymes, a point which is important in the origin of amyloid. An important property of the β-pleated sheet configuration is its insolubility and relative resistance to normal proteolytic digestion; thus amyloid tends to accumulate inexorably and in time inevitably interferes with the normal physiological function of affected organs, with cell death due to the compression.

The nature of the protein deposited in amyloidosis has attracted considerable interest. Amyloid is not a single substance: in a given deposit there is a major protein, which constitutes the fibril, and minor protein components associated with it; among patients, two types of fibril protein can be distinguished and many variants thereof. In primary amyloidosis, the fibril protein consists of part or all of the light chain of an immunoglobulin (antibody) molecule and is referred to as AL (amyloid, light chain) protein; it also occurs in the amyloidosis associated with multiple myeloma (a malignant neoplasm of plasma cells) and is discussed further on p. 97. In the secondary amyloidosis of chronic inflammatory disorders, the major protein of the fibril is not related to immunoglobulin and is called AA (amyloid A) protein. AA is derived from a serum protein, serum amyloid A (SAA), which serves as the protein component (apolipoprotein) of a high density lipoprotein. An important point is that SAA is an *acute phase protein* (p. 42), which accounts for its increased production in inflammatory diseases. Partial proteolysis, perhaps by macrophage enzymes, is required to convert SAA into the

Figure 1.22 Pathogenesis of
amyloidosis.

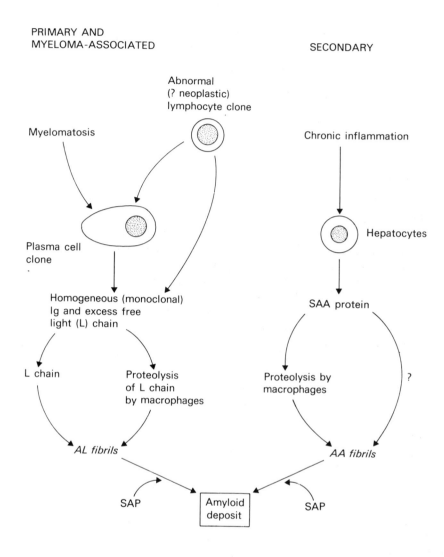

β-pleated sheet configuration of the amyloid fibril. An outline of
the known events in the pathogenesis of amyloidosis is shown in
Figure 1.22.

A minor protein component, called P, is always found in
amyloid deposits, regardless of the tissue site or nature of the
fibrils. Amyloid P component is apparently derived from the
blood, where it is called serum amyloid P (SAP) and is present in
normal serum. SAP shows an intriguing similarity in structure to
C-reactive protein (p. 42) and is also an acute phase protein in
the mouse (but not in man). SAP binds to purified amyloid
fibrils, which presumably accounts for its accumulation in
amyloid deposits. Its physiological role is, as yet, obscure.

67

FURTHER READING

General

Florey H.W. (1970) Inflammation. In Lord Florey (ed.) *General Pathology*, 4th edn, Chapters 2 and 3. Lloyd-Luke (Medical Books).

Mims C.A. (1982) *The Pathogenesis of Infectious Disease*, 2nd end. Academic Press.

Ryan G.B. & Majno G. (1977) *Inflammation*. A Scope publication, The Upjohn Company.

Vane J.R. & Ferreira S.H. (eds.) (1978) *Inflammation* (Handbook of Experimental Pharmacology vol. 50/1). Springer Verlag.

Weissmann G. (ed.) (1980) *The Cell Biology of Inflammation*. (Handbook of Inflammation, vol. 2). Elsevier/North Holland.

Specific topics

Babior B.M. (1978) Oxygen-dependent microbial killing by phagocytes. *New Engl. J. Med.*, **298**, 721.

Franklin E.C. & Gorevic P.D. (1980) The amyloid diseases. In Fougereau M. and Dausset J. (eds.) *Immunology 80*, p. 1219. Academic Press.

Gallin J.I. & Quie P.G. (eds.) (1978) *Leukocyte chemotaxis: methods, physiology and clinical implications*. Raven Press.

Glenner G.G. (1980) Amyloid deposits and amyloidosis. *New Engl. J. Med.*, **302**, 1283, 1333.

Houck J.C. (ed.) (1976) *Chalones*. North Holland.

Houck J.C. (ed.) (1979) *Chemical Messengers of the Inflammatory Process*. (Handbook of Inflammation, vol. 1.) Elsevier/North Holland.

Pepys M.B. (1981) C-reactive protein fifty years on. *Lancet*, I, 653.

Samuelsson B. & Paoletti R. (eds) *Advances in Prostaglandin, Thromboxane and Leukotriene Research Series* (9 vols to 1982). Raven Press.

Snyderman R. & Goetzl E.J. (1981) Molecular and cellular mechanisms of leukocyte chemotaxis. *Science*, **213**, 830.

Wedmore C.V. & Williams T.J. (1981) Control of vascular permeability by polymorphonuclear leucocytes in inflammation. *Nature*, **289**, 646.

Weissman G. (1980) *Prostaglandins in acute inflammation*. A Scope publication, The Upjohn Company.

Introduction

The acute inflammatory response provides a rapid first line of defence against pathogens causing local tissue damage, but for the effective removal of an infectious agent and recovery from disease, the intervention of the immune system is generally essential. Whereas inflammation is a nonspecific response to tissue damage, the key feature of the immune response is its remarkable *specificity*—infection with any particular microorganism leads to an immune response directed solely against that organism (or very closely related organisms). In addition, the immune system possesses the feature of rapid recall or *memory*, enabling a quicker response to be made to a second infection with the same organism, even years after first infection. Efficient immunological memory ensures that, in many cases, we do not suffer from the same infectious disease twice in a lifetime and enables us to provide permanent protection by *vaccination*. Another fundamental aspect of the immune system is its ability to differentiate between '*self*' and '*non-self*'. It is clearly essential that a specific protection system be able to distinguish substances or agents introduced from the outside from the normal body constituents, i.e. to recognise the foreign or non-self. The absolute importance of this distinction is underlined by the instances of *autoimmune disease* which result when for some reason a self component is recognised as if it were foreign and an immune response made to it. Fortunately, the immune system normally makes the distinction between self and non-self with a high degree of reliability. The lack of response to self is termed natural *immunological tolerance* or unresponsiveness. Although the immune system is essential for survival, in so far as it contributes to recovery from disease and provides long-lasting protective immunity, immune responses can also be damaging to host tissues and contribute directly to pathological processes in disease. The term *hypersensitivity* (or *allergy*) is used when immune reactions produce tissue damage and harm the host.

Terminology

A substance capable of stimulating an immune response is referred to as an *antigen*. The immune response to an antigen may take two forms. In the *humoral antibody response*, protein molecules known as *antibodies* (*immunoglobulins*), capable of combining specifically with the antigen, are produced into the circulation. At the same time, in the *cell-mediated immune response* (CMI), lymphocytes proliferate which are capable of specifically recognising the antigen by surface receptors and releasing various mediators known as *lymphokines*. The immune system is thus divided into two distinct, yet closely related, types of response, each of which provides fundamental mechanisms of protective immunity and hypersensitivity.

71

CELLS OF THE IMMUNE SYSTEM

The characteristic cells of the immune system are those of the lymphoid series—small, medium and large lymphocytes, blast cells and plasma cells (Figure 2.1). The small lymphocyte may be considered the basic cellular unit of the system, since immune responses can be transferred with populations consisting solely of small lymphocytes, and by a process of differentiation the small lymphocyte can give rise to the other members of the series. The most important feature of lymphocytes is their ability to recognise and respond to antigens—they are *antigen-sensitive cells*. Despite the vast range of antigens to which the system as a whole can respond, each individual lymphocyte is highly specific—it is only able to recognise one particular antigen. Moreover, the lymphocyte is *precommitted* to that antigen in that it possesses its specificity before it ever meets the antigen. Thus, a population of small lymphocytes consists of cells which, though morphologically identical, are all different with respect to the antigen to which each will respond. It follows that when an antigen is injected into an animal, the antigen must find or *select* the particular lymphocytes in the population which have the potential to respond to it. How this is accomplished is discussed later.

Figure 2.1 *and on facing page.* Cells of the immune system.
(a) Light microscope appearance: (i) small lymphocyte, (ii) large lymphocyte, lymphoblast, (iii) plasma cell, (iv) plasma cell in stained sections.
(b) Fine structure, after electron micrographs: (i) small lymphocyte, (ii) plasma cell.

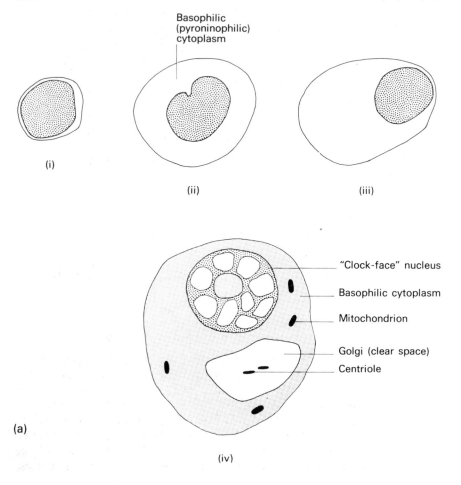

Basophilic (pyroninophilic) cytoplasm

(i)

(ii)

(iii)

"Clock-face" nucleus

Basophilic cytoplasm

Mitochondrion

Golgi (clear space)

Centriole

(a)

(iv)

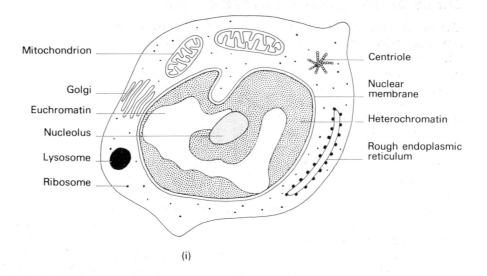

Mitochondrion

Golgi

Euchromatin

Nucleolus

Lysosome

Ribosome

Centriole

Nuclear membrane

Heterochromatin

Rough endoplasmic reticulum

(i)

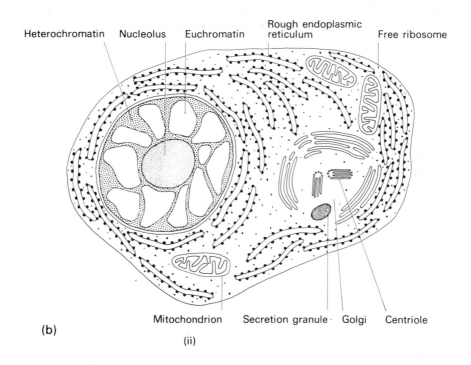

Heterochromatin   Nucleolus   Euchromatin   Rough endoplasmic reticulum   Free ribosome

Mitochondrion   Secretion granule   Golgi   Centriole

(b)

(ii)

T and B lymphocytes and lymphoid organs

The existence of two major types of immune response—cell-mediated and humoral antibody responses—has already been noted. This division results from the presence of two corresponding major classes of lymphocyte, which are called the *thymus-derived* or *T lymphocytes* (*T cells*) and the *bursa-derived* or *B lymphocytes* (*B cells*). All lymphocytes originate from precursor stem cells in the bone marrow (or the liver in the case of the foetus). Some of these precursors migrate to the thymus, a major organ of lymphoid development, in which they multiply and differentiate, finally emerging as mature small T lymphocytes. Other precursors undergo parallel differentiation in another lymphoid organ anatomically identified as the bursa of Fabricius in birds, the equivalent of which in mammals may be the more diffuse gut-associated lymphoid tissue (Peyer's patches and appendix), from which the B lymphocytes are produced. Figure 2.2 shows these pathways of lymphocyte production.

Both T and B lymphocytes are antigen-sensitive cells, but they are fundamentally different in their distribution and range of activities. B cells are the precursors of the antibody-producing cells, the *plasma cells*, into which they differentiate, via a plasmablast stage, after contact with the appropriate specific antigen. Plasma cells are essentially antibody-producing factories, large cells with abundant endoplasmic reticulum and a characteristic 'clock face' nucleus. Each plasma cell produces *only one type* of antibody. The production of humoral antibody is the sole function of the B cell line. T cells, on the other hand, cannot produce antibody, but carry out a variety of other roles, broadly classified as the cell-mediated immune response or CMI. Their principal functions are the following.

1 The major activity of T cells is to provide a defence against microorganisms which survive and grow intracellularly, including viruses, intracellular bacterial pathogens and fungi.

2 T cells are the mediators of *delayed-type hypersensitivity* reactions (p. 163). Some of these are familiar as clinical skin tests for prior or ongoing bacterial, fungal or viral infection, such as the tuberculin, lepromin, candidin and mumps skin tests. While delayed hypersensitivity reflects the T cell defence mechanism against the pathogens, it often plays an important part in the development of pathological lesions in infectious disease (p. 163).

3 T cells participate in graft rejection.

4 T cells play an important part in the recognition and destruction of neoplasms. The role of the immune system in seeking out and destroying neoplastic cells as they arise in the body is expressed in the phrase *'immunological surveillance'*. This

Figure 2.2 The origin of lymphoid cells.

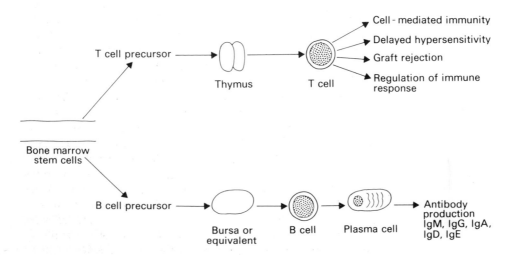

depends on the fact that neoplastic cells express specific antigens on their surface and can therefore be recognised as non-self by antigen-sensitive T lymphocytes. The latter can initiate a process of cell destruction, so that benign as well as malignant cells, which may arise quite frequently by processes of mutation or viral infection, are rejected before they have a chance to establish themselves. This aspect of T cell activity is discussed further in Section 6.

5 Although T cells themselves cannot produce antibody, they are often required to initiate and regulate antibody production by B cells. Some T cells, called *helpers*, have the role of enhancing the antibody response of B cells, while other *suppressor* T cells have an opposite, counterbalancing effect. These regulatory cell interactions between T cells and B cells have excited much interest and are considered more fully on page 110. (Note that helper and suppressor T cells also regulate the other T cells engaged in the cell-mediated responses listed above.)

Experimentally, the role of T cells in the immune response was explored using mice thymectomised shortly after birth and so-called 'nude' mice, the latter being genetically athymic (as well as hairless) mutants. T cell deficient animals such as these are (a) highly susceptible to certain infections, especially with viruses (cf. immunodeficiency in children, p. 78); (b) deficient in certain antibody responses (p. 110); and, perhaps most strikingly, (c) able to accept tissue grafts from animals of different genetic strains and even different species—a hairless mouse with a permanent graft of chicken skin growing feathers is a memorable, if somewhat bizarre, sight!

Besides diverging in their immunological functions, T and B cells show important differences in life-span, distribution, surface markers and physiology. T cells are often long-lived, with a life-span in man of 5–10 years; for this reason they may well be the major contributors to immunological memory. T cells are also mobile and are found circulating in the blood and lymph, where they constitute the majority (70–80%) of small and medium lymphocytes. Mobility is obviously essential to T cell function in cell-mediated immunity. B cells are shorter-lived and relatively more sessile than T cells, remaining in the lymphoid organs, though after antigen stimulation they may enter the lymph and blood in large numbers; there is clearly less requirement for B cells to enter the bloodstream, as they can secrete their circulating product, antibody, from the lymph nodes and spleen.

T and B cells also differ in their distribution in lymphoid tissues. The major lymphoid organs in which immune responses are mounted are the *lymph nodes, spleen* and *gut-associated lymphoid tissue*. The structure of a lymph node is shown diagrammatically in Figure 2.3. T cells are found in the 'thymus-dependent areas', namely the *paracortical areas* of the lymph node and the area around the central arteriole in the white pulp of the spleen. It is in these areas that most cell proliferation occurs during the induction of a cell-mediated immune response. On the other hand, B cells are found in the lymph follicles, germinal centres, corticomedullary junction and the medullary cords of the lymph node, and in the

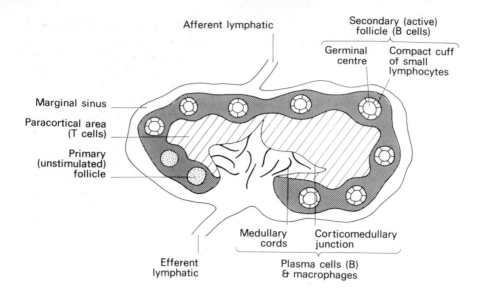

Afferent lymphatic

Secondary (active)
follicle (B cells)

Germinal
centre

Compact cuff
of small
lymphocytes

Marginal sinus

Paracortical area
(T cells)

Primary
(unstimulated)
follicle

Efferent
lymphatic

Medullary
cords

Corticomedullary
junction

Plasma cells (B)
& macrophages

germinal centres and red pulp of the spleen. During a humoral antibody response, germinal centres are prominent in the lymph node follicles, and plasma cells are found particularly at the corticomedullary junction and in the medullary cords. The histology of the active lymph node can thus frequently be a useful indicator of the type of response predominating.

There are various surface markers which enable T and B cells to be distinguished. The most important is the presence of immunoglobulin (antibody) on the surface of B cells and its absence from T cells. T cells in the mouse carry a surface antigen known as Thy-l which is not present on B cells (though, curiously enough, found on some brain cells). T cells of many species also have the property of binding red cells of another species, a phenomenon which is not related to their specificity for antigen; thus, human T cells bind sheep erythrocytes, which provides an

Figure 2.3 Diagram of an immunologically active lymph node, showing T and B cell areas (after H. Cottier *et al.*, 1972).

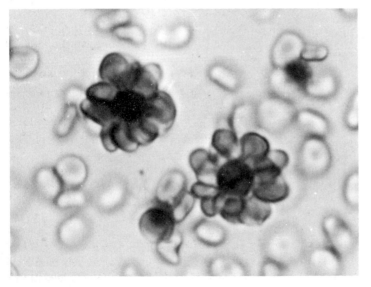

Figure 2.4 Two T cells forming E-rosettes with sheep erythrocytes. To demonstrate this reaction, the lymphocytes and sheep red cells are centrifuged together and gently resuspended; binding of red cells to the T cell surface produces the rosette. (Courtesy of Dr R.M. Binns.)

easy method for T cell enumeration (E rosettes, Figure 2.4). B cells, in common with macrophages and neutrophils, possess surface receptors for fixed C3 (the 3rd component of complement) and the Fc region of IgG antibodies (Figure 2.7); certain types of T cells also have Fc receptors. These receptors can be demonstrated by rosette formation with suitably 'sensitised' red cells, e.g. red cells coated with IgG, for demonstrating Fc receptors, or with C3 for C3 receptors. In addition, various substances capable of stimulating cell division (*mitogens*) can differentiate between T and B cells. Only T cells respond to the kidney bean extract *phytohaemagglutinin* (PHA) or jack bean extract *concanavalin* A (con A) by blast transformation, DNA synthesis and mitosis *in vitro*. This provides a reliable test for T cells, which is useful in various disorders such as immunodeficiency disease. B cells, on the other hand, are stimulated by pokeweed mitogen and the lipopolysaccharide (LPS) of Gram-negative bacteria.

Lymphocyte recirculation

Under normal circumstances, human blood contains $1.5-3.5 \times 10^6$ small lymphocytes per ml and, as noted above, most of these (70–80%) are T cells. Although the number in the blood at any one time is only a small proportion of the total in the body, lymphocytes are constantly entering the circulation, mainly from the thoracic and cervical ducts, at a rate sufficient to replace all those in the blood several times every day; obviously, they must also be leaving the bloodstream at an equivalent rate. The fate of blood lymphocytes was explored experimentally in rats by infusing radiolabelled lymphocytes into the circulation; it was found that such cells left the bloodstream and within a few hours appeared in the thoracic duct. In other words, lymphocytes are constantly *recirculating* between blood and lymph.

There are at least two routes by which blood lymphocytes can return to the lymph nodes. The minor route is by leaving the blood in the tissues and returning to the lymph nodes in the afferent lymph; however, most blood lymphocytes leave the circulation in the lymph nodes themselves by migrating across the walls of post-capillary venules. These blood vessels have a specialised cuboidal epithelium which lymphocytes traverse by passing through intercellular junctions. Most of the cells entering the lymph nodes leave again quite soon (within a few hours) in the efferent lymphatics and in due course complete their recirculation by returning to the blood via the thoracic duct. About 80–85% of thoracic duct lymphocytes are T cells. In addition to this recirculation between blood and lymph nodes (and some other lymphoid tissues), there is a major traffic of more rapid recirculation between blood and the white pulp of the spleen, again involving both T and B cells.

Lymphocyte recirculation is essential to normal immune responses and to the function of T cells. It serves, for example, to bring lymphocytes into contact with antigen trapped in the lymphoid tissues. Antigens drain to the local lymph nodes from the tissues in the efferent lymph and are either phagocytosed by macrophages lining the subcapsular (marginal) or medullary sinuses, or are trapped on the 'interdigitating cells' of the paracortex, or in follicles as complexes with antibody on the surface of 'dendritic' macrophages. Both latter cell types present a particularly large surface area on which antigen is localised to maximise the chances of contact with mobile lymphocytes. Lymphocytes bearing specific receptors bind to the antigen and remain in the lymph node where they are activated to divide and differentiate; after a few days, activated T and B cells leave the node and enter the blood, the former to carry out their roles in the tissues as effector cells of cell-mediated immunity.

Dual nature of protective immune responses

The result of the basic subdivision of lymphocytes into T and B cells is the existence of two parallel types of immune response, the cell-mediated and antibody responses. Both of these patterns of response are important in defence against infectious disease and it is possible to divide microorganisms into two main groups according to the branch of the immune response most involved in protection. Antibody is required mainly for defence against extra-cellular, pyogenic bacteria, such as streptococci, pneumococci, staphylococci, meningococci, etc. One reason for this is that many such organisms protect themselves from phagocytosis by means of an antiphagocytic capsule or wall and must be opsonised by antibody and complement before they can be phagocytosed and destroyed (p. 17). Antibody is also essential in neutralising the toxins of organisms such as *Corynebacterium diphtheriae* and *Clostridium tetani*, the causative agents of diphtheria and tetanus respectively. However, antibody is largely powerless against pathogens which survive and prosper intracellularly, notably viruses and bacterial pathogens such as the tubercle and leprosy bacilli. For these organisms, and also for resistance to fungi, the main immunological defence system is that of T cells, cell-mediated immunity.

Immunodeficiency diseases

The most dramatic illustration of the dichotomy of defence against pathogens comes from observations of immunological deficiency diseases. Primary, congenital immunodeficiency may take the form of a lack of T cells, or B cells, or both; secondary immunodeficiency, which is a result of other disease states, can show a similar subdivision. The most extreme forms of *primary immunodeficiency* in children are (a) the *X-linked infantile (Bruton-type) agammaglobulinaemia*, where there is a complete lack of B cells and antibody production but essentially normal development of T cells; (b) *thymic aplasia* or *Di George syndrome* where, as a result of cogenital absence of the thymus, the T cell system is absent while antibody production is quite well developed; and (c) severe *combined immunodeficiency*, where both T and B systems are deficient due to the absence of stem cells in the bone

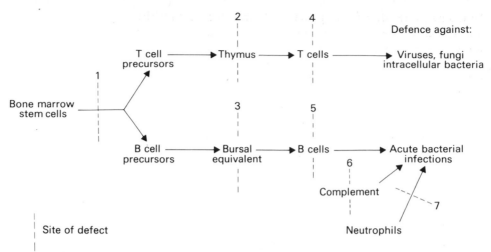

Figure 2.5 Immunodeficiency diseases.

1 Combined immunodeficiency

2 Thymic aplasia (Di George)

3 Agammaglobulinaemia (Bruton)

} Primary immunodeficiencies

4 Secondary T cell deficiency (e.g. Hodgkin's disease)

5 Secondary B cell deficiency (e.g. multiple myeloma)

6 Complement deficiency (primary or secondary)

7 Chronic granulomatous disease (primary immunodeficiency)

marrow (Figure 2.5). Striking patterns of infection are found in the three cases. Children with agammaglobulinaemia show great susceptibility to acute infections with pneumococci, *Haemophilus influenzae*, streptococci, meningococci and *Pseudomonas aeruginosa*, which appear as repeated attacks of sinusitis, skin infections, conjunctivitis, meningitis and pulmonary disease. Yet these children resist infections with fungi, many viruses and the tubercle bacillus very well. In contrast, patients with the Di George syndrome and other conditions involving only T cell deficiency are well able to resist the pyogenic encapsulated pathogens, but succumb to infection with viruses, fungi and acid-fast bacilli. In these patients, for example, common viral infections such as measles and chickenpox are frequently fatal. Attempts to vaccinate against smallpox with vaccinia virus lead to fatal progressive vaccinia (vaccinia gangrenosa), instead of the usual local lesions, and BCG vaccination for tuberculosis results in progressive BCG infection. As expected, patients with combined T and B deficiency are the group most susceptible to all types of infection. Similar patterns are encountered in secondary immunodeficiency states, including those associated with multiple myeloma (B cell deficiency) and Hodgkin's disease (T cell deficiency). Treatment with immunosuppressive drugs in recipients of transplants or in leukaemia patients leads to immunodeficiency which is typically of the T cell type, with the danger of overwhelming and fatal infection by viruses and fungi.

Altogether, the observations in these various conditions underline the striking division of microorganisms into those for which humoral antibody and those for which CMI is required for protection. It is also noticeable that immunodeficiencies of all types are associated with an increased incidence of certain malignant neoplasms, particularly leukaemias and lymphomas, supporting the concept that an immunological surveillance mechanism may normally operate against these neoplasms (see also Section 6, p. 741).

Related to these considerations of immunodeficiency is the fact that, in all individuals, the size of the thymus decreases with age (involutes) so that older persons have but tiny remnants of the organ present at puberty. T-cell dependent responses, including antibody production against certain antigens, often show a significant decline in efficiency with ageing.

ANTIGENS

The first essential characteristic of an antigen is 'foreignness'—in order to provoke an immune response, a substance must differ significantly from normal body components. In addition, although it is difficult to generalise, there are certain minimal requirements of molecular size and complexity which are essential for antigenicity. Among larger molecules there is considerable variation in antigenicity. Proteins are among the most antigenic substances, whereas lipids on their own are non-antigenic. Polysaccharides are antigenic, but may need to be of higher molecular weight than proteins. If a substance is poorly antigenic, it is frequently possible to improve the response to it by mixing or combining it with an *adjuvant*. In experimental work in animals, Freund's complete adjuvant—mineral oil, containing heat-killed tubercle bacilli, which is made into an emulsion with antigen in aqueous solution—is frequently used to bolster weak responses; in human vaccination, toxoids are administered adsorbed onto alum (potassium aluminium sulphate) to improve their antigenicity.

An important concept is that of the *antigenic determinant*. The binding sites on antibody molecules or cell receptors are very much smaller than the antigen molecule itself—an antibody binding site can only accommodate 4–5 amino acids or 5–6 sugar residues. It therefore follows that an antigen molecule consists of many relatively small areas against which specific antibodies or cell receptors may be directed. Each of these small antigenic areas is termed an antigenic determinant; the surface of an antigen molecule may be pictured as a complex mosaic of distinct or overlapping antigenic determinants (Figure 2.6). A single type of antigen molecule can thus stimulate an immune response against tens or even hundreds of determinants present on its surface. The potential complexity of immune responses against structures the size of bacteria or viruses is immediately apparent. (The more recent term *epitope* is synonymous with antigenic determinant.)

Molecules of the size of a single determinant are usually too small to evoke an immune response, but may do so if coupled to an appropriate larger molecule which acts as a carrier. The term *hapten* is applied to such small molecules. Note that the free hapten is capable of reacting in solution with the antibody evoked by the hapten-carrier conjugate. A hapten commonly used in immunological work is the dinitrophenyl group (DNP) (Figure 2.6). Of clinical importance is the fact that drugs such as

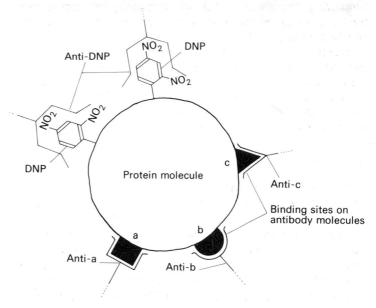

Figure 2.6 Antigenic determinants. Diagrammatic representation of a protein molecule with its determinants *a*, *b* and *c*; a hapten, DNP, has been chemically attached to the protein. Antibody combining sites are shown bound to individual determinants.

penicillin may act as haptens and cause an immune response and hypersensitivity if they, or their metabolised products, become linked to body proteins or cells which act as their carriers.

ANTIBODIES

An antibody is a molecule able to bind specifically to an antigen. Antibodies form a group of structurally related proteins known as γ-globulins, or *immunoglobulins*. In 1937 Tiselius showed that plasma proteins could be separated into four main groups on the basis of their electrophoretic mobility, namely albumin, α-globulin, β-globulin and γ-globulin. Albumin moved the fastest and γ-globulin the slowest towards the anode in electrophoresis. It was subsequently demonstrated that antibodies were present in the γ-globulin fraction. The term 'immunoglobulin' (abbreviated as Ig) is now used, to indicate the immunological function of this group of molecules. Immunoglobulins are divided into five classes, namely IgG, IgA, IgM, IgD and IgE. This division is made on the basis of molecular structure; in addition the Ig classes differ significantly in their biological properties and functions. The characteristic feature of antibody molecules of all classes is the ability to combine specifically with an antigenic determinant—all antibodies possess a *combining site* at which binding to antigen can take place. Antibodies are highly specific, to the extent that each antibody molecule can combine well with essentially only one antigenic determinant. There are thousands of different antigenic determinants in nature, so that there must be a proportionately large number of antibody-combining sites—and therefore thousands of different types of antibody molecules! Since there are only five major antibody classes, it follows that within each class there must exist a tremendously heterogeneous population of molecules, each carrying a different antigen-binding site. Yet, despite the differences in antigen-binding specificity, all the molecules of a certain class share a common structure and common biological properties. This remarkable fact is made possible by the unique features of the antibody molecule.

Structure of antibodies

The work of Porter, Edelman and others revealed the basic unit structure of all antibody molecules, shown diagrammatically in Figure 2.7. One of its striking features is that two functional regions are present on the one molecule. Literally at one end of the molecule are located two identical antigen-combining sites, while the rest of the molecule is concerned with the other biological features of antibody such as activation of the complement system, attachment to various cell surfaces, passage across the placenta, distribution etc. It is the combining sites which differ between antibody molecules, while the biological characteristics are a constant feature of all molecules of the same class.

The basic antibody unit has a molecular weight of 150,000 and is composed of four polypeptide chains—two identical '*light*' chains and two identical '*heavy*' chains. Light chains (mol.wt 22,000) are about half the length of heavy chains (mol.wt 50,000–70,000); the chains are joined together by interchain disulphide bridges. There are two types of light chain known as κ (kappa) and λ (lambda) which are present on all classes of immunoglobulin, though each individual antibody molecule possesses either two κ or two λ chains. There are five main types of heavy chain,

Figure 2.7 (a) Basic structure of the antibody molecule (the molecule shown is human IgG_1). (b) Diagrammatic structures of antibody molecules of different classes. H = heavy chain; L = light chain; J = joining chain; solid line = polypeptide chain; broken line = disulphide bridge. * Note: positions of disulphide bridges are variable and depend on the class.

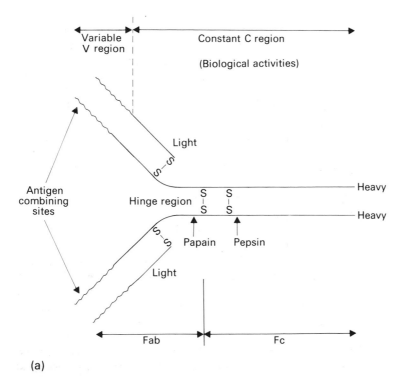

(a)

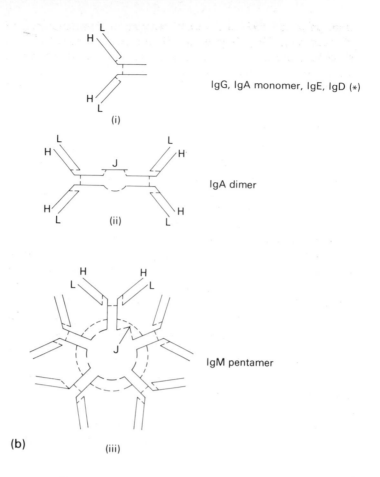

(i)

IgG, IgA monomer, IgE, IgD (∗)

(ii)

IgA dimer

(iii)

IgM pentamer

(b)

corresponding to the five Ig classes, and designated by the Greek letters γ (the heavy chain type of the IgG class), α (IgA), μ (IgM), δ (IgD) and ϵ (IgE). The heavy chains are unique to each Ig class. Thus an IgG molecule could be of chain structure $\gamma_2 k_2$, or $\gamma_2 \lambda_2$; whereas an IgA molecule could be $\alpha_2 k_2$ or $\alpha_2 \lambda_2$, and so on. The two light chain types and the five heavy chain types all differ from each other in amino acid sequence.

A feature of the Ig molecule is that the mid-region is particularly susceptible to enzymatic attack, so that under the right conditions it can be split into two or more fragments—a fact which was a key to elucidating its structure. The two enzymes most used in this respect are papain and pepsin. As shown in Figure 2.7, papain splits the molecule at a site just to the left of the inter-heavy chain disulphide bridge and yields three fragments of approximately equal size. Two of these fragments are identical and each carries one of the two antibody binding sites; they are therefore termed the *Fab fragments*. The third fragment, which crystallises easily, is termed *Fc*. Pepsin attacks the Ig molecule just to the right of the same disulphide bridge and produces one large fragment containing both binding sites, (Fab')$_2$, but also splits the Fc portion into several small fragments. While the Fab fragments contain the antigen-binding sites, shared by all antibody classes, most of the sites concerned with biological activity are carried on Fc. The Fc portion is therefore unique to each antibody class. A small amount of carbohydrate (2–12%) is attached to the heavy chain, so that antibodies are glycoproteins.

Bivalency and binding strength

The function of the antibody molecule depends on its binding reaction with antigen and in this the fact that each molecule possesses at least two identical binding sites is of the utmost importance: bivalency greatly increases the potential binding strength of the antibody molecule when both sites can be used at the same time. Natural antigens, such as the surfaces of micro-organisms, often have antigenic determinants repeated many times over, giving an antibody the opportunity to use both its binding sites simultaneously in attaching to a single particle (Figure 2.8a). Bivalent attachment has a tremendous advantage over single-site binding, being about 10,000 times stronger—i.e. the chance of an antibody molecule detaching is 10,000 times less if both its sites are occupied in binding to the same particle. For the macromolecule IgM, where several sites can be used, the increment due to its multivalency is even greater. The increased binding strength of bivalent or multivalent molecules means that antibodies with individual binding sites of relatively low affinity can still function efficiently. A similar principle will be encountered in the interaction of antibodies with Fc receptors or complement (below). (Note that the term 'affinity' refers to the binding strength of a single antibody-combining site, while the total combining power of the intact molecule with a multideter-minant antigen is called 'avidity'.)

Antibody classes

IgG (γG, 7S)

This is the commonest and most widely distributed anti-body class, comprising about 75% of serum immunoglobulin (~ 12 mg/ml). In structure, it consists of the basic antibody molecule shown in Figure 2.7a, with a molecular weight of 150,000 and with two identical antigen-binding sites per molecule. Like all classes, IgG can carry κ or λ chains, while the distinct heavy chain of the class is γ. Electron microscopy of IgG in combination with antigen has confirmed that the molecule has a Y structure, in which the two Fabs form the arms and Fc the stem of the Y, (Figure 2.9a). The antigen-combining sites are located at the ends of the arms. An important feature is that the point in the molecule where the arms join forms a flexible 'hinge', allowing the angle between the arms to vary. This helps a single IgG molecule to make the utmost use of its two binding sites and to bind to two identical antigenic determinants simultaneously.

In defence against pathogens, IgG antibodies function as opsonins, antitoxins, antiviral antibodies, etc. Their ability to act

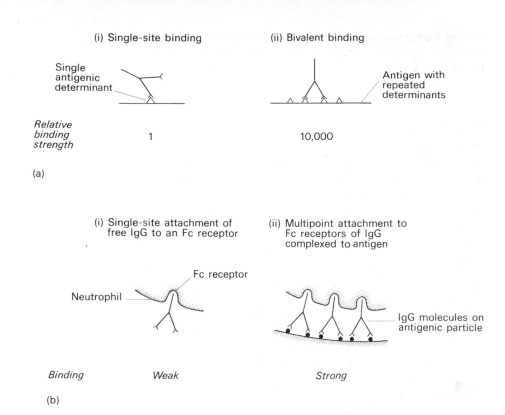

(i) Single-site binding

Single antigenic determinant

(ii) Bivalent binding

Antigen with repeated determinants

Relative binding strength

1

10,000

(a)

(i) Single-site attachment of free IgG to an Fc receptor

(ii) Multipoint attachment to Fc receptors of IgG complexed to antigen

Fc receptor

Neutrophil

IgG molecules on antigenic particle

Binding

Weak

Strong

(b)

Figure 2.8 Illustrations of the increase in binding strength resulting from multivalency. (a) Advantage of bivalency of IgG in reacting with a multideterminant antigen. (b) Advantage of multipoint attachment in binding of antigen-complexed IgG to Fc receptors at the neutrophil surface.

as opsonins derives from the presence on the surface of neutrophils of receptors for the Fc region of IgG complexed to an antigen. Note that neutrophil Fc receptors bind free IgG molecules weakly compared with complexed IgG, and some IgG subclasses not at all in the free state. The reason that complexed IgG is bound strongly at the neutrophil surface illustrates the principle that 'multipoint attachment' greatly increases binding strength (Figure 2.8b). An individual neutrophil Fc receptor has only a relatively poor affinity for a free IgG molecule, but when several IgGs are complexed to an antigenic particle, such as a bacterium, the receptors at the neutrophil surface are presented with a multiple array of several Fc regions which can be bound simultaneously, and this vastly enhances the overall strength of the binding reaction. This effect ensures that neutrophil Fc receptors are never functionally blocked by free plasma IgG. The importance of opsonisation in defence against pyogenic bacteria has been described in Section 1 (p. 16).

IgG is also able to fix complement, which assists its role in opsonisation as the neutrophil also has surface receptors for fixed C3 (p. 30). In order to fix complement, *two* IgG molecules must be bound in close proximity at the antigen surface and to achieve this a relatively high IgG concentration is required in the solution. In this respect, the pentameric molecules of the IgM class (below) are more efficient, since single molecules of bound IgM will fix complement. The reaction with complement is described in more detail on p. 121. It will be recalled from Section 1 that complement plays an important role in acute inflammation, and the ability of antibodies to activate this important biological amplification system is one of their most significant properties.

Another important property of human IgG, in this case unique to the class, is passage across the placenta. A large proportion of the antibodies present in the foetus—and therefore in the newborn—are *maternal* and are obtained by transfer across the placenta. They are essential to the newborn in providing protection at a stage of relative immunological inexperience. All these maternally transferred antibodies are of the IgG class. Ability to cross the placenta is again a function of the Fc of the IgG molecule. In several species other than man, including the cow, pig and sheep, placental transfer of immunoglobulin does not occur and the newborn receives maternal antibodies in colostrum on suckling in the first day after birth.

There are four subclasses of human IgG which differ from each other in heavy chain amino acid sequence and biological properties. They are denoted as IgG_1, IgG_2, IgG_3 and IgG_4. The main differences between them are that IgG_4 does not fix complement and IgG_2 is not transported across the placenta. Interestingly, the response to some antigens seems to favour a particular IgG subclass, e.g. antidextran is often mainly IgG_2 and antibodies to blood clotting factor VIII in a rare form of haemophilia are IgG_4.

IgM (γM, 19S, macroglobulin)

IgM is present at a much lower serum concentration than IgG ($\sim 1.2\,$mg/ml or 7% of serum Ig), yet it is nevertheless of great importance in protective immunity. IgM is a large molecule of molecular weight 900,000 and consists of five of the basic units joined together. A 'joining' or J-chain assists formation of the pentamer (Figure 2.7b). The molecule thus possesses 10 identical

Figure 2.9 Antibody molecules seen by electron microscopy (courtesy of Dr A. Feinstein).
(a) An IgG molecule reacting with two molecules of ferritin. The IgG forms a Y between two ferritin spheres.
(b) IgM molecules in different stages of reaction with salmonella flagella:
(i) an IgM molecule, in face view, bridging two flagella, showing its 5 arms, some of which are seen to be bifid, protruding from the central disc;
(ii) side view of an IgM molecule, again bridging flagella, this time as a cross-linking 'staple';
(iii) two IgM molecules, one attached by one arm to the flagellum, the other using all its arms to form a 'staple'.
(iv) another side view of an IgM 'staple'.

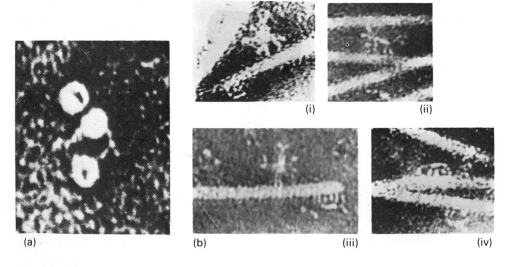

(a)   (b)   (i)   (ii)   (iii)   (iv)

antigen-binding sites and, although it generally uses a maximum of only 5 sites at a time, this gives IgM the ability to bind with tremendous strength to antigens which possess repeating identical determinants—such as most bacterial, viral, or cell surfaces. The use of several binding arms at the same time is clearly shown in the electron micrographs of IgM antiflagellum antibodies reacting with salmonella flagella (Figures 2.9b, 2.10). Note that the arms can move up or down in binding to antigenic determinants.

IgM is the most efficient antibody class in complement activation and complement-dependent cell killing (p. 121). It has been shown that a single IgM molecule at the surface of a cell is sufficient to activate complement leading to lysis, whereas two IgG molecules close together are needed to produce the same effect. Since many hundreds or thousands of IgG molecules would need to be present on a cell surface to provide a reasonable chance of finding two close together, the extent of the increased effectiveness of IgM over IgG is clear. Because of its size, IgM is also the most effective antibody class for agglutination of bacteria or red cells. In the absence of complement, IgM cannot act as an opsonin since neutrophils do not possess an appropriate Fc receptor for the IgM class. However, once IgM has fixed C3 at a bacterial, or other cell surface, opsonisation is accomplished.

IgM is generally produced earlier than IgG in the immune response and, together with complement, often provides an efficient first line of defence against many microorganisms. IgM is also the first class of antibody which can be produced by the foetus as its immune system develops. Thus, although IgM cannot cross the placenta, it is frequently produced by the foetus itself before birth if exposed to infection.

Common examples of IgM antibodies include the naturally

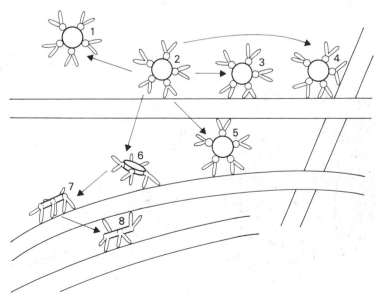

Figure 2.10 Diagrammatic representation of the reaction of IgM with antigen (flagellum), based on electron micrographs such as Figure 2.9b (courtesy of Dr A. Feinstein). The free molecule (1) attaches to a flagellum, at first by one or two arms (2, 3); it may cross-link adjacent flagella (4, 5) or, via a transient intermediate (6), may form a staple on a flagellum (7) or a cross-linking staple (8). Clearly, other sequences are possible and the process is reversible.

occuring ABO red cell isoantibodies; antibodies against the somatic (O) antigen of enterobacteria; and rheumatoid factor, found in the serum in rheumatoid arthritis (p. 190).

IgA (γA)

The IgA class is the second commonest Ig in serum after IgG (serum concentration ~ 3.5 mg/ml, about 20% of serum Ig). In serum, it essentially resembles IgG in structure—a single 4-chain unit of molecular weight 150,000—but carrying the class-specific α heavy chain. Its main role, however, is as the most important antibody class in secretions—intestinal, bronchial and nasal secretions, saliva, tears, colostrum and milk. In secretions it exists as dimers (two 4-chain units) linked together by J-chain (Figure 2.7b), and in addition is linked to a fragment known as transport piece which appears to facilitate its secretion and protect it from intestinal enzymes.

The function of IgA in secretions is to provide *local immunity* against infectious agents in the gut and respiratory tract, by combining with and neutralising them before they can gain entry into the body. For example, IgA in nasal secretion is important in preventing reinfection with the common cold and influenza viruses, while in the intestine IgA provides immunity against enteric microorganisms and polioviruses. In these areas, IgA is produced locally by plasma cells in the mucous membranes and around the exocrine glands—80% of the plasma cells in the duodenal submucosa, for example, are IgA producers. This is an important point for human vaccination, in that for some agents the most effective vaccination is achieved by stimulating local immunity rather than circulating antibody. The attenuated Sabin polio vaccine, which is administered orally, is particularly effective because it gives rise to local IgA formation by lymphoid tissue in the intestine, the normal point of entry of poliovirus into the body; for similar reasons intranasal administration of attenuated influenza viruses has been used successfully for vaccination in Russia and the USA.

IgA is the main antibody class in milk and breast milk provides protection for the suckling infant against enteric organisms. Note that IgA in milk includes antibodies against the mother's own gut flora. A strong case can be made for breast feeding the human infant in view of the protection it affords against organisms gaining access through the gastro-intestinal tract.

IgD (γD)

The IgD class is present in serum in only very small amounts (about 0.03 mg/ml). However, it has been found that over 50% of all B cells carry IgD on their *surface membrane*, where it presumably functions as a receptor for antigen (p. 107). The little IgD there is in serum is either shed from the surface of B cells or secreted by the very small number of IgD-producing plasma cells. IgD is clearly very important to B lymphocytes even though it makes an insignificant contribution to circulating antibody.

IgE (γE, reagin)

The major significance of the IgE class is not in protective immunity but as the mediator of *immediate hypersensitivity* or *anaphylaxis*, including hay fever and allergic asthma, etc. (p. 153). Although present in minute amounts in serum, IgE has the unique ability to bind to the surface of certain cells, notably basophils and mast cells, by means of its Fc. Subsequent combination of antigen—pollen, house dust, etc.—with specific IgE bound to the surface of a mast cell causes immediate degranulation of the cell and release of its stored histamine and other mediators of acute inflammation, resulting in the clinical symptoms of immediate hypersensitivity. IgE-mediated inflammation of this type is also of protective value, particularly in helminth infections. In structure, IgE consists of monomeric 4-chain units and is unusual in being heat-labile, its activity being destroyed by heating to 56°C for 30 minutes.

In summary, antibodies of all classes share the common feature of ability to combine specifically with antigen, a function which is localised in combining sites at the end of the Fab regions of the molecule. At the same time, significant biological differences exist between the classes, resulting in functional diversity. These differences are governed by the distinct heavy chains of each class and are generally associated with the Fc region. Some of the biological activities of antibodies, such as complement activation and binding to neutrophils at Fc receptors, only occur after the reaction with antigen, while others, such as placental transfer, gut transfer and binding of IgE to mast cells, are independent of antigen and are properties of free antibody molecules.

Myeloma proteins

It is clear that antibodies, while sharing basic structural features, are a highly heterogeneous group of molecules. In order to pursue their molecular structure further, therefore, it was necessary to obtain pure, homogeneous preparations of immunoglobulins. The heterogeneity of normal immunoglobulin is such that separation of a single homogeneous species in quantity is virtually impossible. A natural source of homogeneous immunoglobulin is found in the condition of *multiple myeloma* (*myelomatosis*). This is a malignant neoplasm of plasma cells in which the latter grow as tumours in the bone marrow, invading and eroding the bones. The proliferating cells are all descendents of a *single plasma cell*, which at some point underwent a neoplastic change; hence they form a clone of identical cells, all of which produce and secrete an identical (monoclonal) immunoglobulin known as a *myeloma protein*. This is present in the serum of patients in large quantity and it can be of any Ig class. In a closely related condition, known as *Waldenström's macroglobulinaemia*, the infiltrating plasma cells produce IgM rather than other

Ig classes, and do not form the local bone-eroiding tumour masses which characterise multiple myeloma.

In addition to the homogeneous myeloma protein in the serum of patients with multiple myeloma, In addition to the homogeneous myeloma protein in the serum of patients with multiple myeloma, a characteristic protein is often found in the urine. This is the *Bence-Jones protein*, named after its discoverer (1847) who noted its unusual property of coagulating at 60°C and redissolving at around 80°C. Bence-Jones proteins are in fact a pure source of immunoglobulin light chains which are apparently produced in excess by myeloma cells and excreted. They and the serum myeloma proteins have proved invaluable in chemical studies of antibody structure. It is important to note that serum myeloma proteins are normal immunoglobulins in structure, but in homogenous form; several have been shown to have antibody activity when screened against a series of antigens. The fact that neoplastic plasma cells produce a single Ig products is important as it implies that plasma cells are restricted to the production of a single, genetically determined antibody type only.

Variable and constant regions of antibody chains

Amino acid sequencing of Bence-Jones proteins (light chains) revealed the most remarkable feature of immunoglobulin structure. When the amino acid sequences of several κ light chains were compared, it was found that one half of the light chain showed great variability in sequence, whereas the other half was almost completely constant—in other words each light chain possessed a *variable* or V region and a *constant* or C region. It is now clear that possession of a V and a C region is a feature common to all immunoglobulin chains, both light and heavy, as illustrated in Figure 2.7. The V region is of the same length in both light and heavy chains, comprising half the light and a quarter of the heavy chain, while the C region constitutes half the light chain and three-quarters of the heavy chain.

In three-dimensional structure, heavy and light chains are composed of globular regions known as *domains*, each about 110 amino acids in length (Figure 2.11a). Thus, a light chain consists of a variable domain, V_L, comprising the V region, and a constant domain, C_L. Similarly, a heavy chain has a single variable domain, V_H, and three constant domains, C_H1, C_H2 and C_H3 (μ and ϵ chains have an additional domain, C_H4). There is a high degree of similarity (homology) in amino acid sequence and conformation among domains, e.g. between V_L and V_H and among the C-region domains.

The existence of V and C regions gives rise to the two functional parts of the molecule—an antigen-binding region and a class-specific region with other biological activities. Thus, V_L and V_H domains associate with each other to make up the antigen-combining site and are responsible for the individual specificity of each antibody molecule. C domains, on the other hand, play no part in binding of antigen, but are responsible for the biological properties of the different antibody classes; functions such as complement

Figure 2.11 Domain structure of immunoglobulins.
(a) Schematic diagram showing domains of the variable (V) and constant (C) regions of IgG; • = site of attachment of carbohydrate; S–S = disulphide bridge.
(b) Space-filling model of human IgG₁ showing the arrangement of domains. Cγ1, etc. are the C_H domains of the γ chain. Note that the Cγ2 domains cannot pair; Cγ1 and Cγ2 are linked by the flexible hinge region. (From A. Feinstein & N. Richardson (1981), *Monographs in Allergy* **17**, 28).

activation, cytoadherence, placental transfer, etc., are localised to one or other of the C-region domains. Thus, the C_H2 domain of IgG is responsible for binding the first component of complement, while the C_H3 domain interacts with cell surface Fc receptors. Most C domains associate closely with a partner in the native molecule (i.e. C_H1 with C_L, etc.), though not the C_H2 domains of IgG (Figure 2.11b).

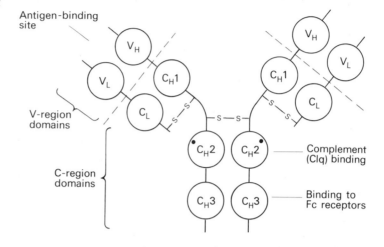

(a)

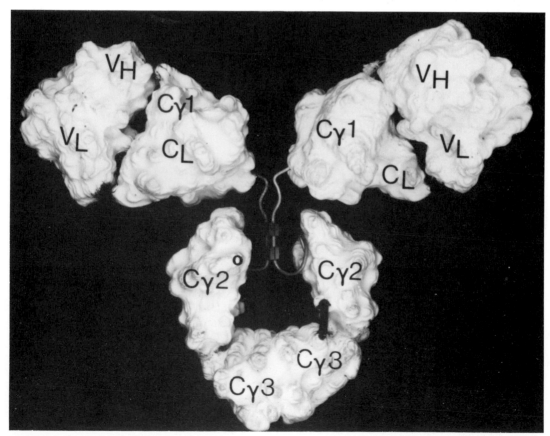

(b)

91

Within light chains, κ and λ have their own distinct V regions (V_k, V_λ), while all heavy chains share the same V regions (V_H). The C regions of the κ and λ chains are distinct (C_k, C_λ), as are the C regions for each heavy chain class (C_γ, C_μ, C_α, C_δ, C_ϵ).

The antigen-combining site

We have noted that the V domains of heavy and light chains associate to form the antigen-combining site of the antibody molecule. The specificity of each binding site is determined directly by the amino acids which are present in it; V region amino acids make contact with the antigenic determinant and by electrostatic, hydrophobic and other interactions they bind the antigen in the site. It follows that antibodies with different specificities possess different V region amino acid sequences. In fact, within the V region itself, certain stretches of the chain are particularly involved in forming the binding site and display an especially high degree of variability, so-called *hypervariable* regions.

The size of the combining site was first determined by inhibiting antigen–antibody reactions with oligosaccharides or peptides of known length (for carbohydrate and protein antigens respectively). For example, the precipitation of the carbohydrate dextran by antidextran antibodies is maximally inhibited by oligomers consisting of six glucose units, and increasing the size above six fails to increase inhibition (Figure 2.12). Hence, most antidextran-combining sites can evidently accommodate six glucose units, though it should be noted that individual sites vary from extremes of two to seven sugars. Similar experiments with antibodies to a polypeptide antigen (polyalanine) showed that the site is filled by 4–5 alanine residues. Note, therefore, that for most antigens one antibody-combining site reacts with only a small area of the antigen molecule (p. 80).

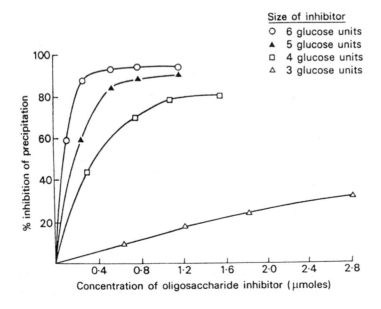

Size of inhibitor
O   6 glucose units
▲   5 glucose units
□   4 glucose units
△   3 glucose units

Figure 2.12 Determination of the size of the antibody-combining site by inhibition of precipitation. Oligosaccharides of increasing length were used to inhibit the precipitation of dextran by antidextran antibodies. Inhibition was maximal with oligosaccharides containing 6 glucose units and was not increased with larger inhibitors (not shown). (After Kabat (1976) *Structural Concepts in Immunology and Immunochemistry*, 2nd edn. Holt, Rinehart and Winston).

Genetics of antibodies

Another remarkable discovery followed on the realisation that antibody chains consisted of V and C regions. It had been considered axiomatic in molecular biology that for a single polypeptide chain there exists in the genome a single stretch of DNA which codes for that polypeptide, the 'one gene—one polypeptide chain' hypothesis. However, genetic studies showed that the heavy and light chains of immunoglobulin are an exception to this basic concept, because the V and C regions of the chains are coded for separately in the genome, i.e. for every heavy and light chain there are *two* genes in the DNA, a V gene and a C gene. It appears that the V gene and C gene are physically quite widely separated in the germ line DNA, but are brought together during B cell development (Figure 2.13). There are three linkage groups of V and C genes on three separate chromosomes: a group for the κ chain (V_κ and C_κ genes), a separate group for the λ chain (V_λ and C_λ genes) and a third for the heavy chains (V_H and C_μ, C_γ, C_α, etc.) (Figure 2.13). The products of the three linkage groups do not intermix; thus the V_κ region cannot become associated with the heavy chain C regions, and so on.

A further major problem is, how many genes are present in the genome to code for the diverse range of antibodies? This question of the genetic origin of antibody diversity has been hotly debated for many years. Two main alternatives have been argued, namely

Figure 2.13 Outline arrangement of immunoglobulin genes in the genome (germ line) and B cells and events involved in the synthesis of an IgG molecule.

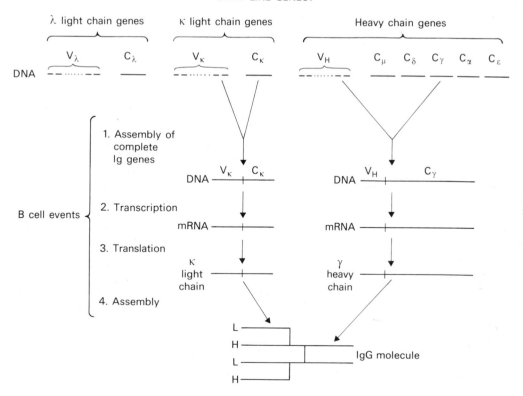

93

the 'germ line' and the 'somatic mutation' hypotheses. According to the germ line theory, each lymphocyte has a large number of Ig genes, carrying the genetic information required for the production of all antibody specificities, and the cell becomes restricted to a single specificity by shutting off the expression of all but a very few genes. In practice, this theory would require each cell to carry a very large number of V genes to code for the whole range of antibody-combining sites, but only a small number of C genes (10–20), sufficient to code for the constant regions of the light and heavy chain classes and subclasses (Figure 2.13). At the other extreme, the somatic mutation model argues that only relatively few genes need be carried by each lymphocyte if mutational events occurred frequently in the genes coding for antibody specificity (the V genes). All the necessary binding sites would be generated in the lymphocyte population by somatic mutation, though each individual lymphocyte would only carry the information for one specificity of binding site. In the last few years there has been considerable progress in solving this problem and it has become clear that, while most of the genetic information of variable regions is in fact encoded by germ line genes, somatic events are important in the generation of diversity in an unexepected way.

Remarkable discoveries were made when the DNA coding for κ light chains was mapped and sequenced. First, it was shown that, as mentioned above, the V and C region genes are quite widely separated in the DNA of all cells *except* B lymphocytes, where they are in close proximity. Secondly, the V_κ region itself was found to be coded by not one but two separate gene segments. One, the V_κ *segment*, codes for 90% of the κ variable region (the first 95 amino acids), while the other codes for the remainder and is called the $\mathcal{J}_\kappa$ *segment* because it joins the variable and constant regions (Figure 2.14a). The germ line contains a large set of V_κ gene segments (about 300 in the mouse) and a small set of 4 J_κ segments. Since a complete κ variable-region gene is a combination of one particular V_κ gene segment and one J_κ gene segment, it becomes possible, in principle, to generate 1200 variable regions from random combinations of V_κ and J_κ segments (300 × 4). In their physical arrangement, the set of V_κ segments is located in the germ line (the DNA as inherited) at a considerable distance from C_κ, while J_κ genes are much closer to C_κ. Thus, during B cell development, a *rearrangement* of the DNA occurs in which the intervening nucleotides separating V_κ and J_κ are removed and a V_κ and a J_κ segment are linked together, as shown in Figure 2.14a (V-J joining).

For heavy chains, the arrangement of the genetic information of the variable region is even more complicated in that it is divided among *three* segments—in addition to V and J, there is another segment called D (for diversity, as it codes for one of the hypervarible stretches of the variable region). Thus, a complete variable-region gene requires the combination of three pieces of DNA—V_H, D_H and J_H—which are brought together by rearrangement of the germ line DNA during B cell ontogeny, again with elimination of intervening DNA (V-D-J joining, Figure 2.14b).

Figure 2.14 Detailed organisation of immunoglobulin genes in germ line and B cell DNA, and events involved in the production of heavy and light chains.
(a) Genes for κ light chain.
(b) Genes for heavy chains.
(Germ line DNA = genetic material as inherited in germ cells.)

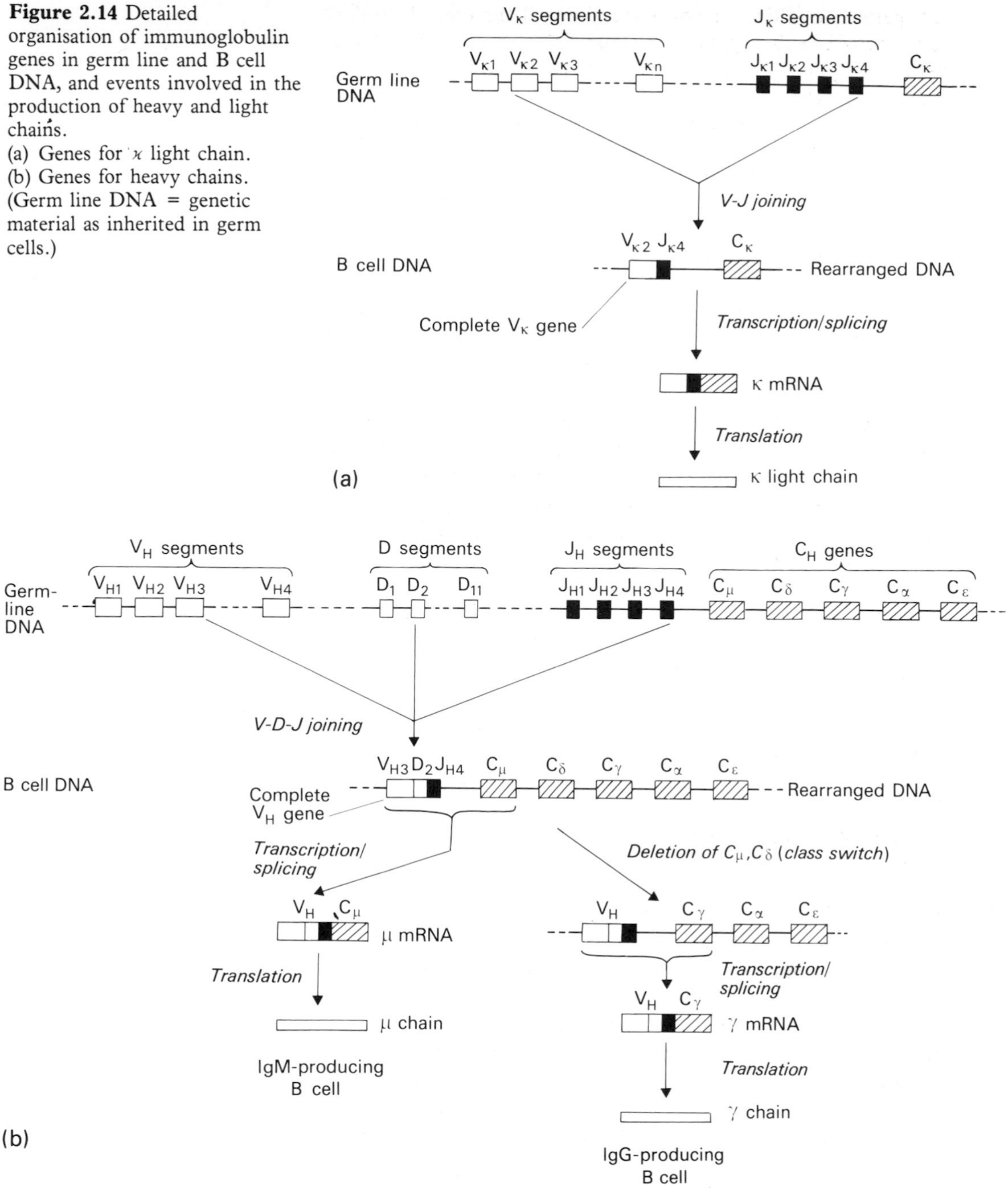

There are about 200 V_H gene segments, a family of 12 D_H segments and 4 J_H segments, giving a possible 9600 combinations; hence, here too the possibility of making random combinations of V, D and J is the somatic basis for developing a very large number of variable regions from the more limited germ line information.

In the heavy chain gene complex, there are also eight constant region genes (C_μ, C_γ, C_α, etc.), corresponding to the classes and subclasses of antibodies, and during B cell maturation one of these becomes associated with the completely assembled V-region gene. The order of C genes in the germ line DNA is shown in Figure 2.14b, with C_μ first, followed by C_δ, the four C_γ genes, etc., in tandem. Initially, all B cells synthesize μ chains, producing IgM which functions as membrane receptor (p. 106); subsequently, when the cell or its descendents make another class—IgG, IgA or IgE—the variable-region gene associates with a C_γ, C_α or C_ϵ gene instead. This is achieved by *deleting* the intervening genes (C_μ, C_δ, etc.), thus bringing the V-region gene close to the appropriate gene for the C region (Figure 2.14b). (Events in the expression of C_δ are rather different, as some B cells make IgM and IgD simultaneously.)

In summary, the diversity of antibody-combining sites is a result of (i) the large number of V gene segments and a smaller number of D and J segments encoded in the germ line, and (ii) the somatic assembly of complete variable-region genes by means of *combinations* of V and J, or V, D and J segments (for light and heavy chains respectively), which increases considerably the potential number of variable regions which can be generated from the germ line information. Moreover, (iii) additional diversity may be generated by somatic mutational events, some of which occur during the process of rearranging gene segments, including 'inaccuracies' in V-J or V-D-J joining; point mutations add further diversity to the hypervariable region information. It should also be borne in mind that the number of antibody-combining sites which can potentially be generated is the product of the number of light chain and heavy chain variable regions; for a mouse this would be about 1200×9600 ($V_k \times V_H$) or over 10^7 binding sites. Even if only 1% of these combinations is functional, the genetically inherited information would generate over 10^5 useful antibodies without invoking somatic mutation at all.

Allelic exclusion is an important phenomenon which occurs in the expression of the genetic information for antibodies in the cell. Animal cells, being diploid, carry a double set of all autosomal genes. In general, where two alleles of a genetic locus are present in the same cell (i.e. in a heterozygote), they can both be expressed simultaneously. For example, the red cell antigens A and B are allelic forms of a single locus and in heterozygotes (constitution AB) both the A and B antigens are expressed on the same red cells. The Ig genes are an exception in that only a single set of the genes for heavy and light chains are expressed in any particular cell. The Ig genes on the homologous (partner) chromosome are essentially silent in that cell. The effect of this allelic exclusion is to ensure the formation of a single antibody product for each cell. As far as is known, the phenomenon is unique to the antibody genes among the autosomes. A somewhat similar situation does exist for the X chromosomes in females, where one of the two is always inactivated in each somatic cell (the Lyon hypothesis: see Section 7). However, there is no suggestion in the case of Ig genes that allelic exclusion affects

96

more of the chromosome than the region containing the antibody genes.

Ig light chains and amyloidosis

The main features of amyloidosis are described in Section 1, from which it will be recalled that the disease can occur as a complication of multiple myeloma; about 10% of all myeloma patients develop amyloidosis. Both in myeloma-associated amyloidosis and in so-called primary amyloidosis, where there is no overt underlying disease, the protein deposited in the tissues consists of part or all of a homogeneous (monoclonal) Ig light chain called *AL protein*. Often only the variable-region domain is deposited, indicating that the light chain has first undergone partial proteolysis. It now seems that in all cases of deposition of AL amyloid there is an overproduction of a single species of light chain by one aberrant clone of plasma cells or lymphocytes. Sometimes these cells are neoplastic and malignant, in which case myeloma is evident, while in primary amyloidosis the cellular disorder is apparently benign. Usually the free light chain is detectable in the serum or urine as a Bence-Jones protein (p. 90); myeloma cells commonly release free light chains in addition to fully assembled immunoglobulin molecules.

An unusual feature of AL proteins is that they are much more often derived from λ chains than κ chains, despite the fact that κ is the predominant class of light chain in normal and myeloma Igs. Experimentally, it is possible to produce precipitates of amyloid-like fibrils by partial enzymatic digestion of certain pure λ chains; V_L domains, or smaller V_L fragments, aggregate spontaneously and form the β-pleated sheet fibril characteristic of amyloid (p. 66). Fibrils produced in this way give a green polarisation colour after staining with Congo red and are indistinguishable under the electron microscope from natural amyloid fibrils. Evidently, the capacity to form a β-pleated sheet fibril is inherent in the variable-region structure of some light chains. It is thought that AL formation is the result of partial proteolysis of free light chains taken up by macrophages, leading to fibril deposition (Figure 1.22).

Hybridomas and monoclonal antibodies

Antibodies have many applications in medical diagnosis, therapy and research. Until recently, all antibodies were produced by inoculating antigens into animals and taking serum some time later. One of the drawbacks of conventional antisera (sera containing antibodies) is that they are invariably heterogeneous mixtures of many antibodies of different specificities, affinities and classes; a sought-after antibody might be present at an inconveniently low concentration in the serum or, because of its heterogeneity, an antiserum might produce unwelcome cross-reactions. For many purposes, the usefulness of an antibody is greatly increased the more it can be purified and thus approach the state of a single molecular species. The latter would in fact be the product of a single B cell clone: since each B lymphocyte and its descendents are restricted to making a single type of antigen-combining site, all the antibody molecules produced by an individual B cell clone are identical in terms of their antigen specificity—a so-called *monoclonal antibody*. During immunisation of animals, a single monoclonal antibody is unlikely to be produced as many B cell clones are activated at the same time (hence the heterogeneity of antibodies raised in this way); nor has it been possible to grow individual B cell clones for more than a few days in culture. Myeloma cells are a source of monoclonal immunoglobulins and grow permanently *in vivo* and in some cases also in culture; however, although myeloma proteins are antibodies, the antigen against which they are directed is usually unknown. Thus, while they have been invaluable in elucidating the structure of antibodies (above), myeloma proteins are of little other practical usefulness. However, in 1975 a method was devised in Cambridge, by G. Köhler and C. Milstein, in which myelomas producing monoclonal antibodies of almost any desired specificity could be 'manufactured' in the laboratory. The principle of the technique is the *fusion* of an antibody-producing B cell with a myeloma cell to produce a 'hybrid myeloma' cell, more commonly called a *hybridoma*. The latter combines the important properties of both its parent cells, namely the ability to produce the specific antibody of the B cell with the permanent growth and high rate of secretion of the myeloma cell. In short, a B cell can essentially be immortalised by fusion with a myeloma; once established, hybridomas grow and secrete their monoclonal antibody indefinitely, the product being pure, homogeneous and highly specific.

When the tremendous potential of monoclonal antibodies as highly specific reagents became appreciated, the hybridoma method, which is highly reliable, was very widely adopted. Indeed, such is the demand for monoclonal antibodies in medical diagnostics and research, and in biological research in general, that many commercial companies have recently sprung up for large scale production and marketing; together with genetic engineering, hybridomas have become a mainstay of the developing industry of biotechnology.

Most hybridomas are of mouse origin, though human hybridomas are also being prepared. The procedure for making a hybridoma cell line is as follows (Figure 2.15).

(i) The method starts with the injection of the antigen of interest, which need not be pure, into a mouse to stimulate an antibody response. Within a few days, antibody-producing cells proliferate and mature in the lymph nodes and spleen; the animal is then killed and a cell suspension prepared from these organs.

(ii) A few days before sacrificing the animal, mouse myeloma cells are seeded into culture medium and grown in suspension to generate the required number by the day of the fusion. In the original experiments, the myeloma cells secreted their own immunoglobulin, but now a variant line (NS0) is used which has lost this ability. An essential feature of the myeloma cells is that they

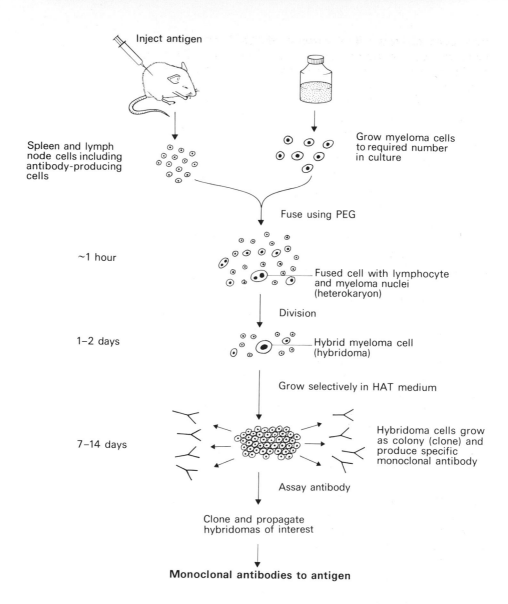

Inject antigen

Spleen and lymph
node cells including
antibody-producing
cells

Grow myeloma cells
to required number
in culture

Fuse using PEG

~1 hour

Fused cell with lymphocyte
and myeloma nuclei
(heterokaryon)

Division

1–2 days

Hybrid myeloma cell
(hybridoma)

Grow selectively in HAT medium

7–14 days

Hybridoma cells grow
as colony (clone) and
produce specific
monoclonal antibody

Assay antibody

Clone and propagate
hybridomas of interest

Monoclonal antibodies to antigen

Figure 2.15 Procedure for
making monoclonal antibodies.
(PEG = polyethylene glycol;
HAT = hypoxanthine-
aminopterin-thymidine)

are specially selected mutants deficient in an enzyme involved in
purine metabolism, namely hypoxanthine-guanine phosphoribosyl transferase (HGPRT); as a result of this deficiency, the cells
die in culture medium containing hypoxanthine, aminopterin and
thymidine, so-called HAT medium. Lymphocytes, like other
normal cells, are HGPRT-positive and so too, therefore, are
hybridomas; thus, HAT medium can be used for the *selective*
growth of hybridoma cells, since only myeloma cells which
receive the HGPRT enzyme through fusing with a lymphocyte or
plasma cell will be able to survive and grow in HAT.

(iii) The lymphoid cell suspension, containing antibody-
producing cells, is now mixed with that of the myeloma cells and
the two are centrifuged into a pellet. A fusing agent is then stirred
into the cell mixture; formerly, Sendai virus was used, but now
polyethylene glycol (PEG) has become the standard fusing agent.

Over the next few minutes, fusion takes place at random to produce multinucleate cells, among which will be a few (binucleate) hybrids resulting from the fusion of a myeloma cell and an antibody-producing cell. When such a hybrid cell divides, the nuclei coalesce to form a mononuclear cell which is at first tetraploid, though subsequently several chromosomes are lost. By this stage, the cells have been distributed into the wells of a tissue culture dish and incubated at 37°C. HAT medium is added to kill any unfused myeloma cells, which would otherwise grow and overwhelm the small number of hybridomas; unfused lymphocytes and plasma cells die of their own accord within a few days. Hence, the only cells to grow out in HAT medium are hybrids; since only about one myeloma cell per thousand fuses to a lymphocyte to give a viable hybrid, HAT selection is essential.

Colonies of hybridoma cells become apparent 7−14 days later and their supernatants are assayed for the presence of an antibody of interest. Potentially useful cells are isolated and *cloned*, e.g. by growing individual colonies from cells seeded onto agar. Clones producing antibody are then grown to large cell numbers in flasks. The antibody produced by cloned hybridoma cells is certain to be homogeneous and is also often made in high concentration; as the cells grow continuously and permanently in culture, a virtually unlimited amount of pure monoclonal antibody can be obtained. Moreover, if the hybridoma cells are transplanted into suitable recipient mice, extremely high levels of monoclonal antibody (5−20 mg/ml) can be found in the serum or ascitic fluid after a few days. Thus, in addition to their purity and specificity, hybridoma antibodies are obtainable in large amounts, making them ideal standard reagents for distribution to many laboratories.

Monoclonal antibodies are being employed in many areas where antisera were formerly used, some obvious applications being as reagents for blood grouping and tissue typing, hormone radioimmunoassay, etc. Some less immediately obvious areas are the following.

(i) Monoclonal antibodies are highly specific probes with which to analyse complex biological systems, ranging from the molecules on cell surfaces to the organisation of whole tissues. Each antibody can be used to determine the presence of an individual component on a cell surface or pinpoint the localisation of molecules within a tissue; a panel of antibodies can be employed to assemble a complete picture. In the nervous system, for example, monoclonal antibodies labelled with a fluorescent dye have been used to explore the localisation of neurotransmitter substances in different parts of the brain or spinal cord.

(ii) Because of its exquisite binding specificity, a monoclonal antibody is the ideal means of isolating a particular substance from a mixture in which it may be only a very small component. A good illustration is provided by the purification of the antiviral protein *interferon* which, when obtained from a mammalian cell source or genetically-engineered bacteria, constitutes less than 1% of total protein. A mouse monoclonal antibody was prepared against interferon and coupled to an insoluble carbohydrate matrix to make a specific 'immunoadsorbent'; when a crude mixture containing interferon is passed over such an adsorbent, the interferon molecules are specifically bound by the antibody while the other proteins are washed away (Figure 2.16). Pure interferon can subsequently be recovered from the adsorbent by elution in acid or alkali, which reversibly unfolds the antibody-ombining site. A single cycle of adsorption and elution leads to a 5000-fold purification of interferon and this method is now in use in the industrial manufacture of interferon. This is an example of

Figure 2.16 Use of monoclonal antibody and affinity chromatography in purification of interferon.
(Secher, D.S. & Burke, D.C. (1980) *Nature* **285**, 446).

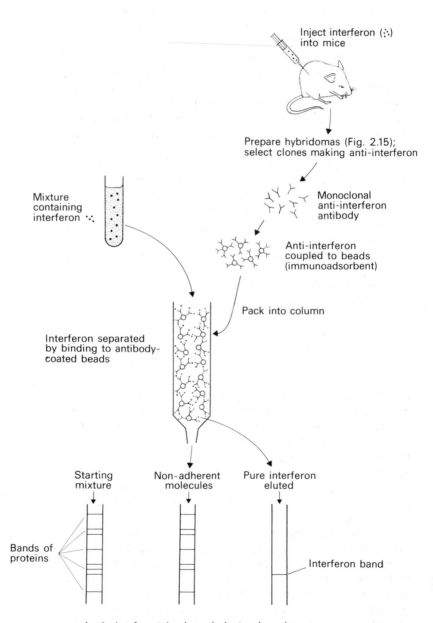

PADDINGTON COLLEGE LIBRARY
PADDINGTON GREEN
LONDON W2 1NB

a general method called *affinity chromatography*, in which substances or cells are isolated by means of their specific binding to insolubilised molecules for which they have affinity; it is often used to isolate antigens or antibodies. In a similar way, monoclonal antibodies can be used to isolate specific surface molecules from microorganisms, molecules which can then be tested for their potential as vaccines; this promises to be especially useful in defining the antigens involved in immunity to parasites.

(iii) The application of monoclonal antibodies in cancer diagnosis and therapy is attracting much attention. As described in Section 6, tumour cells often express specific antigens against which monoclonal antibodies can be prepared. The antibodies can then be used (a) to isolate tumour-specific molecules and hence better understand the nature of neoplastic change; (b) as an aid to diagnosis, by detecting tumour cells in the body; and (c) perhaps therapeutically, by using the antibody to carry a cytotoxic agent directly to the tumour cell surface (see also p. 750).

(iv) A monoclonal antibody can be used to control fertility in animals. Thus, an antibody against the female reproductive hormone progesterone successfully prevents pregnancy if injected into female mice within a few hours after mating. A single dose of antibody produces surprisingly long-lasting effects. This may become a useful method of contraception in dogs and cats, avoiding the need for spaying; however, whether such an immunological approach to birth control will ever be employed in humans, only time will tell.

INDUCTION OF AN IMMUNE RESPONSE

Basic features

When a foreign antigen—microorganism, toxin, etc.—is introduced into the body for the first time, the immune response generally takes between 7–14 days to reach its peak and is often of relatively low intensity and short duration. Such a response is called the *primary* immune response. In contrast, if the same antigen is introduced for a second time a *secondary* response is produced which is considerably more rapid, reaching high levels in about 3–5 days, is often far larger and more persistent than the primary response and requires less antigen for its induction (Figure 2.17). As a result of its initial experience of antigen, the body is said to possess *immunological memory* to that antigen, which enables the secondary response to be more rapid and powerful than the primary. However, instead of an immune response, antigen can in certain circumstances induce a state of specific immunological unresponsiveness or *tolerance*. This situation is most familiar for self antigens, but tolerance can also be produced for non-self antigens if they are introduced into the foetus or newborn or in particularly large amounts in adults.

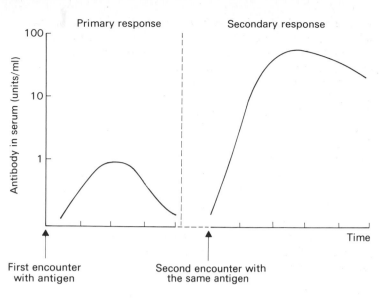

Primary response   Secondary response

First encounter
with antigen

Second encounter with
the same antigen

Figure 2.17 Primary and
secondary antibody responses
(note logarithmic scale for
antibody concentration).

Clonal selection theory

What are the cellular events in the primary and secondary
responses and the induction of tolerance? The basic principles are
contained in the clonal selection theory proposed by Burnet in
1959 (Figure 2.18). As already mentioned, lymphocytes are
antigen-sensitive cells, having the ability to recognise and respond
to antigen. However, individual lymphocytes are highly *restricted*
in respect of the antigen which they can recognise, to the extent
that each can only react well with *one* particular antigenic determinant. Each lymphocyte carries, on its surface, *specific receptors*
for the particular antigen to which it is committed. In the case of
B cells, the receptors are *antibody molecules*, identical in
specificity to those which the B cell will later produce, while the
nature of the T cell receptor is still a matter of research. It is via
its specific surface receptors that a lymphocyte recognises the
presence of antigen.

A primary response occurs when an antigen meets a
population of lymphocytes for the first time. Since lymphocytes
are highly restricted in specificity, the antigen will only be able to
react with the very small proportion of cells which are
precommitted to it and which carry surface receptors for it. In
short, antigen will *select* the appropriate antigen-sensitive cells
from the population. After antigen has combined with the
receptors on a specific lymphocyte, the cell is triggered into
proliferation. The daughter cells which are produced, and which
all share the same specificity, make up a *clone* of cells. Some
members of the clone differentiate into specific antibody-
producing cells in the case of B cells, or into cells carrying out
cell-mediated immunity in the case of a T cell clone. Other cells
in the clone become *memory cells*, small lymphocytes which are
available should the antigen be introduced for a second time.
Thus, after an individual has made a primary response to a
particular antigen, he possesses an increased number of specific
antigen-sensitive cells—memory cells—which are able to react

103

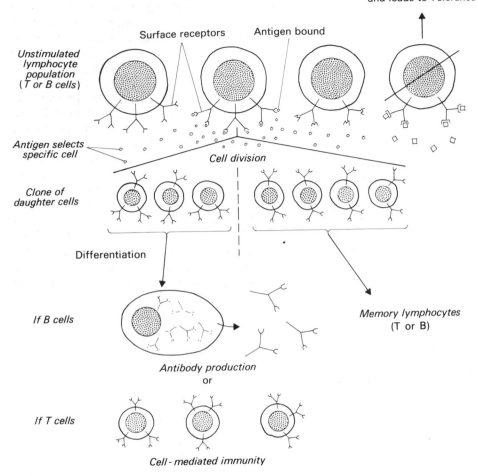

Encounter with
antigen kills cell
and leads to *Tolerance*

Surface receptors   Antigen bound

*Unstimulated
lymphocyte
population
(T or B cells)*

*Antigen selects
specific cell*

Cell division

*Clone of
daughter cells*

Differentiation

If B cells

Antibody production
or

*Memory lymphocytes
(T or B)*

If T cells

Cell-mediated immunity

with the same antigen on future occasions. For this reason, the secondary response will both be more rapid and reach a higher level than the primary.

To account for immunological tolerance, the clonal selection theory proposes that in certain circumstances contact with antigen via specific receptors can lead to death of the lymphocyte rather than its proliferation; in other words, tolerance is a result of the *elimination* of antigen-sensitive cells. At early stages of development of the immune system in embryonic life there is a particular susceptibility to tolerance induction and it is probably then that lymphocytes reactive with self determinants are eliminated.

In summary, clonal selection proposes that antigen selects from the lymphocyte population the small number of cells which are genetically precommitted to react with it. As a result of recognising and reacting with antigen by specific surface receptors the lymphocyte either divides to give a clone of daughter cells, including memory cells, or alternatively is

Figure 2.18 The clonal selection theory of the immune response.

eliminated, thereby giving rise to a state of antigen-specific unresponsiveness.

Although the clonal selection theory has for many years been the accepted framework for thinking about antibody formation, it is only rather recently that a formal experimental proof has been possible of its fundamental postulate, namely the clonal precommitment of each lymphocyte to a single specificity. This has now been achieved for B cells by physically separating those cells bearing receptors for a particular antigen and demonstrating that individual B cells respond uniquely to that antigen in culture. In this experiment, two unrelated antigens were used, namely the haptens nitroiodophenyl (NIP) and fluorescein (FLU). As shown in Figure 2.19, the spleen of a normal mouse contains B cells which are able to respond to each of these haptens in culture. When the cells were passed over an insoluble form of NIP, a very small proportion ($<1\%$) adhered by means of their NIP-specific receptors (another example of affinity chromatography); the $>99\%$ of B cells which did not adhere to NIP were now unable to respond to NIP in culture, but were still responsive to FLU, demonstrating the specific depletion of NIP-reactive cells. In contrast, when the adherent

Figure 2.19 Experimental verification of the clonal selection theory for antibody-producing (B) cells.
NIP = nitroiodophenyl; FLU = fluorescein.

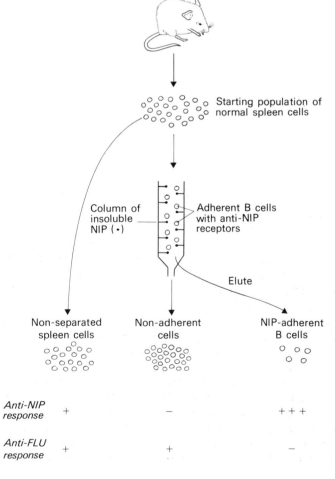

cells were recovered from the NIP-adsorbent, they were found to be highly enriched for responsiveness to NIP but completely unresponsive to FLU; moreover the frequency, among the NIP-selected population, of B cells which could be triggered into anti-NIP production was as close to the 100% predicted by the clonal selection theory as the experimental conditions allowed. Thus, this experiment is a demonstration of the existence of lymphocytes of precommitted specificity and their selection and triggering by antigen, and hence of the essential validity of the clonal selection theory.

B lymphocyte receptors

Lymphocytes must first recognise the presence of antigen before they can respond and this recognition is achieved by means of the surface receptors alluded to above. B cell receptors are antibody molecules and each B cell carries surface Ig of a single specificity (the same specificity that the plasma cells of the clone will later secrete). Since most antibody in serum is IgG, it might be expected that most B cells would have IgG on their surface as receptor, but this is not the case. In fact the distribution of antibody classes on the surface of B lymphocytes is very different

Figure 2.20 (a) B cell immunoglobulin receptors. (b) Distribution of Ig classes (i) in serum and (ii) on B cells.

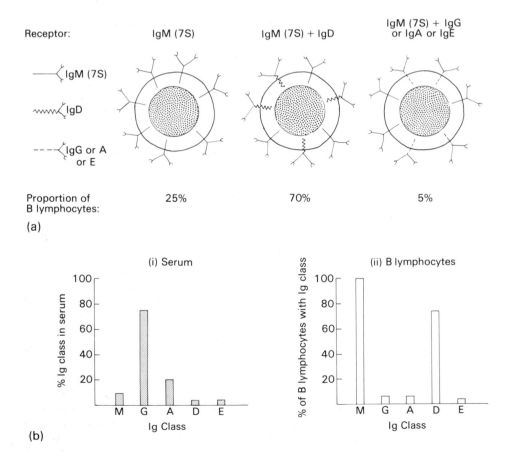

(a)

(b)

106

from that of serum Ig (Figure 2.20b). All small B lymphocytes carry IgM on their surface membrane and in a monomeric form (7S IgM) rather than the pentameric form of serum IgM (19S). Moreover, in addition to surface IgM, many B cells (about 70%) carry a second Ig class as well and this is generally IgD. The discovery that IgD is widely distributed on B cell surfaces came as a considerable surprise, considering the minute amounts of IgD present in serum. It appears that the role of IgD is confined to acting as a lymphocyte receptor rather than being secreted. A few lymphocytes ($\sim$ 5%) do carry IgG, IgA or IgE; these cells always have surface monomeric IgM as well. Thus, the antibody receptors on B cells are of one or two Ig classes (never more than two), of which one class is always IgM while the other is often IgD (Figure 2.20a).

The function of the surface Ig on B cells is to bind sufficient antigen to the specific B cell for it to be triggered along the pathway of B lymphocyte differentiation into plasma cells or memory cells. Each plasma cell, as already noted, secretes a single Ig class only and the question of why lymphocytes express receptors of two classes is at present enigmatic; so too is the particular role of surface IgD. However, the nature of the Ig receptor marks out the future course of the cell, in that B cells which carry IgM alone or IgM and IgD are destined to give rise to plasma cells producing the IgM class, while those carrying IgM and IgG (or IgA or IgE) have 'switched' and will become IgG (or IgA or IgE) producers (below). The relative amounts of the Ig classes in serum reflect the numbers of plasma cells of each class, rather than the class distribution of lymphocytes.

In addition to the receptors by which they recognise antigen, B cells carry receptors for the Fc portion of IgG (Fc receptors) and for fixed complement (C3b receptors). These receptors may play a role in regulating B cell activity.

Distribution of classes in the antibody response

Several factors govern the way in which an antibody response is distributed among the various antibody classes, including the nature of the antigen and whether the response is primary or secondary. One frequent observation concerns the order in which different classes appear. In the primary response, IgM is the first-formed antibody in serum, an initial wave of IgM being followed by a roughly equivalent wave of IgG production (and other classes). In the secondary response, the proportion of IgM may be much less and the bulk of antibody produced in the serum is of the IgG class. There are of course exceptions, including some bacterial antigens such as lipopolysaccharide (endotoxin), polymerised flagellin and pneumococcal capsular polysaccharide, for which the response appears never to pass the IgM stage and for which this is the majority antibody class in both primary and secondary responses. However, for many antigens, including most proteins, an initial IgM response generally gives way to IgG and other classes. The cellular basis for this seems to involve a so-called 'switch' event. It appears that all antigen-sensitive B cells begin life as potential IgM producers. After meeting antigen, they divide to form clones of IgM-producing cells, but during the development of some clones, and even perhaps within individual cells, a switch occurs from IgM production to other classes. In the primary response, this gives an IgM wave followed by IgG, but since many of the memory cells generated will be IgG producers, the secondary response is mainly IgG. It is important to note that even after a switch to a different class has occurred, the specificity of the antibody produced by a given clone continues to be the same, i.e. one clone can only produce one type of antibody binding site, which becomes part of antibody molecules of different classes. In molecular terms, a clone is committed to a single light chain type, and to a single heavy chain V region, but can switch the latter onto heavy chain C regions of different classes (μ, α, γ, etc.) as described on p. 96.

The route by which exposure to antigen takes place can influence the class of antibody produced. A good example is IgA production, which will be most pronounced for antigens presenting in the respiratory and alimentary tracts, where there are the largest numbers of IgA-producing cells. The factors tending towards IgE production are of great clinical significance, since IgE is responsible for immediate hypersensitivity (anaphylaxis, p. 152). There is an important inherited component, with a family tendency to increased IgE levels and specific IgE production to certain antigens such as pollens. Some of the genes causing this tendency are located in the major histocompatibility complex, HLA (p. 180).

Antigen recognition by T cells: the T cell receptor

While B cells use antibody molecules as their receptors for antigen, the molecular nature of the T cell receptor is still uncertain. What is clear, however, is that T cells do not produce surface antibody nor do they become antibody-secreting cells. Moreover, the recognition of antigen by T cells and B cells is fundamentally different. By means of their surface antibodies, B cells can recognise and bind virtually any physical form of an antigen, whether it be free in solution, insolubilised by polymerisation, or present on a cell membrane (Figure 2.21a); thus, specific B cells can be isolated by binding to an adsorbent of insolubilised antigen as in Figure 2.19. In contrast, most T cells *cannot react with free antigens*: it is not possible to demonstrate binding of antigen from solution onto T cells, nor can T cells be specifically trapped on an inanimate antigen adsorbent. The reason for this is that T cells (with the possible exception of suppressor cells) only bind to antigens *associated with cell surfaces*. Thus, certain T cell types, such as helper and lymphokine-releasing T cells, react with antigen 'presented' on the surface of *macrophages*: after phagocytosing the antigen and 'processing' it, probably by partial proteolysis, the macrophage expresses the antigen or fragments thereof on its surface, where recognition by T cells occurs (p. 115). Cytotoxic T cells, on the other hand, recognise antigens on the surface of virally-infected cells,

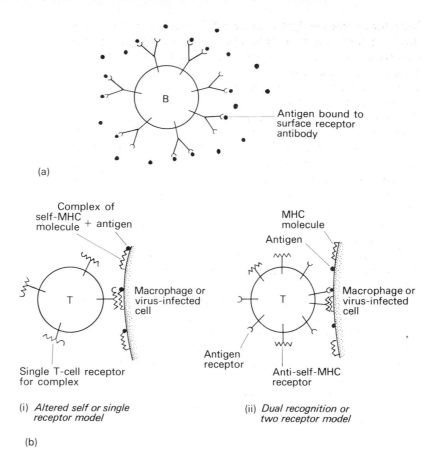

(a)

(b)

(i) *Altered self or single receptor model*

(ii) *Dual recognition or two receptor model*

Figure 2.21 The recognition of antigen by B and T cells.
(a) B cells can recognise free antigen by means of their Ig receptors.
(b) T cells recognise antigen in association with an MHC molecule on the surface of other body cells: alternative models.

neoplastic cells, or the cells of foreign tissue grafts. The limitation of T cell recognition to antigen presented on a cell surface can be understood in relation to the main functions of T cells in cell-mediated immunity, such as direct engagement and killing of virus-infected cells or close-range activation of bacterially-infected macrophages. Since the target of a T cell reaction is always another cell and never a soluble molecule, it would be unproductive or even counter-productive for T cells to be activated by antigens which were not cell-associated.

The question then arises of how a T cell recognises the cell-associated, as opposed to any other, form of an antigen. This is achieved through an ability to recognise simultaneously both the antigen and specific surface molecules of normal body cells. The component of the normal cell surface which the T cell 'sees' is coded by genes in the *major histocompatibility complex* (MHC), a genetic system which specifies several membrane proteins (MHC molecules or antigens) involved in the immune response (the MHC is more fully described on p. 168). In principle, one can envisage two possible ways in which T cells could recognise a foreign antigen and a self-MHC molecule together on a cell surface (Figure 2.21b). (i) The antigen may be physically associated with an MHC molecule and the complex recognised by a *single* T cell receptor (the 'altered self' or single receptor model);

109

alternatively (ii) the T cell may be endowed with *two receptors*, an antigen receptor and an anti-MHC receptor, which recognise these molecules independently (the 'dual recognition' or two receptor model). At present it is not possible to make a definite choice between these possibilities. A further important point is that since unrelated animals show many differences in their MHC molecules, T cells (other than those involved in graft rejection) are often unable to recognise antigens presented on the surface of foreign cells of a different MHC type. This phenomenon is known as *MHC restriction* (self-restriction) of T cell recognition; the MHC molecules are called restricting elements, because unless they are recognised as self the T cell cannot react with the antigen (see also p. 177). The ability of T cells to recognise self-MHC seems to be acquired during their maturation within the thymus.

Role of T cells in antibody production

One of the most exciting developments of recent years has been the discovery that for antibody production to some antigens a cooperative interaction between B and T lymphocytes is essential. Whereas B cells provide the precursors of the plasma cells which produce the antibody, T cells are required in a *helper* capacity, assisting B cells in their proliferation and differentiation towards antibody formation. Thus, mice which have been neonatally thymectomised or are congenitally athymic (nude mice) are found to be unable to produce antibodies to certain antigens, including red cells of other species, proteins, and haptens coupled to protein carriers. Some antigens are more *thymus dependent* than others, and many pathogenically important bacterial antigens such as endotoxin and pneumococcal capsular polysaccharide are *thymus independent*, i.e. thymectomy does not impair the ability of the animal to mount an antibody response. In addition, IgG responses are more thymus-dependent than IgM, and thymus independent antigens stimulate mainly IgM production.

Many of the early experiments designed to investigate the phenomenon of T cell—B cell cooperation utilised heavily irradiated mice as 'living test-tubes'. The irradiation eliminates most of the lymphoid cells of the mouse and thus prevents it from making an immune response of its own. The animal can then be inoculated with lymphocytes of another normal mouse, which will repopulate the lymphoid organs and make an antibody response if antigen is injected. In this way a living, but irradiated and immunologically unresponsive mouse is used to provide the environment in which to follow the responses of the transferred lymphoid cells. An example of a typical experiment is shown in Figure 2.22. The irradiated mice are inoculated with different normal lymphocyte populations—T cells, B cells or T cells *and* B cells—in each case together with a thymus-dependent antigen such as sheep red blood cells (SRBC). A few days later the antibodies to SRBC in the mice are measured and it is found that a good anti-SRBC response is made only in the animals receiving

Figure 2.22 Experiment to demonstrate cooperation between T cells and B cells in the antibody response.

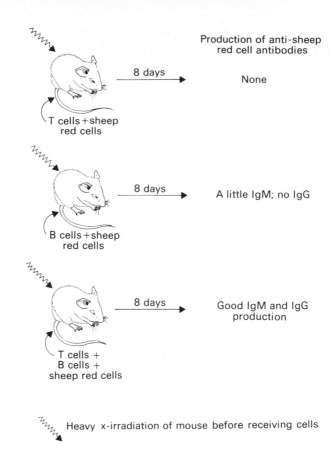

Production of anti-sheep red cell antibodies

T cells + sheep red cells → 8 days → None

B cells + sheep red cells → 8 days → A little IgM; no IgG

T cells + B cells + sheep red cells → 8 days → Good IgM and IgG production

〰 Heavy x-irradiation of mouse before receiving cells

both T and B cells. By using cells with a chromosome marker which can be identified microscopically, it was proved that the antibody is produced exclusively by B cells. Nevertheless the presence of T cells was essential to enable B cells to develop into antibody-producing cells; some cooperative event between T and B cells must therefore occur in order that B cells may proceed to antibody production. It appears that for the thymus-dependent group of antigens it is not sufficient for B cells simply to recognise antigen by their surface immunoglobulin receptors; they must receive an additional signal from T cells to divide and differentiate.

When T and B cells interact, they seem to recognise antigenic determinants on different parts of the same molecule. This was concluded from experiments with hapten-carrier conjugates, e.g. haptens such as DNP linked to protein carriers such as foreign albumin or globulin. It has been known for many years that to stimulate an animal to make a secondary response to, say, DNP, it must receive DNP conjugated to the same protein that was used in the primary response. Thus, as Figure 2.23 shows, a mouse immunised with DNP coupled to bovine serum albumin (DNP-BSA) will make a secondary anti-DNP response on subsequent injection of DNP-BSA, but not to DNP coupled to, say, chicken gamma globulin (DNP-CGG). This phenomenon is called the *carrier effect* and occurs even though the anti-DNP

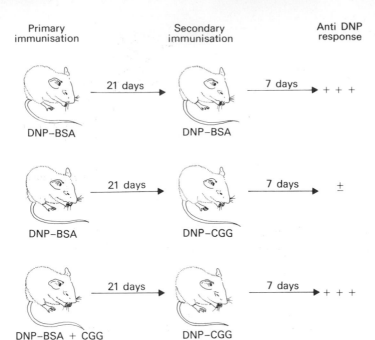

Primary immunisation		Secondary immunisation		Anti DNP response
DNP–BSA	→ 21 days	DNP–BSA	→ 7 days	+ + +
DNP–BSA	→ 21 days	DNP–CGG	→ 7 days	±
DNP–BSA + CGG	→ 21 days	DNP–CGG	→ 7 days	+ + +

Figure 2.23 The carrier effect. DNP = dinitrophenyl, BSA = bovine serum albumin, CGG = chicken gamma globulin.

antibodies are directed only at the hapten and have no carrier reactivity (anti-carrier antibodies, i.e. anti-BSA, are of course also produced); this is illustrated in Figure 2.23. The carrier effect implies that specific immunological recognition of the carrier is required for the antihapten response. Indeed, if the DNP-BSA-immunised mice also receive an injection of unconjugated CGG, they will later respond to DNP-CGG (Figure 2.23). In cellular terms the carrier effect can be explained by the necessary interaction between T and B cells: specific B cells recognise the hapten (DNP) while specific T cells are required to recognise the carrier (BSA or CGG), and only when enlarged populations of both hapten-specific B and carrier-specific T cells have been produced by immunisation can a secondary response to the hapten be obtained. The following experiment proves this point (Figure 2.24). Mice are immunised with DNP-BSA and 3 weeks later their spleens are removed, cell suspensions are prepared and transferred into groups of irradiated recipient mice of the same strain. One group of such recipients is then immunised with DNP-BSA and the cells it has received proceed over the next few days to a secondary anti-DNP response (Figure 2.24, group 1). The next group receives DNP-CGG instead of DNP-BSA and makes hardly any anti-DNP during the same period of time (i.e. the carrier effect is again demonstrated). A third group receives, in addition to spleen cells immunised against DNP-BSA, spleen cells from donors immunised against CGG; in contrast with the second group, they respond well both to DNP-BSA *and* DNP-CGG. Thus the carrier effect is overcome by the CGG-reactive spleen cells. In the final group the CGG-immunised spleen cells are treated before transfer with anti-Thy-1 antibodies which are cytotoxic for mouse T cells in the presence of complement; this

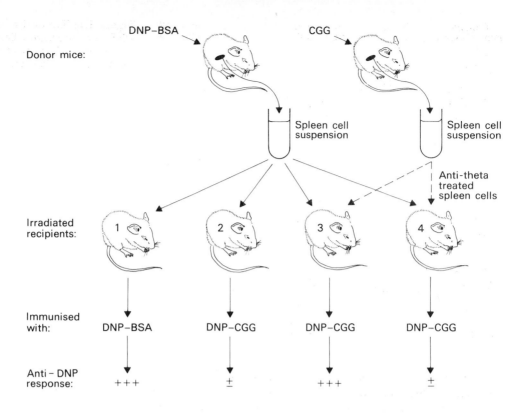

Donor mice:

DNP–BSA

CGG

Spleen cell suspension

Spleen cell suspension

Anti-theta treated spleen cells

Irradiated recipients: 1   2   3   4

Immunised with: DNP–BSA   DNP–CGG   DNP–CGG   DNP–CGG

Anti – DNP response: +++   ±   +++   ±

Figure 2.24 Experiment on the cellular basis of the carrier effect (see text for explanation).

treatment prevents them from helping the response to DNP-CGG. Thus the role of T cells demonstrated in this experiment is to recognise carrier determinants and by so doing to assist the response to a hapten linked to that carrier.

From experiments such as these it was proposed that when T cells help B cells, they are brought into close proximity with them by an antigen 'bridge', T cells binding one determinant and B cells another on the same molecule (Figure 2.25). The close contact between helper T cell and B cell was assumed to lead to proliferation and differentiation of the latter into antibody-producing cells. Subsequently, however, it was found that helper T cells produce soluble substances, termed T cell *factors*, which mediate the interaction with B cells, so that physical contact between T and B cells may be unnecessary. The factors are of two functional types: some show no specificity for antigen and will promote all thymus-dependent antibody responses (e.g. T-cell replacing factor, TRF), while others are strictly antigen-specific. The latter carry a binding site for the antigen, as well as a functional region which enables them to trigger B cells; their relationship, if any, to immunoglobulin is currently under investigation. B cells carry surface sites called *acceptors*, where reaction with the T cell factors takes place. Thus, in a thymus-dependent response, a B cell receives *two signals*, one via its Ig receptors which recognise the specific antigen and a second signal from the binding of T cell factor to the acceptor site. These interactions are shown diagrammatically in Figure 2.26.

113

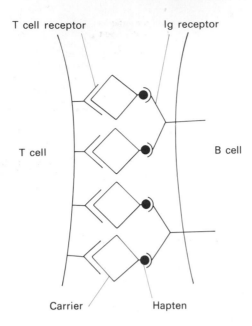

T cell receptor   Ig receptor

T cell   B cell

Carrier   Hapten

Figure 2.25 T cell–B cell cooperation: antigen bridge model. (The more recent finding that the T cell must also recognise an MHC molecule is ignored in this figure.)

Macrophages as antigen-presenting cells in antibody responses

Studies of T cell–B cell interaction *in vitro* revealed that a third cell type was necessary for antibody production, namely the macrophage. Being adherent cells, macrophages are easily separated from lymphocytes by passage over glass beads or incubation on the surface of a plastic culture vessel; lymphocytes depleted of macrophages fail to respond to antigens in culture, while replacement of the macrophages restores the response. The role of the macrophage is elucidated by the following observations. (i) Macrophages which have been incubated with and have phagocytosed antigen, so-called antigen-pulsed macrophages, are an effective source of antigen for T and B cells *in vivo* and *in vitro*. (ii) Antigen-bearing membrane fragments of antigen-pulsed macrophages are highly immunogenic *in vivo*, stimulating more vigorous antibody responses than an equivalent amount of antigen in free form. (iii) Antigen-pulsed macrophages stimulate T cells specific for the antigen to proliferate and release soluble factors; in this reaction, the macrophage and T cell must have certain genes of the major histocompatibility complex in common. Thus, it is often found that T cells are stimulated by antigen associated with syngeneic macrophages (i.e. of the same genetic strain as the T cell), but not by the same antigen associated with macrophages of an unrelated strain *unless* the two strains share certain MHC genes (I-region genes in the mouse H-2 complex, HLA-D-region genes in man, p. 169). (iv) A soluble factor obtained from macrophages, known as *interleukin-1* or IL-1 (formerly called lymphocyte activating factor) is required for stimulation of helper T cells; it is mitogenic for thymocytes and is apparently essential for the response of helper T cells to macrophage-associated antigen.

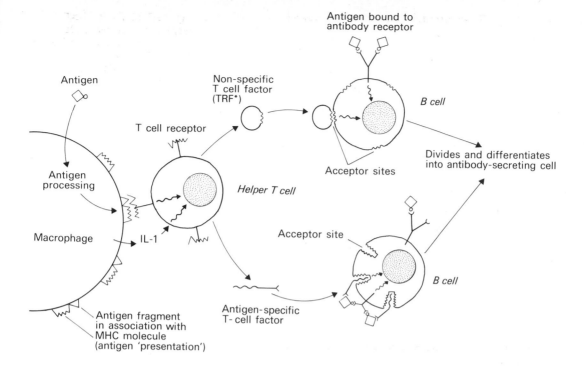

Figure 2.26 Possible pathways of T cell–B cell interaction.
(a) Stimulation of B cell by antigen and nonspecific T cell factor.
(b) Stimulation of B cell by antigen and antigen-specific T cell factor.

Thus, it appears that the initial event in an antibody response to a thymus-dependent antigen is the uptake of the antigen by macrophages. Most of the antigen is evidently degraded within the macrophage, but a small proportion survives, either intact or more likely as antigenic fragments, and is carried to the macrophage surface; there it is 'presented' in association with an MHC molecule to the antigen-specific helper T cell. Only macrophages bearing MHC molecules which the T cell recognises as self are effective in antigen presentation, for the reasons previously described (page 109); the particular MHC molecules involved are known as class II molecules, called Ia in the mouse and HLA-D in man (see p. 170 for further explanation). Release of IL-1 by macrophages is also required for the response of helper T cells; thus, like B cells, helper T cells receive two signals in order to trigger proliferation, namely antigen and IL-1. The helper T cell then proliferates, releasing helper factors which stimulate B cells nearby which have also recognised the antigen.

Macrophages are apparently not required for responses to thymus independent (i.e. T cell-independent) antigens; in fact, macrophages seem to be unable to present them to T cells, thus explaining why the responses to such antigens are limited to IgM and do not progress to the T cell-dependent IgG phase. Thymus independent antigens are characteristically polymeric molecules, in which the same antigenic determinants are repeated many times over; hence they will attach strongly to specific B cells by binding to several surface Ig receptors simultaneously (multipoint attachment). In addition, they have mitogenic properties for B cells. The failure of macrophages to present thymus-independent antigens seems to be related, at least in some cases, to poor digestibility by lysosomal enzymes; e.g. synthetic polymers of D-amino acids, which resist enzymatic degradation in macrophages, are thymus-independent antigens, while their L-amino acid counterparts, which can be degraded, are thymus-dependent.

Helper T cells also help T cell responses

The action of helper T cells is not limited to antibody responses; they are also required in the development of other types of cell, such as the cytotoxic T cells which kill virus-infected cells. We have noted above that helper T cells, having recognised antigen presented on the surface of macrophages and received interleukin-1, respond by releasing a nonspecific factor (TRF) involved in the stimulation of B cells. At the same time, activated T cells produce a second nonspecific factor which promotes the proliferation of T cells in response to antigen; this factor is known as *interleukin-2* (IL-2 or T cell growth factor, TCGF) and seems to be the principal T cell-derived mediator of T cell proliferation. Interleukin-2 acts as a helper factor for cytotoxic T cells and also for helper T cells themselves. It is used experimentally to promote the growth of isolated T cells in culture (T cell clones) and is also attracting medical interest because it accelerates tumour rejection in mice, probably by stimulation of cytotoxic T cells. For these purposes, interleukin-2 is obtained by mitogen stimulation of T cells (e.g. with concanavalin A), or from permanently growing T cell lines, or very recently from genetically engineered bacteria into which the IL-2 gene has been introduced.

We may note here the general point that many lymphocytes require the combined action of two signals for their activation and proliferation during an immune response: one signal comes from the recognition of antigen via specific surface receptors, while the other is provided by a soluble factor released either by a macrophage (IL-1) or a helper T cell (IL-2, TRF, antigen-specific factors). Soluble factors derived from macrophages are called monokines; those from T cells are lymphokines. The role of factors and antigen in the induction of immune responses is summarised in Figure 2.27.

Suppressor T cells

While helper T cells take part in antibody production and CMI by stimulating B cells and effector T cells, other T cells known as *suppressors* exert a balancing inhibitory influence on immune responses. Suppressor T cells prevent responses from becoming excessive by interacting with helper T cells, as well as with T cells participating in cell-mediated immunity and possibly B cells; e.g. one well-recognised mode of suppression is that suppressor T cells 'switch off' helper T cells. They produce suppressive mediator factors analogous to the stimulatory factors produced by helper T cells. It is clear that suppressor T cells occupy an important position as immunoregulatory cells, and they may also be responsible for

Figure 2.27 Role of antigen and soluble factors in induction of responses of T and B cells.

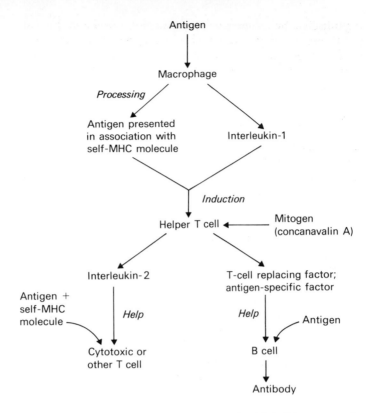

some forms of immunological tolerance (p. 186). Two examples where their activity may be clinically relevant are noteworthy: overactivity of suppressor T cells may be a cause of immunodeficiency, while underactivity may allow the development of autoimmunity.

1   In one type of antibody deficiency, *common variable hypogammaglobulinaemia*, excessive suppressor T cell activity rather than an intrinsic B cell deficiency has been implicated. This type of hypogammaglobulinaemia presents with similar clinical symptoms to the congenital X-linked agammaglobulinaemia (p. 78), but does not become clinically apparent until 15–35 years of age. It has been shown that T lymphocytes from patients with common variable hypogammaglobulinaemia were able to suppress Ig production by normal lymphocytes *in vitro*. Moreover, when patients' B cells were prepared free of T cells, they were able to commence synthesis of immunoglobulin *in vitro* when triggered with mitogenic agents; this Ig production could be completely suppressed by the patients' own T cells. Thus, it seems that excessive nonspecific suppressor T cell activity can lead to certain forms of hypogammaglobulinaemia, in contrast with the X-linked and combined immunodeficiencies where B cells fail to develop as a result of defects in bone marrow stem cells.

2   The possible role of suppressor T cells in maintaining immunological tolerance is discussed at greater length later in this section (p. 186). In brief, there is evidence from certain strains of mice that an early decline in suppressor T cell activity is

accompanied by an increase in production of various autoantibodies (i.e. antibodies reacting with self molecules), indicating
the loss of self-tolerance. Thus it may be that natural tolerance to
the body's own molecules is in some cases dependent on active
suppression of helper T cells and B cells, rather than the specific
elimination of self-responsive cells as proposed in the clonal
selection hypothesis (p. 103).

Differentiated types of T cells

After triggering by antigen there are several possible pathways of
differentiation of T cells, leading to effector cells with distinct
functions. They are summarised in Figure 2.28. Some T cells
become *lymphokine-releasing* cells, able to secrete a variety of
soluble mediators of cell-mediated immunity, with effects on
macrophages, lymphocytes and blood vessels (p. 147). Others
become *cytotoxic* cells, which can kill antigenic cellular targets,
such as virus-infected or neoplastic cells (p. 149). The helper and
suppressor T cell types have been described above; they often
seem to act by release of soluble protein lymphokines (helper and

Figure 2.28 Pathways of T cell
differentiation. (Note that in
reality the antigen would usually
be presented in association with
an MHC molecule on the surface
of a macrophage or target cell.)

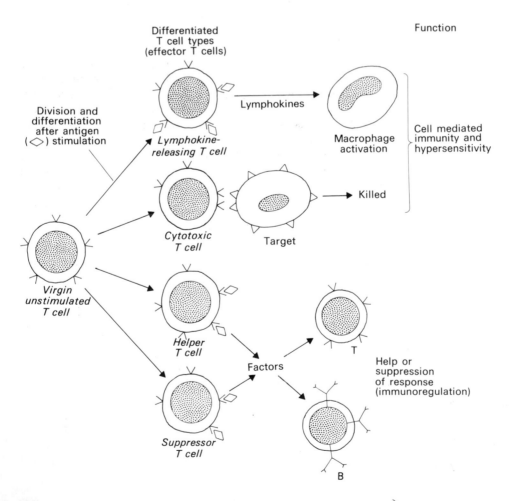

suppressor factors). Note that these regulatory T cells can help or suppress the activities of other T cells as well as B cells. Finally, there are also *memory* T cells responsible for rapid recall of response on second contact with the antigen.

Differentiated T cells can to a certain extent be identified by surface marker molecules, known in the mouse as Lyt (lymphocyte-T cell) antigens (Lyt-1, 2 and 3). Thus, helper T cells and T cells which release lymphokines affecting macrophages are Lyt-1 positive (Lyt-1$^+$) and Lyt-2,3 negative (Lyt-2,3$^-$); suppressor T cells and cytotoxic T cells have the opposite surface phenotype, being Lyt-2,3$^+$ and Lyt-1$^-$. In man, similar markers have been identified with monoclonal antibodies. As noted elsewhere, all T cells, with the possible exception of suppressors, recognise antigen on cell membranes in association with molecules coded by the major histocompatibility complex. For helper T cells and lymphokine-releasing T cells, the MHC molecules are class II molecules (Ia in the mouse and HLA-DR in man, whereas cytotoxic T cells recognise antigen in association with class I MHC molecules (called K and D in the mouse and HLA-A,B,C in man; see p. 169). Thus the differentiated state of a T cell is described by its function, surface markers and MHC restriction molecules.

COMPLEMENT

The complement system is an important part of the body's defence mechanisms against microbial infection, interacting with the antibody response on the one hand and with the 'primitive' processes of inflammation and phagocytosis on the other (Figure 2.29). Complement reactions are initiated *inter alia* by antigen-antibody complexes and the envelopes of Gram-negative bacteria, and assist in defence in three ways, namely (a) triggering of acute inflammation, (b) facilitation of phagocytosis and (c) direct killing of certain microorganisms. However, complement is a double-edged weapon: because of its ability to initiate inflammation, activation of complement can lead to tissue damage and plays an important part in hypersensitivity (p. 161).

In Section 1, the complement system was introduced in the context of inflammation. It will be recalled that there are nine com-

Figure 2.29 Role of complement in bacterial infection.
1 Classical pathway
2 Alternative pathway (certain bacteria)
3 C3a, C5a, C2 kinin, C$\overline{567}$
4 C3b
5 Termination of infection

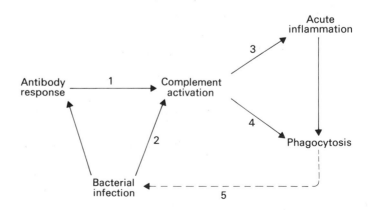

plement components present in inactive form in the blood, that several activated components are enzymes, and that once triggered the system follows a cascade process with one component activating the next in sequence until a final effect is achieved. In common with blood clotting (p. 632) and kinin formation (p. 29), the complement cascade thus allows a small stimulus to be amplified into a significant biological effect. In the following pages, the complement pathways are considered in greater detail.

Designation of components

Complement is abbreviated as C; individual inactive components are numbered from 1 to 9 (C1, C2, etc); activation is indicated by a bar—thus C$\overline{1}$ for activated first component, etc.; factors involved in the alternative pathway are called B, D, P (for properdin) and IF (initiation factor).

Pathways of complement activation

Two convergent pathways are known for complement activation, called the *classical* and *alternative* pathways, and one is again reminded of blood clotting where there are convergent 'intrinsic' and 'extrinsic' pathways leading to thrombin activation (p. 633, Figure 5.5). The complement pathways are shown in Figure 2.30. The classical pathway is triggered by antigen–antibody

Figure 2.30 Pathways of complement activation.
† As complex with C$\overline{42}$ or C$\overline{3b,B}$ and bound to cell membrane.

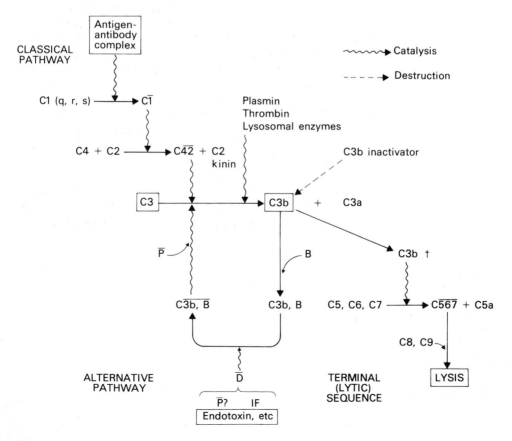

complexes, while the alternative sequence is independent of antibody.

The classical pathway

The reaction of antibody of the IgM and IgG classes (IgG$_1$, IgG$_2$, IgG$_3$) with antigen allows the Fc portion of the molecule to bind the first component of complement, C1. Recently, C1 has been shown to possess a remarkable structure. It is made up of three subcomponents, C1q, C1r and C1s; C1q is the one which binds to the Fc of complexed antibody. In the electron microscope, C1q resembles a 'bunch of tulips' with six globular heads and with the stems joined together (Figures 2.31a, 2.32a). A most unusual feature is that the 'stem' of the molecule closely resembles collagen in structure. C1q reacts with Fc by its globular heads; thus it is easy to see that it will be more effectively trapped by IgM than by IgG, since in the former there are several Fc's close together to which two or more C1q heads can bind simultaneously. This explains the greater efficiency of the IgM class in complement activation; indeed, a single molecule of IgM at a cell surface is sufficient to activate complement and cause cell lysis.

Complement activation via binding of C1q to antibody provides a particularly good illustration of the importance of multivalent attachment (Figure 2.31). Thus, the Fc 'tail' of an individual IgG molecule possesses a C1q binding site on its C$_H$2 domain, but free IgG molecules in plasma or isolated IgG molecules bound to antigen do not activate complement because the affinity of a single IgG Fc site for a single C1q head is very weak (Figure 2.31a). However, when two IgGs come close together on an antigen, two C1q heads can engage simultaneously, with an enormous resulting gain in binding strength, and binding is now strong enough to activate the complement pathway (Figure 2.31b). This raises the question of why free IgM, in which 5 Fc's are associated as a central disc, does not spontaneously activate complement but must first be complexed with an antigen. The explanation is that the C1q sites are not exposed in native IgM; however, on binding to a multivalent antigen, the arms fold away from the disc and IgM adopts its 'staple' conformation (Figure 2.10), an event which renders Fc

Figure 2.31 Activation of the first component of complement by IgG. Two IgG molecules are required close together on the antigen so that strong multipoint attachment of C1q can occur.
(a) Single-site binding is too weak to fix C1q to IgG.
(b) Binding of C1q to two (or more) IgG sites is much stronger and leads to complement activation.

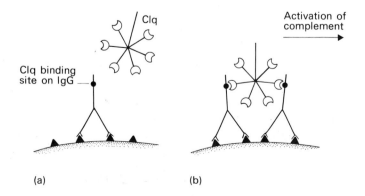

C1q

Activation of complement

C1q binding site on IgG

(a)

(b)

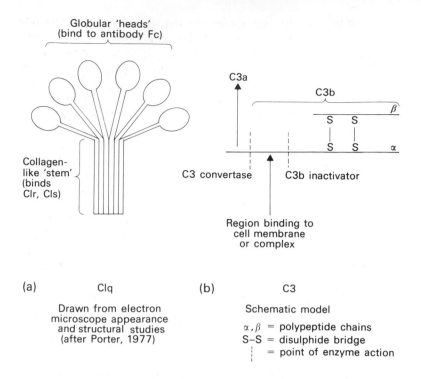

Globular 'heads'
(bind to antibody Fc)

Collagen-like 'stem'
(binds
C1r, C1s)

C3a

C3b

β

S S
| |
S S

α

C3 convertase

C3b inactivator

Region binding to
cell membrane
or complex

(a) C1q

Drawn from electron
microscope appearance
and structural studies
(after Porter, 1977)

(b) C3

Schematic model

α, β = polypeptide chains
S–S = disulphide bridge
$\vdots$ = point of enzyme action

Figure 2.32 Structure of complement components.

sites accessible to C1q. For this reason, binding of IgM to a single antigenic determinant does not activate complement, as there is no associated change in the shape of the IgM molecule. Another molecule which activates complement by the classical pathway, i.e. via C1q binding, is C-reactive protein, the acute phase reactant present at raised levels in the blood during some microbial infections and acute inflammatory diseases (p. 42).

Once the C1q heads have bound, the collagenous tail is able to activate C1r and C1s; the latter, in activated form, is a protease which catalyses the next step in the sequence. The activation of C1 is also the point at which the classical pathway is regulated by C$\bar{1}$ inhibitor. A lack of this inhibitor leads to angio-oedema, as described in Section 1 (p. 41).

C$\bar{1}$s acts on components C4 and C2 to form an active complex, C$\overline{42}$, which attaches itself to cell membranes or to the antigen–antibody complex (Figure 2.30). Activation of C2 is accompanied by release of the inflammatory mediator C2-kinin (p. 30). C$\overline{42}$ is another proteolytic enzyme (C3 convertase) and brings about the central event in the complement sequence, namely the *activation of C3*, the most important complement component and the one present in largest amount in plasma. In this reaction (also called C3 conversion) a small fragment called C3a is released from C3 (Figure 2.32b); C3a or *anaphylatoxin*, has inflammatory properties, including stimulation of histamine release from mast cells and basophils (p. 31). The major fragment of C3 is C3b. C3b possesses a short-lived hydrophobic site which enables it to adhere covalently to proteins or to cell membranes. This is important because complement reactions are frequently initiated at a cell, e.g. bacterial, surface; C3b will then accumulate in quantitiy at the cell surface in the vicinity of the antibody molecules. The significance of the fixation of C3b at microbial surfaces derives from its role in phagocytosis; neutrophils and macrophages are enabled to bind to the organism by means of receptors for fixed C3b at their surface, and engulfment and destruction of the microbe follow (Section 1). C3b also binds to platelets and can initiate the release of inflammatory mediators from them.

The alternative pathway

In this pathway, complement is activated without requirement for antibody or components C1, C4 and C2; like the classical pathway, its main result is the conversion of C3 into C3b. The stimuli which activate this sequence include the lipopolysaccharides (endotoxins) of Gram-negative bacteria, yeast cell wall polysaccharide (zymosan), a factor from cobra venom, and complexes with antigen of antibodies which do not trigger the classical pathway, notably IgA. Its significance is that it provides a defence mechanism against certain bacteria in which direct activation of complement leads to their destruction or removal by phagocytes, without the need to wait for specific antibody production.

The alternative pathway functions as a *positive feedback* system: the major complement product, C3b, is itself incorporated into a convertase enzyme which catalyses C3b production (i.e. conversion of C3). In the absence of classical pathway activity, a small amount of C3b must first be generated, perhaps by continuous low-level breakdown of C3, to set the cycle in motion (Figure 2.30). The factors involved in the alternative pathway are proteins called B, D and P (properdin). C3b binds to factor B in serum to form a complex denoted C3b,B. This is acted on by factor D, to produce the active convertase complex $\overline{C3b,B}$ which catalyses the conversion of C3 to C3b. Factor P serves to stabilise this enzyme complex. Thus, whenever C3b is formed by either pathway or by the direct action of enzymes such as plasmin or thrombin (p. 32), it will enter into the feedback cycle and rapidly generate further large quantities of itself. It is not completely clear how molecules such as endotoxin initiate the alternative pathway; a likely means is via activation of factor D, in the presence of an initiating factor (IF).

In order to prevent the wholesale conversion of C3 into C3b by the feedback circuit, the blood contains an enzyme called *C3b inactivator* which destroys C3b. This eliminates all the activities of C3b, including adherence to phagocytes and feedback amplification. In the absence of C3b inactivator, the complement system fires off spontaneously and C3 can become exhausted. This occurs in patients with a rare inherited C3b inactivator deficiency; the patients' sera lack C3 and protective complement activity. As a result of this *secondary C3 deficiency*, the individuals suffer repeated acute bacterial infections similar to those seen in immunoglobulin-deficient patients and chronic granulomatous disease. However, although these infections are very severe for the first few days, patients with C3 deficiency eventually recover normally, following antibiotic therapy, whereas those with primary antibody or neutrophil deficiencies develop complications. This difference arises because the C3-deficient patient is most disadvantaged during the early, IgM phase of the antibody response, since IgM requires C3 for its opsonic and lytic activity. IgG, which is formed later, can act as an opsonin in the absence of C3 (p. 85) and its production enables the C3-deficient patient to recover. (Note that there is also a rare, inherited, i.e. primary, C3 deficiency.)

The terminal complement sequence

Following fixation of C3b by either classical or alternative pathways, there is a single series of complement reactions leading to lysis of thin-walled cells. C3b activates C5, with release of another anaphylatoxin fragment C5a; the active trimolecular complex $\overline{C567}$ then forms and, as noted in Section 1, both C5a and $\overline{C567}$ are *chemotactic* for neutrophils. Some $\overline{C567}$ is released into solution and can attach itself to neighbouring cell surfaces within a small radius; spread of $\overline{C567}$ in this way may be significant in producing tissue cell damage in some hypersensitivity reactions (Type III, p. 160). Finally, fixation of C8 and C9 leads to damage to the cell membrane and lysis, most familiar as the haemolysis of red blood cells coated with antibody and complement where it is of practical importance in the complement fixation test (p. 136). Cell membrane lesions caused by the terminal complement sequence can be visualised in the electron microscope (Figure 2.33) as pores or holes which take up negative stain. Rupture of the cells follows osmotic swelling. Some thin-walled pathogens, such as trypanosomes and the malarial parasite, are killed in this way by complement, and some Gram-negative bacteria can be killed by complement in conjunction with

Figure 2.33 Lesions produced by complement in a red cell membrane as seen in the electron microscope (courtesy Dr E.A. Munn). The lesion is a darkly staining pore surrounded by a ring, often incomplete, of unstained material (complement). (1 cm = 30 nm)

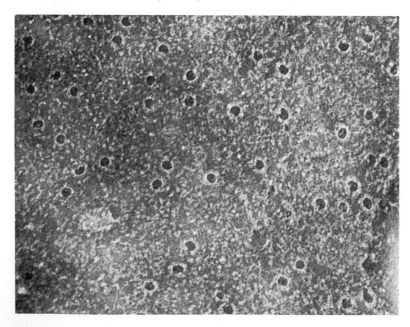

lysozyme. However, complement-mediated lysis is of limited importance as a bacteriocidal mechanism, when compared with phagocytic destruction of bacteria. Inherited deficiencies of the late components of complement (C5-9) are associated particularly with infection by gonococci and meningococci, both species being pyogenic organisms which can survive inside neutrophils and for which complement-dependent killing is evidently important.

Summary of functions of complement

The complement pathways serve to generate a variety of molecules which are required in defence against microbial infection. Some of these molecules promote inflammation by causing mast cells to release histamine (C3a, C5a), by interacting with platelets to stimulate release of mediators (C3b), by acting directly on blood vessels (C2 kinin) or by attracting neutrophil polymorphs (C5a, $\overline{C567}$). The major fixed product C3b enters into adherence reactions via C3 receptors with macrophages and neutrophils to facilitate phagocytosis; its importance is evidenced by the susceptibility of individuals with C3 deficiency to acute bacterial infection (pneumonia, meningitis, septicaemia). Lysis of microorganisms is important for defence against certain pathogens. (See also Section 1 for role of complement in acute inflammation, and p. 161 for its importance in hypersensitivity.)

DETECTION AND ESTIMATION OF ANTIBODIES, ANTIGENS AND COMPLEXES

The following are some of the most widely used methods based on antigen–antibody interaction.

PRECIPITATION

The most characteristic reaction between antigen and antibody is the *precipitin reaction* (precipitin = precipitating antibody). In its various forms this is of great value for the quantitative determination both of antibodies and antigens. A typical procedure for demonstrating precipitation is shown in Figure 2.34a; in Figure 2.34b the precipitin curve is drawn. A series of tubes, each with an equal amount of serum containing antibody (*antiserum*), is set up and antigen in increasing concentration is added to each tube. After a short time, precipitates appear in some tubes and reach a maximum amount at a certain optimal antigen concentration; higher concentrations of antigen are found to inhibit precipitation. Thus the typical precipitin curve, in which weight of precipitate is plotted against antigen concentration, shows a gradual increase to a maximum followed by a falling off as the concentration of antigen increases. Maximum precipitation occurs at *optimal proportions* of antibody to antigen; antigen excess causes inhibition of precipitation. From the weight of precipitate at optimal proportions, the antibody content of the serum can be accurately determined, since all the antigen and antibody are in the precipitate.

(a) *Precipitation test in tubes*

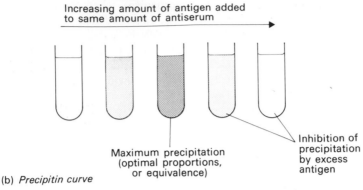

Increasing amount of antigen added
to same amount of antiserum

Maximum precipitation
(optimal proportions,
or equivalence)

Inhibition of
precipitation
by excess
antigen

Figure 2.34 The quantitative
precipitin reaction.
(a) Precipitation in tubes.
(b) Precipitin curve.
  Both illustrate optimal
proportions (equivalence between
antibody and antigen) and
inhibition of precipitation by
antigen excess.

(b) *Precipitin curve*

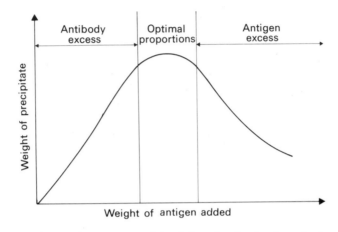

Antibody
excess

Optimal
proportions

Antigen
excess

Weight of precipitate

Weight of antigen added

These observations are explained by the *lattice hypothesis*, shown in Figure 2.35. At optimal proportions, antigen molecules are cross-linked by antibody to form a large, precipitable lattice. Note that precipitation cannot occur with univalent antigens, such as free haptens. When antigen is in excess, antibody combining sites are blocked and cannot cross-link, thus preventing precipitation and causing small soluble complexes of antigen and antibody to be formed instead. Similarly, soluble complexes are also formed in antibody excess, though inhibition of precipitation by excess of antibody is generally harder to demonstrate.

The formation of soluble complexes and inhibition of aggregation in antigen excess is most important in the pathogenesis of several conditions which are classed together as *immune complex diseases* (p. 161). Complexes which form in the circulation are normally removed by the littoral macrophages of spleen and liver. Complexes which fail to be removed in this way, because of their small size or excessive quantity, tend to become deposited in the walls of blood vessels in various sites, particularly in the kidney, joints, heart and skin. Once localised, they initiate the activation of complement, resulting in local inflammation and consequent tissue damage. The main effects which follow are glomerulonephritis, arthritis, myocarditis, valvulitis and diffuse vasculitis. These are present in varying

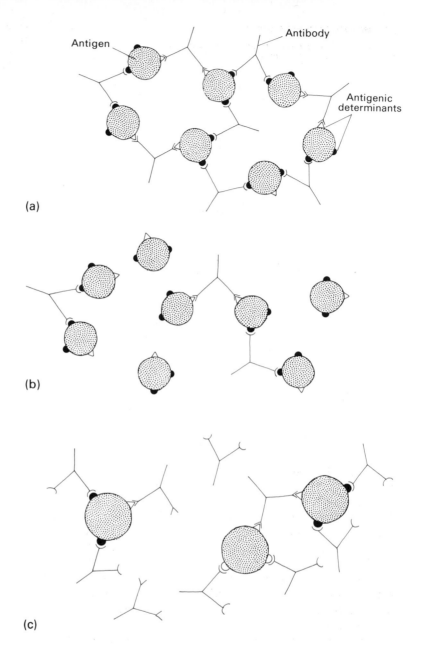

(a)

(b)

(c)

Figure 2.35 Antibody–antigen precipitation: the lattice hypothesis.
(a) Optimal proportions: formation of a lattice.
(b) Antigen excess: soluble complexes.
(c) Large antibody excess: soluble complexes.

degree in serum sickness, rheumatic fever, rheumatoid arthritis, systemic lupus erythematosus and drug hypersensitivities, and may accompany infectious diseases such as malaria, leprosy and streptococcal infection (see p. 161 for details of complex-mediated tissue damage). Methods used to detect soluble complexes in serum are described below.

Various adaptations of the precipitin reaction have been made for diagnostic and analytic tests, the most widely used being those based on precipitation in agar gel. In the basic *Ouchterlony double diffusion* method, antigen and antibody are placed in wells cut a short distance (~1 cm) apart in agar on a glass slide. The reactants diffuse towards each other through the gel and where

127

they meet at optimal proportions a line of precipitate is formed (Figure 2.36). Its final appearance depends on the relative amounts of antigen and antibody in the solutions placed in the wells. When antigen is in excess, the first-formed precipitate gradually redissolves and forms again nearer the antibody well at the diffusing antigen front; as this process is continuous, the precipitate becomes diffuse and moves slowly towards the antibody well (Figure 2.36b). On the other hand, when the reactants are in optimal proportions, the precipitation line is sharp and permanent, both in appearance and position; the same is generally true in antibody excess (Figure 2.36a, c). The position of the line between the two wells depends both on the relative concentrations of the reactants and their relative diffusion co-

Figure 2.36 Precipitation in gel.

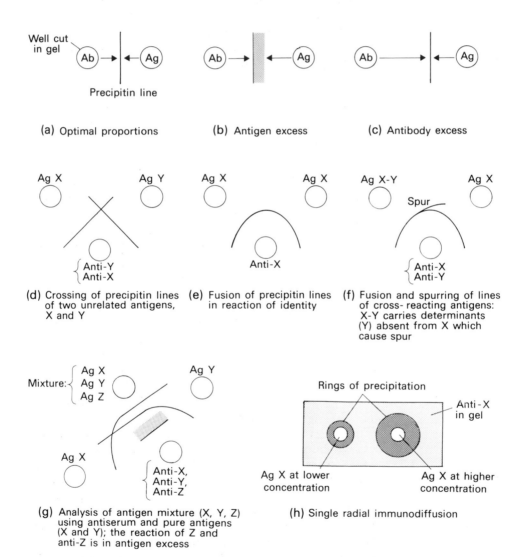

Ab = Antibody
Ag = Antigen

128

efficients, the latter in turn being related to molecular size. Double diffusion in gel can be used to determine optimal proportions and can give an approximate estimate of antibody (or antigen) concentration. It is also a powerful analytical method. For example, it can be used to demonstrate relationships between antigens. Thus, if one antibody well is positioned near to two antigen wells, patterns such as those shown in Figure 2.36d–f are obtained and it is possible to determine whether two antigens are identical, related or independent, according to whether their precipitation lines fuse, spur or cross, respectively. Moreover, a mixture of independent antigens gives rise to multiple lines of precipitation when diffusing towards a well containing the corresponding antibodies (Figure 2.36g). The number of lines indicates the number of independent components in the mixture, each of which may be identified by formation of lines of identity with standards in adjacent wells.

A modification of precipitation in gel, known as *single radial immunodiffusion* is regularly used for accurate quantitative determinations of proteins. In this technique, antibody against the protein is incorporated into the agar gel; holes are cut and test solutions of the protein (antigen) placed in them. After a few hours, rings of precipitate are seen around the wells and gradually grow outwards with a sharp outer edge and diffuse precipitate behind (Figure 2.36h). A ring forms because antigen diffuses into the gel where it precipitates at optimal proportions with the immobilised antibody; with further diffusion from the well, the precipitate dissolves in antigen excess and re-forms further out. The size of the ring at any time is proportional to the antigen concentration in the well. Thus, by placing standard solutions of the protein antigen in some of the wells, the method can be calibrated and used to determine concentrations of the same protein in test solutions. It is routinely used for measurement of immunoglobulin in serum (anti-Ig is then incorporated into the gel), for serum C3 determination (anti-C3 in the gel) and several other proteins to which appropriate antisera are available. The reverse of this method, in which antigen is incorporated into the gel for determination of antibody levels in serum, is less satisfactory as precipitates dissolve with more difficulty in antibody excess.

Another versatile application of precipitation in gel is *immunoelectrophoresis* (Figure 2.37). This enables the identification of proteins in complex mixtures, such as serum, by the separating power of electrophoresis followed by analysis by immune precipitation. The mixture to be investigated is placed in a well in the agar and electrophoresed; in the case of serum proteins, the albumin moves fastest to the anode and immunoglobulins either move towards the cathode (IgG, IgM) or remain around the well (IgA). After electrophoresis, a trough is cut in the gel parallel to the direction of the electrophoretic run and filled with appropriate antiserum. After a few hours, each of the serum proteins is visualised as a discrete precipitation arc and can be identified. Immunoelectrophoresis can be used to detect gross changes in levels of different Ig classes, as in multiple myeloma (p. 89) where myeloma proteins cause arcs of excessively heavy, diffuse pre-

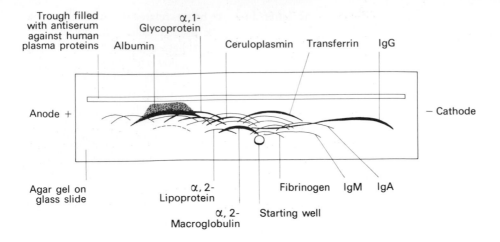

Trough filled with antiserum against human plasma proteins

Albumin

α,1-Glycoprotein

Ceruloplasmin

Transferrin

IgG

Anode +

− Cathode

Agar gel on glass slide

α,2-Lipoprotein

α,2-Macroglobulin

Fibrinogen

IgM

IgA

Starting well

cipitation in one Ig class, or in hypogammaglobulinaemias, where the Ig precipitation arcs are much weaker than normal.

DETECTION OF SOLUBLE COMPLEXES IN SERUM

As noted above, soluble circulating complexes play an important role in some forms of immunological tissue damage. Several methods are employed to detect complexes in serum, though none is completely satisfactory. (Detection of complexes in tissues by immunofluorescent staining is described below.)

Cryoprecipitation

Some complexes are soluble at 37°C but precipitate from sera at 4°C; the proteins in the precipitates which form in the cold are known as *cryoglobulins*. Their isolation provides one of the best opportunities for identifying the antigen and antibody components of the complex, but unfortunately all complexes do not form cryoprecipitates. Among those which do are complexes in which IgG itself is the antigen, the antibody component of the complex being an anti-IgG autoantibody called *rheumatoid factor* which reacts with the Fc region of IgG. Rheumatoid factors can be of either IgM or IgG class and are characteristic of rheumatoid arthritis, but also appear in systemic lupus erythematosus (see p. 190.)

Ultracentrifugation

Complexes can be detected in the analytic ultracentrifuge, though this is a rather insensitive method and does not have wide application.

Polyethylene glycol

Antigen−antibody complexes, but not free immunoglobulin, are precipitated in 2.5% polyethylene glycol. This is of most use in conjunction with the C1q binding test described below.

Figure 2.37 Immuno-electrophoresis of human plasma. A small volume of human plasma was placed in the starting well cut into the agar on a glass slide and electrophoresed. A trough was then cut and filled with antiserum against human plasma proteins. 24 hours later, the complex pattern of precipitin lines appeared, each caused by the reaction of a different plasma protein with its specific antibodies. The identities of some of the human proteins are shown.

Complement (C1q) binding

Soluble complexes containing IgG or IgM will activate the complement system and, as described on p. 94, this reaction begins with binding, to the Fc region of the antibody, of a subcomponent (C1q) of the first complement component (C1). The reaction with C1q can be used in several ways to detect serum complexes. Because C1q is multivalent it will cause precipitation of complexes from solution, or as more commonly performed, in an agarose gel. C1q precipitation is, however, also produced by substances other than complexes, including endotoxins and DNA. A more sensitive and reliable method utilising the same principle is binding of radiolabelled C1q, followed by separation of the complex in polyethylene glycol and counting the radioactivity precipitated.

Raji cell binding

This test utilises the fact that complexes bind to the Fc receptors of certain cells. In the standard procedure, a cell line called Raji is used; Raji cells are human B lymphocytes which grow permanently in culture because they have been transformed by Epstein–Barr virus (p. 792). The cells carry surface Fc receptors. Complexes are detected by their ability to compete with radiolabelled aggregated IgG for binding to the Raji cell Fc receptors.

AGGLUTINATION

Antibody agglutinates (clumps) cells when it reacts with surface antigens, by cross-linking the cells as in lattice formation (Figure 2.38) and agglutination provides a more sensitive method than precipitation for detection of antibodies. Bacterial agglutination is useful in the identification and typing of bacteria as well as in diagnosis. *Haemagglutination*, the agglutination of red blood cells by antibody against antigens on the red cell surface, is especially important in blood transfusion, being the method used in determination of blood groups. The major blood group system of man is the *ABO system*, A and B being antigens on the red cell surface while O is the absence of both A and B (from the German *ohne*, without). Each individual carries 'natural' agglutinating antibodies in the serum directed at the A or B antigens which are absent from his own red cells, these antibodies being called *isohaemagglutinins*. Thus individuals of blood group A have natural serum anti-B antibodies which specifically agglutinate group B red cells; similarly group B individuals have an anti-A, group O individuals have both anti-A and anti-B, while those of group AB have neither. This arises because certain common bacterial polysaccharides, to which all individuals are exposed via gut flora, have A- and B-like structures; self-tolerance restricts the response of each individual to the antigens recognised as foreign or non-self. The existence of antigenic blood groups makes the matching of donor and recipient in transfusions essential, to

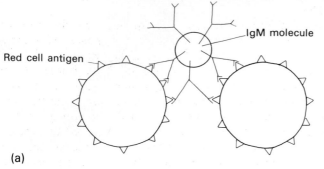

(a)

Figure 2.38 Haemagglutination
by IgM and IgG anti-red cell
antibodies.
(a) IgM: efficient agglutination.
(b) IgG: poor agglutination.
(c) Antiglobulin agglutinates
IgG-coated red cells (Coombs
test).
(d) Inhibition of agglutination by
gross antibody excess (prozone).

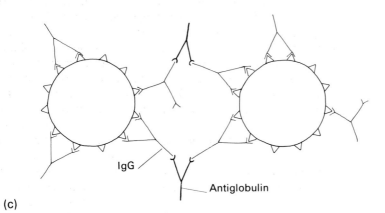

(b)

(c)

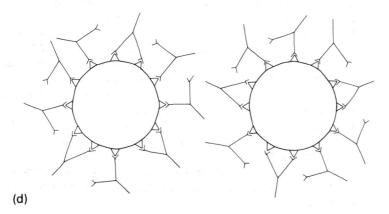

(d)

avoid a reaction against the transfused blood by natural ABO antibodies.

The efficiency of agglutination depends on the class of antibody. While both IgM and IgG will agglutinate bacteria and red cells, less IgM is required because of the ease with which the larger molecule cross-links cells (Figure 2.38). Isohaemagglutinins are IgM. In order to detect IgG which has bound to a cell surface antigen but failed to produce agglutination, the *antiglobulin* or *Coombs test* was introduced. The principle of the test, shown in Figure 2.38c, is to treat the washed IgG-coated cells with a second antibody, namely an anti-human IgG (an antiglobulin prepared by injecting an animal with human IgG). Addition of the antiglobulin now leads to agglutination. The Coombs test is especially important in connection with haemolytic anaemia of the newborn (p. 157), in which a mother who lacks the rhesus (Rh) blood group antigen D (i.e. is 'rhesus negative') reacts against the D antigen on red cells of her Rh-positive foetus. The mother produces anti-Rh (D) antibodies which cross the placenta and cause destruction of foetal red cells. Maternal anti-Rh antibodies which cross the placenta are IgG and do not agglutinate (see p. 159), and the antiglobulin test is used to demonstrate the presence of anti-Rh in maternal serum or on foetal (Rh +) red cells. Similarly, the antiglobulin test is used to detect IgG anti-red cell antibodies in certain forms of autoimmune or drug-induced haemolytic anaemia (p. 196).

Agglutination is used in a variety of other important diagnostic laboratory tests. It is conveniently observed in round-bottom tubes or wells, in which non-agglutinated cells settle as a discrete round 'button' while agglutinated cells spread out over the whole area of the base. In practice, sera being tested are diluted serially and an aliquot of an appropriate cell preparation is added to an equal volume of each dilution. The reciprocal of the highest dilution of serum producing agglutination is called the *titre*. Thus a high titre is equivalent to a high level of antibody in the serum. When antibody is in very large excess it is possible for agglutination to be inhibited because all the antigenic sites on the cell surface become blocked by the excess of antibody and none are available for cross-linking (Figure 2.38d). The failure to agglutinate at high antibody concentrations is called the *prozone*, and it emphasizes the need to titrate the serum under test. Agglutination tests in which the serum reacts against antigens intrinsic to the cell surface are known as *direct* agglutination tests. Alternatively, a soluble antigen can be chemically coupled to the cell or particle; antibody against the coupled antigen then agglutinates the particle, which essentially behaves as an indicator. This is called a *passive* agglutination test. Passive agglutination is inhibited by the presence of free antigen, which combines with the antibody and blocks the reaction. Agglutination inhibition can therefore be used as an assay for soluble antigens.

Some examples of diagnostic agglutination tests are given below. The use of haemagglutination in blood grouping has already been noted.

Rheumatoid arthritis: Rose-Waaler and latex agglutination tests

A characteristic feature of rheumatoid arthritis which we have already noted is the presence in patients' sera of antibodies against IgG (rheumatoid factors). They can be detected by passive agglutination tests in which a red cell or latex particle is first coated with IgG and then exposed to a patient's serum. Agglutination indicates the presence of rheumatoid factor in the serum. In the *Rose-Waaler test*, sheep red cells are treated with rabbit anti-sheep red cell IgG antibody at a dose which is too low to cause agglutination but sufficient to coat the red cells; the latter can then be agglutinated by an anti-IgG antibody. In an alternative test, aggregated human IgG is adsorbed onto latex particles which are then agglutinated by rheumatoid factors. This test is more sensitive, but less specific for rheumatoid arthritis, than the Rose-Waaler test. In these tests, an agglutination titre of 8–16 is considered significantly positive; high titres (512 or over) in the early stages of rheumatoid arthritis are associated with a poor prognosis with respect to mobility of the joints.

Infectious mononucleosis: Paul-Bunnell test

Infectious mononucleosis or glandular fever is a common acute disease characterised by swollen, tender lymph nodes (lymphadenopathy) and spleen (splenomegaly) and the presence of high numbers of lymphoblastoid cells in the blood; it is caused by the Epstein–Barr virus (p. 794). Patients' sera contain a diagnostic IgM antibody called a *heterophile agglutinin*, capable of directly agglutinating sheep red cells. The term 'heterophile' refers to groups of antigens which are shared by the cells of several unrelated animal species and some microorganisms, and which cross-react extensively. Thus, the Paul-Bunnell antibody agglutinates bovine and horse red cells as well as sheep. In the Paul-Bunnell test the titre of this antibody is measured both before and after the serum has been absorbed with bovine red cells or minced guinea-pig kidney. In a positive test, agglutination of sheep red cells by unabsorbed serum occurs, and by serum absorbed with guinea-pig kidney, but not by serum absorbed with bovine red cells. This procedure is necessary to distinguish the agglutinins diagnostic of infectious mononucleosis from red cell agglutinating heterophile antibodies found in conditions such as serum sickness or in normal sera. The latter antibodies react with a different heterophile antigen present on sheep red cells called the *Forssman antigen*, which is shared by guinea-pig kidney cells but not bovine red cells. Hence, by differential absorption the two heterophile antibodies, Paul-Bunnell and anti-Forssman, can be distinguished.

Hashimoto's thyroiditis: tanned red cell haemagglutination test

We have noted above that soluble antigens can be coated onto red cells, which can then be used in passive haemagglutination tests. A common method for coating red cells with proteins is to treat the cells with tannic acid, after which they bind proteins to their surface and are then susceptible to agglutination by antibody against the adsorbed protein. A good example is the test for antibodies against thyroglobulin which occur in the autoimmune thyroiditis called Hashimoto's disease (p. 189). Passive haemagglutination using tanned red cells coated with thyroglobulin provides a sensitive assay for antithyroglobulin antibodies in patients' sera.

Syphilis: Treponema pallidum *haemagglutination (TPHA) test*

This provides a further example of passive haemagglutination using tanned red cells. During the course of syphilis, serum antibodies appear against the causative organism, *Treponema pallidum*; they can be sensitively detected by the agglutination of red cells coated with treponemal antigens. Because of its ease and the possibility of automation, the TPHA test is now widely used in screening for syphilis (see also p. 619).

Serum hepatitis carriers: reverse passive haemagglutination

Hepatitis B virus, the agent of serum hepatitis, is found in large amounts in the blood of carrier individuals with a clinically inapparent (subclinical) infection, as well as sometimes persisting after recovery from the disease. Transfusion of contaminated blood donated by carriers has been an important route of transmission of the virus and it is therefore essential to screen all blood for its presence. This is done by detection of the viral surface antigen which occurs free in the blood (HBsAg, formerly known as Australia antigen), either by radioimmunoassay (p. 140) or reverse passive haemagglutination. In the latter method, antibody to HBsAg is coupled to indicator red cells; such antibody-coated red cells are agglutinated by HBsAg (see Figure 3.53). Detection of HBsAg is an important and routine part of screening of blood before transfusion.

Viral haemagglutination and haemagglutination inhibition

Several viruses possess a surface protein called a *haemagglutinin* which has a binding affinity for a sugar, such as N-acetyl neuraminic acid, found on the membrane of red cells and other body cells; such viruses, of which influenza is an example, agglutinate red cells and this provides a simple method for their assay. Moreover, antiviral antibodies can be demonstrated by their ability to inhibit this reaction—the haemagglutination inhibition or HI test. These procedures are described at greater length on p. 318-9 (Figure 3.38).

Typhoid fever: Widal test

Agglutination of *Salmonella* organisms is used in the diagnosis of typhoid fever (Widal test). The antibody titre rises towards the end of the second week of illness, reaching a peak in the third week. Agglutinins (agglutinating antibodies) react with the somatic O and Vi antigens and with the flagellar H antigens; a rising titre of anti-O agglutinins is significant (other infections can cause a rise in anti-H agglutinins). If the patient has been previously vaccinated with typhoid vaccine (TAB), the Widal test is of less use, since a high agglutinin level is likely before infection. (See also p. 556).

COMPLEMENT-MEDIATED LYSIS

The fixation of complement at the surface of red cells leads to lysis (haemolysis) and is a particularly sensitive indicator of the presence of IgM. It can therefore be used, in the same way as agglutination, to detect antibodies either against red cells themselves or against antigens coupled chemically to the red cell insusceptible to lysis). Lysis, like agglutination, is less sensitive for IgG; some IgG subclasses do not fix complement, while for those which do, fixation requires that two IgG molecules be found close together at the red cell surface, which can only be obtained at relatively high concentrations of antibody in the surrounding solution. Rhesus antibodies either of IgM or IgG classes do not cause lysis even when in high concentration, because the D antigens are too widely separated on the erythrocyte membrane (p. 159).

COMPLEMENT FIXATION TEST

The complement fixation test (CFT) is a highly sensitive and diagnostically important test for serum antibody. The principle of the test is that if an antibody–antigen reaction takes place in the presence of a limited amount of complement, the latter is activated and thereby consumed. An indicator system is then added to detect the presence of remaining complement. The indicator consists of sheep red blood cells coated with anti-sheep red cell IgM antibody at a level insufficient to cause agglutination, but which will cause the red cells to lyse if complement is present. If the complement has been used up by the reaction of antibody and antigen, no lysis of red cells occurs (positive test), and lysis is seen only when the test is negative. A classical diagnostic application of the CFT is the *Wassermann test* for syphilis. The Wassermann antibody is an autoantibody to lipid-containing antigens in the mitochondria of human liver, heart and other tissues; it is produced characteristically in syphilis, but is also found in other chronic diseases such as systemic lupus erythematosus, leprosy, malaria and glandular fever. In the Wassermann test, an extract of pig heart is used as the antigen and tested against the suspected syphilitic serum (see also p. 618).

The advantage of complement fixation in demonstrating antibody (or antigen) is that there is no need to visualise the antigen–antibody complex by precipitation or agglutination. Thus, smaller amounts of antibody can be detected, optimal proportions are not required and there is no inhibition by excess antibody or antigen. As in the case of agglutination and complement-mediated lysis, the usefulness of the CFT depends on the class of the antibody, since not all classes are equally efficient in complement activation (p. 121).

IMMUNOFLUORESCENCE

This is especially useful in detection of antigens, antibodies or complexes in cells or tissues. The method involves the use of antibodies conjugated to fluorochromes, chemicals which fluoresce when excited by short-wavelength, e.g. ultraviolet, light; thus antigen–antibody reactions can be visualised with the aid of the u.v. microscope. The fluorochromes commonly used are fluorescein and rhodamine, which appear green and red respectively in u.v. light. The following are some of the ways in which fluorescent antibodies can be used (Figure 2.39).

Detection of antigens

Antigens in tissues or isolated cells can be detected using specific fluorochrome-conjugated antibodies against the antigen (*direct immunofluorescence*). For tissue slices, a thin section is prepared from frozen tissue with a microtome and dried onto a slide. The fluorescent antibody reagent is applied and after 30 minutes, incubation the excess is washed off and the section viewed under the fluorescence microscope. The distribution of fluorescence within the tissue is that of the specific antigen. Thus, using fluorescent autoantibodies against thyroid antigens (antibodies which appear in Hashimoto's disease), the distribution in thyroid cells of the antigens involved in this autoimmune disorder can be determined. Similarly, cell suspensions can be stained directly with fluorescent antibodies. This can be used on living cells to stain cell surface antigens and on fixed preparations to visualise cytoplasmic antigens. One application is the determination of immunoglobulin classes on B lymphocytes using specific antisera against different Ig classes. Sometimes two reagents conjugated with different fluorochromes are used to investigate the distribution of two antigens simultaneously. Thus, it was shown that many B cells carry both IgM and IgD at their surface, by staining cell suspensions with fluorescein-conjugated anti-IgM (specific for the μ heavy chain) and rhodamine-conjugated anti-IgD (δ-chain specific); the fact that many B lymphocytes showed both green and red fluorescence (distinguished by filters) proved that both antibody classes were present on the same cell.

In the *indirect immunofluorescence test*, the tissue or cell is first reacted with an unconjugated antibody against a specific antigen; visualisation is then achieved by a second antibody, a fluorescent anti-immunoglobulin (antiglobulin, anti-Ig) which reacts with the first antibody fixed in the tissue (Figure 2.39a). (Antiglobulin is raised by injection of an animal with Ig of a different species, e.g. rabbit anti-human Ig; cf. Coombs' test.) The indirect test produces a brighter fluorescence, since for every antibody molecule in the first layer several anti-Ig molecules bind in the

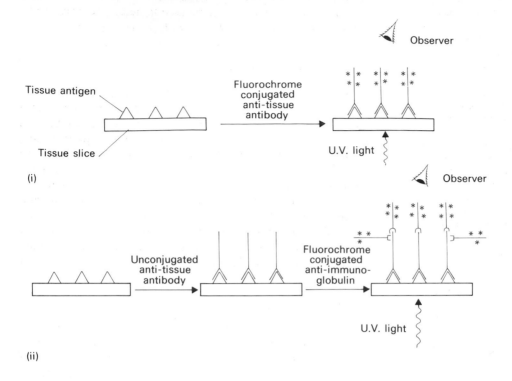

Tissue antigen

Tissue slice

Fluorochrome
conjugated
anti-tissue
antibody

U.V. light

Observer

(i)

Unconjugated
anti-tissue
antibody

Fluorochrome
conjugated
anti-immuno-
globulin

U.V. light

Observer

(ii)

(a)

*indicates fluorescence

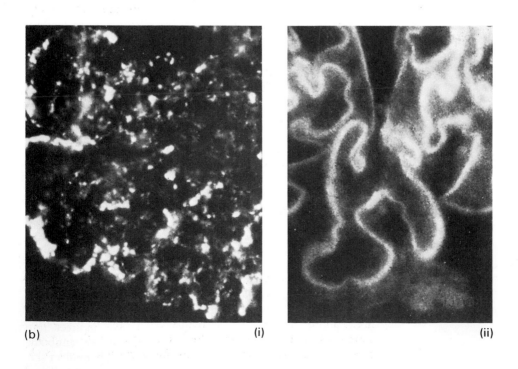

(b)   (i)   (ii)

Figure 2.39 (*opposite*)
(a) Immunofluorescence
techniques.
    (i) Direct immuno-
fluorescence test.
    (ii) Indirect immuno-
fluorescence test.
(b) Immunofluorescent staining
of the kidney glomerulus in
glomerulonephritis (from Michael
et al., 1971).
    (i) 'Lumpy-bumpy' granular
deposition of immune
complexes along the basement
membrane as revealed by
fluorescent anti-
immunoglobulin staining (e.g.
in serum sickness, post-
streptococcal
glomerulonephritis or
systemic lupus
erythematosus).
    (ii) Smooth, linear distribution
of antibody against the
glomerular basement
membrane in Goodpasture's
syndrome, again using
fluorescent anti-
immunoglobulin.

second. It is also more economical and versatile, as a single fluorescent anti-Ig reagent can be used to detect the reaction of a range of unconjugated antibodies with tissues.

Detection of serum autoantibodies

Indirect immunofluorescence is commonly applied in detection of serum autoantibodies against tissue antigens in autoimmune diseases. The serum containing the suspected autoantibody is allowed to react with an appropriate tissue slice; after washing, the fluorescent anti-Ig is applied. If, after further washing, the tissue fluoresces under the u.v. microscope, antibodies against a tissue antigen must have been present in the test serum. The strength of the autoantibody can be measured by titration and determination of the highest dilution at which a reaction is detectable. Circulating autoantibodies against thyroid, stomach, muscle, adrenal, salivary duct and other tissue autoantigens are conveniently measured in this way.

Detection of immune complexes

The immunofluorescence test is also very valuable in detection of immune complexes in tissues, such as the joints and kidneys, in various diseases. As described elsewhere (p. 160) deposition of soluble complexes in and around blood vessels is an important cause of tissue damage. Glomerulonephritis provides a good example: soluble complexes deposited in the basement membrane in post-streptococcal glomerulonephritis, serum sickness, systemic lupus erythematosus or drug hypersensitivities, lead to renal damage, through complement-initiated inflammation and/or neutrophil invasion. Such complexes can be visualised in the glomerular membrane by fluorescent anti-immunoglobulin; complement can likewise be demonstrated with fluorescent anti-C3. Much less often, glomerulonephritis results from autoantibodies reacting directly with the basement membrane (e.g. Goodpasture's syndrome, p. 203), and these can be revealed in the same way. However, the pattern of immunofluorescence observed microscopically is different in the two cases. In immune complex glomerulonephritis, a granular deposit (of complex) is seen along the glomerular capillary wall, sometimes called a 'lumpy-bumpy' distribution; in contrast, anti-glomerular basement membrane antibodies are distributed evenly and continuously along the basement membrane (Figure 2.39b).

Diagnosis in infectious disease

We may also note the diagnostic use of immunofluorescence in infectious disease, where it serves to detect antibodies in patients' sera against microorganisms and parasites. The organisms are immobilised on a slide and the serum suspected to contain antibody to them is applied. Fluorescent anti-Ig is then used to detect human antibodies bound to the organisms. This is the basis of a widely used test for syphilis (fluorescent treponemal antibody or FTA test, p. 618) and similar tests for infection with *Candida albicans*, *Toxoplasma gondii*, *Entamoeba histolytica* and schistosomes.

RADIOIMMUNOASSAY

Among the most sensitive methods for measuring the concentration of antigens and antibodies is to label one of the reactants with a radioisotope such as ^{125}I, ^{3}H or ^{14}C. There are many permutations of radioimmunoassay and they are widely used in sensitive measurement of antigens, such as hormones, drugs, vitamins, etc., and of antibodies of all classes. Such assays are so sensitive that amounts as low as a few nanograms (10^{-9} g) may be detectable. A simple form of the method is the solid phase *primary binding radioimmunoassay*, in which the antigen is insolubilised by covalent attachment to agarose or polyacrylamide beads or non-covalent sticking to the wells of plastic titration plates. The antibody being assayed is then incubated with the immobilised antigen and, after extensive washing, bound antibody is detected with radiolabelled anti-immunoglobulin followed by counting of bound radioactivity (Figure 2.40a). An example of the use of this method is the sensitive determination of IgE levels in sera of individuals with immediate hypersensitivity (the radioallergosorbent test or RAST); specific ^{125}I-labelled anti-IgE is used in the final detection stage. Another application is in the detection of monoclonal antibodies produced by hybridoma cells (p. 97). With slight modification, a primary binding radioimmunoassay can be used to detect and assay antigen. In this case, unlabelled antibody against the antigen is immobilised and used to bind the antigen from serum or other fluid; the bound antigen is then detected by addition of radiolabelled specific antibody (Figure 2.40b). An application of this principle is in screening for hepatitis B viral antigen (HBsAg) in donated blood (Figure 3.53).

Another form of radioimmunoassay measures the concentration of unlabelled antigen by competition with a fixed amount of radiolabelled antigen for binding to a small amount of antibody, the *competitive binding radioimmunoassay*. Assays of this type are widely used and have been developed for almost every type of biological molecule. They vary in the technical details of separation of the antigen bound to antibody from antigen free in solution. Thus, in the solid-phase methods, the antibody is coupled to an insoluble support as already described; labelled and unlabelled (test) antigen are then added and, after incubation and washing, bound radioactivity is counted. The more unlabelled antigen is present, the less radiolabelled antigen will be bound; hence the system is first calibrated and a standard curve constructed with known amounts of unlabelled antigen. In an alternative method, the reaction between antigen and antibody takes place in solution, followed by precipitation of the antibody and bound antigen under conditions in which free (unbound) antigen remains soluble (Farr-type assay).

Figure 2.40 (*opposite*) Radioimmunoassay methods. (a) and (b) are solid phase primary binding radioimmunoassays to estimate antibody and antigen respectively. (c) is a competitive binding solid phase radioimmunoassay to estimate antigen.

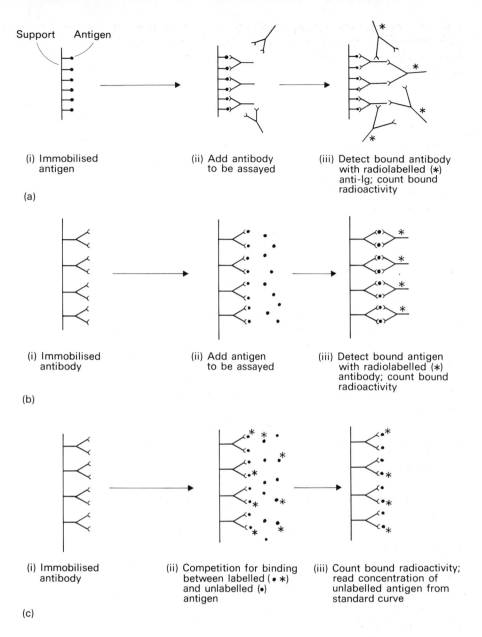

(a)

(i) Immobilised antigen

(ii) Add antibody to be assayed

(iii) Detect bound antibody with radiolabelled (∗) anti-Ig; count bound radioactivity

(b)

(i) Immobilised antibody

(ii) Add antigen to be assayed

(iii) Detect bound antigen with radiolabelled (∗) antibody; count bound radioactivity

(c)

(i) Immobilised antibody

(ii) Competition for binding between labelled (● ∗) and unlabelled (●) antigen

(iii) Count bound radioactivity; read concentration of unlabelled antigen from standard curve

IMMUNOLOGICAL DEFENCE IN INFECTIOUS DISEASE

From the observations on patients with immunodeficiency states already described (p. 78) it is possible to group infections into those for which an antibody mechanism is important in recovery and those for which, in contrast, cell-mediated immunity plays the major defence role. Deficiencies in antibody production lead to inability to deal with the encapsulated, extracellular, pyogenic bacteria, whereas T cell deficiencies are associated with progressive infection with intracellular bacteria, viruses and fungi. In discussing immune mechanisms in infectious disease, we must not overlook the fact that in the crucial early stages of an

141

infection, the most immediate protection is provided by the nonspecific 'natural' defence processes of inflammation and phagocytosis (Section 1); immune responses take several days to develop, unless a state of acquired immunity exists due to previous contact with the same agent or similar antigens. Furthermore, both the specific humoral and cell-mediated immune mechanisms very frequently act in collaboration with the nonspecific inflammatory phagocytic cells, namely neutrophil polymorphs and macrophages. Thus, antibody frequently acts as an opsonin, promoting the phagocytosis of extracellular parasites by neutrophils which then destroy them, while T cells enhance the digestive ability of macrophages, bringing them to the state of activation necessary to kill persistent intracellular organisms. In other cases, antibody or T cells neutralise or kill their target directly without the intervention of phagocytes, as in antibody neutralisation of toxins and viruses, and T-cell killing of virus-infected cells. The following are some examples of antibody and T cell mechanisms in disease.

Antibody-mediated defence (Figure 2.41)

NEUTRALISATION OF TOXINS

In certain bacterial infections, production of a toxin is the major factor in pathogenesis, as in diphtheria (*Corynebacterium diphtheriae*), tetanus (*Clostridium tetani*) and cholera (*Vibrio cholerae*). In such situations, where the symptoms and ultimately death are caused by a single powerful toxin, host defence is dependent on direct neutralisation of the toxin by antitoxin antibodies. Once the toxin has been neutralised, the organism can generally be dealt with relatively easily. Protective immunity in some of these diseases can be established by vaccination with a formalin-inactivated toxin, the *toxoid*, which retains the antigenicity of the toxin without its harmful effects (e.g. diphtheria and tetanus toxoids). In streptococcal and staphylococcal infections, toxins are frequently produced but are generally not the major pathogenic factors; the role of antitoxin is thus less significant.

NEUTRALISATION OF VIRUSES

Antibody neutralises viruses by combining with them in such a way as to prevent their entry into host cells. In general, this is of only minor significance in recovery from primary virus infections, since viruses are obligate intracellular parasites and in a first infection will be inaccessible to antibody by the time the latter is produced. In principle, after release from the cells in which they multiply, viruses can be neutralised by antibody in the blood or extracellular fluid; however, the major part in recovery from viral diseases is often played by CMI (below). On the other hand, antibody can be very significant in preventing reinfection in the immunised individual. In some cases, prophylactic vaccination can be designed to provide neutralising antibody at the site of entry of a virus into the body to provide maximal protection,

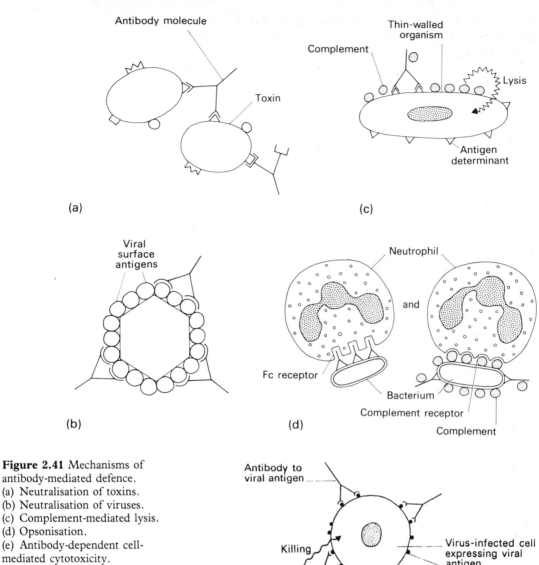

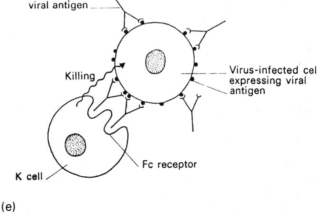

Figure 2.41 Mechanisms of antibody-mediated defence.
(a) Neutralisation of toxins.
(b) Neutralisation of viruses.
(c) Complement-mediated lysis.
(d) Opsonisation.
(e) Antibody-dependent cell-mediated cytotoxicity.

e.g. in the upper respiratory tract for influenza virus and in the intestinal tract for poliovirus. IgA, locally produced and present in secretions of the respiratory and intestinal tract, is the main antibody class involved in these cases and is stimulated by administration of an attenuated strain by the appropriate route. In comparison with bacterial immunity, antiviral immunity is frequently very long lasting, perhaps due to the persistence of a small amount of virus in the body.

143

When antibody reacts with a cell surface and fixes complement, the cell may be killed as a result of the damaging effect of the terminal components of complement, C8 and C9, on the cell membrane. Gram-negative bacteria are often susceptible to the action of antibody and complement; the latter damages the outer membrane of the cell envelope and lysozyme can complete the organism's destruction by acting on the peptidoglycan wall. In contrast, Gram-positive bacteria are not usually killed by complement.

Protozoa, including trypanosomes and plasmodia, are particularly sensitive to lysis by antibody and complement. However, some parasites have evolved means of escaping from the effects of antibodies; a particularly striking mechanism is the *antigenic variation* exhibited by African trypanosomes, which cause sleeping sickness in man as well as a huge loss of cattle (*Trypanosoma brucei gambiense* and *T. brucei rhodesiense*). Trypanosomiasis begins with the introduction of the organisms into the body via the bite of a tsetse fly; thereafter, the number of parasites in the patient's bloodstream shows a regular fluctuation, with periodic waves of parasitaemia (parasites in the blood) over several weeks (Figure 2.42). Each episode of parasitaemia is followed by production of antitrypanosomal antibodies which clear most of the organisms from the blood by lysis or opsonisation; however, a few organisms escape destruction by changing their surface antigens and after a few days these variants establish the next wave of parasitaemia. Many such cycles occur in a single patient, each round of antibody production serving to select variants with new surface antigens.

The mechanism of antigenic variation has been studied in detail. The plasma membrane of the trypanosome is surrounded by an outer coat composed of a single glycoprotein, which is the variant-specific antigen and which evidently serves as a barrier preventing antibodies to the invariant membrane proteins from binding to the parasite. The trypanosomes have the remarkable potential to make many different types of coat glycoprotein and express them in an ordered sequence. Thus, the antigenic form of the trypanosome which is injected by the tsetse

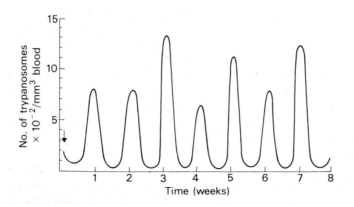

Figure 2.42 Typical waves of parasitaemia in a patient with African trypanosomiasis.

fly vector is always the same one (type A); as antibodies to the type A glycoprotein are made, variant organisms with a completely different coat glycoprotein, type B, are selected and will be followed in successive waves by types C, D, and so on, in a predictable order. In short, the variants are not mutants, but are the result of expression of alternative genes for the surface glycoprotein; evidently many such genes exist and can be 'switched on' in a regular sequence. The variants are only seen in the presence of antibody because of the survival advantage of organisms expressing the next gene in the sequence. Whatever variant the tsetse fly happens to take up from the bloodstream, the trypanosomes are always type A on completing their vector cycle. It is not known how many surface glycoprotein types the trypanosomes can potentially make, but it is at least 20. Antigenic variation has also been described in the malarial parasite, *Plasmodium*.

OPSONISATION BY ANTIBODY AND COMPLEMENT

The opsonisation of pyogenic, extracellular bacteria by antibody directed against the capsule or wall, together with complement, has been described in Section 1. Note that bacteria sometimes counter this mechanism by releasing soluble antigenic capsular material, such as the capsular polysaccharide of pneumococci, which will block the antibody before it reacts with the organism. Once the organisms have been successfully coated, receptors on neutrophils and macrophages for fixed complement (C3) and Fc (of IgG) assist binding to the phagocyte before engulfment (*opsonic adherence*). The great importance of opsonisation in defence is underlined by the frequency of infection with pyogenic organisms in agammaglobulinaemia (p. 79).

ANTIBODY-DEPENDENT CELL-MEDIATED CYTOTOXICITY (ADCC) AND SIMILAR MECHANISMS

In addition to complement-mediated lysis and opsonisation, there is a third way in which cells to which antibody has bound may be killed. This is antibody-dependent cell-mediated cytotoxicity (ADCC) and is mediated in some cases by lymphocytes of uncertain descent called K (killer) cells (Figure 2.41e). K cells carry *Fc receptors* by means of which they bind to IgG antibodies; once brought into contact with a target in this way, a K cell kills nonspecifically. Note that K cells do not recognise antigen—they are distinct from the antigen-specific cytotoxic T cells, nor are they B cells since they lack surface Ig. ADCC may be a means of killing some virus-infected cells: viral antigens are expressed on the surface of the infected cell, which thus becomes a target for IgG and K cells.

Other cells bearing Fc receptors, such as neutrophils, eosinophils and macrophages, may take part in similar cytotoxic reactions. Particularly interesting is the role of *eosinophils* in

145

killing schistosomes, the trematode worms which cause the tropical disease *schistosomiasis* (bilharzia). The principal target of immunity is the invasive larval stage of the parasite, the schisto- somulum, while adult worms are relatively unaffected. One means by which schistosomula are killed is an ADCC-like reaction in which IgG antibodies adhere to the larval surface, followed by binding of eosinophils via membrane Fc receptors. The eosinophils then degranulate, releasing the toxic contents of their granules, such as the major basic protein and eosinophil cationic protein, onto the surface tegument of the organism.

Adult schistosomes have an interesting method of avoiding the antibody response, namely by acquiring a coating of host cell material which masks their antigens and protects them from recognition by host lymphocytes and antibodies. Some of the host molecules appropriated by the worms are those of red cells; they can also acquire MHC molecules, apparently after fusing their outer membranes with those of host neutrophils. Thus, adult schistosomes are evidently 'hidden' by host cell molecules and effectively mistaken for 'self'. In addition, they may cease to produce the antigens recognised by circulating antibodies.

IgE AND HELMINTH INFECTIONS

IgE production is a regular feature of helminth infections. Indeed, infection with *Ascaris lumbricoides* in children is associated with anaphylactic symptoms, such as attacks of urticaria and asthma (p. 153). However, IgE also plays a role in defence against helminths, such as schistosomes; indeed massive production of IgE is a prominent feature of schistosomiasis, as is eosinophilia. We have noted above that IgG-dependent killing of schistosomes is mediated by eosinophils. IgE appears to facilitate eosinophil-mediated killing in several ways. (a) Mast cells take up IgE passively onto their surface at Fc receptors; subsequent contact with the antigen leads to degranulation and release of histamine, with a resulting increase in local vascular permeability (p. 153). It is generally believed that this contributes to immunity simply by increasing the influx of antibody to the area around the parasite. In addition, however, mast cells release two tetrapep- tides which are specifically attractive to eosinophils and comprise the *eosinophil chemotactic factor of anaphylaxis* (ECF-A); thus, IgE ensures that both antibody and eosinophils accumulate at sites of infection. Apparently, ECF-A tetrapeptides not only attract eosinophils but also play an essential role in the killing process by local enhancement of eosinophil killer activity. (b) IgE also appears to participate directly in an ADCC-like reaction against schistosomes very similar to that described above for IgG. Thus, some eosinophils possess Fc receptors for IgE and can therefore bind to IgE-coated schistosomula to carry out a killing reaction as already described.

IgE is also important in defence against intestinal parasites, local histamine release leading to expulsion of worms from the gut.

Cell-mediated immunity, CMI (Figure 2.43)

INTRACELLULAR BACTERIA

One major pattern of protective cell-mediated immunity involves collaboration between specifically sensitised T cells and non-specific inflammatory cells, generally macrophages. This is well exemplified in infection with organisms which can survive intracellularly (Figure 2.43a), such as mycobacteria. The latter are readily phagocytosed but are very resistant to the enzymes of the normal macrophage. As a result they grow and multiply inside the phagocytic cells, and the problem is one of improving the bactericidal activity of macrophages sufficiently for them to kill and destroy the ingested bacteria. Macrophage activation is accomplished by mediators (*lymphokines*) produced by sensitised T cells, as follows. During the course of the infection, specific antigen-sensitive T cells recognise the bacterial antigens in the tissues and lymph nodes draining the site of infection, and undergo proliferation in the thymus-dependent areas of the lymph nodes and spleen. They emerge as effector T cells which, on making contact again with the organism in the tissue, release lymphokines, the molecular mediators of cell-mediated immunity. These cause a local inflammation and the influx of inflammatory cells. In particular, lymphokines such as CF (chemotactic factor), macrophage MIF (migration inhibition factor) and MAF (macrophage activating factor) cause the accumulation and activation of macrophages, with increase in their lysosomal enzyme activity. Note that while the T cells producing the lymphokines are specific for the organism stimulating them, the activated macrophages are nonspecific effector cells, which acquire enhanced microbicidal activity against many organisms.

Activated macrophages are important in disposing of organisms such as *Brucella abortus, Salmonella typhi, Mycobacterium tuberculosis, M. leprae* and *Listeria monocytogenes*. However, even activated macrophages may not be potent enough to deal with exceptionally hardy parasites such as mycobacteria, which even when they are killed can resist complete destruction. When this happens, the organism or its cell wall tends to persist as a source of antigenic stimulation, the influx of phagocytic cells continues and *granuloma* formation results (p. 59). Damage to the host tissue is caused by the continuation of this process and, since this damage is largely the result of the body's own cell-mediated immune response, a state of *hypersensitivity* is said to exist. At the same time, a delayed inflammatory response can be elicited in the skin by injecting the bacterium or its soluble products, such as tuberculin in the case of *M. tuberculosis*. The *delayed hypersensitivity* skin test is a reflection of the process taking place in foci of infection in the tissues. In a non-infected individual, a positive delayed reaction in the skin indicates the presence of cell-mediated immunity as a result of previous infection or immunisation (e.g. Mantoux, lepromin tests, etc; see p. 594). Thus the characteristics of bacterial infection involving cell-mediated immunity are chronicity, because of the persistence of the

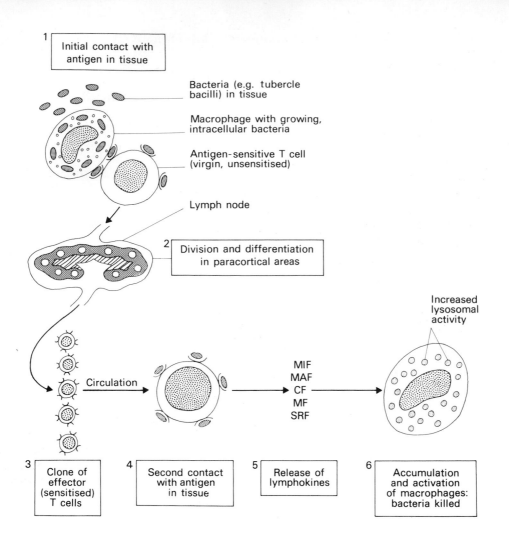

1 | Initial contact with antigen in tissue

Bacteria (e.g. tubercle bacilli) in tissue

Macrophage with growing, intracellular bacteria

Antigen-sensitive T cell (virgin, unsensitised)

Lymph node

2 | Division and differentiation in paracortical areas

Increased lysosomal activity

Circulation

MIF
MAF
CF
MF
SRF

3 | Clone of effector (sensitised) T cells

4 | Second contact with antigen in tissue

5 | Release of lymphokines

6 | Accumulation and activation of macrophages: bacteria killed

organism or its breakdown products, granuloma formation and delayed hypersensitivity. Examples of bacterial diseases in which cell-mediated immunity is involved are tuberculosis, leprosy, brucellosis, syphilis and typhoid.

In some cases, diseases involving cell-mediated immune processes present a 'spectrum' or range of clinical symptoms depending on the degree of T cell response which, as we have seen, determines both the extent of hypersensitivity and killing of the organism. This is particularly well illustrated by leprosy, where two extreme or 'polar' forms exist in different individuals. In the *tuberculoid* form of leprosy, a vigorous CMI response causes the destruction of most of the organisms (*M. leprae*) by activated macrophages and the disease results entirely from hypersensitivity to persistent bacterial products. A positive lepromin test is elicited (a delayed skin reaction to intradermal injection of lepromin, an autoclaved preparation containing leprosy bacilli). At the other extreme, some individuals have an inherited inability to produce a T cell response to *M. leprae*, which multiplies extensively inside the non-activated macrophages and produces the

Figure 2.43 *and on facing page.*
(a) Stages in the development of cell-mediated immunity to intracellular bacteria.
MIF: Macrophage migration inhibition factor
MAF: Macrophage activating factor
CF: Chemotactic factor
MF: Mitogenic factor
SRF: Skin-reactive factor
(b) Stages in the development of cell-mediated immunity against virus-infected cells.

148

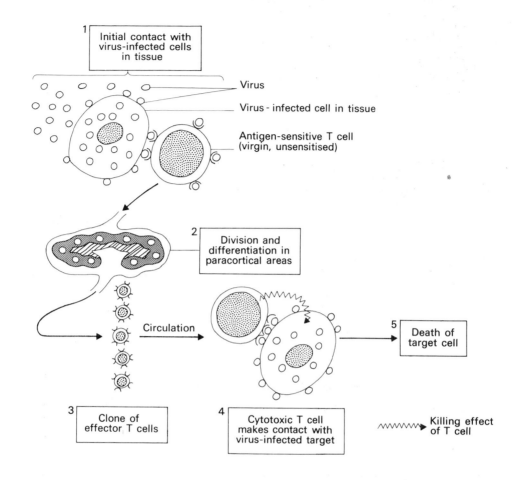

Within the figure:

1 | Initial contact with virus-infected cells in tissue

— Virus

— Virus-infected cell in tissue

Antigen-sensitive T cell (virgin, unsensitised)

2 | Division and differentiation in paracortical areas

Circulation

5 | Death of target cell

3 | Clone of effector T cells

4 | Cytotoxic T cell makes contact with virus-infected target

MMMMM→ Killing effect of T cell

lepromatous form of the disease. In this polar form, neither cell-mediated immunity nor hypersensitivity to *M. leprae* exist and the lepromin test is negative. A large amount of antibody is produced, but is without protective value since the organisms are intracellular. Between these extremes of hypersensitivity and deficiency in response, a wide spectrum of possible situations exists, reflected in the clinical heterogeneity of leprosy patients (see also p. 601).

VIRAL INFECTIONS

In general, recovery from viral disease is dependent on cell-mediated immunity to the virus (Figure 2.43b). As already mentioned, antibody is usually of relatively little importance in a primary virus infection and is principally involved in prevention of reinfection. The importance of CMI is again illustrated by immunodeficiency disease. Children with congenital agammaglobulinaemia recover normally from most viral infections without producing antibody at all; moreover these children have normal, substantial immunity to reinfection, suggesting that antibody is not essential here either. On the other hand, where a T cell deficiency exists (Di George syndrome, dual system immunodeficiency) the children are very susceptible to virus infection. Diseases which normally follow a relatively mild course, such as measles, chickenpox, herpes simplex and vaccinia, may become overwhelming and fatal.

There are several possible ways in which specific T cells can lead to the destruction of intracellular virus, though it is not always clear which mechanisms are most significant. Sensitised T cells cause the accumulation of macrophages at a focus of infection by releasing lymphokines and the macrophages may then phagocytose free virus or kill virus-infected cells. T cells also release the antiviral protein *interferon* which inhibits viral replication (see p. 246). However, probably most important is the fact that T cells themselves engage virus-infected cells and kill them by direct *cytotoxic action* (Figure 2.43b). The recognition of an infected cell is only possible if an alteration of its surface occurs as a result of infection. Virus particles or viral proteins are frequently found on the surface of infected cells, so that the latter can be picked out by circulating sensitised T cells. It has recently been found that in addition to the viral antigens themselves, *histocompatibility (MHC) molecules* at the surface of infected cells are involved in the recognition of the infected target by the T cell. This role of the major histocompatibility complex is discussed at greater length on p. 177. Having discovered an antigenic infected cell, the specific cytotoxic T cell can kill it by a mechanism involving direct membrane contact. The details of how killing is achieved are not yet clear, but surface-bound complement components may play a part. Killing of infected cells before viral replication has been completed will eventually eliminate the infection.

Although cell-mediated immunity is frequently essential for recovery from viral diseases, it may also cause some of the symptoms, notably where cell-mediated hypersensitivity is involved. *Measles* provides a good illustration of the ramifications of immunological processes in viral infection. After one attack there is complete, life-long immunity to further infection, due to the proliferation of T cells capable of killing measles-infected cells and the high levels of IgG anti-measles antibodies, which may persist in the blood for many years. Children with agammaglobulinaemia show a normal measles course with a typical rash and normal immunity afterwards, so it appears that antibody is not essential either for recovery or for protective immunity. The opposite situation is seen when the cell-mediated response is absent, for example in children with primary thymus deficiency such as the Di George or Nézelof syndromes. Measles is an extremely dangerous disease for these patients and follows an unusual course. There is no rash and the children die of a 'giant-cell pneumonia' in which the lung is packed with multinucleate giant cells (cell fusion being a characteristic effect of the measles virus). Normal recovery is impossible, because in the absence of CMI the virus cannot be eliminated. Moreover, the absence of the typical rash indicates that this too is normally caused by the cell-mediated response to the virus and is an inflammatory response, akin to a delayed hypersensitivity reaction, to virus in the skin. In normal patients at the same time as the skin rash, *encephalitis* (inflammation of the brain) of variable degree may occur and this is probably a result of a cell-mediated hypersensitivity response against virus in the brain. Although rather rare (1/1000–2000 cases), encephalitis is a much feared complication with a mortality of about 15%; it may lead to permanent brain damage and is a major reason for the recommended universal vaccination against measles. Protective immunisation is now carried out with a live, attenuated measles virus vaccine. Another later and rarer sequel to measles involving the nervous system is *subacute sclerosing panencephalitis* (SSPE), which can prove fatal even years after the original measles attack. In SSPE it appears that the measles virus continues spreading slowly from cell to cell through the brain and that for some reason cell-mediated immunity is unable to deal with it, perhaps due to the development of T cell unresponsiveness to the virus. The brain is infiltrated with plasma cells and there is anti-measles antibody in the CSF, but this is useless against the virus in the brain cells (see p. 342).

Other viral infections for which CMI is known to be required in recovery include smallpox, chickenpox, herpes simplex and yellow fever. Viruses such as cytomegalovirus, herpes simplex and varicella-zoster are prominent as opportunistic infections which occur when CMI is depressed (below and p. 265).

FUNGAL INFECTIONS

A cell-mediated response is required for immunity against fungi, while anti-fungal antibodies are without protective effect. Fungi are prominent *opportunistic* pathogens, a term describing organisms such as endogenous microflora, which in normal circumstances do not cause clinical disease, unless a disturbance of the host defence mechanism allows them to invade (see also p. 478). Opportunistic infections are of considerable importance today because of the widespread use of therapeutic agents with immunosuppressive or anti-inflammatory properties, such as antimetabolites, corticosteroids and X-irradiation. Depression of the cell-mediated immune response permits the spread and growth of fungi commonly present in the environment, such as *Aspergillus*, *Candida* and *Mucor* species, as well as the viruses mentioned above. Thus, *chronic mucocutaneous candidiasis*, a generalised infection of the skin and mucous membranes with *Candida albicans*, occurs in patients undergoing treatment with immunosuppressive drugs and in infants with deficient thymus function (thymus dysgenesis). Remarkable clinical improvement in candidiasis has been achieved by immunotherapy designed to correct the CMI defect, including administration of normal lymphocytes or transfer factor (p. 164).

HYPERSENSITIVITY (ALLERGY)

Hypersensitivity refers to those immunological reactions which, rather than contributing to recovery, themselves produce tissue damage and form an important and sometimes the major part of the disease process. The terms 'hypersensitivity' and 'allergy' are often used synonymously, though the former is the term of preference and will be used here. Just as protective immunity can be divided into antibody-mediated and cell-mediated responses, so hypersensitivity (allergic) reactions may be classified into those caused by antibodies of different classes and those reactions mediated solely by lymphocytes. Coombs and Gell proposed a classification into four types of reaction, illustrated in Figure 2.44. *Type I* is the immediate or *anaphylactic* reaction, mediated by an antibody class with the special property of tissue-sensitisation (IgE in man) and in which histamine and other mast cell products trigger an acute inflammatory response and constriction of smooth muscle. *Type II* is a *cytotoxic* reaction, in which cells are killed by the direct action of antibody against a cell surface antigen or towards a hapten, such as a drug, attached to the cell surface; complement may be involved in cell destruction. In the *Type III* reaction, soluble antigen–antibody complexes become localised in the walls of blood vessels where a damaging inflammatory response is initiated, usually via complement activation. This underlies *immune complex* disease, with effects on the kidney, joints, heart and skin. Finally, *Type IV* is the cell-mediated *delayed hypersensitivity*, which plays a major role in chronic infectious diseases such as tuberculosis and leprosy, in contact sensitivity and in graft rejection.

TYPE I (ANAPHYLACTIC REACTIONS)

The term *anaphylaxis* was introduced by Charles Richet in 1902 to describe the severe and sometimes fatal reactions of animals to a second injection of a foreign protein, which in Richet's original observation was the reaction of dogs to a second injection of sea anemone toxin. Anaphylaxis was defined as the opposite of prophylaxis—the first injection caused the animal to become hypersensitive rather than producing protective immunity. The reaction may be local or general. *General anaphylactic shock* is readily demonstrated in the guinea-pig, an animal particularly sensitive to anaphylaxis. A guinea-pig injected with an antigenic protein such as egg albumin for the first time experiences no ill effect, but if reinjected intravenously 10–14 days later with even very small amounts of the same protein, will quite likely die within a few seconds from asphyxia caused by intense constriction of the bronchioles. Other symptoms are those of intense generalised shock. Fortunately, anaphylactic shock on this scale is rare in man, but does sometimes occur if an antigenic drug such as penicillin enters the circulation of a hypersensitive individual, or following an insect sting, or during desensitisation with pollen extracts (below). *Local* Type I reactions on the other hand, are very common, and include hypersensitives to pollen, house dust, animal dander and food, which are familiar as hay fever, allergic asthma and urticaria (local weal-and-flare reactions in the skin). Local anaphylaxis is caused by an antigen–antibody reaction in the tissue at the surface of *mast cells*, followed by their release of histamine and other mediators such as leukotrienes, with pharmacological effects on smooth muscle (contraction) and blood vessels (increased permeability); general anaphylaxis is initiated by the release of these mediators into the circulation from *basophils*.

The basis of the anaphylactic response in man is as follows. In certain individuals, contact with the antigen (pollen, etc., also termed the 'allergen') stimulates the production of an antibody of the IgE class, which has the ability to adhere to mast cells in tissues and basophils in the circulation. The antibody is termed *homocytotropic*, since it can only sensitise cells of the species in which it is produced; it is also termed *reagin*. IgE fixes to the mast cell or basophil by the binding of its Fc portion to membrane Fc receptors; this leaves its antigen-combining sites free to combine with antigen (Figure 2.44). When an individual sensitised in this way makes contact with the same antigen on a later occasion, the antigen combines with IgE at the surface of local mast cells and this reaction triggers the cell into immediate degranulation (secretion of granule contents).

The mechanism of IgE-mediated degranulation has been studied experimentally using rat mast cells. Binding of antigen to IgE at the mast cell surface causes *cross-linking* of Fc receptors, which triggers a complex cascade of biochemical events. An important change in the membrane is an increase in permeability to Ca^{2+} ions; the influx of calcium (or mobilisation of intracellular calcium) is essential for degranulation. The precise role of calcium is unknown, but it operates intracellularly via the calcium-binding protein *calmodulin* to activate a number of enzymes, including adenylate and guanylate cyclases. A transient rise in cyclic AMP is necessary for degranulation, though a larger rise is inhibitory. The granule contents are then secreted, releasing stored mediator substances, including *histamine*, the vasoactive amine *serotonin* (5-hydroxytryptamine, 5-HT) in species other than man, *platelet activating factor* (PAF) and *eosinophil chemotactic factor of anaphylaxis* (ECF-A), which attracts eosinophils to the scene. Membrane changes also activate phospholipase A_2 and lead to production of another important mediator, *slow reacting substance of anaphylaxis* (SRS-A), a potent bronchoconstrictor and inflammatory agent (below).

Since IgE sensitises mast cells in all tissues, the results which follow depend on the mode of entry of the antigen into the body. At the mucosal surfaces of the eye, nose and respiratory tract there is respectively conjunctivitis, rhinorrhoea, swelling of the tongue, laryngeal oedema and asthma. In the gastrointestinal tract

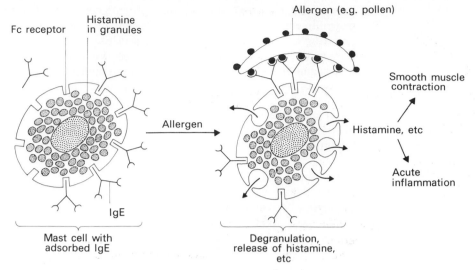

Fc receptor
Histamine in granules
Allergen (e.g. pollen)
Allergen
IgE
Smooth muscle contraction
Histamine, etc
Acute inflammation
Mast cell with adsorbed IgE
Degranulation, release of histamine, etc

Type I (anaphylactic)

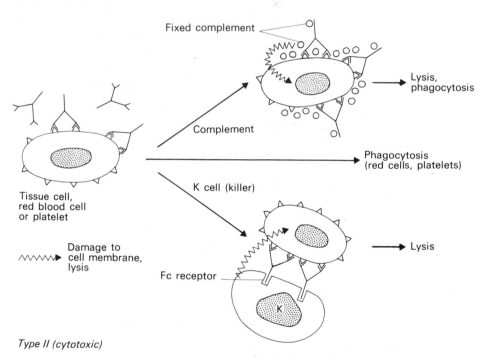

Fixed complement
Complement
Lysis, phagocytosis
Phagocytosis (red cells, platelets)
K cell (killer)
Tissue cell, red blood cell or platelet
Damage to cell membrane, lysis
Fc receptor
Lysis
K

Type II (cytotoxic)

the reaction is one of vomiting and diarrhoea, while in the skin it takes the form of urticaria. A sensitised individual will also give an immediate (i.e. peaking within 15–20 minutes) weal-and-flare reaction if the antigen is pricked into the skin, and the skin test finds important diagnostic use in ascertaining precisely the antigen involved and the state of sensitisation.

While histamine has for many years been the most familiar mediator molecule in immediate hypersensitivity in man, it is now thought that the molecules which comprise slow reacting substance (SRS) may be equally important, especially in the lung.

Figure 2.44. Hypersensitivity reactions.
(Abbreviations as in Fig. 2.43a)

154

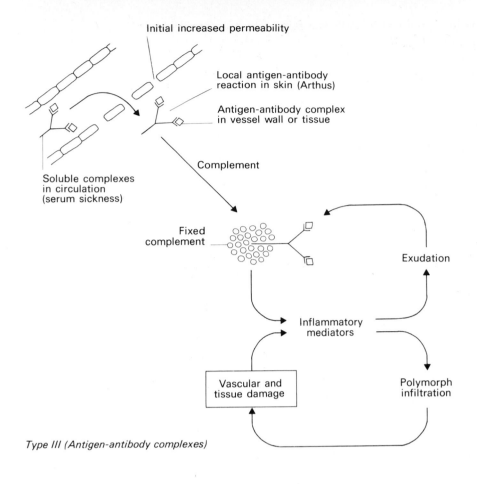

Initial increased permeability

Local antigen-antibody
reaction in skin (Arthus)

Antigen-antibody complex
in vessel wall or tissue

Soluble complexes
in circulation
(serum sickness)

Complement

Fixed
complement

Exudation

Inflammatory
mediators

Vascular and
tissue damage

Polymorph
infiltration

Type III (Antigen-antibody complexes)

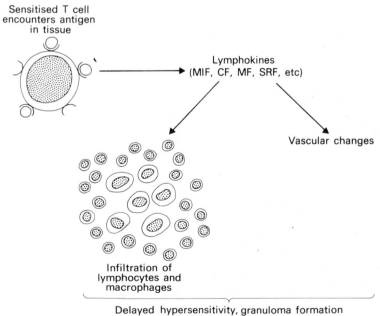

Sensitised T cell
encounters antigen
in tissue

Lymphokines
(MIF, CF, MF, SRF, etc)

Vascular changes

Infiltration of
lymphocytes and
macrophages

Delayed hypersensitivity, granuloma formation

Type IV (delayed)

155

SRS was first described in 1938 as a factor which appeared in perfusates of guinea-pig lung following treatment with cobra venom (which contains phospholipase A_2); the factor caused a contraction of smooth muscle (guinea-pig ileum) which was of slower onset and more sustained than that produced by histamine, and was hence named 'slow reacting substance' (the designation SRS-A being used for immunologically released SRS). Subsequent studies, in which it was produced by human asthmatic lung exposed to pollen, indicated that SRS-A is an important mediator of allergic bronchial asthma; a role in other anaphylactic reactions is also likely. Recently, considerable excitement was generated by the finding that SRS belongs to the newly discovered family of bioactive substances called *leukotrienes* (LTs) which, like prostaglandins, are metabolic derivatives of arachidonic acid (p. 34). SRS-A is a mixture of three leukotrienes, the principal and most potent one being LTC_4, with varying amounts of LTD_4 and LTE_4. Evidently, triggering of the mast cell by antigen activates phospholipase A_2, which generates arachidonic acid from membrane phospholipid; arachidonic acid is then oxidised by the lipoxygenase pathway as described on p. 36, to give rise to leukotrienes. Experimentally, SRS can be generated from mouse mastocytoma cells (neoplastic mast cells which grow in culture) by stimulation with the ionophore A23187, an agent which increases membrane permeability to Ca^{2+} ions. In the lung, mast cells exposed to IgE and antigen have been shown to be the major producers of SRS-A. The leukotrienes which comprise SRS-A are extremely potent in causing contraction of human bronchial smooth muscle and play an important role in the *bronchoconstriction* of allergic asthma; their activity in this respect exceeds that of histamine by more than a hundredfold. In addition, they cause increased vascular permeability (intradermal injection produces a weal-and-flare reaction) and may thus also mediate oedema in the respiratory submucosa.

Eosinophils are frequently associated with anaphylactic inflammatory reactions and sensitive individuals may show eosinophilia. Eosinophils move to the site of the reaction as a result of chemotaxis, being attracted both by histamine itself and by ECF-A, which consists of two tetrapeptides (Val-Gly-Ser-Glu and Ala-Gly-Ser-Glu) which bind to eosinophils. The role of eosinophils in anaphylaxis is to control the reaction by destroying mediators released from mast cells. They are a source of histaminase, the enzyme which inactivates histamine, and other enzymes which destroy SRS-A and PAF (aryl sulphatase B and phospholipase D, respectively).

To relieve the acute symptoms of anaphylactic reactions antihistamines, β-adrenergic agents and corticosteroids may be used. Specific treatment may involve *desensitisation*, the object of which is to stimulate production of antibodies of the IgG or IgA class to compete for the antigen and effectively block the reaction between antigen and IgE. The procedure involved, which is of only variable success, takes the form of repeated subcutaneous injections of the antigen, such as pollen antigens in hay fever, in small but gradually increasing doses (to prevent a general anaphylactic reaction). As many as 50 inoculations, at intervals of 1–3 weeks, may be required. An agent which has found widespread use in treatment of allergic bronchial asthma is *disodium cromoglycate* (cromolyn, DSCG, Intal), which inhibits mast cell degranulation. It is believed that cromoglycate prevents triggering of the mast cell by Ca^{2+} ions, since experimentally it prevents the uptake of radioactive calcium (^{45}Ca) by mast cells.

Unfortunately, it is not known what factors cause the preferential production of antibodies of the IgE class in some individuals in the first place, though genetic mechanisms are certainly involved since there is a strong familial disposition. The genes involved are linked to the major histocompatibility gene complex, HLA (see page 180).

TYPE II (ANTIBODY/CELL SURFACE REACTIONS)

These involve direct damage to cells caused by antibody, usually of the IgM or IgG classes, directed against the cell surface or against a small molecule which becomes attached to the cell surface. The target for such reactions is frequently the red cell, which after reacting with antibody may be lysed by fixed complement or removed by phagocytes, as in haemolytic anaemias and transfusion reactions. *Haemolytic disease of the newborn* (erythroblastosis fetalis) caused by rhesus (Rh) incompatibility between mother and foetus provides a good example of Type II hypersensitivity. Rhesus (Rh) is a group of red cell antigens unrelated to the ABO or other red cell systems, so called from its discovery in rhesus monkeys by Landsteiner and Wiener in 1940. About 85% of Caucasians possess the Rh (D) antigen and are called rhesus positive (Rh +), the remainder being rhesus negative (Rh −).* Genetically, the Rh antigen has dominant expression, so that Rh + individuals can be either homozygous or heterozygous for the gene *D* determining the Rhesus antigen (*DD* or *Dd*); Rh − individuals are homozygous for the recessive allele *d*, i.e. of constitution *dd*. (See Section 7 for explanation of genetic terms.) The problem of haemolytic disease of the newborn arises when an Rh − mother carries an Rh + foetus, the latter having inherited the Rh antigen from its Rh + father (Figure 2.45). If foetal red cells enter the maternal circulation in sufficient quantity, they act as an antigenic stimulus and anti-Rh antibodies are produced. IgG antibodies are able to cross the placenta into the foetal circulation, where they react with the Rh antigen on foetal red cells. These opsonised cells are then removed by macrophages in the foetal liver and spleen and destroyed, giving rise to the haemolytic anaemia; they are *not* lysed by complement. In practice, the first pregnancy of an Rh − mother with an Rh + foetus is not usually affected; although

---

* There are other rhesus antigens, but D is the one of major importance; the terms 'Rh antigen' and 'Rh antibody' as used here refer to D and anti-D.

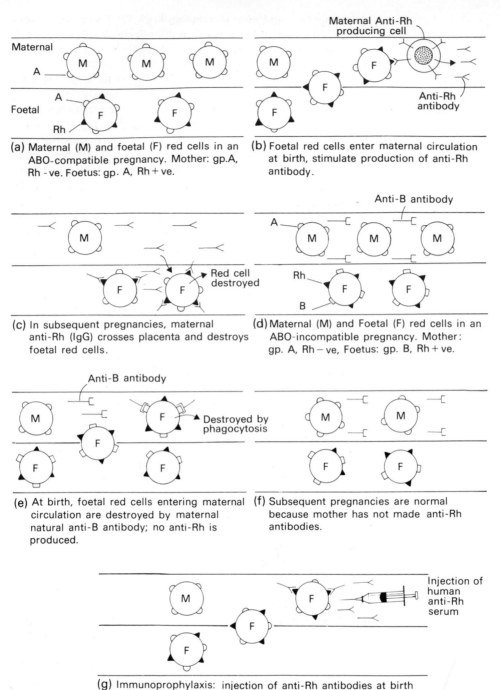

(a) Maternal (M) and foetal (F) red cells in an ABO-compatible pregnancy. Mother: gp.A, Rh - ve. Foetus: gp. A, Rh + ve.

(b) Foetal red cells enter maternal circulation at birth, stimulate production of anti-Rh antibody.

(c) In subsequent pregnancies, maternal anti-Rh (IgG) crosses placenta and destroys foetal red cells.

(d) Maternal (M) and Foetal (F) red cells in an ABO-incompatible pregnancy. Mother: gp. A, Rh − ve, Foetus: gp. B, Rh + ve.

(e) At birth, foetal red cells entering maternal circulation are destroyed by maternal natural anti-B antibody; no anti-Rh is produced.

(f) Subsequent pregnancies are normal because mother has not made anti-Rh antibodies.

(g) Immunoprophylaxis: injection of anti-Rh antibodies at birth prevents stimulation of maternal antibody production, similar to (e) and (f), hence avoids subsequent haemolytic anaemia.

foetal red cells are introduced into the mother's circulation throughout pregnancy, the dose is too low to sensitise until the transplacental haemorrhage at parturition. Thus anti-Rh antibodies (IgM and IgG) are usually produced only in the weeks

Figure 2.45 Basis of haemolytic disease of the newborn and its immunoprophylaxis.

following the birth of the first Rh+ child. Subsequent Rh+ foetuses are then affected because the trickle of foetal red cells into the maternal circulation during pregnancy is able to elicit a secondary response of IgG antibody.

The properties of anti-Rh antibodies in agglutination and complement fixation differ in some important respects from those of antibodies to the ABO system. While IgM anti-Rh antibodies do agglutinate Rh+ red cells, IgG antibodies normally fail to do so even when provided at high concentration; anti-Rh IgG agglutinates directly only by various expedients, such as in high albumin concentration or after partial digestion of the red cell surface by proteases, and is usually demonstrated indirectly by the *antiglobulin (Coombs) test* (p. 133, Figure 2.38c). This contrasts with IgG antibodies against ABO antigens which do produce agglutination, though less efficiently than IgM. Another important feature is that *neither* IgM nor IgG anti-Rh causes lysis of Rh+ red cells by complement fixation; once again this is contrary to expectation based on ABO antibodies. The probable explanation for these differences lies in the Rh antigen rather than in the antibodies, in particular its relatively *low concentration* on the surface of Rh+ cells. The density of Rh molecules on the red cell membrane is such that it is probably impossible to bind a sufficient number of anti-Rh IgG molecules to cause agglutination—there are only about $1-3 \times 10^4$ Rh molecules per Rh+ cell, compared with $3 \times 10^5-10^6$ ABO molecules. Moreover, the Rh molecules are too far apart from each other, and the red cell membrane insufficiently fluid, to enable two IgG molecules to come close together on the red cell surface, a necessary condition for complement fixation by IgG (p. 121). The low density of Rh antigen also prevents IgM from activating complement, since, as we have noted on p. 121, IgM only does so in its 'staple' conformation, attained by folding the antigen-binding arms away from the central Fc disc, and this requires multipoint attachment of the IgM molecule to two or more determinants simultaneously (Figure 2.10). Since the distance between two Rh molecules is greater than the diameter of an IgM molecule, the latter can use only *one* of its ten binding sites at a time in attaching to the Rh+ red cell surface and so does not undergo the requisite conformational change.

Haemolytic disease of the newborn provides a major example of *immunoprophylaxis* and can now be prevented by immunological methods. The key to this was the observation that anaemia was significantly less common when, in addition to the Rh incompatibility, there was also an incompatibility of ABO antigens; in short, ABO incompatibility between mother and foetus protected against haemolytic disease of the newborn. The reason lies in the presence of maternal natural isohaemagglutinins, IgM antibodies directed at those ABO antigens which the mother does not possess (p. 131). Where there is an ABO incompatibility between mother and foetus such that the mother possesses natural antibodies against foetal ABO antigens, the foetal red cells are destroyed before they can stimulate anti-Rh production (Figure 2.45d–f). This also explains why ABO incompatibilities do not lead to serious haemolytic foetal disease. (Note that there are no 'natural' anti-Rh antibodies in Rh − women before exposure to the foetal Rh antigen.) Thus it is possible to suppress primary Rh sensitisation by ensuring rapid removal of foetal red cells from the maternal circulation at parturition. This can be accomplished in every case by inoculation to the Rh − mother of *anti-Rh antibodies* shortly after giving birth. It has now become routine to give this passive immunisation by intramuscular injection of 200–300 µg anti-Rh (purified gamma globulin, obtained from Rh-immunised donors) at the time of birth to all Rh − mothers. This procedure has strikingly reduced the incidence of haemolytic disease of the newborn, and represents one of the most significant contributions of immunology to medical practice.

Other examples of Type II reactions against red cells are the *autoimmune* and *drug-induced haemolytic anaemias*. In the former, autoantibodies are produced which react with antigens on the individual's own red cells, causing them to be lysed or removed by phagocytes. (A full description can be found on page 195.) In the drug-induced haemolytic anaemias, exemplified by that associated with *penicillin*, the drug or one of the reactive products of its metabolism or degradation (e.g. penicilloic acid) functions as a hapten and becomes attached to the red cell membrane. Antibody against the drug or drug derivative then leads to destruction of the red cell. Platelets may also be affected, as in the *thrombocytopenic purpura* which complicates therapy with Sedormid and other drugs (p. 196).

Autoantibodies, reacting with antigens on the surface of body cells, provide further instances of Type II hypersensitivity. Thus, diseases of the thyroid (*thyroiditis, thyrotoxicosis*, pp. 196–7) involve production of antibodies against surface antigens of thyroid cells, while in *myasthenia gravis* antibodies are produced against the acetylcholine receptors of the muscle cell motor endplate (p. 198). *Thyrotoxicosis* (hyperthyroidism, Graves's disease) provides an unusual instance of an antibody which stimulates cellular activity (secretion of thyroxine) rather than causing cell damage. Thyroid epithelial cells are normally regulated by thyroid stimulating hormone (TSH) produced in the pituitary gland and carry a surface receptor for this hormone. In thyrotoxicosis, an autoantibody against the TSH receptor is produced and mimics the action of TSH itself on thyroid cells by triggering the receptor. This leads to oversecretion of thyroxine and the syndrome of hyperthyroidism (see p. 197 for further details).

Antibody-dependent cell-mediated cytotoxicity (ADCC), mediated by K cells, provides another mechanism whereby antibody can cause cell damage (p. 145).

TYPE III (TISSUE DAMAGE BY ANTIGEN–ANTIBODY COMPLEXES)

Antigen–antibody complexes exert a toxic effect when they become localised in and around the walls of blood vessels and initiate a damaging inflammatory response as a result of the activation of complement and infiltration of neutrophils (Figure 2.44). This is seen most frequently when complexes form in the circulation and subsequently become deposited in the walls of blood vessels in several tissues, producing acute vasculitis, chiefly in the joints, kidney, skin and heart. It plays an important role in the pathogenesis of several conditions known collectively as *immune complex diseases*. *Serum sickness* serves as the prototype for these conditions. It was a frequent sequel to the administration of large amounts of horse antitoxin serum when this was used to provide passive immunity in the treatment of diphtheria and tetanus. The condition is unrelated to the antitoxin content of the serum and can be produced in response to normal horse or other foreign serum in man and animals. The foreign serum proteins are, of course, antigenic and stimulate antibody production. When the response is sufficiently large, antigen–antibody aggregates are formed which are rapidly cleared by phagocytosis. However, during the early phase of the response, the level of antibody is moderate in comparison with the antigenic load, and antigen remains in *excess*; reference to the precipitin curve (p. 126) shows that in these circumstances, precipitation is inhibited and small soluble complexes form. These circulate for several days and give rise to the inflammatory lesions of serum sickness, which include painful swelling of the joints (arthritis), transient albuminuria or more severe renal failure, periorbital oedema, carditis, skin lesions (vasculitis) and fever. These lesions are produced when complexes escape from the circulation. Antibody in the complexes is mainly IgG and IgM. However, complex deposition is facilitated by IgE production; the interaction of antigen with IgE, on basophils or on mast cells, is followed by histamine release which increases vascular permeability and allows soluble complexes to enter the vessel wall. Once deposited there, the complexes activate complement and hence cause acute inflammation (p. 30). As a result of the production of chemotactic factors during complement activation, neutrophils are attracted into the area and are responsible for subsequent tissue damage.

As described in Section 1, the lysosomes of neutrophils contain enzymes and cationic proteins which, when released, encourage further inflammation; moreover, the lysosomal enzymes include proteases, collagenases, elastase and cartilage-degrading enzymes which together lead to tissue damage. Enzyme release is partly a passive process following the death *in situ* of the short-lived neutrophils. In addition, antigen–antibody complexes cause an active enzyme release, akin to secretion, in which lysosomal enzymes are shed selectively without the release of cytoplasmic contents. This process, called 'reverse endocytosis', is triggered by the interaction of complexes with the neutrophil at surface Fc receptors, which bind IgG after its combination with antigen, and at C3 receptors that recognise fixed C3b. The perturbation of the neutrophil surface, caused by movement and bridging of Fc or C3b receptors, triggers the fusion of lysosomal with plasma membranes and release of the lysosomal contents to the outside (see also p. 25 and Figure 1.8b).

Immune complex disease, with its characteristic features of

vasculitis, arthritis, glomerulonephritis and carditis, sometimes accompanies infections by viruses, bacteria and parasites, auto-immune disorders and immune reactions to drugs. *Glomerulonephritis* provides a good illustration of one of its common manifestations. Antigen–antibody complexes trapped at the glomerular basement membrane initiate inflammation. Complement is activated, but may not always be essential since neutrophils can make contact with the basement membrane at endothelial fenestrations and bind directly to trapped complexes; also complexes alone can disturb renal function without neutrophil involvement. Immunofluorescence techniques (p. 137) and electron microscopy show antibody and complement in irregular, granular deposits, often outside the basement membrane, sometimes called a 'lumpy-bumpy' distribution. This contrasts with the smooth, linear deposition of antibodies reacting directly with antigens of the glomerular basement membrane itself (p. 139, Figure 2.39b). The granular form of deposit characteristic of complex damage is seen in 70–80% of all forms of immunologically produced glomerulonephritis. Renal damage of this type is a late complication of infection by streptococci in post-streptococcal glomerulonephritis; by *Treponema pallidum* and *Salmonella typhi* in the nephritis of syphilis and typhoid fever respectively; by plasmodia in the nephrotic syndrome which develops in malaria; and by viruses such as hepatitis B, measles and Epstein-Barr. Production of autoantibodies against DNA in systemic lupus erythematosus (SLE) and thyroglobulin in Hashimoto's thyroiditis also lead to glomerulonephritis by complexes.

Arthritis is another prominent symptom of immune complex disease. Examples include drug hypersensitivities (below), SLE, and following recovery from certain infections, as in rheumatic fever after streptococcal throat infection. In rheumatoid arthritis, IgG itself is recognised as an antigen; anti-IgG antibodies (rheumatoid factors) are formed and are present in the circulation both free and as IgM– and IgG–anti-IgG complexes. However, although such complexes are responsible for damage to the joints which characterises this disease, they are formed in this case *in situ* in the joint, rather than deposited from the circulation (see p. 207). Rheumatoid factors are also found in the serum in other chronic diseases including SLE and leprosy.

Immune complex lesions in the skin are seen as the cutaneous vasculitis known as *erythema nodosum leprosum* of lepromatous leprosy, and as part of drug hypersensitivity. Drugs such as penicillin, penicillamine, sulphonamides and streptomycin can all produce serum sickness-like syndromes. The drug or one of its derivatives or metabolic products first becomes attached as a hapten to a body protein to induce an antibody response. The antibody and the drug-protein conjugate are then deposited as a complex. Sometimes, hypersensitivity is induced by a contaminant in the drug and does not occur if the drug can be sufficiently purified.

A different method of inducing local immune complex inflammation is by injection of antigen into the skin of an animal which has a high circulating antibody level against it. A haemorrhagic, oedematous reaction occurs in the skin, which takes 2–8 hours to develop and persists for 12–24 hours or results in tissue necrosis which can be serious. The necrosis is due to destruction of small blood vessels by thrombi (p. 640). This is the *Arthus reaction*, named after its discoverer (1903). Since the complexes form locally in the tissue, they can occur in equivalence as well as antigen excess. The details of the inflammatory response and its dependence on complement and neutrophils are as described above. At one time, when antitoxin or antibacterial sera were administered repeatedly to provide passive immunity (p. 167), the Arthus reaction was seen regularly. Today it is much less common clinically, but can be seen after frequent immunisation with toxoids, in intradermal injection of fungal antigens in pulmonary aspergillosis and as a response to thermophilic actinomycetes in 'Farmer's lung'. Sufferers from this latter condition experience severe respiratory difficulties 6–8 hours after exposure to dust from mouldy hay and this is probably an intrapulmonary Arthus-type reaction.

TYPE IV (CELL-MEDIATED OR DELAYED HYPERSENSITIVITY)

The term *delayed hypersensitivity* refers to the inflammatory response which develops in a sensitised individual 24–48 hours after contact with antigen, especially in the skin, and for which the prototype is the *tuberculin reaction*. The recognition of delayed hypersensitivity dates from Koch's studies on tuberculosis. In the tuberculin test itself, either tuberculin, obtained from cultures of *Mycobacterium tuberculosis*, or its purified protein derivative (PPD) is injected in various dilutions intradermally. The reaction begins after a few hours and reaches a peak at about 48 hours, taking the form of an erythematous induration (a red, hard swelling). Histologically, there is an intense infiltration by mononuclear cells, 80–90% of which are lymphocytes and 10–20% macrophages, which surround and pack the small capillaries and venules and are also found in the connective tissue. Neutrophils are generally absent in the reaction in man. This is in contrast with the Arthus reaction, which develops more rapidly (2–8 hours), is predominantly oedematous rather than indurated and in which neutrophils predominate.

The fundamental difference between the Arthus-type and tuberculin reactions is that the former is antibody-mediated while the latter is cell-mediated. Unlike the Arthus reaction, tuberculin sensitivity can be transferred from a sensitive to a non-sensitised individual by cells, but not by serum. Interestingly, if sensitivity is transferred in this way and a reaction stimulated in the new host with tuberculin, 90% of the cells participating in the transferred reaction are *host* in origin and less than 10% are derived from the donor inoculum. Therefore, most of the cells in the delayed hypersensitivity response are not the specifically sensitised lymphocytes, but have been attracted to and trapped in the area non-specifically. The process whereby this occurs is essentially the same as that already described for cell-mediated immunity (p. 147). A population of sensitised T cells is produced following initial contact with the antigen or organism (e.g. infection with *M. tuberculosis* in the case of tuberculin reactivity). These T cells circulate in the blood and on making contact again with the antigen locally in the skin release lymphokines (p. 147) which cause the non-specific accumulation of further lympho-cytes and macrophages. Lymphokines can be obtained by cultur-ing sensitised T cells with antigen *in vitro* and if injected into the skin will themselves produce an inflammatory response re-sembling delayed hypersensitivity. The major lymphokines include macrophage migration inhibition factor (MIF), which causes the accumulation of macrophages, a monocyte chemotactic factor, a skin-reactive factor, which can initiate an increase in vascular permeability and cell exudation, and a blastogenic factor stimulating proliferation of lymphocytes.

It is clear that delayed hypersensitivity involves the same processes as cell-mediated immunity to bacterial, viral and fungal infection, and generally both appear at the same time. In pro-tective immunity, the accumulated macrophages are activated to deal with persistent intracellular parasites. The reaction swings towards tissue damage when the antigenic stimulus is large or unusually persistent or where the host is highly sensitive. Damage is then caused by the massive infiltration of mononuclear cells, leading to local tissue ischaemia (p. 648), and perhaps direct cell killing by lymphocytes (cytotoxic T cells) and macrophages.

Cell-mediated immunity and the delayed hypersensitivity response can both be transferred, as already described, with sensitised lymphocytes. In man, sensitivity can also be transferred with a cell-free agent known as *transfer factor* (TF), obtained as an extract from sensitised T cells by freezing and thawing. It is claimed that the sensitivity which is transferred in this remarkable way is specific for the antigen against which the donor was sensitised; moreover, it is long-lasting and resembles much more the active sensitisation produced by antigen itself than that transferred passively by living cells. Transfer factor appears to be a most unusual molecule. It is *dialysable*, and therefore of low molecular weight (less than 10,000), yet seems to confer on a normal, apparently non-sensitive individual, specific reactivity to the antigen against which it is produced. However, transfer factor has engendered a long-standing scepticism, centred around the nature of its specificity. Thus, while it is claimed that donor sensitivity is transferred specifically with the extract, an alternative view is that transfer factor acts in a non-specific fashion and merely amplifies a pre-existing, low level sensitivity in the recipient. This issue remains unresolved, but is funda-mental to understanding the action of transfer factor at a molecular level. On the other hand, what is less disputed is its possible value as a therapeutic agent in immunodeficiency states affecting cell-mediated immunity. Thus, transfer factor has been used with some success in treatment of candidiasis and lepromatous leprosy and to prevent life-threatening chickenpox in childhood leukaemia.

Besides the familiar tuberculin test, delayed hypersensitivity can be elicited with other microbial antigens: with viruses, for example, as in the reaction of immunity to vaccinia virus (p. 281); with protozoal antigens in the Montenegro test for cutaneous leishmaniasis; in tests with fungal extracts such as histoplasmin and coccidiomycin; and in the pseudo-Schick reaction to diphtheria toxoid (p. 577). Insect bites such as mosquito and flea bites are also often delayed reactions, though reactions to bee and wasp stings are frequently anaphylactic. Simple chemical compounds can induce a state of *contact sensitivity* (contact dermatitis), which is also a typical delayed hypersensitivity response. Sensitisation generally depends on binding of the chemical to skin epidermal proteins. Sensitivity is seen to metals such as mercury, nickel and chromium; to potassium dichromate among workers in the cement industry; to many dye-stuffs; and to products of plants such as Primula and poison ivy. Dinitrochlorobenzene and picryl chloride are sensitising agents which are sometimes used to test for an individual's ability to make a cell-mediated response where this is in question. The rejection of tissue grafts is also primarily a cell-mediated response, akin to delayed hypersensitivity (p. 173).

Finally, the way in which the cell-mediated response can lead to granuloma formation has been described in Section 1. Cell-mediated hypersensitivity plays a major role in the pathogenesis of chronic bacterial infections such as tuberculosis and leprosy (p. 591). It can be associated with tissue necrosis, as almost always occurs in clinical tuberculosis. This is essentially analogous with the necrosis produced by a large antigenic challenge in a sensitised individual, as when using too high a concentration of tuberculin intradermally in testing a patient with active tuberculosis for sensitisation to tubercle bacilli, or on inhalation of material from a liquefied tuberculous lesion. In the clinical disease, the tissue necrosis is due in large part to the massive immigration of macrophages into the focus following the local release of lymphokines. The accumulation and enlargement of activated macrophages leads to local tissue ischaemia. The necrosis which follows injection of antigen is probably due in part to cell adsorption of tuberculin and killing directly or indirectly by lymphocytes. This mechanism probably also plays a role in the clinical lesion.

ACQUIRED IMMUNITY

Specific immunity to infectious microorganisms may be acquired actively or passively. *Active* immunity can be either *natural*, following recovery from infection, or *artificial*, following prophylactic vaccination. Active immunity depends on immunological memory, the ability to specifically and rapidly recall a response, and is therefore usually long-lived, often permanent. *Passive* immunity, on the other hand, is acquired by transfer of antibodies, either naturally from mother to foetus across the placenta, or artifically by inoculation of immune serum. It lasts only as long as the transferred antibodies survive in the circulation. Table 2.1 summarises the different types of acquired immunity.

Active immunisation: vaccination

Effective prophylactic immunisation against infectious disease involves the preparation of a suitable *vaccine*—a form of the organism or its toxins which retains the antigens of the original but lacks its harmful effects. The major methods used are the following.

Toxoids

Toxins which have been inactivated by formaldehyde without destroying their antigens are called toxoids. They are clearly of use only where the pathogenic effects of the organisms are wholly toxin-produced, as in diphtheria and tetanus. The 'triple vaccine' which is often the first vaccine administered to babies, contains diphtheria and tetanus toxoids (combined with pertussis vaccine against whooping cough). Toxoids are generally adsorbed onto alum for greater efficiency in immunisation; this extends the stimulus by delaying antigen release and acts as an adjuvant (p. 80).

Bacterial polysaccharides

The purified capsular polysaccharides of pneumococci, meningo-cocci and *Haemophilus influenzae* are effective vaccines. They stimulate production of anticapsular antibodies which act as opsonins in infections with these organisms.

Killed organisms

Killed bacteria and inactivated viruses may be safely used for vaccination, but are frequently less effective than living attenuated strains. They have to be used if attenuation (below)

Table 2.1 Acquired immunity.

	Active	Passive
Natural	Infection: subclinical or recovery from disease.	Maternal antibody.
	Lasts for years or permanently.	Lasts several months.
Artificial	Administration of toxoid, killed organisms, attenuated organisms. Lasts for years or permanently.	(a) Administration of antibody from same species: lasts for several months. (b) Antibody from different species: on first contact lasts 1–3 weeks, on second contact lasts 2–6 days.

results in loss of the antigens which stimulate protective immunity. Examples are TAB vaccine (typhoid combined with paratyphoid A and B), cholera vaccine and pertussis vaccine.

Attenuated organisms

These possess the advantages of multiplication in the body to produce a larger antigenic stimulus, and of following in mild form the course of the natural disease. This, together with the correct route of administration, is frequently important in building up the necessary local immunity—e.g. in the intestinal or respiratory tracts. Cell-mediated immunity is also much better established by living organisms than with killed vaccines, unless the latter are incorporated in Freund-type adjuvants (not possible in human vaccination). The disadvantage of attenuated strains is that they may occasionally revert to a virulent form. Among the most widely used attenuated organisms is BCG (Bacille Calmette et Guérin), the avirulent attenuated strain of bovine *Mycobacterium tuberculosis* used in vaccination against tuberculosis and which also provides protection against leprosy. Attenuated viruses in common use include the Sabin polio vaccine, measles, rubella, smallpox, influenza and yellow fever vaccines. Route of administration is important. The Sabin vaccine is administered orally to promote local IgA production in the intestinal tract and influenza vaccine is most effective when given as a nasal spray. Very similar to an attenuated strain is the use of a strain which is virulent in another species but avirulent in man. The classic example of this was the use of cowpox to protect against smallpox in man, introduced by Jenner in 1798 and enshrined in the word 'vaccination' (Latin *vacca*, a cow).

Several specific examples of vaccines can be found in Sections 3 and 4; for a discussion of the advantages and disadvantages of living and inactivated organisms, see e.g. p. 293.

Passive immunisation

Administration of antitoxin-containing sera, raised in horses, was widely used in the past in treatment of diphtheria and tetanus. However, the use of foreign sera is attended by several risks, summarised in Table 2.2, including serum sickness and other hypersensitivity reactions. Nowadays when it is essential to administer antiserum, human antitoxin is preferred as it is free of these side-effects; unfortunately human anti-diphtheria toxin is not available. Since the advent of active immunisation using toxoids, cases of diphtheria and tetanus have become rare in developed countries. The duration of passive immunity depends on the species from which the serum is obtained. Human antibodies will persist for several months after transfer in man, but foreign sera will be cleared, by the immune response against them, about 2 weeks after first inoculation and 2–6 days after second administration. The important use of passive administration of human Rh antibody to Rh − mothers at parturition in

Table 2.2 Risks of administration of foreign antigen e.g. horse serum.

First contact with the antigen	Serum sickness 6–14 days after administration: occurs in antigen excess as antibodies are produced.
Second contact with the antigen	Serum sickness 2–6 days after administration; occurs in antigen excess as antibodies are produced.
	Anaphylaxis (immediate); occurs only with low titre circulating antibody so that antigen can react with cell-adsorbed IgE.
	Arthus reaction (local tissue necrosis); occurs with high titre of complement-fixing antibody.
	Massive complement activation occurs if antigen is given intravenously and there is a high titre of complement-fixing antibody.

prevention of haemolytic disease of the newborn is discussed on p. 159.

TRANSPLANTATION AND THE MAJOR HISTOCOMPATIBILITY COMPLEX

Graft rejection

The rejection of tissue grafts is one of the most important practical problems in contemporary immunology. While the transplantation of organs or tissues from one individual to another is surgically often straightforward, grafts between unrelated individuals do not normally survive for more than a few days before showing signs of being rejected by the recipient. That rejection is an immunological process is shown by the specific increase in speed of rejection of a second graft compared with an initial graft from the same donor (*second set* versus *first set* rejection). This is due to the stimulation of the more rapid secondary response in second set rejection. Why is grafted tissue rejected? In brief, it is because the recipient's circulating lymphocytes enter the graft and recognise antigens on the transplanted tissue which are foreign, i.e. not present on the recipient's own tissues. A cell-mediated response develops against these antigens which eventually leads to the death of the graft.

A graft between two individuals of the same species is termed a *homograft*. If, as is generally the case for man, the individuals are not genetically identical, the term *allograft* is also used.

THE MAJOR HISTOCOMPATIBILITY COMPLEX (MHC)

The antigens which are recognised in the rejection reaction are called *histocompatibility antigens*; it is the fact that the graft donor and recipient differ in these antigens that leads to rejection. Histocompatibility antigens are inherited and are determined by a number of genetic loci, each with considerable polymorphism. (*Polymorphism* of a genetic locus is the occurrence in a population of two or more alleles with an appreciable frequency, i.e. at least 1%; see also p. 863.) Although each individual possesses a large number of histocompatibility antigens (more than 20 histocompatibility systems have been discovered in mice), one set of antigens is paramount in determining the rate at which grafts are rejected. These are called the *major* histocompatibility antigens and they are coded by genes in a region known as the *major histocompatibility complex* or MHC. In man this complex is called HLA, an abbreviation of *H*uman *L*eucocyte antigen system *A*, havin been first discovered on leucocytes by Dausset in 1954; the equivalent system in the mouse, where a great deal of the basic research has been done, is termed *H-2* (*H*istocompatibility-*2*). The HLA complex is located on chromosome 6 and H-2 on mouse chromosome 17. Genetic maps of HLA and H-2 are shown in Figure 2.46. The important antigens in transplantation reactions are the products of loci termed A, B, C and D in HLA and K, I and D in H-2. (I and HLA-D are in fact genetic regions rather than single loci). Since each individual is diploid, eight distinct major histocompatibility antigens can be present on tissue cells (two each of the A, B, C and D antigens in man).

Figure 2.46 Arrangement and function of genes of the major histocompatibility complex (a) in the mouse (H-2) and (b) in man (HLA).

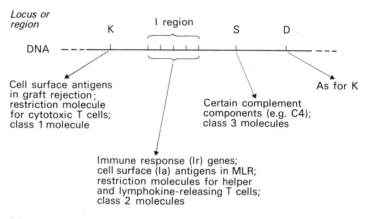

(a)

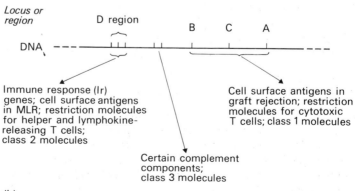

(b)

Because of the high degree of polymorphism in the system, with many alleles at each locus, it is very unlikely that two unrelated persons will be HLA-identical; hence unhindered acceptance of a graft between unrelated individuals will be a very rare occurrence. HLA antigens are present on most tissue cells, but not on red blood cells. The molecules encoded by the H-2 K and D loci and HLA-A,B,C are structurally similar glycoproteins composed of a polypeptide chain of 44,000 mol.wt together with a smaller chain of 12,000 mol.wt; they are known as *class I MHC molecules*. The small chain, called β_2-microglobulin, is not coded in the MHC and is common to all class I molecules. The molecules coded by the I-region of H-2 or the HLA-D region likewise resemble each other; they consist of two polypeptide chains of 34,000 and 29,000 mol.wt and are termed *class II MHC molecules*. The MHC also contains the genes for certain complement components (e.g. C4); the latter are *class III molecules*.

The significance of HLA antigens in human transplantation is demonstrated by grafting between HLA-identical as compared with non-identical siblings (brothers or sisters). Skin, kidney and bone marrow grafts all show greatest survival where graft donor and recipient are HLA-identical. For skin grafts, the survival period between unrelated individuals or HLA-different siblings is about 12 days; where siblings are HLA-identical, the grafts survive for up to 20 days. Note, however, that unless donor and recipient are identical twins, rejection always occurs and the survival time between perfectly HLA-matched siblings is only about twice that observed between unrelated individuals. It follows that other, non-HLA antigens are also important in graft rejection; they are known as *minor* histocompatibility antigens, to indicate that their strength is less than that of HLA antigens. Grafts of kidneys between HLA-matched siblings survive much better than skin, with 90% surviving for one year as opposed to only 60% between HLA-different siblings and 50% between unrelated, HLA-different individuals. Note that when siblings are HLA-matched, *all* their HLA antigens will necessarily be identical, through inheritance of the same HLA chromosomes; identity of matching of unrelated individuals to this degree is probably impossible by present typing methods. Hence, HLA matching has less effect on graft survival when the donor and recipient are unrelated. Nevertheless, here too there is a significant correlation between completeness of HLA matching and graft survival and it is usual to match donor and recipient as far as possible in clinical transplantation. However, for long-term survival, *suppression* of the immune response is always essential.

HLA typing is carried out serologically. Cells, usually lymphocytes, taken from the individual being typed, are tested with a range of specific antibodies against different HLA antigens. A positive reaction occurs if the cells are killed by a particular serum in the presence of complement. The individual is then known to carry the HLA antigen which the antibodies in the typing serum recognise. Typing antisera are obtained from multiparous women, who produce antibodies against paternal HLA antigens on foetal cells; from multiple blood transfusion recipients; or from planned immunisation programmes. However, antisera are now being replaced by monoclonal antibodies to individual HLA antigens, which are the ideal typing reagents for reasons discussed on p. 100.

While products of all the HLA loci (A, B, C, D) can now be detected serologically, the HLA-D region antigens can be tested for by other means, namely by the *mixed lymphocyte reaction* (MLR). This test is performed by mixing the blood lymphocytes of two individuals in culture. If they differ in HLA-D antigens, the lymphocytes respond by developing into blast cells and proliferating. The proliferation is measured as uptake of tritiated thymidine by the dividing cells. Absence of reactivity in MLR indicates that the individuals are identical at the HLA-D region. The lymphocytes responding in the MLR are T cells, while those which carry the HLA-D antigens and therefore stimulate the reaction are B cells. The strength of MLR does not necessarily correlate with speed of graft rejection, because the MLR does not detect HLA-A, B, C antigens and it is the latter that are the targets recognised by cytotoxic lymphocytes when grafts are rejected. However, HLA-D antigens are also involved in the rejection process, so that for complete matching at HLA it is necessary to detect and match the products of all four HLA loci. In practice the time required for the MLR test (96 hours) precludes its use in most cases of transplantation in man, and the availability of antisera and monoclonal antibodies to HLA-D antigens has made their rapid serological detection possible.

IMMUNOSUPPRESSION

In order to secure the long-term survival of a graft, even where HLA-matching is complete, it is necessary to actively suppress the immune response against the graft. Several different types of agent with immunosuppressive properties are in clinical use; some are drugs with cytostatic properties which were originally used in cancer therapy. Combinations of the following agents are commonly used to suppress graft rejection.

Base analogues, in particular *6-mercaptopurine* (6-MP) and its imidazole derivative *azathioprine*, are among the most widely used immunosuppressive agents. 6-MP and azathioprine are analogues of guanine which interfere with DNA synthesis in several ways, principally by competing with normal bases in metabolism or for incorporation into DNA. Hence their main effect is to prevent cell division; in addition they also exert an anti-inflammatory effect.

Alkylating agents also interfere with nucleic acid synthesis and thereby inhibit mitosis. The principal example in clinical use is *cyclophosphamide*, a relative of nitrogen mustard, which binds to guanine in DNA (see p. 769 for details).

Some antibiotics, especially *actinomycin C* and *D*, are also in use as immunosuppressants, in conjunction with azathioprine. Actinomycin binds to DNA and blocks RNA polymerase and hence protein synthesis.

Corticosteroids (e.g. *prednisone*) are powerful anti-inflammatory agents and this seems to be the basis of their immunosuppressive action. Although in high doses they can kill lymphocytes of some species, this is not believed to be significant in their action in man. Part of their anti-inflammatory effect is due to stabilisation of lysosomal membranes, hence inhibiting release of enzymes from neutrophils. Besides their suppression of general immunity, there are serious side-effects to their use, e.g. Cushing's syndrome, perforation of peptic ulcer and activation of latent tuberculosis.

Cyclosporin A (CyA) is the most recent immunosuppressive drug to be introduced and, while evaluation in clinical trials has only recently been completed, its promise is such that it is certain to be extensively employed in organ transplantation in the future. It is a fungal product discovered in 1972 during screening for new antibiotics; although it had little antimicrobial action, CyA was found to inhibit lymphocyte proliferation and subsequently to be a powerful immunosuppressant in all species tested, including man. In clinical trials, it has been shown to produce exceptionally good survival of kidney and heart grafts: the use of CyA as sole immunosuppressive agent in recipients of unmatched kidney grafts has secured a survival rate of about 80%, which is better than other drugs in current use. Its particular advantages lie in its selective action on T lymphocytes and its low toxicity for recipient bone marrow cells, myelotoxicity being a problem which limits the use of all other immunosuppressants; CyA also lacks the side-effects of steroids noted above. Its most serious side-effect still to be overcome completely is nephrotoxicity; kidney function is impaired, apparently as a result of damage to the renal tubules.

Among lymphocytes, CyA seems to act exclusively on T cells, with B cells remaining unaffected. An important virtue is that secondary antibody responses are not inhibited, so that opportunistic bacterial infections by organisms already experienced are relatively infrequent (see below). CyA prevents the activation of T cells by interfering with the production or action of the interleukins IL-1 and IL-2 (p. 116). An exciting observation is that grafts in animals may survive almost indefinitely after cessation of CyA administration, i.e. CyA seems to allow a permanent state of tolerance to the graft to be induced, a goal which has been the ultimate objective of much transplantation research (p. 182). Thus the use of CyA holds out the possibility of taking patients off immunosuppression altogether after a certain time; at present, drugs must be continued indefinitely even though the doses are reduced with time.

Antilymphocyte serum (ALS) obtained from horses (or other animals) injected with human lymphocytes provides an approach different from the use of immunosuppressive drugs. ALS contains antibodies against human lymphocytes and by killing them prevents graft rejection. The main effect seems to be on T cells. In practice, the IgG fraction is purified (antilymphocyte globulin, ALG) and administered to the graft recipient; use of ALG minimises the risk of serum sickness (the antibody response is only partially suppressed by ALS). Nevertheless, being a foreign protein, ALG can also have unpleasant and occasionally fatal side-effects in sensitive individuals.

Immunosuppressive regimens involve the combined use of some of the above agents. Because of their dangerous side-effects, the dose of these agents is strictly regulated, e.g. the maximally tolerated dose of azathioprine is often given together with the minimum necessary dose of prednisone, and in some centres cyclosporin A is being used in conjunction with steroids. The major drawback of chemical immunosuppression is that it destroys the patient's ability to deal with infection; this is especially true of the corticosteroids. Infections with opportunistic organisms, frequently of endogenous origin, are a major cause of death among transplant patients (see p. 271). There is also the risk of uncontrolled proliferation of hepatitis virus in the recipient who then infects all his contacts. In uncontrollable infection, it is necessary to stop immunosuppression altogether and risk loss of the graft, to enable the patient's immune system to recover. Because of the low toxicity of cyclosporin A for bone marrow and B cells, neutrophil activity and secondary antibody responses are spared (the latter are less affected than primary responses by suppression of T cells); thus bacterial infection is less common in patients receiving CyA than other drugs and viral infections also seem to be less of a serious problem. In patients on long-standing immunosuppression, there is also an increase in the risk of certain malignant neoplasms, particularly lymphomas, which in the under-50 age group may be as much as a hundred times higher than normal. Such tumours are often due to Epstein-Barr virus (EBV), which is carried in latent form in some B cells of many normal adults. This virus is the cause of infectious mononucleosis in adolescents and young adults, but otherwise persists permanently in B lymphocytes without clinical manifestation. EBV is oncogenic (p. 792), but the tendency of occasional B cells to transform is normally controlled by cytotoxic T cells specific for EBV-infected cells, which eliminate neoplastic B cell clones as they arise; suppression of T cell activity evidently allows neoplastic B cells to grow and develop into lymphomas. Early small-scale trials with cyclosporin A suggested that patients receiving this agent developed lymphomas with an alarming frequency (about 10% of recipients), but more extensive use indicates that the risk is in fact considerably less. Cyclosporin A is not itself carcinogenic and the development of lymphomas seems to be solely a result of immunosuppression; note, however, that some of the other drugs in use, such as base analogues and alkylating agents, are carcinogenic as well as immunosuppressive.

MECHANISMS OF GRAFT REJECTION

The process of graft rejection can involve both cell-mediated reactions and antibody production against antigens on the grafted tissue. When an individual receives a graft for the first time and is not treated with immunosuppressive agents, acute rejection usually occurs after about 12 days and is mediated by T cells. On the other hand, if the individual has pre-existing circulating antibodies to antigens in the graft or receives immunosuppressive therapy, antibody-mediated processes are involved.

T cell-mediated rejection

There is little doubt that the classical *acute rejection* which occurs in untreated recipients 10–14 days after primary grafting is a cell-mediated process. Thus, animals which lack T cells, such as neonatally thymectomised and nude (athymic) mice, or children with thymic deficiencies, accept permanently grafts from unrelated donors. The ability to reject can be transferred to athymic mice by lymphoid cells, but not by serum from animals immunised against the graft antigens. Furthermore, grafts undergoing rejection are infiltrated with mononuclear cells (lymphocytes and macrophages), but neutrophils are not involved. T cells mediating rejection are of both the cytotoxic and lymphokine-releasing types.

After initial contact with cell-bound antigen in the graft, or with soluble antigens released from the graft and trapped in the local lymph nodes, T cells proliferate in the paracortical areas of the nodes and develop into effector cells, as shown in Figure 2.47. They then enter the graft, some killing tissue cells by direct cytotoxicity while others release the soluble mediators which cause accumulation of macrophages. Rejection occurs as a result of T cell killing of grafted cells, together with ischaemic necrosis caused by occlusion of arterioles by leucocyte-fibrin masses. The presence of antibody, far from being necessary for acute rejection, can be a hindrance by interfering with the recognition of antigens by T cells. Thus, transfer of antibodies against graft antigens into transplant recipients can prolong graft survival time, an effect known as *immunological enhancement*. Reference to Figure 6.16 of Section 6 shows how this may come about, either by antibody

Figure 2.47 Processes involved in acute rejection of a renal allograft.
1 Antigen (HLA) is released (shed) from kidney cells and carried to regional lymph nodes.
2 Antigen stimulates formation of antibodies and sensitised T cells.
3 Antibodies and cytotoxic T cells enter the graft which is then rejected. T cells are particularly important in acute rejection.

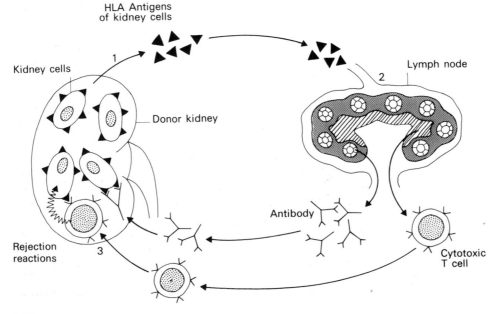

HLA Antigens
of kidney cells

Kidney cells

1

Lymph node

2

Donor kidney

Antibody

Rejection
reactions

3

Cytotoxic
T cell

'blocking' the antigen at the surface of grafted cells and interfering with the access of T cells, or by binding to T cells themselves as a complex with soluble antigen. Some attempts have been made to enhance graft survival in man by anti-HLA sera, but so far the results have not suggested that it will be possible to replace nonspecific immunosuppression by specific enhancement.

Antibody-mediated rejection

The different forms which antibody-mediated rejection processes can take are well illustrated by experience with kidney transplants. Very rapid *hyperacute rejection* can take place within a matter of minutes of grafting if the recipient has circulating antibodies against antigens in the graft, either as a result of ABO incompatibility or due to previous contact with the transplantation antigens through blood transfusion or previous attempts at grafting. The antibodies bind to antigens on the graft endothelium and initiate complement- and neutrophil-mediated damage to the endothelium (Type II hypersensitivity). Platelets then adhere to the damaged vessel wall and the vessels are occluded by platelet/fibrin thrombi (p. 640). (Hyperacute rejection should not be confused with second-set rejection, the accelerated rejection reaction which occurs after 5–7 days in animals receiving the same grafted antigens for a second time and which is T cell-mediated.)

Antibodies are also a cause of rejection of grafts in individuals receiving immunosuppression. The commonly used combination of azathioprine and prednisone is effective at suppressing T cell responses, but some antibody production may continue. If it does, a delayed rejection may occur 2–6 weeks after grafting (*acute late rejection*). Vascular changes are prominent, the most characteristic being *fibrinoid necrosis* of arterioles, so called because the vessel walls stain intensely with eosin, a characteristic of fibrin (see p. 203), and fibrosis of the endothelium of larger arteries. IgG, IgM and complement are present in the vascular lesions. Platelets aggregate in the glomerular capillaries, probably as a result of binding to antigen–antibody complexes on the vessel walls, and they eventually block the vessel as thrombi.

Finally, *chronic rejection*, which can occur months or years after kidney transplantation, is also an antibody-mediated hypersensitivity reaction. It seems that antibody production gradually escapes from immunosuppression in these cases. Anti-HLA antibodies are produced which bind to antigens on the surface of endothelial cells. Activation of complement leads to a condition similar to glomerulonephritis. The antibody and complement are revealed by immunofluorescence in a smooth, continuous distribution on the glomerular basement membrane rather than the 'lumpy-bumpy' appearance produced by accumulation of complexes infiltrated from the circulation as in serum sickness (p. 139). Glomerular damage leads to loss of renal function.

Clearly, the process of rejection depends on vascularisation of the graft, both for recognition of the antigens and attack by lymphocytes. If a graft remains avascular, it may well survive even though it carries foreign HLA antigens. This underlies the special survival of corneal transplants, the majority of which are not rejected despite the presence of HLA antigens on corneal cells. It seems that since the cornea remains avascular, sensitisation of host lymphocytes does not occur. However, it is possible for the cornea to be rejected if the recipient has been previously sensitised to HLA antigens on corneal cells.

Graft-versus-host reaction

Bone marrow grafts are of special significance in transplantation because the transplanted tissue itself contains immunocompetent cells. The purpose of such a graft is often to repopulate the immune system of infants with severe combined immunodeficiency, caused by absence of lymphoid stem cells in the bone marrow (p. 78). Since these infants are unable to mount immune responses and hence cannot reject grafts, it might be thought that any donor bone marrow could be used as it could not fail to be accepted. However, although the graft cannot be rejected, it contains lymphoid cells which can themselves recognise the antigens on the tissues of the *recipient*. Thus, unless the donor and recipient are perfectly matched, a *graft-versus-host* (GVH) reaction will develop (in contrast with the usual host-versus-graft reaction) in which host tissues are attacked by transplanted T lymphocytes. In this reaction, the attacking T cells multiply in the spleen and liver, which become enlarged; there follow exfoliative dermatitis, diarrhoea, maladsorption, loss of weight, pneumonia and thrombocytopenia (platelet deficiency). Uncontrolled GVH disease is rapidly fatal. Hence the requirement for HLA matching is extremely important, and the best results are achieved when the bone marrow is donated by an HLA-identical sib. An alternative approach to avoiding a GVH reaction is to kill T cells in the donor bone marrow using specific antibodies and complement; this is now becoming a practical possibility using monoclonal antibodies against human T cell antigens.

Besides immunodeficiency, bone marrow grafting is also used to replace haematopoietic tissue in aplastic anaemia and leukaemia. Many cases of severe combined immunodeficiency have now been successfully treated by bone marrow grafting, the children developing full immunocompetence with repopulation of previously depleted lymphoid organs. Similarly, the Di George syndrome (p. 78) has been treated by thymus transplantation. Once a lymphoid or haematopoietic graft has taken, the leucocytes and red cells which the individual carries in the circulation are of the donor rather than the recipient type. An individual carrying foreign cells without rejecting them is called a *chimera*.

The physiological role of the MHC

While the great importance of the major histocompatibility complex as the strongest system of transplantation antigens is now well recognised, the true role of the MHC and its products in the body have until recently remained a mystery. The rejection of foreign tissue grafts is a contemporary phenomenon of considerable inconvenience, but it was clearly not the rationale for the evolution of the system. Nonetheless, the main role of the MHC does have to do with a type of rejection reaction, namely the removal from the body of 'abnormal' cells, including those which have become infected by intracellular parasites such as viruses or which have undergone a neoplastic change to a tumour cell. Indeed, it is becoming evident that the MHC occupies a central position as part of the immunological defence system in combating infection and cellular abnormality. In addition, the MHC region contains genes which code for certain complement components, such as C2, C4 and factor B of the alternative pathway. There are also genes which play an important role in regulating immune responses, known as the *immune response genes* (Ir genes), of which more will be said below. Thus a very close relationship exists between the MHC and the protective function of the immune system. The HLA-A, B, C and D loci are polymorphic, each having several alleles which occur at frequencies of 5%–20% in the population. As a result, most individuals are heterozygous at all loci and, as noted above, the probability that two unrelated individuals will be completely HLA-identical is very small. The complement and Ir genes also show polymorphism. Polymorphism in the MHC is probably not fortuitous, but is closely related to its physiological role as part of the immune system. A summary of present understanding of the role of the MHC follows.

INTRACELLULAR INFECTION

When cells are infected with pathogens such as viruses or intracellular bacteria, it is necessary for the existence of the infection to be recognised by the immune system, particularly by T lymphocytes, so that a cell-mediated immune response can be initiated. One of the functions of MHC molecules on the surface of infected cells is to take part in the interaction between the T cell and the infected target. The following experiment illustrates this role. When mice of a particular H-2 type are infected with a virus, cytotoxic T cells develop which are capable of specifically killing virus-infected cells on contact, hence enabling the animal to recover, as described on p. 149. The cytotoxic T cells can be isolated from the animal and *in vitro* can be shown to kill mouse cells infected with the same virus. However, they will only kill infected target cells which carry the *same H-2 antigens* as the infected mouse from which the T cells were obtained; target cells of a different H-2 type are not killed, even though the virus infecting them is the same. In short, a *restriction* is placed on the reaction between a cytotoxic T cell and its target by the MHC. The restriction molecules involved are class I MHC molecules, i.e. those of the K and D loci in the mouse H-2 complex, the equivalent in man being those coded by the A, B or C loci of HLA (Figure 2.46). Two possible types of explanation for this experimental result have been proposed, and are illustrated in Figure 2.48. In the first, called the *altered-self hypothesis*, it is suggested that a molecular complex is formed on the surface of the infected cell between an MHC molecule and a virus or viral antigen, creating a new antigenic determinant (altered self-MHC) which is then recognised by a T cell (Figure 2.48(i)). Note that according to the altered-self theory, the T cell has a *single* receptor which recognises the MHC-viral antigen complex. Alternatively, the cytotoxic T cell may carry *two receptors*, one for the viral antigen at the cell surface and a separate receptor for an unaltered self-MHC molecule; this *dual recognition hypothesis* is illustrated in Figure 2.48(ii). Whichever theory turns out to be correct, it is clear that MHC molecules are central to the mechanism of elimination of infected cells. Other abnormal cells, such as tumour cells, may also be recognised by similar mechanisms.

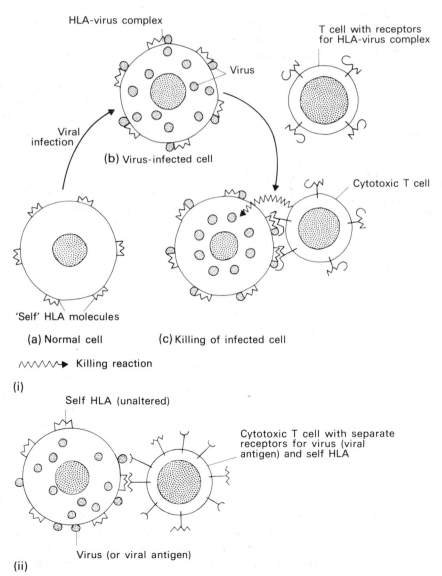

178

A long-standing puzzle, which the altered-self theory goes some way to solving, has been that T cells recognise foreign (non-self) major histocompatibility antigens more strongly than other antigens such as foreign proteins. This is due to the surprisingly large number of T cells capable of recognising foreign MHC determinants. If it is true that T cells pick out infected self cells by reacting with altered MHC molecules on their surface, the high number of T cells reacting with foreign MHC antigens becomes less surprising; in other words, according to this hypothesis, graft rejection occurs because foreign MHC molecules resemble the complexes of self-MHC and antigen which T cells are adapted to recognise. Note that the reaction of a cytotoxic T cell with a foreign target cell is the one occasion where such a T cell does not recognise antigen in association with self-MHC, a situation which is difficult to explain by a two-receptor or dual recognition model. In general terms, graft rejection itself reflects the important role of the MHC in signalling cellular abnormality to the immune system.

Similar events occur in infections with intracellular bacteria, for example, recognition by T cells of macrophages infected with mycobacteria or brucellae. In such cases the T cells respond by release of lymphokines and development of delayed hypersensitivity, rather than cytotoxicity which would only serve to release viable bacteria. In contrast with cytotoxic T cells, lymphokine-releasing and other T cells recognise antigen at the surface of infected cells in association with class II MHC molecules, i.e. coded by genes in the I-region of H-2 (Ia molecules) or in the D region of HLA.

Thus, the involvement of MHC molecules seems to extend to most, if not all, T cell recognition processes. We have noted elsewhere the general principle that T cells recognise antigens only on the surfaces of other cells and in association with a self-MHC molecule (p. 109). The fact that different self-MHC molecules are recognised by different T cell types reflects a division of the latter into two broad groups, namely those which destroy their target cells (cytotoxic T cells) and those which release soluble mediators and activate or suppress other lymphocytes or macrophages (helper T cells, suppressor T cells, lymphokine-releasing T cells). Cytotoxic T cells recognise antigens in association with class I MHC molecules (H-2 K and D, HLA-A, B, C), while the other T cells recognise antigen in association with class II molecules (Ia, HLA-D). Thus, MHC molecules can be thought of as recognition 'guides' for T cells of each category, homing them onto their targets so that the appropriate reaction occurs.

REGULATION OF THE IMMUNE RESPONSE

The *immune response (Ir) genes* located in the MHC control the levels and type of response made to specific antigens. They are polymorphic and the variation in Ir genes can be recognised in the population by inherited differences between individuals in the way they respond to different antigens. In extreme cases, some

Figure 2.48 (*opposite*) The possible role of histocompatibility (HLA) molecules in killing of virus-infected human cells.
(i) The altered-self hypothesis.
　(a) Normal cell carries 'self' HLA molecules.
　(b) After viral infection, HLA molecules combine with virus or viral antigen on cell surface to form a new antigenic complex. T cells with appropriate receptors are stimulated.
　(c) Cytotoxic T cells engage and kill infected target cell.
(ii) The dual recognition hypothesis. The cytotoxic T cell carries two independent receptors, one for the viral antigen, the other for 'self' HLA.

individuals are *high responders* to a certain antigen, while others are *low responders*. Note that the phenomenon of low responsiveness controlled by Ir genes is antigen-specific and not a generalised immune deficiency. A good example of the influence of an Ir gene in man has been found in the development of immediate hypersensitivity to ragweed pollen (ragweed hay fever). The predisposition is inherited, due to an Ir gene which determines the level of the IgE response to the ragweed antigen. Thus, high responders will have a greater tendency to develop hypersensitivity than low responders. In families, the Ir gene for ragweed sensitivity segregates with HLA type, though in the population at large there is no association with any particular HLA antigen. It is clear that inherited variations in immune response could have an important influence on all aspects of immunity, reflected in individual differences in ability to combat pathogens or in tendencies to hypersensitivity or autoimmunity. Many Ir genes have been discovered in mice, originally by the use of synthetic polypeptide antigens and later with proteins in low doses, viruses and indeed all categories of antigen under appropriate conditions.

In the mouse, the Ir genes are located in the I (for immune response) region of the H-2 complex, while in man they probably occur in the HLA-D region. Their protein products are the class II molecules (Ia, HLA-D molecules) found on the surface of certain cells, especially macrophages and B cells; as we have noted above, these are the self-MHC molecules which, in association with antigen, are 'seen' by helper and lymphokine-releasing T cells. A general explanation of Ir-gene determined low responsiveness, therefore, would be that some antigens cannot associate 'correctly' on the macrophage surface with the class II molecules inherited by certain individuals. Such antigens would not then be presented to helper T cells and as a result would be unable to induce antibody or other immune responses. The low responder trait would be inherited with the class II molecules coded by the Ir genes. There is also experimental evidence that the interaction between antigen-specific T cell factors and their cell-bound acceptors (Figure 2.26) is controlled by Ir genes and is ineffective in low responder animals. However, it will be difficult to formulate a precise molecular theory for Ir gene action until the details of recognition of antigens on macrophages and other cell surfaces are better understood.

COMPLEMENT

The HLA complex contains some of the genes which code for complement components, including C2 and C4, as well as factor B of the alternative pathway. Inherited deficiencies of complement components are sometimes found and several families have been observed in which some members lack C2. This particular deficiency is associated with development of certain immune complex diseases, including systemic lupus erythematosus (SLE). C2 deficiency is inherited with HLA type within the family.

The intimate relationship between the major histocompatibility complex and the immune system seems to extend to the structure of some MHC molecules. In particular, the class I molecules, products of the HLA-A, B and C or H-2 K and D loci, are structurally intriguingly similar in some respects to immunoglobulins. They possess a 2-chain structure on the cell surface, with a larger chain of molecular weight 44,000 and a smaller chain of 12,000 mol.wt, the latter known as β_2-microglobulin (β_2-m). There is an obvious parallel with the heavy and light chains of antibody molecules, and isolation of class I MHC molecules from cell surfaces by detergent yields a dimeric Ig-like structure. Moreover, both the large chain and β_2-m show similarities with Ig chains in structure and amino acid sequence. β_2-microglobulin is similar in size, sequence and conformation to a single Ig domain (p. 90). The large chain for its part has three regions, each similar in their folding to Ig domains, two with intrachain disulphide bridges; the second HLA domain shows a highly significant sequence homology with Ig C-region domains. A diagrammatic view of the molecular structure of a class I molecule is shown in Figure 2.49. Note that only the large chain is coded by MHC loci and carries the polymorphic antigenic determinants recognised in grafting; β_2-m is encoded separately, on chromosome 15 in man, and is invariant in all class I molecules in the species. It is likely that the MHC class I genes and the Ig genes evolved from a common precursor, which may well have been the β_2-m gene. However, despite these similarities, there is no evidence for sites on MHC molecules akin to the binding sites of antibodies.

Class II (Ia, HLA-DR) molecules are structurally different from class I but nevertheless also show some sequence homologies with them and with Ig. Each molecule has two polypeptide

Figure 2.49 Structure of a class I MHC molecule. (After Strominger J.L. (1980). In Fougereau, M. & Dausset, J. (eds) *Immunology 80*, 541. Academic Press)
CHO = carbohydrate
S-S = disulphide bond

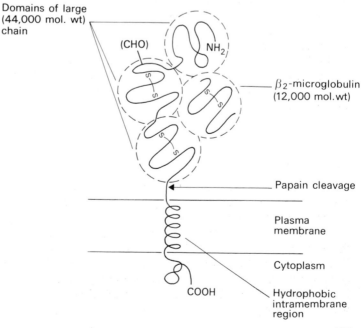

181

chains, α and β, of sizes 34,000 and 29,000 mol.wt respectively, in non-covalent association; both chains are MHC-coded. In addition to their presence on the surface of B cells, macrophages and certain other cell types, class II molecules or chains form part of the antigen-specific helper and suppressor factors released from the respective T cells; thus, class II molecules are involved in cellular interactions (immunoregulation) as well as in recognition of antigen by T cells.

HLA and disease susceptibility

One of the most significant recent findings in immunology has been the association between some HLA types and certain diseases, many of which involve autoimmunity. These include ankylosing spondylitis, myasthenia gravis, systemic lupus erythematosus, multiple sclerosis, and several others. This discovery has not only enhanced understanding of these disorders, but may well prove to be of diagnostic and therapeutic usefulness. A detailed description of the association between HLA and these diseases and its interpretation can be found under *autoimmunity* (p. 187 ff.) and in Section 7 (p. 880).

IMMUNOLOGICAL TOLERANCE

Sometimes, encounter with antigen, rather than leading to antibody production or cell-mediated immunity, produces a state of antigen-specific unresponsiveness known as *immunological tolerance*. This underlies the ability of the immune system to distinguish self from non-self, for in normal circumstances the body does not respond to its own constituents (natural tolerance) and will only do so when the tolerant state is broken to a specific body molecule. (Note that for some 'self molecules', tolerance is apparent rather than real, as tissue-specific or intracellular components may never normally make contact with lymphocytes and therefore induce neither immunity not tolerance; see p. 187.) The loss of self-tolerance is one of the causes of *autoimmunity* in which antibodies or T cells are produced which are able to combine with or react against body molecules. Autoimmunity is involved in the pathogenesis of a variety of important diseases, some of which are discussed below; it can also develop as a consequence of infection with certain microorganisms. To understand the possible mechanisms which are involved in auto-immune disease, we must consider the experimental induction and breakage of tolerance.

Induction of tolerance

Neonatal animals

Some of the earliest experiments in tolerance induction were concerned with transplantation antigens; indeed practical interest in tolerance derived largely from the development of transplantation and the search for methods to overcome graft rejection. In what are now classic experiments, Medawar and his colleagues demonstrated that tolerance to foreign tissues could be easily induced in newborn animals of some species: exposure of neonatal mice to antigen produced tolerance, whereas exposure of adults to the same antigen led to an immune response. For example, when neonatal mice of the CBA strain were injected with cells taken from the unrelated A strain, they would later, as adults, accept skin grafts from the A strain which would otherwise have been rapidly rejected. The unresponsiveness to A skin was specific, as shown by unimpeded rejection of skin from a third party, unrelated strain. It has since been found to be generally the case that tolerance is more readily induced in very young, immunologically immature animals than it is in adults. It seems that during their early development, lymphocytes pass through a stage in which they are especially easily tolerised, thereby ensuring that those with the ability to recognise self are rendered unresponsive before completing their maturation into potentially reactive cells. The ease with which very young animals are tolerised can also be a disadvantage: the introduction of microorganisms of low pathogenicity into the foetus or newborn may lead to tolerance and hence overwhelming disease rather than stimulate a protective immune response. This seems to be the case in intra-uterine infections such as rubella (German measles), with consequent serious damage to the foetus. The early contact of mice and chickens with some tumour viruses leads to a permanent state of infection and later to the appearance of neoplasms (Section 6).

Adult animals

Tolerance can also be induced in mature animals, though it often requires special conditions such as extremes of antigen dose. Thus for many antigens, very high (superimmunogenic) doses will produce tolerance rather than immunity. Tolerance induction can be encouraged to occur in adults if, at the time of giving antigen, the lymphocyte population is partially depleted, e.g. by administration of cyclophosphamide or antilymphocyte serum. Such measures in effect return the system to its immature and tolerance-sensitive stage, by forcing the regeneration of the lymphocyte pool. The physical state of the antigen can also promote tolerance over immune response. For example, proteins from which macromolecular aggregates have been removed by centrifugation or phagocytosis, are able to produce adult tolerance at doses which would normally stimulate an antibody response. The uptake of antigenic material by macrophages is an essential step in immune induction for these antigens and if this is avoided, by deaggregation of the antigen, tolerance ensues instead. Antigens which are difficult for lysosomal enzymes to degrade, including pneumococcal capsular polysaccharide and polymers of D-amino acids such as the capsular protein of *Bacillus anthracis*, are also able to produce tolerance efficiently at low doses in adults. (Pneumococcal polysaccharides stimulate an antibody response at doses even lower than those which produce tolerance.)

Surprisingly, normal adults can be tolerised by very low (sub-immunogenic) as well as very high doses of proteins such as foreign albumins and globulins. Mitchison was the first to demonstrate the existence of two dosage zones of tolerance induction; doses between the high and low extremes led to antibody formation. In his experiments, mice were injected repeatedly with bovine serum albumin (BSA) in solution at different doses and subsequently subjected to a standard immunisation procedure or 'challenge' with BSA in Freund's adjuvant, which would normally lead to anti-BSA production. At doses of about 1 µg or above 1 mg per mouse, tolerance to BSA was established, while intermediate doses led to antibody formation (Figure 2.50.) The tolerant states induced by the two extreme dose ranges are called *low zone* and *high zone* tolerance respectively. The discovery of the two zones of tolerance proved to be very important in understanding the cellular basis of tolerance and its breakdown in autoimmunity, as described below.

Cellular basis of tolerance

According to the clonal selection theory (p. 103), tolerance results from the death of antigen-sensitive cells (*clonal elimination*). Self-tolerance is envisaged as being the result of purging all self-reactive lymphocytes from the system at an early stage by contact with self molecules; surviving lymphocytes should therefore be responsive only to non-self (foreign) antigens. For some antigens, including those recognised in transplantation reactions, clonal elimination seems to be the true basis of tolerance. However, the discovery of two types of lymphocyte (T cells and B cells) with

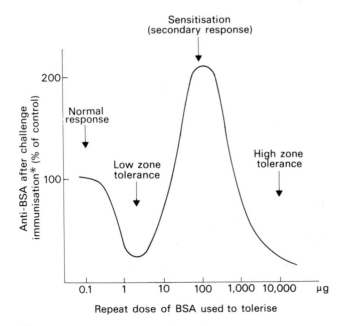

Figure 2.50 High and low zone tolerance to BSA in mice.

Groups of mice were injected repeatedly with different doses of BSA in solution, then given a single 'challenge' immunisation of BSA in Freund's adjuvant. Anti-BSA production was measured a few days later. Note the two zones of tolerance separated by a zone of increased (i.e. secondary) response.

*with BSA in Freund's adjuvant

specialised functions brought to light additional complexities in relation to tolerance. For example, the antibody response to many antigens is dependent on the interaction of T and B cells, as described on p. 110. Theoretically, therefore, functional tolerance could result from elimination of either T cells or B cells or both, for a particular antigen. It appears that T cells are more readily and permanently tolerised than B cells and that for at least some self molecules, tolerance is 'T cell tolerance' only. Thus, it has been found that low zone tolerance to protein antigens involves unresponsiveness of the T cells only, whereas in high zone tolerance both T and B cells are rendered inactive (Figure 2.51a–c). The overall result for the animal is the same, namely lack of antibody production; the important difference is that in low zone tolerance, potentially reactive B cells are still present in the animal. The triggering of those B cells provides a possible pathway to the *breakage of tolerance*, and hence induction of

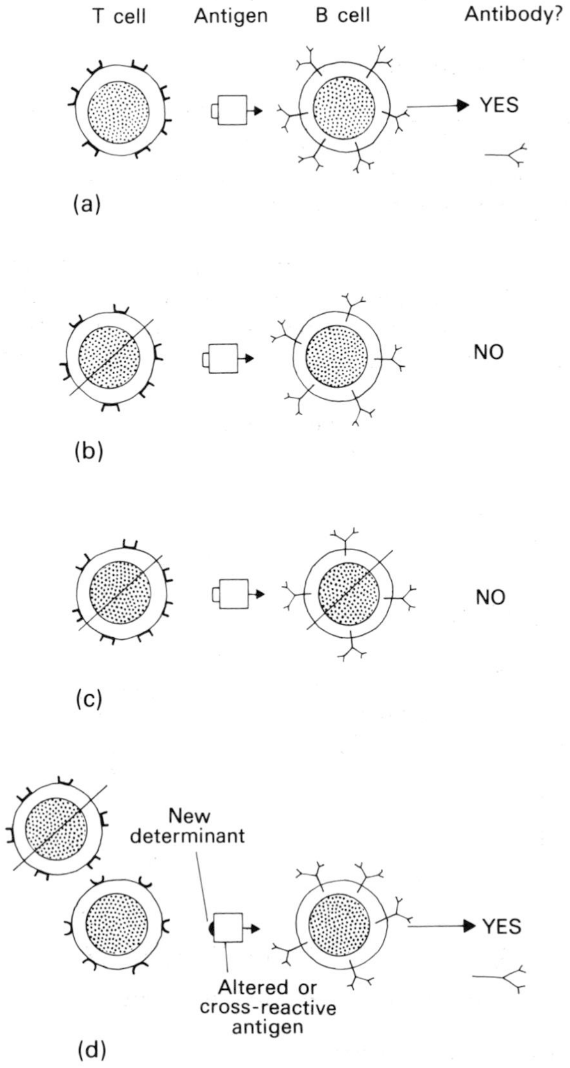

Figure 2.51 Cellular basis of tolerance.
(a) Normal T cell–B cell cooperation.
(b) Low zone (T cell) tolerance.
(c) High zone (T and B cell) tolerance.
(d) Breakage of low zone tolerance by bypass of tolerant T cells.

antibodies to some self antigens, i.e. autoimmunity. In order to break low zone tolerance, it should be sufficient partially to alter the tolerated antigen, introducing a few new determinants while leaving others unaltered. As Figure 2.51d shows, tolerant T cells are thereby effectively bypassed: helper T cells are available to recognise the new (i.e. non-tolerated) carrier determinants on the molecule and stimulate antibody production by B cells. Note that the antibodies produced by breakdown of tolerance in this way will react with the *native*, unaltered molecule. Experimentally, low zone tolerance to BSA can indeed by broken by injection of cross-reacting albumins of different species. A clinically relevant example is the breakdown of natural tolerance in rabbits to the thyroid protein thyroglobulin by the injection of thyroglobulin altered by conjugation with sulphanilic acid. The rabbits respond by production of an autoantibody which binds to the animals' own native thyroglobulin and leads to a destructive autoimmune inflammation of the thyroid (thyroiditis) which resembles *Hashimoto's disease* in man (p. 197). The breakdown of natural tolerance by partial alteration of self molecules is of importance in autoimmunity in man; the bypassing of tolerant helper T cells may also explain why certain bacteria such as group A streptococci, which cross-react antigenically with some human tissues, induce formation of autoantibodies in diseases such as *rheumatic fever* (p. 192).

In some cases, tolerance is caused by an active *suppression* of the immune response by suppressor T cells (p. 116) rather than by elimination of specific antigen-sensitive clones. This is indicated by the successful transfer of tolerance from one animal to another with T lymphocytes. Suppressor T cells produce nonspecific as well as antigen-specific factors (not antibodies) which can maintain a state of permanent suppression. In one important animal model, self-tolerance appears to depend on suppressor T cells rather than on clonal elimination; here the decline in T cell activity with ageing is accompanied by the appearance of auto-immune disorders resembling some seen in man. The animals belong to strains of mouse called New Zealand Black (NZB) and New Zealand White (NZW); the former develop a spontaneous haemolytic anaemia, while the hybrids (NZB × NZW) suffer from a murine equivalent of systemic lupus erythematosus (SLE) with production of autoantibodies against DNA. It is possible that the increase in autoantibody production in man which occurs with age is also due to some falling off in the regulation of the antibody response by T cells.

Finally, we should note that for some tissue-specific molecules, tolerance may not in fact exist. The lack of response against self can result equally well if the relevant antigens are inaccessible to lymphocytes as by elimination or suppression of reactive cells. Many tissue antigens probably never make contact with lymphocytes, either because of tissue/blood barriers as in the nervous system, or because of lack of vascularisation, as for the cornea and lens of the eye, or because of an intracellular localisation. Tissue damage by external agents, accompanied by inflammation, may lead to the first contact between the antigen and the immune system and is then more likely to produce auto-immunity than tolerance. Antigens which are targets for auto-immune disease and which may be revealed to the immune system in this way include the basic protein of myelin; the glomerular and lung basement membrane; intraocular proteins; spermatozoal antigens; acetylcholine receptors; islet cell, thyroid, stomach and adrenal cell cytoplasmic antigens; and nucleic acids, mitochondria and microsomes (see Table 2.3). On the other hand, for antigens present in the circulation, such as those on the surfaces of leucocytes and red cells and on proteins such as immunoglobulins or thyroglobulin, a breakdown of natural tolerance must occur in autoimmunity. Specific examples of the processes involved are discussed below.

AUTOIMMUNITY

Immunological responses against self take the forms both of antibody production and cell-mediated immunity. Since *autoanti-bodies* (i.e. antibodies reacting with self molecules) are readily detected by serological examination or tissue staining techniques (p. 137), a great deal more is known about their occurrence, both in health and disease, than about T cell responses against body components. Table 2.3 is a summary of the antigens against which autoreactive antibodies are found in various clinical conditions and in the following pages some of the processes by which such antibodies may arise are described. The association of autoantibodies with a particular disease does not necessarily provide information on the role which they may play in patho-genesis. Many autoantibodies, though very useful diagnostically, may play no part at all in pathogenesis, being secondary to pathological changes in the tissues, while others are directly involved in cell damage and complex-mediated hypersensitivity; still others appear in normal individuals or in chronic diseases where they appear to cause no harmful effect. In many autoimmune diseases, cell-mediated reactions are as important, if not more so, than damage by antibody.

It is possible to distinguish two major categories in auto-immune disorders, namely those reactions and pathological changes which are *organ-specific* and those which are *non-organ-specific*. The former are exemplified by disorders of, *inter alia*, the thyroid, stomach, adrenals, blood cells and skin, and involve antigens specific for the organ or tissue in which the disease occurs. The non-organ-specific disorders, which include *systemic lupus erythematosus* (SLE) and *rheumatoid arthritis*, involve immune reactions against antigens which are either normally present in or released into the circulation, such as IgG or DNA, or widely distributed in tissues. The lesions of this class are not restricted to any single organ and are often associated with connective tissue. Some disorders occupy an intermediate position in which the effects are localised to a single organ, but the autoantibodies are non-organ-specific, e.g. primary biliary cirrhosis, where the antibodies are against mitochondrial antigens but the disease is localised to the bile duct.

Table 2.3 Self antigens in autoimmunity.

Antigen	Disease
(a) *Soluble, circulating*	
Immunoglobulin (IgG)	Rheumatoid arthritis, SLE, Sjögren's disease, scleroderma
Thyroglobulin	Hashimoto's thyroiditis, thyrotoxicosis
Clotting factors	SLE
Complement (C3b)	Rheumatoid arthritis
(b) *Soluble, non-circulating*	
Intrinsic factor	Pernicious anaemia
(c) *Cell surfaces (excl. receptors)*	
Erythrocytes	Autoimmune haemolytic anaemia
Platelets	Idiopathic thrombocytopenia
Leucocytes	Idiopathic neutropenia, SLE
Thyroid cells	Thyroiditis, primary myxoedema
Cardiac muscle	Rheumatic fever
Spermatozoa	Infertility
Zona pellucida of ovum	Infertility
(d) *Cell surface receptors*	
TSH receptor	Thyrotoxicosis
Acetylcholine receptor	Myasthenia gravis
Insulin receptor	Insulin-resistant diabetes
(e) *Extracellular*	
Salivary gland ducts	Sjögren's disease
Glomerular and alveolar basement membrane	Goodpasture's syndrome
Epidermal basement membrane	Bullous pemphigoid
Desmosomes	Pemphigus vulgaris
Reticulin	Coeliac disease
(f) *Intracellular*	
Nucleic acid, nucleoprotein	SLE, rheumatoid arthritis
Mitochondria	Primary biliary cirrhosis, Sjögren's disease
Microsomes	Thyroiditis, pernicious anaemia
Thyroid colloid	Thyroiditis
Adrenal cytoplasm	Addison's disease
Islet cell cytoplasm	Juvenile diabetes, polyendocrine syndrome of females
Skeletal muscle A-band (actin, myosin)	Myasthenia gravis
Smooth muscle (actin)	Active chronic hepatitis
Cardiolipin	Syphilis, leprosy, malaria

There is frequently a tendency for more than one type of auto-antibody to appear in the same individual and for autoimmune diseases to *overlap*. Thus the organ-specific conditions of the thyroid, stomach, parathyroid, adrenals, ovaries and pancreatic islet cells show a close association, e.g. in the polyendocrine syndrome which occurs especially in young and middle-aged females. There may be shared genetic factors, and an HLA-linkage of autoantibody production against these organs occurs in families. The association between thyroid and stomach auto-immunity is particularly impressive: 30% of patients with

Hashimoto's thyroiditis show antibodies against stomach antigens and conversely, 50% of cases of stomach autoimmunity (pernicious anaemia) have antibodies to thyroid antigens. This overlap occurs even though the antibodies in each case are strictly organ-specific and show no cross-reactivity. Several examples of overlap between non-organ-specific diseases, such as SLE and rheumatoid arthritis, are quoted below. It is interesting that the organ-specific diseases overlap much more among themselves than with non-organ-specific diseases. Thus, Hashimoto's thyroiditis does not usually present with antibodies to DNA or IgG, both of which occur in SLE and rheumatoid arthritis. On the other hand, SLE patients may have antibodies against red cells and leucocytes, thyroglobulin (though without thyroiditis) and muscle elements as in myasthenia gravis.

Familial predisposition often plays a significant role in autoimmunity. Recently, its genetic basis has been shown in some cases to depend on the HLA gene complex, as indicated by an association of certain autoimmune disorders with particular HLA antigens in the population and a linkage in families. The relationship between HLA and autoimmune disease is discussed below and in Section 7.

Processes involved in formation of autoantibodies

Alteration of self molecules

Changes in the structure of body molecules can have two immunological consequences, namely (i) breakdown of existing tolerance leading to antibody production against the native molecule, and (ii) induction of antibodies against the new antigenic determinants. Both possibilities are seen in autoantibody production. A good example of tolerance breakdown is provided by antibodies to native *thyroglobulin* which are found in the sera of patients with thyroid diseases, particularly *Hashimoto's thyroiditis* and *primary myxoedema*. Thyroglobulin is the storage protein for thyroid hormones (thyroxine and triiodothyronine) in the thyroid follicles and constitutes over 75% of the protein of the colloid. It is not totally sequestered in the gland, but is also present in low concentrations in normal blood and lymph of most individuals. Normally a state of natural tolerance to thyroglobulin exists and is probably confined to T cells; indeed the presence of B cells capable of binding thyroglobulin has been demonstrated. T cell tolerance is sufficient to prevent antibody production, since thyroglobulin is a T-dependent antigen requiring cell cooperation for induction of an antibody response. The injection of normal thyroglobulin into animals, therefore, does not cause autoantibody production. Experimentally, tolerance can be broken, as we have noted above, by injection of thyroglobulin altered by conjugation to sulphanilic acid; the new 'carrier' determinants are recognised by T cells which act as helpers for B cells. The latter are in consequence triggered to antibody production against thyroglobulin determinants as shown in Figure 2.51d. These antibodies, as expected, bind to normal

189

thyroglobulin. A similar course of events may occur in man. The source of altered thyroglobulin in Hashimoto's disease is speculative; it may be that partial degradation of the molecule by lysosomal enzymes reveals new antigenic groups which behave as carrier determinants and stimulate helper T cells. The anti-thyroglobulin antibodies may play a role in the lesions in the thyroid, though the latter are probably mainly the result of a cell-mediated hypersensitivity reaction (p. 197). It is noteworthy that autoantibodies to thyroglobulin are found in 4% of normal individuals, and also occur in unrelated immunological diseases such as SLE where there is no evidence of thyroid disease.

Another important type of autoantibody, the stimulus to which may be an alteration in a body protein, is the *rheumatoid factor* (RF) found in *rheumatoid arthritis*. In this case, the antigen is the IgG molecule itself; rheumatoid factors are therefore *antiglobulins*. RFs are a heterogeneous group of autoantibodies, both with respect to their class and to the antigenic specificities they recognise. Most RFs in serum are IgM molecules, though some are IgG and occasionally even IgA, while in the diseased joints themselves RFs are mainly IgG. The antigens recognised by RFs are present on the Fc piece of IgG. RFs react much more strongly with IgG which has been complexed to an antigen or denatured (aggregated) by heat than with native IgG. This may be because of the possibility of making multivalent attachment to aggregated IgG, hence increasing the binding strength of RF (cf. p. 84); alternatively, the production and binding of RF may depend on an alteration in the Fc region of the IgG molecules following their reaction with an antigen. The latter is shown in Figure 2.52a, though there is little evidence that such Fc conformational changes actually occur. Some of these antigens are genetically determined and present on IgG of some individuals but not others; they are termed *Gm types*. The detection of RFs in serum is by agglutination either of latex particles coated with human IgG, or of sheep red cells complexed with rabbit anti-sheep red cell IgG, the latter being the Rose-Waaler test, p. 134. (Note that, despite the vast excess of free IgG in plasma, the binding sites of RFs are not blocked, because binding to normal IgG is very weak.) The ability of human RFs to react with IgG of different species, such as rabbit, makes the Rose-Waaler test possible. RFs in sera are often in the form of IgM–IgG and IgG–IgG complexes which precipitate from sera held at 4°C; they are therefore called *cryoglobulins*. RFs can be detected at a low level in some normal sera and also appear in some non-rheumatoid diseases such as SLE, subacute bacterial endocarditis and leprosy.

RFs may well play an important role in the pathogenesis of rheumatoid arthritis (p. 207); they can be found in diseased joints, where they initiate immune complex hypersensitivity. A large proportion of the complexes in joints are formed by IgG rheumatoid factors. Here a particularly interesting situation arises in which the RF, being itself an IgG molecule, acts both as antibody and antigen. Figure 2.52b shows how IgG RF molecules can associate with each other: one antigen-combining site of each

Figure 2.52
(a) Possible stages in the
production of rheumatoid factor.
(b) Self-association of two IgG
rheumatoid factor molecules.

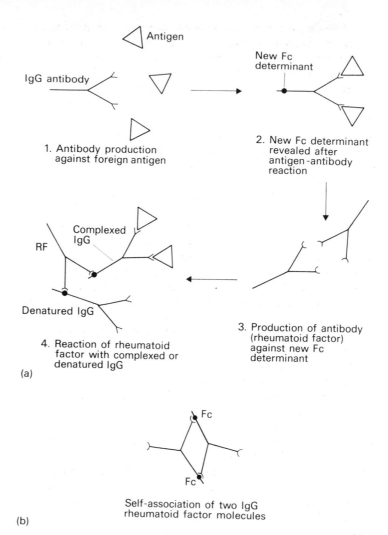

Antigen

IgG antibody

New Fc
determinant

1. Antibody production
against foreign antigen

2. New Fc determinant
revealed after
antigen-antibody
reaction

RF

Complexed
IgG

Denatured IgG

4. Reaction of rheumatoid
factor with complexed or
denatured IgG

3. Production of antibody
(rheumatoid factor)
against new Fc
determinant

(a)

Fc

Fc

Self-association of two IgG
rheumatoid factor molecules

(b)

molecule reacts with a determinant on the Fc region of an
adjacent molecule, to form a cyclic or 'head-bites-tail' structure
which is the first stage in formation of a larger complex. In
diseased joints, such complexes are located both intracellularly
within local RF-synthesizing plasma cells, as well as extracellularly. After release from the cell, the complexes activate complement, hence initiating inflammation (p. 207).

Immunoconglutinin is an autoantibody directed against a complement component, fixed C3 (C3b). This is a further example of
antibody production against new determinants, in this instance
revealed by enzymatic cleavage of C3, rather than a breakdown of
natural tolerance. In general, immunoconglutinin does not react
with the native C3 molecule. It is most frequently encountered in
diseases such as rheumatoid arthritis and chronic cold haemagglutinin disease, where chronic complement fixation occurs as
part of the hypersensitivity reaction.

Another way in which self molecules or cells can be altered
and rendered immunogenic is by conjugation with reactive

191

molecules administered to the body: the metabolic products of drugs are good examples of small reactive chemicals which conjugate readily to body proteins. We have already noted that some drugs induce hypersensitivity reactions by behaving as haptens: antibodies against the drug or one of its metabolites are produced, which then react with cell surfaces to which the hapten has bound and lead to cell damage by complement activation (p. 160). Thus *haemolytic anaemia* may follow penicillin therapy in sensitised individuals, because penicillin products, e.g. penicilloic acid, combine with red cells which thus become the targets of lysis by antipenicilloyl antibodies. In such instances, autoimmunity is not involved because the antibodies are directed towards the hapten, not the native red cell. However, it is also possible for autoantibodies to be induced under similar circumstances. For instance, α-methyldopa, a drug used in treatment of hypertension, induces autoimmune haemolytic anaemia in which antibodies against native red cell rhesus antigens are produced. Tolerance breakdown can again be understood in terms of bypassing tolerant T cells; after forming a complex with the drug or one of its metabolic derivatives, conjugated red cell proteins are recognised by T cells and thus act in effect as carriers for the Rh molecules on the same cell. Other drugs, notably hydralazine, procainamide and practalol compounds, induce an SLE-like syndrome in which autoantibodies against DNA and histone proteins are produced. It is possible that the drug or its products react with DNA and thereby break T cell tolerance in the manner already described.

Cross-reactive antigens introduced from the outside

Autoantibodies can be induced in response to foreign antigens which are cross-reactive (i.e. show antigenic resemblance) with body components. The best examples are provided by cross-reactivity between bacterial antigens and human tissues. In *rheumatic fever*, antibodies formed against *Streptococcus pyogenes* react with human heart because of similarities between antigens in the streptococcal wall and determinants present on cardiac muscle cells and heart valves (Figure 2.53). Thus antistreptococcal antibodies include autoantibodies against the heart which, by activating complement, initiate an inflammatory reaction (carditis, valvulitis) leading to damage to the heart valves and even heart failure. There may be permanent residual heart damage in the form of mitral stenosis. After elimination of the streptococci, autoantibody production ceases, but may recur on further streptococcal infection or even surgical manipulation of the heart. Autoantibody production in rheumatic fever may represent a breakdown of tolerance by mechanisms outlined above, namely presentation of antigens resembling self on the foreign streptococcal carrier (Figure 2.53). Equally, it is possible that true tolerance to cardiac muscle does not exist and that infection with streptococci represents the first occasion on which heart muscle antigens are 'seen' by lymphocytes. (For further discussion of the immunological hypothesis of heart damage in rheumatic fever,

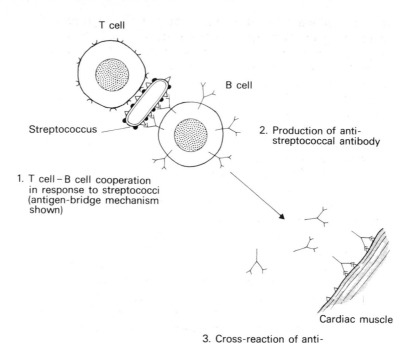

T cell

B cell

Streptococcus

2. Production of anti-
   streptococcal antibody

1. T cell – B cell cooperation
   in response to streptococci
   (antigen-bridge mechanism
   shown)

Cardiac muscle

3. Cross-reaction of antistreptococcal antibody
   with cardiac muscle

Figure 2.53 Cross-reaction between antistreptococcal antibodies and heart antigens in rheumatic fever.

see p. 504). Another example of bacterial cross-reactivity with human tissue antigens is found in *ulcerative colitis*, where autoantibodies against the colon cross-react with *Escherichia coli* O14.

Antigens revealed by tissue damage

We have noted that some tissue-specific antigens are unlikely ever to come into contact with the immune system, due to intracellular sequestration in tissue cells or because of blood-tissue barriers. When tissue damage occurs, perhaps through bacterial or viral infection, such tissue components make contact with lymphocytes for the first time and an autoimmune response ensues. This may account for the success in producing autoimmune disorders experimentally in animals by injection of extracts of normal tissues, such as testis, brain, liver, adrenals, etc. An adjuvant, such as Freund's (p. 80), is required to induce the autoimmune response. While some tissue components may have become altered and hence immunogeneic by this procedure, others are probably being presented to the immune system for the first time. Clinically, it is likely that responses against intracellular components such as microsomes and mitochondria, against the cytoplasmic antigens of pancreatic islet cells and adrenal cortex cells, or against myelin and sperm (Table 2.3) arise after the antigens have been made accessible following tissue damage.

Autoantibodies in infectious diseases

Chronic infectious diseases, particularly those involving granulomatous inflammation, are frequently accompanied by the presence of autoantibodies in the blood. A classic example is the *Wassermann antibody* found in syphilitics, the detection of which is one of the important diagnostic tests in this disease. This antibody reacts with an antigen known as *cardiolipin*, present in extracts of heart muscle (and other tissues); cardiolipin is a lipid component of mitochondrial membranes (diphosphatidyl glycerol). The antibody is not thought to play an active role in the disease. Besides its characteristic appearance in syphilis, the Wassermann antibody is sometimes found in other diseases, such as leprosy, malaria, hepatitis, pneumonia, glandular fever and SLE, and this can be a cause of false-positive reactions in testing for syphilis (see p. 618). Rheumatoid factor can also be found in about 10% of syphilitic patients.

Other chronic granulomatous diseases in which autoantibodies occur are lepromatous leprosy and chronic tuberculosis. In the former, antibodies are produced against thyroglobulin, IgG (rheumatoid factor), cardiolipin (Wassermann) and DNA (antinuclear factor, p. 204); a wide range is also detected in sera of patients with tuberculosis. It is assumed that many of these antibodies are a result of nonspecific stimulation of the antibody response, an explanation which is especially plausible in the case of mycobacterial infections. The adjuvant properties of these organisms are well known and exploited in complete Freund's adjuvant (p. 80). Indeed, to induce autoimmunity experimentally, organ extracts are commonly administered together with this adjuvant. Many normal individuals have low levels of serum autoantibodies (below), and it is these which are raised in chronic bacterial diseases.

Occurrence of autoantibodies in normal sera

It should be noted that a wide range of autoantibodies occurs in low concentration in the circulation of normal individuals, apparently without harmful effects. The occurrence of these 'natural' autoantibodies increases with age; as in many other autoimmune phenomena, there is a strong female predominance. About 30% of women over 60 years of age possess antibodies to one or more of several antigens, including rheumatoid factors, antinuclear factors, and antibodies against thyroid, adrenal or gastric cells or intracellular organelles such as microsomes and mitochondria. These antibodies may in fact serve a useful function, namely to assist as opsonins in the removal of debris of dead cells when large numbers of cells have been destroyed. The increase in autoantibody level with ageing may reflect a decline in regulatory controls which keep autoimmune responses in check, especially suppressor T cells. The extent and rate at which such suppressor activity declines may determine the tendency in the individual to autoimmune diseases, a tendency in which there is sometimes a genetic predisposition. Note, however, that most autoimmune diseases occur in early and middle life, rather than old age. Control of suppression may be one mode of action of the HLA-linked genes which are involved in some autoimmune phenomena, as discussed elsewhere (p. 206).

Mechanisms of autoimmune tissue damage

Autoreactivity, in the forms of autoantibody production and sensitisation of T cells against self, can lead to tissue damage by the processes of hypersensitivity already described (p. 152 ff.). The mechanisms are (a) reaction of autoantibodies with cell surfaces, producing either a cytotoxic effect, blockade of cell receptors or, in one case, stimulation of cellular secretion (Type II hypersensitivity); (b) reaction of autoantibodies with excess soluble antigen to produce soluble complexes which lead to tissue damaging inflammation initiated by complement fixation in and around blood vessels (Type III); and (c) cell-mediated tissue damage (Type IV). In short, all hypersensitivity mechanisms are represented with the exception of anaphylaxis. The organ-specific disorders involve either Type II or Type IV mechanisms; Type III hypersensitivity is characteristic of non-organ-specific conditions, though cell-mediated mechanisms are important in these as well.

DIRECT EFFECTS OF AUTOANTIBODIES

Cytotoxicity or opsonisation of target cells

(i) *Blood cells* Destruction of blood cells by autoantibodies provides the best example of autoimmune cytotoxicity. The targets are red cells in autoimmune haemolytic anaemias, platelets in idiopathic thrombocytopenia, and occasionally leucocytes (autoimmune leucopenia).

In the *autoimmune haemolytic anaemias*, autoantibodies reacting with red cell antigens may cause haemolysis by fixing complement at the red cell surface; however, the anaemia is more often due to *opsonisation*, i.e. uptake of red cells coated with antibody and complement by macrophages of the spleen and liver. The antibody can be of the IgM or IgG class. An interesting phenomenon associated with these antibodies is an unusual division into 'warm' and 'cold', the former reacting better with red cells at 37°C than in the cold, while the latter react best at low temperatures and may elute at 37°C. The IgM antibodies are frequently *cold agglutinins* and cause visible agglutination of the patient's red cells if the blood is cooled below 28–32°C. They account for a quarter of the cases of autoimmune haemolytic anaemia. Red cell destruction only occurs if parts of the body are cooled to about 20°C, which is easily achieved in the skin; the IgM causes C1 and C4 complement components to fix to the red cells in the cold periphery and, as the blood returns to 37°C in the general circulation, further complement components attach to the red cell membrane. Although the IgM itself may then elute, enough C3 is fixed to facilitate removal of red cells by macrophages and there is also significant intravascular haemolysis.

There is one case of a cold IgG anti-red cell antibody, called the *Donath–Landsteiner* antibody; it reacts with red cells in the cold, but elutes from them at 37°C. This antibody is particularly associated with tertiary syphilis and is also a rare complication of virus infections (idiopathic cases also exist). It causes a syndrome called *paroxysmal cold haemoglobinuria*. As with the IgM cold agglutinins, reaction with red cells *in vivo* takes place when the patient is exposed to cold; after an interval of a few minutes to several hours, the symptoms which follow appear on rewarming and include the passage of dark urine, uncontrollable shivering (rigors) and backache. They are due to massive intravascular haemolysis which follows complement fixation (note the difference with IgM agglutinins and warm antibodies which cause much less lysis in the circulation). The paroxysmal attack usually lasts for a few hours, after which the anaemic patient may become jaundiced and the spleen enlarges due to uptake of red cells. As in cold haemagglutinin disease (above) the symptoms are worse during winter months. Most IgG anti-red cell antibodies, in contrast, react better at 37°C than in the cold and are called *warm antibodies*. They do not directly agglutinate red cells, but can be demonstrated by the antiglobulin (Coombs) test (p. 133). The majority of patients with autoimmune haemolytic anaemia have this type of antibody. Once again, opsonisation is the chief cause of anaemia, though complement is fixed and can cause haemolysis.

Red cell autoantibodies are directed against blood group antigens on the patient's red cells. The IgG warm antibodies often have anti-rhesus specificity, while IgM cold agglutinins react with antigens called big 'I' and little 'i'. The Donath-Landsteiner antibody is directed against the P red cell antigens. Autoimmune haemolytic anaemias are *primary* (idiopathic) in about two thirds of cases and *secondary* to other diseases in the remainder. The association of Donath–Landsteiner antibody with syphilis has been noted. Infection with *Mycoplasma pneumoniae* (primary atypical pneumonia) is a cause of appearance of IgM agglutinins, which are also found in viral pneumonia, glandular fever, infective hepatitis and some malignant lymphomas. Warm autoantibodies are seen in chronic lymphocytic leukaemia, SLE, chronic active hepatitis and Hodgkin's disease. The α-methyl-dopa-induced haemolytic anaemia is of this type also. In most cases, the reasons for autosensitisation against red cells are obscure though there is often major pathology or malignancy in the lymphoid system. It is worth noting that autoantibodies to red cells are present at low concentrations in many normal sera.

Idiopathic thrombocytopenic purpura is a disease caused by destruction of platelets by a specific antiplatelet antibody. Coating with antibody leads to removal of platelets by phagocytic cells in the liver and spleen. This disease is discussed more fully in Section 5 (p. 638). IgG antiplatelet antibodies can cross the placenta and cause thrombocytopenia in the newborn. Leucocyte-reactive autoantibodies are found in some children with polymorph deficiency who suffer from defective immunity to bacterial infection as a result (agranulocytosis, neutropenia). Such antibodies may also occur in SLE.

(ii) *Thyroid* Some antibodies against thyroid antigens are cytotoxic for thyroid cells *in vitro* and are found in the sera of patients with *Hashimoto's thyroiditis*. They are distinct from the antithyroglobulin antibodies and react with thyroid epithelium microsomes. However, it is unlikely that antibodies play the main role in the aetiology of thyroiditis. The histological features of infiltration by lymphocytes and macrophages, with replacement of the typical glandular thyroid structure by lymphoid tissue, are strongly indicative of cell-mediated hypersensitivity. Further, the mere presence of antibody in the circulation does not lead to the disease, for example in babies born to mothers with Hashimoto's disease. Experimentally, an autoallergic thyroiditis resembling that of man can be induced in animals by immunisation with thyroid tissue in adjuvant. This disease cannot be transferred with serum, but has been transferred with lymphocytes. Thus, thyroiditis is likely to be a 'T cell disease' with antibodies playing a secondary role, if any.

(iii) *Spermatozoa* Antibodies against spermatozoal antigens cause sperm agglutination and are present in some infertile males. Agglutination and immobilisation of sperm in the ejaculate prevent them from penetrating the cervical mucus. The level of agglutinins in the seminal fluid does not always correlate with that in serum and there may be some local production of IgA antibodies in the genital tract. Serum IgM agglutinins will not enter the seminal fluid, though IgG does. Spermagglutinins may also be a cause of female infertility. It seems that the local sperm stimulus can provoke antibody production in the female with both serum antibody and local secretion in cervical mucus. Spermagglutinins have been found in a number of women with otherwise unexplained infertility.

Reaction of antibodies against cell surface receptors

Autoantibodies which bind to receptors for hormones or transmitter substances inhibit the reaction of physiological ligands with cell surfaces. Sometimes the antibody mimics the action of the normal ligand, as in the case of thyroid-stimulating antibodies in thyrotoxicosis; elsewhere antibodies abolish the activity of the receptors, as exemplified by inhibition of acetylcholine receptors in myasthenia gravis.

(i) *Thyroid. Thyrotoxicosis (Graves's disease, hyperthyroidism)* is a disease in which the thyroid hormones are secreted excessively, raising the body metabolic rate; characteristic symptoms are nervousness, restless overactivity, tremor, weight loss, heat sensitivity and exophthalmos (protrusion of the eyeballs). Despite the difference in clinical symptoms from thyroiditis, where the association is with hypothyroidism, lymphoid infiltration of the gland and production of antithyroglobulin occur in both. The reason for the overactivity of the thyroid in thyrotoxicosis lies in the production of autoantibodies unique to this disease which stimulate thyroxine secretion by thyroid cells. The first thyroid-stimulating antibody (TSAb) to be discovered was the 'long-acting thyroid stimulator' (LATS), so called because its stimulation of the thyroid was considerably prolonged in comparison with the thyroid-stimulating hormone (TSH) produced by the pituitary gland. TSH, the physiological thyroid stimulator, acts via TSH receptors on the surface of the thyroid epithelial cells; TSH binding leads to intracellular production of cyclic AMP, which triggers release of stored thyroxine. LATS is an IgG antibody which also reacts with the TSH receptor and stimulates thyroxine secretion by the same pathway as TSH. LATS is able to stimulate the thyroid cells of different species. Its presence in thyrotoxic serum is assayed by injection of the serum into mice, followed by measurement of the release of radioactive iodine (^{131}I) from prelabelled mouse thyroid. Good evidence that LATS is the immediate cause of thyrotoxicosis is the transient hyperthyroidism produced in babies born to mothers with the disease, which lasts as long as maternal IgG persists in the infants' circulation. A finding which suggested that there was another cause of the same disease was the absence of LATS from at least 40% of thyrotoxic patients. However, it has now been discovered that LATS-negative patients possess a different TSAb, which does not react in the standard assay in mice. The second type of TSAb is specific for human thyroid and is present in all patients; it also reacts with the TSH receptor, prevents TSH binding and stimulates thyroxine release.

(ii) *Muscle* Another example of autoantibody production against a receptor molecule, with direct involvement in pathogenesis, occurs in *myasthenia gravis*. Here the antibodies interfere with neuromuscular transmission by binding to acetylcholine receptors of the motor endplate. The characteristic feature of myasthenia is the easy fatiguability of certain groups of voluntary muscles upon repetitive use; the muscles return to function with rest or administration of appropriate drugs and do not often atrophy. Weakness of the orbital muscles causes a typical diplopia (double vision) and ptosis (drooping of the eyelids); other muscle groups affected are those of the jaw, respiratory system, neck, shoulder and hip. Some cases are rapidly fatal due to respiratory failure, while in others the life-span is little affected. In addition to muscular weakness, there are frequently pathological changes in the *thymus*, with hyperplasia in 65% of patients, while in 10% of cases a thymoma is present. The close involvement of the thymus with myasthenia is also shown by the significant clinical improvement in the muscular symptoms afforded by thymectomy.

The fundamental changes leading to muscle weakness in myasthenia gravis are in neuromuscular transmission; the disease has been treated for over 40 years with anticholinesterases, drugs which prolong the activity of acetylcholine (ACh) at the neuromuscular junction. The deficiency in myasthenia occurs on the postsynaptic side of the neuromuscular junction, the amount of ACh released at the presynaptic surface being normal (Figure 2.54). Electrophysiological recordings show that the miniature end-plate potentials at the motor end-plate are smaller than normal, and ultrastructural investigations reveal severe degeneration of the postsynaptic folds and loss of the normally close apposition of pre- and postsynaptic surfaces. Most significant, however, is the decrease in the number of postsynaptic ACh receptor sites, which average 80% below normal.

The *ACh receptor* itself seems to be the principal target of autoimmune attack in myasthenia. Antibodies to the ACh receptor protein have been demonstrated in over 80% of patients, both in serum and bound to the postsynaptic clefts of biopsied muscle, but not in normal subjects or patients with other neuromuscular diseases. Furthermore, myasthenic sera can produce transmission defects if injected into mice and reduce the sensitivity of human muscle cells to ACh in tissue culture. The aetiological role of the antireceptor antibodies has been strongly suggested by the development of an animal model for myasthenia induced by active immunisation with the receptor protein (experimental autoallergic myasthenia gravis, EAMG). A considerable breakthrough was achieved with the isolation of purified ACh receptors from the electric organ of electric fish, which has the structure of a large motor end-plate. This was accomplished using the venom of a snake, *Bungarus multicinctus*; α-bungarotoxin binds specifically to the ACh receptor protein and can be used to isolate the receptors from electric organs of the eel *Electrophorus electricus* or the ray *Torpedo californica*. Immunisation of several species, including mice, rats, rabbits and monkeys, with the purified receptor protein leads to muscular symptoms which resemble myasthenia in man. The degeneration of the postsynaptic clefts is similar to that seen in the human disease. Antibodies to the ACh receptor appear in the animals' sera and can be used to transfer the disease passively to normal animals. Recently, highly specific monoclonal antibodies against the ACh receptor have also been shown to produe passive EAMG, which would

Figure 2.54 The neuromuscular junction.

Acetylcholine is released from vesicles at the release sites on the presynaptic surface and reacts with acetylcholine receptors on the postsynaptic surface. Acetylcholinesterase in the clefts hydrolyses acetylcholine. The acetylcholine receptors are the target of antibody attack in myasthenia gravis. (After Drachman 1978).

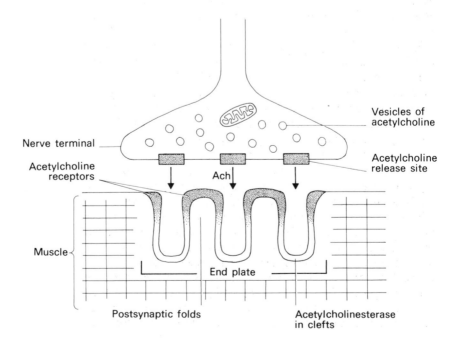

seem to put the role of antibody in this disease beyond doubt. The production of myasthenia by antibody could be via blocking of ACh receptors, complement-mediated membrane damage, or acceleration of receptor degradation.

It should be noted that other autoantibodies are also found in myasthenic sera: antibodies reacting with the A bands of striated muscle occur in many patients and can be identified by immuno-fluorescent staining of muscle. Lymphocytic infiltration of the muscle also occurs, suggesting a cell-mediated reaction. However, the evidence so far, including the occurrence of neonatal myasthenia and improvement after plasmapheresis, indicates that humoral immunity is the more important.

The aspects of the disease which have not been reproduced experimentally in EAMG are those of the thymus; thymic changes are probably involved in the initiation of myasthenia in man, but not in the effector phase which is induced in EAMG. The origins of autosensitisation against the ACh receptor are indeed as yet obscure; they seem to involve the thymus and have a genetic basis. The beneficial effects of thymectomy have been noted above; there is immediate transient remission in most patients and 30% stable remissions within one year. These changes occur too rapidly to be accounted for by depletion of the long-lived pool of recirculating thymocytes. The level of autoanti-bodies is also substantially lower after thymectomy. It has therefore been suggested that the thymus is the source of antigen in myasthenia. Thymus cells possess ACh receptors and might express them in immunogenic (? altered) form during thymic disease. The genetic influence is shown by a familial predis-position in 5% of cases and an association in the population with HLA antigens (p. 878). Individuals carrying the HLA-B8 antigen have an approximately 40-fold increased risk of developing myasthenia over the rest of the population. Mice appear to show a similar genetic susceptibility to EAMG controlled by the H-2 complex. It may be that the association with HLA in man is due to genetic control of the type or level of the antibody made to the ACh receptor protein. In common with several other auto-immune disorders, myasthenia shows a higher incidence in females than males.

Antibodies against active secreted molecules: pernicious anaemia

Antibodies which inhibit a biologically active secreted molecule are found in *pernicious* (*Addisonian*) *anaemia*, an anaemia which results from insufficient uptake of vitamin B_{12} by the stomach. The underlying condition is a chronic inflammation of the stomach mucosa (*atrophic gastritis*) in which the mucosa atrophies and hydrochloric acid and pepsin fail to be produced due to destruction of parietal and chief cells. The normal absorption of vitamin B_{12} depends on a mucoprotein called *intrinsic factor*, secreted by the parietal cells of the gastric mucosa. Intrinsic factor in the gastric juice binds vitamin B_{12} specifically and the complex is then absorbed by the intestinal epithelium. In pernicious anaemia the destruction of parietal cells reduces the amount of

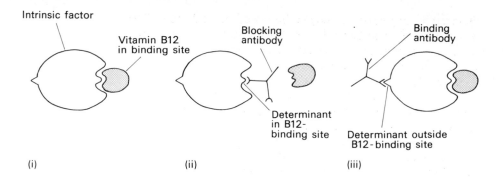

Intrinsic factor

Vitamin B12 in binding site

Blocking antibody

Binding antibody

Determinant in B12- binding site

Determinant outside B12-binding site

(i)   (ii)   (iii)

Figure 2.55 Autoantibodies against intrinsic factor.

intrinsic factor available in the stomach. In addition, autoantibodies against intrinsic factor are present in the serum and, more importantly, in the gastric juice itself. The antibodies are of two types. The commonest (*blocking antibodies*) react with the binding site for vitamin B_{12} on intrinsic factor and prevent the combination of vitamin B_{12} with the factor, while others found more rarely (*binding antibodies*) react with intrinsic factor but do not prevent vitamin B_{12} binding. There are, therefore, two antigenic determinants (at least) on the intrinsic factor, one of which is in or close to the vitamin B_{12}-binding site, while the other is elsewhere on the molecule (Figure 2.55). The second type of antibody might prevent uptake of the B_{12}-factor complex by the intestinal mucosa.

Antibodies against intrinsic factor are only part of the autoimmune response in this disease. Another antibody reacts with the parietal cells themselves, which are responsible for production of hydrochloric acid as well as intrinsic factor. The anti-parietal cell antibody reacts with microsomal rather than surface antigens and it has not been shown to be toxic for parietal cells. Atrophy of the gastric mucosa probably results from a combination of the action of the parietal cell autoantibodies and specifically sensitised T cells. The mucosa is infiltrated with lymphoid tissue containing germinal centres indicative of local antibody production as well as cell-mediated hypersensitivity. Antibodies against intrinsic factor, when present in the gastric juice, would accelerate the development of anaemia by inhibiting factor produced by surviving parietal cells.

One of the interesting features of autoimmune stomach disease is its overlap with organ-specific autoimmune disorders, particularly of the thyroid and adrenals. The thyroid association, as already noted, is especially striking: about 10% of patients with thyroiditis have pernicious anaemia and up to half have antibodies against intrinsic factor or parietal cells. Similarly, up to 30% of pernicious anaemia patients have levels of thyroid antibodies indicative of active thyroiditis. Indeed, there are also parallels in the courses of the diseases themselves. In both there is production of autoantibodies against a strictly organ-specific secreted product (intrinsic factor, thyroglobulin) and, in addition, antibodies to organ-specific microsomal antigens. In both atrophic gastritis and thyroiditis the organ is infiltrated with lymphocytes, plasma cells and macrophages, and there is frequent appearance of germinal centres in the organ with destruction of specific secretory cells. Finally, both diseases are more common in females than males and show a familial incidence. The overlap of these disorders is suggestive of shared aetiological factors, one of which may be a common genetic predisposition.

Antibodies reacting with non-circulating extracellular antigen: glomerular basement membrane (GBM)

Damage to the kidney can be produced by autoantibodies reacting with extracellular connective tissue of the basement membrane. Anti-GBM antibodies are one of two pathways to immunological renal damage, the other and more common being deposition of antigen–antibody complexes from the circulation (as described on p. 160). Only about 5% of all cases of *glomerulonephritis* are caused by anti-GBM antibodies. The basement membrane is an important structural element in the glomerulus. It is in contact with the fenestrated endothelium of the glomerular capillary on one side and on the other with the foot processes of the epithelial cells which line the glomerular cavity. Proteins are free to pass though the fenestrae of the endothelium; the basement membrane prevents passage of proteins of molecular weights over about 65,000 (including albumin), while filtration of smaller proteins depends on slits between the foot processes resting on the basement membrane. Inflammatory reactions initiated at the basement membrane lead to proteinuria and eventually to renal failure. The basement membrane is composed of collagen and non-collagenous proteins; the latter are the antigens with which anti-GBM antibodies react. The antibodies become attached to the basement membrane as a uniform linear deposit which can be demonstrated by immunofluorescence using anti-human IgG conjugated to a fluorescent dye (p. 137 and Figure 2.39). It is important to note the difference between the fluorescence pattern seen in glomerulonephritis caused by anti-GBM antibodies and that which results from trapping of immune complexes. Complex deposition appears as an irregular granular deposit along the basement membrane (usually on the epithelial side) and individual deposits are often distinct enough to be counted, the so-called lumpy-bumpy distribution (Figure 2.39b).

Anti-GBM antibodies are a direct cause of renal damage, either as a result of complement-mediated inflammation or by direct binding of neutrophils to the Fc regions of antibodies attached to the basement membrane. The adherent neutrophils can displace the endothelial lining and penetrate the GBM. Release of lysosomal enzymes from neutrophils is an important cause of glomerular damage. The glomerulonephritis is generally severe and rapidly leads to fatal renal failure. The causative role of anti-GBM antibodies has been confirmed by eluting antibodies from the kidneys of patients and passively transferring the disease with them to monkeys. Similarly, experimental glomerulonephritis can be produced in animals by active immunisation with

GBM and the sera of such animals will transfer the disease to normal animals, a model known as nephrotoxic serum nephritis. In man, anti-GBM antibodies appear in a condition known as *Goodpasture's syndrome*, where in addition to renal disease there occurs pulmonary haemorrhage caused by antibodies reacting with the alveolar basement membrane. Goodpasture's syndrome occurs in half the cases of renal damage by anti-GBM antibodies. The antibodies responsible for lung and kidney damage appear to be the same. The mortality in patients with this unusual syndrome is high, death being due to uraemia or pulmonary haemorrhage. The original stimulus to production of the autoantibody against basement membrane is obscure; in Goodpasture's syndrome it may be a viral infection such as influenza, or inhalation of noxious substances such as hydrocarbon solvents.

TISSUE DAMAGE BY ANTIGEN–ANTIBODY COMPLEXES

Type III hypersensitivity, mediated by antigen–antibody complexes and complement, is characteristic of the non-organ-specific autoimmune disorders, the presence in the circulation of complexes containing autoantibodies being associated with inflammation in several tissues. Several of these disorders are classified together as *connective tissue diseases*, because they affect the tissues containing collagen, reticulin and elastin fibres, including cartilage and bone. However, the lesions are focal, joints and vessels being frequently affected. A characteristic connective tissue lesion is *fibrinoid necrosis*, consisting of an increase in ground substance with swollen, fragmented collagen fibres and necrosis, resulting in a structureless eosinophilic area resembling fibrin in appearance. (Fibrinoid necrosis is not exclusive to this group of diseases but is also seen in small arterioles in malignant hypertension, p. 675, and other conditions.) The main diseases involving autoimmunity in the connective tissue group are *systemic lupus erythematosus* (SLE), *rheumatoid arthritis* and *rheumatic fever*. Complex-mediated hypersensitivity is intimately involved in the tissue damage in both rheumatoid arthritis and SLE, though for neither are the initiating causes known.

Systemic lupus erythematosus

SLE is a rather rare disease, with an incidence of about 1 in 2000 among all women, though considerably more common among Negro women (1 in 275); it is nine times more frequent in females than males, and the age of onset is usually between 20 and 40 years. It is a multiorgan disease with lesions in the skin (erythematous rash), joints (polyarthritis) and kidney (glomerulonephritis), which will be recognised as characteristic of immune complex diseases of the serum sickness type (p. 161). The common skin lesion is a symmetrical rash in areas exposed to u.v. light; the classical 'butterfly' rash is sometimes seen on the face and there is erythema of the fingertips and palms. Ninety percent of SLE patients have arthritis which is symmetrical and can affect almost any joint. Renal involvement, which can be life-threatening, occurs as a result of deposition of complexes in the glomeruli in a focal 'lumpy-bumpy' distribution as revealed by immunofluorescent staining (p. 139). In the classical (but uncommon) 'wire loop' lesion, there is focal brightly eosinophilic thickening of glomerular vessels, reminiscent of a bacteriologist's wire loop. However, the morphological changes in the kidney in this disease are extremely varied, often with lymphocyte rather than neutrophil involvement.

The unusual feature of autoantibodies in SLE is specificity for DNA; indeed the antibodies against double-stranded DNA are unique to this disease in man and some animal equivalents, and are very difficult to induce experimentally (antibodies to single-stranded DNA are more widespread). These are not the only antibodies to nuclear components which occur in SLE sera. Other *antinuclear antibodies* are directed against nucleoproteins (including histones), single-stranded DNA and other nuclear antigens. The antinuclear antibodies themselves are not SLE-specific, but are sometimes found in a variety of other conditions; however, in SLE they are found in high titre and are present in 95% of patients. They cause a characteristic phenomenon which is used as a routine diagnostic test for SLE, called the *LE cell phenomenon*. The LE cell is a phagocyte, usually a neutrophil, which has engulfed the nuclear material of another cell (Figure 2.56). This is essentially an *in vitro* phenomenon, produced when heparinised blood of an SLE patient is allowed to incubate for 30–60 minutes at 37°C. During this period, some leucocytes are inevitably damaged, allowing antinuclear antibodies to penetrate the cell and bind to nuclear antigens. The nucleus swells through

Figure 2.56 The LE-cell phenomenon.
Drawing of blood cells of SLE patient after incubation showing LE cell.

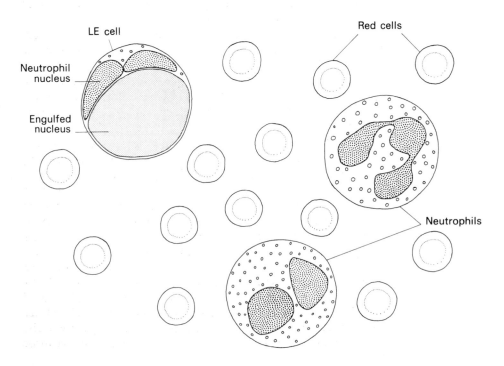

water uptake (lysis) and its chromatin pattern is destroyed. The DNA is extruded as a large homogenous mass which is then phagocytosed, having been opsonised by a coating of IgG antinuclear antibody and complement. The LE-cell phenomenon is positive in 75% of SLE patients and in 15% of patients with rheumatoid arthritis. The antibody responsible is an IgG with specificity for nucleoprotein. Although LE cells are not commonly observed in freshly drawn blood, there is an *in vivo* equivalent, namely the *LE body* or *haematoxylin body*, a globular nuclear mass which stains bluish purple with haematoxylin and is found in the tissues at the periphery of areas of necrosis in the heart, kidneys, lungs, synovial membranes, etc. LE bodies are usually extracellular and may form large masses, especially in lymph nodes. They presumably represent the effect of antibody and complement on nuclei of dead or damaged cells.

The anti-DNA antibodies are responsible for the immune complex disease symptoms in the kidneys, joints and skin. DNA-antibody complexes are difficult to demonstrate in the circulation, but can sometimes be detected by activation of C1q (p. 131). They can be eluted from the kidney and demonstrated in skin lesions and inflamed joint fluid. Antibodies against both single-stranded as well as double-stranded DNA are found; the former also sometimes occur in rheumatoid arthritis and chronic active hepatitis, while the latter are unique to SLE. The level of anti-DNA antibody mirrors quite well the progress of the disease. A range of other autoantibodies may appear, including anti-red cell (haemolytic anaemia), antileucocyte, antiplatelet (thrombocytopenia), anti-IgG, antibody to clotting factor VIII, and occasionally antibodies to thyroid and stomach. Wassermann antibodies in SLE give rise to false-positive reactions for syphilis. This range may well reflect an underlying disturbance of the regulation of the antibody response by T cells (see below).

Progress in understanding the aetiology of SLE has come from the occurrence of similar diseases in animals, notably in the hybrids of New Zealand Black (NZB) with New Zealand White (NZW) mice (the hybrids are designated NZB/W); there is also an SLE-like disease in dogs. The animals develop antinuclear and anti-DNA antibodies, LE cells and immune complex glomerulonephritis. Three main points of interest emerge from the SLE-like disease of NZ mice and dogs. (a) Its regular occurrence in NZB/W hybrid mice indicates the importance of genetic factors, which include an ability of the NZW parent and the hybrid to produce large amounts of antibody after immunisation with DNA. An important point is that the SLE-like disease does not occur in either the NZB or NZW parent strains; its appearance in the NZB/W hybrid therefore implies that at least *two genes* are required for development of murine SLE, one donated by each parent (complementation). (b) There is strong evidence for the involvement of a virus in the disease. Both NZB and NZB/W mice carry a murine (Gross) leukaemia virus (p. 798) and much of the Ig in immune complexes in the glomeruli consists of antibody to the antigens of this virus. Similar antigens have been discovered in the canine equivalent of SLE. Moreover, cell-free filtrates of the spleens of dogs with SLE-like disease induce antinuclear antibodies when injected into mice, some of which also develop lymphomas. The latter carry C-type particles characteristic of RNA tumour viruses. Further, antibodies made against these particles show some reactivity against a small proportion of lymphocytes of human SLE patients, but not normal individuals. Antinuclear factors have also been found in the sera of families of owners of dogs with SLE. These startling findings suggest a role for an RNA virus, apparently murine leukaemia virus, in murine, canine and human SLE. (c) A characteristic feature of the immunology of NZB/W mice is an early decline in suppressor T cell activity, already demonstrable at one month of age. One consequence is the excessive antibody responses which these mice make on immunisation, a tendency which may also underlie autoantibody production. Autoantibodies to nucleic acid and lymphocyte surface antigens appear at about 3 months in NZB/W mice and are followed from 5 months onwards by immune complex disease. The tendency to autoimmunity seems to be acquired from NZB mice, which regularly develop spontaneous autoimmune haemolytic anaemia. Gross defects in cell-mediated immunity appear at about 8 months. In older animals, malignant B-cell lymphomas, some producing IgM (macroglobulinaemia) appear. There is an interesting parallel here with another human disease, Waldenström's macroglobulinaemia (p. 89). It is believed that these events are caused by a genetically controlled deficiency in suppressor T cells and their regulation of B cells, together with environmental agents, notably viral infection.

It is possible to find parallels between the aetiology of SLE in the NZB/W mouse and factors involved in the human disease. Thus, in man there is a genetic predisposition to SLE, indicated by familial occurrence and twin concordance (SLE has been found in at least five pairs of identical twins). Moreover, there is an association in the population between SLE and a certain HLA antigen (HLA-BW15), suggesting that genes in the HLA complex may determine susceptibility, an increasingly common finding for autoimmune disorders (p. 880). Genetically determined complement deficiencies also predispose to SLE. Environmental agents also play a role. A suggestion of viral involvement has been made above. Virus-like tubular structures resembling nucleocapsids of paramyxoviruses (p. 335) occur in various tissues in SLE, especially in the glomerular endothelium, though their significance is not known and they also occur in other autoimmune disorders. Antibodies to paramyxoviruses occur at a raised level in SLE patients. An SLE-like disease can also be induced in susceptible individuals by certain drugs, particularly hydralazine, practalol, procainamide and certain anticonvulsants; these drugs induce formation of antinuclear antibodies and a positive LE cell test. A breakdown of tolerance to nucleoprotein may be involved here, resulting from reaction of a drug or its metabolites with histones or other nuclear components.

In summary, the underlying causes of SLE appear to be a combination of an infectious or other external agent and a genetic predisposition related to control of the immune response. The details are only speculative. A virus may introduce cross-reactive antigens or reveal nuclear antigens in immunogenic form as a result of cell damage. HLA-linked genes may determine both a general tendency to autoimmunity, via the level of suppressor T cell activity, as well as a specific control of immune responses to particular viral or self antigens. It will be apparent that similar combinations of environmental and genetic factors, the latter often HLA-linked, have been invoked to explain several disorders involving autoimmunity (see e.g. myasthenia gravis, p. 198, multiple sclerosis, p. 883, juvenile diabetes, p. 872, etc.).

Rheumatoid arthritis

Rheumatoid arthritis is a chronic inflammatory disease of the joints which is one of the most widespread causes of disability in the population. About 1–2% of all populations are affected and, like many autoimmune disorders, it is more frequent in women (the ratio of females : males affected is about 3:1). Typically there is symmetrical involvement of small joints of the hands and feet, wrists, elbows and ankles, though any—or all—of the 187 synovial joints in the body may be affected. In addition to the joint lesions, there is a characteristic granulomatous swelling known as the *rheumatoid nodule* which is found subcutaneously over pressure points. In severe cases, rheumatoid nodules also occur in the viscera.

Hypersensitivity mediated by antigen–antibody complexes is an important part of the process leading to joint damage in rheumatoid arthritis, while cell-mediated reactions are also involved. The interplay between these two forms of hypersensitivity is not altogether clear and the initiating events are also speculative. In outline, the processes involved are the following (Figure 2.57). Complexes of IgG and anti-IgG antibodies (*rheumatoid factors*, p. 190) are formed *in situ* in the joint and by activation of complement are responsible for neutrophil exudation into the joint space and subsequent damage to the collagen of the articular surfaces by release of lysosomal enzymes. At the same time, sensitised T lymphocytes against an as yet unidentified antigen in the joint are responsible for cell-mediated (Type IV) hypersensitivity, with accumulation of lymphocytes and macrophages in the synovial membrane; damage is caused by release of enzymes from activated macrophages. Chronic, irreversible erosion of the cartilage and bone in the joint is associated with a growth of inflamed synovial tissue over the surfaces of the joint; this tissue, which replaces the articular cartilage, is called *pannus*. Pannus is able to invade and destroy cartilage and bone, principally by release of destructive enzymes from macrophages and factors from lymphocytes.

Figure 2.58 illustrates the general anatomical features of a synovial joint and the changes which occur during rheumatoid arthritis. In the normal joint, the articular surfaces are covered by a layer of avascular cartilage; a capsule composed of fibrous tissue encloses the joint and all the non-articular surfaces are lined by synovial tissue, which produces the lubricant and nourishing

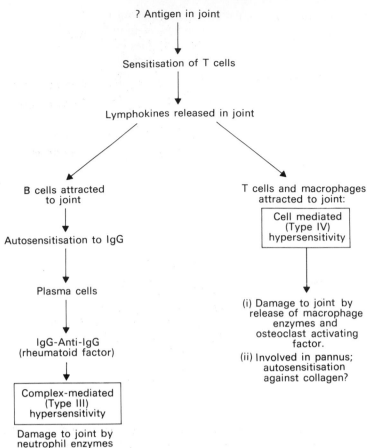

Figure 2.57 Possible aetiology of rheumatoid arthritis.

? Antigen in joint

Sensitisation of T cells

Lymphokines released in joint

B cells attracted to joint

Autosensitisation to IgG

Plasma cells

IgG-Anti-IgG (rheumatoid factor)

Complex-mediated (Type III) hypersensitivity

Damage to joint by neutrophil enzymes

T cells and macrophages attracted to joint:

Cell mediated (Type IV) hypersensitivity

(i) Damage to joint by release of macrophage enzymes and osteoclast activating factor.
(ii) Involved in pannus; autosensitisation against collagen?

synovial fluid. The latter is normally clear, pale yellow and highly viscous, and contains less than 10^3 cells/mm^3, mostly small lymphocytes. The early events in rheumatoid arthritis involve inflammation of the synovial tissue (synovitis); finger-like villi develop at the synovial surface, the outermost (intimal) layer of which becomes hypertrophied. The synovial tissue is infiltrated by lymphocytes, plasma cells, macrophages and neutrophils; lymphocytic cells become organised into follicles near the joint surface and are responsible for the production of immunoglobulins, including rheumatoid factors. The colonising cells may come to synthesize Igs at a rate comparable with that of a lymph node. The synovial fluid increases in amount and becomes an acute inflammatory exudate, with an increase in cell number to over 5×10^3/mm^3, most of the cells now being neutrophils. The fluid becomes increasingly cloudy and almost watery in consistency; the presence of fibrinogen may lead to clotting if fluid extracted from the joint is allowed to stand. The neutrophils can be shown to have phagocytosed immune complexes, such as IgG-rheumatoid factor complexes; one of the consequences of such uptake is the release of lysosomal enzymes from neutrophils, including collagenase and elastase capable of breaking down cartilage (p. 25). This is

Figure 2.58
(a) A normal synovial joint.
(b) Changes in the joint in rheumatoid arthritis. Erosions and 'cysts' occur when pannus extends into marginal and sub-articular bone respectively.

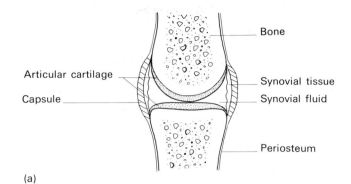

(a)

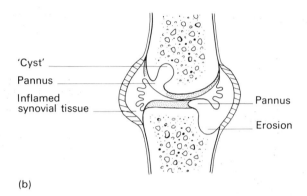

(b)

doubtless an important early contribution to articular damage. An interesting recent finding is a raised level of β_2-microglobulin (p. 181) in synovial fluid. During periods of acute inflammation, the joint is swollen and painful and in consequence movement is limited.

As inflammation continues, tongues of inflamed synovial villi adhere to the margins of the articular cartilage and creep progressively over its surface as the *pannus*: the articular cartilage is destroyed and the pannus takes its place (Figure 2.58b). Pannus is a vascular inflammatory granulation tissue containing fibroblasts, lymphocytes and macrophages. In its destructive invasiveness of cartilage and bone it has been likened to a malignant neoplasm, to indicate its progressive, erosive nature. Collagenases are released from activated macrophages in the pannus, and lymphocytes produce a factor which activates osteoclasts, the cells responsible for bone resorption; the loss of bone gives rise to the radiologically visible erosions which are characteristic of the disease. The origin of the inflammatory cells of the pannus may lie in sensitisation of T cells to collagen itself, following damage to the articular cartilage by neutrophil enzymes. In time, the pannus extensively replaces articular cartilage and is itself converted into fibrous tissue, which binds together the articular surfaces and restricts the movement of the joint (fibrous ankylosis). In severe cases, the joint becomes unstable and subluxation and dislocation are then common.

The characteristic serum autoantibodies of rheumatoid

arthritis, the rheumatoid factors (RFs), have been described at length above (p. 190). However, although they are present as IgM-IgG and IgG-IgG complexes in the circulation, the complexes responsible for inflammation in the joint are formed *in situ*, by plasma cells in the synovial membrane itself, rather than by deposition from the blood. Indeed, the joints are the main source of RF in serum. RFs, as already discussed, are anti-IgG antibodies made in response to determinants on the Fc portion of the molecule; one possibility is that such determinants are revealed when antibody IgG combines with antigen. However, the identity of any antigen involved in rheumatoid arthritis, other than IgG itself, is as yet only speculative. Several possible sources have been suggested, including chronic infection with bacteria, mycoplasmas or viruses, though there is no conclusive evidence in man for their aetiological involvement. Mycoplasmas produce arthritic diseases in animals, notably pigs, and sometimes have been isolated from the joints of rheumatoid patients. Similarly, rubella virus (German measles) is arthrotropic and can cause arthritis in man. The question of the identity of foreign antigens in rheumatic joints is important because at least half the plasma cells in the synovium are producing antibodies which are not RFs. Their specificity is unknown, but potentially complexes between antibodies and antigens other than IgG could be as important in joint inflammation as those involving RFs themselves.

Although serum RFs are mainly of the IgM class, a large proportion of the RF in joints is IgG anti-IgG. The unusual feature of such a molecule, in that it is at the same time antibody and antigen, and its resulting ability to self-aggregate have been described previously (p. 190) and illustrated in Figure 2.52b. Such aggregates are found within RF-producing plasma cells in the synovial membrane, as well as extracellularly; the complexes secreted by the plasma cell activate complement and initiate inflammation. The formation of intracellular aggregates may interfere with the normal feedback regulation of IgG synthesis in the plasma cells and could explain why they produce IgG RF at an apparently uncontrolled rate. The local formation of IgG–anti-IgG complexes makes the rheumatoid joint akin to the site of an *Arthus reaction* (p. 163), rather than a serum sickness-type reaction where soluble complexes are deposited from the circulation. The resulting inflammation is, of course, much the same.

The role of T cells and macrophages in rheumatoid arthritis may be no less significant than that of antigen–antibody complexes. Indeed, rheumatoid arthritis can occur in congenitally agammaglobulinaemic boys, where complexes presumably play no role at all. T cells and their lymphokine products are both demonstrable in rheumatic joints and injection of lymphokines into normal joints stimulates an inflammatory response. T cells and macrophages with cytotoxic properties for synovial cells have been found in patients' blood. Furthermore, depletion of circulating lymphocytes from patients by cannulation of the thoracic duct has a beneficial effect on joints and can lead to disappearance of rheumatoid nodules. This has been held to support a role for circulating T cells in the disease; although both T and B cells are depleted by this procedure, T cell functions are more rapidly and profoundly depressed. The stimulus to the initial involvement of T cells in the joint is unknown, but it could be one of the infectious agents previously mentioned. Once collagen has been damaged, it may itself become immunogenic for T cells. Cell-mediated mechanisms are probably involved in the erosive activity of the pannus. Activated macrophages are a source of lysosomal enzymes, including collagenases; in addition a T-cell lymphokine, *osteoclast activating factor*, causes bone resorption by stimulating osteoclastic activity. Cell-mediated hypersensitivity is also probably responsible for the granulomatous *rheumatoid nodule*. Histologically, this consists of a central area of necrosis surrounded by a 'palisade' layer of histiocytes arranged with their long axes perpendicular to the centre; peripheral to the palisade is an infiltrate of lymphocytes, macrophages and plasma cells, suggestive of a cell-mediated response.

It is evident that the scheme of Figure 2.57 is partially speculative and leaves some important questions unanswered, in particular the nature of the antigenic stimulus which starts the process off. Lymphocytic infiltration is assumed to begin with recognition of antigen in the joint by specifically sensitised T cells; chemotactic factors, MIF and other lymphokines would then account for further lymphocyte, plasma cell and monocyte accumulation. The site of autosensitisation against IgG, i.e. in the joint itself or in the periphery before entry into the joint, is also a matter of conjecture.

CELL-MEDIATED HYPERSENSITIVITY IN AUTOIMMUNITY

The likely involvement of Type IV hypersensitivity, mediated by T cells sensitised against autoantigens, in autoimmune tissue damage has been noted for several disorders including thyroiditis (p. 197), atrophic gastritis (p. 201), rheumatoid arthritis (p. 207), multiple sclerosis (p. 882) and juvenile diabetes (p. 873) among others. The infiltration of organs and tissues by lymphocytes and macrophages is indicative of a cell-mediated response, though it cannot be assumed that the lymphocytes observed histologically are necessarily always T cells; some may be K cells interacting with localised antibody. In some instances, autosensitised cytotoxic or lymphokine-producing T cells can be obtained from patients. The role of T cells can also be inferred from the beneficial effects of agents which inhibit T cell activity; for example, prednisone administration can restore gastric mucosal cells and production of acid and intrinsic factor in patients with pernicious anaemia.

Experimental autoallergic disease against organs such as the thyroid, stomach, testis and nervous tissue is also characterised by cell-mediated organ damage. Although autoantibodies appear in the sera of affected animals, the disease can often only be transferred to normal animals by lymphocytes and not by serum, though sometimes this may reflect the amount of antibody required. Further, the failure to induce experimental auto-immune disorders in neonatally thymectomised animals indicates cell-mediated reaction as a pathogenic mechanism, although thymectomy will also decrease autoantibody production to thymus-dependent autoantigens. In man, most organ-specific autoimmune diseases are probably the combined outcome of anti-body and cell-mediated hypersensitivity reactions, as discussed in the preceding pages.

FURTHER READING

General

Alexander P. & Good R.A. (1978) *Fundamentals of Clinical Immunology*. Holt Saunders.

Bach J.F. (1978) *Immunology*. John Wiley.

Benacerraf B. & Unanue E.R. (1979) *Textbook of Immunology*. Williams and Wilkins.

Fougereau M. & Dausset J. (eds.) (1980) *Immunology 80: 4th International Congress of Immunology, 1980*. Academic Press.

Fudenberg H.H., Stites D.P., Caldwell J.L. & Wells J.V. (eds.) (1980) *Basic and Clinical Immunology*, 2nd edn. Lange Medical Publications.

Golub E.S. (1982) *Cellular Basis of the Immune Response*, 2nd edn. Sinauer Associates.

Holborow E.J. & Reeves W.G. (eds.) (1983) *Immunology in Medicine: A Comprehensive Guide to Clinical Immunology*, 2nd edn. Academic Press.

Hood L.E., Weissman I.L. & Wood W.B. (1978) *Immunology*. Benjamin/Cummings.

Lachmann P.J. & Peters D.K. (eds.) (1981) *Clinical Aspects of Immunology*, 4th edn. Blackwell Scientific Publications.

Miescher P.A. & Muller-Eberhard H.J. (eds.) (1976) *Textbook of Immunopathology*, 2nd edn. (2 vols.). Grune and Stratton.

Roitt I. (1980) *Essential Immunology*, 4th edn. Blackwell Scientific Publications.

Talal N. (ed.) (1977) *Autoimmunity: Genetic, Immunologic, Virologic and Clinical Aspects*. Academic Press.

Thompson R.A. (1978) *The Practice of Clinical Immunology*, 2nd edn. Edward Arnold.

Turk J.L. (1978) *Immunology in Clinical Medicine*, 3rd edn. W. Heine-mann Medical Books.

Specific topics

Amos H.E. (1976) *Allergic Drug Reactions*. Edward Arnold.

Asherson G.L. & Webster A.D.B. (1980) *Diagnosis and Treatment of Immunodeficiency Diseases*. Blackwell Scientific Publications.

Bloom B.R. (1979) Games parasites play: how parasites avoid immune surveillance. *Nature*, **279**, 21.

Butterworth A.E. *et al.* (1982) Studies on the mechanisms of immunity in human schistosomiasis. *Immunological Reviews*, **61**, 5.

Cox K.O. & Howles A. (1981) Induction and regulation of autoimmune haemolytic anaemia in mice. *Immunological Reviews*, **55**, 31.

Cushley W. & Owen M.J. (1983) Structural and genetic similarities between immunoglobulins and class-1 histocompatibility antigens. *Immunology Today*, **4**, 88.

Dahlen S.E. *et al.* (1980) Leukotrienes are potent contrictors of human bronchi. *Nature*, **288**, 484.

Dick G. (1978) *Immunisation*. Update Books.

Dodd B.E. & Lincoln P.J. (1975) *Blood Group Topics*. Edward Arnold.

Drachman D.B. (1978) Myasthenia gravis. *New Engl. J. Med.*, **298**, 136.

HLA and disease susceptibility. *Immunological Reviews* (1983), 70.

Immunological tolerance. *British Medical Bulletin* (1976), **32**, no. 2.

Immunoparasitology. *Immunological Reviews* (1982), **61**.

Immunosuppressive agents. *Immunological Reviews* (1982), **65**.

Interleukins and lymphocyte activation. *Immunological Reviews* (1982), **63**.

McMichael A.J. & Fabre J.W. (eds.) (1982) *Monoclonal Antibodies in Clinical Medicine*. Academic Press.

Milstein C. (1980) Monoclonal antibodies. *Scientific American*, **243**, No. 4, 56.

Models of Autoimmune Diseases. *Immunological Reviews* (1981), 55.

Molgaard H.V. (1980) Assembly of immunoglobulin heavy chain genes. *Nature*, **286**, 657.

Pernin L.H. *et al.* (1981) Inhibition of *P. falciparum* growth in human erythrocytes by monoclonal antibodies. *Nature*, **289**, 301.

Piper P.J. (ed.) (1981) *SRS-A and Leukotrienes*. (Prostaglandins Research Series, vol. 1). John Wiley.

Receptors, Antibodies and Disease. *Ciba Foundation Symposium*, (1982), **90**.

Salaman M.R. (1982) The state of transfer factor. *Immunology Today*, **3**, 4.

Samuelsson B. & Paoletti R. (eds.) (1982) *Leukotrienes and other lipoxygenase products* (Advances in Prostaglandin, Thromboxane and Leukotriene Research Series, vol. 9). Raven Press.

Secher D.S. (1980) Monoclonal antibodies by cell fusion. Immunology Today, **1**, 22.

Steinberg A.D. *et al.* (1981) The cellular and genetic basis of murine lupus. *Immunological Reviews*, **55**, 121.

Tan E.M. (1982) Autoantibodies to nuclear antigens (ANA): their immunobiology and medicine. *Advances in Immunology*, **33**, 167.

Taussig M.J. (1980) Antigen-specific T cell factors. *Immunology*, **41**, 759.

The HLA system. *British Medical Bulletin* (1978), **34**, no. 3.

Theofilopoulos A.N. & Dixon F.J. (1979) The biology and detection of immune complexes. *Advances in Immunology*, **28**, 89.

Tonegawa S. (1983) Somatic generation of antibody diversity. *Nature*, **302**, 575.

Unanue E.R. (1981) The regulatory role of macrophages in antigenic stimulation. Part two: symbiotic relationship between lymphocytes and macrophages. *Advances in Immunology*, **31**, 1.

Weigle W.O. (0980) Analysis of autoimmunity through experimental models of thyroiditis and allergic encephalomyelitis. *Advances in Immunology*, **30**, 159.

White D.J.G. & Calne R.Y. (1982) The use of cycolsporin A immuno-suppression in organ grafting. *Immunological Reviews*, **65**, 115.

Zinkernagel R.M. & Doherty P.C. (1979) MHC-restricted cytotoxic T cells: studies on the biological role of polymorphic major transplantation antigens determining T cell restriction. Specificity, function and responsiveness. *Advances in Immunology*, **27**, 52.

SECTION 3 INFECTION: VIRUSES

Introduction

Viruses are responsible for many of the important acute diseases of man, from influenza and the common cold to the familiar childhood infections of mumps, measles and chickenpox, to highly dangerous diseases such as yellow fever, lassa fever and smallpox. At the other end of the temporal spectrum, viruses cause some of the chronic disorders of tissue growth known as neoplasms or tumours (Section 6), including the common wart and quite probably some cancers. These extremes reflect two of the effects of viruses on eukaryotic cells. The acute diseases result because viruses can kill tissue cells directly or cause the immune system to do so; tumours, on the other hand, arise when viruses induce cells to undergo uncontrolled proliferation. Viral infections do not necessarily lead to disease, however; indeed the majority go unnoticed, doing no apparent harm to the host. Viruses are not cellular organisms, but consist essentially of genetic material (nucleic acid) protected from the environment by a protein coat; they are thus quite distinct from even the simplest prokaryotic organisms. In lifestyle, they are obligate intracellular parasites. Before describing the processes of viral disease, we shall consider the characteristic features which distinguish viruses from other microbial groups, followed by details of their structure and replication.

THE NATURE OF VIRUSES

The first distinguishing feature of viruses to be discovered was their extremely small size, shown by their passage through bacteria-retaining filters and their invisibility under the optical microscope. In addition, unlike most other organisms, they proved impossible to culture on artificial media. Subsequently, their relative chemical simplicity was recognised—many viruses contain only protein and nucleic acid, and while others have a lipid outer membrane, free polysaccharides are universally lacking. The discovery in 1935 that a virus could be crystallised raised further philosophical questions about the definition of life and whether viruses qualified as living organisms at all.

A summary of the chief characteristics of viruses is given in Table 3.1. Not all the features listed are unique. A quality such as *small size*, for example, contains an area of overlap between the largest viruses, just visible by light microscopy (poxviruses), and the smallest prokaryotic cells (chlamydiae, mycoplasmas). For the most part, however, viruses are only visible using the electron microscope, and the maximal dimension (usually diameter) of animal viruses ranges between 20 and 300 nanometres (nm; $1\,nm = 10^{-3}\,\mu m$); for comparison, the diameter of a cell of *Staphylococcus aureus* is about 1000 nm. (Note that if a virus is, say, 1/10th of the diameter of a bacterial cell, it is 1/1000th of the volume.) *Chemical composition* is also highly variable, and while the smallest viruses (parvoviruses, picornaviruses) are indeed chemically very simple and possess only three or four different proteins associated with their small nucleic acid genomes, the

Table 3.1 Summary of characteristic or unique properties which distinguish viruses from other microorganisms.

---

  1 Small size (20–300 nm); pass through filters which retain bacteria.

*2 Simplicity of chemical composition; some are only nucleic acid plus very few proteins.

*3 Subunit construction; strict geometric structure; icosahedral or helical symmetry.

*4 Genetic information as DNA or RNA; only one type of nucleic acid present; genome may be segmented.

  5 Replication intracellular only.

*6 Eclipse period; no binary fission; assembly from independently synthesized protein and nucleic acid components.

  7 No ribosomes[+]; no mitochondria or other organelles; no ATP production.

  8 No rigid cell wall or muramic acid.

  9 Unaffected by most antimicrobial drugs.

*10 Sensitive to interferon.

*11 May be crystallisable.

---

* properties unique to viruses

[+] exception—arenaviruses

largest viruses code for several dozen proteins. The structural feature common to nearly all, however, is that their nucleic acid is surrounded by a protective protein coat made up of repeating *subunits* in precise *symmetrical arrangement*. The geometry of viral design falls into just two basic types, namely either *helical* or *icosahedral* (20-sided) structures. Viruses are particles rather than cells: they lack characteristic intracellular structures such as ribosomes (arenaviruses, which carry some host cell ribosomes, excepted), and are devoid of mitochondria and other organelles. The particle is often surrounded by a lipid membrane called the *envelope*, but unlike even the most rudimentary prokaryotic cells, there is never an outer wall structure nor peptidoglycan containing muramic acid.

In common with all other organisms, the genetic information of viruses is carried in the form of nucleic acid. Thus, in some cases, naked (i.e. protein-free) viral nucleic acid is itself infectious and able to replicate complete virus particles. However, whereas all cellular organisms possess both DNA and RNA, viruses contain only *one type of nucleic acid*, which may be either DNA or RNA: hence the major subdivision in viral classification is into DNA- and RNA-containing viruses. The RNA viruses are in fact the only organisms to have their genome in this form. Another feature unique to some RNA viruses (reoviruses, bunyaviruses, orthomyxoviruses) is that the genome consists of several fragments or segments of RNA, rather than a continuous thread; each fragment often consists of a single gene.

Viral replication is also unique. In the first place, the lack of protein-synthesizing apparatus and energy-producing systems means that viruses are *obligate intracellular parasites*, entirely dependent for their replication on the synthetic and metabolic machinery of the cells they infect. In reply to the question, 'are viruses alive?', one could reply that inside their host cells they can reproduce and therefore possess the fundamental criterion of life; extracellularly they are purely chemical entities, incapable of replication or any of the other activities associated with living organisms. In itself, an intracellular existence is not particularly unusual, being shared by several bacteria and eukaryotic parasites. However, the replication of such cells takes place by binary fission; viruses are incapable of this process—they do not grow and divide. Once the virus is inside the host cell, viral nucleic acid is released from its protein coat and directs the synthesis of viral proteins as well as its own replication. During this phase, no virus particles can be obtained from the infected cell, and the virus is said to be in the *eclipse period*. Thus, whereas cells retain their recognisable identity during replication, viruses lose theirs. Protein and nucleic acid components are synthesized independently and are ultimately assembled into identical mature virus particles, which can then be released from the cell. Because they are all identical and do not grow, they can aggregate into crystal-like arrays which can often be seen in infected cells.

Finally, we may note that viruses are generally not affected by antibiotics and chemotherapeutic drugs used against other infections; such agents can specifically prevent, for example, bacterial division, but it is evident that it would be much more difficult to devise substances capable of distinguishing viral from host cell replication. Nevertheless, some very promising antiviral agents are emerging, especially nucleoside analogues active against herpes simplex virus (p. 268). Viral multiplication is also specifically inhibited by proteins known as *interferons*, which are released by the virus-infected cells themselves and can act on other cells to protect them from viral infection. Interferons hold great promise in the treatment of certain viral diseases and are also under intensive study as possible anticancer agents (p.246).

VIRUS STRUCTURE

The mature virus particle is referred to as a *virion* and, as already noted, this consists principally of DNA or RNA surrounded by protein. Each group of viruses has one of four possible types of nucleic acid, namely double-stranded DNA, single-stranded DNA, double-stranded RNA or single-stranded RNA; the first and last of these categories are the most common. Table 3.2 gives the types of nucleic acid found in the different families of animal viruses. In most cases there is a single continuous piece of nucleic acid, but in three families of RNA viruses the genome is *segmented*, i.e. present in several pieces: reoviruses have ten fragments of double-stranded RNA, while bunyaviruses and orthomyxoviruses have three and eight respectively of single-stranded RNA. Each fragment of RNA in the reoviruses and orthomyxoviruses represents a single gene. In retroviruses, such as the Rous sarcoma virus, there is the unusual feature of two complete copies of the RNA genome.

The protein forms a covering known as the *capsid* around the

Table 3.2 Types of nucleic acid found in animal viruses.

Type of nucleic acid	Family
Double-stranded DNA	Papovaviridae, Adenoviridae, Herpetoviridae, Poxviridae
Single-stranded DNA	Parvoviridae
Double-stranded RNA	Reoviridae
Single-stranded RNA	Picornaviridae, Togaviridae, Orthomyxoviridae, Paramyxoviridae, Arenaviridae, Rhabdoviridae, Coronaviridae, Bunyaviridae Retroviridae

nucleic acid (Lat. *capsa*, box). The capsid is composed of subunits called *capsomeres* (or capsomers), which can be discerned by electron microscopy. In *icosahedral viruses*, the capsomeres form a rigid 20-faced box which encloses the nucleic acid, while in *helical viruses* they are arranged as a cylinder around the nucleic acid. The package of nucleic acid within its capsid is called a

Figure 3.1 Basic viral forms.
(a) Icosahedral non-enveloped.
(b) Icosahedral enveloped.
(c) Helical, rigid, non-enveloped.
(d) Helical, flexuous, enveloped.
Inset—'herring-bone' appearance of nucleocapsid sometimes seen in electron microscope.

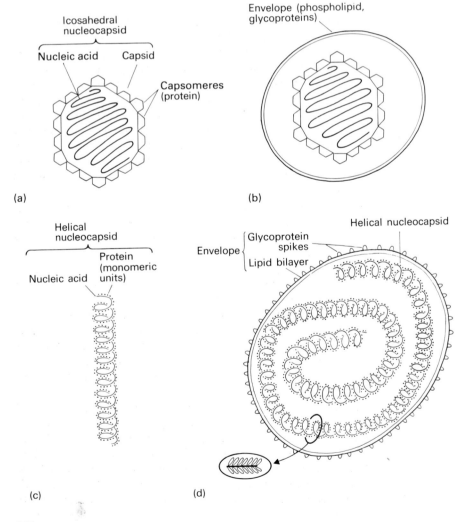

Table 3.3 Structural forms of animal viruses.

Architecture	Nucleic acid	Family
Icosahedral, non-enveloped	DNA	Papovaviridae, Adenoviridae, Parvoviridae
	RNA	Picornaviridae, Reoviridae
Icosahedral, enveloped	DNA	Herpetoviridae
	RNA	Togaviridae
Helical, non-enveloped		None
Helical, enveloped	RNA	Orthomyxoviridae, Paramyxoviridae, Rhabdoviridae, Coronaviridae
Helical and icosahedral, enveloped	RNA	Retroviridae
Complex	DNA	Poxviridae

nucleocapsid. This may be surrounded by a loose membrane or *envelope* consisting of a lipid bilayer derived from the host cell membrane into which viral (but not host cell) glycoproteins are inserted. Small *spikes* can often be seen projecting from the envelope and consist of organized aggregates of viral glycoproteins. The different viral structures are illustrated diagrammatically in Figure 3.1; and Table 3.3 and Figure 3.2 summarise the distribution of these structural forms among the families of animal viruses. Note that (a) with the exception of the poxviruses, all DNA viruses are icosahedral; all helical viruses are RNA viruses; (b) RNA viruses may be icosahedral or helical; and (c) while some icosahedral viruses are enveloped and others not, all helical animal viruses are enveloped. Also, most families of DNA viruses are non-enveloped (herpesviruses are the main exception), while most RNA viruses are enveloped (except picornaviruses and reoviruses).

To a first approximation, icosahedral viruses appear to be spherical, but close examination by high resolution electron microscopy confirms their true geometric symmetry (Figure 3.3a). A regular icosahedron has 20 faces, which are equilateral triangles, and 12 vertices or corners (Figure 3.4a). The capsomeres can commonly be seen to be hollow hexagonal or pentagonal structures; the former, called *hexons* or (hexamers), are disposed over the faces of the icosahedron, while the latter, *pentons* (pentamers), are found at the vertices. The shape of the hexons and pentons arises because they are themselves composed of *protein subunits*, six and five respectively. Each hexon has six neighbouring capsomeres, while pentons have five. These features can be seen in the model of the adenovirus icosahedron (Figure 3.4b). In this virus, the capsid is composed of 1500 protein subunits, arranged into 240 hexons and 12 pentons; each penton is marked by a protruding fibre (unique to adenoviruses).

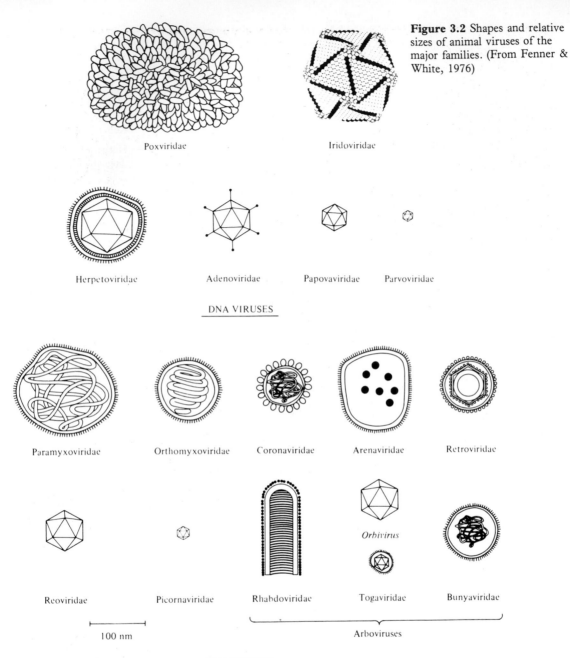

Figure 3.2 Shapes and relative sizes of animal viruses of the major families. (From Fenner & White, 1976)

Poxviridae

Iridoviridae

Herpetoviridae

Adenoviridae

Papovaviridae

Parvoviridae

DNA VIRUSES

Paramyxoviridae

Orthomyxoviridae

Coronaviridae

Arenaviridae

Retroviridae

Reoviridae

Picornaviridae

Rhabdoviridae

Orbivirus

Togaviridae

Bunyaviridae

100 nm

Arboviruses

RNA VIRUSES

The pentons, hexons and fibres are composed of different proteins. The number of protein subunits and capsomeres is a characteristic of each virus.

The structure of helical viruses is essentially filamentous; the capsomeres are arranged in helical symmetry to form a hollow cylinder along the inside of which the nucleic acid is wound (Figure 3.1c, d). Each capsomere is a single protein unit only. In their envelopes, these viruses usually appear roughly spherical as

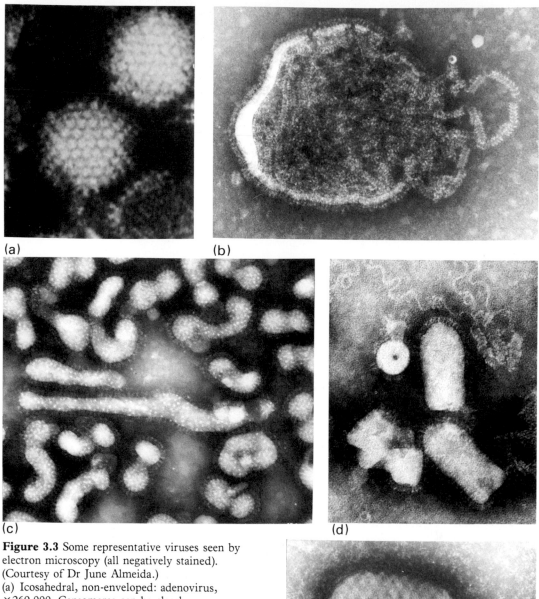

(a)

(b)

(c)

(d)

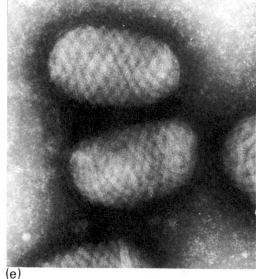

(e)

Figure 3.3 Some representative viruses seen by
electron microscopy (all negatively stained).
(Courtesy of Dr June Almeida.)
(a) Icosahedral, non-enveloped: adenovirus,
×260,000. Capsomeres can be clearly
distinguished.
(b) Helical, enveloped: parainfluenzavirus 1,
×215,000. The herring-bone appearance of the
helical nucleocapsid is evident where it emerges
from the disrupted envelope.
(c) Influenza virus, ×125,000, showing
pleomorphic particles and spikes projecting from
the envelope.
(d) Vesicular stomatitis virus, ×180,000,
characteristic bullet-shaped rhabdovirus particles
with surface spikes.
(e) Orfvirus, a poxvirus (contagious pustular
dermatitis group), ×110,000. Note the ovoid
particle shape and the criss-cross arrangement of
surface strands or tubules.

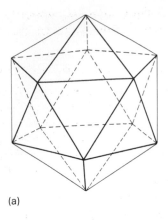

(a)

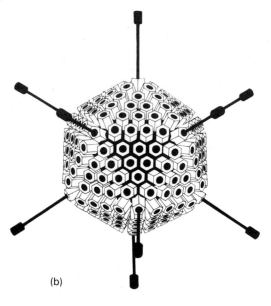

(b)

Figure 3.4
(a) A regular icosahedron (20 triangular faces, 12 apexes, 30 edges).
(b) A model of the adenovirus capsid, based on electron microscope and other evidence (e.g. Figures 3.3a and 3.23a). The virus has 240 hexagonal prisms located on the faces and edges of an icosahedron, 12 pentagonal prisms at the apexes, and 12 spike structures linked to the pentagonal prisms. (Courtesy of Professor R.W. Horne.)

the nucleocapsid is flexible enough to coil up within the loose-fitting lipid membrane (e.g. orthomyxoviruses, paramyxoviruses; Figures 3.1d; 3.3b, c); if the envelope is disrupted, however, the filamentous nature of the capsid becomes more apparent (Figure 3.3b). One group with a more rigid structure is the rhabdoviruses, which are uniquely bullet-shaped (Figure 3.3d); the regular cross-striations which can be seen are the closely fitting coiled helical nucleocapsid.

There are two structures which are more complicated. In the retroviruses (RNA tumour viruses), the helical nucleocapsid is super-coiled into the form of a hollow sphere, which is surrounded by an icosahedral shell, and the whole structure is further enclosed in an envelope. In the poxviruses, the largest animal viruses, the particles are ovoid or brick-shaped and their structure is 'complex', with neither icosahedral nor helical symmetry (Figure 3.3e).

Finally, we may note that not all the virion proteins are structural capsid components or envelope glycoproteins; often there are virion-associated enzymes, generally required for transcription or replication of the viral nucleic acid.

CLASSIFICATION AND NOMENCLATURE

The criteria employed in viral classification include the nature of the nucleic acid (DNA or RNA, double-stranded or single-stranded), the symmetry of the virion (icosahedral, helical, or other), its size and the number of capsomeres, the presence of an envelope, and antigenic characteristics. The major grouping is the *family*, the name of which ends in the suffix *viridae*; a family is subdivided into genera (suffix *virus*) and species, the latter often named after a particular disease. There may be further subdivision into types, subtypes, etc., on the basis of serology, and this aspect of classification has recently been greatly improved by the unique specificity of monoclonal antibodies (p.97).

A valuable 'supergrouping' is now commonly used, known as the *Baltimore classification* after its proposer. In this system, families are grouped into *classes* on the basis of the expression of their genetic material, in particular the pathway of synthesis of messenger (m) RNA. This is shown schematically in Figure 3.5.

Figure 3.5 The Baltimore classification of viruses. Messenger (m) RNA and strands of identical sequence to mRNA are designated '+'; viral DNA and RNA strands complementary to mRNA are designated '−'. Double-stranded nucleic acid is denoted '±'. Arrows show route of arriving at mRNA.

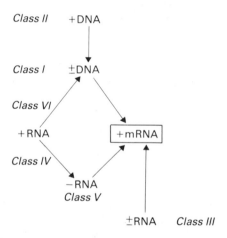

All mRNA is designated as 'positive'; accordingly viral DNA or RNA strands can be either positive, if they have the same base sequence as mRNA, or negative, if their base sequence is complementary to mRNA. Six classes are recognised, as follows. *Class I*: viruses with a double-stranded DNA genome; mRNA may be transcribed from either of the two strands, depending on the gene (as in cells). *Class II*: single-stranded DNA genome; where this is a positive strand, it is converted to double-stranded DNA and mRNA is transcribed from the new negative strand. *Class III*: double-stranded RNA genome; the genome is segmented and mRNA is transcribed from the negative strand of each segment. *Class IV*: positive single-stranded RNA genome; the genome itself can act as mRNA, and complementary negative strands are also synthesized which act as the templates for *de novo* mRNA

Table 3.4 Classification of viruses infecting man.

Family/genus	Structure	Species	Disease
Class I. Double-stranded DNA genome			
Herpetoviridae/Herpesvirus	Icosahedral; enveloped; 180–200 nm; DNA $50–90 \times 10^6$	Herpes simplex virus, type 1	Gingivostomatitis Cold sores (fever blisters) Keratitis
		Herpes simplex virus, type 2	Genital herpes ? Cervical carcinoma
		Varicella-zoster virus	Chickenpox Zoster (Shingles)
		Cytomegalovirus	Congenital abnormalities (CMID) Mononucleosis Hepatitis
		Epstein–Barr virus	Infectious mononucleosis Burkitt's lymphoma Nasopharyngeal carcinoma
Adenoviridae/Adenovirus	Icosahedral; non-enveloped; 70–90 nm; DNA $20–30 \times 10^6$	33 serotypes	Pharyngitis Acute respiratory disease Conjunctivitis Acute pharyngoconjunctival fever
Papovaviridae/Papillomavirus	Icosahedral; non-enveloped; 45–55 nm	Papillomavirus	Warts in man and other species
Poxviridae/Orthopoxvirus	Complex; several layers; 220×370 nm; DNA $130–240 \times 10^6$	Variola major virus Variola minor virus Vaccinia virus Cowpox virus	Smallpox Alastrim Complications of vaccination Cowpox
Unclassified	Icosahedral; enveloped; 42 nm (Dane particle); DNA 1.6×10^6	Hepatitis B	Serum hepatitis
Class II. Single-stranded DNA genome			
Parvoviridae/Parvovirus	Icosahedral; non-enveloped; 18–26 nm; DNA $1.5–2.2 \times 10^6$	May include Norwalk virus and similar agents	Gastroenteritis

Class III. Double-stranded RNA genome

Reoviridae/Rotavirus	Rotavirus (3 types)	Icosahedral; double-walled; non-enveloped; 60–80 nm; RNA $10–16 \times 10^6$, (10–12 segments)	Gastroenteritis

Class IV. Single-stranded (+) RNA genome

Picornaviridae/Enterovirus	Poliovirus (3 types)	Icosahedral; non-enveloped; 20–30 nm; RNA 2.5×10^6	Poliomyelitis (infantile paralysis)
	Coxsackievirus (29 types)		Aseptic meningitis Herpangina Hand, foot and mouth disease Epidemic myalgia Myocarditis in newborns Common cold
	Echovirus (32 types)		Aseptic meningitis Boston fever Common cold Gastroenteritis
	Enterovirus 70		Acute haemorrhagic conjunctivitis
Rhinovirus	Rhinovirus (113 types)		Common cold
Coronaviridae/Coronavirus	229E OC43	Helical; enveloped with sparse spikes; 70–120 nm; RNA 9×10^6	Common cold Common cold
Togaviridae/Alphavirus	see disease name	Icosahedral; enveloped; 40–70 nm; RNA 4×10^6	Eastern, Western, Venezuelan equine encephalitides Chikungunya O'nyong-nyong; etc.
Flavivirus	see disease name		Yellow fever Dengue Japanese encephalitis Tick-borne encephalitis, etc.

continued

Table 3.4 *continued*

Family/genus	Structure	Species	Disease
Continued			
Rubivirus		Rubella virus	Rubella (German measles) Congenital rubella syndrome
Class V. Single-stranded (−) RNA genome			
Orthomyxoviridae/Influenzavirus (types A, B, C)	Helical; enveloped; 100 nm; RNA 4×10^6, in 8 segments (7 in type C)	Influenza virus subtypes (A0, A1, A2, A3)	Influenza
Paramyxoviridae/Paramyxovirus	Helical; enveloped; 150 nm; RNA $5-8 \times 10^6$, (non-segmented)	Parainfluenza virus	Acute laryngotracheobronchitis (infantile croup) Acute respiratory infections
		Mumps virus	Mumps
Morbillivirus		Measles virus	Measles (rubeola) Subacute sclerosing panencephalitis
Pneumovirus		Respiratory syncytial virus	Lower respiratory tract disease in infants
Rhabdoviridae/Lyssavirus	Bullet-shaped; helical; enveloped; RNA 4×10^6	Rabies virus	Rabies
Bunyaviridae/Bunyavirus	Helical; enveloped; 100 nm; RNA 6×10^6, segmented	see disease name	Bunyamwera Manituba
Arenaviridae/Arenavirus	Capsid symmetry unknown; 50−300 nm; contain ribosomes; RNA $3.5-5.5 \times 10^6$ in 5−7 segments.	Lymphocytic choriomeningitis virus	Lymphocytic choriomeningitis
		Lassa virus	Lassa fever
Unclassified			
	Icosahedral; non-enveloped; 27 nm; single-stranded RNA	Hepatitis A	Infectious hepatitis

production. *Class V*: negative single-stranded RNA genome, from which mRNA is copied directly. *Class VI*: positive single-stranded RNA genome, but with a *DNA* intermediate both in replication and mRNA synthesis.

The classification and nomenclature of the major families of animal viruses are given in Table 3.4, together with the principal diseases they cause.

VIRAL REPLICATION

Viruses infect cells in order to replicate by making use of the cellular machinery which they, the viruses, lack, most obviously the protein synthesis apparatus of ribosomes and associated enzymes. From the pathological viewpoint, virus replication is important because it frequently leads directly to cell death, usually as a result of the shut-down of the cell's own macromolecular synthesis. The classical experimental design employed in studies of virus replication in bacterial or animal cells is called the *one-step growth experiment*, developed initially with bacteriophages (viruses which infect bacterial cells). In this experiment, a single cycle of replication is initiated by synchronous infection of all the cells in a culture, followed by

Figure 3.6 Virus replication: one-step growth curves.

Hypothetical growth curves for an animal virus which matures intracellularly and is released efficiently by lysis.
Key: (a) — Intracellular virus
    (b) --- Extracellular virus
    1. Adsorption and penetration.
    2. Eclipse period.
    3. Maturation.
    4. Latent period.
    5. Lytic release.

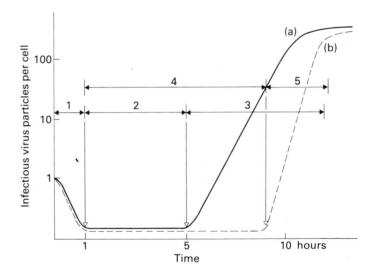

periodic sampling for the progress of viral replication, either by artificial lysis of the cells at regular intervals after infection or by following the appearance of extracellular virus released from the cells into the medium. Typical one-step growth curves for a virus which matures fully inside its host cell before release are shown in Figure 3.6. The curve obtained when the cells are lysed artificially (Fig. 3.6a) shows a period, of varying length, during which no virus particles can be detected intracellularly. This is the *eclipse period* and represents the phase of disassembly of the infecting virion and synthesis of viral components prior to assembly of mature particles. As noted, an eclipse period is unique to the replication of viruses. It may be as short as a matter of minutes in the case of bacteriophages, or last some hours for animal viruses. It ends when mature, infectious particles are first detected; their number steadily increases, the yield being from a few dozen up to several thousand particles per cell. If the experiment is conducted by waiting for virus to appear extra-cellularly, a curve such as that in Figure 3.6b is obtained. In this case there is a *latent period*, followed by the sudden, rapid appearance of virus in the cell culture fluid. Latent periods vary in length from 30 minutes for T2 bacteriophage to several hours (generally 5–10) for animal viruses, and for viruses which mature intracellularly the latent period is always longer than the eclipse period since it includes the time when mature virions are collecting in the cell cytoplasm. The viral yield in this case is called the burst size. For viruses which mature as they leave the cell, i.e. by budding from the cell membrane, the eclipse and latent periods are the same.

The stages in the replication of animal viruses can be sum-marised thus. (1) *Adsorption (attachment)*, in which the virions adhere to receptors on the host cell membrane, is followed by (2) *penetration* of the virion through the membrane and entry into the cell cytoplasm, and (3) *uncoating* of the particle, in which the capsid proteins are removed and viral nucleic acid is released. (4) *Transcription* of mRNA from viral nucleic acid, using either host cell or viral enzymes, is followed by (5) *translation* of mRNA into viral proteins, structural and non-structural, on host cell ribosomes in the cytoplasm. (6) *Replication* of nucleic acid commences as soon as the necessary viral polymerases, etc. are available and may be nuclear or cytoplasmic. (7) When both viral nucleic acid and capsid proteins have been synthesized, *assembly* of particles into their icosahedral or helical structures occurs; assembly too may be nuclear or cytoplasmic, depending on the

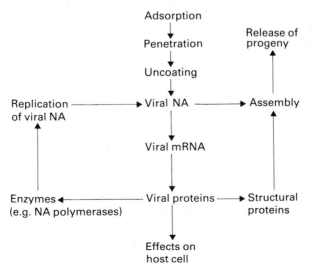

Figure 3.7 Scheme of events in viral replication.
(NA = nucleic acid)

virus. (8) Finally, *release* of mature virions from the cell takes place, either by cell lysis or by budding through specifically prepared sites in the membrane. In the latter case, the virus acquires its envelope of cell membrane lipid and viral glycoprotein as it leaves the cell. These events are shown schematically in Figure 3.7 and are now considered in more detail.

ADSORPTION (ATTACHMENT)

A virus can gain access to the interior of a cell only if it can bind to the outside of the cell membrane, and this requires a binding protein on the virus and a corresponding cell membrane receptor. If the receptor is lacking, the cell cannot be naturally infected by the virus, and this is one basis for the cell selectivity which some viruses show, with consequent species specificity and preferential infection of certain tissues in the host body. Poliovirus provides an illustration: cells without the poliovirus receptor are not susceptible to infection, but if the virus is introduced artificially into such cells it replicates normally. Influenza is an example where the adsorption process is well understood. The envelope of the virus carries a glycoprotein called *haemagglutinin*, from its ability to cause agglutination of red blood cells; it is present as spikes projecting from the envelope surface. The haemagglutinin binds specifically to N-acetylneuraminic acid (NANA) residues on cell membrane glycoproteins. Treatment of the cells with neuraminidase removes NANA, thereby destroying the receptor sites for influenza virus and preventing infection. Less is known about the receptor sites for other animal viruses.

PENETRATION

After attachment, a non-enveloped virion may be taken into the cell by a process called *viropexis*, which resembles phagocytosis (Figure 3.8a). It thus enters the cytoplasm enclosed in a membrane-bound vesicle, to be released subsequently, probably by fusion of the vesicle with an intracellular membrane. Enveloped viruses can fuse their lipid membrane with that of the host cell, releasing the nucleocapsid immediately into the cytoplasm (i.e. virus envelope does not enter the cell, Figure 3.8b). Enveloped viruses can also enter cells by viropexis.

UNCOATING

This is the term for the removal of capsid proteins leading to release of viral nucleic acid. The process varies for different viruses; for example, poliovirus uncoating begins as soon as the virion binds to the cell receptor, with the loss of a capsid protein while the virus is adherent to the membrane and still extracellular. For other non-enveloped, as well as for enveloped viruses, uncoating occurs intracellularly in the cytoplasm. In some cases, e.g. reoviruses, uncoating is never complete and the viral nucleic acid remains in a nucleoprotein core from which template

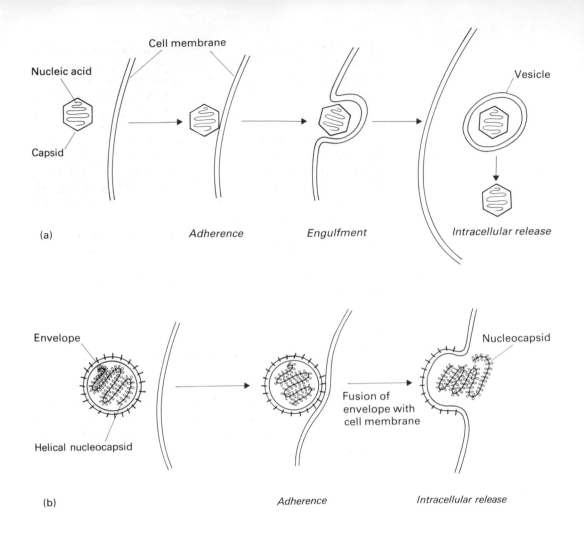

Nucleic acid

Cell membrane

Capsid

(a)   Adherence   Engulfment   Intracellular release

Vesicle

Envelope

Helical nucleocapsid

(b)   Adherence   Intracellular release

Fusion of
envelope with
cell membrane

Nucleocapsid

copies are extruded. In general, however, viral nucleic acid, together with associated enzymes, is released from the protein capsid.

Figure 3.8 Stages in the entry of viruses into cells.
(a) Viropexis of a non-enveloped icosahedral virus.
(b) Fusion of an enveloped helical virus.

PROTEIN SYNTHESIS AND NUCLEIC ACID
REPLICATION

Subsequent stages in replication may take place in the host cell nucleus or cytoplasm, depending on the virus. For DNA viruses other than the poxviruses, which confine themselves to the cytoplasm, DNA is both transcribed into mRNA and replicated in the nucleus (where the necessary host cell polymerases are located); virion proteins are synthesized in the cytoplasm and then enter the nucleus for assembly. In contrast, most RNA viruses complete all the stages of transcription, replication and assembly in the cytoplasm (they carry and/or code for their own polymerases); influenza viruses are the exception here, resembling DNA viruses in replicating in the cell nucleus. For some viruses, enzymes carried in the virus particle itself are essential for steps such as the generation of messenger (i.e.

positive strand) RNA; for example, the negative-strand RNA viruses (class V) must be copied by their own RNA-dependent RNA polymerase as this enzyme is unknown in animal cells. Retroviruses (class VI) require their own unique enzyme, RNA-dependent DNA polymerase (reverse transcriptase) as a first step in both replication and mRNA generation. On the other hand, virion-associated polymerases are not required for positive-strand RNA viruses (class IV)—their RNA acts directly as messenger without prior copying—nor for most double-stranded DNA viruses (class I), which are transcribed into mRNA by host cell polymerases. For these two groups, the naked nucleic acid itself is often infectious if taken up by cells, and is capable of generating complete virions, an observation which was fundamental in proving the nucleic acid to be the sole repository of viral genetic information.

It is now convenient to describe the subsequent events for DNA and RNA viruses separately.

DNA viruses

With the exception of poxviruses, which replicate in the cytoplasm, replication of double-stranded DNA viruses is partly or wholly dependent on host cell polymerases and other enzymes and takes place in the nucleus. The replication of papovaviruses, such as SV40, provides a well-studied model which in essence is shared by others, including adenoviruses and herpesviruses (Figure 3.9). Transcription occurs in two stages, generating

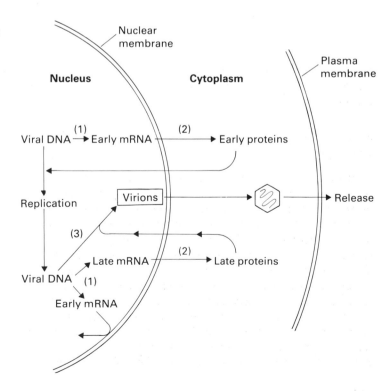

Figure 3.9 General scheme for replication of a DNA virus, after entry and uncoating (based on papovavirus replication).
(1) Transcription
(2) Translation
(3) Assembly

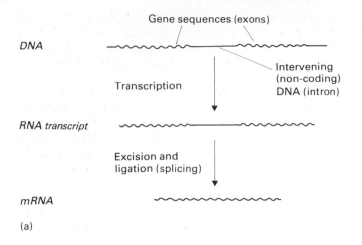

DNA

Gene sequences (exons)

Intervening
(non-coding)
DNA (intron)

Transcription

RNA *transcript*

Excision and
ligation (splicing)

mRNA

(a)

mRNA

Complementary
base pairing

Gene DNA
(exon)

'R loop'
(non-coding DNA, intron)

(b)

Figure 3.10 Transcription of adenovirus DNA.
(a) Production of mRNA from non-contiguous gene sequences.
(b) Demonstration of non-coding (intron) DNA after hybridisation of DNA with mRNA; schematic electron microscope appearance. (After Primrose and Dimmock, 1980)

mRNA designated 'early' and 'late', according to the time of its appearance. Early mRNA is copied from the DNA by a host DNA-dependent RNA polymerase and migrates to the cytoplasm, where it is translated on cell ribosomes into 'early' proteins. These are not capsid proteins, but are required for DNA synthesis and may include a viral DNA polymerase. Replication of viral DNA then ensues and is semi-conservative (i.e. each daughter molecule has one newly-synthesized strand and one derived from the parent molecule) as for cellular DNA. It is followed by transcription of the 'late' mRNA (early mRNA is, in fact, also synthesized again, but at this stage only late mRNA can leave the nucleus). The late proteins are the structural virion components (capsomere subunits) and once they have been synthesized they too enter the nucleus where the particles are assembled. DNA viruses tend to accumulate in the cell before eventual release, e.g. by cell lysis. The envelope of herpesviruses is acquired by budding through the nuclear rather than the plasma membrane (Figure 3.13a; cf. enveloped RNA viruses, p. 238); herpesviruses leave the cell gradually via the endoplasmic reticulum.

Poxviruses are the only DNA viruses to replicate in the cytoplasm, in so-called 'factories' which become visible as characteristic inclusion bodies. They are also the only ones to carry their own DNA-dependent RNA polymerase within the virion. Their genomes, with up to 200 genes, are many times larger than those of the small viruses and code for all the enzymes required for transcription and replication; the host cell principally provides a closed environment, the machinery of protein synthesis and raw materials such as amino acids and nucleotide triphosphates.

The process of transcription of DNA viruses may involve more than mere copying of the template strand of DNA into mRNA by a polymerase, due to the fact, recently discovered in adenoviruses and SV40, that some viral genes are not continuous, i.e. in the DNA, gene coding sequences (exons) are interrupted by sequences of non-coding DNA (introns), splitting the gene into non-contiguous segments (Figure 3.10a). The initial RNA transcript is thus longer than the final messenger, and to produce functional mRNA the non-coding regions are excised and the coding segments rejoined (ligated). This process (splicing) does not occur in bacteria, where DNA gene sequences are not interrupted, but is common in eukaryotic cells, where genes are often 'split' (p. 473). If adenovirus mRNA is annealed (heated and recooled) together with its DNA, it hybridises with complementary DNA sequences, and under the electron microscope the non-coding DNA is revealed as a loop (Figure 3.10b). Among the DNA viruses, there are also cases where a given DNA sequence can specify more than one protein, depending on how the primary RNA transcript is spliced. This 'multi-choice' splicing appears to be confined to viruses.

RNA viruses

The replication of RNA viruses involves unique processes, since in normal cells copying of RNA does not occur. Consequently the virions are expected to carry, and/or code for in their genomes, the enzyme necessary for transcription and replication, namely *RNA-dependent RNA polymerase*, and this is indeed the case for all except the retroviruses, which have an alternative mechanism. The generation of messenger (positive) RNA depends on whether the infecting virus itself is positive-or negative-stranded (Baltimore classes IV or V). For a class IV virus such as poliovirus, the viral RNA, being a positive strand, acts as mRNA and is translated directly into proteins, including the polymerase. Negative-strand class V viruses must first be copied by their virion-associated RNA polymerase to generate mRNA (Figure 3.11 a and b).

Replication of single-stranded RNA, i.e. for production of progeny virus, follows a similar course for both class IV and class V viruses, with two stages of copying by polymerase, as summarised in Figure 3.11, (a, b). For class IV viruses, the infecting positive RNA is copied to make negative RNA strands; these in turn act as templates for synthesis of further positive strands, some of which are used as mRNA while others are destined for progeny viruses (Fig. 3.11a). In class V viruses, the starting point is the negative strand of the infecting virion, which is copied into positive RNA strands; the latter can then be either

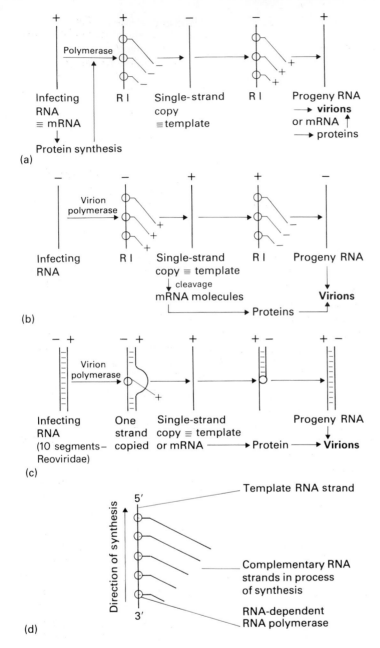

Figure 3.11 Replication schemes of different RNA viruses.
(a) Positive single-stranded RNA genome (class IV).
(b) Negative single-stranded RNA genome (class V).
(c) Double-stranded RNA genome (class III).
(d) Structure of replicative intermediate.
O = polymerase molecule
RI = replicative intermediate

mRNA molecules or templates for progeny (Fig. 3.11b). At each step, synthesis of several copies of mRNA can take place simultaneously at a single template, and macromolecular forms called *replicative intermediates* are isolable (Fig. 3.11d).

For the majority of RNA viruses, replication is cytoplasmic. The orthomyxoviruses (influenzaviruses) are unique in replicating their RNA in the nucleus, which is also the site of their assembly, similar to DNA viruses described above. Another unusual feature of influenzaviruses is that replication is prevented by actinomycin D, an inhibitor of *DNA* transcription which does

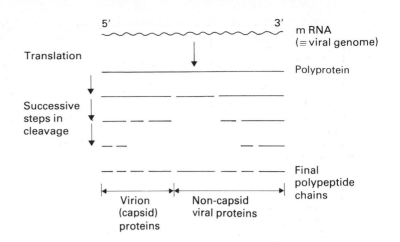

Figure 3.12 Translation of the poliovirus genome with post-translational cleavage.

5′   3′   m RNA (≡ viral genome)

Translation

Polyprotein

Successive steps in cleavage

Final polypeptide chains

Virion (capsid) proteins   Non-capsid viral proteins

not affect replication of other RNA viruses (except retroviruses, p. 782). Thus, a functioning cell nucleus is essential to influenza-virus replication, whereas other RNA viruses can multiply in enucleated cells.

The replication of double-stranded RNA viruses (class III, reoviruses) is unexpectedly different from that of their DNA counterparts in that it is not semi-conservative, i.e. the parental RNA is totally conserved during replication and both progeny RNA strands are newly synthesized (Figure 3.11c). One of the RNA strands is copied first and is then used as template for the complementary strand.

There are important differences between class IV and class V viruses in the nature of the mRNA and its translation into protein. For the class IV viruses, the mRNA is polycistronic (several genes in continuity on one mRNA molecule) and is not divided into separate messages before translation. In the well-studied example of poliovirus protein synthesis, a very large polyprotein is made which must be cleaved by a series of precise enzymatic steps to generate individual protein molecules (Figure 3.12). *Post-translational cleavage*, as this process is called, in fact begins before synthesis of the polyprotein is completed, but by inhibiting protease activity the single large molecule can be isolated. For class V RNA viruses, proteins are always synthesized from *monocistronic* mRNA, perhaps derived by cleavage of an original polycistronic message. Where the genome is segmented, as in orthomyxoviruses and reoviruses, the mRNA is monocistronic *ab initio*.

For some RNA viruses, it is necessary for positive-strand RNA molecules destined to be mRNA to be distinguished from those which may be either progeny virus RNA (class IV viruses) or templates for synthesis of a negative strand (class V) (Figure 3.11). For example, with poliovirus, positive RNA strands could in principle serve either as messengers or be packaged into new virions (Fig. 3.11a), and to avoid this confusion a small polypeptide (VPg) is attached to all positive RNA strands, but removed from those which function as mRNA. Similarly, in the case of orthomyxoviruses, with eight genome segments, monocistronic mRNA must be differentiated from the positive RNA to be used as template (Fig. 3.11b). This is achieved by omission of a short sequence of bases from the end of mRNA molecules so that they are unable to serve as templates for replication of complete genome sequences.

The retroviruses (class VI) form a group in which replication is completely different from that of other RNA viruses. The events are decribed fully in Section 6, in connection with their tumour-causing properties (p. 781). In brief, the distinguishing feature is that they replicate via a *DNA intermediate*. Instead of being copied directly into RNA, they are first copied into DNA by the unique enzyme, *reverse transcriptase* (RNA-dependent DNA polymerase). The DNA replicate is then integrated with the host chromosomal DNA as a 'provirus' from which messenger and virion RNA are both transcribed. Proviral integration is an essential step in the ability of retroviruses to change the nature of the cell.

The final steps in replication of RNA viruses are assembly and release. While most are assembled at cytoplasmic sites, orthomyxoviruses are assembled in the nucleus. The non-enveloped icosahedral viruses, such as the picornaviruses, are released by lysis. Many RNA viruses, however, including all the helical viruses, are enveloped and are released by *budding* from the plasma membrane. Special areas of membrane are prepared for the budding process by replacement of host membrane proteins by viral glycoproteins, organised into visible spikes, e.g. haemagglutinin (Figure 3.13b). The inside of the membrane is in some cases lined by a matrix (M) protein which may function as an attachment site for the completed nucleocapsid. The latter associates with the prepared area and, as it buds off, becomes enclosed in the lipid envelope. For viruses with segmented genomes, one representative of each nucleocapsid segment (eight for orthomyxoviruses, ten for reoviruses) must be brought together at the budding point; precisely how the appropriate complete set of segments is assembled together is not yet understood.

ABERRATIONS IN VIRAL REPLICATION

Virus replication is far from completely efficient and it is not unusual to find that many progeny particles are empty capsids lacking nucleic acid. The electron microscope invariably shows that a virus preparation contains a larger number of particles than can be accounted for as infectious units in biological assay, often several hundred incomplete particles for every infectious virion. Occasional spontaneous mutation also inevitably accompanies replication of viral nucleic acid—point mutations, frame shifts, deletions, etc.—and several types of mutant are recognised from the resulting changes in viral behaviour. Some mutations are lethal, i.e. prevent viral replication. Sometimes, however, a mutation is only lethal under certain defined conditions in which replication fails to occur; a virus with this type of defect is called a *conditional lethal mutant*. An important example is the

Figure 3.13 The process of viral budding.
(a) Stages in the budding of herpes simplex virus from the nuclear membrane into the cytoplasm. N = nucleus. Electron micrographs of thin sections, ×85,000. (From Shipkey *et al*, 1967, *Exp. Molec. Path.*, **6**, 39.)
(b) Budding of a helical virus.

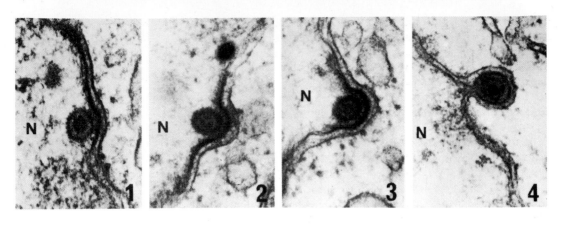

(a)

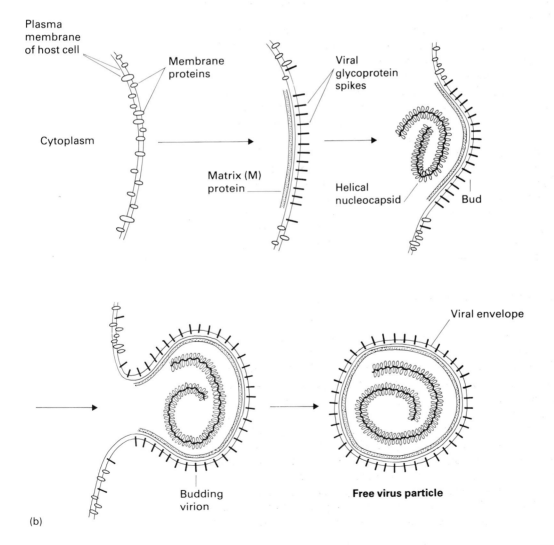

Plasma membrane of host cell

Membrane proteins

Cytoplasm

Viral glycoprotein spikes

Matrix (M) protein

Helical nucleocapsid

Bud

Viral envelope

Budding virion

Free virus particle

(b)

temperature sensitive (ts) type of mutant which is able to replicate and produce progeny virus at some low 'permissive' temperature, but not at a higher 'restrictive' one at which the normal virus would grow. Temperature sensitive mutants have been very important in biochemical and genetic studies. The explanation for their behaviour is that a base change in the viral nucleic acid has caused an amino acid substitution in a viral protein, such that the protein cannot maintain its correct shape and function above a certain temperature. These mutants can also be useful as attenuated strains for viral vaccines; e.g. a *ts* mutant of influenza virus which cannot multiply above 33°C is restricted to the cooler regions of the upper respiratory tract and therefore produces a much milder disease than normal, while at the same time stimulating protective immunity against influenza.

A virus which cannot complete its replication is called a *defective virus*, and changes in the genetic material such as mutation and deletion are the causes of such particles. A defective virus may be able to absorb to and penetrate the host cell and direct the synthesis of proteins and nucleic acid, but cannot complete its replicative cycle because of a defect in a crucial protein. Nevertheless, it can replicate completely if rescued by the simultaneous presence in the cell of a *helper virus*, which provides the defective particle with its missing component. An example of such an interaction occurs between adenoviruses and a defective parvovirus (a small, single-stranded DNA virus) called adeno-associated virus or AAV, which electron microscopy shows often to be present in adenovirus preparations. Replication of AAV is absolutely dependent on the adenovirus, though the precise function supplied by the latter is unknown. It is noteworthy that the replication of the adenovirus itself is inhibited when it gives help to the AAV, and this is an instance of a phenomenon known as *viral interference*, in which the presence of one virus species in a cell suppresses the replication of another species co-infecting the cell. Where a defective particle causes interference, it is termed a *defective interfering* or DI virus. Interference by a DI virus is essentially a form of competition in which the defective virus uses up a protein produced by the helper and, by completing its own replication more rapidly, thereby inhibits the latter's multiplication. DI particles usually lack some part of the normal genome, e.g. through deletion.

An interesting example of interference occurs in the replication of influenzavirus if cells are infected at a high virus : cell ratio (high multiplicity). The influenzavirus genome consists of eight separate RNA segments and during replication there is a tendency to exclude from the progeny the largest and slowest replicating segment, hence giving rise to defective viruses which lack this gene. The defective particles can subsequently interfere with the replication of complete influenza virions by competing in the cell for RNA polymerase—the excess of the seven RNA segments of the defective virus effectively reduces the amount of the enzyme available to copy the vital eighth segment. Hence the apparent paradox that a high multiplicity of infection leads to a lower viral yield. Since under these conditions influenza

240

virus is inhibiting its own replication, the effect is called *autointerference* (the von Magnus phenomenon). Another mechanism of interference, namely production by the infected cell of the inhibitory protein interferon, is described below (p.246).

PATHOGENESIS OF VIRAL DISEASE

Once a virus has entered the body, the disease process can be divided into four overlapping stages: (a) effects of virus on individual cells, including cell death, virus replication, etc.; (b) the cellular antiviral response, namely production of the antiviral protein interferon; (c) effects of virus on the host, including the route of acquisition of infection, the dissemination of virus in the body, clinical manifestations of disease, etc.; and (d) the host defensive reactions against the virus and infected cells, notably the immune response.

EFFECTS OF VIRUSES ON HOST CELLS

The infection of a cell by a virus can have one of several possible consequences for either partner and the following categories are not all mutually exclusive. They are usually observed in cells in tissue culture. (i) The commonest outcome is for the virus to replicate and the cell to die, a *lytic* or *cytocidal* infection. (ii) Cell death is not an inevitable consequence of viral replication, however, and a *persistent* infection may ensue in which virus is continuously produced and the cell remains alive. (iii) Alternatively, the virus may fail to replicate, but instead integrate its genome into that of the host cell as a *latent infection*. (iv) An infected cell may enter uncontrolled proliferation, an event known as *transformation*, which may be accompanied by either persistent or latent infection. Finally, (v) an infection may be *abortive*, in that replication starts but cannot be completed, as in the case of defective viruses; abortive infections may nevertheless damage cells.

Cytocidal (lytic) infections

The death of a virus-infected cell may be the consequence of lytic release of progeny virions, but frequently occurs much earlier as a result of the 'shut-down' of host cell macromolecular (protein and nucleic acid) synthesis, caused either by certain viral proteins or by competition between viral and cellular mRNA for ribosomes. Sometimes cell death results from the intracellular release of lysosomal enzymes. The term *cytopathogenic effect (CPE)* describes the adverse cellular consequences of viral infection (including cell fusion, below), which culminate in cell death.

A cytocidal outcome of infection is widely used in assaying the presence and concentration of viruses, as in the *plaque assay* (Figure 3.14a). In this method, a suspension of susceptible cells is prepared by trypsinisation of appropriate animal tissue and allowed to form a monolayer on the surface of a culture dish. A

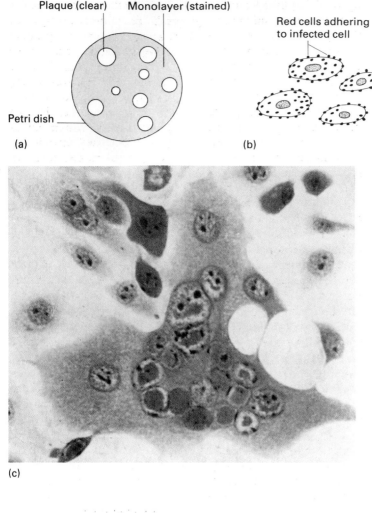

Plaque (clear)   Monolayer (stained)

Red cells adhering
to infected cell

Petri dish

(a)   (b)

(c)

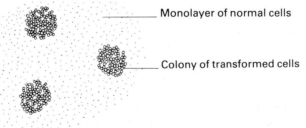

Monolayer of normal cells

Colony of transformed cells

(d)

Figure 3.14 Results of
interactions between viruses and
animal cells in culture.
(a) Cytolytic virus: plaque assay.
(b) Haemadsorption.
(c) Fusion and inclusion bodies.
A multinucleate giant cell in a
culture of ox kidney cells infected
with bovine mamillitis virus (a
herpesvirus). A large, Cowdry
type A inclusion body is present
in several nuclei, separated by a
clear halo from marginated
chromatin. (From Buxton &
Fraser, 1977)
(d) Transformation.

dilution of the virus preparation is poured over the monolayer
and after a brief period, during which the virus adheres to the
cells, the monolayer is covered with a layer of viscous medium,
such as methylcellulose, to prevent virus released from an
infected cell from spreading further than its immediate
neighbours. After 24–48 hours incubation, the monolayer is
stained with a vital dye, such as neutral red, which is only taken

up by living cells, so that areas of cell death become visible as circular, clear, unstained 'plaques'. Each plaque originates through the infection of one cell by a *single* particle, the progeny of which spread to and kill neighbouring cells until a macroscopic area of cell death if produced. The concentration of the virus preparation can be expressed as the number of plaque-forming units (pfu's) per ml, which is equivalent to infectious units of virus. We have already noted that this is much smaller than the particle count by electron microscopy, as many are non-infectious empty capsids. The advantage of a plaque, or 'focal', assay is that it is quantitative; however, with many viral species it is not successful, in which case the cessation of metabolic activity, indicated by a lack of acid production by infected cells in culture, can be used as an alternative assay. Such assays are 'quantal' (i.e. all or nothing) and the viral *titre*, the highest dilution affecting 50% of the cultures, is not a precise measure of the number of infectious units.

It may take some time for infected cells to die and during this period there can be characteristic *alterations in cell membranes*. For viruses which leave the cell by budding from the plasma membrane, viral glycoproteins, destined for the envelope, are inserted into the membrane while the virus is replicating. Since one common envelope protein is the *haemagglutinin*, an infected cell may be able to bind red cells of certain species at its surface, a phenomenon known as *haemadsorption* (Fig. 3.14b). If a virus is not cytocidal during a reasonable time interval, haemadsorption can be used to detect infected cells, especially for the orthomyxoviruses, paramyxoviruses and togaviruses.

Some viruses promote *cell fusion*, in which membranes of adjacent cells coalesce to produce multinucleated giant cells (syncytia, polykaryons; Figure 3.14c). This CPE is typical of paramyxoviruses, such as measles virus, and some herpesviruses, such as herpes simplex virus.

An intracellular indication of infection is the appearance of one or more *inclusion bodies*, nuclear or cytoplasmic structures with characteristic *staining properties*, which generally occur at the site of virus multiplication (Figure 3.14c). They may be accumulations of completed virions, capsids or other components, sometimes in crystalline array. Note that an inclusion body can sometimes be an artefact of staining, as in cells infected by herpes simplex virus, where the inclusion body usually observed is not a real structure under natural conditions. The site, shape and staining properties of the inclusion body may be highly characteristic of a particular virus and in some diseases may be an important part of diagnosis; the Negri body of rabies is a good example. The typical appearance of some inclusion bodies is shown in Figure 3.15. Some inclusion bodies may be cytotoxic.

Persistent (steady-state) infections

Certain viruses, such as paramyxoviruses, produce infections in cell cultures in which almost all cells are infected, but none are killed. In fact, the cells continue to multiply and produce virus

Virus	Schematic appearance	Location	Staining	Name
Vaccinia	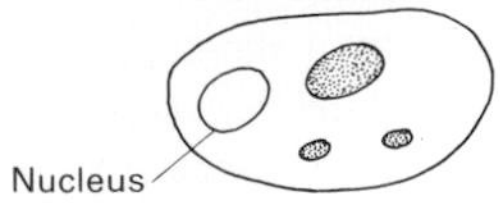 *(Nucleus)*	Cytoplasm	Acidophilic	Guarnieri body
Herpes simplex	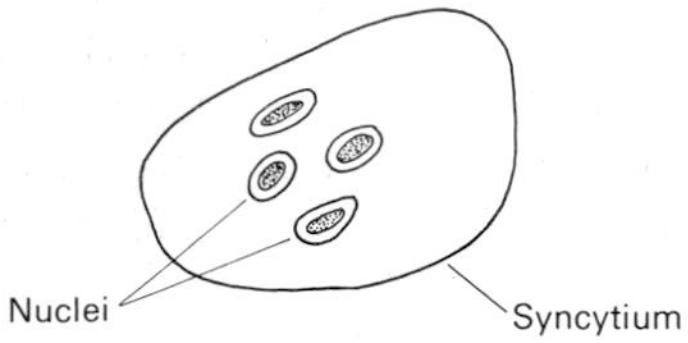 *(Nuclei; Syncytium)*	Nuclei of syncytia	Acidophilic	Cowdry type A
Reovirus	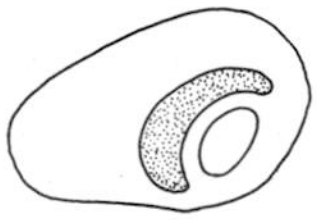	Cytoplasm, perinuclear	Acidophilic	
Adenovirus	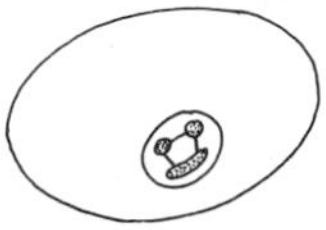	Nucleus	Basophilic	
Rabies	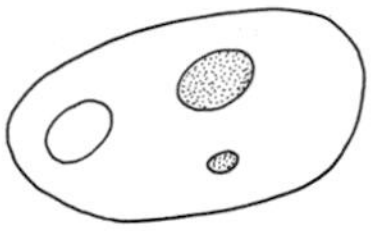	Cytoplasm	Acidophilic	Negri body
Measles	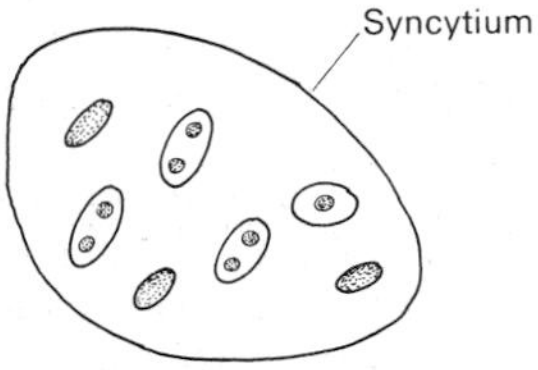 *(Syncytium)*	Nuclei of syncytia; and cytoplasm	Acidophilic	
Cytomegalovirus	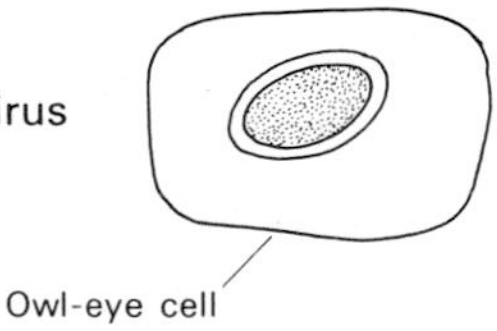 *(Owl-eye cell)*	Nucleus	Eosinophilic	

Inclusion body   *Nucleus*

Figure 3.15 Viral inclusion bodies.

through several generations, apparently because the virus is unable to disrupt the cell or inhibit its synthetic processes. Another example occurs in those neoplastic (tumour or transformed) cells which continuously produce and release RNA tumour viruses as they proliferate (p. 779). In some cases, a cytocidal virus only infects and kills a fraction of the cells in a culture while the majority escape infection and continue to grow; e.g. the presence of a small amount of antibody or interferon may limit viral multiplication to the extent that most cells in the culture are spared while a few are infected and killed, a model which may resemble persistent infections in the body. Co-infection of the cell with a DI particle can also encourage infections to become persistent, by limiting through interference the yield of infectious virions.

Latent (integrated) infections

These occur when viral *information* (i.e. nucleic acid) persists in the cell, but mature viral particles are not detectable. A prime example is the disappearance of DNA tumour viruses from the cells which they infect and transform, viral nucleic acid being integrated into the host DNA as a provirus. No viral replication inside the transformed cells occurs, but the continuous presence of viral genes is required for the maintenance of the abnormal state of the cell. Viral proteins may be demonstrable as antigens, and the integrated genome can be detected by nucleic acid hybridisation (p. 779). Moreover, production of virus may be reactivated by fusing or co-culturing the neoplastic cell with a cell susceptible to lytic (productive) infection. Important examples of latency in more commonplace diseases occur in infections with the herpesviruses, herpes simplex (cold sores) and varicella-zoster (chickenpox), which become latent in sensory nerve ganglia. Latent infections are non-cytocidal during the period of latency.

Transforming infections

Tumour viruses *transform* susceptible cells in culture, that is they change the behaviour of a cell and cause it to proliferate free from the normal restraints on division. Such restraints include *contact inhibition*, whereby cells cease dividing when a critical number of contacts with neighbouring cells has been established and hence tend to form monolayers on culture dishes. Loss of contact inhibition is characteristic of transformed cells, which grow in culture as colonies composed of cells heaped on one another in irregular fashion (Figure 3.14d). Transformation is a rare cellular event, the equivalent of tumour induction *in vivo*; transformed cells will often grow as tumours if transplanted. A more detailed account can be found in Section 6.

DNA tumour viruses only transform cells which they are unable to infect productively (i.e. with viral replication), as their replication is cytocidal; as noted above, they become latent by integrating their genome into a host cell chromosome. RNA tumour viruses (oncornaviruses), on the other hand, continue to replicate in the cells they transform, establishing a persistent infection and budding from the cell surface. Nevertheless, their genome is also integrated with the host DNA, an essential part of transformation for all tumour viruses. For the oncornaviruses, this is achieved by reverse transcription, the synthesis of DNA from the single-stranded RNA template of the infecting virus. The DNA copy, in double-stranded form, is inserted into a cell chromosome and directs both transformation of the cell and replication of progeny virus (p. 779).

Abortive infections

Sometimes a virus fails to replicate fully in the cell it infects, either due to an apparent incompatibility between the two or to an intrinsic viral defect. An example of the former is the inability of adenoviruses to multiply in monkey cells, in which they are thus essentially defective; interestingly, they can be rescued by co-infection with a simian papovavirus (SV40) or a simian adenovirus, which act as helpers. Infection of glial cells by herpes simplex virus is also abortive: progeny particles are released, but either lack a nucleic acid core or are non-enveloped, and in both cases are therefore non-infectious. True defective viruses, which lack a part of the normal virus genome, also give rise to abortive infections and are rescued by helper viruses—the example of adeno-associated virus has already been cited (p. 240).

Another mechanism of abortive infection occurs when the progeny, rather than the original infecting virus, are defective because of a missing host cell enzyme. Thus, in some cells influenza virus infection gives rise to non-infectious progeny because of the failure of an enzymatic cleavage step to complete the structure of the haemagglutinin, the molecule which the virus uses to adhere to other cells. The defect can be corrected by addition of a little trypsin to the cultures, whereupon normal infectious virus is produced (see also p. 316).

Even an abortive infection can still exert a cytopathogenic effect, as part of the replicative cycle of the virus occurs; since there are no mature progeny, however, the damage cannot spread to other cells.

THE CELLULAR ANTIVIRAL RESPONSE: INTERFERONS

The term interferon denotes a family of related protein and glycoprotein molecules which are produced principally by virus-infected cells and have the property of preventing virus multiplication. Interferon is at present the object of intense experimental and clinical scrutiny for two reasons, firstly as a potential agent in the treatment or prevention of viral disease, and secondly to assess its possible use in the therapy of certain cancers. It is now under industrial production, where it has benefited from recent major advances in genetic engineering and monoclonal antibody research. Large-scale production is vital in obtaining sufficient interferon for clinical trials, several of which are in progress. Quite soon the likely usefulness (or otherwise) of interferon as a chemotherapeutic agent will become clearer.

Discovery

The initial discovery of interferon by Isaacs and Lindenmann in 1957 was in connection with studies on viral *interference*, the phenomenon in which multiplication of one virus type inhibits that of a second virus usually added subsequently to the same cell culture (and also demonstrable in animals and plants *in vivo*). They infected fragments of chick chorioallantoic membrane with UV-inactivated influenza virus and, after incubation, found that

246

the virus-free culture fluid inhibited the growth of normal influenza virus in fresh pieces of membrane. The implication was that the infected cells had produced a soluble substance, which was termed 'interferon', capable of inhibiting viral multiplication in other cells. Interferon accounts for many examples of viral interference. It is now known that it is not a single substance, but a group of small proteins, of molecular weights 15,000–40,000, and that different members of the family may be produced by different cell types. Also, viral infection is not the only means of stimulating its production; for example, interferon can be obtained by treating cells with synthetic polyribonucleotides, and some types of interferon are products of activated T-lymphocytes following stimulation by antigen or mitogens (cf. lymphokines, p.147).

Terminology

Understandably, there has been some confusion in the nomenclature of interferons, but a standard terminology has now been agreed internationally (Table 3.5). The accepted abbreviation is IFN. Until recently, interferon from virus-infected cells was called Type I, and that from antigen-stimulated T cells Type II. An indication of the cell of origin was also added, namely leucocyte or fibroblast, these being cells in common use for large scale production; but although interferons from different cell sources are known to differ antigenically, these terms are misleading because leucocytes and fibroblasts can each produce both types of interferon when infected. The new nomenclature does away with all these designations in favour of a classification

Table 3.5 New and old nomenclatures for interferons.

New	Old
IFN-α	Type I, leucocyte, pH2 stable
IFN-β	Type I, fibroblast, pH2 stable
IFN-γ	Type II, immune, pH2 labile

based on antigenic specificities as defined by antisera. Three major types are recognised in this way and denoted IFN-α, IFN-β and IFN-γ (Table 3.5). Note that these three types may themselves be groups of related molecules rather than homogeneous proteins: in man there are at least eight different forms of IFN-α and possibly more than one of IFN-β. All three types of interferon and mixtures thereof have been used in clinical trials.

Characteristics of action

Interferons, as noted, are relatively low molecular weight proteins, some but not all of which are glycoproteins; IFN-α and IFN-β are stable at acid pH (pH2). One purification method makes use of their strong binding to certain polyribonucleotides (poly(I) or poly(U)). A standard assay is to measure the effect of interferon on production of plaques by a sensitive virus such as vesicular stomatitis virus: 1 unit of interferon is the amount required to cause 50% inhibition in the standard test. Interferons are extremely potent agents and 1 mg is equivalent to about 10^9 units; as little as $10-20$ molecules can confer resistance on a cell, making them among the most powerful drugs known (in terms of dose-response). The activity assay may soon be replaced by immunoassays using monoclonal antibodies.

An important feature is that the interferon induced by one virus is active against the whole range of other viruses, i.e. it is non-virus-specific. There is species restriction, however, and it acts best on cells of the species which made it, though interferon from monkey kidney cells is effective in human cells and some human interferons act on cells of other mammalian species. For experimental studies and therapy in man, human interferon is used. Most animal cells appear to be able to produce interferon on infection.

Sources and purification

Although interferon is a highly potent substance, clinical trials and therapeutic applications have been hampered by the small amounts available, and it is only recently that the supply of human interferon has approached adequacy in meeting the relatively huge requirements for clinical trials in cancer patients. Large-scale production from virus-infected cells uses one of three cellular sources, namely leucocytes, fibroblasts or lymphoblastoid cells. *Leucocytes* used for interferon production are obtained by separation from blood used in transfusion; they are then infected with Sendai virus. Production on a large scale from *fibroblasts* has been made possible with the advent of new bulk culture methods for growing adherent cells on microcarrier beads. *Lymphoblastoid cell lines*, on the other hand, can be grown to high concentration in suspension and in large volumes and, being neoplastic, they continue to grow indefinitely. A lymphoblastoid line called Namalwa is used industrially and the cells are infected with live Sendai virus to stimulate interferon production.

However, the most important source for large-scale commercial interferon production will soon be bacteria into which human interferon genes have been introduced by 'genetic engineering' (recombinant DNA technology). The techniques involved are described at greater length on p. 470. In essence, copies of the human gene are integrated into loops of bacterial DNA called plasmids, which are taken up by receptive organisms such as *Escherichia coli*. As the plasmids are replicated with the bacterial cell each time it divides, individual human genes can soon be grown to high yield and cloned. In some cases, interferon being one, the human gene is expressed functionally in the bacterial cell and its protein product can be obtained (Figure 4.38). Although the amount of interferon produced by such engineered organisms is at present small, the yield per bacterium is certainly capable of improvement and is compensated by the rapid generation time of *E. coli* (~ 30 minutes) vs. lymphoblastoid cells (~ 18 hours).

There has also been an important step forward in isolation and purification of interferon from culture fluids of all cellular sources, namely *monoclonal antibodies* against interferon (see also p.100). They are homogeneous and thus absolutely specific for interferon and moreover can be produced in unlimited amount. They are thus ideal reagents for separating interferon from the myriad other components of culture fluid, a particularly important point when one considers the neoplastic nature of some of the cells used. The anti-interferon antibody is complexed to a solid support such as cellulose beads or agarose, to make an 'immunoadsorbent' which will specifically bind interferon; the latter is recovered from the beads by elution with low pH buffer, thus purifying and concentrating in one operation (Figure 2.16). The exquisite specificity of these antibodies will enable separation of α and β IFNs on the basis of their antigenic differences and should thereby also clarify the potential uses of each.

Biological activity

The biological activity of interferons can be divided into two stages: (i) induction, either in virus-infected cells (α, β) or sensitised T lymphocytes (γ), followed by (ii) stimulation of an anti-viral state in target cells, as well as various effects on the immune response.

Induction of interferons

The molecule of central importance in the induction of α and β interferons in virus-infected cells is *double-stranded (ds) RNA*. Originally, it was noticed that synthetic dsRNAs (polyribonucleotides) and the dsRNA genome of reoviruses were excellent inducers of interferon, both in animals and tissue culture; one of the most effective is the polyribonucleotide poly(I:C) (polyriboinosinic acid : polyribocytidilic acid). Double-stranded RNA can be produced intracellularly during infection either by DNA or by RNA viruses, e.g. as a result of transcription of both strands of viral DNA or when RNA viruses form double-stranded replicative intermediates. The requirement for dsRNA means that, except for reoviruses which have a dsRNA genome, interferon cannot be induced until viral replication has begun. By an unknown process, dsRNA activates the interferon genes (the gene for IFN-β is on chromosome 9 in human cells) with production of mRNA followed by interferon synthesis. Thus, good inducers are viruses which do not cause early inhibition of host cell protein synthesis or exert a rapid cytocidal effect. Interferon induction is summarised in Figure 3.16a. Most of the interferon synthesized by the cell is concentrated into vesicles and exported; its principal action is to protect surrounding cells rather than the one in which it was made.

As noted above, IFN-γ is a product of T lymphocytes and is released in the manner of a lymphokine following reaction of the sensitised T cell with its specific antigen via the T cell receptor. It

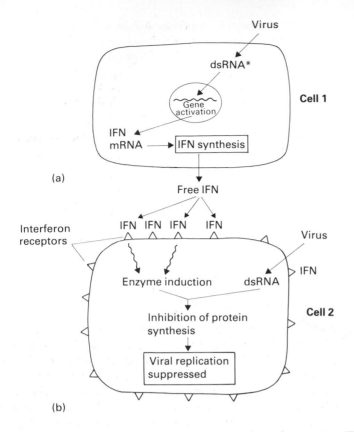

Figure 3.16 Mechanism of action of interferon (IFN).
1. Outline of events.
(a) Induction of IFN.
(b) IFN stimulates antiviral state in target cell.
*ds = double-stranded

is also produced by mitogen-activated T cells, e.g. after treating T cells with plant lectins such as concanavalin A.

Mechanism of action

Interferons act via cell-surface receptors and probably do not enter their 'target' cells (Figure 3.16b); thus, interferon immobilised by binding to beads is said to be as effective in protecting cells as free interferon. The receptors are (or contain) gangliosides (p. 855); genes on human chromosome 21 are involved in determining the receptor, and cells of individuals with Down's syndrome, in whom each cell has three copies of this chromosome instead of two (p. 815), are particularly sensitive *in vitro* to interferon. An *antiviral state* is produced within the cell following binding of interferon at the cell membrane; there are two pathways whereby this state is achieved, and both lead to *inhibition of translation* of viral protein from mRNA (Figure 3.17). Both involve an increase in the activity of certain intracellular enzymes. In the first, a *protein kinase* is stimulated, which inhibits protein synthesis by phosphorylation of the initiation factor eIF$_2$. The second pathway is rather more complicated. Interferon-treated cells contain an increased level of an adenine trinucleotide called '*2-5A*' from its unusual 2'-5' phosphodiester linkage (pppA2'p5'A2'p5'A); interferon evidently activates the synthetase for 2-5A. In intact cells and cell-free systems, 2-5A has been shown to activate a *ribonuclease*

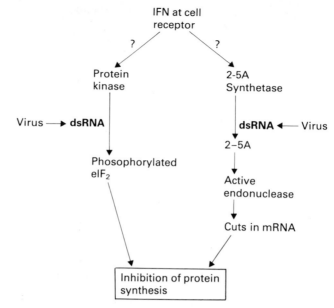

Figure 3.17 Mechanism of action of interferon (IFN). 2. Pathways of induction of antiviral state in target cells.
ds = double-stranded
? = coupling pathway unknown

(endonuclease), RNase F, which destroys certain viral messenger RNAs. Both the kinase and the 2-5A synthetase also require the presence of dsRNA for their activity, so that these translation-inhibiting pathways are only activated during viral infection of the cell, thus safeguarding normal cells from damage. Note that dsRNA is the signal for the presence of viral infection both at the stages of interferon induction and its activity. Figure 3.17 shows the biochemical processes involved in the action of interferon. Due to its mode of action via cell-surface receptors, interferon cannot protect the cell which produces it until secreted; even then, the producer cell may not be affected because interferon has little influence on viral synthesis that is already in progress.

We have noted that normal cells are generally shielded from interferon-induced inhibition of protein synthesis; even in the infected cell there is a certain selective effect on viral protein synthesis. However, the host cell is not always spared; its death would often be no disadvantage, as it also halts viral spread (cf. the cytotoxic action of T cells). On the other hand, this may contribute to a disease process (cf. hypersensitivity), as demonstrated in experimental infection of mice with lymphocytic choriomeningitis (LCM) virus. Injection of anti-interferon serum to these mice *alleviates* their symptoms, while increasing the level of virus in the circulation.

IFN-γ induces the same antiviral activities as described above. It differs antigenically from the α and β molecules and is more labile in acid. One of its advantages is that it is available during viral infections which switch off host cell mRNA or protein synthesis too rapidly for the other interferons to be made.

Significance of interferon

Although we have concentrated on its anti-viral role, interferon also has effects on the immune response, while at high doses it may be a cytotoxic agent.

Antiviral role: This is the major protective function of interferon, but its success depends on the dynamics and timing of infection— for example, the relative concentrations of virus and interferon may be critical; also interferon needs to influence a cell *before* it is infected for maximal effect. Advantages of interferon include its wide range of action and its rapid appearance—more rapid than a primary immune response.

Immunomodulatory role: Several effects of interferon on the immune system are coming to light. It tends to suppress antibody production, while enhancing both T cell and NK cell activity; this produces a shift in the response from antibody to cell-mediated immunity and probably contributes to interferon's antitumour properties.

Cytotoxicity: Interferon is not toxic to normal cells or animals at moderate doses and there are no side effects of treating viral diseases with interferon. At high doses, however, it can inhibit cell proliferation *in vitro*, while *in vivo* the production of platelets and leucocytes by the bone marrow is depressed; this is, in fact, one of the problems in cancer patients treated with very large doses of interferon (others include hair loss, fever, nausea and lethargy). This cytotoxicity may also be important in the action of interferon on neoplastic cells.

Present and potential therapeutic uses

In principle, interferon should be the ideal antiviral agent, having a wide spectrum of action, high potency, poor antigenicity and no side effects at therapeutic doses. In practice, its promise in therapy of virus diseases has not yet been realised. In clinical trials, interferon has been shown to prevent the common cold and reduce the severity of other respiratory diseases such as influenza. Delivery in these cases is local, by intranasal drops or respiratory spray, and to be effective the interferon must be given before symptoms arise and preferably before infection. Local and systemic treatment with interferon can also be used in herpesvirus infections, e.g. to reduce the spread of herpes simplex (cold sores, genital herpes) and to treat zoster in cancer patients and chickenpox in immunosuppressed children with cancer (p. 270). There has also been some success in treating individuals with chronic hepatitis B (HBV) infection, and in some cases permanent eradication of HBV has been achieved with prolonged interferon therapy.

It is the antitumour properties of interferon which are understandably attracting the most interest at the moment. Some animal and human cancers have been treated successfully. In patients there were at first encouraging results with osteosarcomas (bone cancers), though the numbers treated were small. Larger scale trials are currently under way, but at present interferon does not seem to be any more effective than established chemotherapeutic agents in treating diverse cancers such as lymphoma, myeloma, melanoma and breast cancer. Out of 82 patients in the

American Cancer Society programme, some 25-40% showed a favourable response, but permanent remissions were only obtained in a few cases. At the high doses used, interferon side effects were a problem (above). It is too early for a final judgement, but, at the time of writing, interferon appears less of a breakthrough in cancer treatment than early dramatic results in individual cases suggested.

EFFECTS OF VIRUS ON THE HOST

The interaction between a virus and the body—as opposed to individual cells—of its animal host begins with the acquisition of infection. The virus may then establish itself purely locally or spread away from the initial site of infection via lymphatics and the bloodstream to infect distant tissues. Finally, symptoms of disease may be produced, though this is by no means always the case as many infections are asymptomatic; the distinction between *infection* and *disease* should be noted.

Routes of infection

The principal routes of entry of a virus into the body are via the epithelial surfaces of the skin, the respiratory tract, and the oropharynx and alimentary tract. There are also examples of invasion of the mucous membranes of the genital tract and conjunctiva, as well as transplacental infection. In animals, genetic transmission, i.e. of viral information incorporated into the genome, is also known.

Skin

The skin may be penetrated by viruses as a result of (i) mechanical trauma, as in cowpox, molluscum contagiosum, warts or venereal acquisition by males of genital herpes; (ii) by injection, as in transmission of hepatitis B virus on contaminated syringe needles or in infected blood; (iii) by the bite of an infected insect, as in arbovirus diseases such as yellow fever; or (iv) by the bite of an infected mammal, the classic example being rabies. In many of these cases the virus does not multiply locally, but is carried away in the bloodstream (hepatitis B, arboviruses) or migrates along nerves (rabies). Local infection is only established for those noted under 'mechanical trauma'.

Respiratory tract

This is a major route of invasion, not only for viruses causing local respiratory infections, such as the common cold, influenza and parainfluenza viruses, but also for many others, which cause an asymptomatic initial infection of the respiratory tract followed by generalised spread around the body (e.g. smallpox, mumps, chickenpox, and some enteroviruses). The virus is transmitted by *droplet infection* in the aerosol or dispersion of droplets which results from sneezing, coughing, singing or merely talking. The size of droplet is crucial to successful transmission, as the very small (0.3 μm diameter) droplets dry rapidly and the very large ones (10 μm diameter) fall rapidly, so that only the intermediate sizes transmit the infection in some diseases. Droplet size also influences the local site of infection, as larger droplets are trapped in the nasal baffles while smaller ones may be carried into the lungs.

Droplet dispersion is encouraged by the nasal secretions which often accompany respiratory tract infections. Not all infected individuals are able to transmit virus effectively and, experimentally, respiratory transmission is often hard to demonstrate; probably only particular individuals will produce both sufficient virus and nasal secretion to enable spread to occur. Upper respiratory tract diseases are typically associated with cold weather, but this seasonal restriction probably has to do more with crowding of people in poorly ventilated rooms than with temperature *per se*.

Alimentary tract and oropharynx

Faecal-oral transmission, as a result of poor personal or community hygiene or imperfect sanitation, is responsible for spreading viruses which multiply in or pass through the intestinal tract. Important examples are Norwalk virus and rotaviruses, which are agents of acute gastroenteritis, poliovirus and other enteroviruses, and hepatitis A, all of which are non-enveloped, icosahedral viruses (the infectivity of enveloped viruses being destroyed by the bile, which dissolves the lipid envelope). At first sight, it would be thought that improved standards of hygiene would reduce the incidence of the diseases spread by the faecal-oral route, but paradoxically the opposite is sometimes the case. For instance, in the days before vaccination against poliomyelitis, epidemics of paralytic disease were typical of countries with a high standard of living and rare in densely populated countries with poor hygienic conditions, where the disease was endemic rather than epidemic. This was because the severity of poliomyelitis is related to age and, despite its common name 'infantile paralysis', is in fact far more likely to be paralytic in adolescents and adults than in infants. With improvments in sanitation, etc., young children, in whom the disease is usually mild, were shielded from infection and an individual's first exposure was delayed until an age when the effects were more likely to be severely crippling. The disappearance of polio from developed countries was only achieved by vaccination, which began in the 1950's. A similar situation occurs in infectious mononucleosis (glandular fever), which is essentially a disease of young adults from higher socio-economic groups who do not come into contact with the Epstein–Barr virus at an early age. In contrast, in areas of lower standards of living, primary infection occurs in children and is often asymptomatic, persists for life and induces immunity.

Viruses present in the saliva can be spread by direct contact, e.g. kissing, or via contaminated eating and drinking utensils;

examples include mumps, Epstein–Barr and herpes simplex viruses.

Transplacental transmission

Rubella and cytomegalovirus are important examples of infections occurring *in utero* as a result of transmission from mother to foetus across the placenta. Both are major causes of congenital abnormalities; while they may cause foetal death, the fact that they are of relatively low pathogenicity means that the infected foetus often survives with congenital defects.

Localisation and spread of virus within the body

Having penetrated the epithelial surface, a virus may remain *localised* at or near the site of initial infection, or may be *disseminated* around the body with or without multiplying locally first. Purely local infection is seen in the skin in warts and vaccinia lesions and in the respiratory tract in influenza and the common cold. However, many viruses are carried in the blood-stream and ultimately infect a particular target organ(s) which may be the skin, CNS, liver or elsewhere. Bloodstream dissemination, or *viraemia*, is usually preceded by multiplication of virus at the site of entry and/or in local lymphoid tissue (unless virus is introduced directly into blood); in the circulation itself, the virus may be either free (poliovirus, yellow fever virus) or associated with leucocytes (Epstein–Barr, smallpox, measles viruses) or red blood cells (Colorado tick fever virus).

Figure 3.18 is a general scheme for diseases involving systemic spread of virus, showing that initial rounds of replication at the site of the local lesion and in draining lymph nodes are followed

Figure 3.18 General scheme for infections with systemic spread of virus.

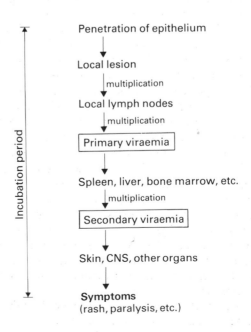

by an early or *primary* viraemia, then further multiplication in organs such as the spleen and liver (partly because of phagocytosis by macrophages), and *secondary* viraemia before the target organ is infected. Up to this point, the disease may be symptomless and the period of silent viral multiplication and distribution, ending with the appearance of symptoms, is called the *incubation period*. Thus an infection is often in progress for several days or weeks before the host is aware of its existence. For generalised infections of this type, the incubation period is usually relatively protracted (10–20 days or more), being much shorter when the disease process is entirely local (e.g. 1–3 days for upper respiratory tract infections). There are exceptions, however, as in the short incubation periods of 3–6 days in infections by arboviruses (e.g. yellow fever) which are introduced directly into the blood by insect bite; conversely, warts are an example of a local infection with a prolonged incubation period. Extreme examples of long incubation periods occur in 'slow virus' infections where the interval between infection and appearance of symptoms may be many months. During the incubation period, probably very soon after the start of infection, the immune response is stimulated and may contribute to disease symptoms, such as skin rashes, through hypersensitivity.

It is apparent that, quite apart from differences in transmission and localisation of virus, there are important variations in the

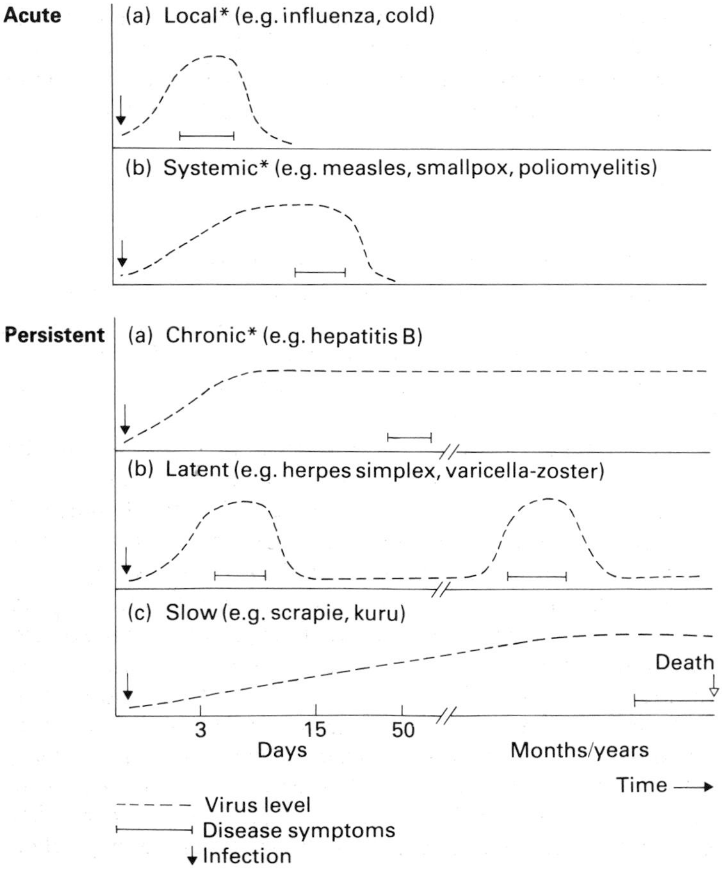

Figure 3.19 Types of viral infection.
* = may be asymptomatic (subclinical)

256

pathogenesis of viral diseases, including time course, the extent to which symptoms are produced and the clearance or persistence of virus. The following patterns are recognised (see also Figure 3.19).

Acute infections

Many viral infections fall into the category of acute febrile diseases (e.g. smallpox, yellow fever, measles, poliomyelitis, influenza, common cold), with an incubation period of from 2 to 20 days, followed by symptoms resulting from either local or widespread cell death and tissue damage and, within a relatively short time (2–3 weeks), the elimination of the virus or death of the host. Often, however, an acute infection is *inapparent* (asymptomatic or subclinical) and indeed the same virus may produce clinical disease in one individual yet be inapparent in another. The tendency for subclinical infection to occur is dependent, in general, on the infecting dose and on host 'reactivity' (in its widest sense). Overall, inapparent infections are the commonest type. Acute inapparent infections follow the same course, including duration and recovery, as acute diseases and, while clinically silent, they also stimulate immunity (which is the proof that they occurred). They are important epidemiologically as a means of covert dissemination of the virus in the population. Sometimes infections are symptomless in a virus's natural host, but severe or lethal in a different host; for example, yellow fever is a harmless and inapparent infection of Old World monkeys, but a severe disease in man. This doubtless reflects an adaptation of the virus to its natural host, which is to the virus's advantage.

Persistent infections

On recovery from an acute infection, virus is completely cleared from the body by the humoral and cell-mediated immune responses. In contrast, persistent infections are those in which the virus survives for months or years, in large quantity in some instances, in barely detectable amounts in others. There are four categories, namely *latent, chronic, slow* and *oncogenic* infections.

Latent infections Here an acute infection (which can be asymptomatic) is followed by apparently complete recovery, but a minute amount of virus remains sequestered in a small number of body cells and is able to cause a recurrence of the acute symptoms after an interval of months or years. The classic examples are found in infections with the herpesviruses, herpes simplex (cold sores, genital herpes) and varicella-zoster virus (chickenpox, shingles). After the acute stage of these conditions, the herpesvirus travels along sensory nerve fibres (intra-axonal transport) to the appropriate dorsal root ganglion, where it remains dormant in ganglion cells. During this latent stage, infectious virus is not detectable, but can be recovered by growing ganglion fragments in tissue culture. Using labelled probes, viral nucleic acid can be demonstrated to be in the nuclei of ganglion cells, but whether in free form or integrated into the cell DNA is not known. For a certain period of time, re-emergence of the virus is prevented, at least in part, by host cell-mediated immunity, but when this wanes or is suppressed the acute infection may reappear. Experimentally, however, immunosuppression of mice, e.g. by X-irradiation, does not stimulate reactivation, suggesting that other factors are also involved. One could envisage that molecular control mechanisms determine reactivation of viral DNA, while the level of the immune response then influences the recurrence of disease. In the case of cold sores, herpes simplex type 1 virus becomes latent in cells of the trigeminal ganglion; recurrences at intervals of a few months are common, the virus passing back down the sensory nerves to the skin around the mouth. Reactivation of the virus can be triggered by a number of disparate factors, including sunlight, menstruation and respiratory tract infections (p.262). Similarly, genital infections with herpes simplex type 2 virus recur from time to time; in this case the virus lies dormant in the sacral ganglion. Following childhood chickenpox, varicella-zoster virus remains latent for many years and spontaneously recurs in adults as zoster (shingles), the local skin lesions of which are located around the sensory nerve endings from which the virus has reappeared. In summary, a latent virus is present in *very small amount* and is *non-cytocidal* during its period of latency.

Chronic infections Sometimes viruses persist in quantity in the body over a long period of time, with or without a history of disease; chronically infected individuals, who are often symptomless carriers, are an important source of infection for others. The fact that virus is *continuously detectable* is the main difference between chronic and latent infection; also chronic infections may be cytocidal. Hepatitis B (serum hepatitis) provides a major example. After recovery from acute hepatitis, up to 30% of patients continue to carry the virus in their bloodstream for months or years; there are also many carriers in whom the infection has been inapparent throughout. Altogether there are estimated to be over 100 million carriers of hepatitis B virus in the world. Transmission can occur by injection of virus into the bloodstream, either by transfusion of infected blood or contamination of needles or syringes, so that careful screening of donor blood for hepatitis B virus is an essential and now universal practice. Cytomegalovirus and Epstein–Barr virus are herpes-viruses which regularly establish asymptomatic chronic infections, though they can also cause acute diseases such as mononucleosis (both) or foetal infection (cytomegalovirus); in the latter, virus continues to be excreted in urine or saliva for a long period after birth. Rubella is another foetal infection in which virus is present over a long period. Infected infants may shed virus continuously for one or two years and the apparently normal infant carrier excreting virus is a dangerous source of infection.

Chronic infections, particularly those acquired *in utero*, may be due to partial immunological tolerance. Infant carriers of cytomegalovirus or rubella virus are able to make antibodies, and virus persists despite the presence of high levels of serum IgM and IgG against it. However, depression of cell-mediated immunity, or tolerance, may be responsible for long-term infection. Asymptomatic persistence of cytomegalovirus and Epstein–Barr virus can occur in lymphocytes, evidently without elimination of the infected cells.

Infections of rodents by arenaviruses, such as lymphocytic choriomeningitis (LCM) virus, provide excellent animal models of chronic infection and immunological tolerance. LCM virus is indigenous in the house mouse (*Mus musculus*), being transmitted from generation to generation by transplacental infection. Mice acquiring the virus *in utero* carry it as a life-long infection with viraemia and viruria; most of the cells in the body are infected, but there are no major cytopathic changes and for most of their lives the mice experience no harmful effects. The early exposure to the virus leads to tolerance of viral antigens, which is evidently complete for cell-mediated immunity; antibody production is depressed but not wholly absent, as antibody–virus complexes are found in the circulation, though free antibody cannot be detected. The lack of cell-mediated (T cell) response allows the virus to establish a persistent infection which remains asymptomatic, except in old age when sufficient immune complexes may be formed to cause glomerulonephritis (p. 162). Other arenaviruses, such as Lassa virus, also cause chronic, silent infections in rodents, in the latter case in rats (p. 352).

Slow infections This term applies to a group of rare diseases, many of the central nervous system, which have an unusually long incubation period lasting for months or years. ('Slow' applies to the development of the disease and not necessarily to the rate of replication of the agent.) Another characteristic feature is their gradual, but inexorable progression to the death of the host. One such disease, subacute sclerosing panencephalitis (SSPE) is a late consequence of measles; others in man and animals are not caused by recognised viruses, but by so-called 'unconventional agents' which include those of certain degenerative brain diseases such as scrapie in sheep and kuru and Creutzfeldt-Jakob disease in man. These agents may be extremely small virus-like entities, but there is also reason to suggest that they may be a novel type of infectious particle which contains protein but lacks nucleic acid altogether (p. 371). In infection by these agents, the absence both of a host immune reponse and interferon production allows the disease process to continue unchallenged. This is not the case in SSPE, where plasma cells infiltrate the brain and there are high levels of antimeasles antibody; there may nevertheless be a contributory defect in cell-mediated immunity.

Oncogenic infections A fourth type of persistent infection occurs with tumour viruses. In the discussion of transformation, it was noted that the maintenance of the neoplastic state requires the continuous presence of the virus in the cell and in fact demands the integration of viral genetic information into a host cell chromosome. DNA viruses remain in a latent state in their tumour cells; nevertheless, progeny virus may still be produced by productive infection of a few cells, as in Burkitt's lymphoma (Epstein–Barr virus). In contrast, RNA viruses (other than those which are defective) are continuously replicated in and released from their tumour cell hosts, budding from the surface without damaging the membrane. Genetic and developmental factors are important in determining whether a particular virus is tumourigenic in a given animal, e.g. inbred strains of mice show different susceptibilities and very young, immunologically immature or otherwise immunodeficient animals may be especially sensitive. Thus, as in other examples of viral persistence, the effectiveness of the host immune response is a major factor in determining the pattern of disease. Although virus-induced tumour cells are more than merely virus-infected cells, some of the ways in which they avoid immunological destruction—the presence of interfering or 'blocking' antibodies for example—may be relevant to other persistent virus infections (see p. 746).

In summary, the mechanisms of persistence in virus infection are often due to properties both of the virus and the host. The former may be able to sequester itself into a cell safe from immune attack, or it may either suppress the immune reponse or lack antigenicity. Infection of the foetus or neonate can lead to a partial state of tolerance, especially in the vital cell-mediated immune reponse, while in the adult the production of certain types of antibody can interfere with the recognition of infected cells by cytotoxic T cells. Finally, we can note that there are many instances in which the same virus causes different types of infection depending on the state (age, immunological competence, etc.) of the individual host. Three examples are rubella infection in adults or foetuses (p. 310); poliovirus in infants or adults (p. 290); and infection by Epstein–Barr virus in different age groups and geographical locations (p. 792). Others will be found in the rest of this Section.

HOST IMMUNE RESPONSE

The details of the types of immune reaction relevant to viral infection have already been described in Section 2. Here we will briefly summarise a few points. The response consists of both antibody and cell-mediated immunity. The role of antibody is to *neutralise* virus in the blood and extracellular fluid, by reacting with viral proteins required for adherence to cell surfaces, as well as to encourage uptake of viral particles by phagocytic cells. Antibody is important both in the bloodstream, where it will be effective against viraemic spread, and on mucosal surfaces such as the gut and respiratory tract, where in the form of IgA it provides vital local immunity against enteric and respiratory viruses. Maternal IgG, acquired either across the placenta (in humans) or in the milk, and milk-borne IgA play a major role in passive protection of the newborn at a stage of immunological immaturity. (Most of the infective agents which threaten the newborn derive from the mother herself, who coincidentally

260

transfers the passive immunity which allows the infant to survive to produce its own immune defence, illustrating the importance of breast feeding.) Antibodies are of course only useful once present at the required level in the blood or at a tissue surface; in a primary infection the time for this to occur may be too long to prevent the occurrence of disease. Thus, in general, antibodies are of greatest use in prevention of *reinfection*, i.e. in establishing long-lasting immunity; at a mucosal surface, antibody has the power to prevent a virus entering the body altogether, while in the bloodstream access to internal target organs can be blocked.

Recovery from primary infections often requires cell-mediated immunity in the form of cytotoxic T cells, production of lymphokines (which include interferon) and recruitment/ activation of macrophages. Examples have already been cited of the persistence of viruses in the face of quantities of antibody, underlining the central role of cell-mediated processes. A principal protective function of T cells is indeed precisely to seek out and destroy virus-infected cells, and in dealing with intracellular infection T cells are more effective than antibodies, despite the ability of the latter to cause lysis via complement fixation or K cells. The rapid secondary T cell response is also important in protective immunity.

The rate of induction of the immune response versus the length of the incubation period is a major factor determining the outcome of infection. In diseases with a long incubation period, the primary immune response must be delayed, otherwise disease would not occur; the delay may be due to the fact that many viruses infect lymphoid tissue during the incubation period, which may interfere with its function. The increased speed of the secondary over the primary response is crucial in ensuring that many diseases occur only once in a lifetime.

Where a virus species exists in a number of types differing in their surface antigens (serotypes), it is often found that immunity is *type-specific*, despite the fact that different types may be similar in many respects and share some common group antigens. The reason is that immunity must usually be directed either against viral structures involved in adherence to cells (in the case of antibody) or against viral proteins which appear on the surface of infected cells (for T cells), and it is these viral structures which show variation between serotypes precisely as a result of the selective pressure of host immunity. This is particularly important in the common cold (over 100 types of rhinoviruses), respiratory infections due to adenoviruses (33 types), poliomyelitis (3 types), and influenza (strains changing regularly).

Finally, we should note the contribution of hypersensitivity mechanisms to the symptoms and severity of viral disease. This ranges from Type III (immune complex) damage due to deposition of virus-antibody complexes, e.g. in the kidney in hepatitis B, to the role of Type IV (cell-mediated) hypersensitivity in the dermal manifestations (skin rashes) of exanthematous diseases. A classic illustration of hypersensitivity mechanisms in a viral infection is lymphocytic choriomeningitis (LCM) of mice, noted above as an example of a chronic infection when acquired in *utero*. Intracerebral inoculation of LCM virus into normal (i.e. uninfected) adult mice leads to LCM disease, with massive infiltration by (note) lymphocytes and macrophages throughout the meninges, ependyma and choroid plexus and death within two weeks due to cerebral oedema. It seems clear that this is a T cell response against localised viral antigen, as might be suspected from the histology; thus, mice can be protected from the disease by various forms of immuno-suppression, including X-irradiation, anti-Thy-1 serum, neonatal thymectomy or cyclophosphamide, all of which treatments eliminate T cell responses. Moreover, LCM-reactive T cells can transfer the disease to infected, immunosuppressed mice, while there is no evidence that antibody is involved. Thus, Type IV hypersensitivity is responsible for LCM in adult mice. It should be noted that inoculation of the virus by the same route either in newborn mice or in chronically infected adult carrier mice does *not* lead to LCM disease: these animals are immunologically tolerant to LCM virus as a result of their exposure to viral antigens at a very early age. As noted above, they carry the virus as a benign infection in all their tissues and are unable to make the T cell response necessary to clear it—or to cause the disease. Interestingly, in mice with chronic LCM infection, an immune complex disease may eventually occur; tolerance in antibody production is not complete, and complexes of virus and antibody are present in the circulation throughout life. In old mice (over 10 months) the complexes may accumulate sufficiently in the kidneys to cause death through chronic glomerulonephritis. Another animal viral infection involving Type III hypersensitivity is Aleutian disease of mink (p. 369). Here too, kidney damage due to deposits of virus-antibody complexes is a prominent pathological feature.

VIRUS FAMILIES INFECTING MAN

Thus far we have considered the general principles of the nature of viruses and their interaction with the host at the level of infected cells and the body as a whole. Specific examples of viral diseases of man to illustrate these principles are now described.

HERPETOVIRIDAE

The herpesviruses comprise a large group of very widely distributed DNA (class I) viruses which cause a number of common diseases as well as inapparent infections. The major members affecting man are the *herpes simplex viruses* (the agents of cold sores and genital herpes); *varicella-zoster virus* (chickenpox and shingles); *cytomegalovirus* (an important cause of congenital abnormalities and a major opportunistic pathogen); and *Epstein–Barr virus* (glandular fever). Two of these are also strong candidates for human cancer viruses, namely herpes simplex type 2 (cervical carcinoma) and Epstein–Barr virus (Burkitt's lymphoma and nasopharyngeal carcinoma), while others are oncogenic in animals (p. 791). A property common to all is the ability to

Table 3.6 Persistence in herpesvirus infections.

Virus	Disease	Type of persistence	Conditions for reactivation
Herpes simplex type 1	Gingivostomatitis Cold sore Keratitis, etc.	Latent in sensory ganglia with many acute recurrences of disease	Fever; menstruation; stress; sunlight; naturally depressed CMI; immunosuppressive drugs
Herpes simplex type 2	Genital herpes	Ditto	? local trauma
Varicella-zoster virus	Chickenpox Zoster	Latent in dorsal root ganglia after childhood chickenpox; usually single recurrence in adult as zoster	Ageing; naturally depressed CMI; immunosuppressive drugs, etc; spinal injury; trauma
Cytomegalovirus	Cytomegalic inclusion disease of the newborn Congenital defects Mononucleosis with hepatitis	Chronic infection of salivary glands and kidney, with shedding in saliva and urine	Immunosuppressive drugs, etc.; pregnancy
Epstein–Barr virus	Infectious mononucleosis Burkitt's lymphoma Nasopharyngeal carcinoma	Chronic production in oropharyngeal secretions; latent in lymphocytes and tumour cells	Immunosuppression

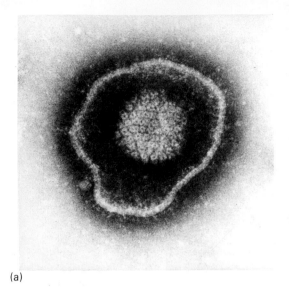

(a)

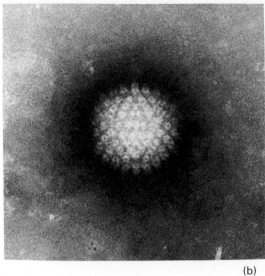

(b)

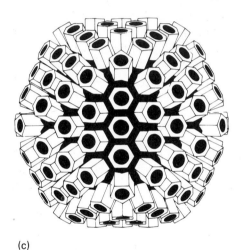

(c)

Figure 3.20 Structure of herpesviruses.
(a) Electron micrograph of enveloped particle, ×200,000; negative staining.
(b) Naked capsid, ×200,000; negative staining.
(c) Drawing of a herpesvirus capsid (cf. electron micrographs. The icosahedron is viewed along a 2-fold symmetry axis. The capsid is composed of 150 hexagonal prisms (hexons) at the faces and edges of the icosahedron with 12 pentagonal prisms (pentons) at the apexes.
(d) Diagrammatic cross-section of a herpesvirus.
((a) and (b) by courtesy of Dr June Almeida; (c) by courtesy of Professor R.W. Horne)

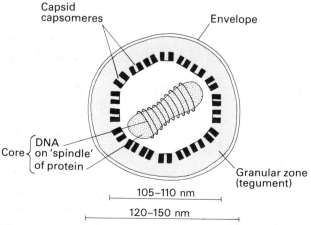

Capsid capsomeres

Envelope

Core { DNA on 'spindle' of protein

Granular zone (tegument)

105–110 nm

120–150 nm

(d)

establish *persistent infections*, which may be of the latent, chronic or oncogenic types (Table 3.6); infections are probably always lifelong, with recurrent episodes of acute symptoms in some. A persistent herpesvirus infection can often be reactivated into an acute disease by suppression of cell-mediated immunity, and as a result they are frequently seen as troublesome opportunistic infections in patients receiving immunosuppressive treatment to prevent graft rejection, or in cancer therapy, etc.

Structure (Figure 3.20)

The virions are quite large, and among DNA viruses are second only to the poxviruses in size. The icosahedral capsid, 105–110 nm in diameter, is composed of 162 hollow hexagonal and pentagonal capsomeres (150 hexons and 12 pentons) and is surrounded by a lipid envelope containing viral glycoproteins. Between the capsid and the envelope there is a granular zone or tegument which contains several viral globular proteins. The overall diameter of the particle is 120–150 nm. The virion contains 25–30 major proteins and the DNA probably codes for at least 50 polypeptides altogether, including several enzymes (e.g. thymidine kinase and DNA polymerase, which are useful targets for specific antiviral agents, p. 268). Like other enveloped viruses, herpesviruses are inactivated by lipid solvents (chloroform, ether).

Replication and cellular infection

Replication follows the pattern of most class I viruses, the DNA being replicated in the nucleus while capsid proteins are synthesized in the cytoplasm and enter the nucleus for virion assembly (p.233). Infected cells often show characteristic intranuclear (Cowdry type A) inclusion bodies which are initially basophilic, as viral DNA is synthesized and accumulates, and later eosinophilic when they are the remains of viral replication areas after the progeny virions have migrated into the cytoplasm. The inclusion body fills the nucleus, pushing the (basophilic) chromatin to the margin, as shown in Figure 3.14c. The viral envelope is unusual in that it is acquired by budding through the *nuclear* membrane, rather than the plasma membrane as in enveloped RNA viruses (Figure 3.13a). Nevertheless, during infection, herpesvirus glycoproteins appear in both the nuclear and plasma membranes, rendering the cells susceptible to lysis by either antibody and complement, antibody and K cells, or cytotoxic T cells.

Herpesvirus infections are generally cytocidal when accompanied by replication. Latent, non-cytocidal cellular infections are common, notably by herpes simplex and varicella-zoster viruses in sensory nerve ganglia, cytomegalovirus in salivary glands, and Epstein–Barr virus in lymphocytes. As part of their cytopathogenic effect, herpes simplex and varicella-zoster viruses induce cell fusion, with formation of characteristic multinucleated giant cells (Figure 3.14c). Such syncytia, with their intranuclear inclusions, can be useful diagnostically when obtained from scrapings of the skin vesicles caused by these viruses.

Transmission

Transmission takes several forms, depending on the virus species. Herpes simplex and Epstein–Barr viruses require close personal contact, e.g. kissing (cold sores, glandular fever), or venereal spread (genital herpes); varicella-zoster virus is spread by the respiratory route; and cytomegalovirus can be acquired by transplacental passage or during birth (as well as by more conventional routes). Infections are frequently established in childhood and persist for life; they are often symptomless, but serological studies testify to their ubiquity. Most herpesviruses are species-specific, but herpes simplex is unusual in that, while man is the only natural host, it can infect a variety of animals, including mice, guinea-pigs and rabbits; these are useful animal models for the study of its pathogenicity.

Herpes simplex viruses (HSV)

Infection with herpes simplex viruses is very widespread. There are two related types, distinguishable by their specific antigens. Both cause vesicular lesions on the skin and mucous membranes. (A *vesicle* is a fluid-containing cavity within or beneath the epidermis and less than 5mm in diameter; if larger-it is called a *bulla*.) *Type 1* virus is responsible for cold sores (fever blisters) which occur around the mouth, one of the commonest human diseases, while *type 2* is the agent of genital herpes, a venereal disease of increasing prevalence. The generality of infection is indicated by serological surveys which show that more than 80% of the population over the age of 30 years have serum antibodies and cell-mediated immunity to type 1 virus. Although infection is inapparent in many, a sizeable proportion of those infected suffer from cold sores. Both types establish latent infections and over a period of years the acute phase of the disease may recur many times.

Type 1 virus. Infection is often acquired in infancy at 6–18 months, less often in adults, and persists for life. 10–15% of babies develop the primary disease, which may be dismissed as 'teething', occurring inside the mouth and on the gums (*gingivostomatitis*). It may also affect the eye (*keratitis*, inflammation of the cornea) and occasionally spreads to the CNS where infection of the meninges and brain leads to meningitis or encephalitis; the latter has a high mortality and causes mental defects in survivors. The commonest recurrent form is the *cold sore* which occurs around rather than inside the mouth, and on the mucocutaneous junction of the lips and skin (also known as herpes labialis) or nose. The inflammatory vesicles are painful, occur in clusters and are filled with clear fluid; after a few days they ulcerate, crust over and heal. Multinucleate giant cells with intranuclear inclusions can be obtained from the base of the vesicles. Cold sores always recur at the same site in any one individual. Recurrences are induced by certain febrile illnesses such as influenza, malaria or meningococcal infection, by emotional or physical stress, menstruation, sunlight or cold wind, or certain drugs. Keratitis is also recurrent and, because of gradual corneal scarring, is a major infectious cause of blindness.

Type 2 virus. The lesions of genital herpes have similar characteristics to cold sores—they are initially vesicular, then ulcerate to give raw, painful areas. In females, they occur on the labia, vagina and cervix; in males, on the glans and shaft of the penis or around the anus. Aided by frequent recurrences, genital herpes has become a major venereal disease. Infection can be acquired by the newborn during birth, if acute lesions are present in the birth canal, and an overwhelming, possibly fatal, disseminated herpes infection may result. There is also evidence associating type 2 infection in women with cervical cancer, as discussed on p. 796, and it is noteworthy that the cervix is a site commonly affected by the virus.

As described above, herpes simplex viruses remain in the body as latent infections during the quiescent periods between acute symptomatic phases. They are not present in the skin at these times, but lie hidden in the trigeminal or sacral nerve ganglia (type 1 and type 2 viruses repectively), reached by travelling within the axoplasm of sensory nerve fibres. The viruses remain latent in ganglion cells until reactivated. In about 2% of carriers, type 1 virus is present during the latent phase in the saliva, which can be a source of infection.

Recovery from the acute phase of HSV infections is due to a cell-mediated immune reaction against infected cells; high levels of antibody are also present, and while this may prevent viraemic spread, it does not seem to be important in recovery. The recurrence of the acute symptoms is apparently due to a diminution in the effectiveness of T cell immunity, coupled with the factors noted above. The virus then re-emerges down the sensory nerves into the epidermis, and the repetition of this pathway accounts for the identical localisation of vesicles at each recurrence. The importance of CMI in controlling the disease is underlined by the severe *disseminated* form of reactivated herpes simplex seen in immunosuppressed patients.

Chemotherapy. Herpesvirus infections are among the few viral diseases for which specific chemotherapy (i.e. more effective against the virus than toxic for host cells) is available, using base or nucleoside analogues which interfere with DNA synthesis. The iodinated derivative of deoxyuridine, *iododeoxyuridine* ('idoxuridine', IUdR) is used in treatment of herpetic keratitis. Although toxic if administered systemically, it is used in the eye by local application, but with some toxic side-effects; it is less successful in treatment of cold sores or genital lesions. *Adenine arabinoside* ('vidarabine', Ara-A) is a nucleoside analogue in which arabinose replaces deoxyribose; it also has specific antiviral properties and is useful in treating severe disseminated

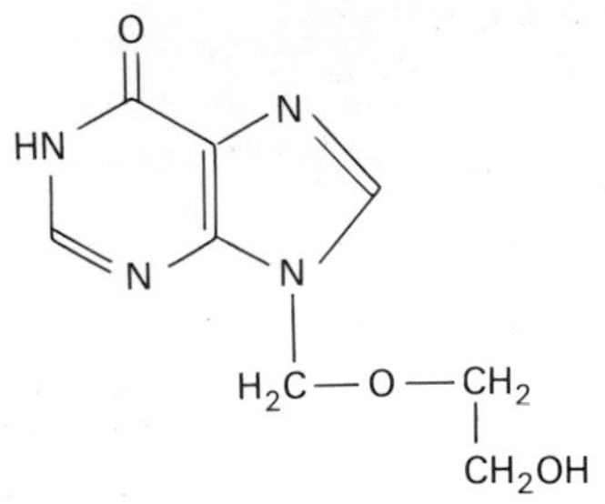

Figure 3.21 Acyclovir.

herpesvirus infections, e.g. in immunosuppressed patients. The drawbacks of Ara-A are not so much toxicity as its rapid deamination to an inactive form, and its low solubility which necessitates a large fluid dose to the patient.

A recently developed agent of great promise is another nucleoside, 9-(2-hydroxyethoxymethyl)guanine ('*acyclovir*' or '*zovirax*'; Figure 3.21), which is active against both type 1 and type 2 herpes simplex viruses and has the advantage of much lower toxicity. The reason for the latter lies in its high degree of selective action for HSV infected cells. The basis of its selectivity lies in the fact that acyclovir is inactive until phosphorylated, and activation is brought about uniquely by the *viral* enzyme thymidine kinase. Thus, the active form of the drug is only present in virus-infected cells. Thereafter, activated acyclovir specifically inhibits the action of viral DNA polymerase to suppress viral replication. Recent clinical trials on recipients of heart, liver or bone marrow grafts, as well as cancer patients, all suffering from herpes simplex activated as a result of their immunosuppression, have been encouraging and acyclovir will probably be the drug of choice in such cases. A topical ointment preparation is also available for more general use against cold sores *and* genital herpes. However, acyclovir does not eliminate the latent form of the virus since thymidine kinase is not expressed during latency; thus, in the clinical trials, the disease recurred after termination of treatment. A problem which is already attracting attention is the possibility of acyclovir-resistant mutants of herpes simplex which may arise with widespread use. Acyclovir itself is only active against HSV, but it is likely to be the first member of a family of virus-selective drugs acting on similar principles.

Varicella-zoster virus (VZV)

One of the common major exanthematous (i.e. with skin rash) diseases of childhood, *chickenpox (varicella)* is contracted by most children in their first six to eight years. In contrast, *herpes zoster (shingles)* is a much less familiar disease of adults, generally over 50 years of age; adults do not acquire zoster from each other, and if infection is transmitted to a non-immune individual from a zoster patient, it leads to chickenpox. The viruses of chickenpox and herpes zoster are *identical*, and zoster is in fact the result of reactivation in the adult of the varicella-zoster virus which has persisted in the body since recovery from chickenpox in child-

Figure 3.22 Pathogenesis of infection by varicella-zoster virus.
(a) Chickenpox.
(b) Herpes zoster.

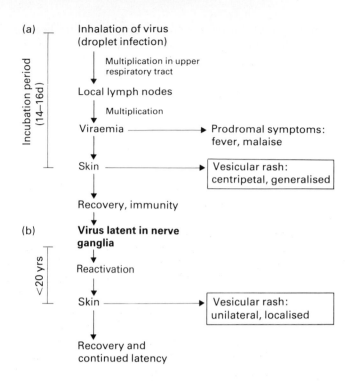

(a) Inhalation of virus (droplet infection)

Incubation period (14–16d)

Multiplication in upper respiratory tract

Local lymph nodes

Multiplication

Viraemia ⟶ Prodromal symptoms: fever, malaise

Skin ⟶ Vesicular rash: centripetal, generalised

Recovery, immunity

(b) **Virus latent in nerve ganglia**

<20 yrs

Reactivation

Skin ⟶ Vesicular rash: unilateral, localised

Recovery and continued latency

hood. The virus thus resembles herpes simplex in its latency and lifelong infection of the individual. After a child's recovery from chickenpox, the virus enters into its latent phase in spinal or cranial sensory nerve ganglia, but unlike herpes simplex, recurrence usually occurs only once as zoster, and that after many years latency (further recurrences are possible, but uncommon). Once again, a decline in CMI allows the virus to reappear, and zoster is a frequent complication of immunosuppressive treatments (drugs, radiotherapy) for cancer or following organ transplantation. Injury to, or irradiation of, the spine also encourages reactivation.

Chickenpox is acquired by the respiratory route, in infected droplets from the nose and throat. It is one of the most communicable viral diseases, with epidemics in the winter or early spring every three or four years (the time it takes for a susceptible population of children to build up). Its pathogenesis is that of a typical generalised virus infection and is summarised in Figure 3.22. After multiplying in the upper respiratory tract and local lymph nodes, viraemic dissemination distributes VZV to the skin and other organs. The incubation period lasts 14–16 days, when a *prodromal* fever (i.e. just preceding the main symptoms) is soon followed by the *generalised* vesicular skin rash. This occurs on the trunk, neck and proximal areas of the limbs in 'centripetal' distribution, sparing the face and extremities. The vesiculated skin lesions occur in *successive crops* over a period of a few days, fresh vesicles arising as older ones are crusting over and healing, so that different stages of lesion can be seen in the same area of skin (cf. smallpox, p. 279). Each lesion progresses from macule (flat spot) to papule (small solid raised lesion) to fluid-filled vesicle in 24–48 hours; the vesicles rupture and crust, or become pustular as a result of secondary infection, before healing. The rash itches, but is otherwise painless. Recovery occurs in 8–14 days. Chickenpox is much more severe and even fatal in children with impaired CMI, e.g. those undergoing treatment for leukaemia with cytotoxic drugs or corticosteroids, or with congenital immunodeficiency disease.

In zoster, the lesions, which are much more painful than in chickenpox, are principally *localised* to the area of skin around the sensory nerve endings from which the virus emerges, with perhaps some scattered individual vesicles elsewhere (disseminated zoster). Thus the main lesions are unilateral, usually on the trunk or face, and end sharply at the midline. *Ophthalmic zoster* is an eruption around the eye following the distribution of the ophthalmic division of the 5th nerve; the cornea is only affected if the nasociliary branch of the nerve is involved, indicated by a lesion on the tip of the nose. Keratitis may then be severe, with corneal ulceration and scarring (cf. herpes simplex). Immunity to zoster is usually permanent and a recurrence is rare; nevertheless, the varicella-zoster virus continues its latent existence for the lifetime of the patient.

Cytomegalovirus (CMV)

This is perhaps the most widespread member of this widely distributed family, up to 80% of adults having antibodies indicative of exposure to the virus; infection is again persistent. Cytomegalovirus is so called from the grossly enlarged cells, with their characteristic outsize inclusion body lying in an enlarged nucleus, which are found particularly in the salivary glands and renal tubules (Figure 3.15; the inclusion body is an accumulation of virus particles). The 'haloed' appearance of the inclusion body has given them the name 'owl-eye cells'. Despite its universal occurrence, CMV rarely causes disease in adults and the vast majority of its infections are asymptomatic. Infection may be chronic, with virus in saliva, urine, blood, salivary glands, kidney and liver; or latent, when the virus is sequestered in lymphocytes. Saliva and urine are the likely common sources for spread. The significance of CMV is twofold: (a) as a cause of disease in newborns and infants through congenital infection, and (b) as an opportunistic pathogen in immunosuppressed patients.

Congenital infection with CMV can result either from infection of the foetus *in utero*, the virus crossing the placenta, or during birth, if virus is present in the mother's genital tract at that time (10–15% of pregnant women excrete CMV in the third trimester). Again, infection is usually silent and perhaps as many as 10% of all healthy infants will excrete virus for the first year or more, serving as an important source of dissemination. In a small proportion, there is disease of varying degree. At one extreme, intra-uterine infection leads to abortion or stillbirth; 10% of stillbirths show CMV lesions. Alternatively, the baby may have a severe and possibly fatal syndrome called *cytomegalic inclusion disease of the newborn* (CMID), in which there is liver damage, thrombocytopenic purpura and haemorrhage, anaemia, mental

270

retardation and microcephaly (abnormally small head, of which CMV is the chief cause in neonates). Blindness and deafness may develop and CMV is now regarded as surpassing even rubella as cause of congenital defects. Owl-eye cells are found in many organs. Even if there is no obvious disease at birth, varying degrees of neurological or mental impairment may subsequently become apparent, such as deafness, mental retardation or low intelligence. Placental transfer requires that the mother be infected for the first time (primary infection) during her pregnancy, and subsequent pregnancies are not affected even though she may still be carrying the virus. This is probably because of the transience of viraemia and the subsequent protective effect of maternal IgG antibodies. The possibility of vaccination using attenuated strains of the virus is being studied.

Cytomegalovirus infection can also be a hazard of transfusion of whole fresh blood, as it may be present either free in the donor blood or in leucocytes. This can give rise to a post-transfusion syndrome resembling infectious mononucleosis in its haematological picture, with a large number of atypical large lymphocytes, but from which it can be differentiated by a negative Paul–Bunnell test (p. 794). Hepatitis of variable degree may also be present. It has been troublesome where large volumes of blood are transfused, as in open heart surgery.

We have noted that CMV infection is very common and usually silent. As with other persistent herpesvirus infections, the infection is maintained in subclinical (as opposed to disease) state by the cell-mediated immune response; impairment of CMI allows the virus to grow and promotes the appearance of disease. Cytomegalovirus is indeed an important opportunist and, like varicella-zoster virus, appears in patients with neoplastic disease or organ grafts subjected to immunosuppressive drugs such as corticosteroids, etc. It is rapidly emerging as the most feared infection in certain types of immunocompromised host, being a ruthless killer in recipients of kidney, heart and bone marrow transplants. It occurs typically 6–7 weeks after grafting, and pulmonary, hepatic, gastrointestinal and renal lesions may occur. What makes CMV infection an especially dangerous complication is the complete absence of effective chemotherapy.

Epstein–Barr virus (EBV)

This herpesvirus was first discovered in the lymphoblastoid cells of the tumour known as *Burkitt's lymphoma*, and was subsequently found to be the cause of *infectious mononucleosis (glandular fever)*, a common disease of adolescents and young adults; EBV is also associated with another neoplasm, *nasopharyngeal carcinoma*. The feature common to all three conditions is the neoplastic transformation produced by the virus. Since they are described at length in Section 6 (p. 791–6), we will merely point out here some similarities with other herpesvirus infections.

Like the other members of this family, EBV is widespread throughout the world; depending on the country and local conditions, 50–95% of adults have antibodies to the virus. Infection is also often acquired in childhood, especially where housing and hygienic conditions are poor, and it is then symptomless; infectious mononucleosis only results from infection later in life. Another familiar property is that of persistent infection; after childhood infection or recovery from mononucleosis, chronic production of virus may continue for a long period in pharyngeal and oral secretions, and in fact up to 20% of normal individuals secrete the virus in this way. Latent infection is also present in lymphocytes, and infected cells from carriers can be grown as continuous transformed lines in culture. Like other persistent herpesviruses, production of EBV is greater in immunosuppressed patients (see cyclosporin A, p.173). The virus is transmitted in oral secretions; infectious mononucleosis is the 'kissing disease', perhaps reflecting the requirement for a large infecting dose.

It is an oncogenic virus and is almost certainly the cause of Burkitt's lymphoma; it is probably the only virus for which the evidence of an oncogenic role in man is convincing. This aspect of its behaviour is discussed on p. 792. Note that in Burkitt's lymphoma cells there is latent infection of the transformed cells but also some chronic infection, as there are always some productively infected cells releasing virus.

ADENOVIRIDAE

The adenoviruses were first discovered in 1953 in normal human adenoids and tonsils, where they are often present as a *latent infection*; they are widespread, 50–80% of healthy people harbouring an adenovirus in this asymptomatic way. However, there are 33 types of adenovirus known to date, and some are responsible for important inflammatory diseases of the *respiratory tract* and *conjunctiva*. A small but significant proportion, estimated as 4–5%, of all human respiratory illness is caused by adenoviruses, typically as acute *pharyngitis* in children and as a syndrome called *acute respiratory disease*, which is common among military recruits. In the summer months, there are often outbreaks of *pharyngoconjunctival fever* among children in schools and holiday camps, a condition in which pharyngitis is combined with conjunctivitis. There has been much interest in the oncogenic properties of these viruses, as some types of human adenovirus give rise to tumours in rodents and transform rodent cells in culture. However, this seems to be a case where a virus only causes tumours in a host other than its natural one, and there is little evidence to associate adenoviruses with human neoplasms.

Structure and properties

Adenoviruses have a unique appearance in the electron microscope (Figure 3.23a). They are icosahedral and non-enveloped, with unusual fine fibres projecting from the corners of the virion, each with a knob-like termination. The capsid is composed of 252 capsomeres, of which 240 are hexons and 12

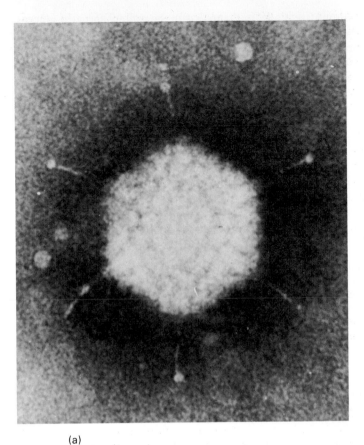

(a)

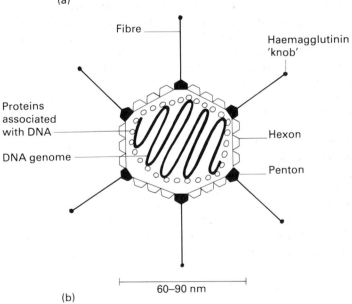

(b)

Figure 3.23 Structure of adenoviruses.
(a) Electron micrograph, negative staining, ×700,000
(from Valentine and Pereira (1965) *J. Mol. Biol.* **13**, 13)
(b) Diagrammatic section.
(see also Figure 3.4b)

pentons (see model in Figure 3.4b); the pentons form the apices of the icosahedron and the fibres are attached to them. Distinct proteins are present in the hexons, pentons and fibres; altogether there are ten different virion proteins. At the fibre tip is a *haemagglutinin*, which gives adenoviruses the ability to agglutinate red cells of various species by cross-linkage; isolated fibres bind to red cells, but do not agglutinate.

The capsid encloses the core of DNA and its associated histone-like protein; adenovirus DNA has less than half the genetic information of a herpesvirus. The lack of envelope means that adenoviruses are resistant to lipid solvents, including bile salts, enabling them to survive in the gut. Adenovirus preparations often contain a second, much smaller particle, the *adenoassociated virus* (AAV), a defective *parvovirus* which is dependent on the adenovirus as a helper in its replication (p.240).

Classification

Adenoviruses can be divided into four subgroups on the basis of the type of red cell they will agglutinate (rhesus monkey or rat) and their oncogenicity in rodents. Within these subgroups, altogether 33 serotypes are distinguishable by specific antibodies against the haemagglutinin and capsid hexons; they are designated numerically 1–33. Haemagglutination-inhibition (p. 319) and virus neutralisation tests are used in identification of a serotype.

Cellular infection

Adenoviruses adhere to cells by means of the haemagglutinins, which attach to sugar residues on membrane glycoproteins, and the particles are subsequently taken up by the cell. A puzzling finding is that antibodies against the haemagglutinin are much less effective at neutralising adenovirus infectivity than antibodies to the hexon capsomeres, suggesting that capsid proteins play a role in adherence or penetration. Inside the cell, replication follows the general pattern described for DNA viruses (p.233), with synthesis of DNA and viral assembly taking place in the nucleus. There are some unusual features, however. One is that rather little (10–15%) of the DNA and protein which is synthesized is actually incorporated into progeny virions; most of it remains in the nucleus in characteristic basophilic inclusion bodies composed of viral capsomeres, fibres and DNA. Another peculiarity is that less than 1% of the mature virus present in the cells after replication is actually released; instead, in many cells, all the progeny remain in the nucleus where they appear in crystalline array in inclusion bodies.

The viruses exert a cytopathogenic effect on cultured cells, which are ultimately killed by inhibition of their protein and nucleic acid synthesis. This toxicity is due to the penton and its fibre. The purified fibre itself blocks cellular synthesis of macromolecules, inhibits mitosis and causes interference with replication of other viruses. The penton base is also toxic, causing cells to detach from their culture dishes. However, adenoviruses are not cytolytic, and apparently do not damage the cell membrane, so that metabolic activity continues in the cytoplasm for some time and even increases.

We have noted that adenovirus infection is usually *latent* in normal human adenoids and tonsils. By this is indicated the fact that virus cannot be demonstrated in homogenates of fresh tissue, but only by culturing adenoid cells for some weeks, whereupon a cytopathogenic effect due to the growing virus is seen. It appears that a few cells (about 1 in 10^7) in the adenoid carry virus in their nuclei and that latency occurs because of the failure of virus to be released. In addition, antibodies may prevent intercellular spread of such virus that is released.

A final oddity is that adenoviruses fail to grow in cultures of monkey cells, but will do so if a simian virus such as SV40 co-infects the cells. In effect, the adenovirus behaves as if it were defective in simian cells and SV40 acts as its helper virus (p.240). Among the progeny of such double infection are some *hybrid viruses*, e.g. adenovirus capsids carrying SV40 DNA or in which the genetic information of both is recombined. The production of adenovirus-SV40 hybrids is of more than academic interest (considerable in itself), since SV40 is oncogenic in rodents and can transform human cells in culture, and growth of adenovirus in monkey kidney cells has been used for vaccine production. The inevitability of SV40 contamination of such vaccines and the risk of producing a hybrid virus with oncogenic potential in man made it necessary to abandon this method, and vaccine virus is now grown exclusively in human cells. (See p. 295 for a similar problem in poliovirus vaccine.)

Transmission

Adenoviruses are acquired by the respiratory route or by swimming in virus-contaminated water; faecal-oral spread may also occur (adenoviruses can be isolated from faeces and have been linked with gastroenteritis).

Adenoviral disease

Not all 33 serotypes are associated with disease, and some only produce latent infections. Of those which are known to be pathogenic, different types have different manifestations and epidemiologies. Characteristically, adenoviral diseases are localised inflammations of the mucous membranes of the respiratory tract or conjunctiva or both. Infection with certain serotypes, e.g. 1,2,5 and 6, is endemic and causes the most wide-spread condition, namely an acute febrile respiratory disease of children, in which pharyngitis is usually prominent; this is more prevalent during the winter months. Other types produce epidemic infections: types 3,4,7 and 21 are responsible for the syndrome known as *acute respiratory disease* (ARD) syndrome, an influenza-like condition with nasopharyngitis and cough, which occurs chiefly in military camps among new recruits. Type 4 virus in fact only occurs among the military and hardly ever produces disease among civilians; the reason for this unique state of affairs is a mystery.

The other epidemic adenovirus disease is *acute pharyngo-conjunctival fever*, which also occurs among children (and thence spreads to other family members) but in the summer months; clinically there is a triad of symptoms, viz. pharyngitis, conjunctivitis and fever, though conjunctivitis may be present alone in the parents of affected children. The condition, which is caused by serotypes 3 and 7, is often spread in swimming-pool water ('swimming-pool conjunctivitis'). The conjunctivitis is without harmful consequences. In contrast, type 8 virus causes a *keratoconjunctivitis* which can lead to corneal opacity and impaired vision. This occurs in factory or shipyard workers involved in jobs such as welding, in which dust or small particles cause corneal irritation ('shipyard eye').

Type 11 adenovirus can produce a serious urinary condition in children, *acute haemorrhagic cystitis* (cystitis—inflammation of the bladder); this is the rarest adenoviral disease. Adenoviruses have also been incriminated in gastroenteritis, though their significance as enteric viruses is uncertain.

Interestingly, people may carry a latent infection with the defective adenoassociated virus (p. 283), waiting for an adenovirus infection in order to start its own replication and returning to a latent state thereafter. No disease is connected with AAV.

Vaccination

The occurrence of ARD among military personnel is sufficiently important to warrant vaccination. Formalin-inactivated viruses have not proved very effective and live types 3,4,7 and 21 viruses are now used with success. These are not attenuated strains, but the normal 'wild-type' viruses given orally in a protective capsule which prevents inactivation by stomach acid and avoids pharyngeal infection. In principle, a vaccine could be made from the purified hexon capsomeres and fibre proteins, and would thus avoid the risk of oncogenicity which, though minimal, might be carried by live viruses. Immunity following natural infection or vaccination is type-specific and permanent.

POXVIRIDAE

For thousands of years, *smallpox (variola)* was one of the world's most dreaded diseases, with a toll of death and disfigurement in millions. Even as recently as the early 1970's, epidemics still occurred in parts of Africa (Ethiopia, Somalia) and the Indian subcontinent. Today, smallpox has been totally eradicated and the variola virus no longer exists, except in the few laboratories around the world which are permitted to store it for reference or research purposes. This remarkable achievement ends a saga going back to time immemorial with attempts to protect against the disease by *variolation* (p. 280); a major medical landmark occurred in 1796, when the Gloucestershire doctor Edward Jenner experimentally protected a boy from smallpox by artificial

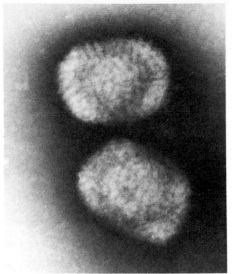

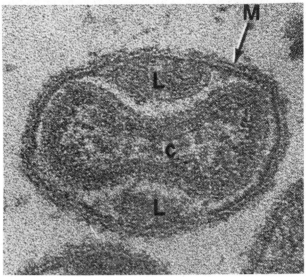

(a)

(b)

Figure 3.24 Structure of poxviruses.
(a) Electron micrograph of vaccinia virus, negative staining, ×125,000. (Courtesy of Dr June Almeida.)
(b) Electron micrograph of thin section of vaccinia virus, ×300,000. M = outer membrane, L = lateral body, C = core. (From Pogo & Dales (1969) *Proc. Nat. Acad. Sci. USA,* **63**, 820)
(c) Diagrammatic section of vaccinia virus.

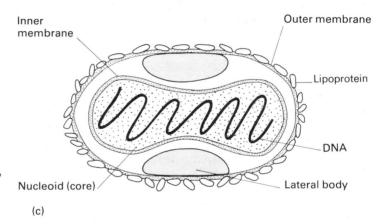

Inner membrane

Outer membrane

Lipoprotein

DNA

Nucleoid (core)

Lateral body

(c)

infection with the related bovine disease *cowpox* and thereby discovered *vaccination* (L. *vacca*, cow).

Smallpox (initially so called to distinguish it from syphilis, the 'large pox') is restricted to man, but similar diseases occur in many species (fowlpox, sheeppox, cowpox, mousepox, etc.); among other important poxvirus diseases of animals is *myxomatosis* of European rabbits (myxoma virus). Some poxviruses produce proliferative, tumour-like, rather than destructive lesions, including those of *molluscum contagiosum* (a skin condition resembling warts) and benign tumours in animals (e.g. Shope fibroma virus and myxoma virus in rabbits, and Yabavirus in African monkeys).

Here we will principally be concerned with the viruses associated with smallpox: variola virus itself occurs in two very similar strains, one of which (variola major) is the agent of severe smallpox, while the other (variola minor) causes a much milder form (alastrim); vaccinia virus is the related strain used in immunisation and now differs significantly from that of natural cowpox. The genus Orthopoxvirus includes these as well as other mammalian poxviruses.

Structure

The poxviruses are the largest animal viruses and the only ones visible by light microscopy. In surface view, under the electron microscope, they are quasi-rectangular, 'brick-like' or oval forms, with dimensions of 250–390 nm × 200–260 nm, lacking the icosahedral symmetry of other DNA viruses; in fact no particular geometric symmetry is apparent in their structure, which is described as 'complex'. The outermost layer is a 'membrane' of tubular lipoproteins which in vaccinia virus have a seemingly random arrangement (Figure 3.24), and a more regular lattice-like appearance in others (e.g. orfvirus of sheep, Figure 3.3e). A thin-section reveals a dumbbell-shaped core or nucleoid (DNA and protein) surrounded by its own 'membrane' (lipoprotein), with two 'lateral bodies' in the concavities (the significance of which is unknown), all enclosed by the outer membrane (Figure 3.24b, c). Note that the lipid in these membranes is not derived from the host cell membrane, but incorporated during the assembly of the virion. There are at least 17 protein components in the particle, some of which are nucleoid-associated enzymes, such as the DNA-dependent RNA polymerase (p.234). Vaccinia and variola have a surface haemagglutinin (for chicken red cells), but this is not involved in adherence to mammalian cells.

The poxviruses are very stable and resistant to drying, an important factor in transmission of smallpox; active variola virus can be recovered from dried pock crusts stored for a year at room temperature.

Cellular infection

Cellular infection has been studied in detail with vaccinia virus. After adhering to a cell by an unknown receptor, the virus is taken up in a phagosome. Uncoating occurs in two stages: the outer viral membrane is enzymatically removed within the phagosome, and the nucleoid, in its membrane but without the lateral bodies, is released into the cytoplasm. While still thus enclosed, viral DNA is transcribed by the virion-associated DNA-dependent RNA polymerase into 'immediate early' mRNA. This is extruded and codes for some of the early proteins, including a protease which completes the process of uncoating by digesting the nucleoid membrane and releasing viral DNA. All stages in replication and assembly are *cytoplasmic*, but otherwise resemble the pattern described for other DNA viruses, with production of early proteins followed by DNA replication, late (structural) protein synthesis and finally assembly. The 'factories' where replication takes place are seen as inclusion bodies (*Guarnieri bodies*), consisting of viral particles and proteins, which can be useful in diagnosis. The translation of late viral mRNA is specifically inhibited by the drug methisazone (N-methylisatin-β-thiosemicarbazone) and this has been of prophylactic use in smallpox and complications of vaccination. After the complex process of assembly, mature virions are released either by cell lysis, which occurs slowly, or more probably through surface microvilli. Most of the particles fail to be released, at least from cultured cells.

As viral mRNA takes over the ribosomes, host cell protein synthesis ceases and host DNA replication is inhibited. Vaccinia infection is thus cytocidal and can be demonstrated in culture by the plaque assay; haemadsorption of chicken red cells can also be used, as viral haemagglutinin is inserted into the plasma membrane. With variola virus, infected cells are induced to proliferate before they die so that hyperplastic foci can be counted instead of plaques. The ability to induce *hyperplasia* is quite characteristic of poxviruses; indeed, as noted above, some cause benign tumours in animals.

Pathogenesis of smallpox

Smallpox is a severe exanthematous disease with a mortality of up to 50%; the less severe form of the disease, alastrim, has a mortality of less than 1% and occurs predominantly in South America. The characteristic skin lesions are *pocks*, pustules ultimately distributed all over the body; in fatal cases of smallpox they become haemorrhagic, but this complication is absent in alastrim.

Infection with variola virus is acquired by the respiratory route, either in droplets from nasopharyngeal secretions of patients or in dust from infected clothing, bedding, etc. (the virus is very resistant to drying). Smallpox is highly contagious, but less so than influenza, measles or chickenpox. During the incubation period of 12–16 days, the infection follows the course described in Figure 3.18. In brief, after multiplying in local lymph nodes of the respiratory tract, a transient *primary viraemia* distributes the virus to cells of the reticulo-endothelial system (e.g. macrophages) around the body in which further multiplication occurs. Its release from these cells leads to a more intense *secondary viraemia*, which is marked by the abrupt onset of prodromal symptoms — chills, fever, prostration, etc., resembling severe influenza. The viraemia is brief and virus disappears from the blood by the second day of fever, by which time it has been taken up by epithelial cells of the skin. There it continues to multiply and after 3 days the beginnings of the skin rash appear. The pocks progress from macules to papules to vesicles and then pustules in 4–5 days. They first appear in 'centrifugal' distribution, i.e. on the face and extremities of the limbs, before spreading in about 24 hours to the trunk. Typically, there is a *single* crop of lesions and all become pustular simultaneously. These features helped to distinguish smallpox from chickenpox in doubtful cases (cf. p. 269). The pocks contain the virus, and purulence is not the result of secondary bacterial contamination. By a further 3–4 days, they rupture, crust over and begin to heal; healing is gradual and takes up to two weeks, with widespread scarring. There may be loss of hair, eyebrows and nails. In the fatal cases, the fever, which subsides with the appearance of the rash, returns and the pocks become haemorrhagic; death occurs in 3–4 days. It is not clear why this fatal progression does not occur in variola minor, as the variola major and minor viruses are virtually indistinguishable.

Recovery from smallpox is dependent on cell-mediated immunity. This has been studied experimentally using *ectromelia (mousepox)* as a model. Under conditions of infection which kill 5% of control mice, almost all T-cell depleted mice will die, but can be protected by infusion of normal T cells. Antibody and interferon appear to play little part in recovery from ectromelia. In man, the severity of the normally benign vaccinia in children with thymic deficiency is noted below. Cell-mediated reactions probably also contribute to the development of the lesions themselves; studies in rabbits have shown that the characteristic pustules do not form in immunosuppressed animals.

Confirmation of *diagnosis* of smallpox can be achieved most rapidly (in two hours) by electron microscopy of pustular smears negatively stained with phosphotungstic acid. If electron microscopy is not available, identification of Guarnieri bodies or immunoprecipitation tests for viral antigens in lesion exudates are used.

Prevention of smallpox: vaccination

Immunisation against smallpox had been practised for centuries before Jenner, in the form of *variolation*. It was well recognised that recovery from smallpox conferred lifelong protection from the disease; the principle of variolation was to acquire smallpox artificially in a (hopefully) mild form, e.g. by ingesting crusts or by inoculating fluid from pocks into the skin. In the latter form it was introduced into England from Turkey in 1717 by Lady Mary Wortly Montague, wife of the British ambassador, who had both her sons inoculated and started an enthusiasm for variolation throughout Europe. Variolation was nevertheless hazardous and in about 1% of those treated produced the full-blown disease (alastrim crusts, which were safer, were also sometimes used and might justifiably be regarded as the first example of what we now call a vaccine). It was, in fact, while carrying out variolation in his local village practice that Jenner realised that dairymaids and other country people, who had experienced the harmless condition of *cowpox*, could not be infected with smallpox through variolation. (Cowpox is acquired by milking cows with lesions on their teats; the pocks remain localised on the milker's hands.) After many years' patient observation, he undertook a famous experiment for the first time in 1796, when he inoculated a boy (Phipps) with fluid taken from the hand of a milkmaid who had been infected by a cow. A pustule developed on the boy's arm and then disappeared, after which Jenner was unable to transmit smallpox to him by variolation. Jenner submitted a report of his discovery to the Royal Society and it is disappointing to note that he was politely rebuffed, with the advice that his paper could injure the reputation he had established by his former work—on the cuckoo. Thus was one of the great advances in medical science received! Happily, Jenner persisted and quite soon convinced the world that in vaccination he had found a safe means of preventing one of mankind's severest afflictions. Nearly a century later, Pasteur, in homage to Jenner, called his own work—on protecting chickens against chicken cholera—'vaccination', since when the term has been used for all examples of artificial immunisation with micro-organisms or their products.

Vaccinia virus, used in present-day smallpox vaccination, is no longer identical with that of natural cowpox and is believed to be an attenuated form of variola virus, though its precise origin is uncertain. It is still generally maintained by time-honoured means in animals, alternately transferring pustular material from the skin of an inoculated rabbit to that of a calf or sheep, and back again from the new pustule; this appears to keep its virulence at a constant level. Live virus is required for immunisation as the protective antigens are destroyed if it is inactivated. In preparing the vaccine, scrapings of lesions from the calf or sheep's skin are homogenized and suspended in 40% glycerol to ensure stability until inoculated.

The immunisation procedure is to puncture gently the epidermis under a drop of vaccine. One of three types of reaction may occur, depending on the individual's state of immunity. In a non-immune person, a 'primary take' occurs, a local lesion developing into a single pustule in 8–10 days and then healing with a crust and, when this falls off at about 21 days, a scar. Normally the virus remains localised at the site of inoculation. In a person with partial immunity, e.g. one vaccinated some years before, the lesion becomes pustular more rapidly and the reaction is called *vaccinoid*. In recently immunized individuals with solid immunity, the response takes the form of a delayed-type hypersensitivity reaction; a papule develops by 48 hours (i.e. more quickly than above) and does not become a vesicle or pustule. This is sometimes called the *reaction of immunity* and indeed generally is such, but may also be an immune response to contaminants in the vaccine. Protection with vaccinia lasts from 3 to 7 years and boosters are required for continuing protection. With the disappearance of smallpox from most parts of the world, routine vaccination and boosting ceased to be a mandatory measure in many Western countries, except for travellers to areas of disease and others at risk.

Today, when smallpox has been finally eradicated, the risks of the vaccination procedure itself no longer justify its perpetuation. In the USA, for example, there has been no natural disease since 1948, but an average of seven deaths annually as a result of vaccination. The possible complications are as follows. (a) *Progressive vaccinia* is an alarming local spread of the primary take with destruction of surrounding skin and muscle, and is ultimately fatal (*vaccinia gangrenosa*). It occurs in children with thymic deficiencies who are unable to make a cell-mediated immune response to the virus, and is very rare (1–2 per million vaccinees). Methisazone has been valuable in treating this condition; extracts of immune leucocytes (transfer factor) have also been successful in halting the necrosis, presumably by inducing the development of the child's T cell immunity (see p. 164). (b) *Generalised vaccinia* (~ 1 per 100,000) is a result of viraemic spread of the vaccinia virus with multiple skin lesions around the body. This is seen in children with agammaglobulinaemia, who fail to make an antibody response; it is again severe, with 30–40% mortality. These 'experiments of nature' indicate that CMI is responsible for healing of the local lesion and restricting it to a pustule, but that antibody is important in preventing viraemic spread. (c) *Postvaccinial encephalitis* (~ 1 per 50,000) is another severe complication with high mortality. Encephalitis is accompanied by demyelination and a perivascular infiltration of mononuclear cells in the brain, indicative of hypersensitivity, probably autoimmunity. Paralysis and death follow. (d) *Eczema vaccinatum*: in children with eczema (dermatitis) vaccinia can spread over the eczematous area and then to healthy skin; this too may prove fatal. A similar condition occurs in eczematous individuals infected with herpes simplex virus, which spreads over existing skin lesions; this together with eczema vaccinatum is called *Kaposi's varicelliform eruption*. (e) *Foetal vaccinia*: vaccinia virus has been known to cross the placenta and produce abortion; hence vaccination in pregnancy is also avoided.

The worldwide eradication of smallpox through vaccination was possible because the disease is restricted to man and there is no animal reservoir. The WHO Smallpox Eradication Campaign began in 1966, at which time the disease was endemic in 30 countries. It proved impracticable for logistical reasons to immunise the entire populations of countries in Africa and Asia; surveillance and containment were therefore the main approaches, with isolation of cases and vaccination of all their contacts. By 1978 smallpox had been eliminated, barring laboratory accidents (e.g. Birmingham, 1978). As vaccination is no longer common practice, a steadily increasing proportion of the world's population is unprotected; this situation is safe as long as the virus does not accidentally reappear, and laboratory stocks have indeed been reduced to prevent such an occurrence.

Molluscum contagiosum

This is a widespread, harmless skin infection, more prevalent in children than adults and more common in some localities than others. The lesions, called mollusca, are not pock-like, but waxy, white, painless papules, 2–5 mm in diameter, found particularly on the face and trunk and in the genital area; they are contagious and acquired by direct contact, which may be venereal. Each molluscum has a central depression from which a white, pasty material can be extruded; when stained this is seen to contain cells with huge inclusion bodies (molluscum bodies), which are also found free and which the electron microscope shows to be composed of typical poxvirus particles. The paste consists of accumulated dead cells and their breakdown products. The main interest of these lesions is that they are cellular proliferations and may be likened to benign tumours such as warts (p. 789). As in the latter, the basal layer of the epidermis proliferates excessively, but is free of detectable virus; presumably the basal cells are transformed by virus integrated into the cell DNA. Those cells just above the basal layer contain small inclusion bodies, and the further towards the surface of the lesion, the larger these become, until the nucleus is confined to the edge of the cell. As with warts, mollusca regress spontaneously after a few months. Molluscum contagiosum is a good example of the proliferative effect of poxviruses already noted for variola and also seen in benign tumours of animals (myxoma virus, Shope fibroma virus).

PAPOVAVIRIDAE

These are tumour-causing DNA viruses which in man include the agents of *warts* (*papillomaviruses*) and the very widespread *polyomaviruses* JC and BK. For description see pages 368 and 789.

PARVOVIRIDAE

The parvoviruses are very small viruses (Lat. *parvus*, small) with a single-stranded DNA genome and are the only class II viruses to infect animals. The amount of genetic information they carry is sufficient only to code for the capsid protein, and one of the two genera—*Adeno-associated virus* (AAV)—is defective in replication. As already mentioned (p.240) AAV is only replicated in cells which are coinfected by an adenovirus to act as helper. AAV infection in man is common, apparently always in association with an adenovirus, and with no pathological consequences. The other genus, *Parvovirus*, is not defective, but only replicates during the S phase of the host cell cycle (i.e. during host cell DNA synthesis). Candidates for inclusion in this genus are viruses causing acute infectious gastroenteritis known as the *Norwalk virus* and Norwalk-like viruses. However, although they resemble parvoviruses in physical characteristics, these agents have not been fully studied, owing to difficulties in propagating them in culture, and their definitive classification awaits analysis of the nucleic acid. (Should it turn out that they have an RNA rather than a single-stranded DNA genome, an alternative grouping would be in the *Calicivirus* genus of the Picornaviridae.)

Norwalk virus, Norwalk-like agents and gastroenteritis. Acute infectious non-bacterial gastroenteritis ('winter vomiting disease') is very common during colder months in many parts of the world; indeed, it is second in frequency only to acute viral respiratory tract infections. Outbreaks may be confined to individual families or institutions, or be wide epidemics involving entire communities. The Norwalk virus was isolated during an epidemic of gastroenteritis in the town of that name (Ohio, USA) in 1968; it was demonstrated in faeces by immunoelectron microscopy (p. 354) and produced the disease when ingested by volunteers. Other agents, similar in physical properties but antigenically distinct from the Norwalk virus, have since been isolated during outbreaks of non-bacterial gastroenteritis in Hawaii and Ditchling (England). The Norwalk agent itself is widely distributed and has been responsible for outbreaks of food poisoning in Australia, associated with the consumption of oysters, and for epidemics on both sides of the Atlantic. About 70% of adults in the 30–40 year age group have antibodies to the virus. Its role in tropical countries, where diarrhoea in infants is a major problem, is not yet known.

Gastroenteritis due to these viruses is generally a benign, self-limiting condition which affects all ages, most commonly adults and older children (non-bacterial gastroenteritis in young children is more likely to be a rotavirus infection, p. 365). After a brief incubation period (about 48 hours), the main symptoms are diarrhoea and vomiting, which last for 24–48 hours. The infection is evidently confined to the upper part of the small intestine, the mucosa of which becomes inflamed and invaded by neutrophils and mononuclear cells; villi are shortened and crypts hypertrophied, a picture also seen in gastroenteritis due to other viruses. Stools do not contain blood or leucocytes. Deaths, although rare, may occur in the very young or old or in the debilitated and undernourished. Antibodies appear in the blood and intestine, but immunity is short-term and volunteers reinfected a few months after primary infection experienced a further bout of diarrhoea. Transmission is by the faecal-oral route, including person-to-person spread and via contaminated food (e.g. seafood, above).

PICORNAVIRIDAE (ENTEROVIRUSES, RHINOVIRUSES)

The picornaviruses derive their name from the fact that they are 'pico (small)—RNA—viruses' and indeed, together with the parvoviruses, are the smallest animal viruses. They are an important family of human and animal pathogens, including the agents of poliomyelitis and the common cold in man, and foot and mouth disease in animals. They are divided as shown in Figure

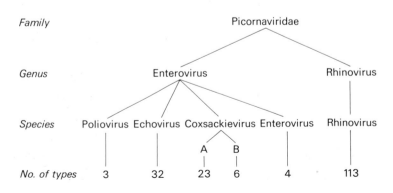

Figure 3.25 Picornaviridae: enteroviruses and rhinoviruses.

3.25 into two genera, *Enterovirus* and *Rhinovirus*, and then into species and types.

The *enteroviruses* are a diverse group which have in common the ability to infect the alimentary tract and, in addition to the polioviruses themselves, the group includes viruses discovered in faeces during studies initially concerned with poliomyelitis. The distinction between the 29 *coxsackieviruses* and the 32 *echoviruses* is now felt to be an artificial one, being based solely on the fact that only the former are pathogenic in newborn mice; hence newly discovered enteroviruses are no longer assigned to these groups, but are referred to simply as numbered enteroviruses. *Poliovirus* is the most familiar enterovirus species, having been the cause of one of mankind's most feared afflictions; happily, it has been banished from many countries by highly effective vaccination programmes, but is still prevalent in some parts of the world. The other enteroviruses cause a range of illnesses, many in children, from the relatively mild such as herpangina and 'hand, foot and mouth disease', to more serious heart disease in the newborn (myocarditis) and aseptic meningitis (see Table 3.4). Despite their name, they do not seem to be major causes of viral gastroenteritis, which is more likely to be caused by a rotavirus; nor are they restricted to the gastrointestinal tract, but are also involved in mild upper respiratory tract infections (colds) in children. The *rhinoviruses*, of which over 100 serotypes are known, are the major—but not the only—agents of the common cold and are restricted to the upper respiratory tract. Some general properties of picornaviruses are compared in Table 3.7.

Structure, etc.

The particles are very small icosahedrons, 20–30 nm in diameter, and are non-enveloped (Figure 3.26). The poliovirus capsid, which has been studied in the most detail, consists of 60 identical capsomeres arranged around the centres of the 20 faces of the icosahedron, and not of hexons and pentons as elsewhere; there

Table 3.7 Features of picornaviruses.

Group	Stability at pH3	Optimum growth temp.	Route of transmission	Sites of infection in man
Poliovirus	Stable	37°C	Faecal-oral	Gastrointestinal tract; CNS
Echovirus	Stable	37°C	Faecal-oral; respiratory	Gastrointestinal tract; upper respiratory tract; CNS; skin
Coxsackievirus	Stable	37°C	Faecal-oral; respiratory	Gastrointestinal tract; upper respiratory tract; CNS; muscle
Rhinovirus	Unstable	33°C	Respiratory	Upper respiratory tract

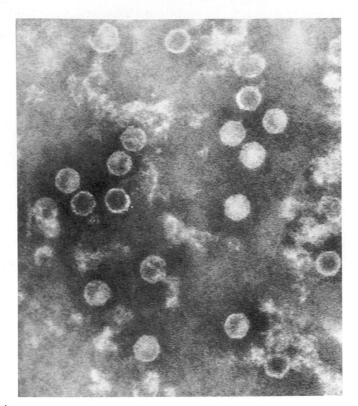

(a)

Figure 3.26
(a) Poliovirus capsids as seen by electron microscopy, ×260,000. (Courtesy of Dr June Almeida.)
(b) Large crystalline array of poliovirus from a thin section of a tissue culture cell (×75,000). (From Dales *et al* (1965) *Virology*, **26**, 379)

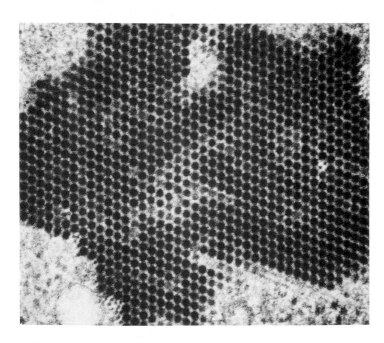

(b)

are 180 protein subunits in the capsid. There are five types of virion protein, termed VP (viral protein) 1, VP2, VP3, VP4 and VPg; VP1–4 are present in the capsid, while VPg is associated with the nucleic acid. The VP4 protein is involved in cellular attachment. The capsid encloses a single positive strand of RNA, which is commensurately small (molecular weight of 2.5×10^6, or 7500 bases).

The other enteroviruses and rhinoviruses appear to have a similar structure. The latter can be distinguished by their higher buoyant density on ultracentrifugation in caesium chloride (their capsids are permeable to caesium) and their inactivation in acid, infectivity being lost within an hour at pH3 and 37°C, whereas this treament does not affect enteroviruses (Table 3.7). All species of picornaviruses exist in several antigenically distinct serotypes.

The enteroviruses are among the stablest animal viruses and are well suited to survival in the gut. Since they are non-enveloped, they can withstand bile and other lipid solvents; they also resist acid and intestinal enzymes. Infectivity is retained for several weeks in sewage and water, but is destroyed by moist heat at 50–55°C and pasteurisation. The rhinoviruses, as noted, are less acid-resistant and do not infect the intestine.

Cellular infection and replication

Poliovirus serves as the model for replication of picornaviruses. A major step forward in the study of animal viruses occurred in 1945 when Enders, Weller and Robbins showed that poliovirus could be grown in cultured non-neural cells, namely monkey kidney cells; this was the first time an animal virus had been grown *in vitro* and opened the way to research on the cytopathogenic effects of viruses, plaque assays, and ultimately

Figure 3.27. Replication of poliovirus.
Stages represented:
1. Attachment.
2. Penetration.
3. Uncoating.
4. Translation of viral RNA.
5. Single polypeptide product.
6. Post-translational cleavage.
7. Assembly of procapsid.
8. Synthesis of negative RNA templates and
9. Replication of positive RNA strands, both using RNA-dependent RNA polymerase (a product of stage 6).
10. Some positive RNA strands are used as messenger RNA.
11. Others are incorporated into capsids.
12. These may accumulate intracellularly in crystalline arrays.
13. Release of progeny by lysis of the cell.

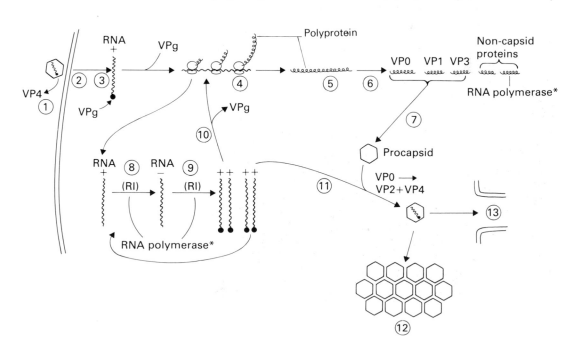

287

production of vaccines, including that for poliomyelitis itself. Besides simian cells, poliovirus is grown in human tissue cells and lines including HeLa cells.

Cellular infection by poliovirus (Figure 3.27) begins with attachment to specific cell receptors, which have not been identified but contain glycoprotein and lipid. Attachment requires the capsid protein VP4; this is removed from the virion at the membrane prior to penetration, and at this point many particles also lose their RNA and detach from the cell. The remainder are taken up by pinocytosis and released into the cytoplasm. The loss of VP4 is the first stage in uncoating (unusual in being extracellular), which is completed in the cytoplasm with release of viral RNA. Replication follows the lines described on p. 235 and Figure 3.11a, and is cytoplasmic, taking place near the nucleus, though nuclear functions are not required. Viral RNA, being a positive strand, is immediately translated as a single polygenic message on host polysomes into a giant polypeptide, with subsequent post-translational cleavage into viral capsid proteins and non-structural proteins such as the essential RNA-dependent RNA polymerase (p. 237, Figure 3.12). With this enzyme, virion RNA molecules are transcribed to give complementary negative strands, which function as templates for production of further positive strands via replicative inter-mediates. Some of the positive strands are required as mRNA, while others are destined for the capsids of progeny virions. The two types of RNA (messenger and progeny) are of identical sequence and need to be distinguished. This is achieved by the VPg polypeptide; it is attached to the 5' terminal oligonucleotide of all newly snythesized RNA molecules, but subsequently removed from those (about half) required as messengers.

Although there are four capsid proteins (VP1–4), post-translational cleavage only produces three, namely VP1, VP3 and a protein called VP0 from which VP2 and VP4 are generated later. VP0, VP1 and VP3 are assembled into immature procapsids, into which the RNA molecues are packaged; only then is VP0 cleaved into VP2 and VP4. The mature progeny virions are now ready for release from the cell, which they leave by lysis, several hundred being produced per cell.

Picornavirus infections are cytocidal. Toxic effects begin after the virus has been uncoated; translation of host proteins is inhibited as viral RNA occupies cell ribosomes, and a viral protein inhibits transcription of host DNA. Cytopathological changes become visible during the course of viral replication, the nucleus first shrinking and then becoming pyknotic with chromosomal fragmentation; the cell retracts, becomes rounded or balloons, and dies. During this process, a large eosinophilic inclusion body develops at the site of viral assembly near the nucleus; crystalline arrays of assembled particles can be seen (Figure 3.26b). Release of virus completes the cytopathogenic effect by lysing the cells.

The replication of other enteroviruses and rhinoviruses follows the same pattern and is also cytocidal. A unique feature of rhinoviruses is their need for a lower growth temperature, namely

33°C, a fact which delayed their discovery for many years since cell cultures are routinely set up at 37°C. The lower temperature reflects that of their natural nasal habitat.

Transmission and epidemiology

Picornaviruses which infect man occur naturally only in humans, with no animal reservoirs; the distribution of all species is worldwide. Infections are acute and there is no long-term carrier state. The enteroviruses are rapidly disseminated where conditions of hygiene and sanitation are poor—they are excreted in faeces and recoverable from sewage. While the major route is faecal—oral, respiratory transmission in droplets is also significant, especially for echoviruses and coxsackieviruses, which can cause cold-like infections. For polioviruses, the alimentary route is predominant; virus is excreted in quantity in the faeces for up to five or six weeks after infection and can be easily transferred on the hands to food or eating utensils to complete the cycle. Explosive epidemics have resulted from contamination of water by sewage; although poliovirus does not survive modern methods of water purification employed for piped supplies, it can be acquired from untreated water, for instance during summertime swimming. Similar considerations apply to echoviruses and coxsackieviruses, and all enteroviruses are most likely to be contracted in the summer and autumn. For example, coxsackievirus infections such as 'hand, foot and mouth disease' (virus types A5 and A16) and aseptic meningitis (A7) are sometimes summer epidemics which originate in swimming pools, while outbreaks of herpangina occur in children under five years of age in day nurseries and kindergartens. Echoviruses can be detected in the faeces of infants soon after birth, and in underdeveloped countries are present in faeces of 80% of children (cf. 2–3% in New York City). Epidemics of undifferentiated 'summer febrile illness' in children are often due either to echoviruses (4,6,9,16) or coxsackieviruses (A9,16,23,B1–5). Nevertheless, it should be borne in mind that the vast majority of enterovirus infections pass unnoticed; even during epidemics of poliomyelitis, only 1% of infections gave rise to clinical manifestations. We may also note an enterovirus (species 70) which is spread directly to the eye and is the cause of acute haemorrhagic conjunctivitis. An enormous epidemic spread through Asia and Africa between 1969 and 1974, with some half a million cases in Bombay alone.

While enteroviruses are able to be transmitted by the faecal-oral route due to their high degree of stability and resistance to acid and bile, rhinoviruses are restricted to respiratory transmission. The common cold is indeed the commonest of man's viral afflictions and, like other upper respiratory tract infections, is transmitted principally in droplets, especially during the first two days of coryza. A very small dose—no more than a few particles—is all that is required to transmit a cold. The association with cold and inclement weather is indirect. Experiments on volunteers at the Common Cold Research

Establishment in England showed that chilling and wet conditions did not influence individual susceptibility; more likely to be responsible is the tendency for people to congregate in poorly ventilated surroundings during the winter months. The common cold, like influenza, is of tremendous economic significance, with the loss of millions of working days each year. Most people can expect to have from two to six colds annually, a situation which arises because of the large number of *antigenically distinct* rhinovirus types. These are probably a result of 'antigenic drift' as for influenza, with continuous generation and selection of variants (see p. 326). The difference between the cold viruses and influenza viruses is that all rhinovirus variant types coexist together, whereas a new influenza subtype replaces its predecessors. There are 113 known serotypes of rhinoviruses; in addition, several other virus species can cause the common cold syndrome in the winter (coxsackieviruses, coronaviruses, paramyxoviruses, etc.), so that the chances of avoiding infection are slender—unless one can totally avoid other human beings during the autumn and winter months!

Whereas cold viruses affect all age groups with roughly equal severity, enteroviruses are (a) more common in children than in adults, and (b) more likely to produce asymptomatic infections in infants and young children and become more severe in older children and adults. This was particularly apparent in the epidemiology of poliomyelitis before vaccination was introduced in 1954. During the nineteenth century, poliomyelitis was endemic throughout the world; most infections occurred in children under five years of age, with only sporadic cases of infantile paralysis, and epidemics were unknown. The vast majority of infections produced only mild disease or were totally inapparent. A major change occurred towards the end of the nineteenth century, initially in Scandinavia and the USA, when poliomyelitis became an epidemic disease which increasingly affected older children, adolescents and even adults, with a greater incidence among them of severe paralytic disease. Ironically, this shift could be accounted for by the improvements in hygiene and sanitation which 'protected' small children from the relatively insignificant early infection and thus prevented the natural induction of immunity. Older age groups soon came to lack protection and susceptible individuals accumulated, and since poliomyelitis becomes clinically more severe with age, it took on an epidemic form. (A similar contemporary situation exists for infectious hepatitis, which is also spread by the faecal-oral route, p. 356). Vaccination has now totally eradicated natural poliovirus infection from many parts of the world, including Europe, the USA, Australia, etc., but has been rather less successful in some tropical countries, where the disease remains endemic and outbreaks occur throughout the year.

PICORNAVIRAL DISEASE

Polioviruses and poliomyelitis

There are three antigenically distinct types of poliovirus: type 1 is responsible for most epidemics, type 2 is commonly involved in endemic infections, while type 3 is occasionally associated with epidemics. There is little cross-protection between the three strains and all three must be incorporated when vaccines are prepared. Before protective immunisation programmes were introduced in the 1950's, poliomyelitis was one of the most feared of all diseases, despite the fact that paralysis was an infrequent complication of an otherwise very common trivial infection. The sight and prospect of permanently crippled children, some of whom had to be kept alive in 'iron lung' respirators, filled parents with horror. Happily, it has become one of the great success stories of prophylactic vaccination.

The affinity of poliovirus for nervous tissue is one of its outstanding characteristics: poliomyelitis literally means 'inflammation of the grey matter of the spinal cord' (Gk. *polios*, grey, *muelos*, spinal cord). Another is its natural restriction to man; although chimpanzees can be infected artificially, man is the only source of the virus. As we shall see below, this is a vital consideration in the possible elimination of the virus from the world by vaccination (cf. smallpox).

Pathogenesis (Figure 3.28). Infection is generally acquired by the faecal–oral route, though there is occasional respiratory transmission and person-to-person spread in oropharyngeal secretions. The virus invades the mucosal cells of the oropharynx and small intestine, but its main replication occurs in the tonsils and Peyer's patches of the ileum. From this time on, it

Figure 3.28 Pathogenesis of poliomyelitis.

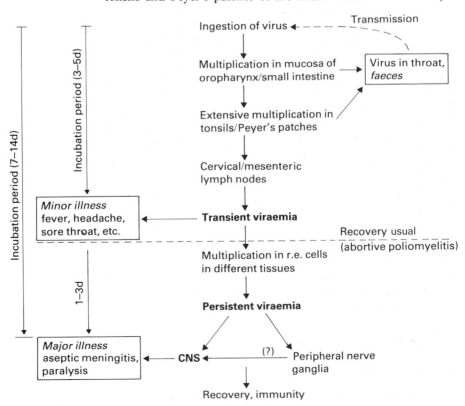

291

can be found in the throat and faeces; faecal excretion can continue for several (3–6) weeks and is the major source of virus for spread to others (there is no prolonged carrier state). From its tonsillar and ileal sites, where large amounts are produced, virus is carried to the local lymph nodes (deep cervical, mesenteric) and thence into the bloodstream, creating a transient viraemia in which it is spread to other extraneural tissues. This process, the incubation period, takes 3–5 days. Viraemia is generally accompanied by a *minor illness* with symptoms such as slight fever, sore throat, headache and vomiting, but it may be so slight as to go unnoticed. The majority (90%) of poliovirus infections do not proceed beyond this stage, which is then called *abortive poliomyelitis*. In the remaining 10% or so, viraemia becomes persistent as blood is replenished with virus from reticulo-endothelial cells, and the virus may then make its appearance in the CNS, probably by infection from the bloodstream.

Infection of the CNS presages the clinical appearance of the *major illness*, which begins 1–3 days after the minor stage; thus the full course is biphasic. Commonly it takes the form of *aseptic meningitis* (so called because no bacteria can be isolated), with fever, stiff neck and muscular pain; unlike bacterial meningitis, glucose and protein levels in the CSF are normal. Ultimately, but again in a minority, the virus invades the grey matter of the spinal cord and the medulla and motor cortex of the brain, with neuronal necrosis, viral destruction of the *anterior horn cells* of the spinal cord, and *encephalitis*. Since anterior horn cells give rise to the motor fibres of peripheral nerves, their destruction is accompanied by flaccid paralysis of limb muscles. In the most serious state, *bulbar (medullary) lesions* lead to paralysis of respiratory muscles. A paralytic state affects only about 0.1% of those infected, though the figure is higher in older children and young adults. The extent of paralysis is also influenced by other factors, such as tonsillectomy, which, even if performed some time before, predisposes to the bulbar form; recent injections (often the triple vaccine), which encourage paralysis of the inoculated limb; pregnancy; and vigorous exercise, which also exacerbates the disease in the limbs used. The reasons are not clear, but these factors seem to facilitate entry of virus into the CNS. Mortality overall of paralytic poliomyelitis is 2–3%, but is higher in adults and if there is bulbar involvement.

Recovery from paralysis is possible, depending on the degree of neuronal destruction; initial paralysis may be due to neuronal injury from inflammation and oedema as well as direct infection of cells, so that some recovery occurs when the inflammation resolves. Compensatory muscular hypertrophy can also eventually occur providing there is still some innervation. However, paralysis remaining after a few months is likely to be permanent. Recovery from all forms of infection—subclinical, minor or major illness—is accompanied by permanent immunity (both IgG and local IgA) to the infecting viral type.

Diagnosis is by recovery of the virus from the throat (during the first 10–14 days), or the faeces (for 3–6 weeks) and inoculation

292

into cultures of monkey kidney cells. If a CPE develops, the virus can be positively identified by neutralisation (loss of infectivity) with type-specific antisera.

Vaccination. Until 1955, the annual incidence of diagnosed poliomyelitis in the USA and western Europe was about 15 per 100,000 population. In the USA in that year there were approximately 30,000 diagnosed cases of which 7,000 led to residual paralysis; in 1964, there were 122 cases in all, and in the five years to 1974 only 110. In Finland and Sweden, where the rate was formerly among the highest in the world, there has been not a single case for 15 years. This remarkable turnabout was achieved through the use of two highly effective vaccines, the inactivated virus vaccine (Salk) and the living attenuated strains (Sabin vaccine). Since man is its only host, there is also the possibility, as for smallpox, of eradicating the virus itself on a world-wide scale through vaccination.

Vaccine development began with the discovery in the 1940's that poliovirus could be grown in non-neural tissue cultures. Funded by the 'March of Dimes'—a highly successful appeal for money from the general public—Salk, Sabin and others competed to be the first to develop a vaccine. In the event, Salk was successful with a mixture of the three poliovirus types inactivated with formaldehyde. Initially there were difficulties with large-scale production, particularly in securing complete inactivation. In one unfortunate incident, 260 children contracted poliomyelitis after receiving the Salk vaccine, of whom 10 died. These problems were fortunately only temporary and the vaccine was widely used during the late 1950's; in Scandinavia it has been in continuous use ever since and, as noted above, has had great success. Most of the rest of the world, however, adopted the Sabin preparation in the early 1960's. This consists of attenuated strains of the three serotypes, mixed together in proportions which avoid mutual interference. They infect the body, but are incapable of multiplying in or damaging nervous tissue, even when injected intracerebrally (in chimpanzees). In warm countries, among crowded communities where enteroviral infection can be widespread in the summer months, interference with the replication of the vaccine strains in the gut can occur through the simultaneous presence of other viruses. Immunisation with the Sabin vaccine is therefore best carried out in winter and spring, at which times this is less likely to be a problem.

There are several reasons for preferring the living to the inactivated vaccine, though it must be said that in terms of poliomyelitis prevention they have been equally effective. Table 3.8 summarises the relative merits of each. A first consideration is the method of administration. Salk vaccine is administered by subcutaneous inoculation whereas Sabin is given orally (usually on a lump of sugar). It is not merely that the latter is more pleasant to take; it is also far easier, quicker and cheaper to immunise a large number of people if inoculations, with attendant requirements for sterility, are not needed. Secondly, a much lower dose (in terms of viral particles) is required for the live virus, since it is amplified naturally by replication in the

Table 3.8 Considerations in use of live (attenuated) or inactivated poliovirus vaccines.

Vaccine	Advantages	Disadvantages
Inactivated (Salk)	Totally safe Totally effective Stable	More complicated to administer (inoculation) Boosters required High dose of virus needed Serum antibody only Wild-type virus remains in the population
Living, attenuated (Sabin)	Very safe Low dose of virus Rapidly and totally effective Simple administration (oral) Prolonged antigenic stimulation Long-term immunity Local and serum antibody Eradication of virus Herd immunity Transmission of vaccine strains to non-immune contacts	Sporadic cases of paralysis Interference by other enteroviruses Cannot be used in immunodeficiency Contaminating live viruses Transmission of revertants to contacts Limited stocks of seed strains and new attenuated strains proving difficult to make

intestine just like the native virus. About 10^4 times more particles are needed for immunisation with the inactivated form, so that the Salk vaccine is more expensive and requires larger scale (as well as more complicated) production methods.

A more important biological point is that by giving a living virus by the oral route, the course of natural infection is imitated; the attenuated strains multiply in the gut, remain for a few weeks and provide a plentiful immunogenic stimulus which leads to rapid and long-lasting immunity. Moreover, the antibody response consists of local IgA production in the gut as well as IgM and IgG in the blood, so that the immunised individual has both a barrier to the entry of virus into the intestinal mucosa and the ability to neutralise viraemia. This prevents altogether the replication of poliovirus in the gut, which not only protects the individual but also breaks the chain of transmission of the wild-type virus. In addition, vaccine strains are excreted faecally and provide a natural, harmless infection for others. As a result, the use of Sabin vaccine has led to the virtual disappearance of wild polioviruses in human sewage in Europe and the USA and their replacement by the attenuated strains. Thus, the attenuated virus vaccine also protects the community even before the entire population has been treated, so-called *herd immunity*. In contrast, the killed viruses, given parenterally, provoke serum antibody but not gut IgA; this is sufficient to prevent individual disease by interrupting viraemia, but does not prevent infection by, and faecal excretion of, wild polioviruses. Hence it does not contribute to herd immunity, making it essential to immunise the entire population. Inactivated virus is also a less immunogenic stimulus and boosters are needed at five-year intervals to maintain immunity.

However, there is another side to the picture, namely the matter of safety rather than efficacy. The Salk vaccine is now totally safe and, apart from the early incidents mentioned, has never given rise to clinical disease. In contrast, many of the admittedly rare cases of paralytic disease which have occurred in the USA and Europe since 1961 have been caused by the Sabin vaccine itself, due to the tendency for the attenuated type 3 strain to revert to a virulent form. While this only occurs once in every three million vaccinees, it is nevertheless a significant problem, the more so as the revertant virus is transmissible. There is sufficient concern on this point to warrant a search for a safer type 3 strain.

A problem affecting all vaccines produced in monkey cell cultures is that of contaminating simian viruses, which may persist in a viable state even in formaldehyde-treated preparations. *SV40 virus* is one example of a simian virus which is oncogenic in rodents and which contaminated early preparations of both the Salk and Sabin vaccines, fortunately without harmful consequences (p. 790). Others include the *Marburg virus* and *B virus*. The former infected laboratory workers handling tissues and cultures from imported African green monkeys in Marburg and elsewhere in 1967; there were seven deaths. B virus, or herpesvirus simiae, resembles herpes simplex and, while it gives rise to latent infections in monkeys, it can cause encephalomyelitis in man. There have been about 20 cases in as many years among those handling monkeys and their kidney cells for commercial poliovirus vaccine production. These dangers have led to the abandonment of simian cells in favour of human cell lines such as WI38, though fears of contamination by human 'cancer viruses' have also been expressed, probably unnecessarily.

Despite what has been said above, poliovirus vaccination has been less than completely successful in tropical and under-developed parts of Africa, Asia, Central and South America. Nevertheless, the continuation of mass immunisation throughout the world could lead to the complete disappearance of polio-viruses, as it has for the variola virus, providing the practical problems involved in such a large enterprise can be overcome.

Coxsackieviruses

These enteroviruses were first isolated from the stools of two children in the town of Coxsackie, New York State, in 1948, by inoculation of faecal extracts into newborn mice; this particular method was chosen after the demonstration that togaviruses, such as yellow fever virus, were more pathogenic in newborn than in adult mice. They were the first enteroviruses to be discovered after the polioviruses. The ability to cause disease in newborn mice and hamsters turned out to be a major characteristic, distinguishing the coxsackieviruses from other enteroviral species; adult mice suffer only an inapparent infection. The selectivity for newborn over adult mice may be related to the lack of interferon production by the former in response to coxsackieviruses; cortisone, which inhibits interferon synthesis, increases adult mouse susceptibility.

Twenty-nine types have been isolated, divided into two groups according to the murine manifestations of disease. *Group A viruses* cause skeletal muscular damage only, culminating in a flaccid paralysis of the hind limbs which is ultimately fatal (but, note, not due to CNS involvement); there are 23 serotypes, numbered A1–22 and A24 (type A23 is identical with another enterovirus and the designation has been dropped). *Group B viruses*, on the other hand, infect a variety of internal organs, including the myocardium, pancreas, liver, brain, skeletal muscle, etc.; there are 6 serotypes (B1–6). Interest has been shown in the fact that some produce a diabetes-like syndrome on inoculation into mice (B4 virus). This stimulated interest in a possible association of coxsackievirus infection with human diabetes, in particular with the juvenile onset form of the disease (p. 870). However, a follow-up study in the USA of 120 children infected with coxsackie B3 and B4 viruses produced no evidence of diabetes; nor was there any evidence of increased prevalence of diabetes after an extensive outbreak of these same viruses on an arctic island. Nevertheless, a recent report points to the existence of a diabetogenic variant of coxsackie B4 virus. Such a virus was isolated from the pancreas of a ten-year-old child who died in the acute phase of sudden-onset diabetes; inoculation of the agent into mice led to T-cell necrosis and diabetes. (See p. 872 for further discussion of the possible role of viruses in diabetes.)

In man, coxsackievirus infections are similar in several respects to those of polioviruses. They are world-wide in distribution and man is the only natural host; spread is by the faecal-oral route or oropharyngeal secretions. The majority of those infected are young children duing summer and autumn epidemics, though most infections remain subclinical or mild. The viruses replicate in the throat and intestine before viraemic dissemination to internal organs. Like polioviruses, some produce aseptic meningitis, though this rarely leads to paralysis. The commonest manifestations of group A viruses include herpangina; hand, foot and mouth disease; and a summer influenza-like fever. *Herpangina* (virus types A2, 4–6, 8 and 10) is an ulcerating infection of the tonsils and soft palate, accompanied by fever and pains in the neck and abdomen. *Hand, foot and mouth disease* (type A16), not connected with the animal disease of similar name, is a stomatitis similar to herpangina, with a rash on the hands and feet; epidemics occur in the summer, often centered around swimming pools.

Group B viruses cause, *inter alia*, infections affecting muscles and the CNS. *Epidemic myalgia* (or *Bornholm disease* after the Danish island in which it was first recognised) is characterised by severe stabbing pains in the lower chest and upper abdomen (epigastrium, hypochondrium), especially in children, and is caused by all group B viruses. *Myocarditis* is a group B infection which, though uncommon, has serious consequences both in children and adults. Newborns are particularly susceptible (cf. mice) and may acquire the virus *in utero*; disease becomes noticeable as dyspnoea (laboured breathing), tachycardia (rapid heart beat) and cyanosis (anoxic blueing of the skin). There may be permanent heart damage and mortality is high. Like rubella virus, coxsackieviruses are an important cause of congenital heart defects. It is also possible that some cases of 'cot death' (sudden infant death syndrome) are due to coxsackieviral heart disease.

Aseptic meningitis can be due to either A or B group viruses; it is clinically indistinguish able from the acute stage of poliomyelitis, but rarely leads to encephalitis or paralysis. Type A7 infections, however, do tend to cause paralysis and in recent years epidemics with this strain have occured in Scotland and the USSR. Finally, both groups may be involved in mild respiratory diseases, akin to the common cold, which occur particularly in infants.

Echoviruses

Much of what has been said above about coxsackieviruses also applies to echoviruses, with the exception of pathogenicity in the mouse. Indeed, they are so similar that with newly discovered enteroviruses the distinction is no longer made (p. 285). The echoviruses were discovered in normal human faeces during epidemiological studies connected with poliomyelitis, and demonstrated by their cytopathogenic effect on cultured cells. 'Echo' is an acronym of 'enteric cytopathic human orphan', the 'orphan' indicating lack of an associated disease. They are specific to man, but similar to enteroviruses occurring in different species. Echoviruses are widely disseminated and are regularly found where hygiene is inadequate, generally without adverse effect. They are common, often harmless, passengers in the human gut; most are no longer 'orphans', but recognised agents of a variety of enteroviral diseases, including aseptic meningitis, some paralytic disease, infantile gastroenteritis, and minor respiratory disease. In general these conditions tend to be less severe than the coxsackievirus equivalents. Epidemics may occur, such as *Boston fever* (echovirus 16), a sharp fever with abdominal pains and a pink rash on the face, chest and back, named after the city of its first occurrence.

Although they are occasionally isolated from cases of diarrhoea in infants, echoviruses (and enteroviruses in general) are not a major cause of gastroenteritis. Acute infectious non-bacterial gastroenteritis, one of the commonest and most important illnesses among children, is generally due to a rotavirus (p. 365) or parvovirus-like agents not yet fully characterised, such as the Norwalk agent (p. 283).

Rhinoviruses and the common cold

The rhinovirus genus comprises (to date) *113 types* of related picornaviruses which cause the mild upper respiratory tract condition known as the common cold (acute coryza). As we have already noted, they are not the only cold viruses (but are the largest single group); others include enteroviruses, adenoviruses, coronaviruses, influenzaviruses, parainfluenzaviruses and respiratory syncytial virus. They are distinguished from the enteroviruses by their survival at 50°C, their acid-lability and their requirement for an unexpectedly low culture temperature (33°C). They can be transmitted to chimpanzees but not to other animals, so that cell cultures are the main means of studying their behaviour. Rhinovirus types can be divided into groups according to whether they infect human cell cultures only (H strains), human and monkey cells (M), or only organ cultures of human embryo respiratory epithelium (O). Replication and cytopathogenic effect are much as described above for polioviruses. Antisera are used for identification of individual types.

In temperate climates, colds due to rhinoviruses occur throughout the year but are relatively more common in early autumn and late spring, and are less associated with the winter months than those due to other cold viruses. The common cold begins with infection, via droplets, of the ciliated nasal epithelium. During the 24–48 hour incubation period, the virus multiplies locally; cilia are immobilised and then degenerate with the cells. The first symptoms are of clear, watery nasal discharge (rhinorrhoea), sneezing and malaise, but fever is usually absent except in infants and small children. The discharge later becomes purulent, often due to secondary bacterial contamination, which is also responsible for infection of nasal sinuses (sinusitis) and the middle ear (otitis media). Other parts of the respiratory tract may also be involved; a hacking (harsh, dry) cough and hoarse voice may develop, with tonsillitis, laryngitis and tracheitis, and there may be exacerbation of existing chronic bronchitis and asthma. The virus remains localised to the nasal mucosa throughout, at least in part because the temperature restriction noted above means that rhinoviruses only multiply in the cooler parts of the upper respiratory tract. Recovery generally takes 4–10 days.

Specific local immunity to the infecting strain is provided by IgA antibodies, while serum IgG also develops. These antibodies do not prevent subsequent and frequent reinfection by other rhinoviruses, and local type-specific immunity itself only lasts for about two years. There is a period of about four weeks of non-specific resistance to reinfection which is probably due to interferon. With so many antigenically distinct types of cold virus, the problems of developing a useful composite vaccine are obviously enormous. While a preparation of all 113 rhinoviruses is impractical, it may be possible to find cross-protection between certain strains which would enable a less complex yet effective vaccine to be developed. Interferon can prevent colds, and may be generally available for this purpose in the forseeable future (p.252). Large doses of vitamin C (up to 2 g per day) have not been protective in controlled clinical trials.

CORONAVIRIDAE

We have noted above that viruses of several families can cause the common cold. While rhinoviruses are responsible for the largest number of colds, coronaviruses are the second most frequent agents, being responsible for at least 10–15% of colds and at times considerably more. In temperate climates, colds due to coronaviruses are particularly prevalent in winter and early spring ('winter colds'), at which times rhinovirus infections are relatively few. As well as those inhabiting the respiratory tract, there are also enteric coronaviruses; they may be a cause of human gastroenteritis, but this remains to be established. It would not be very surprising, however, as they are well-known agents of enteric disease in animals, e.g. transmissible gastroenteritis of piglets. There are many other animal coronaviruses, among them one which causes avian infectious bronchitis of chickens. Difficulties in growing human coronaviruses in culture has made progress in studying this group rather slow.

Structure, etc. Coronaviruses resemble influenza viruses in the electron microscope, with a roughly spherical or pleomorphic appearance, and surface spikes projecting from an envelope which encloses a helical nucleocapsid. The spikes are distinctive, however, being larger, more widely spaced and club-shaped; the halo of spikes is reminiscent of a solar corona, whence the name of the family. The viral genome is single-stranded (+) RNA (class IV). While coronaviruses from animals can be grown relatively easily in culture, human strains have been much more difficult to grow due to their strict host-cell specificity, so that very few have been isolated. The prototype human coronavirus is known as 229E and was isolated in human embryo cell culture; other strains, such as OC43, can only be grown in organ culture of human respiratory epithelium from nasal or tracheal tissue of aborted foetuses. These two strains are the best studied, but there are doubtless several yet to be identified.

Coronaviral infection. The clinical features of upper respiratory tract infection by coronaviruses are indistinguishable from the common cold syndrome of other viruses. Volunteers inoculated intranasally develop colds with acute coryza after 2–3 days. The virus multiplies in the nasal epithelium. Occasionally the infection spreads to the lower respiratory tract, and coronaviruses may be responsible for a substantial proportion of cases of bronchiolitis and pneumonia in children. Little is known about mechanisms of immunity, but reinfection is possible despite the presence of neutralising antibody in the blood; presumably the waning of local IgA immunity allows reinfection to occur. The same strain does not seem to recur in successive years, however, but returns regularly after a few years' absence. Laboratory diagnosis of a coronavirus infection depends on a rising titre of serum antibody, usually measured by complement fixation (p.136) or, more recently, by enzyme-linked immunoassay (ELISA).

ARBOVIRUSES (TOGAVIRIDAE)

The term 'arbovirus' literally means viruses which are

'arthropod-borne', i.e. transmitted to man and other animals by the bite of blood-sucking (haematophagous) arthropod vectors, such as mosquitoes, ticks, gnats or sandflies. Thus, it is an epidemiological rather than a taxonomic grouping, and includes viruses from at least five different families—Togaviridae, Bunyaviridae, Reoviridae, Rhabdoviridae and Arenaviridae—all of which are RNA viruses. A huge number of arboviruses have been discovered—over 350 species—of which only a fraction are pathogenic in man. Among them are the agents of major tropical and subtropical diseases, including dengue, yellow fever, other haemorrhagic fevers and encephalitides (encephalitic diseases), some of which are among the most dangerous of all the viral diseases of man. The major family of human pathogens is the *Togaviridae*, all of which (except for rubella virus) are arboviruses.

An essential point in the definition of an arbovirus is that the arthropod does not merely provide mechanical transportation of virus from one infected animal or human being to another, but is a *true host* in which the virus multiplies before its transmission to its other, vertebrate host. (Purely mechanical transmission by insects does occur for some viruses, such as myxoma virus in rabbits, but they are not classified as arboviruses, nor do they infect man.) Both hosts are essential to the survival of the virus, since direct transmission between individual members of the same species does not occur (other than transovarial transmission in ticks, p. 304). The natural vertebrate host is often a wild or domestic animal in which the infection is harmless, reflecting a high degree of mutual adaptation of parasite and host. Human disease arises because man is an *unnatural host*, usually intruding accidentally into the normal life cycle of the virus. Thus, with the exception of the urban forms of dengue and yellow fever, most human arboviral diseases are *zoonoses*: infections primarily of animals but transmissible to man. A selection of arboviruses infecting man is shown in Table 3.9.

Classification and structure

The togaviruses are class IV viruses, with a single-stranded 'positive' RNA genome. They are small (40–70 nm) particles with an icosahedral capsid and close-fitting envelope (whence the name, from the *toga* worn by citizens of ancient Rome). Projecting from the envelope are short glycoprotein spikes which are haemagglutinins for certain red cells (goose, pigeon); antibodies can thus be usefully assayed by haemagglutination inhibition (p. 319). As the envelope is required for infectivity, togaviruses are inactivated by lipid solvents and bile salts. Two main subdivisions (genera) of the family can be distinguished serologically, the *alphaviruses* (formerly called group A) and the *flaviviruses* (formerly group B). Individual species are named both after the disease they cause and the geographical location where they were first isolated or where the disease is endemic (Table 3.9). Extensive biochemical studies have been carried out with two, the Sinbis and Semliki Forest viruses, which are not usually pathogenic in man.

Table 3.9 Some important arboviruses.

Family	Genus	Clinical syndrome	Vector	Species/Disease
Togaviridae	Alphavirus	Fever, encephalitis	Mosquito	Eastern equine encephalitis Western equine encephalitis Venezuelan equine encephalitis
		Fever, arthralgia, rash, etc.	Mosquito	Chikungunya O'nyong nyong Semliki Forest Sindbis
		Fever, haemorrhage	Mosquito	Chikungunya
	Flavivirus	Fever, encephalitis	Mosquito	Japanese encephalitis St Louis encephalitis Murray Valley encephalitis
			Tick	Powassan Tick-borne encephalitis Russian spring-summer encephalitis Louping-ill (sheep) Kyasanur Forest disease
		Fever, arthralgia, etc.	Mosquito	Dengue
		Fever, haemorrhage, etc.	Mosquito	Dengue Yellow fever
			Tick	Omsk haemorrhagic fever Crimean–Congo haemorrhagic fever
Bunyaviridae	Bunyavirus	Encephalitis	Mosquito	California encephalitis Tahyna
		Fever	Mosquito	Bunyamwera; Bwamba
		Fever, myalgia, conjunctivitis	Phlebotomus	Sandfly fever
Reoviridae	Orbivirus	Fever, myalgia	Tick	Colorado tick fever

The *Bunyaviridae* are class V viruses—'negative' single-stranded RNA genome—which are helical and enveloped; the RNA is divided into three segments. Some bunyavirus diseases are summarised in Table 3.9, but are not further specifically described here, though the same principles apply to their transmission.

Replication and cellular infection

The replication of togaviruses differs in some important details from that of poliovirus (p.234–7), e.g. only a part of the RNA genome is translated immediately. However, post-translational cleavage again occurs. A major difference is that they acquire an envelope, budding through either the plasma membrane (alphaviruses) or cytoplasmic vacuoles (flaviviruses). They multiply in a variety of vertebrate cells in culture, where infection is cytocidal; they replicate in, but do not kill, cultured mosquito cells, which

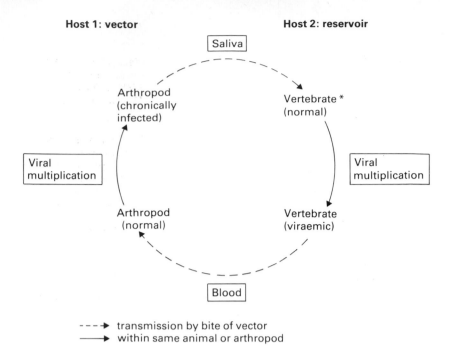

Host 1: vector   Host 2: reservoir

Saliva

Arthropod (chronically infected)

Vertebrate * (normal)

Viral multiplication

Viral multiplication

Arthropod (normal)

Vertebrate (viraemic)

Blood

- - -▶ transmission by bite of vector
——▶ within same animal or arthropod

may explain why no apparent harm is done to their vector hosts. Infected cells may develop characteristic inclusion bodies, such as the intranuclear Torres bodies in liver cells infected with yellow fever virus.

Figure 3.29 Basic transmission cycle of an arbovirus.
* = wild or domestic bird or animal, or man

Transmission and epidemiology

By definition, arboviruses have two hosts, an arthropod and a vertebrate. The former is the *vector* which transmits the infection in its saliva directly into the vertebrate circulation during the course of a blood meal. The vertebrate, for its part, is a *reservoir* of infection for acquisition by uninfected arthropods, and hence transmission to other animals in a cyclical manner. The basic events in this life cycle are shown in Figure 3.29. The arthropod is unharmed by the virus and retains a chronic infection for its short lifetime; virus is taken up during feeding, penetrates the arthropod gut wall and multiplies in tissue cells, finally entering the salivary glands ready for transmission. In the vertebrate host, the virus multiplies in vascular endothelium and reticulo-endothelial cells before causing a short (2–3 day) viraemia; the role of the vertebrate in the cycle can only be effected during this brief viraemic period, when it must be bitten again and infected blood taken up by another arthropod, and so forth. Only animals in which a sufficiently high number of virus particles are present in the blood can take part in the cycle; for this reason some 'unnatural' hosts, including man and the horse, will often be 'dead-ends' as far as transmission is concerned.

The principal vectors for tropical infections are mosquitoes of the genera *Aedes*, *Haemagogus* and *Culex*; in temperate regions, ticks and sandflies (*Phlebotomus*) are also important. In temperate

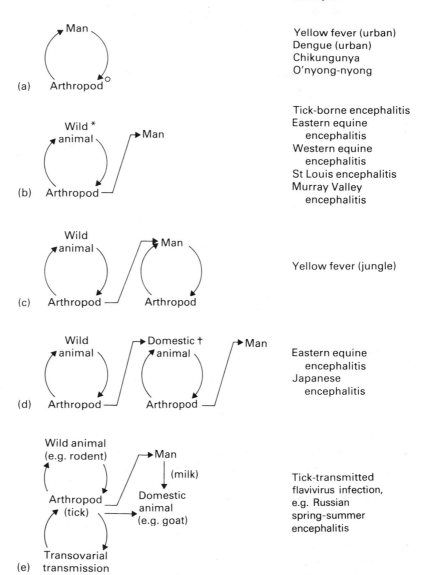

(a)	Yellow fever (urban) Dengue (urban) Chikungunya O'nyong-nyong

(b)	Tick-borne encephalitis
	Eastern equine
	  encephalitis
	Western equine
	  encephalitis
	St Louis encephalitis
	Murray Valley
	  encephalitis

(c)	Yellow fever (jungle)

(d)	Eastern equine
	  encephalitis
	Japanese
	  encephalitis

(e)	Tick-transmitted flavivirus infection, e.g. Russian spring-summer encephalitis

Figure 3.30 Transmission cycles of arbovirus infections of man.
° = mosquito, tick, sandfly, etc.
* = birds, or mammals such as rodents, monkeys, etc.
† = fowl, pigs, etc.

climates the vector may be absent in the winter months and it is not always clear how the virus survives; some mosquito-borne viruses survive by transovarial transmission and overwintering in mosquito eggs, while for others overwintering may be achieved in the blood of birds, hibernating bats or snakes. Tick-borne arboviruses survive during the cold seasons in their hardy, overwintering arthropod hosts. The distribution of the vector obviously determines that of the disease and depends in turn on climatic conditions. Thus arbovirus infections are endemic in tropical jungles and rain forests where mosquitoes abound, while in subtropical areas epidemics appear after heavy rainfall has led to an increase in the vector population. By the same token, artificial control of the vector can be the key to eradicating the disease, as with urban yellow fever.

A variety of possible *transmission cycles* occurs and those involving man are shown schematically in Figure 3.30. It is unusual for man to be a reservoir of infection, but this is the case in a few major diseases, including yellow fever and dengue in their urban cycles, and the African diseases Chikungunya and O'nyong-nyong (Figure 3.30a). More commonly, man is a terminal, 'tangential' host, unable to transmit the infection further (Figure 3.30b, d). Thus, in the encephalitides, such as Eastern equine encephalitis, etc., the natural cycle is between a wild animal, often a bird, and a mosquito. Sometimes a domestic species (fowl, pig) is an intermediate host and plays an important role in amplifying the amount of virus in the vicinity of man (Figure 3.30d); e.g. in Japanese encephalitis, the wild reservoir is a heron and the domestic one a pig, with man as an ultimate 'blind alley' and the only host in which clinical disease occurs. Ticks have an additional feature as vectors in that they are able to transmit virus *transovarially* to the next generation, thus serving both as vector and reservoir (Figure 3.30e). Some tick-borne viruses may find their way to man by an indirect route, viz. in the milk of domestic goats, as in Russian spring-summer encephalitis (Figure 3.30e). Transovarial transmission can also occur for bunyaviruses in mosquitoes and may be a means of overwintering the months when the vectors do not breed.

Isolation

Over 350 arbovirus species are known; they are discovered by isolation from the arthropods themselves, which are macerated and extracts injected intracerebrally into newborn mice (the most sensitive hosts) or introduced into cell cultures. Sometimes mice or chickens are used as 'sentinels', which are left overnight in areas infested with mosquitoes, etc., to encourage a natural infection from which a virus can then be isolated. 'New' viruses are subjected to serological tests for classification. Only a fraction of the arboviruses discovered by these methods are of significance to man.

Pathogenesis

The vast majority ($\sim 90\%$) of arbovirus infections of man are subclinical, while the remainder can vary from transient fever to severe, often fatal conditions. A generalised scheme for their pathogenesis is shown in Figure 3.31. Virus in the saliva of a mosquito or tick is introduced directly into a capillary; thereafter there is a short incubation period (3–7 days) during which viral replication takes place in vascular endothelium and cells of the reticulo-endothelial system in lymph nodes, spleen, etc., culminating in the short-lived viraemia. Clinical symptoms are often *biphasic*, the first phase coinciding with viraemia and manifested in fever, nausea, headache, muscular pain, etc. At this point, the disease may either terminate completely or enter a short period of remission of a few days during which the fever subsides, only to be followed by the

304

second symptomatic phase. Fever then recurs, so that the patient's temperature curve is sometimes called 'saddle-back'. In addition, there are manifestations of disease in one or several organs, depending on the distribution of the virus. (a) In the *encephalitic diseases*, inflammatory and necrotic lesions occur in the brain, leading at first to headache and stiff neck, and progressing to stupor, coma and paralysis; some, such as Eastern equine encephalitis and Japanese encephalitis, have a high mortality. (b) In other arboviral diseases, the CNS is not involved, but joints and muscles are often painfully affected (myalgia, arthralgia) and there may be a skin rash; dengue is a good example. (c) In the *haemorrhagic fevers*, bleeding occurs into the skin and mucous membranes throughout the body and from every orifice, e.g. haematemesis (vomiting of blood); death is from hypotensive shock. This is a diverse group, some of which, like dengue haemorrhagic shock syndrome, can be highly lethal. Haemorrhage probably results from thrombocytopenia (platelet deficiency, p. 638) following destruction of megakaryocytes

Figure 3.31 General scheme for pathogenesis of arboviral diseases.

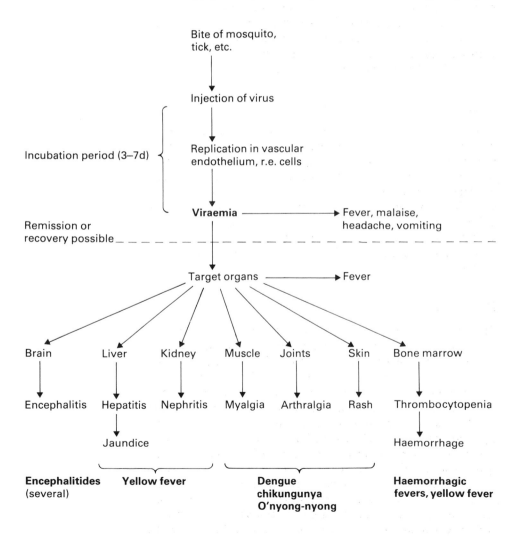

(the platelet progenitor cells) by virus in the bone marrow. (d) In the most wide-ranging syndrome, the liver and kidney are also infected, with hepatitis and nephritis as well as haemorrhage, a potentially lethal combination seen only in yellow fever.

Note that Figure 3.31 represents all the possible stages in arboviral disease, but all are not always seen. Thus, instead of the complete biphasic progression, there may be only the early phase of fever, etc., coincident with viraemia, then recovery; or alternatively this phase may be inapparent and only the later, post-viraemic syndrome occurs. Recovery from infection is accompanied by permanent immunity.

Some specific examples of togavirus diseases are now described more fully.

Encephalitides

Several togaviruses cause encephalitic disease in man. The *equine encephalitis* group are alphaviruses which, as their name suggests, also infect horses. Both horse and man are generally dead-end hosts which do not transmit the infection further, while the natural cycle is between wild birds and mosquitoes, as in Figure 3.30b. Three important examples are found in North or South America, namely the Eastern, Western and Venezuelan equine encephalitides. *Eastern equine encephalitis* (EEE) is the most severe in man, with mortality of up to 75%, inapparent infection being rare. It occurs in the eastern part of the USA, Canada and South America, and is particularly serious in infants where, when not fatal, it leaves permanent mental deficiency and paralysis. It is transmitted by *Culiseta* mosquitoes between wild birds; domestic chickens may be an intermediate reservoir prior to transmission to man (Figure 3.32).

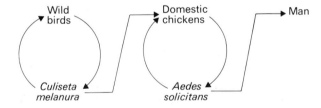

Figure 3.32 Spread of Eastern equine encephalitis in New Jersey, 1959.

Western equine encephalitis (WEE) is less severe and only some 0.1% of human infections are clinically apparent. Formerly more prevalent west of the Mississippi, it now occurs throughout the United States, again often in children under one year of age. Both EEE and WEE cause *epizootics* (the animal equivalent of epidemics) in horses in the USA and Latin America, which may be very damaging; e.g. in 1938, nearly 200,000 horses were infected, with a high rate of mortality. The horse, like man, is not a reservoir, because the viraemia is not sufficently great. *Venezuelan equine encephalitis* is also mild in man and is primarily a major equine disease in the USA, Central and South America. In this case, in addition to birds, the horse is a reservoir for transmission. A huge epizootic in Texas and Mexico killed thousands of horses in 1971 before it was halted by vaccination and strict quarantining; mild disease occurred in over 100 people at that time.

Flaviviruses also cause human encephalitis in the USA, the most important being *St Louis encephalitis*, which occasionally breaks out in considerable epidemics in different parts of the country. The most recent was in 1975, when 140 deaths occurred out of 1815 cases. Birds are again the main reservoir. *Japanese encephalitis* is a major encephalitic flavivirus disease, widely distributed throughout Asia from eastern Siberia to Malaysia and particularly in Japan. About 0.2% of infected individuals develop a severe encephalitis, similar to EEE, with a very high mortality (up to 90%) or permanent mental damage and paralysis. The incidence in Japan used to be quite high, with several thousand people affected in epidemics in cities such as Tokyo, but has fallen dramatically with the now routine vaccination of children and pigs with formalin-inactivated virus. It provides a good illustration of a domestic animal link between the wild reservoir and man, which amplifies the amount of virus in circulation. Birds, especially herons and egrets, are the primary hosts, with *Culex* and *Aedes* mosquitoes as vectors. The herons breed near Tokyo in late summer and mosquitoes spread the virus to domestic pigs (which are widely kept in Japan) and hence to man, the terminal host and the only one in which disease occurs (Figure 3.33).

Figure 3.33 Japanese encephalitis in Tokyo.

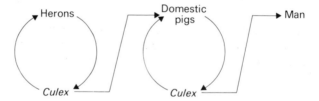

Dengue

This is the most prevalent arboviral disease of man in the world, being endemic throughout the tropics and subtropics; the agent is a flavivirus. It is representative of those arboviral syndromes which do not involve encephalitis but have instead other systemic manifestations, in this case intense pain in the muscles, joints and back (hence its familiar name of 'breakbone fever'). In a sense, it is atypical in that it is not a zoonosis, being transmitted in urban environments from person to person by the domestic mosquito *Aedes aegypti*, with no animal reservoir involved (Figure 3.30a). However, a jungle form with an animal reservoir does also exist. Dengue usually shows the characteristic biphasic development and saddle-back temperature curve described above. After an incubation period of 5–8 days, fever is accompanied by the painful symptoms; 2–3 days later, the fever falls and there is temporary respite for 24 hours, after which a second rapid rise in temperature occurs, together with a muculopapular skin rash described as 'morbilliform' (i.e. measles-like).

Despite the pain, dengue is not a dangerous condition and

there is no significant mortality. However, there is a more perilous form of infection, a haemorrhagic fever called the *dengue shock syndrome* (DSS). Its appearance on a large scale is relatively recent, and it became suddenly more prevalent in the 1950's among children in areas where dengue is endemic; it has since spread rapidly and is now seen mostly in children in the Philippines, Malaysia, Vietnam, Thailand and India. Bleeding occurs as purpura (haemorrhagic rash) and bruising in the skin (petechiae, ecchymoses, p. 638), and as haematemesis and epistaxis (nosebleed); hypotensive shock occurs after 2–6 days and in 10–30% of cases is fatal, especially in infants less than one year old. There is evidence that the shock syndrome is a hypersensitivity reaction of the immune complex type, involving complement activation and release of vasoactive fragments such as C3a (p.31). One theory is that it stems from reinfection with a related dengue virus serotype in a child who has recently made an antibody response to a dengue infection, and that antigenic cross-reaction with the second virus leads to formation of a large amount of non-neutralising antibody, immune complexes, complement activation and shock. It is not certain that this picture is correct, though C3 levels are markedly depressed in the individuals concerned; however it is very important to settle the possible role of antigen–antibody complexes before starting programmes of vaccination with attenuated virus. In the meantime, dengue control consists of the eradication of the mosquito and the isolation of patients under mosquito netting until their fever has subsided.

Yellow fever

For 200 years, from the beginning of the eighteenth century, yellow fever, with its gruesome symptom of black (bloody) vomiting, was one of the great plagues of the world. Its major centres were in the tropical and subtropical areas of West Africa (the supposed area of its origin), Central and South America, and with the opening up of the American continent by European colonisation there were devastating epidemics in the growing cities of Latin America, the West Indies and the southern states of the USA. In the nineteenth century, outbreaks spread as far north as Boston, and even to Europe. Its history is linked with that of the Panama canal (the spread of lethal yellow fever among French workers being one of the factors which caused construction to be abandoned in 1889) and with the names of Carlos Finlay and Major Walter Reed. Finlay was a Cuban physician who, in 1881, was the first to suggest that yellow fever was transmitted by the mosquito now known as *Aedes aegypti*. This was firmly established in 1900 by the brilliant pioneering observations and experiments of Reed and the Yellow Fever Commission of the US Army, despatched to Cuba to study the disease because of its disastrous effect on US troops in the Spanish–American war. Reed not only proved that *Aedes* mosquitoes were indeed the vectors, but also showed for the first time that a filterable agent was the cause of a human disease. Thus yellow fever has been of considerable historical importance both to mankind and to virology.

Since the 1930's, the eradication of *Aedes aegypti* and related mosquitoes from tropical cities has eliminated urban yellow fever which, like dengue, is transmitted in the simplest possible cycle from person to person via the mosquito (Figure 3.30a). However, this progress revealed the existence of a second type of cycle in tropical jungles and forests (sylvatic cycle) where the virus is endemic in several species of monkey and transmission is by mosquitoes of the forest canopy such as *Haemogogus*. The monkeys are usually only subclinically infected. Man is liable to acquire infection when he intrudes into the jungle, e.g. for road building, tree felling (*Haemagogus* is especially numerous around newly-felled trees), etc., and might then take the disease back to a village or town where human outbreaks can ensue (Figure 3.34). As it is impossible to eradicate the jungle vectors and reservoirs, yellow fever remains endemic in Central Africa and parts of South and Central America, and may occasionally erupt

Figure 3.34 Two types of transmission cycle for yellow fever virus.
(a) Urban yellow fever.
(b) Jungle yellow fever.

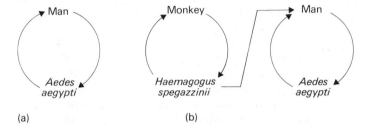

(a)   (b)

into epidemics; as recently as 1960–62, thousands died in an epidemic in Ethiopia.

The pathogenesis of yellow fever is that of a haemorrhagic fever with the additional complications, in severe cases, of hepatitis and nephritis due to excessive viral multiplication in the liver and kidneys (as well as in the bone marrow). Its severity is quite variable. In the full-blown disease, symptoms again follow a biphasic course. The first phase of fever starts abruptly after a brief incubation period of 3–6 days (prodromal symptoms are absent) and coincides with viraemia; there is nausea, vomiting and a pulse rate which is slow for the degree of fever (Faget's sign). After a period of remission, during which the fever falls rapidly, the major manifestations of the disease occur in the second phase or 'period of intoxication'. Fever recurs, liver damage leads to jaundice (hence 'yellow fever') and kidney damage to extreme albuminuria and acute renal failure, while bleeding into the stomach is responsible for the characteristic 'black vomit' (haematemesis). Finally, delirium, convulsions and coma presage death in about 10% of cases. The liver shows distinctive midzonal hyaline necrosis, with preservation of its basic architecture; fused dead cells form eosinophilic hyaline masses called *Councilman bodies*. Recovery from yellow fever confers lifelong immunity to reinfection.

The elimination of urban yellow fever depended firstly on the eradication of the domestic mosquito, greatly aided by the introduction of insecticides such as DDT, and secondly on *immunisation*. A live vaccine is required as inactivation destroys the protective antigens. The *17D strain* is an avirulent variant attenuated by successive passage through mice, tissue cultures and embryonated eggs; it is a highly effective vaccine, partly because there is only one antigenic type of the yellow fever virus. Vaccination is essential to prevent sylvatic outbreaks, since the eradication of jungle yellow fever by mosquito control, other than in restricted areas, is a practical impossibility.

Rubella virus

Rubella virus is a member of the Togaviridae, but as it is the only one that is not an arbovirus, it is discussed separately. It does not share antigens with other togaviruses and is classified in a separate genus, namely *Rubivirus*. Rubella, or German measles, is a fairly innocuous disease, primarily of children, resembling a mild form of measles without its major complications. However, it has one property which elevates it in significance to one of the most notorious of infections, namely the ability to infect the foetus *in utero* and cause a range of severe congenital defects known as the *rubella syndrome*. For many years, rubella was the major infectious cause of abnormalities in the newborn, but since 1970 the policy of vaccination of children and susceptible women has led to a progressive decline in its incidence to current low levels.

Structure and replication

Like the other togaviruses, rubella virus is enveloped, with a positive single-stranded RNA genome (class IV) within a probably icosahedral core. There is an envelope haemagglutinin, in the form of projecting spikes, which has specificity for membrane lipid rather than glycoprotein (cf. influenza); there is no neuraminidase. Replication is as described for other togaviruses.

Cellular infection

In several types of cell culture, a cytopathogenic effect may not be apparent, but cellular alterations without lysis develop slowly in primary human cell cultures. Infection is best demonstrated either by haemadsorption or by *interference* with the replication and CPE induced by a picornavirus with which the culture (of monkey kidney cells) can be superinfected. Rubella virus often establishes a *persistent infection* in culture in which there is continued production of virus without obvious cell damage; this reflects similar events in infections in newborns, from whom chronically infected cells can be isolated.

Epidemiology

As in measles, transmission of rubella is via droplets of infected respiratory secretion. It is less contagious than measles and, although it causes epidemics among children, up to 20% of young adult women would escape infection and be susceptible were it not for vaccination. The disease is mild and indeed often goes unnoticed. Minor outbreaks occur every year or two and major epidemics at six- to nine-year intervals; before vaccination was introduced, about one pregnant woman in every thousand would be infected in non-epidemic years, rising to 20 per thousand in epidemics. Of such pregnancies, 40% were affected in some way, either with foetal death (10–15%) or with congenital rubella (25%). In the last major epidemic in the USA in 1964, about 20,000 babies were born with congenital rubella. The risk is critically dependent on the extent to which pregnancy has progressed at the time of infection. If infection occurs during the first month, the rate of malformation is up to 50%, falling to 25% in the second month, 17% in the third, and decreasing to zero after the fifth. Thus rubella in an expectant mother during the first trimester of her pregnancy would be grounds for termination. Since vaccination became widely practised, the number of cases of rubella in women and the congenital syndrome have been very markedly reduced. Nevertheless, serological tests for *antirubella antibodies* in pregnant women exposed to infection are still essential. The assay is by haemagglutination-inhibition (p. 319); a high titre indicates immunity, but if low the woman may be at risk; rubella is confirmed by an antibody titre rising over four

Figure 3.35 Pathogenesis of rubella.

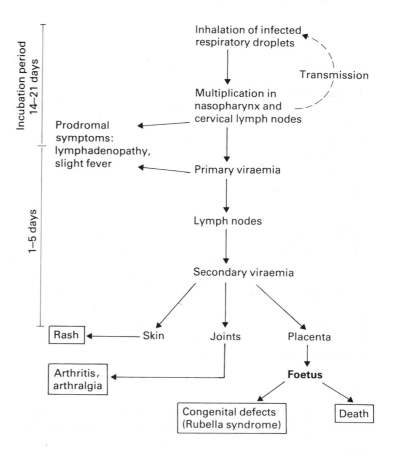

weeks. (In performing the haemagglutination-inhibition test, care must be taken to remove serum lipoprotein inhibitors by adsorption with dextran sulphate–CaCl$_2$.)

Pathogenesis (Figure 3.35).

Rubella is much milder and has fewer complications than measles, which it otherwise resembles (p. 340). The virus multiplies at first in the upper respiratory tract (nasopharyngeal mucosa) and then in local lymph nodes; postauricular lymphadenopathy (swollen 'glands' behind the ears) is a characteristic of the prodromal phase which precedes the rash. During the incubation period, virus is disseminated via the circulation to other lymph nodes for further replication, finally causing a macular 'rubelliform' skin rash of relatively brief duration (about three days). The commonest complications occur in the joints with pain (arthralgia) and stiffness, and occasionally arthritis in adults; this is transient and is not thought to be a prelude to chronic joint disorders.

Congenital rubella

Congenital rubella is a severe syndrome which, as noted above, is more likely to result the earlier in pregnancy infection is contracted. Principal damage occurs in the *ears* (deafness), *eyes* (cataracts, retinopathy) and the *cardiovascular system* (patent ductus arteriosus, in which the foetal communication between the aorta and pulmonary artery fails to close; atrial and ventricular defects in the heart). However, rubella infection affects many organs, and hepatitis, jaundice, splenomegaly, pneumonia, microcephaly, thrombocytopenia and skeletal defects are all common. Death may occur *in utero* or subsequently. On the other hand, in about half of all infected foetuses the infection remains subclinical and the child is born apparently normal; there may, nevertheless, be persistent production of virus for some time and such infants are an important source of infection in hospitals.

The question arises of why the seemingly innocuous rubella virus should be endowed with such teratogenic potential, apart from the fact that the virus can cross the placenta and cause a generalised infection. It is not possible to give a complete answer. Partly it is because rubella is not an aggressively cytocidal virus—a more toxic agent would probably kill the foetus outright—and tends to establish mild but chronic infections which lead to chromosomal abnormalities and a slowing of the rate of division. Thus, early in foetal life, differentiation of infected tissues is profoundly disrupted at a critical stage. A second point concerns the foetal immune response. Infection of the early foetus will occur at a time of immunological immaturity and can be expected to progress unchallenged for some time; nor can the foetus make interferon. Contrary to expectation, complete tolerance is not established despite the chronic nature of the infection, and newborns can have significant levels of antirubella IgM in the blood; the ineffectiveness of antibody in recovery is shown by the fact that the same newborns may continue to shed virus for several months. However, the cell-mediated immune response, which is almost certainly instrumental in recovery, is probably suppressed or tolerated. Such a state, in which only one 'limb' of the immune response is depressed, is sometimes called 'split tolerance'.

Vaccination

Rubella immunisation is unique in that its aim is to protect not children or adults, but a generation yet to be conceived. Since their introduction in 1970, attenuated virus vaccines have successfully reduced the incidence of infection and prevented major epidemics. As a precaution, pregnant women are excluded as far as possible from the vaccination programme, so that in addition to the usual requirements of efficacy and general safety, these vaccines should not be transmissible to contacts (which could include pregnant women), and must be free of teratogenic effects (in case of inadvertent immunisation in pregnancy). In this way, there should be no possibility of accidental production of foetal disease through vaccination. The viral strains used appear to meet the necessary criteria, especially the Cendehill strain developed in Belgium; there are two others, one of which (HP77) produces arthritic reactions and cannot be used in adults. The antibody response to all three is up to 5–10 times lower than after natural infection, and protection declines significantly after a few years; consequently reinfection is about ten times more common after artificial than natural immunisation.

Two different approaches to the vaccination programme have been adopted. In the UK and Australia, girls are vaccinated in their early teens, but children are *not* vaccinated; maximal use is thereby made of the longer-lasting protection which follows natural infection, while ensuring that all women of childbearing age have adequate antibody levels. In contrast, in the USA, *all* children are immunised, from infants upwards. Here the rationale is both to eliminate the source of infection to which pregnant women are commonly exposed (infected children) and in the long term to eliminate the virus from the population altogether, there being no reservoir other than man. This method has the potential drawback that immunity may decline to such an extent by adulthood as to make reinfection possible during pregnancy; moreover, if the virus is made to disappear, the opportunity for natural boosting of immunity through adult infection disappears as well. Since mass vaccination started only relatively recently, it is too early to say which approach has been the more successful in preventing congenital rubella. In both schemes, non-immune women of the appropriate age group are also immunised and should not conceive for two months after vaccination; *postpartum* immunisation is a simple way of ensuring this.

ORTHOMYXOVIRIDAE (INFLUENZA VIRUSES)

The prefix 'myxo' means mucus, and the name myxoviridae was originally given to a group of viruses with certain common properties, including an affinity for and presence in respiratory mucus, and an ability to bind to cell membrane glycoproteins, which they also attack enzymatically. Influenza viruses were the first to be isolated, followed later by parainfluenza, measles, mumps and others. It then emerged that the properties of influenza viruses were sufficiently distinctive to warrant splitting the myxoviruses into two families, the Orthomyxoviridae (influenza viruses) and the Paramyxoviridae (parainfluenza viruses, etc.). The families have several shared features—they are negative single-stranded RNA viruses which possess surface haemagglutinins and neuraminidase—but differ in aspects of their structure, replication and epidemiology (see Table 3.11, p. 333).

Huge worldwide outbreaks (pandemics) of influenza as well as more localised epidemics have taken millions of lives over the centuries. The most costly in terms of life was the pandemic of 1918, which affected half the population of the world and is estimated to have killed 20 million people—more than the First World War which had just ended—but those of 1889–90 and 1743 were by all accounts little less terrible. At one time it was thought that epidemics were governed by astrology—whence, from the Italian for 'influence', the name influenza was derived. At the end of the nineteenth century, bacteria were held to be responsible, particularly the 'influenza bacillus' *Haemophilus influenzae*, isolated in 1890 by Pfeiffer. It was not until 1933, when Smith, Andrewes and Laidlaw showed that a filter-passing agent present in nasal washings of influenza patients could transfer the disease to ferrets, that its viral nature was established. (Bacterial invasion, which is the usual cause of death, is a secondary complication.) Subsequent major developments were the growth of the virus in chick embryos (Burnet), which became the principal system for studying viral replication until cell culture methods for polioviruses were introduced in the late 1940's; and the discovery of viral haemagglutination (Hirst), an invaluable assay method both for virus and antiviral antibodies.

The key problems in influenza concern its epidemiology. How is the virus able to cause epidemics more or less regularly throughout the local population every 2–3 years? Why are there occasional worldwide pandemics of increased severity on the average once in every generation? And why is individual immunity apparently unable to prevent reinfection? Much has to do with the unique and fascinating genetic variation of the influenza viruses.

Structure

Freshly isolated influenza virus takes a number of forms when viewed by the electron microscope (pleomorphism), some roughly spherical, others filamentous (Figure 3.3c, 3.36a); filamentous forms are long enough ($1-2\,\mu$m) to be visible by light microscopy after silver staining or by dark-field. The typical rounded/ovoid particle has a diameter of about 100 nm and is composed of an outer lipid envelope, with short protruding spikes, surrounding the nucleocapsid (Figure 3.36a, b). The latter consists of single-stranded RNA and associated protein (ribonucleoprotein, RNP), coiled into a helical core (see also p. 222–4). The exact structure of the RNP is not known; there is no evidence from electron microscopy for a particular arrangement of capsomeres (cf. the 'herringbone' appearance of paramyxovirus nucleocapsids and others) and the RNA is accessible to RNase and therefore cannot be completely enclosed. In addition to the nucleocapsid protein, NP, which is a single polypeptide species, there are three other polypeptides associated with the core in small amounts, denoted PB_1, PB_2 and PA (for basic 1, basic 2 and acidic). PB_1 and PB_2 appear to constitute the enzyme *RNA-dependent RNA polymerase*

Figure 3.36 Structure of influenza virus.
(a) Influenza virus A, showing internal coil of nucleocapsid and surface spikes; negative staining; ×200,000. (Courtesy of Dr June Almeida.)
(b) Diagrammatic section.
(c) Schematic diagram to indicate the segmented nature of the influenza virus genome. For identification of segments see text p.313. (Note: P_1, P_2, P_3 are now known as PB_1, PB_2, PA.)

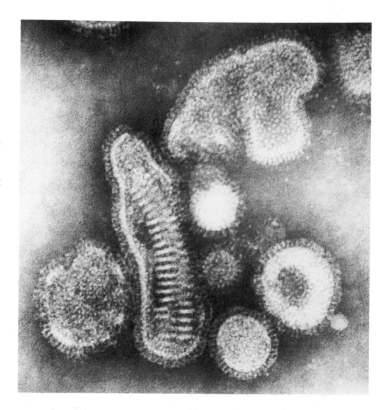

(a)

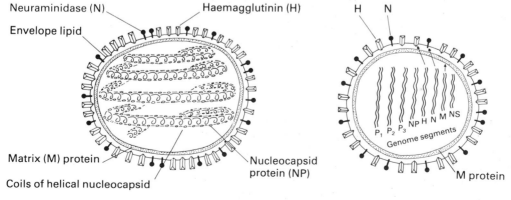

(b)

(c)

315

(RNA transcriptase) required for copying viral RNA, while PA may also be involved in replication.

The envelope is a lipid bilayer derived from the plasma membrane of the cell in which the virus was replicated, and carries two viral glycoproteins, the *haemagglutinin* and *neuraminidase*. They form the closely-packed spikes, 10–14 nm long, which have different morphologies: the haemagglutinin spikes are rod-shaped and triangular in section, while the neuraminidase spikes are mushroom-shaped (Figure 3.36b). The haemagglutinin protein is enzymatically 'nicked' during viral maturation into two chains (HA$_1$ and HA$_2$) which remain linked by a disulphide bond (the 'nicking' is essential to viral infectivity, p.246). Each haemagglutinin spike consists of three sets of HA$_1$-HA$_2$ polypeptides, while the neuraminidase spike is composed of four neuraminidase molecules. Haemagglutinin and neuraminidase are both involved in the infectivity of influenza viruses *in vivo*. The haemagglutinin has a specific binding site for *N-acetyl-neuraminic acid (NANA)*, a sugar residue widely distributed on cell membrane glycoproteins and glycolipids, and is responsible for the attachment of the virus to cell membranes which leads both to cellular infection and, *in vitro*, agglutination of red cells. Neuraminidase is an enzyme with the same specificity as haemagglutinin; its role is to help release of the virus from infected cells after budding, by removing NANA residues from cell surface glycoproteins to which the haemagglutinin otherwise attaches (Figure 3.37). Thus, neuraminidase-negative mutants remain attached to cells and each other in long chains. It has also been suggested that neuraminidase assists passage of the virus through mucus by destroying inhibitory glycoproteins. Between the envelope and the core is a layer of matrix or membrane (M) protein, closely associated with the inner surface of the lipid bilayer, which imparts stability to the envelope. The filamentous forms of the virus appear to be aggregates of spherical subunits which originate through a defect in the budding process.

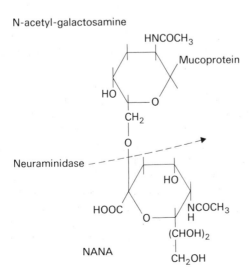

Figure 3.37 Removal of NANA from glycoprotein (mucoprotein) by neuraminidase.

The viral RNA is a negative strand, i.e. of complementary sequence to messenger RNA. An important point is that it is not a single continuous thread, but consists of eight *segments*, each surrounded by capsid protein and each a single gene. In the major influenza viruses, types A and B, there are eight segments and ten viral proteins, namely: PB_1, PB_2, PA, nucleocapsid (NP) protein, M protein, M2 protein (non-structural), haemagglutinin (H), neuraminidase (N), and two other non-structural proteins (NS_1 and NS_2) which are only found inside infected cells (nucleus and cytoplasm respectively). An additional polypeptide, M3, which is only nine amino acids long, has not yet been isolated, although there is plenty of mRNA for it in infected cells. The segments are of different sizes, and their protein products have been assigned as shown in Figure 3.36c. (The fact that there are ten or eleven products but only eight gene segments is explained on p. 321).

Classification (see Table 3.10)

Based on the internal antigens of the M and nucleocapsid proteins, three independent noncross-reacting influenza virus *types* are recognised, *A, B and C*, which have now been given the status of genera. Strains of influenza type A virus are found in man and animals (pigs, horses and several avian species including chickens), while B and C viruses are restricted to man. Types A and B viruses are both associated with epidemics, while type C gives rise only to sporadic mild infections. Distinct *subtypes* (species) of the A virus with *radically different* haemagglutinin, and sometimes also neuraminidase, molecules appear every 10–20 years and their arrival may lead to pandemics, of which those of 1889, 1918, 1957 and 1968 were the most dramatic examples; this type of variation, called *antigenic shift*, does not occur in B or C viruses. The haemagglutinin (H) and neuraminidase (N) of each A subtype is indicated numerically; those known to date in man are H0, H1, H2, H3, Hsw, N1 and N2 (Hsw is apparently identical to the haemagglutinin of swine influenza). Thus, the first influenza virus isolated in 1933 was type A, subtype H0N1 (originally termed the A0 subtype); it was the cause of all influenza A infections between 1929 and 1947, when a new subtype appeared, H1N1 (or A1) with a different haemagglutinin, H1, but the same neuraminidase as the A0 subtype. In 1957 there was a huge pandemic caused by the 'Asian' influenza subtype, H2N2 (A2), with both new haemagglutinin and neuraminidase, while the 'Hong Kong' virus, H3N2 (A3) which caused the 1968 pandemic had yet another haemagglutinin. Note that (i) all the A virus subtypes share the same *internal* antigens; (ii) while the haemagglutinin and neuraminidase of the various subtypes differ markedly in terms of their antigens and primary protein structure (amino acid sequence), they all retain binding site specificity for N-acetyl neuraminic acid; and (iii) only *one* subtype ever exists in a population at one time, i.e. as a new one appears, the previous subtype disappears.

Table 3.10 Classification of Orthomyxoviridae.

Genus/type	Species/subtype*	Host	Year of isolation in man
Influenzavirus A	H0N1 (A0)	Human	1933
	H1N1 (A1)	Human	1946
	H2N2 (A2)	Human	1957
	H3N2 (A3, AHK)	Human	1968
	HswN1	Swine, human	1976
	HeqN (2 species)	Equine	
	HavN (8 species)	Avian	
Influenzavirus B	†	Human	
Influenzavirus C	†	Human	

*According to the recently revised nomenclature, there are now only three human influenza virus A subtypes, namely H1N1, H2N2 and H3N2. H0 and Hsw are regarded as variants of H1 with a high degree of antigenic drift. For details see Bulletin of the World Health Organisation (1980) vol. 58 (4), pp. 585–591, 'A revision of the system of nomenclature for influenza viruses: A WHO memorandum' However, in this text the 'old' nomenclature, as in Table 3.10, has been retained.
† Insufficient information to classify subtypes.

Within each subtype/species there are individual virus *strains*, which show *minor changes* in H and N antigens and give rise to local epidemics at 2–3 year intervals. Strain variations are the result of point mutation and selection, a process called *antigenic drift*, which occurs in all three influenza virus types. Individual strains are numbered. In order to define a strain precisely, its characteristics are indicated in the following order: type (A,B,C)/host species (omitted if human)/geographical origin/strain number/year of isolation and finally (H,N) subtype. Thus the Asian influenza virus of 1957 is designated A/Singapore/1/57 (H2N2), while the Hong Kong virus of 1968 is A/Hong Kong/1/68 (H3N2), and so on.

Haemagglutination

Influenza viruses agglutinate the red cells of a number of mammalian and avian species, including human red cells. Agglutination occurs because of the presence of NANA on the red cell membrane, enabling cross-linking by viral haemagglutinin to occur (Figure 3.38a). This reaction is a very important method for detection and quantification both of virus and antiviral antibody, not only for influenza viruses but for several other haemagglutinating viruses as well. The *haemagglutination test* (Figure 3.38e) is carried out in wells of a titration plate by making serial dilutions of an influenza virus suspension, (such as the allantoic fluid of embryonated eggs inoculated with virus), followed by addition of 1% human or guinea-pig red cells for type A and B viruses, or chicken red cells for type C. The reaction is allowed to occur at 4°C and agglutination observed after 30–60 minutes; the viral *titre* is the highest dilution of the suspension to cause visible red cell agglutination. The temperature at which the test is done is critical for influenza and other viruses which possess a surface neuraminidase; at 4°C the enzyme is prevented from acting, but at higher temperatures it splits off NANA residues from the cell surface and thereby prevents agglutination. Indeed, if red cells agglutinated by influenza virus at 4°C are brought to 37°C for one hour, the virus *elutes* and the red cells return to their non-agglutinated state (Figure 3.38b); since their surface NANA has been removed, they cannot be reagglutinated by lowering the temperature again, although the eluted virus can still agglutinate freshly added red cells.

Antiviral antibodies can be assayed by their ability to inhibit haemagglutination, following binding to viral haemagglutinin. In the *haemagglutination-inhibition (HI) test* (Figure 3.38c, e), serial dilutions of antibody are prepared in the titration plate and an equal amount of virus added to each well, sufficient to cause agglutination of red cells but not excessive (e.g. four times the minimal agglutinating dose). One per cent red cells are then added: in wells containing sufficient antiviral antibody, no haemagglutination occurs and the titre of inhibition indicates antibody concentration. When using HI to detect antibodies in serum (or other body fluids), it is necessary to destroy any naturally occurring glycoproteins which carry NANA groups and could spuriously inhibit agglutination (Figure 3.38d). They can be removed either by treatment of the test serum with a neuraminidase from *Vibrio cholerae*, or a mixture of trypsin and potassium periodate, or by adsorption with kaolin.

The HI test has several applications: (a) to detect antibodies in patients' sera, when a titre rising over a few days can confirm diagnosis; (b) to determine the identity of a virus type, subtype or strain using antibodies of known specificity; and (c) to study the antigenic relationship of the haemagglutinins of newly-isolated epidemic or pandemic strains to known human strains.

Replication

The events in replication of influenza viruses are outlined in Figure 3.39. They present some unusual features for an RNA virus, principally the requirement for a functioning cell nucleus; moreover, viral RNA is apparently transcribed and replicated, and the nucleocapsids assembled, in the nucleus rather than the cytoplasm.

Adsorption of virions to the host cell membrane occurs, as already noted, by the binding of viral haemagglutinin spikes to

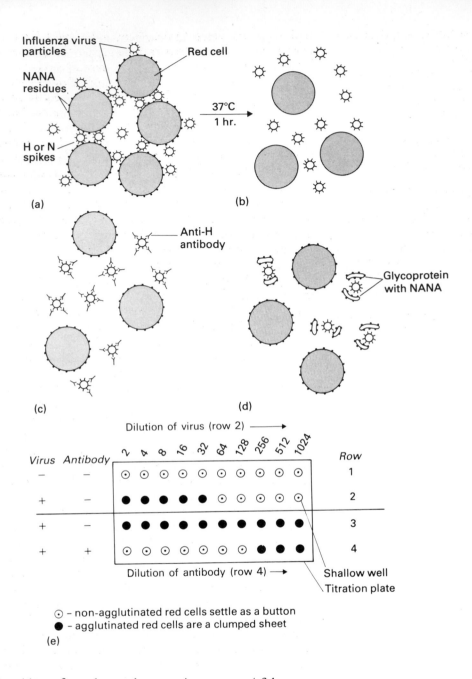

Influenza virus particles

NANA residues

H or N spikes

Red cell

(a)

37°C
1 hr.

(b)

Anti-H antibody

(c)

Glycoprotein with NANA

(d)

Dilution of virus (row 2) ⟶

Virus	Antibody	2	4	8	16	32	64	128	256	512	1024	Row
−	−	⊙	⊙	⊙	⊙	⊙	⊙	⊙	⊙	⊙	⊙	1
+	−	●	●	●	●	●	⊙	⊙	⊙	⊙	⊙	2
+	−	●	●	●	●	●	●	●	●	●	●	3
+	+	⊙	⊙	⊙	⊙	⊙	⊙	⊙	⊙	●	●	●	4

Dilution of antibody (row 4) ⟶

Shallow well
Titration plate

⊙ – non-agglutinated red cells settle as a button
● – agglutinated red cells are a clumped sheet

(e)

NANA residues of membrane glycoprotein receptors (cf. haemag-glutination). This initial stage can be prevented either by anti-haemagglutinin antibody or by treating the cell surface with *Vibrio cholerae* neuraminidase (also, therefore, called 'receptor destroying enzyme', RDE). The viral envelope fuses with the cell membrane, releasing the nucleocapsid segments into the cytoplasm; uncoating liberates the negative-strand viral RNA, which probably then enters the nucleus. Both transcription of viral RNA ($-$) to mRNA ($+$) and replication of viral RNA by copying of $+$ RNA templates are (probably) *intranuclear* events and require the virion RNA-dependent RNA-polymerase. What

Figure 3.38 Haemagglutination by influenza virus and its inhibition.
(a) Haemagglutination (at 4°C).
(b) Elution of virus at 37°C.
(c) Inhibition of haemagglutination by antiviral antibody.
(d) Inhibition by NANA-bearing glycoproteins.
(e) Appearance of wells in haemagglutination and haemagglutination-inhibition tests. *Rows 1 and 2*: haemagglutination test. In row 1, no virus is present, so no agglutination occurs; in row 2, virus is present with a titre of 32. *Rows 3 and 4*: haemagglutination-inhibition test. In row 3, no antibody is present, so there is no inhibition of agglutination, but in row 4 antiviral antibody is detected to a titre of 128.

is also unusual is that the *functioning of host cell DNA* is required during the phase of transcription; apart from RNA tumour viruses, no other RNA viruses are known to require host cell DNA and indeed will replicate in enucleated cells, which influenza viruses cannot. Replication is blocked by *actinomycin D*, which inhibits DNA transcription. This is not because the virus needs a host cell protein, but because it utilises cellular mRNA strands as sources of nucleotide 'caps' for its own RNA molecules; the caps, found at the 5′ termini, increase the rate of translation of messenger and act as primers for viral transcription.

The eight species of transcribed + RNA molecules which act as messengers are translated into their respective viral proteins in the cytoplasm on cell ribosomes. Recently, the fascinating discovery has been made that the genetic information for the M protein (segment 7) *includes* that of two other products, the M2 protein and M3 polypeptide; the mRNAs for M2 and M3 are obtained by 'splicing' the complete M message (p. 235). Similarly, the NS_2 information is part of the NS_1 gene (segment 8). This explains how ten (or eleven) proteins are generated from the eight RNA segments. Newly synthesized haemagglutinin, neuraminidase and M protein molecules move to the plasma membrane in preparation for budding, while the nucleocapsid protein re-enters the nucleus. During this time, other molecules of + RNA act as templates for replication of the viral − RNA; the latter then associates with the capsid protein to assemble the segments of helical nucleocapsid. It will be appreciated that there are two species of + RNA, namely mRNA and template RNA; they are differentiated by the fact that mRNA molecules are polyadenylated at the 3′ end and lack a sequence of 17 nucleotides at the 5′ end, which effectively prevents them from acting as replication templates (see also p.237).

The nucleocapsid segments migrate from the nucleus to the cell membrane where they accumulate at the sites prepared for budding as described on p. 238 and in Figure 3.13b. The means by which the eight different segments are brought together is not known. It is not totally efficient, but is remarkable for its accuracy, as experiments show in which a single cell is infected by *two* influenza strains of the same type but with distinguishable RNA segments. The progeny virions replicated in such co-infected cells never have two copies of the same gene, e.g. haemagglutinin genes from both virus types do not become associated in the same particle. Thus the 'packaging' process is strictly controlled. It is possible, however, for segments to be omitted, causing the appearance of defective viruses; the auto-interference phenomenon described on p.240 is an example of this. The final release of budding virus may require the participation of envelope neuraminidase to prevent adherence to membrane NANA. This is suggested by the finding that anti-neuraminidase antibodies inhibit release, although this may perhaps be due merely to antibody linking the virion, at the moment of its release, to neuraminidase molecules at the membrane, since monovalent Fab fragments of anti-neuraminidase are not inhibitory. Budding continues for several hours,

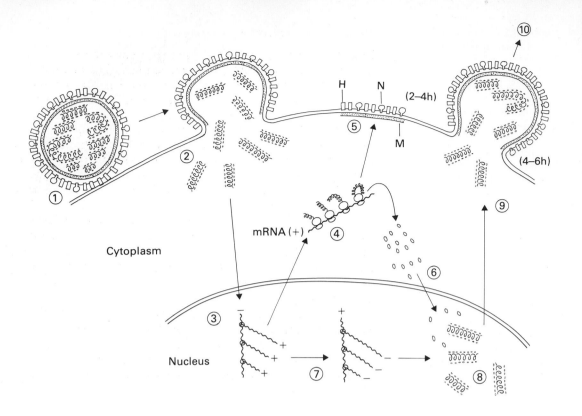

mRNA (+)

Cytoplasm

Nucleus

apparently without harming the cells, but eventually they die as a result of the infection.

The segmented nature of the influenza virus genome, with its eight pieces of RNA nucleocapsid, leads to a most important implication, namely: if two different influenza viruses coinfect a cell, it is possible for RNA segments of the two viruses to become mixed, giving rise to *hybrid virus* progeny with some properties of one virus strain and the remainder of the other. Thus, new genome combinations are produced and, if they are infective, new viral strains or even species (Figure 3.40). This possibility is called *genetic reassortment* or recombination, the former term being preferable as it more accurately describes the process of independent association of separate segments of two viral genomes. In the extreme case of two viruses which differ in all eight genes, reassortment could theoretically lead to 256 gene combinations, of which two would be the original parental types and the remainder hybrids. Reassortment only takes place between viruses of the same type and not, for example, between type A and B viruses. We will return to this phenomenon, which has important epidemiological implications, in more detail below.

In culture, influenza viruses can be grown in monkey kidney cells and this is used in diagnosis. The cytopathogenic effect is often minimal, but after 3–7 days the cells show haemadsorption, at 4°C, due to the presence of viral haemagglutinin in the plasma membrane.

Figure 3.39 Stages in the replication of influenza virus. Stages represented:
1. Adherence of virion to cell membrane.
2. Fusion of viral envelope with cell membrane and release of nucleocapsid segments into the cytoplasm.
3. RNA segments are transcribed into mRNAs in the nucleus.
4. mRNAs are translated into proteins in the cytoplasm on host cell ribosomes.
5. Haemagglutinin (H), neuraminidase (N) and matrix (M) proteins are incorporated into the cell membrane.
6. Capsid and other internal proteins enter the nucleus.
7. Replication of viral (−) RNA from + templates.
8. Assembly of nucleocapsid segments.
9. Segments migrate to budding sites.
10. Release of mature particles by budding.

Pathogenesis of influenza

Influenza is the most important viral respiratory disease of man and one which may have fatal complications. The infection is *localised* to the respiratory tract and viraemia is very unusual. Virus is acquired by droplet spread of infected respiratory secretions or by person-to-person contact, and settles on the mucous membrane lining the nose, pharynx, trachea and bronchi. In order to attach to epithelial cells, it must pass through the lining layer of mucus and in so doing comes into contact with secreted glycoproteins (mucoproteins) which, because they contain NANA, could inhibit binding. The role of viral neuraminidase may be to remove NANA residues from these molecules and thereby prevent them from acting as inhibitors; influenza virus is then free to attach to the cells of the respiratory epithelium. After a brief incubation period of 24–48 hours, the death of these cells and the resulting desquamation of the epithelium and inflammation lead to the familiar symptoms of influenza. They appear suddenly, with fever and chilliness, headache, sore throat and generalised muscular aches and pains. Respiratory symptoms then dominate the clinical picture, with coryza (discharge of nasal mucus) and a cough which may become severe. The more generalised symptoms are probably due to distribution in the bloodstream of cellular breakdown products.

Figure 3.40 Generation of hybrid viruses by genetic reassortment during replication of two influenzaviruses.

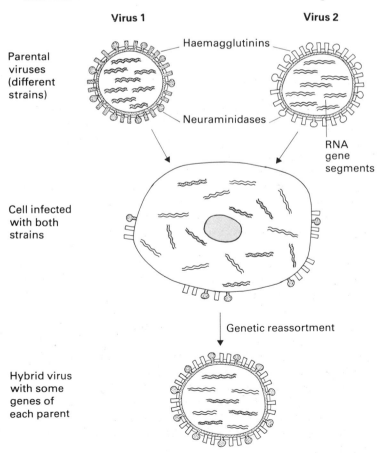

323

Fever and other acute symptoms usually subside in two or three days, but sometimes the infection spreads to the lower respiratory tract, causing viral pneumonia. This can be fatal, with haemorrhage and oedema in the lungs, which become hugely distended with exudate and blood. However, the chief complication of influenza is pneumonia due to *secondary bacterial infection* which, before the era of antibiotics, was often fatal and is still hazardous in the elderly or very young. The vast majority of the 20 million deaths which occurred during the 1918–1919 pandemic were due to bacterial pneumonia, including, rather surprisingly, millions of healthy young adults. The organisms chiefly responsible are *Staphylococcus aureus, Streptococcus pneumoniae, Strep. pyogenes* and *Haemophilus influenzae.* Influenza encourages bacterial invasion partly because of the destruction of ciliated epithelium and partly through inhibition of neutrophil phagocytosis. We may also note that, in contrast, influenza virus infections are also often mild or asymptomatic. Individuals infected subclinically may be important in disseminating the virus.

The immune response occurs both as antibody (local IgA plus serum antibodies) and cytotoxic T cells. Both locally secreted IgA and antibody in exudate will neutralise virus released from infected cells. While T cells are doubtless important in recovery, they also contribute to the severity of respiratory damage. Experimental influenza infection in mice is more severe in normal mice than in animals whose T cells have been depleted by anti-Thy-1 serum. Thus once again we see evidence of the dual effect of CMI, being essential for recovery but also playing a part in cell or tissue damage.

Immunity to reinfection by a given strain is provided by antibody, especially IgA in mucous secretion, and persists for 1–2 years; as it wanes, infection by variant strains, but probably not by the identical strain, becomes possible. Protection is principally due to *antihaemagglutinin* antibody; antineuraminidase does not prevent infection, but since it depresses the release of virus probably plays a part in recovery and immunity. The pre-eminent role of antihaemagglutinin is demonstrated by the following experiment using a hybrid virus, created by recombination between parental strains with antigenically distinct haemagglutinin and neuraminidase molecules (Figure 3.41). The hybrid carried the haemagglutinin of one parent virus and the neuraminidase of the other, and was used to immunise mice which were then experimentally infected with either of the parent viruses. As Figure 3.41 shows, the latter would encounter antibodies either to their haemagglutinin or their neuraminidase, but not to both. Only in mice with the appropriate anti-haemagglutinin could the infection be neutralised; antineuraminidase did not prevent infection although, as described above, it reduced the viral yield. Thus changes in haemagglutinin will be more critical to viral survival in the presence of limited antibody, accounting for the fact that antigenic variations (drift and shift, below) principally occur in this molecule.

An interesting phenomenon is that the antibodies made in

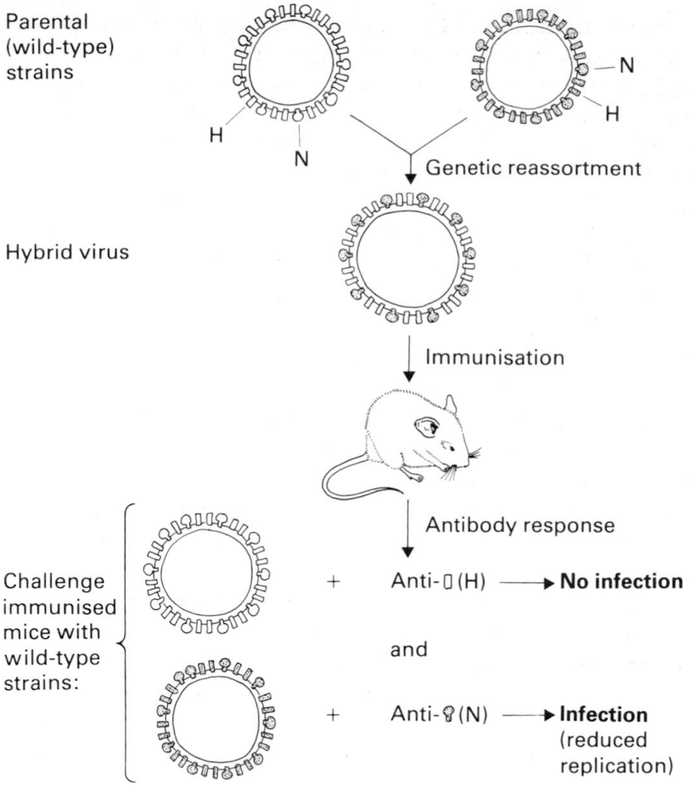

Figure 3.41 Protective role of antihaemagglutinin antibody in experimental influenza virus infection. (See text for explanation.)
H = haemagglutinin
N = neuraminidase

Parental (wild-type) strains

Genetic reassortment

Hybrid virus

Immunisation

Antibody response

Challenge immunised mice with wild-type strains:

+ Anti-□(H) ⟶ **No infection**

and

+ Anti-♀(N) ⟶ **Infection** (reduced replication)

response to subsequent infection with related, cross-reacting (but non-identical) strains or subtypes react better with the first virus ever encountered rather than with later ones. Thus, the anti-influenza antibodies made in childhood tend to be dominant throughout life, even though viral strains are gradually changing and even if new subtypes appear. This phenomenon goes by the colourful name of 'the doctrine of original antigenic sin' and is probably due to preferential restimulation of memory cells produced in the very first infection.

Where necessary, the diagnosis of influenza can be confirmed by inoculation of nasal or throat washings into ten-day-old embryonated chicken eggs; after 2–3 days the harvested virus can then be demonstrated by haemagglutination and identified precisely by HI with strain-specific antisera. Alternatively, the virus can be grown on monkey kidney cell monolayers and detected by haemadsorption.

Epidemiology of influenza and genetic variation of influenza viruses

The unusual epidemiology of influenza is the most fascinating aspect of this disease and one which is still not completely understood. The main facts are quite familiar: (a) in any given geographical region, epidemics occur every 2 to 4 years during the winter, with smaller outbreaks in intervening years; (b) at longer time intervals, 10 to 20 years or more, influenza spreads throughout the world, generally from the East, in the form of pandemics which in the past have been associated with a huge mortality; and (c) an individual who suffers the disease in one epidemic is not protected in the next, and during his life may have influenza several times. One has only to consider the epidemiology of other viral diseases described in this Section to appreciate the uniqueness of these phenomena. The reasons are several; some lie in the nature and mutability of the virus, while others have to do with individual and population immunity.

A fundamental factor is the *genetic variability* of influenza viruses. Each regular epidemic is caused by a viral strain which is slightly, but demonstrably, different from that of the one before. The nature of the virus, by which we mean the nature of its *surface antigens*, is in a continuous state of flux, in which variants arise and are regularly selected in the human population; this process of gradual minor change is called *antigenic drift*, a term introduced by Burnet. Such variation in haemagglutinin can be demonstrated by HI tests, which show that strains of the same subtype isolated over several years are progressively less able to react with a reference antihaemagglutinin serum (Figure 3.42). A more dramatic major change coincides with pandemics, or with epidemics on a larger than usual scale. In such outbreaks, the existing haemagglutinin, and sometimes also the neuraminidase, is replaced by a new haemagglutinin (or neuraminidase) molecule which is antigenically sharply different from its predecessor. This is *antigenic shift* and, as Figure 3.42 shows, has occurred more or less regularly over the 50 years since the virus was discovered, with four shifts since 1933. The difference in mechanism between antigenic drift and shift can be summed up by saying that drift is the result of point mutations in the existing haemagglutinin gene and single amino acid substitutions in the protein, followed by selection of the minor variants; shift, on the other hand, is the replacement of the haemagglutinin (or

Figure 3.42 Antigenic drift and antigenic shift in influenza type A virus. The axis shows the viral subtypes and the year of their appearance; the abscissa is an indication of antigenic similarity to the original 1933 isolate. (The appearance of HswN1 in 1976 is omitted.) The vertical lines are points of antigenic shift; the gradual downward slope between them is antigenic drift.
H = haemagglutinin
N = neuraminidase
(Simplified from original results.)

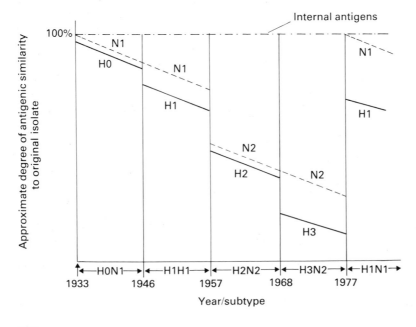

326

neuraminidase) gene by a different gene, so that multiple changes in amino acid sequence in the molecule and several antigenic changes appear suddenly. Thus, drift produces a new viral strain, but shift produces a new subtype (species). Note that while drift occurs with both influenza virus A and B types, only type A undergoes antigenic shift and gives rise to pandemics (type C virus is non-epidemic).

Viruses which cause epidemics require a susceptible host population, which can arise in different ways. It may, for example, be a particular age group, as in epidemics of chickenpox or poliomyelitis among children; alternatively, a hitherto unknown virus may be introduced into a virgin population, which occurred with measles in Greenland and myxomatosis in Australian rabbits; or an unprotected group may be removed to a centre of infection, as in the migration of Europeans to areas where yellow fever was endemic in the nineteenth century. For influenza, the fact that variants arising from antigenic drift or shift become established in epidemic fashion is due to a combination of the nature of the infection and the individual immune response to it. The infection is localised to the surface of the respiratory tract; viraemia is necessary neither for the production of disease, nor for transmission of the virus. The principal protection against reinfection is provided by secretory IgA present in the respiratory mucus. Because the IgA levels at the surface tend to be low, this protection is limited compared with that provided by circulating antibodies against viraemic infections, such as those of polioviruses or measles virus. In fact in many people, after a year or two, virus-specific IgA is still adequate to protect against the original infecting virus, but insufficient to deal with a cross-reactive variant, even though it be partially bound by the same antibody. This reflects the lower *affinity* of binding between the surface IgA and the variant virus, compared with that of the same antibody with the original inducing strain; and when the binding affinity is reduced, a larger amount of that antibody would have to be present to successfully neutralise variant particles. Thus, in effect the IgA level becomes a selective pressure which will allow infection by mutants differing antigenically from the previous strain to become established, and this 'immunoselection' is the basis of antigenic drift (Figure 3.43). That antibody can enable drift to

Figure 3.43 Selection of antigenic mutants as a function of population antibody.

New pandemic viral subtype H3 transcends barrier of antibody to unrelated previously prevalent virus H2 and readily infects the population (antigenic shift). When a critical percentage of the population has been infected with H3, survival of H3 is impeded, and antigenically changed mutant H3'- and later H3"—have survival advantage (minor antigenic variation or antigenic drift). (From Kilbourne, 1979)

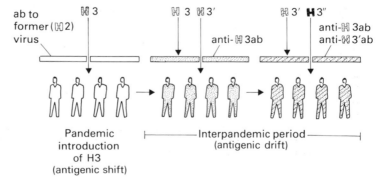

327

occur has been demonstrated experimentally by passing influenza virus repeatedly through mice, chick embryos or tissue cultures in the presence of antibody at a 'critical' concentration, i.e. just insufficient to neutralise the virus completely. After only a few passages, mutants had been selected by their growth advantage over the initial virus in the presence of antibody 'pressure'. The mutants can be shown to have significantly different haemagglutinins from the starting virus.

In short, the IgA in respiratory secretion is a crucial factor in determining the susceptibility of individuals to reinfection by new strains, and hence that of the population to epidemics. Two further factors which are relevant are the very short incubation period (1–2 days), which is more rapid than the secondary antibody response, so that the local IgA levels cannot be boosted to an effective concentration in time; and the large doses of virus which are present in droplets from infected individuals. The latter include many in whom infection is subclinical.

We have indicated above that both the major and minor antigenic changes in type A viruses occur predominantly in the haemagglutinin, to a lesser extent in the neuraminidase, and not at all in the other virion proteins, all of which are internal. The reason for this is not hard to find: selection by antibody can only act on those viral proteins which play a role in the infectivity of the virus and since antihaemagglutinins are the principal neutralising antibodies, it is the haemagglutinin mutants which are the most likely to be selected. Antibodies to neuraminidase decrease viral yield but do not inhibit infection altogether, so that variants with altered neuraminidase would be expected to be less frequently encountered, and this is the case. Internal proteins will obviously be irrelevant, since antibodies to them do not affect viral survival in any way. If we now refer to the composition of virus A subtypes affecting man, we see that there have been five distinct haemagglutinins in the five subtypes isolated since 1933 (H0, H1, H2, H3 and Hsw), but only two neuraminidases (N1 and N2). Indeed, the pandemic of Hong Kong influenza of 1968 was caused by the H3N2 (A3) subtype which differed from its predecessor, the Asian H2N2 (A2) subtype, only in its haemagglutinin; thus while alternations from N1 to N2 also occur regularly, and must contribute to the spread of new subtypes, they are evidently not essential to production of a new pandemic species.

A unique and unexplained facet of influenza virus variation is that *no two subtypes (or strains) exist together* in a population. Thus, when the Asian H2N2 subtype arrived in 1957, it displaced the existing H1N1 species, which in a rather short time was no longer detectable; similarly, in 1968, H2N2 was itself replaced by the Hong Kong virus. This phenomenon, which also applies to individual strains within the subtype, is unknown for other viruses, even those in which similar antigenic changes and selective pressures exist, such as the rhinoviruses (p. 290).

It seems that the number of possible major variants of the haemagglutinin and neuraminidase molecules is limited to those which have appeared since 1933. It is possible to trace back the

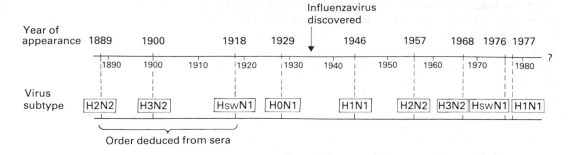

Figure 3.44 An influenza virus cycle? The order of appearance of influenza virus A subtypes since 1889.

type of virus prevalent before 1933 by studying the antibodies in stored sera of individuals who experienced influenza many years before; rather like a 'fossil record', the virus has left its mark in the serum of each person it infected. In this way, it has become evident that the subtypes which have been seen over the last 50 years have mostly been experienced by the world's population before, and there is a suggestion that they reappear in a particular sequence or cycle, as shown in Figure 3.44. Thus, the pandemic of 1889 was apparently caused by a type A virus with the same haemagglutinin and neuraminidase as Asian influenza of 1957, H2N2; it was followed in 1900 by a rather less dangerous pandemic, due to a 'new' subtype, H3N2, which turns out to be identical to the Hong Kong virus of 1968.

At this point one might begin to think that the order of appearance is in some way prescribed and that subtypes would recur at intervals of about 60 years; the possibility of a predictable recurrence would be highly welcome in production of vaccines for future use. Accordingly, it was anticipated that the 1918 subtype, which was apparently identical to swine influenza HswN1, would be the next to reappear, a possibility viewed with some trepidation as the 1918 pandemic was the most disastrous on record. Thus, when in 1976 a local outbreak of influenza at Fort Dix, New Jersey, with 200 infections and one death, was found to be due to the swine virus, there was an immediate rush in the USA to prepare vaccine for mass immunisation against a possible impending pandemic. President Nixon allocated $135 million for this programme and by December 1976 over 35 million individuals had received swine influenza vaccine. Contrary to the predictions, however, the swine virus did *not* become a pandemic or even an epidemic strain, and there was the misfortune that the vaccinations themselves produced some cases of paralytic illness (Guillain-Barré syndrome) in a small number of vaccinees. Another surprise was that in 1977 a different subtype reappeared, on a large epidemic scale, the so-called Russian influenza; this time it was the 1946 subtype, H1N1, apparently out of order, the 'cycle' having missed H0N1. This could not possibly have been predicted, which must make the notion of an orderly cycle rather suspect. The sequence is probably determined in some way by the susceptibility of the world population rather than by a subtle 'biological clock' of the virus's own natural history. At first, a periodicity of 60–70 years, i.e. an average life-expectancy, was indicated by the H2N2

(1889/1957) and H3N2 (1900/1968) species, but the rapid reappearance of H1N1 (1946/1977) suggests that 30 years is sufficient time in which to accumulate a susceptible population.

We have seen that gradual antigenic drift can be understood as mutation and selection, but what explanations can be found for the discontinuous changes in haemagglutinin and neuraminidase of antigenic shifts? Three theories have been advanced. (a) The viruses might persist in animal hosts and re-emerge when a suitably susceptible human population containing a critical number of non-immune individuals has come into existence. The genetic similarity between human and animal type A viruses would support this possibility. Such a situation, if it exists, raises the interesting question of how an apparently mutable virus could survive for many years and countless rounds of replication and re-emerge apparently unaltered. (b) The viruses responsible for shift may on some occasions be primarily animal viruses which have acquired the ability to infect man. This would account for the appearance of the subtype with swine virus characteristics in 1918 and 1976. (c) The model which has received most attention is that 'new' viruses can be generated by genetic recombination during viral replication. This requires the simultaneous presence in the same cell of two viruses of different subtypes, e.g. an animal type A virus and a human type A virus. Under these conditions, hybrid viruses with various combinations of parental genes can be produced as described on page 322. Let us imagine that a human A virus replicates in the same cell as an animal A virus; hybrids may be produced in which the human virus haemagglutinin and/or neuraminidase gene has been replaced by that of the animal virus (cf. Figure 3.40). Thus, in a single step, a virus could be produced with the genes to enable it to multiply in human cells, but with new (i.e. animal) surface molecules enabling it to resist existing antibodies in the human population. Hybrid strains of this nature have been produced experimentally by coinfection of animals with two independent type A species and it is envisaged that a rare event of this sort in man, birds, pigs or other species susceptible to infection could be the point of creation of new pandemic subtypes. However, it will be difficult, if not impossible, to prove that this is responsible for new species of human type A viruses, although the hypothesis is attractive.

Vaccination

The changing antigenic nature of influenza viruses creates a serious problem in the production of vaccines, namely the absolute need to have available the current strains in vaccine form, as well as making regular revaccination necessary. The protection afforded by immunisation with one strain on exposure to a subsequent strain is only partial, and to a new subtype arising by antigenic shift is negligible. Emerging strains are therefore closely monitored throughout the world by surveillance laboratories established by the World Health Organisation. Because of the time it would take to develop avirulent variants of each new strain, *inactivated virus vaccines* have been the most widely used.

330

The viruses are grown in embryonated chicken eggs, isolated from the allantoic fluid by high speed centrifugation and inactivated with formaldehyde. It is usual to make a concentrated mixture of the current A and B type strains and to administer the vaccine subcutaneously or intramuscularly.

The inactivated vaccines have a number of drawbacks. Firstly, their effectiveness is quite variable; different studies have suggested that protection of a population can vary from 70% at best to nil at worst. In part, this is because subcutaneous immunisation predominantly stimulates *circulating* antibody, while prevention of the disease is most likely to be mediated by *local* immunity, viz. secreted IgA. A local respiratory route of administration, such as a nasal spray, would be advantageous, but its efficacy has not yet been fully evaluated with inactivated vaccines. Secondly, immunity is relatively short-lived and even against the immunising strain wanes after a few months, so that annual boosters are necessary. It can be improved by adjuvants, such as light mineral oil or peanut oil, but these are not recommended for use in man. The short incubation period and large infecting dose make it especially important to maintain as high an antibody level as possible. Thirdly, there may also be side-effects of vaccination, including a pyrogenic reaction commonly encountered in children, hypersensitivity reactions to egg proteins contaminating the preparation, and (though not unique to influenza vaccination) the rare development of a serious neurological disease, the Guillan-Barré syndrome, which was associated with the use of killed swine influenza vaccine in 1976 (354 cases and 28 deaths out of 35 million vaccinees).

Subunit vaccines, consisting of the semipurified haemagglutinin and neuraminidase proteins rather than whole viruses, are being widely used with success. They are also administered subcutaneously, but a larger specific dose of these antigens can be given and the toxic side-reactions are minimised.

The problem with attenuated influenza viruses has been one of preparing and testing avirulent forms of new strains and subtypes quickly enough to prevent epidemics. One method of attenuation is to make a *temperature sensitive (ts) mutant* (p. 240) by passaging the virus at low temperatures, e.g. 33°C instead of 37°C. The *ts* strains are unable to replicate at 37°C or above and therefore become restricted to the uppermost (nasal) regions of the respiratory tract, where the disease is much milder. The local infection, administered by nasal spray, stimulates IgA in respiratory secretions. Such mutants are widely used in the USSR and elsewhere. An important advance which can accelerate production of a *ts* mutant from a newly isolated strain or species makes use of *genetic recombination*. Since the vaccine virus must combine the haemagglutinin, and perhaps the neuraminidase, of the new virus strain with the *ts* characteristic of the avirulent virus, it is possible to make a hybrid by coinfecting an embryo or culture with both the new strain and an established *ts* mutant. As previously described, reassortment of genes of the two viruses in single cells leads to production of hybrid viruses (Figure 3.40), some of which will have the desired combination of properties. It seems likely that in time there will be a switch over to the use of living attenuated viruses engineered by these methods. The recombination approach is also useful in production of virus for inactivated vaccines, since it is possible to build into a newly isolated strain the ability to grow more rapidly in chick embryos (a *high yield* characteristic) and hence greatly improve the speed with which large quantities of vaccine can be made available. This is particularly important with strains which do not grow well under laboratory conditions and was used to hasten the production of the HswN1 virus for mass vaccination in the United States in 1976. Finally, the fact that there is a limited number of influenza virus subtypes in man enables some advance preparation of vaccine for the major species to be made, even if the order of their appearance is not as predictable as it once seemed.

We may also note the prophylactic use of *amantadine* (adamantanamine), an agent which inhibits an early event in influenza replication, probably uncoating. During epidemics it can be given to individuals at special risk, such as non-vaccinated family members or other close contacts of the patient, and ideally to all non-vaccinated persons pending immunisation.

PARAMYXOVIRIDAE

The paramyxoviruses resemble the orthomyxoviruses in some important properties, such as binding to cell surface glycoproteins and agglutinating red cells, the possession (by some) of neuraminidase, and infectivity for the respiratory tract. They are also negative-strand RNA viruses with a helical nucleocapsid and lipid envelope. On the other hand, there are significant differences in structure, replication and cellular effects which are summarised in Table 3.11. Two notable characteristics of their interactions with cells which are not found in orthomyxoviruses are: (a) the ability to cause *cell fusion*, giving rise to typical multinucleate 'giant cells' or syncytia *in vivo* and *in vitro*, a property utilised in laboratory studies on cell hybrids; and (b) the establishment of persistent infections in culture, in which infected cells survive for long periods while virus is continuously replicated (carrier cultures).

These viruses particularly affect children. *Parainfluenza viruses* and *respiratory syncytial virus* are major causes of lower respiratory tract disease, while *measles* and *mumps* are among the commonest childhood infections. There are also important animal diseases, such as *Newcastle disease* of birds, especially chickens, *canine distemper* and *rinderpest* of cattle.

Classification

The family is divided into three genera which can be distinguished by the presence or absence of surface haemagglutinin and neuraminidase (Table 3.12). The genus *Paramyxovirus* is the one most similar to the influenza viruses in possessing both haemagglutinin and neuraminidase with NANA specificity; its

332

Table 3.11. Comparison of Orthomyxoviridae and Paramyxoviridae.

	Orthomyxoviridae	Paramyxoviridae
Major viruses	Influenza	Parainfluenza, mumps, measles, respiratory syncytial virus, Newcastle disease
Nucleic acid	Negative single-stranded RNA; 7–8 segments; helical nucleocapsid	Negative single-stranded RNA; 1 molecule; helical nucleocapsid
Envelope	+	+
Particle size	80–100 nm	120–250 nm
Diameter of capsid	9 nm	18 nm
Haemagglutinin	+	+[a]
Neuraminidase	+	+[b]
Haemolysis	−	+[a]
Cell fusion	−	+
Replication in enucleated cells	−	+
Actinomycin D inhibits replication	+	−
Genetic recombination	Common	Rare
Prominent cytoplasmic inclusions	−	+
Syncytia	−	+
Persistent infection *in vitro*	−	+
Antigenic drift/shift	Frequent variations	Stable

a: not respiratory syncytial virus
b: not measles or respiratory syncytial virus

species behave in much the same way in haemagglutination except that at 37°C they cause *haemolysis*. This group includes the parainfluenza and mumps viruses. *Morbilliviruses*—the measles, canine distemper and rinderpest group—possess a haemagglutinin for monkey red cells, but lack a neuraminidase. Moreover, the specificity of their haemagglutinin is evidently not for NANA, as the red cell receptors are not destroyed by *Vibrio cholerae* neuraminidase. They also cause haemolysis. The *Pneumovirus* genus is quite distinctive in its lack both of haemagglutinin and neuraminidase; it is also non-haemolytic. The

Table 3.12 Properties of Paramyxoviridae.

Genus	Species	HA*	Haemolysis	NA*	Serotypes
Paramyxovirus	Parainfluenza virus	+	+	+	4
	Mumps virus	+	+	+	1
Morbillivirus	Measles virus	+	+	−	1
Pneumovirus	Respiratory syncytial virus	−	−	−	1

* HA: haemagglutinin; NA: neuraminidase.

representative species is respiratory syncytial virus. All paramyxoviruses cause cell fusion.

Structure, etc. (Figures 3.3b, 3.45a)

The typical paramyxovirus particle is an irregular shape, often roughly square under the electron microscope, with filamentous forms also common. The size of the basic particle is about twice that of an influenza virus. The outer envelope, which seems loose-fitting and is easily ruptured, encloses a helical nucleocapsid, less tightly and regularly packed than that of influenza viruses (Figure 3.3b). The nucleocapsid consists of a continuous thread of negative single-stranded RNA enclosed by its capsomeres in typical helical arrangement. An RNA polymerase is associated with the capsid. The envelope is the familiar lipid bilayer with projecting spikes; these are of two types which cannot be distinguished morphologically. One spike is the haemagglutinin, and where neuraminidase is present it is carried on the *same* (HN) spike. In fact, there seems to be only one HN protein to account for both haemagglutinin and neuraminidase activities. The other projection is the F glycoprotein, which is responsible for lysis of red cells and fusion of other cells. A matrix (M) protein is associated with the inside of the lipid bilayer and maintains its form and integrity. The principal antigens of most paramyxoviruses are the haemagglutinin (H) or haemagglutinin-neuraminidase (HN) glycoproteins; the haemolysis/fusion (F) glycoprotein and the nucleocapsid protein (NP).

The fragility of the envelope makes paramyxoviruses easily destroyed by storage or freezing and thawing; partially disrupted forms are often seen in the electron microscope (Figure 3.3b). The viruses are rapidly inactivated by organic solvents (such as ether), detergents or surface-acting agents, all of which dissolve the envelope and liberate the nucleocapsid. Respiratory syncytial virus is particularly fragile and difficult to preserve.

Replication and cellular infection

The pattern of replication of all paramyxoviruses is essentially the same and is typical of class V, negative-strand RNA viruses. Adherence to cells is via the reaction of the HN spike (or

Figure 3.45 Paramyxoviruses. (a) Diagrammatic section. (b) Cytopathogenic effect of measles virus. (i) Multinucleate giant cell formed after infection of human kidney cells in culture. Each nucleus has a prominent inclusion body surrounded by a pale rim. (From Enders *et al* (1959) *New Engl. J. Med.*, **261**, 875) (ii) Electron micrograph of section through an intranuclear inclusion body, showing that it is an aggregate of 'viral tubules' (helical nucleocapsids); ×70,000. (From Nakai *et al* (1969) *Virology*, **38**, 50)

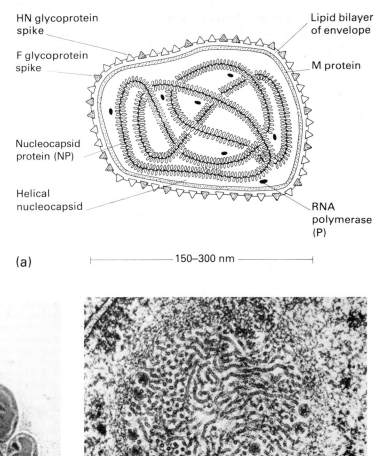

HN glycoprotein spike

F glycoprotein spike

Nucleocapsid protein (NP)

Helical nucleocapsid

Lipid bilayer of envelope

M protein

RNA polymerase (P)

(a)

150–300 nm

(b) (i)

(ii)

haemagglutinin in the case of measles) with a membrane receptor; penetration seems to require the F glycoprotein, as viruses with an inactive F molecule are non-infectious (the F glycoprotein is only active after cleavage from a larger precursor by a cellular enzyme during viral maturation). Replication is cytoplasmic, does not require a functioning cell nucleus, will occur in enucleated cells and is not inhibited by actinomycin D (cf. influenza viruses). The viral RNA-dependent RNA-polymerase transcribes the − viral RNA strand into large + strands, which are made in considerable excess and which are copies (transcripts) of the entire viral genome. Some of these are then cleaved into seven or eight separate molecular species of mRNA, each of which is translated into a single viral protein. Other complete + strands act as the templates for replication of − strands of virion RNA (Figure 3.11b). As the envelope proteins are translated they migrate to the plasma membrane where the haemagglutinin-neuraminidase and fusion proteins form their spikes, and the matrix protein becomes associated with the eventual budding areas. The capsomere protein monomers (a single molecular species) and viral RNA assemble into the helical nucleocapsids; relatively few of these mature into virions, the remainder accumulating in the cell as prominent eosinophilic *inclusion bodies* (Figure 3.45b, c). These are cytoplasmic and sometimes also nuclear (e.g. measles). Those particles which do mature complete the process at the cell membrane, where budding occurs. The cell remains intact during viral release.

Cytopathic changes develop slowly in culture and infected cells are most readily detected by haemadsorption with guinea-pig or other appropriate red cells. The most characteristic CPE is cell fusion (Figure 3.45b and below); this leads to formation of large multinucleated cells (syncytia) containing cytoplasmic or nuclear inclusion bodies. Although some cells die, paramyxoviruses readily establish carrier cultures in which most cells remain viable and continue to multiply for some time even though practically all are infected. Such persistent infections *in vitro* may be a relevant model for viral persistence *in vivo*, of which the most striking instance is subacute sclerosing panencephalitis, a late sequel of measles in which the virus spreads slowly through brain cells years after recovery from the original infection. There is also the possibility that long-term paramyxovirus infections are involved in multiple sclerosis (measles, p. 882), though this now seems unlikely, and systemic lupus erythematosus (parainfluenza virus, p.206).

Cell fusion

We have noted that cell fusion is a property common to all paramyxoviruses. Both fusion and haemolysis depend on the F glycoprotein spike in the viral envelope. The precise role of the F protein is not elucidated, but it presumably interacts in some way with membrane lipids. When virus is bound to the surface of a red cell by its haemagglutinin, the interaction between F and the membrane leads to lysis; on the other hand, when membranes of two juxtaposed cells are physically linked by a paramyxovirus, cell fusion results instead. The virus most widely used in studies of this phenomenon is *Sendai virus*, a murine parainfluenza virus strain (named after the Japanese city in which it was discovered). Sendai virus has been of particular usefulness in making *cell hybrids*, by fusion of cells of different tissue or species origin. Figure 3.46, for example, shows the result of fusing a human tumour cell (HeLa) with a chicken red cell; the hybrid cell shown is a *heterokaryon*, i.e. contains more than one type of nucleus. Often the nuclei eventually fuse to form a mononuclear, polyploid cell. Cell hybrids have found a wide variety of applications in genetics, tumour biology, immunology, developmental biology, etc. For example, since 1971 inter-species hybrids have been invaluable in mapping human chromosomes. This is possible through 'chromosome segregation', the fact that a hybrid between, say, a human and a mouse cell preferentially loses human chromosomes as it grows. It is possible to correlate the

336

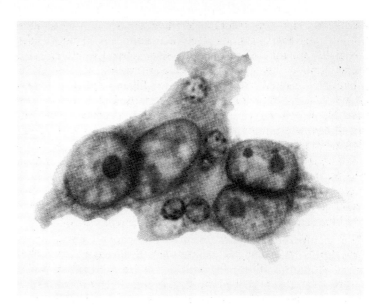

Figure 3.46 Cell fusion with Sendai virus.

This multinucleate cell, a heterokaryon (i.e. with different types of nuclei) was formed by fusing HeLa cells (large nuclei) with chicken nucleated erythrocytes (small nuclei). (From Bolund, Ringertz & Harris, (1969), *J. Cell Sci.*, **4**, 71.)

properties of the cell—presence or absence of certain human proteins, enzymes, etc.—with the retention or loss of certain specific chromosomes and hence to assign the genes coding for those proteins to their correct chromosomes, leading eventually to a map of the human genome. This technique is called *somatic cell genetics* as it achieves by a cellular method what would otherwise be possible only through analysis of inheritance, if at all. Other applications of cell hybrids are in making monoclonal antibodies (p. 97), in the analysis of cancer cells (p. 730) and in studies of genetic disease (p. 774). In some, Sendai virus has been replaced by chemical fusion agents such as polyethylene glycol.

Parainfluenza viruses

There are four serologically distinct types of parainfluenza viruses (types 1–4), the main distinguishing antigens being the HN and F envelope proteins and the internal NP protein. All four types cause infections of the respiratory tract resembling the common cold or influenza. In adults they tend to be mild and confined to the upper respiratory tract; they are more severe in young children, however, in whom they invade the lower respiratory tract also. Of all lower respiratory tract infections in children, 20% are due to parainfluenza viruses, with outbreaks in nurseries, schools and paediatric wards of hospitals. The most dangerous manifestation is *acute laryngotracheobronchitis* or *croup*, which occurs in children infected with type 1 or type 2 viruses. Respiratory obstruction may be life-threatening in this condition and require tracheotomy. Type 3 viruses also spread to the lungs, giving rise to bronchitis or bronchopneumonia, but these are rarely, if ever, fatal.

Like influenza, the viruses remain localised and there is no viraemia. Immunity is again dependent principally on anti-haemagglutinin IgA and is not long-lasting; thus reinfection with the same virus type in children and adults is not uncommon, but antigenic changes do not seem to occur or be necessary for reinfection. Protection does improve with repeated exposure, which is probably why adults experience much milder disease than children. Parainfluenza virus infections tend, unlike influenza, to occur in all seasons, with epidemics of type 1 more likely in the autumn and of type 3 in the summer.

In culture, the viruses often establish persistent non-lytic infections, as well as causing formation of syncytia through cell fusion. The multinucleate cells have eosinophilic inclusion bodies. Sendai virus, the archetypal fusion agent, is a murine parainfluenza virus corresponding to type 1.

Mumps

The mumps virus closely resembles the parainfluenza viruses, both structurally and antigenically, with envelope HN and F antigens and the ability to agglutinate and lyse red cells, as well as to cause cell fusion. There is only one antigenic type and man is its only natural host. Mumps is one of the major childhood diseases; unlike chickenpox and measles it is not exanthematous, its most characteristic symptom being *parotitis* (inflammation of the parotid gland). It is easily recognised by the intense oedematous swelling below and in front of the ears, accompanied by pain on touch, chewing or swallowing; fever and headache are also present. It is less infectious than chickenpox or measles, and while most children in the 5–10 year age group will contract the disease, many do not. This is important, because infection in adolescent or adult life has the severe consequence of *orchitis* in males, following viral infection of the testis; not only is this very painful, but it may lead to testicular atrophy, though not often to sterility as it is usually unilateral. In post-pubertal females the ovaries may be involved, with *oöphoritis*.

The pathogenesis of mumps is outlined in Figure 3.47. The virus is present in patients' saliva and respiratory secretions, and is either acquired from salivary contamination of objects or in droplets. It was previously thought to enter the parotid gland directly via Stensen's duct, but the evidence now makes it probable that the virus replicates first in the pharynx and upper respiratory tract, followed by the cervical lymph nodes, before establishing an initial (primary) viraemia; thus the salivary glands are infected via the bloodstream. There is a lengthy incubation period and it may take up to 24 days for the parotids to become swollen; usually the swelling is bilateral, but sometimes only one gland is infected. The sublingual and submaxillary glands may also be involved. Parotitis is accompanied by fever. In uncomplicated mumps, the swelling subsides and disappears in a matter of days. However, viraemic spread to several other organs occurs and thus leads to complications, the commonest of which is seen in the CNS, as *aseptic meningitis* or *meningoencephalitis*, 4–7 days after salivary swelling. This is presaged by headache, one of the major symptoms of mumps. Mumps is probably the commonest single cause of meningitis. Fortunately CNS involvement is less severe than in measles and permanent disability unusual, though

Figure 3.47 Pathogenesis of mumps.
(Orchitis and oöphoritis are complications of adolescent or adult patients only.)

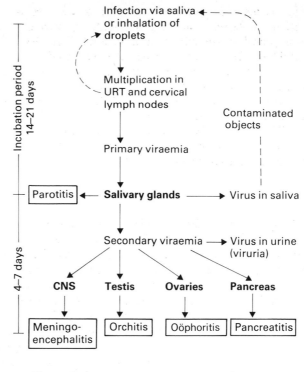

unilateral deafness or facial paralysis can occur. The involvement of the testes or ovaries in post-pubertal patients has been mentioned. Sometimes the pancreas is also infected, with nausea, vomiting and abdominal pain, but no permanent ill-effects; and several other organs (heart, prostate, kidney, joints, lacrymal glands) are also occasionally inflamed. During the disease, virus is present in urine as well as in blood and saliva.

Mumps is endemic in heavily populated areas throughout the world. In addition to sporadic cases, there are epidemics in the late winter and spring, where susceptible individuals are crowded together. Twenty to thirty per cent of infections remain sub-clinical, which is more than in other childhood infections. An effective live vaccine is available, an attenuated strain grown in chick embryos, and vaccination is now a routine procedure for children and infants over 15 months. The occurrence of orchitis in young men warrants immunisation of susceptible groups such as military recruits. As viraemia is involved in its pathogenesis, injection of the vaccine is an effective route of administration; alternatively it can be sprayed into the mouth. Delayed hypersensitivity to the virus develops during infection and a skin test can be performed with inactivated virus; although it indicates immunity it is not considered reliable in diagnosis. Immunity is permanent, through antibodies to the haemagglutinin-neuraminidase.

Before the introduction of routine measles vaccination in the 1960's, this was perhaps the most familiar of the major diseases of childhood, virtually all children being infected before the age of ten. It is one of the most contagious of all diseases, so much so that 98% of the population would have experienced the infection by adulthood, and most as children. The virus itself resembles the other paramyxoviruses, but although it agglutinates monkey and guinea-pig red cells, it does not elute from them at 37°C and does not possess a neuraminidase; as noted above, the specificity of measles haemagglutinin differs from the other viruses of the family in not being directed towards neuraminic acid. Cell fusion is the characteristic cytopathogenic effect, and very large multinucleate cells are found in measles-infected tissues and nasal secretions, with *intranuclear* as well as cytoplasmic eosinophilic inclusion bodies (Warthin-Finkeldy giant cells, Figure 3.45b). The inclusion bodies are arrays of nucleocapsids (Figure 3.45c). There is only one antigenic type and humans and monkeys are the only natural hosts.

In the vast majority of children in Europe and the USA measles is a benign condition, with fever, respiratory symptoms and conjunctivitis, culminating in the generalised skin rash, then complete recovery. However, there are two particular complications which lent urgency to the development of a vaccine. The first is *encephalomyelitis*, which affects about one in every 1000 patients and can lead to serious CNS impairment and death; the other is a much later sequel called *subacute sclerosing panencephalitis* (SSPE) which develops a few years after recovery from measles. SSPE is due to a chronic infection of brain cells with measles virus and a gradual destruction of the cerebral cortex. Vaccination has been successful in eliminating measles encephalomyelitis, and the indications are that it has very much reduced the incidence of SSPE. The latter is classified as a 'slow virus' disease (p. 367).

Epidemiology. In Western urban communities, measles used to occur in winter and spring epidemics every 2–3 years in young children (peak incidence at 5–7 years of age), with smaller outbreaks in the intervening years. Infants are protected by maternal (transplacental) antibodies for the first year and are susceptible thereafter. In parts of Africa and South America, it is still an important cause of infant mortality, primarily because of complicating secondary bacterial infection of the lung (bronchopneumonia), coupled with the effects of malnutrition. In some isolated communities, such as those on islands, the virus was unknown and its introduction led to a very severe epidemic throughout the population; a catastrophic outbreak of this nature occurred in Greenland in 1951, while in Fiji in 1875 the 'new' disease caused the death of 20–25% of the entire population. This was partly due to the fact that measles is more severe in adults.

Pathogenesis. The disease begins with the transmission of virus in infected droplets to the respiratory tract and conjunctiva, the main source being children with catarrhal symptoms before the appearance of the rash. It follows a course similar to that of other generalised exanthemas such as chickenpox and smallpox (Figure 3.48). Early replication takes place in the upper respiratory tract, local lymph nodes and conjunctiva, followed by a brief primary viraemia which distributes virus to reticulo-endothelial cells in different organs, including the liver, spleen and lymph nodes, etc. Warthin-Finkeldy giant cells can be found in the liver, spleen, tonsils, Peyer's patches, appendix, lymph nodes and lungs; their presence in nasal secretions is diagnostic. The virus multiplies in macrophages and lymphocytes, which has some significant effects, such as: assisting the dissemination of virus in the body; production of a leukopenia typical of the prodromal phase; chromosomal aberrations in a high proportion of leucocytes, which have been suggested as preliminary to leukaemia; and a temporary suppression of cell-mediated immune reactions with loss of tuberculin sensitivity and exacerbation of clinical tuberculosis (although it does not seem to interfere with development of CMI to measles virus itself).

After an incubation period of 9–12 days, the prodromal (pre-rash) symptoms appear, notably coryza, hacking cough, conjunctivitis and fever. A diagnostic sign is the appearance of *Koplik's spots* on the mucous membrane on the inside of the cheek, tiny white specks surrounded by an areola of inflammation; they contain multinucleate giant cells with viral nucleocapsids. At this stage, virus is present in respiratory secretions and, since the rash is not yet evident, this early shedding promotes the rapid spread of infection. A more persistent viraemia then distributes the virus to the skin, where the typical 'morbilliform' *maculopapular rash* appears three days after the prodromal syndrome, spreading from the face and neck to the trunk and extremities. The rash is accompanied by a continuation of the respiratory and other symptoms described, with swelling around the eyes (periorbital oedema), photophobia and high fever. In the skin, viral antigens in cell membranes become the target of immune attack by cytotoxic and other T cells, leading to inflammation and the appearance of the rash. In Section 2 (p.150) the immunological aspects of measles were discussed and it was pointed out that immunodeficient children, who cannot make a CMI (T cell) response, do not experience the rash. The disease in such rare children is often fatal, due to a *'giant-cell pneumonia'*.

After three days, the rash and accompanying symptoms rapidly disappear. *Secondary bacterial infection* is common, however, with otitis media (inflammation of the middle ear) and pneumonia, paricularly in infants. *Encephalomyelitis* is the most severe complication in Western countries and occurs a few days after the onset of the skin rash. The virus does not seem to be present in the brain, which shows perivascular haemorrhage and infiltration by lymphocytes; demyelination is seen later in the brain and spinal cord. The histological picture resembles that of experimental allergic encephalitis, a reaction induced by injection

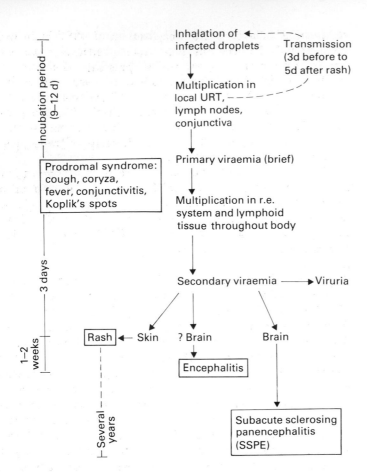

Figure 3.48 Pathogenesis of measles.

URT = upper respiratory tract

Inhalation of infected droplets

Transmission (3d before to 5d after rash)

Multiplication in local URT, lymph nodes, conjunctiva

Primary viraemia (brief)

Prodromal syndrome: cough, coryza, fever, conjunctivitis, Koplik's spots

Multiplication in r.e. system and lymphoid tissue throughout body

Secondary viraemia ⟶ Viruria

Rash ← Skin   ? Brain   Brain

Encephalitis

Subacute sclerosing panencephalitis (SSPE)

Incubation period (9–12 d)

3 days

1–2 weeks

Several years

of brain tissue in animals (p. 882), and this, together with the lack of evidence for viral infection in the CNS, has been taken to indicate an autoimmune process. In any event, it does seem to be a T cell response against antigens in the brain, either viral or 'self'. Mortality of measles encephalomyelitis is about 10%, with permanent mental or physical disability in a large proportion of survivors.

Subacute sclerosing panencephalitis. In contrast with encephalomyelitis, SSPE does not seem to be due to an allergic or autoimmune response, but rather to the localisation of virus in the brain and its very gradual spread. It is a rare, chronic, progressive illness seen in children and young adolescents (usually boys from country areas) a few years after measles infection, with deterioration of intellectual faculties, convulsions and motor abnormalities; it is generally fatal after 6–12 months. There is perivascular infiltration of lymphocytes and plasma cells, and demyelination of the white matter of the cerebral cortex. The association with measles was established by, *inter alia*: the presence of measles antibodies in the CSF; measles antigens in brain lesions, as demonstrated by immunofluorescent staining; cytoplasmic and intranuclear inclusion bodies, containing structures identical to measles nucleocapsids, in brain cells; and the isolation of live virus by cocultivation of SSPE brain with indicator cells (i.e. the virus in the brain is genetically complete, but its replication is apparently suppressed). Moreover, the incidence of SSPE in children who have received measles virus vaccine is only about 15% of that in children contracting the natural infection. The evident lack of an effective T cell response to measles virus in SSPE brains is puzzling, the more so since plasma cells do infiltrate the brain and presumably produce anti-measles antibody, though to no avail.

Because of its long latency and inexorable spread through the brain, culminating in death, SSPE is included in a group of diseases called *slow virus infections* which share these characteristics; they are described further on p. 366. The evidence linking measles with another chronic CNS disease, multiple sclerosis, is discussed on p. 882.

Vaccination. Because of the possibility of serious consequences of measles infection, development of a vaccine was a high priority after isolation of the virus in culture by Enders in 1953. Both formalin-inactivated and attenuated live virus vaccines were developed (cf. poliomyelitis). The former proved unsuitable on several grounds, notably the brevity of the period of protection and the finding that subsequent natural infection was sometimes abnormally severe (see also respiratory syncytial virus for a similar phenomenon, below. The first live vaccine (Enders's Edmonston strain) was insufficiently attenuated and produced a significant disease, with rash and fever, in most recipients, so that antimeasles antibody had to be administered simultaneously to diminish the reaction. The strains now used are more attenuated and produce a very mild, usually subclinical infection, with fever and rash in only about 10% of vaccinees. Most importantly, there are no CNS complications and the living vaccine is extremely effective, inducing neutralising antibodies at a similar level to natural infection. The vaccine strain does not spread to susceptible contacts.

The incidence of measles in Western Europe and the USA has been dramatically reduced and epidemics have disappeared since vaccination for all children was introduced in the 1960's. In the USA, for example, the incidence fell from about half a million annual cases before vaccination to 35,000 in 1976 (this residual number being to a large extent in children who, due to parental apathy or ignorance, were not vaccinated). It is estimated that between 1963 and 1972, 24 million cases of measles were prevented by vaccination, 2,000–3,000 lives saved and 8,000 cases of serious neurological complications avoided. The possibility that the vaccine might induce SSPE was of great concern. It now seems that there is a slight risk, but significantly less than that following natural infection (about one in 10^6 vaccinees as against about seven in 10^6 natural measles cases). Measles virus is often given in combination with other attenuated virus vaccines, notably mumps and rubella, at about 15 months of age, i.e. soon after the disappearance of maternal antibodies. Live vaccine cannot be given to children with immunodeficiency, either congenital or acquired by therapeutic measures; they must rely on passive immunity with antimeasles globulin for protection. Since there is no animal reservoir, measles is another infection for which both the virus and the disease could be eliminated by vaccination (cf. smallpox and poliomyelitis).

Respiratory syncytial virus (RSV)

Although this virus resembles the other paramyxoviruses in structure and behaviour, it is in several ways distinct. For example, it is the only one to lack both haemagglutinin and neuraminidase; while it fuses cells in culture, they do not show haemadsorption. The envelope does, however, have typical surface spikes (though the specificity of its receptors is unknown). It is also the only myxovirus which cannot be grown in embryonated eggs. Its chief importance is as the agent of severe and life-threatening lower respiratory tract disease in infants and children, particularly serious under the age of six months. In adults, infection is milder and confined to the upper respiratory tract (a common cold), though it is also a significant cause of viral bronchopneumonia and induces secondary bacterial pneumonia and exacerbations of existing chronic bronchitis. Seventy per cent of children over five years and 95% of adults have antibodies, indicating the ubiquity of infection.

Respiratory syncytial virus is probably the most important cause of serious lower respiratory tract infection in infants, with sharp annual epidemics in spring and winter. Sudden infant death (cot death), especially with signs of respiratory disease, can sometimes be attributed to the virus. The common symptoms are dyspnoea, wheezing and cough, with *bronchiolitis* and *bronchopneumonia* as prominent manifestations. There is good reason to implicate *antibody-mediated hypersensitivity* in the special severity in babies under six months. Thus, during this period, the infant still has circulating maternal IgG antibodies, but lacks the important local protection of IgA. The clue that IgG could contribute to the disease came from experience with a formalin-inactivated vaccine given to newborns; a good serum antibody response was induced, but during subsequent epidemics the respiratory disease was unexpectedly more severe in vaccinees than in normal unvaccinated babies. It seems likely that local formation of IgG-virus complexes in the lung exacerbates the inflammation, a Type III reaction akin to allergic pulmonary conditions such as 'Farmer's lung' (p.163). Needless to say, this type of killed vaccine, given by parenteral inoculation, was withdrawn. There is still a need for a vaccine and attenuated strains are being developed; the most promising are temperature-sensitive mutants which would be restricted to the upper respiratory tract (cf. influenza, p. 331). A live virus could be administered locally to stimulate IgA immunity rather than IgG. However, as with other respiratory viral diseases, local immunity following natural infection is disappointingly short-lived. Thus, illness due to respiratory syncytial virus can recur in all age groups and, since there is only one clinically relevant serotype, the indication is that immune protection against reinfection in the respiratory tract is poor. This, together with the relatively poor responses made by newborn babies to antigenic stimulation, casts some doubt on the likely usefulness of live vaccines even when they do become available.

RHABDOVIRIDAE

This is a large family of negative-strand RNA viruses, which infect vertebrates, invertebrates and plants; only one, the *rabies virus*, infects man naturally, while another, the *Marburg virus*, is a simian virus which has caused accidental infections in man. *Rabies (hydrophobia)* is the most lethal of all viral diseases and until relatively recently there were hardly any recorded examples of recovery from overt disease. It acquired its name from *rabidus*, the Latin for madness, as it dramatically turns normally quiet animals, especially dogs, into vicious, biting beasts; the bite of a rabid dog or cat is the usual means by which rabies is transmitted to man. It is characterised by a frequently lengthy incubation period and the spread of the virus along nerves from the wound site to the CNS, causing a fatal encephalitis. Rabies represents a historical milestone in that it was the first virus disease for which a man-made vaccine was prepared, another of Pasteur's great medical achievements.

Structure

The rhabdoviruses are distinguished by their unique bullet-shaped appearance, cylindrical particles having one rounded and one flattened end (Figure 3.49). The regular striations which are sometimes visible are the tightly wound coils of the helical nucleocapsid. In most respects, their structure is similar to that of the other class V viruses such as orthomyxoviruses and paramyxoviruses. Thus, there is an outer envelope with short knoblike spikes of glycoprotein, which is a haemagglutinin for goose red blood cells and the means of attachment to cell membranes; the envelope is stabilised by an inner layer of matrix (M) protein and encloses the helical nucleocapsid of negative single-stranded RNA and its repeating units of capsomere protein (N). Like other class V viruses, the virion also carries an RNA-dependent RNA polymerase required during replication. Infectivity, as for other enveloped viruses, is destroyed by lipid solvents; it also deteriorates on drying, a fact which enabled Pasteur to develop an attenuated preparation for vaccination (p. 349). There is only one antigenic type known.

Replication and cellular infection

The details of replication are much as for the paramyxoviruses. The virus attaches to cells by means of its haemagglutinin and the nucleocapsid enters the cytoplasm after the viral envelope has fused with the cell membrane. The RNA polymerase transcribes the virion's − RNA genome into + mRNA without requiring uncoating of the capsid, and a polygenic message is probably cleaved into individual mRNA molecules. Replication is cytoplasmic. As the virus multiplies, its sites of replication become apparent as inclusion bodies, called *Negri bodies* after their discoverer; they are particularly conspicuous and in the brain cells of infected animals or humans are diagnostic of rabies.

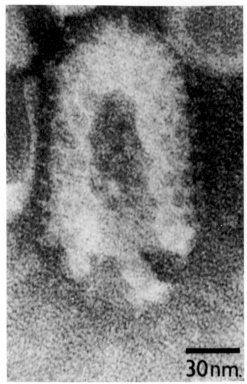

50nm

30nm.

(a)

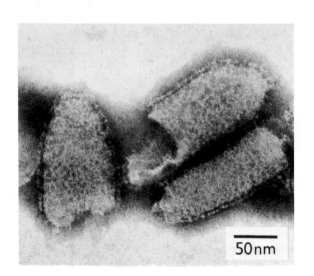

Helical nucleocapsid

Glycoprotein spikes (haemagglutinin)

130–240 nm

Matrix (M) protein layer

Lipid envelope

70–80 nm

Figure 3.49 Structure of rabies virus.
(a) Electron micrographs, negative staining. (Courtesy of Drs. F. Brown and C. Smale.)
(b) Diagrammatic section.

The nucleocapsid amassed in the Negri bodies can be demonstrated by immunofluorescent staining. Final assembly of the mature virion is by budding from the membrane; during this process the characteristic particle takes shape, the flattened end being due to collapse of the region where the particle is sealed.

Cytopathic changes due to the virus in cultured cells are either minimal or absent altogether. Thus, as the virus continues to multiply, persistently infected carrier cultures are readily initiated.

Epidemiology

Rabies is a *zoonosis*; it is principally a disease of warm-blooded animals and all mammals seem to be susceptible, birds rather less so. Infection is via the bite of a rabid animal, the virus being present in its saliva, and man is therefore a terminal (dead-end) host since human-to-human transmission does not normally occur. About 30–50% of people bitten by a rabid animal develop the disease if untreated. The main sources for human infection are domestic animals, principally dogs and cats. In Europe, the USA and Australia, it is a very rare disease in man, both because of its control in the domestic canine population and because it can uniquely be prevented from developing after infection by vaccination. However, elsewhere in the world, about 1,000 human rabies fatalities are recorded annually by the World Health Organisation and this certainly represents only a fraction of its true incidence. In the UK, there have been only eight cases of human rabies since 1946, all fatal and all acquired abroad. In the USA, the annual incidence dropped from 20–30 cases in the 1940's to 1–2 since 1960. Important control measures in domestic animals include registration and leash laws for dogs, destruction of strays, and compulsory vaccination of dogs and cats. Cattle are now the most commonly infected domestic animals in the USA. In islands such as Britain, Australia and New Zealand, strict quarantine laws have prevented the importation of rabies and thus allowed local eradication measures in both domestic and feral species to be completely effective. In Britain, for example, a period of six months quarantine of imported canines and felines was introduced in 1886; this length of time is necessary because the incubation period can be very long and it may take several months for the disease to become apparent in dogs. Today, quarantine is combined with mandatory vaccination.

Apart from these islands, rabies remains enzootic in wild animals in much of the world. In the USA, foxes, coyotes, skunks and raccoons are common sources, with the risk of infection of domestic animals, especially in rural areas; during the 1970's, 2,000–3,000 cases among wild animals were recorded, and 500–600 in domestic species. In mainland Europe, its spread among wolves and foxes is similarly a cause for concern and continued vigilance. In South America, vampire bats are an important source, particularly as bats are the one mammalian species in which infection is persistent and often inapparent (rather than quite rapidly fatal after the incubation period); through their blood-sucking activities, they cause widespread fatal infection among cattle. There have even been two cases of respiratory transmission to man in poorly ventilated caves infested with millions of guano bats. A certain degree of wildlife control is possible through trapping, but in the main it is impracticable and most efforts go into protecting domestic species.

Pathogenesis of rabies (Figure 3.50)

After the bite and deposition of saliva of an infected animal, the virus multiplies locally in the wound for a few days before migrating in the axoplasm of peripheral nerves to the CNS—an example of *neurotropism*, the virus being called neurotropic. This process can take a considerable period of time, determined by the infecting dose and the distance of the wound from the brain; thus, bites on the head and face show the shortest incubation period. The rate of migration along the nerves is 42 mm per day (the same as for herpes simplex virus and poliovirus). The incubation period can vary from as little as 10 days to as much as 2 years, and on the average is 30–50 days in man. This has two important implications: (a) artificial immunisation can be started *after* the infection has been acquired with a good chance of success, and (b) periods of quarantine of imported animals must last several months to be sure they are free of disease. Transmission of virus to the CNS via the bloodstream has been demonstrated experimentally, but does not seem to be relevant to pathogenesis. Thus, if the peripheral nerves are severed, the virus is prevented from causing disease. From a wound other than on the head, the route of migration is via the appropriate dorsal root ganglion and thence to the posterior horn of the spinal cord and gradually to the brain. Infection of the brain leads to *encephalitis*. Neurones in the brain and cord degenerate and contain the diagnostic cytoplasmic Negri bodies. Other histological changes are perivascular accumulation of lymphocytes, and punctate haemorrhages. The hippocampus and cerebellum are the main areas affected in the brain.

Early symptoms of rabies are malaise, headache and intense apprehension; they are followed by high fever, a restlessness progressing to uncontrollable nervousness and excitement (delirium), generalised convulsions and, most characteristic of all, painful spasms of the muscles of the larynx and pharynx when swallowing is attempted. This is the condition of *hydrophobia* (lit. fear of water) in which it becomes impossible to drink and the very sight of water induces the contractions. During this period of clinical disease, the virus is also present in saliva, having reached the salivary glands along efferent nerves. Once clinical signs have developed, a fatal outcome is usually inevitable within a few days, though there have now been some instances of recovery after vigorous supportive treatment. Death is from asphyxia, general paralysis or exhaustion.

In dogs, rabies can take one of two forms, either *furious rabies*,

Figure 3.50 Pathogenesis of rabies.

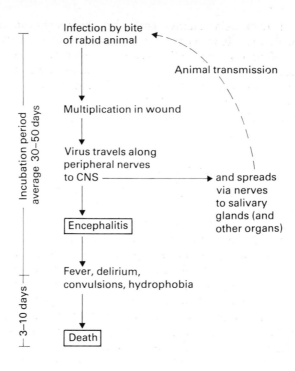

in which the animal becomes uncontrollably aggressive and bites viciously, or *dumb rabies*, when there is paralysis of head and neck muscles and the dog cannot even chew its food. If an animal has bitten but is otherwise asymptomatic, it is kept for veterinary observation for ten days; if it remains healthy it will not have been infectious at the time of the bite and the patient is in no danger, since there is no prolonged, subclinical, infectious carrier state (except in bats). However, if the animal shows signs of rabies at the time of biting or thereafter, it is killed and the brain examined for proof of infection. Traditionally this has been by detection of Negri bodies in the cytoplasm of brain cells, but is now superseded by immunofluorescent staining for viral antigens using labelled antirabies antibodies. It is also possible to isolate the virus from the animal's saliva or brain tissue by intracerebral inoculation into infant mice; after 6–21 days, the mice develop paralysis and rabies is confirmed as above. These measures are obviously essential as the patient cannot be diagnosed until characteristic symptoms appear—by which time it is too late.

Vaccination

The history of immunisation against rabies goes back to Pasteur's vaccine which, as he demonstrated, prevented the disease when given after the bite of a rabid dog. Realising that rabies had an unusually long incubation period, Pasteur attempted to prepare a vaccine strain which would be both milder than the wild type, so-called 'street virus', and have a shorter incubation period, so that it could 'overtake' the natural infection when given to a person who had already been bitten. Following his experience with swine erysipelas vaccine, he passaged the rabies agent serially through rabbits, each time injecting an emulsion of the spinal cord of a previously infected rabbit, and after 50 such passages had succeeded in reducing the incubation period to seven days. Unfortunately the virulence had increased at the same time, so the passaged virus was not usable as a vaccine strain. However, by drying the spinal cords of rabbits infected with the new strain, called 'fixed virus', its virulence was reduced in proportion to the time of drying. We would now recognise this as a means of inactivating, rather than attenuating, the virus, as enveloped viruses such as rabies are usually susceptible to inactivation in this way. Pasteur showed that daily inoculations of the most highly dried spinal cord preparations protected dogs from both the wild type rabies infection and also his own more virulent variant in less well dried cords; most importantly, the immunisation could be commenced after a dog had been bitten by another, rabid dog.

The first human patient whom Pasteur protected, in 1885, was Joseph Meister, a nine-year-old boy who had received 14 bites from a rabid dog. Starting three days after being bitten, Meister was given 13 injections, over ten days, of emulsions of rabbit spinal cord containing the rabies agent, the cords having been dried for successively shorter periods. There were no ill-effects and rabies did not develop, either from the original bites or from the virulent virus being given in the later inocula. After Meister (who was to become gate-keeper at the Institute Pasteur in Paris), Pasteur successfully treated a shepherd, Jupille, who had been bitten while protecting some children from a rabid dog. Thus the principle, uniquely applicable to rabies, of treating the disease by active, post-exposure immunisation was established, against the accepted medical opinion of the day.

The use of a similar vaccine, consisting of rabbit spinal cord inactivated with phenol, continued up to about 20 years ago (the Semple vaccine); however, this carried the serious hazard, in about 0.01% of recipients, of *allergic encephalomyelitis*, an autoimmune reaction to nervous system proteins such as myelin, making it imperative to develop safer effective vaccines. It was replaced by virus grown in embryonated ducks' eggs and inactivated with β-propiolactone, which was effective and safe, but required a course of 21 daily injections as well as boosters after a further 10 and 20 days, due to its weak immunogenicity. This protocol led to the complication of hypersensitivity reactions at the site of inoculation (Arthus reaction, p.163). Since 1980, a new vaccine has been licensed, which is more immunogenic and requires only 3–5 injections over a 10-day period, as well as producing fewer adverse reactions; it is grown in a human diploid fibroblast cell line and is also inactivated with β-propiolactone. This vaccine is now widely used in Europe and the USA and will probably become the choice worldwide. A future vaccine may contain only the purified haemagglutinin glycoprotein, which induces protective neutralising antibodies (a subunit vaccine).

There are several attenuated strains of rabies virus, but unfortunately they fail to multiply sufficiently in man to provide an adequate immune stimulus. However, in animals they are used successfully, notably the Flury LEP (low egg passage) strain for dogs, and the HEP (high egg passage) strain, which is more attenuated and used in more sensitive animals such as cats. They have been highly effective in restricting transmission of rabies in domestic animals, even where it is endemic in the wild.

In treating a possible rabies infection, the wound is first thoroughly cleaned and then infiltrated with antirabies serum; antiserum is also injected (passive immunisation) to provide immediate protection until the antibody response has been stimulated by inoculation of vaccine. The action of the vaccine is apparently to stimulate enough antibody to prevent the virus entering nerves from its site of replication in the wound. Evidently, although the process of incubation is long and slow, the development of the antibody response to natural infection is even slower, either because of poor immunogenicity of the virus or more probably the low dose which actually reaches local lymph nodes. Provided treatment is initiated promptly, clinical rabies rarely occurs in man.

ARENAVIRIDAE

The viruses of this family are unusual both in structure and in their relationship to their hosts. Their most marked property is the tendency to cause chronic, silent infections in rodents (the natural hosts) and severe, potentially lethal diseases in man. One arenavirus, lymphocytic choriomeningitis (LCM) virus, has already been cited as providing a classic model of chronic infection due to immunological tolerance (p.259) and of hypersensitivity mechanisms in viral disease (p.261). LCM virus can infect man, in whom it causes a severe meningoencephalo-myelitis. The other species of medical importance are Lassa, Junin and Machupo viruses, respectively the agents of Lassa fever and Argentinian and Bolivian haemorrhagic fevers (Table 3.13). All are *zoonoses*, with man an accidental host, acquiring the virus from rodents (mice or rats); only in Lassa fever is person-to-person transmission known. A distinctive aspect of their pathology in man is viral damage to capillary endothelium, leading to haemorrhages and hypovolaemic shock, with damage to many organs.

Structure, etc. In electron microscope appearance, arenaviruses are enveloped, round, oval or pleomorphic particles, generally 110–130 nm in diameter, though sometimes much larger (up to 350 nm). The surface is covered with club-shaped projections. The genome is of negative, single-stranded RNA (class V), but the symmetry of the capsid is unknown. The term 'arena' (from Latin, *harena*, sand) refers to unique 'sandy' granules, 20–30 nm in diameter, which are visible inside the virions and appear to be *ribosomes*. Highly purified arenaviruses have been shown to carry 18S and 28S ribosomal RNA. The ribosomes, apparently derived from the host cell, are not required for replication. The latter process is cytoplasmic and the envelope is acquired by budding from the plasma membrane. However, many details of arenavirus/host cell interaction are yet unknown.

Table 3.13 Arenaviruses infecting man

Species	Natural host	Disease in man
Lymphocytic choriomeningitis virus	House mouse (*Mus musculus*)	Lymphocytic choriomeningitis
Lassa virus	Multimammate rat (*Mastomys natalensis*)	Lassa fever
Junin virus	Field mouse (*Calomys* sp.)	Argentinian haemorrhagic fever
Machupo virus	Field mouse (*Calomys callosus*)	Bolivian haemorrhagic fever

Lymphocytic choriomeningitis (LCM)

LCM was first discovered in the 1930's as an asymptomatic infection in mice used during studies of St. Louis encephalitis. The house mouse (*Mus musculus*) is the natural reservoir of LCM virus, in which species its occurrence is worldwide. Besides wild and laboratory mice, infection has been reported in other animal species including guinea-pigs, hamsters and monkeys. We have already described how LCM virus is a chronic, life-long, mostly benign infection in wild (immunologically tolerant) mice (p.259) which may terminate in immune complex disease (p.261), whereas in mice infected as adults, rapid LCM disease occurs due to a cell-mediated response against viral antigens in the brain (p. 262). In man, LCM is rare and usually acquired from mice, probably via urine and faeces, often in laboratories. Infection may be inapparent or cause influenza-like symptoms; CNS involvement (aseptic meningitis, meningoencephalitis) may follow, of which there have been a few severe and even fatal cases. In general, however, LCM infection is benign. A chronic carrier state—as in mice—does not occur in man.

Lassa virus

Lassa fever made its first, dramatic appearance in Nigeria in 1969, when an American nurse contracted the hitherto unknown disease at a mission station in Lassa township, and died soon afterwards. The highly transmissible nature of this lethal infection soon became apparent when two other nurses, both of whom had attended the first patient in hospital, became ill. One died after 11 days, while the other was flown to the USA, where she eventually recovered in intensive care after a severe illness. Lassa virus was first isolated from her blood at Yale University, where a virologist and later a laboratory technician also contracted the disease, the latter dying of it. Further outbreaks in Africa followed in hospitals in Nigeria and Liberia, with a fourth (non-hospital centered) in Sierre Leone in 1970–72. Sporadic outbreaks have continued in West Africa, and by 1978 there had been 386 cases and 105 deaths. In these days of rapid air travel, the possibility of Lassa fever must be considered whenever a patient from the endemic area in West Africa presents with an unexplained, febrile illness of relatively slow onset.

The incubation period is from 6–20 days. Clinically, the disease is characterised by high fever (lasting for 7–17 days), pharyngitis, diarrhoea, vomiting, muscular pain and prostration. In fatal cases, there is a sudden deterioration during the second week, and death is due to hypovolaemic shock, anoxia and cardiac arrest. Lesions occur in many organs (liver, spleen, kidney, heart, brain) with oedema and haemorrhage due to increased capillary permeability. It is not clear whether tissue damage is due to a direct effect of the virus or to hypersensitivity; there is an indication that antigen–antibody complexes may be involved.

The natural host and reservoir of Lassa virus is the multi-mammate rat *Mastomys natalensis*, a common domestic and peridomestic species in West Africa. The animals acquire the virus *in utero* or at birth and, as with other arenavirus infections, become tolerant, life-long carriers suffering no ill effects. They excrete the virus in urine, which is probably the source of primary human infection. The mode of transmission from person to person, however, is not yet clear. Subclinical infection in man is apparently quite common in certain areas; in endemic areas of Sierra Leone, about 10% of individuals have anti-Lassa antibodies. Because of its dangerous nature, few laboratory studies have been carried out with live Lassa virus, and no vaccine is yet available.

Junin and Machupo viruses

These viruses, which occur only in South America, are part of a group of eight arenaviruses known as the 'Tacaribe complex'. Seven of these were isolated in South America, and one, Tamiami virus, in Florida; Tacaribe virus itself was isolated from bats. The Junin and Machupo agents are responsible for haemorrhagic fevers in Argentina and Bolivia respectively. *Argentinian haemorrhagic fever* occurs as annual outbreaks in the area known as the wet pampas, with between 100 and 3,500 cases each year among agricultural workers and a mortality of around 10%. In the most severe cases, there is bleeding from the nose and gums, haematemesis, haematuria and melaena (passage of black stools after bleeding into the bowel). The disease invariably coincides with the maize harvest, between April and July, when the carrier rodent populations are at their peak. The main hosts are field mice (*Calomys* sp.) which live in the maize fields and are disturbed by the harvesting activity. They are chronically infected and excrete the virus in their urine.

The closely similar *Bolivian haemorrhagic fever* also occurs in annual, localised epidemics, mainly in the Beni region of N.E. Bolivia; a notable outbreak occurred in San Joaquin township in 1962–4 when 700 people were affected and 125 died. Once again, the rodent reservoir is a field mouse in which the infection is persistent and benign. Neither of these haemorrhagic fevers shows person-to-person spread.

HEPATITIS VIRUSES

A number of viruses cause acute hepatitis (inflammation of the liver), among them rubella virus as part of the congenital rubella syndrome, cytomegalovirus following blood transfusion, and yellow fever in the tropics. However, most viral hepatitis in temperate climates is due to one of three viruses, denoted *hepatitis A, hepatitis B* and *non-A, non-B* (the latter almost certainly includes more than one agent). These viruses are not related to each other and do not form a family, nor have they been assigned to any of the known virus families; the only feature which they share is their association with liver infection. The disease due to hepatitis A is often termed *infectious hepatitis* (though all three forms are infectious), while hepatitis B and non-A, non-B constitute the agents of *serum hepatitis*, indicating their most familiar mode of transmission in blood and blood products. Most of what follows will deal with hepatitis A and B; non-A, non-B viruses have only been recognised recently and there is still little information available.

Hepatitis is the only major viral disease which is actually increasing in incidence, partly due to the absence of vaccination, partly to changing social conditions. The difficulty in growing these viruses in cultured cells has hampered their study and vaccine development. In the absence of a convenient animal model, experimental investigations of the pathogenesis of the disease have been made in human volunteers, a noted centre being Willowbrook State School in New York, though susceptible monkeys (marmosets, chimpanzees) are now also used. As a result, many of the details of structure, replication, etc. are still quite sketchy compared with other viruses. Despite the gaps in our knowledge, it is perfectly clear that hepatitis A and B infections differ in practically all repects other than the affected organ and clinical symptoms, and accordingly they are described separately below. The chief differences are summarised in Table 3.14 and Figure 3.51.

Besides the acute disease, hepatitis B is also important for its long-term effects. A persistent viraemia can be established with a chronic carrier state which may last for years. In some individuals this can lead to chronic hepatitis and ultimately cirrhosis; there is also reason to link the virus with carcinoma of the liver.

Hepatitis A

Structure, etc. The hepatitis A virus was first detected in 1973, by electron microscopic study of patients' faecal extracts treated with antibody (immunoelectron microscopy). It is a small (27 nm), icosahedral, non-enveloped particle, now known to have a single-stranded RNA genome. In physical and chemical characteristics it is closest to the enteroviruses (Picornaviridae), such as poliovirus. Studies of replication have been delayed by difficulties in culturing the virus, but it can now be grown with a small yield in foetal Rhesus monkey kidney cells or marmoset liver cultures. It is one of the stablest human viruses and resists treatment with

Table 3.14 Comparison of Hepatitis A and B.

Feature	Hepatitis A	Hepatitis B
Virion	27 nm; non-enveloped; RNA; resembles enterovirus	42 nm; enveloped; DNA; unique
Transmission	Faecal-oral	Parenteral injection and other
Incubation period	15–40 days	50–180 days
Occurrence	Autumn and winter	Throughout the year
Epidemics	Yes	No
Age incidence	Highest in children and young adults	All ages
Disease characteristics	Acute onset; fever > 38°C common; jaundice, etc.	Insidious onset; fever > 38°C uncommon; jaundice, etc; immune complexes; more severe than A
Fulminant hepatitis	Yes	Yes
Chronic active hepatitis and cirrhosis	No	Yes
Virus in faeces	From incubation period to 1–2 weeks after recovery	Absent
Virus in blood	ditto	From incubation period to months or years after recovery
HBsAg	Absent	In blood 30–50 days after infection; persists for 60 days to years
Value of γ-globulin for prophylaxis	Good	Ineffective unless high titre of anti-HBs, when good
Possible cause of liver cancer	No	Yes

lipid solvents (there is no envelope) and many disinfectants, and can withstand 56°C for 30 minutes.

Transmission/Epidemiology. Infectious hepatitis is a major public health problem in many Western countries; in the USA, for example, there are about 50,000 cases annually, mostly occurring in the autumn and winter. It has in the past generally been associated with small children, in whom it is often subclinical, but over recent years the prevalence of sporadic disease among older children and young adults has increased; over 25% of

355

healthy adults have antibodies to hepatitis A virus, indicating the widespread nature of asymptomatic infection. It provides a good example of the *faecal-oral* route of transmission. The virus is present in the faeces from about the middle of the incubation period until two weeks after recovery from jaundice, and regularly spreads to other family members through person-to-person contact, probably the most important method. Contaminated water, milk and food are also sources of infection and epidemics result from faecal contamination of water used for drinking, or through eating raw shellfish (oysters, clams) from estuaries contaminated with sewage. The preparation or handling of food or milk by viral carriers is another danger and one which is difficult to prevent, because viral excretion precedes the symptoms and the infection may remain silent. Faecal-oral transmission is encouraged both by the prevalence of subclinical infection and by the unusual stability of the virus, including its resistance to normal concentrations of disinfectants, such as chlorine, in water. As hepatitis A virus is present in the blood towards the end of the incubation period, there is also the possibility of transmission via blood transfusion, though in practice it constitutes only a small proportion of cases of post-transfusion hepatitis.

The disease is endemic and common in many parts of the world where communal hygiene and sanitation are inadaquate (Africa, Asia, South America), but, as noted above, it is also prevalent and increasing in Western countries. The latter seems puzzling at first, but the situation is similar to that of poliomyelitis before universal vaccination (p. 290). Infection in early childhood, which is often asymptomatic but provides immunity, is no longer so common where standards of hygiene are high. Thus, many children and adults may have no protective immunity; since infection in these older groups is more likely to be accompanied by disease, the increasing incidence of clinically apparent hepatitis can be understood.

Prevention. In the absence of a vaccine, the maintenance of high standards of sanitation and personal hygiene are the principal safeguards against the disease. Administration of normal pooled gamma globulin (which contains antibody to hepatitis A) is effective as a prophylactic measure and is used to protect family contacts or high risk groups such as the military; e.g. American troops serving in Vietnam received normal human gamma globulin on arrival and at six-month intervals thereafter.

Pathogenesis. This is outlined in Figure 3.51a. After ingestion of the virus, there is an incubation period of 2–6 weeks, during which it is believed to multiply in the gut epithelium before being carried in the blood to the liver. Before symptoms appear, infected individuals are a dangerous source of virus, which is present both in faeces and blood. The virus multiplies in the cytoplasm of liver parenchymal cells, but the mechanism of liver damage is unknown. Prodromal symptoms appear abruptly, with fever, vomiting and malaise; anorexia (loss of appetite) is the most

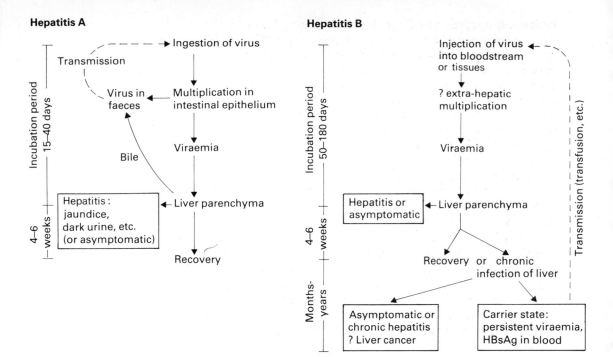

Figure 3.51 Comparison of the pathogenesis of hepatitis A and B.

prominent symptom and smokers lose interest in tobacco. After a few days, the signs of liver damage are seen in excretion of dark urine and *jaundice*. Both are due to the escape of conjugated bilirubin from the liver into the blood (*hyperbilirubinaemia*), which in turn results from interference with the flow of bile along the liver canaliculi (*cholestasis*). Excretion of conjugated bilirubin leads to dark-coloured urine, and when bilirubin stains the skin (and other tissues) yellow, the appearance of jaundice is seen. Stools are pale as there is less bilirubin in the gut. The jaundice fades gradually in about two weeks and full recovery takes a further 2–4 weeks, though weakness or depression may persist for some time after. Hepatitis A infection is less severe than hepatitis B and the mortality from massive liver necrosis is only about 0.1%. The virus continues to be found in faeces during early convalescence, but does not persist once recovery is complete. Thus the infectious carrier state in relatively short. There is *no chronic disease* following hepatitis A.

Diagnosis. During the prodromal phase, incipient liver damage can be detected by an increase in the serum levels of *transaminases*, namely serum glutamic-oxalacetic transaminase (SGOT) and serum glutamic-pyruvic transaminase (SGPT). These are often used as indicators of liver disease, and though not specific (raised levels also occur in myocardial infarction, muscular injury and CNS disease) they are nevertheless of value in routine screening. SGPT is probably the more liver-specific of the two. The presence of specific IgM antihepatitis A antibody in the serum is a good indicator of *recent* infection; confirmation of hepatitis A requires the isolation of virus from faeces and identification by electron microscopy.

Structure and antigens (Figure 3.52). Although it has not yet been possible to grow the virus in cultured cells, its structure has been studied in detail using particles present in high concentration in the blood of patients and chronic carriers. It differs in several repects from the other DNA viruses and could be considered the prototype of a new (unnamed) family. The virion itself, known as the *Dane particle,* is a small enveloped icosahedron, 42 nm in diameter, with a 'double-shelled' appearance by electron microscopy: the outer layer is the envelope or coat surrounding the inner (27 nm) icosahedral capsid, often called the core. The core contains the viral DNA, which is unusual firstly because it is circular and very small—a mere 3,600 base pairs— and secondly because it is part single-stranded and part double-stranded, the two DNA strands being of unequal length (Figure 3.52b). Another unusual feature is the presence of a DNA polymerase in the core. Dane particles are usually considerably outnumbered in serum by smaller, spherical particles about 22 nm in diameter, which are aggregates of the envelope protein(s) together with lipid; because they are detected serologically the small particles are referred to as *hepatitis B surface antigen* or HBsAg (formerly known as *Australia antigen*). Filamentous forms are also plentiful and are aggregates of HBsAg particles. Neither the 22 nm particles nor the filaments contain DNA. The relationship between these forms is shown schematically in Figure 3.52. Two other antigens are present on the virus, namely the core antigen (HBcAg), which is the capsid protein, and an antigen designated 'e' (HBeAg). Antibodies to all three appear during the course of infection or convalescence.

The HBsAg particles can be found in huge quantity in the sera of patients and carriers, up to 100–200 μg per ml. As many as 10^{13} particles per ml have been recorded, with about 10% that number of filaments and 0.1% of complete virions. Thus, there is both viraemia and intense *antigenaemia* in such individuals.

Replication. Information is incomplete as replication cannot be studied in culture, but it seems to resemble the pattern of other DNA viruses, with viral cores detectable by electron microscopy and immunofluorescence in the nuclei of infected hepatocytes. Surface antigen and enveloped virions are found in the cytoplasm, and while the envelope is probably acquired by budding the details of this are still obscure. HBsAg is made in great excess of the envelope requirement and 'exported', leading to the large amount in the blood.

Transmission/Epidemiology. The important feature of hepatitis B infection is the *persistence* of virus in the blood, either following recovery from hepatitis or as a completely subclinical infection; thus infected blood and blood products are a major starting point for spread of the virus—whence the term 'serum hepatitis'. Until recently, blood transfusion was a principal mode of transmission,

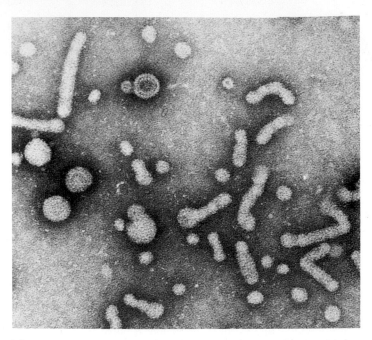

(a)

Figure 3.52 Structural forms of hepatitis B virus in the blood.
(a) Electron microscope appearance, negative staining, ×230,000. (Courtesy of Dr June Almedia.)
(b) Description of forms.

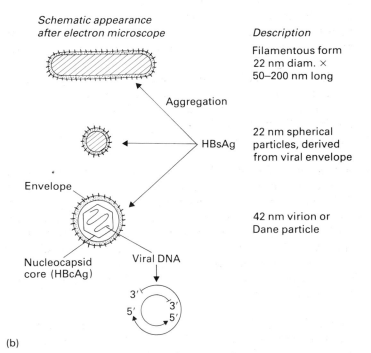

Schematic appearance after electron microscope

Description

Filamentous form 22 nm diam. × 50–200 nm long

Aggregation

HBsAg

22 nm spherical particles, derived from viral envelope

Envelope

42 nm virion or Dane particle

Nucleocapsid core (HBcAg)

Viral DNA

3'
3'
5'
5'

(b)

but since HBsAg can now be detected by serological tests which have become routine in all blood banks (below), transmission in this way is much less common today (non-A non-B viruses are currently the major agents of post-transfusion hepatitis). However, other means of parenteral inoculation can equally well spread infection, e.g. needles and syringes which have been used by more than one person and inadequately sterilised, leading to a prevalence of serum hepatitis among heroin addicts, while dental surgery, vaccination, ear piercing and tattooing can also be similarly hazardous. Apropos of vaccination, we may mention that 30,000 cases of hepatitis were caused among American servicemen in the 1940's by the use of yellow fever vaccine which had been stabilised with normal human serum; this risk could have been minimised by not pooling the serum samples used. Note that passive immunisation with pooled gamma globulin does not carry a risk of hepatitis because the virus is not present in purified Ig or albumin fractions, though other serum fractions can be contaminated. Hepatitis B infection is a particular hazard of renal haemodialysis, with the sharing of machines for extra-corporeal circulation (screening of patients reduces this risk considerably). Interestingly, infection is also an occupational hazard among the staff of dialysis units. Indeed, the occurrence both of sporadic cases and, more often, asymptomatic carriers among individuals with no recent history of injection has made it clear that other routes of transmission are also important. Faecal-oral spread is unlikely as the virus is not usually found in faeces; oral or sexual routes are suggested by the finding of virus in saliva and semen, but the predominant mode is not yet certain. A high frequency of serum hepatitis is found among male homosexuals.

The carrier rate for hepatitis B in Europe and the USA is generally put at about 0.1%, though this depends on the sensitivity of the method used for detection of HBsAg and may well be an underestimate. In parts of Asia and Africa, the rate is much higher (5–20%) and among hard drug addicts, sharing non-sterile syringes and needles, can exceed 50%. Hepatitis B virus also infects subhuman primates, and chimpanzeees are used in experimental work; they are so susceptible that they sometimes contract hepatitis from their human handlers.

Detection of carriers. Hepatitis B antigen was first detected fortuitously by Blumberg in 1963, in the serum of an Australian aborigine. Blumberg had been looking for 'new' antigens in human blood, as an indication of protein polymorphisms, using antibodies present in the sera of haemophiliacs who had received multiple blood transfusions (and thus would be expected to have made antibodies to antigens of polymorphic human plasma proteins). The 'Australia antigen' was then also found in individuals who had received several blood transfusions and the connection with serum hepatitis was soon made.

Detection of HBsAg is now an important part of screening of blood prior to transfusion and a variety of immunological methods are used. Two of the most sensitive are shown in Figure 3.53. In the *solid-phase radioimmunoassay* (Fig. 3.53a) antibody to

HBsAg (anti-HBs) is bound to a plastic surface such as a tube or the well of a titration plate, and a small volume of the plasma (or serum) under examination is added; after incubation, the plasma is washed away and a sample of the anti-HBs antibody radioactively labelled with iodine (^{125}I) is put on (sandwich method). If HBsAg from the plasma has bound, the 'second stage' radiolabelled antibody also binds and can be detected in a gamma counter. A slightly less sensitive method is *reverse passive haemagglutination* (Fig. 3.53b) in which the anti-HBs is coupled to indicator red cells; these will be agglutinated by the presence of HBsAg in the test plasma. Both techniques can be modified to detect antibody instead of antigen.

If HBsAg is present in a plasma or serum sample, it is also useful to test for the HBeAg, as this is only found when there is active viral replication and liver damage; thus, the presence of HBeAg is closely associated with transmission of infection.

Figure 3.53 Sensitive techniques for detection of HBsAg.
(a) Solid-phase radioimmunoassay.
(b) Reverse passive haemagglutination.

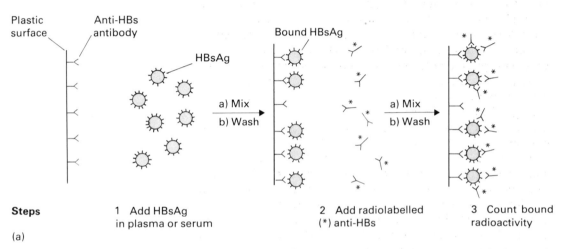

Plastic surface   Anti-HBs antibody   HBsAg   Bound HBsAg

a) Mix
b) Wash

a) Mix
b) Wash

Steps

1 Add HBsAg in plasma or serum

2 Add radiolabelled (*) anti-HBs

3 Count bound radioactivity

(a)

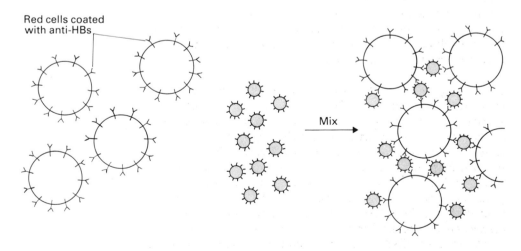

Red cells coated with anti-HBs

Mix

Steps

1 Add HBsAg in plasma or serum

2 Read agglutination

(b)

Screening of blood for HBsAg before tranfusion has not reduced post-transfusion hepatitis as dramatically as had been hoped, due to the widespread occurrence of non-A, non-B viruses for which no simple serological tests are available.

Pathogenesis. The symptoms of hepatitis B are indistinguishable from those of type A, with jaundice, dark urine, light stools, etc., but the disease is often more severe and post-transfusion hepatitis has a significant mortality (occasionally as high as 10–20%) due to the high infecting dose and other disease in the patient. Overall, the mortality of hepatitis B is about 1%. (Note, however, that fulminant hepatitis can be either A or B). The incubation period is considerably longer (50–180 days) and onset more gradual than in infectious hepatitis. Serum transaminase levels tend to be high for a longer period. HBsAg is present in the blood towards the end of the incubation period and in most cases disappears completely after clinical recovery (Figure 3.54). The first antibody to appear in patients' sera is directed at the core antigen (anti-HBc), but is without protective value; strangely enough, antibody to the surface antigen (anti-HBs), which is protective, only appears during convalescence and increases over a long period, providing permanent immunity against reinfection (Figure 3.54).

Recovery is probably dependent on cell-mediated immunity to viral surface (envelope) antigens expressed on the membrane of infected hepatocytes. It seems that the death of liver cells is also principally due to this response and that hepatitis is therefore a result of cell-mediated damage (or Type IV hypersensitivity). Thus, in chronically infected carriers the virus multiplies continuously in liver cells without necessarily damaging the liver; CMI to hepatitis B in such individuals is depressed. Furthermore, in recipients of immunosuppressive treatments for graft rejection or leukaemia, the virus often multiplies rampantly, with persistent viraemia but without disease, a rare example of an

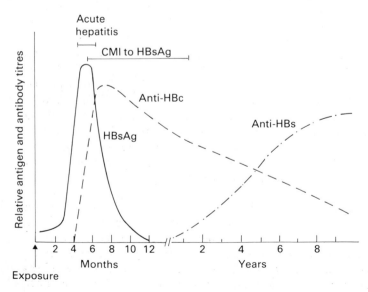

Figure 3.54 Time course of appearance of antigen and antibodies in the circulation, and cell-mediated immunity, in hepatitis B infection.

infectious disease which is less severe during immunosuppression. In short, left to its own devices, the virus seems to establish a chronic but silent (non-cytocidal) infection of the liver; the intervention of the immune response eliminates the virus, but in so doing contributes to the disease process. (cf. lymphocytic choriomeningitis infection of mice, p.261.) The high levels of antigen and antibody in the blood during the disease also lead to hypersensitivity reactions, but of the immune complex (Type III) variety, including arthritis, urticaria, glomerulonephritis and polyarteritis nodosa.

In 20–30% of adults and a rather higher proportion of children, HBsAg and Dane particles do not disappear from the circulation on recovery, but persist for several months; about half of these people become chronic carriers with antigenaemia and viraemia lasting for up to several years. Sometimes this state is established completely asymptomatically; as noted above, virus then continues to multiply in liver parenchymal cells without causing necrosis. In explanation, it is necessary to invoke a form of suppression of the immune response or tolerance, and this is supported by the weak CMI activity to HBsAg in these individuals and the absence of anti-HBs antibodies, but the cellular mechanisms of this suppression are as yet obscure. Persistent hepatitis B virus infection of the liver, however, is not always a benign state, and about half of those chronically infected have evidence of liver damage (*chronic active hepatitis*) which without treatment may progress to *cirrhosis*.

Hepatitis B and liver cancer. There is growing evidence that hepatitis B virus is an important aetiological agent of liver (hepatocellular) carcinoma. The epidemiological data can be summarised as follows. (a) The geographical distribution of chronic viral carriers and liver cancer patients show a close correlation. (b) Hepatitis B infection and associated cirrhosis often precede liver cancer, and HBsAg is found in the sera of liver cancer patients with very high frequency (80–90%) even when the incidence of infection in the general population is low. (c) In an animal model, namely the woodchuck, a North American rodent, natural infection with a very similar virus occurs and leads to chronic hepatitis; there is an impressive association with liver carcinoma. This evidence is now supported by the findings that hepatitis B virus DNA is *integrated* into the chromosomes of liver carcinoma cells, just as that of the Epstein–Barr virus is integrated into the DNA of Burkitt's lymphoma cells. While this does not constitute proof in itself, it is precisely what would be predicted if hepatitis B were an oncogenic virus for liver cells (see also p. 796).

Vaccination. The serious nature of serum hepatitis and its possible long-term consequences make the search for a vaccine an urgent matter. In fact, although the virus cannot be grown in culture—normally today a prerequisite to vaccine development—nature has already provided a vaccine in the form of the HBsAg found in such huge amounts in carrier serum. When separated from Dane particles, the antigen provides protection against serum hepatitis in humans and chimpanzees (anti-HBs is responsible for immunity). A human source might be unsuitable for mass use, because of the presence of human lipids and perhaps glycoproteins in HBsAg (the viral envelope) and the consequent risk of autoimmunity. Nevertheless, there have been two major controlled trials with formalin-treated HBsAg—one in New York homosexuals, the other in French health care personnel—both of which showed a high degree of protection and minimal side-effects. Efforts have been made to introduce the viral gene coding for the surface antigen into *E. coli* cells by recombinant DNA technology, i.e. integrated into a plasmid (p. 471). This has now been achieved, with production of the HBsAg by the 'engineered' bacterial clones. In time, this method should be able to provide the pure antigen in the quantity required for large-scale vaccination. Gamma globulin containing a high level of anti-HBs is of some use in prophylaxis of serum hepatitis, but normal gamma globulin is less effective than for hepatitis A.

Non-A, non-B hepatitis viruses

These are now responsible for most (~ 75%) of the cases of post-transfusion hepatitis. Using immune electron microscopy, a particle rather similar to hepatitis A virus has been identified, a non-enveloped icosahedral virion, 27 nm in diameter. However, it does not share antigens with either the A or B type viruses. There is undoubtedly more than one agent of this type. Non-A, non-B viruses are also associated with chronic hepatitis and cirrhosis, but a connection with cancer is uncertain.

REOVIRIDAE

The designation 'reo' is an acronym of 'respiratory, enteric, orphan', indicating that the viruses of this family were initially isolated from the respiratory and alimentary tracts and were not at first associated with disease ('orphans'). The name has been retained, despite the fact that some members are by now well-known pathogens. The family consists of class III viruses, with a segmented, double-stranded RNA genome (see p. 237 and Figure 3.11c for replication). Members of three genera—*Reovirus*, *Orbivirus* and *Rotavirus*—infect man, of which only the last two cause serious disease. Orbiviruses are arboviruses (p. 300) responsible for Colorado tick fever. Rotaviruses, with which we are principally concerned here, have achieved great importance since the recognition in the 1970's that they are major agents of severe diarrhoea in infants and young children, in both developed and developing parts of the world.

Gastroenteric diseases are a major cause of paediatric illness throughout the world and, in the developing countries, of infant mortality. In the USA, acute infectious gastroenteritis (of all causes) accounts for over 15% of all illnesses, making it the second most prevalent disease, while in Asia, Africa and Latin America it has been estimated that in a single year the number of

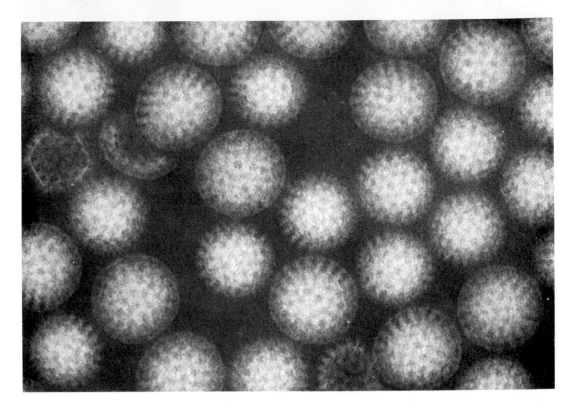

Figure 3.55 Rotavirus particles as seen in the electron microscope, showing 'rough' internal capsids and 'smooth' complete virions; ×200,000. (Courtesy of Dr June D. Almeida.)

cases of diarrhoea would be of the order of 450 million, resulting in the deaths of some 10 million children. In non-epidemic periods, bacterial agents are responsible for about a quarter of the cases, and a large proportion of the rest are probably due to rotaviruses and other viruses such as the Norwalk agent (p. 283).

Rotaviruses

In common with the other reoviruses, the rotaviruses have the unusual feature of a double-layered capsid. Complete particles have a sharply-defined, wheel-like shape (Lat. *rota*, wheel), the smooth outer capsid appearing to rest on 'spokes' projecting from the 'rough' internal capsid (Figure 3.55). The double-stranded RNA genome consists of 11 segments, each corresponding to a single gene. Humans are infected by at least three different serotypes. Rotaviruses were first discovered in 1973 in duodenal biopsies from children with gastroenteritis; electron microscopy subsequently showed them to be present in enormous quantity in the faeces of such patients. It has proved difficult (but not impossible) to grow rotaviruses in culture and their demonstration in stools usually depends on immunological methods, such as radioimmunoassay or enzyme-linked immunoassay (ELISA), or electron microscopy.

Pathogenesis. Most victims of rotaviral gastroenteritis are children under six years of age, the majority between 6 and 24 months; it is less common among adults (cf. Norwalk virus, p. 283). For some reason, infants up to 3 months of age can carry the infection without diarrhoea; this may be a protective effect of IgA antibodies in maternal colostrum and milk, but in that case it is puzzling that asymptomatic infection nevertheless occurs. Rotaviruses are found in the stools of some 50% of children hospitalised with diarrhoea and in a small proportion of healthy children (subclinical infection). Transmission is faecal-oral. The virus multiplies only in the columnar epithelial cells of the tips of the villi in the small intestine; the infected cells cease absorption of sugars from the lumen and this seems to be the chief cause of diarrhoea. After an incubation period of 1–3 days, the clinical signs are vomiting and diarrhoea, the latter being the more persistent and lasting 4–5 days in all. Dehydration frequently necessitates hospitalisation of infants and young children; if severe and untreated it may well be fatal, but oral rehydration is life-saving in most cases. The disease is more severe if it occurs simultaneously with infection by enteropathogenic *E. coli* (p. 547), a combination which is strikingly common.

Epidemiology. Rotaviruses are ubiquitous. The incidence of infection appears to be much the same in Western countries and in the tropics, though the effects are likely to be more severe in the latter, with greater probability of dehydration and often poorer health care. Throughout the world, children are infected at an early age, often as babies. It is interesting that the effects of improvements in hygiene on, say, poliovirus infection, namely to postpone infection to an older age (p. 290), have not been seen in rotavirus infection, though there is little evidence for transmission by a route other than the faecal-oral. IgA antibodies to rotaviruses are present in colostrum and milk, but whether breast-feeding prevents rotavirus infection is controversial. The seasonal distribution of rotaviral diarrhoea is interesting. In temperate climates, infections predominantly occur during the winter months (January–March) and are rare in summer; in other parts of the world, they may also be seasonally restricted or occur throughout the year. Strangely, in West Australia the peak occurrence is in the winter among non-Aborigines, but in the summer in Aborigines. The reasons behind these seasonal patterns are not known.

Given their importance as a cause of diarrhoeal illness in children throughout the world, there is an urgent need for a rotavirus vaccine. This is not yet available, however; the difficulty in growing the virus in culture is a stumbling block to development of an attenuated human strain.

Rotaviruses are also a cause of diarrhoea in newborn animals, including calves, piglets, lambs, kittens and puppies, but there is no evidence for transmission from animals to man.

SLOW VIRUSES

The features common to slow virus diseases are that they have very long incubation periods, often of several years, and that once the symptoms have appeared they progress gradually but inexorably to death. The term 'slow virus' is in many cases a misnomer as a description of the agent, however, for (a) it may not always be a true virus, in the generally understood usage of the word, and (b) its replication may not be any slower than that of other viruses. Moreover, by using the length of the incubation period as the criterion, viruses of several different families are included, as well as the more obscure agents. Thus, as Table 3.14 shows, some slow virus infections are due to 'conventional' viruses, such as paramyxoviruses, retroviruses, etc., whereas others are due to agents which for the moment are called 'unconventional'. The properties of the latter are so unusual that a more suitable collective term will soon have to be found. Table 3.14 also shows that slow virus infections occur both in man and animals, and that in man they are all diseases of the central nervous system. The conventional virus group includes *subacute sclerosing panencephalitis* (SSPE), which we have already discussed as a late complication of measles (p. 342), and *progressive multifocal leucoencephalopathy*, while the unconventional agents cause rare degenerative disorders of the brain, which, because of their similar and unusual histology, are grouped together as the *spongiform encephalopathies*. The latter comprise kuru and Creutzfeldt–Jakob disease in man, scrapie of sheep and transmissible mink encephalopathy. There is a possibility that other chronic neurological disorders of unexplained origin—such as multiple sclerosis, Parkinson's disease and Alzheimer's senile dementia—will also turn out to be slow virus diseases, not to mention some 'unsolved' chronic conditions such as rheumatoid

Table 3.15 Slow virus infections in man and animals.

Agent/family	Disease	Host species	Site of infection
A. *Conventional* Paramyxoviridae			
—measles virus	SSPE	Man	CNS
Retroviridae	Visna	Sheep	CNS
	Maedi	Sheep	Lung
Papovaviridae	PML	Man	CNS
Parvoviridae	Aleutian disease	Mink	Kidney, RES
B. *Unconventional*	Spongiform encephalopathies:		
	Kuru	Man	CNS
	CJD	Man	CNS
	Scrapie	Sheep	CNS
	Transmissible mink encephalopathy	Mink	CNS

SSPE: subacute sclerosing panencephalitis
PML: progressive multifocal leucoencephalopathy
CJD: Creutzfeldt–Jakob disease

arthritis, systemic lupus erythematosus (SLE) and diabetes mellitus.

Conventional slow viruses

The two disorders which affect man are SSPE and progressive multifocal leucoencephalopathy (PML). SSPE, described at greater length on p. 342, is associated with measles virus and is evidently due to the slow spread through the brain of virus retained after recovery from childhood infection. In this disease, viral replication seems to occur without maturation of completed particles (normally formed by budding); thus, infectious measles virus cannot be obtained directly from SSPE brains and is demonstrable only by coculturing brain cells with susceptible indicator cells such as HeLa cells or African green monkey kidney cells.

PML is a rare, progressive, demyelinating disease, which has only been seen under conditions of *immunosuppression*, being associated with Hodgkin's disease, leukaemia and the use of cytotoxic drugs in cancer therapy. As the name suggests, there are multiple foci of degeneration in the white matter of the brain. Papovaviruses (p. 283) of the *Polyomavirus* genus, related to SV40, have been isolated. Initially, in 1965, arrays of virus particles were seen in nuclei of oligodendrocytes from brain tissue of PML patients, and a papovavirus known as *JC virus* (after the patient) was subsequently recovered by inoculating cultures of human foetal astrocytes with dispersed PML brain cells. SV40 virus itself has also been found in the brains of a few patients with PML. A third papovavirus, known as *BK virus*, also related to but distinct from SV40, was first demonstrated in the urine of transplant recipients undergoing immunosuppression, but has not been associated with any disease. The current hypotheses for the origin of PML are that it is either the result of reactivation of JC or SV40 viruses which have remained latent in the host since early life, or an infection by these viruses newly acquired during a period of immunosuppression. What is especially noteworthy is the remarkably widespread ocurrence of the JC and BK viruses in man. Antibodies to BK are practically universal in the USA and Western Europe—in one study, 100% of schoolchildren were seropositive by age 10–11, indicating early infection. Similarly, 50% of infants had anti-JC antibodies by the age of three years, and 65% were seropositive in their teens. Thus, both JC and BK are very common early infections which, to judge from the large number of seropositive adults, probably persist for life. Both viruses are specific for man, but apart from PML and JC virus, have no other known connections with human disease.

Among slow viruses of animals are *visna* and *maedi* in sheep, both of which are due to *retroviruses*, a group more familiar as RNA tumour viruses (p. 777); thus, the virions carry reverse transcriptase and their replication takes place via a DNA intermediate. Visna is a CNS disease (meningoleucoer cephalitis), while maedi is a slowly progressive pneumonia. Both were discovered in Iceland and shown to be transmissible with incubation periods of several years. *Aleutian disease of mink* is a chronic infection of the commercially valuable Aleutian mink caused by a small DNA virus (a *parvovirus*). It was first recognised in the 1940's when 'blue' mink became fashionable, the term 'Aleutian' referring to a mutant with the highly prized bluish fur colour. Although other breeds of mink are also susceptible, the disease is most severe in Aleutians and is currently one of the most serious infectious diseases among ranch-raised mink throughout the world. Like other slow virus infections, it is a condition which gradually worsens over a period of months or even years and is invariably fatal. The infection is persistent and the immune response fails to clear the virus. It is of particular pathological interest because of the occurrence of immunological abnormalities including autoimmunity and an immune complex syndrome. Most prominent is glomerulonephritis due to deposited complexes of virus and antibody; the renal damage is often fatal. However, there are also indications of a general breakdown of the control over B cells and antibody production, with plasmacytosis, hypergammaglobulinaemia and autoantibodies against red cells, all of which suggest that the virus has interfered with the activity of suppressor T cells. If it is an appropriate model, it would lend support to theories of a viral causation for chronic autoimmune disorders such as SLE and rheumatoid arthritis.

Unconventional slow viruses: spongiform encephalopathies

There are four examples of the chronic degenerative brain disease known as spongiform encephalopathy, two in man (*kuru* and

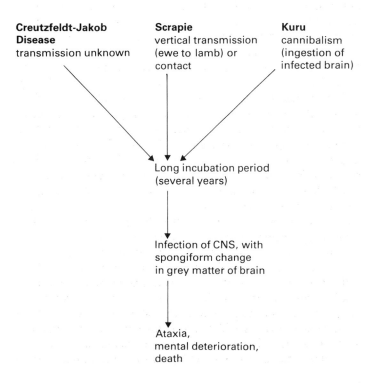

Figure 3.56 Pathogenesis of infections by 'unconventional' slow viruses.

Creutzfeldt-Jakob Disease
transmission unknown

Scrapie
vertical transmission (ewe to lamb) or contact

Kuru
cannibalism (ingestion of infected brain)

Long incubation period (several years)

Infection of CNS, with spongiform change in grey matter of brain

Ataxia, mental deterioration, death

Creutzfeldt–Jakob disease) and two in animals (*scrapie* and *transmissible mink encephalopathy*), Figure 3.56. Histological changes in the brain in all four are very similar, with vacuolation of neurones, proliferation and hypertrophy of astroglia (astrogliosis) and a 'spongiform' change in the grey matter. There are no inflammatory lesions. Furthermore, they are all caused by infectious agents, the properties of which challenge the notion that they are true viruses, in their apparent lack of nucleic acid and their extremely small size. Evidence is accumulating to suggest that they may be an altogether novel type of particle, which has not yet been seen by the electron microscope nor grown in cell culture. A consistent feature of these infections is the total absence of a host immune response, either protective or auto-immune; nor is there induction of interferon. The reasons why the agents are so poorly immunogenic will become clear only when their nature is better understood. Lack of antibodies has been a further obstacle to their characterisation.

Scrapie, the disease of sheep, is the most thoroughly studied of the group, and the mysterious properties of the scrapie agent have been much debated. The disease has been recognised since 1913, its characteristic symptoms being pruritus (itching, which causes the sick animal to scrape or scratch itself against objects) and locomotor ataxia. Its infectious nature and its extraordinary resistance to formalin were shown by its inadvertant inoculation into sheep in Scotland in the 1940's. 18,000 sheep were vaccinated against louping-ill, an ovine encephalomyelitis, using a formalin-treated preparation of sheep brain containing the louping-ill virus, but which was unwittingly contaminated with the scrapie agent. Two years later, 1,500 sheep developed scrapie. Studies on scrapie have been hampered by (a) the absolute requirement for animal assays, cell culture methods having been unsuccessful, (b) the extreme length of the incubation period, and (c) the lack of serological reagents (antibodies). Fortunately, the scrapie agent can be grown in rodents, but it still takes several months for the disease to develop in mice and 60–70 days in hamsters. In murine infections, it has been found that the agent multiplies as rapidly over the first 20 days as many viruses which cause acute infections; its multiplication occurs first in the spleen and then in the brain, though it has a wide tissue distribution, especially in lymphoid tissue (but not liver). After 3–4 months, the brain contains the largest amount and signs of cerebral degeneration become apparent, the clinical signs correlating with the amount of agent in the brain.

Kuru achieved significance as the first human degenerative CNS disorder for which an infectious agent was isolated. Its story is one of the most bizarre in medicine. The disease is restricted to a single Melanesian tribe, the Fore people of the Eastern Highlands of Papua New Guinea; when first described, in 1957, kuru was the major cause of death among all Fore women, was also present in children and young adults of both sexes, but spared older men and outsiders. Indeed, the tribe had at that time only one-third as many women as men. The manifestations are tremor (*kuru* means shivering or trembling in the local language), ataxia, disturbed balance and gait, and a gradual progression to death about a year after onset. Degeneration, with the characteristic histology described above, mainly affects the cerebellum.

At first, a genetic hypothesis for the aetiology of kuru was proposed, but two observations illuminated its true origins. First, in 1965, Gajdusek transmitted the disease to chimpanzees by intracerebral inoculation of extracts of brains of dead patients, demonstrating its infectious nature. Second, since 1957 the incidence of kuru has showed a marked decline; it no longer appears in children and the average age of onset in women has increased by one year every year. In all probability it will soon become extinct. These peculiarities are in fact the result of its unique mode of transmission, namely by *cannibalism*, in the custom of eating the brains of the dead as a mark of respect, practised by Fore women and children but not by men. It appears that this habit was introduced into the tribe between 1910 and 1920, but was suppressed in 1957 with Australian administration. Thus, there is no inherited basis to the disease, merely (to coin a new term) a 'socio-infectious' one. On the basis of an incubation period of up to 30 years, the disappearance of kuru can be anticipated this decade; the origins of the kuru agent, however, remain a mystery.

Creutzfeldt–Jakob disease (CJD) is a very rate (1 per 10^7 population), fatal dementia of the middle aged (a pre-senile dementia) which is worldwide in distribution and strikingly similar in histology to kuru. It can be transmitted to chimpanzees, guinea-pigs and cats. Goats inoculated with CJD brain extracts develop a neurological disorder 3–4 years later which is indistinguishable from scrapie. It was also once transmitted accidentally in man by corneal grafting, indicating that the agent is not restricted to the brain. The similarities between the agents and pathology of CJD and kuru are such as to suggest that CJD may be the 'natural' form of kuru. So far there is no epidemiological evidence to link scrapie with human disease.

Nature of the uncoventional slow viruses

The scrapie agent is the best studied of the group, though all seem closely similar. (They can, however, be distinguished by their host range, as chimps are susceptible to CJD and kuru, but not to scrapie). The remarkable properties of the scrapie agent which have provoked much discussion and speculation in recent years are principally its extreme resistance to inactivation by many physical, chemical and enzymatic procedures which normally destroy proteins and nucleic acids. For example, it resists 90°C for 30 minutes, exposure to acid (pH2), proteases, DNase, RNase, X-irradiation and u.v. irradiation; nor can it be inactivated by formaldehyde or β-propiolactone, the alkylating agents which destroy the infectivity of practically all viruses by reacting with their protein and nucleic acid. Many speculative ideas on its nature have been put forward, the most widely canvassed of recent years being that it is a viroid-like agent; viroids are particles of naked RNA, free of protein, which to date are only known with certainty to infect plants. Another view was that it is a poly-saccharide with the ability to replicate and associated with cell membranes. Recently, however, its relative purification from hamster brain has enabled a careful evaluation of these properties to be made. There is recent evidence, for example, that the scrapie agent contains *protein* essential for its infectivity, including its inactivation by the enzymes proteinase k and trypsin, by the protein-denaturing agents sodium dodecyl sulphate and urea, and by chaotropic salts which disrupt hydrogen bonds in proteins, such as guanidinium thiocyanate. The protein seems to be particularly hydrophobic in nature, suggesting that its role might be to assist passage across cell membranes or the blood–brain barrier. Alternatively, it might be an enzyme such as a polymerase required for replication of associated nucleic acid as in negative-strand RNA viruses.

A major surprise has been the difficulty in demonstrating nucleic acid in the semipurified preparations. Thus, a variety of procedures which destroy nucleic acid fail to inactivate the scrapie agent. These include nuclease digestion, u.v. irradiation at 254 nm wavelength, hydrolysis by divalent cations (Zn^{2+}), chemical modification by hydroxylamine, and reaction with psoralens (substances which associate with nucleic acids and form stable covalent linkage on photoactivation). It is possible to imagine that the nucleic acid is protected from some of these agents by a protein coat or shell, so the presence of DNA or RNA may not yet be totally excluded; nevertheless if nucleic acid be present, it must be in a different form from that found in true viruses, none of which are similarly resistant to all these procedures.

Perhaps most remarkable of all is the extremely small particle size associated with infectivity. We have noted that it has not been visualised by electron microscopy. Evidence from molecular sieving now indicates that particles as small as 50,000 mol. wt are infectious; this is about the size of a typical monomeric protein such as serum albumin and smaller than the most diminutive known viruses or viroids. If correct, the scrapie agent would easily be the smallest infectious agent known. As far as nucleic acid is concerned, a 50,000 mol. wt particle with a protein coat could enclose only about 32 nucleotides at most, or much less than would be required to code for a protein, so that other, non-template functions would have to be envisaged. This is of fundamental importance, for if the nucleic acid—which may yet be present—does not code for the coat protein, it would represent the major distinction between the unconventional agents and true viruses.

What structures for these agents can be envisaged in the light of this information? Firstly, although their characterisation cannot be completed until they have been purified to homo-geneity and their chemical structure determined, it is already clear from the foregoing that they are distinct from the familiar viruses, viroids and plasmids. Secondly, it is possible to rule out the suggestions that they are composed entirely of polysaccharide, of membranes or of nucleic acid, and the 'replicating poly-saccharide' and viroid hypotheses can be discarded. Instead, we can consider three possibilities. (i) These agents are very small particles which resemble viruses in having a nucleic acid genome surrounded and protected by a protein coat coded for by the genome. The particular properties of the protein could account for resistance to the denaturing and enzymatic procedures described above. (ii) The particles consist of protein and an oligonucleotide which is too small to code for the coat protein; instead the protein component is a product of the *host cell* and the role of the nucleic acid is to activate the relevant host cell genes. This regulatory rather than coding function for the nucleic acid would, as noted above, remove these agents from the realm of true viruses. (iii) The agents consist of *infectious proteins*, altogether devoid of nucleic acid; the term 'prion' (for proteinaceous infectious agent) has been suggested for such particles. In order to account for their replication, it would again be necessary for the protein to be host cell coded and, in addition, self-regulated in that it would activate (derepress) its own transcription. This process would be one of 'auto-induction' rather than true replication, and could be indirect, e.g. acting via a cell-surface receptor, or a more immediate interaction with elements controlling DNA expression. Such events can be contemplated because of physiological parallels in the regulation of pro-tein synthesis and gene expression; however, speculations that an infectious protein might code for its own replication by a pathway of 'reverse translation' or by directing its own synthesis are, for the present, solidly in the realm of science fiction. In any event, models (ii) and (iii) in which the protein component is host-derived might explain the absence of immune response against these agents, on the grounds of self-tolerance. An interesting parallel can also be drawn with the oncogene hypothesis for the cellular origin of RNA tumour viruses (p. 805).

Finally, while the spongiform encephalopathies themselves are very rare in man, we should remember that there is a range of chronic neurological disorders for which the aetiology has been sought in vain, from other pre-senile dementias to amyotrophic lateral sclerosis, Parkinson's disease and multiple sclerosis. The possible role of these unusual agents in such conditions will doubtless be investigated in coming years.

RETROVIRIDAE (ONCORNAVIRUSES)

For an account of these RNA viruses, many of which are tumour-causing (oncogenic), see Section 6, p. 776.

FURTHER READING

General

Buxton A. & Fraser G. (1977) *Animal Microbiology*, vol. 2. Blackwell Scientific Publications.

Davis B.D., Dulbecco R., Eisen H.N. & Ginsburg H.S. (1980) *Microbiology*, 3rd edn. Harper and Row.

Duguid J.P., Marmion B.P. & Swain R.H. (eds.) (1978) *Mackie and McCartney's Medical Microbiology* Volume 1: Microbial Infections, 13th edn. Churchill Livingstone.

Evans A.S. (ed.) (1978) *Viral infections of humans*. John Wiley.

Fenner F.J. & White D.O. (1976) *Medical Virology*, 2nd edn. Academic Press.

Fraenkel-Conrat H. & Kimball P.C. (1982) *Virology*. Prentice Hall

Horne R.W. (1978) *The Structure and Function of Viruses*. Institute of Biology's Studies in Biology no. 95. Edward Arnold.

Joklik W.K., Willett H.P. & Amos D.B. (eds.) (1980) *Zinsser, Microbiology*, 17th edn. Appleton Century Crofts.

Luria S.E., Darnell J.E.Jr., Baltimore D. & Campbell A. (1978) *General Virology*, 3rd edn. Wiley.

Metselaar D. & Simpson D.I.H. (1982) *Practical virology for medical students and practitioners in tropical countries*. Oxford University Press.

Nayak D.P. (ed.) (1977) *The Molecular Biology of Animal Viruses*. Marcel Dekker.

Primrose S.B. & Dimmock N.J. (1980) *Introduction to Modern Virology*, 2nd edn. Blackwell Scientific Publications.

Rowson K.E.K., Rees T.A.L. & Mahy B.W.J. (1981) *A Dictionary of Virology*. Blackwell Scientific Publications.

Volk W.A. (1978) *Essentials of Medical Microbiology*. J.B. Lippincott.

Specific topics

Almedia J.D. & Brand C.M. (1975) A morphological study of the internal component of influenzavirus. *J. Gen. Virol.*, **27**, 313.

Barry R.D. *et al.* (1978) Structure and function of the influenzavirus genome. In Mahy B.W.J. & Barry R.D. (eds.) *Negative Strand Viruses and the Host Cell*, p.1. Academic Press.

Blacklow N.R. & Cukor G. (1981) Viral gastroenteritis. *New Engl. J. Med.*, **304**, 397.

Blumberg B.S. (1977) Australia antigen and the biology of hepatitis B. *Science*, **197**, 17.

Buchmeier M.J., Welsh R.M., Durko F.J. & Oldstone M.B.A. (1980). The virology and immunobiology of lymphocytic choriomeningitis infection. *Advances in Immunology*, **30**, 275.

Caspar D.L.D. & Klug A. (1962) Physical principles in the construction of regular viruses. *Cold Spring Harbor Symp. Quant. Biol.*, **27**, 1.

Epstein M.A. & Achong B.G. (eds.) (1979) *Epstein–Barr Virus*. Springer Verlag.

Epstein M.A. (1982) Persistence of Epstein–Barr infections. *Symp. Soc. Gen. Microbiol.*, **33**, 97.

Feinstone S.M. & Purcell R.H. (1978) Non-A, non-B hepatitis. *Ann. Revs. Med.*, **9**, 359.

Fenner F.J. (1977) The eradication of smallpox. *Prog. Med. Virol.*, **23**, 1.

Fenner F.J. (1979) Portraits of viruses: The poxviruses. *Inter. Virol.*, **11**, 137.

Field H.J. & Wildy P. (1981) Recurrent herpes simplex: the outlook for systemic antiviral agents. *Brit. Med. J.*, **282**, 1821.

Gajdusek D.C. (1977) Unconventional viruses and the origin and disappearance of kuru. *Science*, **197**, 943.

Kilbourne E.D. (1979) Molecular epidemiology—influenza as archetype. *Harvey Lectures*, Series 73, 225.

Maugh T.H. (1979) Virus isolated from juvenile diabetic. *Science*, **204**, 1187.

Mims C.A. (1982) Role of persistence in viral pathogenesis. *Symp. Soc. Gen. Microbiol.*, **33**, 1.

Pereira M.S. (1982) Persistence of influenza in a population. *Symp. Soc. Gen. Microbiol.*, **33**, 15.

Pruisner S.B. (1982) Novel proteinaceous infectious particles cause scrapie. *Science*, **216**, 136.

Stewart W.E.II (1979) *The Interferon System*. Springer Verlag.

Szmuness W. (1978) Hepatocellular carcinoma and the hepatitis B virus. Evidence for a causal association. *Prog. Med. Virol.*, **24**, 40.

ter Meulen V. & Carter M.J. (1982) Morbillivirus persistent infections in animals and man. *Symp. Soc. Gen. Microbiol.*, **33**, 133.

ter Meulen V. & Katz M. (eds.) (1977) *Slow Virus Infections of the Nervous System*. Springer.

Tyrrell D.A.J. & Burke D.C. (eds.) (1982). Interferon: twenty five years on. *Philosoph. Transact. Roy. Soc.* B. **299**, 1–144.

Wildy P., Field H.J. & Nash A.A. (1982) Classical herpes latency revisited. *Symp. Soc. Gen. Microbiol.*, **33**, 133.

Work T.H. (1976) Exotic viral diseases. In Hunter G.W., Schwartzwelder J.C. & Clyde D.F. (eds.) *Tropical Medicine*, 5th edn., p.1.

This section deals firstly with the properties of bacteria in relation to their *pathogenicity*, including their structure, the nature of their products, and their genetics. Thereafter, some of the major groups of pathogenic bacteria of medical importance and the mechanisms of the diseases they cause are discussed in detail.

INTRODUCTION TO BACTERIAL PATHOGENICITY

The pathogenicity of a microorganism, defined as its ability to cause disease, is a complex quality dependent both on the properties of the organism (structure, toxic products), and on the capacity of the host to protect itself (natural barriers, defensive cells, immune response); in short, pathogenicity resides in the balance of the parasite–host relationship. For example, in circumstances in which a host's defensive mechanisms are sufficiently incompetent or damaged, many normally harmless organisms display some degree of pathogenicity; indeed, we shall be much concerned later with such *opportunistic pathogens* which require some impairment of host defence as a prelude to causing disease. However, our principal interest will initially be in those attributes which enable bacteria to cause disease in a previously healthy body. Two properties of pathogenic organisms which are shared by non-pathogens are *transmissibility*, the transfer of organisms to a host from another host or reservoir of infection, and *infectivity*, the ability of an organism to colonise (infect) its host, which for non-pathogens is restricted to a body surface such as the skin or mucous membranes of the gut, respiratory tract, etc. *Infection*, however, is clearly not synonymous with *disease*—thus the body is permanently infected, without deleterious consequences, by the many harmless commensals which make up the natural flora.

When disease occurs, infection is followed by tissue damage, pathological changes and clinical symptoms, which occur because pathogens possess one or both of two additional basic qualities lacking in non-pathogenic species, namely *invasiveness* and *toxigenicity*. Moreover, an organism may initiate tissue damage via the immunological consequences of its infection, in the form of *hypersensitivity* reactions (Section 2). Pathogenicity is ultimately dependent on the organism's ability to survive in the host (invasiveness); toxins may play a part in this. Once the hurdle of survival has been passed, damage to the host depends on toxigenicity (mostly in acute diseases) or hypersensitivity (mostly in chronic diseases).

INVASIVENESS

Invasiveness is the ability to pass through the natural barriers of skin or mucous membranes and establish growth in a body tissue, while at the same time resisting the cellular defence mechanisms of the host. This last point is crucial and usually implies that the organism has the means successfully to avoid destruction by the phagocytic cells (neutrophils, macrophages) which are the body's immediate defence when a tissue is invaded (Section 1). In the encounter with the phagocyte, a pathogen may have evolved one or more of three 'tactics': (i) avoidance of uptake by means of antiphagocytic surface properties associated with the cell wall or capsule which prevent endocytosis by neutrophils; (ii) avoidance of uptake through production of leucocidic toxins which kill phagocytic cells; and (iii) resistance to intracellular destruction, which is also often a result of the particular character of the cell wall and can lead to long-term survival of organisms in macrophages. Organisms which are adapted to avoid uptake are usually susceptible to destruction once successfully phagocytosed by a neutrophil; their life-style must therefore be one of *extracellular parasitism*. Moreover, since an antibody response leads to opsonisation (p. 145), the diseases caused by such organisms are often *acute* (e.g. pyogenic cocci). In contrast, bacteria which can resist the normal enzymatic and oxidative killing processes are *intracellular parasites* which may have no resistance to uptake at all (e.g. mycobacteria); they usually establish *chronic* diseases in which cell-mediated immunity is required for recovery. An additional factor which assists bacterial invasiveness, in the sense of spread through a tissue, is the production of *enzymes* which digest connective tissue, dissolve fibrin barriers, liquefy viscous pus, etc.

TOXIGENICITY

Toxigenicity is the ability to produce injurious substances known as *toxins*, which damage cells or interfere with their vital functions. Toxins may be extremely powerful poisons, such as those responsible for severe and lethal illnesses, including diphtheria, tetanus, cholera and anthrax, often acting at sites distant from the focus of infection. Toxins such as these are the major attribute conferring pathogenicity, without which the organism is harmless. On the other hand, there are also many less toxic molecules which act mainly as local accessories to invasion, such as the leucocidic toxins referred to above, and which may be relatively minor factors in pathogenicity. Two types of toxin are recognised, namely *exotoxins*, which are soluble proteins released by the organisms as they grow, and *endotoxins*, complex lipopolysaccharides which are a structural part of the outer envelope of Gram-negative bacteria and tend to be shed after the organism's death. A wide range of molecular mechanisms is involved in the action of toxins on cells, from intracellular enzymatic activity to effects on cell membranes or synaptic transmission.

The blend of invasiveness and toxigenicity varies from species to species, from organisms which are wholly invasive to others which are purely toxinogenic and may not even need to invade the body at all. Furthermore, within a species, variations exist between strains in the extent to which pathogenicity attributes are expressed. Clearly some indication of the *degree* of pathogenicity of different pathogenic organisms is required, and this is called *virulence*. It is reflected in the number of organisms required to cause disease—the smaller the number, the greater the virulence —and this forms the basis of experimental virulence tests such as the LD_{50} (the dose of organisms or toxin which will kill 50% of inoculated animals in a given time).

BACTERIAL STRUCTURE AND PATHOGENICITY

The structure of bacteria is fundamental to their pathogenicity and for many organisms one or more structural components are primary factors in disease production; even for organisms which derive their virulence through secretion of powerful toxins, structural considerations are often highly relevant. Structure determines the survival of organisms outside and inside the body, influences the mode of transmission, and often contributes to invasiveness, toxigenicity and development of host hypersensitivity.

The major elements of bacterial cells are shown schematically in Figure 4.1. Bacteria are *prokaryotes* with a *rigid cell wall* surrounding the cytoplasmic membrane. The wall itself may be covered with another outer layer, the *capsule*, and projecting from

Figure 4.1
(a) Structural elements of bacterial cells.
(b) Detail of Gram-positive and Gram-negative cell envelopes.

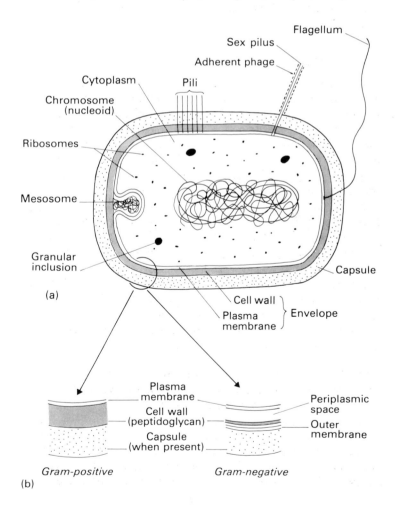

383

the surface may be appendages such as *flagella*, responsible for motility, or hair-like processes called *pili*. Other features of prokaryotic cells are the lack of a nuclear membrane around the DNA (nucleoid) and the absence of intracellular membranous organelles such as mitochondria, endoplasmic reticulum, Golgi apparatus and lysosomes. However, here we will be concerned less with the internal cellular details than with the outer structures which are of key importance in determining an organism's survival and its interaction with body cells and defence mechanisms.

The following are some important ways in which bacterial surface structures contribute to pathogenicity. (i) The cell envelope, which includes the wall, provides many organisms with the ability to survive adverse environmental conditions outside the body, such as drying, heat, disinfectants, etc. An extreme example is the specialised integument of bacterial spores. (ii) Pili are *adherence structures* which enable some organisms to bind to and colonise specific host tissues. (iii) In the encounter with phagocytes, particularly neutrophils, the capsule and/or cell wall often have important *antiphagocytic properties* which help the organisms to avoid being engulfed. (iv) Survival within phagocytic cells may derive from the resistance of certain bacterial envelopes to enzymes and oxidative mechanisms. (v) The wall may be sufficiently thick or have other properties which cause it to resist the damaging action of antibody and complement. (vi) Bacterial surface components are antigens and stimulate a host immune response, which may lead to damaging hypersensitivity, as well as to protective immunity. Sometimes, the tendency to hypersensitivity is promoted by certain *adjuvant* properties of the cell wall; in others it is due to *autoimmunity* resulting from cross-reactivity between cell wall antigens and body tissues. Where the antigens associated with virulence factors can be isolated they may be useful as vaccines; sometimes, however, there is so much antigenic diversity within a pathogenic species that immunity to reinfection is almost unattainable. Specific examples illustrating these points can be found in Table 4.1 and are described at greater length later in this section. In the pages which follow, bacterial structure is described in more general terms, relationships to disease being noted *en route*.

Morphology and staining properties

BACTERIAL FORM

Figure 4.2 shows the shapes of the common pathogenic species discussed later in the section as they appear under the light microscope. There are three main morphological forms, namely (a) spheres (*cocci*), (b) straight rods (*bacilli*), and (c) curved rods, which range from the comma-shaped vibrios to the rigid or flexuous spirals of spirilla and spirochaetes. Size also covers a wide range: cocci usually have a diameter of about 0.5 μm, bacilli range from 0.5 to 10 μm in length and 0.3 to 1.0 μm width, and spirochaetes may be up to 20 μm long and are exceedingly

Table 4.1 Bacterial structures associated with pathogenicity

Structure	Organism	Nature	Role
Capsule	Streptococcus pyogenes	Hyaluronic acid	Antiphagocytic
	Strep. pneumoniae (pneumococcus)	Polysaccharide	Antiphagocytic
	Haemophilus influenzae	Polysaccharide	Antiphagocytic
	Klebsiella pneumoniae	Polysaccharide	Antiphagocytic
	Pseudomonas aeruginosa	Polysaccharide	Antiphagocytic
	Neisseria meningitidis	Polysaccharide	Antiphagocytic
	Bacillus anthracis	Poly-D-glutamic acid	Antiphagocytic
	Salmonella typhi	Vi antigen (glycolipid)	Resistance to intracellular destruction
	Treponema pallidum	Mucopolysaccharide	Antiphagocytic?
Cell wall	Streptococcus pyogenes	M protein	Antiphagocytic
	Staphylococcus aureus	Protein A	Antiopsonic
	Mycobacterium tuberculosis, M. leprae	Wall lipids	Resistance to intracellular destruction
		Cord factor (glycolipid)	Damages mitochondria; adjuvant effect
		Sulphatides	Prevent lysosomal fusion
		Muramyl dipeptide	Adjuvant effect
Outer membrane	Escherichia coli, Salmonellae, Shigellae, Neisseriae, Pseudomonas	Lipopolysaccharide	Endotoxin; antiphagocytic
Pili	Neisseria gonorrhoeae	Protein	Adherence to genito-urinary epithelium; antiphagocytic
	Escherichia coli	Protein	Adherence to epithelium of small intestine

385

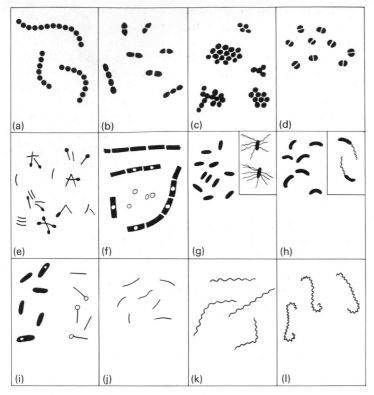

Figure 4.2 Bacterial morphology.
(a) Streptococci—1 μm diameter; chains.
(b) Pneumococci—1 μm diameter; pairs (diplococci) or short chains.
(c) Staphylococci—1 μm diameter; clusters.
(d) Neisseriae—0.8 μm diameter; bean-shaped diplococci.
(e) Corynebacteria—3 μm × 0.5 μm; club-shaped rods; Chinese-letter arrangement.
(f) Bacilli—4–8 μm × 1–1.5 μm; rectangular rods; central spores; some free spores shown.
(g) Enterobacteria—3–5 μm × 0.5 μm; rods; *inset*, flagella stain (e.g. *Salmonella*).
(h) Vibrios—1.5–3 μm × 0.5 μm; curved rods; *inset*: flagella stain.
(i) Clostridia—left, *Cl. perfringens*, 5 μm × 1 μm, rods, subterminal spores; right, *Cl. tetani*, 5 μm × 0.5 μm, rods, terminal spore, drumsticks.
(j) Mycobacteria—3 μm × 0.3 μm; rods, slightly curved.
(k) Treponemata—6–14 μm × 0.1 μm; flexuous, spiral (helical) filaments.
(l) Leptospirae—6–20 μm × 0.1 μm; finely coiled filaments with hooked ends.

narrow. Bacterial form is not related to the Gram staining reaction (below).

STAINING

The stain most widely used in bacterial identification is the *Gram stain*. This is of fundamental importance in classification as it is a differential stain used to distinguish two large categories of bacteria, *Gram-positive* and *Gram-negative*, depending on whether or not they retain the complex of methyl violet and iodine formed in the staining procedure. The reason Gram-reactivity is so important is that it correlates with the two major types of bacterial wall structure, and therefore also with other biological properties (Figure 4.1). In brief, Gram-positive organisms have a much thicker cell wall than Gram-negatives, are more susceptible than the latter to the antibacterial action of penicillin, acids, iodine, basic dyes and lysozyme, but less susceptible to alkalies, proteolytic enzymes or antibody and complement; Gram-negative walls are not only very much thinner and weaker, but are surrounded by an outer membrane which contains the toxic molecule endotoxin.

In the method, which was introduced in 1884 by the Danish bacteriologist Christian Gram, a heat-fixed bacterial smear on a slide is first stained with the basic dye, methyl violet (or crystal violet), which is taken up in equivalent amounts by both Gram-positive and Gram-negative cells; the smear is then treated with Gram's iodine solution (3% I_2-KI) to mordent (fix) the stain as a *dye-I₂ complex*, washed with alcohol or acetone and counterstained with a dye of a different colour (neutral red, safranin). Gram-positive organisms retain the original stain (resist decolourisation) and appear violet, while Gram-negatives are decolourised by alcohol or acetone and are stained pink by the counterstain. The complex is trapped inside Gram-positive cells as a result of the reduction in permeability of the thick wall that occurs on washing with the organic solvent (the wall itself does not stain), whereas the thin wall of Gram-negative cells and the probable discontinuities in the wall at sites of membrane adhesion (p. 394) allow the staining complex to be extracted. This explains why old or dead Gram-positive cells, in which the wall becomes more permeable as a result of autolysis, often stain Gram-negative.

A few bacterial species, notably mycobacteria, have walls which are unusual for their extremely high content of lipids (up to 60% of the dry weight of the wall). These organisms, which include the tubercle and leprosy bacilli, have a characteristic staining property known as *acid-fastness*, in which once stained they resist decolourisation in strong acids which remove stains from all other organisms. The procedure used, the *Ziehl–Neelsen method*, is described on p. 592.

Structure of the cell wall and envelope

The cell wall, which is present in all bacteria except mycoplasmas and certain halophilic organisms, is a rigid structure which determines the characteristic shapes of different bacteria and is responsible for their resistance to osmotic lysis, bacterial cells having a high internal osmotic pressure. Enzymatic removal of the wall in osmotically stabilising solutions (sucrose) converts Gram-positive cocci and rods into spherical 'protoplasts' and Gram-negative cells into 'spheroplasts' (which retain the outer membrane). Both are osmotically fragile and must be kept in hypertonic (0.2–0.5M) sucrose or salt solutions. (*L-forms* are variants, similar to protoplasts and spheroplasts, which have lost the ability to synthesize the wall.) The wall surrounds the cytoplasmic membrane and in Gram-negative organisms there is another lipid membrane outside the wall. The membrane(s) and cell wall are together known as the *envelope*, a term which is particularly appropriate for the complex outer structure of Gram-negative cells. Both Gram-positive and Gram-negative cells may be enclosed by a gel-like outer capsule.

Bacterial envelopes can be divided into three types on the basis of structure and composition, namely Gram-positve, Gram-negative and acid-fast, correlating with the staining criteria outlined above. The essential component of all bacterial cell walls is a giant molecule called *peptidoglycan* (also known as murein or mucopeptide), which consists of linear polysaccharide chains cross-linked by short peptides and is laid down in sheets around the cytoplasmic membrane. While the peptidoglycans of most organisms are of remarkably similar structure, the three types of envelope differ in the proteins, polysaccharides and lipids present, as well as in ultrastructure. The most notable distinguishing features are: (i) the unique outer membrane of Gram-negative organisms; (ii) the presence of polymers linked to the peptidoglycan, such as the teichoic acids of Gram-positive walls and the arabinogalactan of acid-fast cells, for which there are no equivalents in Gram-negative envelopes; and (iii) the complex lipids which are unique to the walls of acid-fast and related bacteria.

CELL WALL MOLECULES

Peptidoglycan

This huge, bag-shaped macromolecule forms the main structure of the cell wall. Its two components are long, linear chains of polysaccharides and short peptides, the latter being attached to and cross-linking the polysaccharide chains. The glycan component always consists of two acetyl-amino sugars, namely N-acetyl-D-glucosamine and N-acetylmuramic acid (the latter being unique to bacteria); they occur as a *repeating β-1,4-linked disaccharide*, the basic unit of the polysaccharide chains (Figure 4.3). Each muramic acid residue is also linked to a *tetrapeptide*, which is thus regularly repeated down the length of each chain; the composition of the tetrapeptide is often L-alanine, D-glutamine, L-lysine or D,L-diaminopimelic acid (meso-DAP), and D-alanine. The alternation of L- and D-amino acids adds

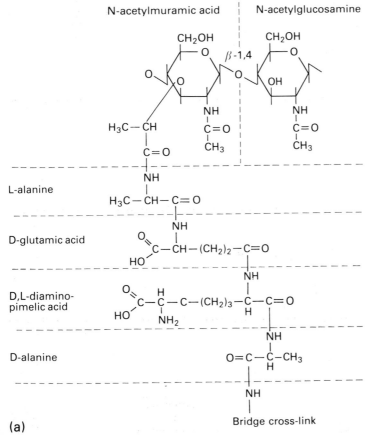

(a)

Figure 4.3 Structure of peptidoglycan.
(a) Repeating unit of *E. coli* peptidoglycan.
(b) Structure of peptidoglycan of *Staphyloccus aureus*.
   NAM = N-acetylmuramic acid;
   NAG = N-acetylglucosamine;
   a = L-alanine,
   b = D-glutamic acid,
   c = L-lysine,
   d = D-alanine,
   g = glycine.
(c) Structure of peptidoglycan of *E. coli*.
   Symbols as above, except
   c = D, L-diaminopimelic acid.

388

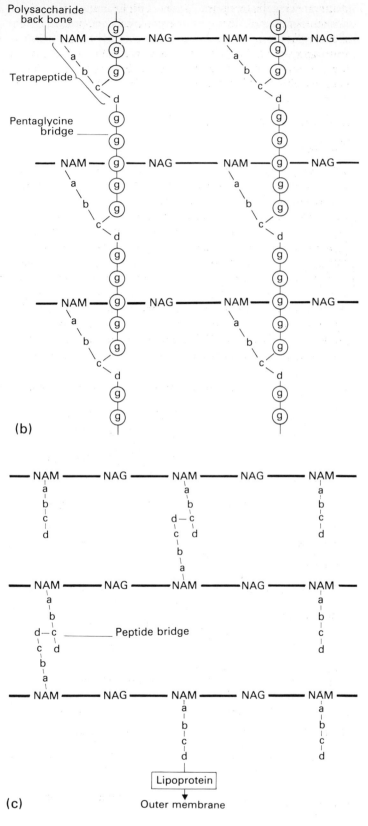

Polysaccharide back bone

Tetrapeptide

Pentaglycine bridge

(b)

Peptide bridge

Lipoprotein

Outer membrane

(c)

structural strength to the molecule. The D-amino acids are an unusual feature, as they are never found in proteins. The tetrapeptides cross-link adjacent polysaccharide strands in one of two main ways, either via a pentaglycine bridge connecting the lysine of one tetrapeptide and the D-alanine of another, or by a direct peptide bond between these same amino acids. The alternative structures are illustrated in Figure 4.3(b,c). The former is found in *Staphylococcus aureus* and streptococci, the latter in *Escherichia coli* and all other Gram-negative bacteria, as well as in *Corynebacterium diphtheriae* and the acid-fast mycobacteria. Note that in the *Staph. aureus* type of peptidoglycan, practically all tetrapeptides are cross-linked, while in the *E. coli* type, cross-linkages are sparser (30–70%).

The peptidoglycan molecule thus forms a two-dimensional molecular sheet which surrounds the cell; the wall of Gram-positive cells may consist of up to 40 such sheets layered in concentric fashion around each other, whereas in a Gram-negative wall there are only 1–3 peptidoglycan layers (a single layer in *E. coli*). There are also bridges between the sheets, as the layers do not peel apart in isolated walls. A feature of the peptidoglycan of Gram-negative cells is the covalent attachment of lipoproteins, which project into the outer membrane and anchor it to the cell wall.

Peptidoglycan is sensitive to degradation by several enzymes, which either attack the polysaccharides (glycosidases) or the peptides (endopeptidases) or cleave the junction between the tetrapeptides and muramic acid residues (amidases). Some of these enzmes are responsible for bacterial autolysis, such as the amidase which causes lysis of pneumococci in stationary cultures (p. 511). *Lysozyme* is an important glycosidase which hydrolyses the glycosidic bond between N-acetylmuramic acid and N-acetyl-glucosamine (Figure 4.4). It is thus bactericidal for many organisms, causing them to lyse, as discovered by Fleming in 1922. Through its presence in tears, saliva, nasal secretions, plasma and neutrophil granules, lysozyme functions as an important first line of defence against infection, though susceptibility is variable. Gram-positive organisms are generally more sensitive than Gram-negatives because the cell wall of the latter is relatively protected by the outer membrane; however, Gram-negative cells are probably destroyed by lysozyme after phagocytosis and/or the action of complement (which damages the outer membrane). Susceptibility is greater in bacteria which are in the rapid, log phase of growth, than in the stationary phase when peptidoglycan is thicker. Some important pathogens develop *lysozyme-resistant* mutants which have modifications of their peptidoglycan structure. Thus in resistant strains of *Staph. aureus*, N-acetylmuramic acid residues are O-acetylated, and in variants of *Strep. pyogenes* the N-acetyl groups are missing from N-acetylglucosamine; both these changes protect the wall from the action of lysozyme.

The cell wall peptidoglycan is also the site of action of certain antibiotics, most notably *penicillin*, which blocks the cross-linking reaction (transpeptidation) during peptidoglycan synthesis.

Figure 4.4 Action of lysozyme on the polysaccharide chains of peptidoglycan.

Lysozyme hydrolyses the (1–4) glycosidic bond between N-acetylmuramic acid (NAM) and N-acetylglucosamine (NAG) residues. (R: lactyl group of NAM, linked to tetrapeptide). (After Stryer, 1981)

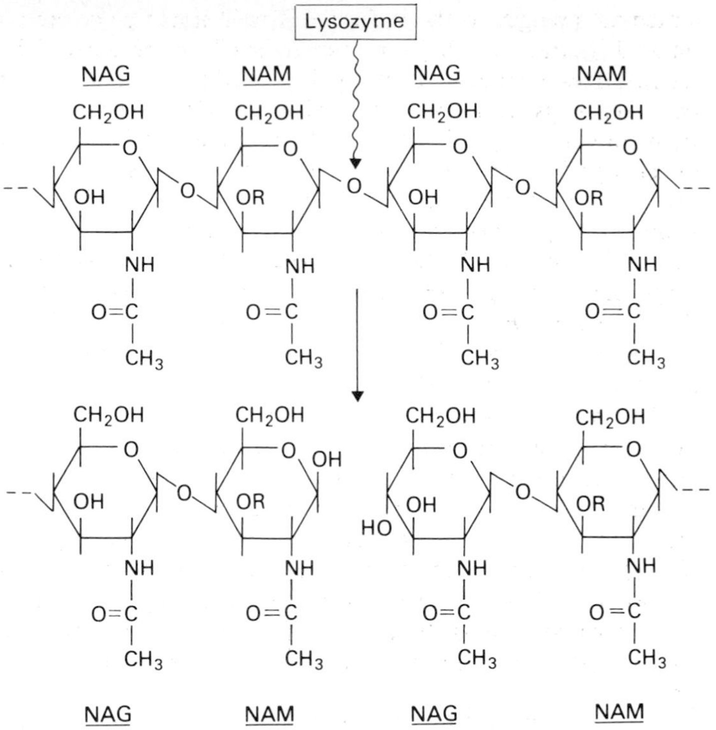

Proteins

Proteins may form part of the cell wall of Gram-positive organisms. A good example is the *M protein* of the pathogenic group A β-haemolytic streptococci, where it is present in the form of fine processes called fimbriae on the surface of the wall (see Figure 4.42). Together with the capsule, M protein is responsible for virulence by protecting the organisms from phagocytosis. As is often the case with such virulence components, there are a great many different types of M protein among group A streptococci, all antigenically distinct, and this forms the basis of serological identification of different strains using anti-M antibodies (p. 495). Another protein bound to peptidoglycan is *protein A* of *Staph. aureus*; it may also be released from the cell. Protein A binds the Fc region of IgG and may therefore assist in pathogenicity by competing with neutrophil receptors for the Fc of opsonising antibodies (p. 521). We have already noted the lipoprotein which is covalently linked to peptidoglycan of Gram-negative cells; other proteins are found in the outer membrane (p. 396).

Teichoic acids

Teichoic acids are acidic polymers which are found in the walls of Gram-positive, but not Gram-negative, bacteria and are linked to the peptidoglycan; they may comprise a large part (10–50%) of the dry weight of the wall. Teichoic aids are present on the cell surface where they are often important antigens (e.g. in streptococci and staphylococci). They are polymers of glycerol or ribitol linked by phosphodiester bridges, with the available hydroxyl groups coupled to sugars (eg. glucose) and/or esterified to D-alanine residues (Figure 4.5). The presence of so many repeating phosphate groups makes them highly acidic, negatively-charged molecules, and it is thought that their main function is in binding cations such as magnesium (Mg^{2+}) which can then be taken into the cell (Mg^{2+} being required for the action of many enzymes and the integrity of ribosomes).

Teichoic acids are found in the walls of most Gram-positive organisms, though lacking in a few species. Also usually found are closely related molecules called *lipoteichoic acids*; these are typical glycerol teichoic acids which are linked to a glycolipid in the cytoplasmic membrane rather than peptidoglycan. They extend through the wall and are present on the surface as antigens. The capsules of many pneumococci consist of teichoic acid-like polymers which appear to be cell-bound; they function as antiphagocytic structures.

Figure 4.6 (*opposite*) Cell envelopes of Gram-positive and Gram-negative bacteria.
(a) Gram-positive.
(b) Gram-negative.
(c) Detailed structure of Gram-negative bacterial envelope.
*A capsule is not always present, nor invariably polysaccharide.

Structure of the Gram-positive cell wall (Figure 4.6a)

The 'typical' Gram-positive wall is a thick layer of peptidoglycan closely associated with the cytoplasmic membrane; teichoic acids and lipoteichoic acids are found on the surface and in some cases there is an outer protein layer (e.g. group A streptococci). There may also be other cell wall carbohydrates (not shown), such as the group-specific C-carbohydrate of streptococci (p. 497). The wall may be surrounded by a capsule.

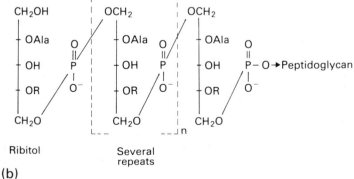

Figure 4.5 Structure of teichoic acids.
(a) Glycerol teichoic acid. R = glucose or D-alanine.
(b) Ribitol teichoic acid. Ala = D-alanine, R = glucose.

392

Structural layer   Composition

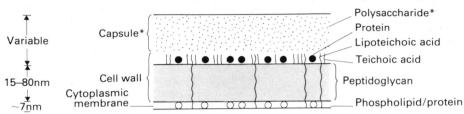

(a)

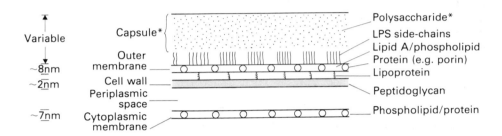

(b)

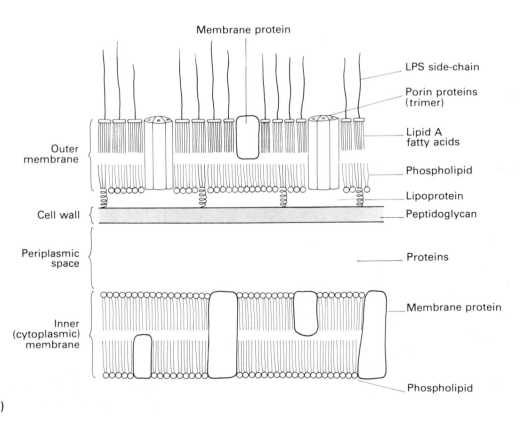

(c)

The envelope of Gram-negative cells (Figure 4.6b).

The envelope of Gram-negative cells is more complex in ultra-structure and composition. Four layers can usually be discerned by electron microscopy; starting on the inside, they are (a) the cytoplasmic membrane, (b) a structureless *periplasmic space*, (c) the very thin peptidoglycan cell wall, and (d) the outer membrane, usually closely associated with the cell wall. The outer membrane contains the *lipopolysaccharide* (LPS) character-istic of Gram-negative bacteria, phospholipid, and *matrix proteins* which act, *inter alia*, as receptors and molecular pores (porins) for the non-selective passage of small molecules in solution. The periplasmic space contains several hydrolytic enzymes and specific transport proteins (periplasmic binding proteins), which are also involved in chemotaxis; they can be released by cold osmotic shock, which damages the cell wall and outer membrane. There are many sites of adhesion between the outer membrane and the cytoplasmic membrane (Bayer's patches), which can break up the continuity of the peptidoglycan layer.

STRUCTURE OF THE OUTER MEMBRANE

Figure 4.6c shows the components of the outer membrane; its outer surface is composed of LPS and protein, while the inner surface is phospholipid and protein. Thus, like cytoplasmic membranes, it is essentially a lipid bilayer with interspersed proteins, but whereas both layers of the cytoplasmic membrane contain equal amounts of phospholipid, the outer membrane is an asymmetric structure in which all the LPS is on the outside and most of the phospholipid is on the inside. The outer membrane is tightly organised and its proteins have less freedom of movement than those in other membranes.

Lipopolysaccharides

Lipopolysaccharides are fundamental to many of the biological properties of Gram-negative bacteria, as well as to their membrane structure. As the name suggests, they are composed of lipid and polysaccharide; the molecules are toxic and are the *endotoxins* present in most Gram-negative organisms. (The term endotoxin is used to indicate a heat-stable, polysaccharide-like toxin bound to the cell, in contrast with the heat-labile, secreted, protein exotoxins found in cell-free culture fluids; see p. 438.) Like other membrane molecules, LPS is *amphipathic*, i.e. has both hydrophobic and hydrophilic parts. Thus, in aqueous solution it forms large micelles with the lipid on the inside, which have a molecular weight of over 10^6; the micelles can be disrupted into individual units by detergent.

The structure of LPS is shown in Figure 4.7a. It is a complex molecule ($\sim 10,000$ mol.wt) which has three regions, known as lipid A, core oligosaccharide and O side-chain. *Lipid A* consists of six saturated fatty acid chains linked to two glucosamine residues;

Figure 4.7

(a) Schematic structure of the lipopolysaccharide (LPS) molecule.
GlcN = glucosamine
P = phosphate.
(b) Composition of the core oligosaccharide and side chain of LPS of *Salmonella typhimurium*.

Abe = abequose
EtN = ethanolamine
Gal = galactose
Glc = glucose
GlcN = glucosamine
GlcNAc = N-acetylglucosamine
Hep = heptulose
KDO = 2-keto-3-deoxygoctonate
Man = mannose
Rha = L-rhamnose.

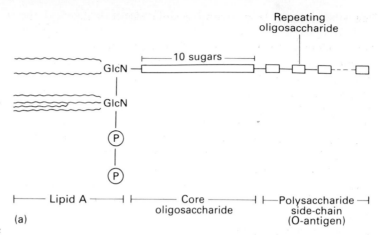

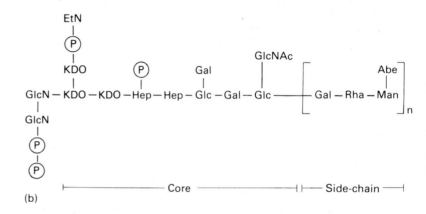

it is these fatty acids which form the outer layer of the membrane. The core oligosaccharide is a short, branched chain attached to one of the glucosamines and consisting of ten sugar units, among them the unusual 8-carbon sugar, 2-keto-3-deoxyoctonate (KDO), and the 7-carbon sugar, heptose (both unique to bacteria). The core region is acidic, due to phosphorylation of the sugars. Attached to the end of the core is a long polysaccharide *side chain*, which consists of up to 40 repeated oligosaccharide units of 3–4 sugar residues each; among them are also found some unusual sugars, such as rhamnose and abequose. In contrast with lipid A, the core and side chain are very hydrophilic and project outwards in whisker-like fashion from the membrane into the aqueous surround. The length of the side chains (i.e. the number of oligosaccharide repeats) is variable, even on the same cell. The side chains are the important *somatic O antigens* against which antibodies are made during infection and which are invaluable in classification of salmonellae and *E. coli*. There is a great diversity among O antigens, due to the numerous possible different sugar combinations in the side chains. As with streptococcal M proteins, this diversity is an advantage to pathogenic species as it enables a strain or type to avoid antibodies resulting from previous infection by a related strain. While the lipid of endotoxin is much the same among all Gram-negative genera, the core composition is characteristic of a genus, with species or strain individuality occurring in the side chains.

As *endotoxin*, LPS is an important factor in the toxigenicity of pathogenic Gram-negative bacteria (e.g. neisseriae, enterobacteriaceae). The effects of endotoxin and its contribution to pathogenesis are described on p. 438; they range from production of fever, as in typhoid, to the fatal consequences of Gram-negative septicaemia (septic shock). A significant part of its action is the activation of complement via the *alternative pathway* (p. 123), which may lead to death of the bacterial cell, since fixed complement damages the outer membrane and encourages uptake by neutrophils. Complement activation in the bloodstream during septicaemia has important pathological consequences (p. 445). The toxic activities of LPS are due to lipid A.

As far as *invasiveness* is concerned, LPS contributes to virulence by causing resistance to phagocytosis. This is demonstrated by the decrease in virulence of mutant (rough) organisms which lack the O side-chains. A series of mutations occurs on subculturing a pathogenic strain, accompanied by a stepwise change in the form of the colonies growing on agar, from the 'smooth' colonies of virulent organisms to a 'rough' or granular appearance. Rough organisms cannot be agglutinated by anti-O sera and at the same time lose their invasiveness, being more readily engulfed by neutrophils. The antiphagocytic effect of LPS can be attributed to the very hydrophilic nature of the O side-chains.

Porins and permeability

The outer membrane acts as a molecular sieve which is non-specifically permeable to hydrophilic molecules of up to about 600 mol.wt; in this respect it differs from the cytoplasmic membrane, which is highly selective in the molecules which can pass through it. The permeability of the outer membrane is due to transmembrane matrix proteins called *porins* (mol.wt 37,000); these assemble as trimers to form channels, regular arrays of which can be seen by electron microscopy. Each channel is approximately 10Å in diameter and about 10^5 channels cover the surface of the membrane. In addition, there are specific transport proteins for the uptake of larger metabolites such as maltose oligosaccharides, vitamin B_{12} and nucleosides, which diffuse too slowly through the porin channels. The outer membrane is much less permeable to hydrophobic or amphipathic molecules, probably because the pores are lined with polar groups and filled with water. In consequence, Gram-negative cells are generally less sensitive to antibiotics than Gram-positives and this has contributed to their increased prominence as pathogens since the widespread use of antibiotics (p. 484). Thus, the outer membrane acts as a *selective barrier* to external molecules, as well as preventing the loss of proteins and enzymes from the periplasmic space, a compartment which seems to have no equivalent in Gram-positive cells.

The outer membrane and the peptidoglycan are closely attached, remaining adherent to each other after mechanical disruption of the wall. Attachment involves both divalent metal ions (e.g. Mg^{2+}) and specialised *lipoproteins*. The latter consist of a small protein covalently attached to fatty acids; the protein moiety is linked to the peptidoglycan while the fatty acids are inserted into the outer membrane. Thus the lipoproteins anchor the outer membrane to the cell wall, as well as imparting stability (Figure 4.6c). The lipoproteins have an unusual composition and structure. The protein consists of only 58 amino acids and contains no histidine, proline, phenylalanine or tryptophan; it forms a *highly ordered α-helix*, linked at the C-terminus to diaminopimelic acid residues on the peptidoglycan. Attachment of the lipid to the protein includes a thoiether bond to a diglyceride. There is one lipoprotein molecule for every 10–12 peptidoglycan disaccharide units.

The wall of acid-fast bacteria

The cell wall of mycobacteria differs from those of Gram-positive and Gram-negative organisms in containing a very high proportion of characteristic *lipids* linked to sugar residues (glycolipids). The unusual composition of the wall gives these organisms the distinctive acid-fast staining property, in which they resist decolourisation with acid. The only other organisms to show acid-fastness are some species of nocardiae; however, similarities in wall composition are shared by the corynebacteria, and the three genera are therefore sometimes grouped together (the CMN group). The waxy, hydrophobic wall is responsible for many of the characteristic features of mycobacterial growth and pathogenicity (more fully discussed on p. 590); most important among the latter is their high degree of resistance to intracellular killing and degradation by phagocytes, which enables them to survive and grow inside normal macrophages and become a persistent stimulus to the immune system.

Much of the lipid is in the form of esterified *mycolic acids*, which occur both bound to cell wall polysaccharide and as unbound glycolipids important in virulence, called *cord factors*. While mycolic acids occur in all three CMN genera, they are only bound to the cell wall in mycobacteria and nocardiae. There is also a characteristic polysaccharide composed of arabinose and galactose in the wall of CMN organisms (*arabinogalactan*); teichoic acids are apparently absent.

MYCOLIC ACIDS

These are long-chain, branched, β-hydroxy fatty acids (Figure 4.8a); mycobacteria, nocardiae and corynebacteria each produce a characteristic mycolic acid of different chain length. The synthesis of mycolic acid in *Mycobacterium tuberculosis* is inhibited by *isoniazid*, the drug used in treatment of tuberculosis.

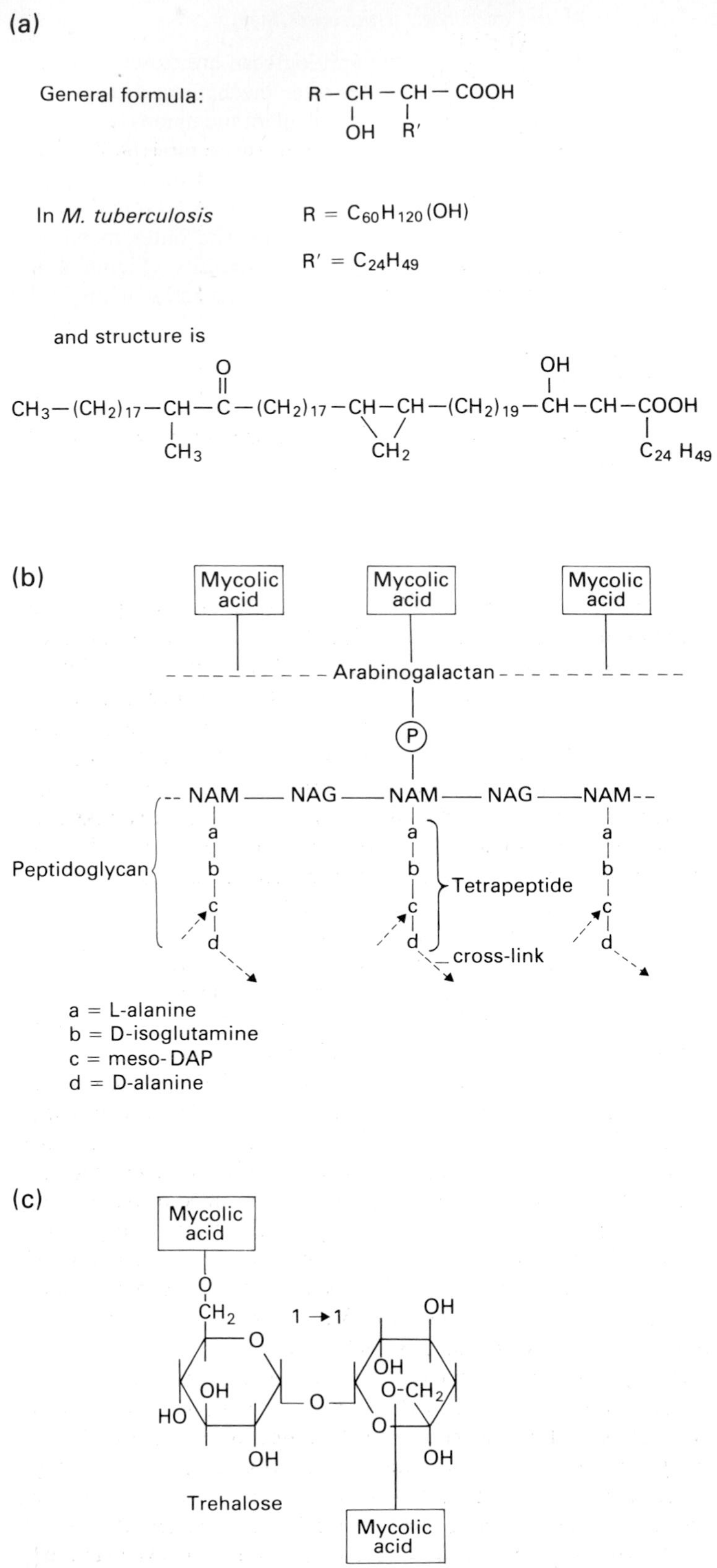

(a)

General formula: $R - CH - CH - COOH$

  with OH, R' below

In *M. tuberculosis* $R = C_{60}H_{120}(OH)$

$R' = C_{24}H_{49}$

and structure is

$$CH_3-(CH_2)_{17}-CH-\overset{O}{\overset{\|}{C}}-(CH_2)_{17}-CH-CH-(CH_2)_{19}-\overset{OH}{CH}-CH-COOH$$

with CH_3 , CH_2 , $C_{24}H_{49}$ below

Figure 4.8 Structural components of cell walls of mycobacteria.
(a) Mycolic acid.
(b) Wax D (cell wall).
(c) Cord factor (Trehalose-6, 6'-dimycolate)
(d) Muramyl dipeptide.

(b)

Mycolic acid | Mycolic acid | Mycolic acid

- - - - - - - - - Arabinogalactan - - - - - - - - -

(P)

-- NAM —— NAG —— NAM —— NAG ——NAM--

Peptidoglycan

a = L-alanine
b = D-isoglutamine
c = meso- DAP
d = D-alanine

Tetrapeptide

cross-link

(c)

Mycolic acid

CH_2 $1 \rightarrow 1$ OH

Trehalose

Mycolic acid

(d)

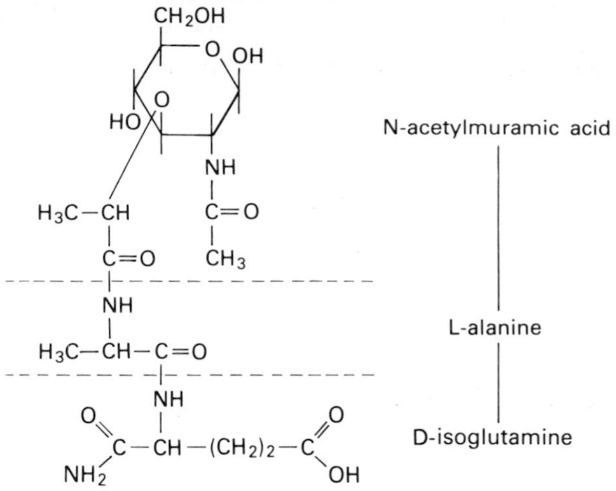

CH_2OH

O OH

HO O

NH

H_3C-CH C=O

C=O CH_3

NH

$H_3C-CH-C=O$

NH

O

C—CH—$(CH_2)_2$—C

NH_2 OH

O

N-acetylmuramic acid

L-alanine

D-isoglutamine

In mycobacteria, mycolic acids are linked to the peptidoglycan via arabinogalactan, which is coupled by phosphate residues to muramic acid (Figure 4.8b). When the wall is extracted with chloroform, a fraction known as *wax D* is isolatable, which consists of this basic wall structure (i.e. a mycolic acid—arabinogalactan—peptidoglycan complex); wax D is now known to be a degradation product of the wall, resulting from partial autolysis of dead cells. (Chemically, it is not a true wax as the mycolic acid is linked to sugars, whereas in a wax, fatty acids are coupled to higher alcohols.) At one time there was a great deal of interest in wax D as it retains the adjuvant (i.e. immunostimulating) properties of mycobacteria, which lead to development of the vigorous cell-mediated immune response in tuberculosis and leprosy. However, it is now clear that neither mycolic acids nor arabinogalactan are required for adjuvanticity, which resides in the structure of the peptidoglycan (see muramyl dipeptide below).

Besides being linked to the cell wall itself, mycolic acids are found as free glycolipids, namely *trehalose-6, 6'-dimycolates* (cord factor). Trehalose is a disaccharide of glucose and, in the cord factor molecule, one mycolic acid is esterified to each glucose residue (Figure 4.8c). The cord factors are so called because when they are present in the wall the organisms grow in serpentine cords. They show a close correlation with the virulence of mycobacteria; purified cord factors have toxic properties and induce granulomatous reactions (tubercles) in the lungs when injected into mice (see also p. 593). Mycolic acids also occur in *sulphatides (sulpholipids)*, conjugates of trehalose sulphate similar in structure to cord factor. These substances also show a correlation with virulence and are thought to prevent the fusion of lysosomes with phagosomes in macrophages, thus assisting mycobacteria in their intracelluar survival. Sulphatides are responsible for binding of neutral red by mycobacteria.

Another type of complex glycolipid found in mycobacterial

walls is called a *mycoside*. Mycosides are non-toxic, non-immunogenic, type-specific molecules which influence colony form and susceptibility to bacteriophages, for which they act as receptors; however, they show no relationship to pathogenicity.

MURAMYL DIPEPTIDE

A great deal of importance in the pathogenicity of mycobacteria is attached to their immunostimulating or adjuvant properties (p. 591); these are also exploited experimentally in *complete Freund's adjuvant*, a suspension of killed mycobacteria in mineral oil which enhances cell-mediated and antibody responses when made into an emulsion with an antigen in aqueous solution (p. 80). It was shown in 1958 that wax D could replace whole mycobacteria in this adjuvant, but since then the portion of the degraded wall required for immunostimulation has been progressively better defined. The minimal structure is now known to be a fragment of peptidoglycan called *muramyl dipeptide* (MDP), consisting simply of N-acetylmuramic acid linked to L-alanine and D-isoglutamine (Figure 4.8d). Interestingly, this structure is present in the peptidoglycan of many bacteria (Figure 4.3) and it is therefore perhaps not the only factor in the immunostimulating action of mycobacteria. MDP also enhances non-specific immunity to bacterial infection, demonstrable in mice by their relative resistance to challenge with *Klebsiella pneumoniae* after MDP administration.

Bacterial capsules and slimes

Many Gram-positive and Gram-negative cells are surrounded by a thick, viscous, gel-like material adherent to the wall, known as a *capsule*; when it is only loosely associated with the wall and easily washed off, it is called a *slime layer*. Capsules can be seen in the light microscope by 'negative staining' in which the organism is suspended in India ink, the capsule standing out as a halo-like border. Capsules are of variable thickness; those of klebsiellae and pneumococci can be particularly copious (up to 10 μm), while the *microcapsules* of *E. coli* and salmonellae are too thin to be visible by light microscopy and are only detected by antisera. The capsule has no particular ultrastructure discernable with the electron microscope. Capsular and slime material is soluble and can often be detected in culture filtrates (hence the term 'specific soluble substance', SSS); soluble material diffuses from the surface or is released by partial hydrolysis.

The presence of a capsule or slime is never essential for viability and in this respect it can be considered dispensable. Thus, within a given species there may be encapsulated and non-encapsulated strains, and variants of the former which have lost the ability to synthesize capsular material as a result of mutation. This is reflected in the morphology of colonies growing on agar. The colonies of organisms with well-developed capsules or slime layers are either *mucoid* (glistening, confluent appearance) or *smooth* (firm, uniform texture), whereas non-encapsulated organisms form *rough* (granular) colonies. A mutation leading to capsular loss is thus accompanied by a change in colonial morphology, from mucoid or smooth to rough. Note that these terms are also used in reference to the organisms themselves, e.g. smooth or 'S' forms of pneumococci are encapsulated, while rough or 'R' forms are non-encapsulated variants.

While the capsule is not necessary for the growth of organisms in culture, it is very often essential to the survival of bacteria in the body and is of major importance in the invasiveness of extracellular pathogens. Its role is usually to prevent phagocytosis (uptake) by neutrophils and for several invasive organisms this is the most important factor in pathogenicity. Thus, smooth encapsulated pneumococci resist phagocytosis and are virulent, while their rough non-encapsulated variants are harmless, being easily phagocytosed and destroyed (p. 513). Other examples of antiphagocytic capsules are listed in Table 4.1.

Capsules and slimes are chemically diverse in composition, but are mostly *acidic polysaccharides*; the acid groups are usually glucuronic acid or phosphate. There are a few examples of non-carbohydrate capsules, such as the poly-D-glutamic acid of *Bacillus anthracis* and the protein capsule of *Yersinia pestis*. Some examples of capsular composition are given in Table 4.2. The polysaccharides of pneumococci, *Klebsiella pneumoniae* and *Strep. pyogenes* are composed of repeating oligosaccharide units; each unit comprises two to four monosaccharides, one of which is a uronic acid. Thus, hyaluronic acid (*Strep. pyogenes*) consists of repeating units of glucuronic acid and N-acetylglucosamine, while type 3 pneumococcal polysaccharide is a polymer of glucuronic acid and glucose (cellobiuronic aid, Figure 4.9). Some capsules are teichoic acids (e.g. type 6 and type 8 pneumococci).

Table 4.2 Chemical composition of some bacterial capsules.

Organism	Capsule	Composition*
Streptococcus pyogenes	Hyaluronic acid	N-acetylglucosamine, glucuronic acid
Streptococcus pneumoniae (pneumococcus)	Type 2 polysaccharide	Glucose, L-rhamnose glucuronic acid
	Type 3 polysaccharide	Glucose, glucuronic acid
	Type 6 teichoic acid	Galactose, glucose, L-rhamnose, ribitol phosphate
Klebsiella pneumoniae	Polysaccharide	Glucose, fucose, glucuronic acid, pyruvic acid
Neisseria meningitidis	Serogroup A polysaccharide	N-acetyl-O-acetylmannosamine
	Serogroup B polysaccharide	N-acetylneuraminic acid
	Serogroup C polysaccharide	N-acetyl-O-acetylneuraminic acid
Bacillus anthracis	Polypeptide	D-glutamic acid

* (sugars are D isomers unless otherwise indicated)

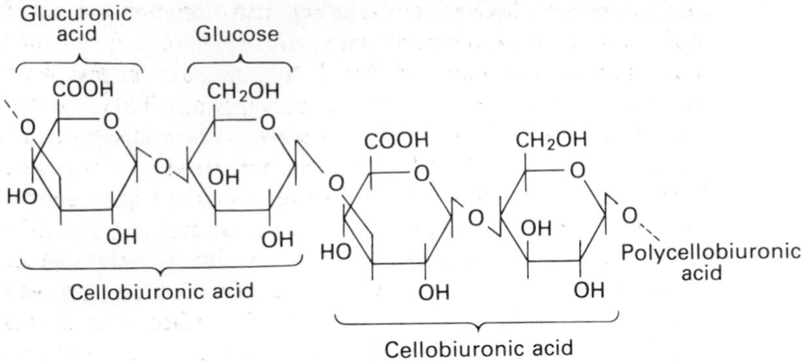

Figure 4.9 Structure of type 3 pneumococcal capsular polysaccharide (after Willett, H.P., in Joklik *et al* 1980)

In general, capsular material can be 'washed' off the cell and is not covalently attached to the wall, although the teichoic acids of pneumococci are probably bound to peptidoglycan. The hydrophilic, acidic nature of capsular material is probably responsible for its antiphagocytic properties, making it difficult for the membrane of the neutrophil to interact successfully with the organism's surface.

Capsules are usually antigenic (an important exception is the hyaluronic acid of *Strep. pyogenes*) and stimulate antibody production; the antibodies are opsonins which overcome the antiphagocytic action of the capsule by acting, together with complement, as a link between the organisms and Fc or C3b receptors on the neutrophil surface (Figure 2.41). Soluble capsular material released into solution from the bacterial surface can block opsonising antibodies and hence prolong an organism's extracellular survival (e.g. that of pneumococci during lobar pneumonia, p. 514). Anticapsular antibodies can be very useful in bacterial identification. Thus, some species produce a wide range of structurally, and therefore antigenically, distinct capsular polysaccharides, each of which gives rise to corresponding specific antibodies; the latter can then be used to assign individual organisms to a group or type. For example, there are over 80 distinct pneumococcal polysaccharides, each produced by a different pneumococcal 'type' and recognisable by a specific antibody. *Haemophilus influenzae* and *Klebsiella pneumoniae* also have several type-specific polysaccharides. Each polysaccharide is genetically determined and hence a permanent characteristic of the type (unless lost through mutation). The reaction between anticapsular antibody and the organism can be recognised microscopically as a reaction of capsular swelling or 'quellung', in which the capsule becomes larger and more distinct (refractile) after treatment with specific antiserum (Figure 4.46).

Pili

The electron microscope reveals the presence of fine hair-like filaments called pili (or fimbriae) on the surface of many Gram-negative bacteria; up to 200 may be present on a cell of *E. coli*, evenly distributed over the entire surface (Figure 4.52c). In contrast, nearly all Gram-positive organisms are non-piliated. In addition to these abundant *common pili*, cells of *E. coli* (and other conjugative bacteria) may possess 1–4 specialised *sex pili*, which are much longer and involved in conjugation. They are only present on 'male' (donor) cells and serve both to attach them to 'female' (recipient) cells and probably as channels for the passage of DNA (p. 458). Sex pili have receptors for bacteriophages; the latter can be seen along their length in electron micrographs (Figure 4.52b). Pili function as *adhesive structures* which enable bacteria to adhere to the surface of tissue cells or, in the case of sex pili, to each other; they bind to sugar residues on cell surface glycoproteins and for this reason piliated cells cause agglutination of red cells. Haemagglutination by *E. coli* is inhibitable by D-mannose and α-D-methylmannoside. In addition, pili sometimes have anti-phagocytic properties (e.g. gonococci).

The adherence properties of pili play a vital pathogenic role for some organisms, enabling them to bind to the surface of a host tissue as a prelude to colonisation or invasion (*colonisation factors*). Good examples are (i) the pili of gonococci (*Neisseria gonorrhoeae*), without which infection of the genito-urinary tract in gonorrhoea cannot occur (p. 533), and (ii) those of entero-pathogenic (diarrhoeal) strains of *E. coli*, which enable the organisms to adhere to the surface of the small intestine of man, piglets and calves, where they cause diarrhoea by secretion of enterotoxins (p. 544). The pili of enteropathogenic *E. coli* can be identified by specific antigens and, in human strains, by haemag-glutination which is resistant to inhibition by mannose. Note that the term 'fimbriae' is also applied to the very fine whisps of M protein on the surface of *Strep. pyogenes*; however, these are much finer and shorter than the pili of Gram-negative cells.

Flagella

Many species of bacteria, both Gram-positive and Gram-negative, are *motile* due to the presence of flagella—long, thin, helical filaments attached to the cell surface. They are composed of repeating subunits of a 53,000 mol.wt protein called *flagellin* and are structurally much less complicated than eukaryotic flagella or cilia; a flagellum can be dissociated into flagellin subunits in mild acid (pH3) and is spontaneously reconstituted on neutralisation. The number and arrangement of flagella varies among different species and may be single or multiple, *polar* (found at one or both ends of the cell) or *peritrichous* (randomly distributed over the surface) as shown in Figure 4.10a. They are often several times longer than the cell itself (up to 12 μm), but are too thin to be seen by ordinary microscopy without staining. They are rendered visible by coating with special stains precipitated onto the surface to increase their diameter; alternatively, they can be seen with dark-field microscopy. Each flagellum has a fixed, helical shape, accounting for its wavy appearance in two dimensions, the wavelength being a species characteristic.

The mode of insertion of a flagellum into the cell envelope is shown in Figure 4.10b, c. The filament is attached to a 'hook' at the

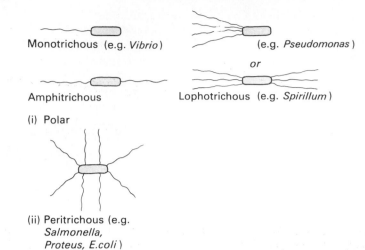

Monotrichous (e.g. *Vibrio*)

(e.g. *Pseudomonas*)

or

Amphitrichous

Lophotrichous (e.g. *Spirillum*)

(i) Polar

(ii) Peritrichous (e.g.
   *Salmonella,
   Proteus, E.coli*)

(a)

Figure 4.10 Bacterial flagella.
(a) Types of flagellation
(b) Model for the structure of the
insertion region of the *E. coli*
flagellum. L, P, S, M are rings
attaching the flagellum to
membranes or peptidoglycan
(after Adler (1976) *Scientific
American*, **234**(4), 46.)
(c) Electron micrographs of
flagella showing (i) filament
attached to envelope fragment
(1 cm : 100 nm); (ii) filament and
hook (1.3 cm : 50 nm); and
(iii) basal body with anchorage
rings inserted into the envelope
(2.3 cm : 50 nm). (Courtesy of Dr
E.A. Munn.)
(d) Appearance of peritrichous
flagella during bacterial
movement.

Filament

Hook

L ring

Outer membrane

Peptidoglycan

P ring

Basal body

Rod

S ring

Periplasmic space

Cytoplasmic
membrane

M ring

(b)

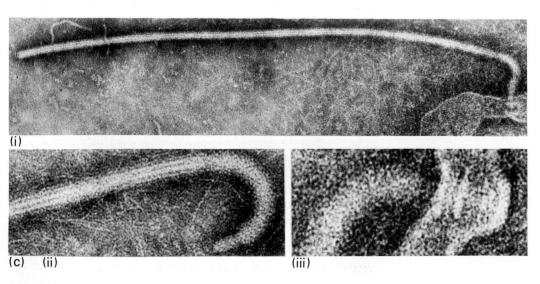

(i)

(c) (ii) (iii)

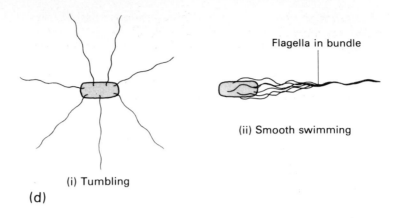

Flagella in bundle

(ii) Smooth swimming

(i) Tumbling

(d)

cell surface, the hook in turn being attached to a 'basal body'. In *E. coli*, the basal body comprises four rings, an outer pair (L, P) associated with the outer membrane and peptidoglycan, and an inner pair (S, M) anchoring to the plasma membrane. The hook and rings consist of different specialised proteins.

The basal body is the 'motor' which drives the flagellum in a rotatory motion; i.e. flagella spin around their long axis rather than beat up and down. Multiflagellated bacteria such as *E. coli* or salmonellae show two kinds of movement, a directional *smooth swimming* in a more-or-less straight line, alternating with a random *tumbling*. These two motions are determined by the direction of rotation of the flagella: when they rotate anticlockwise, the filaments form a single, coordinated bundle which drives the cell along (Figure 4.10d), but clockwise rotation disrupts the bundle, causing the filaments to separate and, since each then pulls the cell in a different direction, tumbling occurs. Typically, *E. coli* swims in a single direction for about 1 second at a time and then tumbles, changing course as a result.

Motile bacteria demonstrate *chemotaxis*, directional movement towards an attractive substance or away from a repellent one, and in this the frequency of tumbling is very important. Bacteria are usually attracted by nutrients (sugars, amino acids) and repelled by toxic or excretory products (fatty acids, hydrophobic amino acids, acid or alkaline pH). When swimming towards an attractant (*positive chemotaxis*), tumbling is less frequent, allowing the organism to swim smoothly for a longer time; and vice versa, when moving away from a repellent (*negative chemotaxis*) tumbling occurs more often.

During positive chemotaxis, organisms move along gradients of concentration of attractive substances; the bacterial cell must therefore possess some means of detecting individual attractants and coordinating flagellar movements accordingly. Detection of specific molecules depends on *chemoreceptors* of which at least twenty have been identified in *E. coli*; they are proteins located in the periplasmic space and besides being involved in chemotaxis are also the specific transport proteins for the nutrient concerned. Thus the chemoreceptor for a particular sugar, such as galactose or glucose, is at the same time the trigger for chemotaxis towards that sugar and responsible for its uptake into the cell. The transfer of information from periplasmic chemoreceptors to flagella takes place via intermediate proteins known as methyl-accepting chemotaxis proteins (MCPs), which undergo *reversible methylation* (Figure 4.11). Three distinct MCPs are known, products of bacterial genes called *tsr*, *tar* and *trg*. The degree of methylation of these proteins is increased after binding of attractants to chemoreceptors and decreased by repellants. The high or low methylation state of MCPs is somehow transmitted to other proteins, products of genes called *che*, which determine in an unknown way the direction of rotation (clockwise or anticlockwise) of the flagella and hence the proportion of its time the organism spends tumbling or swimming.

Flagella are not required for viability, nor do they often seem to be involved as virulence factors, even though flagellated organisms have the advantage of chemotactic movement in searching for nutrients or avoiding poisons. In general, there is little evidence that flagellated pathogens are more invasive than non-motile ones; however, *Vibrio cholerae* probably depends on its motility to penetrate intestinal mucus, as non-motile variants fail to adhere to intestinal epithelium.

Flagella are important *antigens* (H antigens), because of the high degree of variation among flagellins, and are very useful in the serotyping of organisms such as *E. coli* and salmonellae (p. 543). Flagellated cells give a loose, flocculent agglutination with anti-H sera. Individual salmonellae can produce alternately one of two flagellin molecules, and thus possess two distinct flagellar antigens (phase 1 and phase 2) at different times. This phenomenon, known as *phase variation*, is described on p. 543.

Spirochaetes are highly motile, helical organisms, but instead of flagella projecting from the cell surface, they produce filaments which are coiled around the cell body itself, so-called *axial fibrils* (*axial filaments*). The fibrils resemble flagella in length, diameter and membrane attachment. The motion of these organisms is described on p. 607.

Figure 4.11 Information flow during bacterial chemotaxis.

The lines represent the pathways of information flow (left to right); each of the empty boxes (left) represents a different kind of chemoreceptor. The arrows at the bottom indicate where the flow of information is interrupted in various mutants used to deduce the sequence. (From Springer *et al* (1979) *Nature*, **280**, 280.)

Bacterial spores

Two genera of medical importance, namely *Bacillus* and

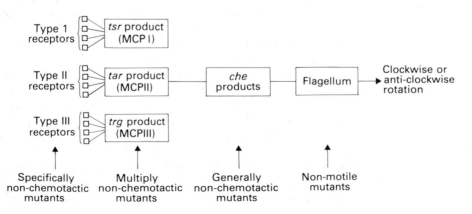

Clostridium, form highly resistant *endospores* which enable them to survive under adverse environmental conditions, often for very long periods of time. Endospores are formed within the vegetative cell. *Sporulation* (spore formation) is not a means of reproduction, since one vegetative bacterial cell gives rise to one spore and this in turn forms one cell on germination; it is simply a means of long-term survival. Spores are highly *dehydrated* structures which have a high degree of resistance to conditions such as drying, heat, freezing, toxic chemicals (disinfectants) and radiation. They are often present in soil. Thus, when a pasture has been contaminated by spores of the anthrax bacillus (*Bacillus anthracis*) it can remain a source of infection for 20–30 years, the spores entering the body of an animal by ingestion; clostridial spores of the gas gangrene and tetanus organisms (*Clostridium perfringens*, *Cl. tetani*) can be introduced on soil particles into wounds where they may germinate and cause disease. Contamination of food by spores of *Cl. perfringens* or *Cl. botulinum* can lead to food poisoning (in the latter case botulism) because the spores resist normal cooking procedures, including boiling water, and are induced to germinate by heating. The spores of botulism bacilli are particularly resiliant, so that extreme precautions are taken in canning factories to make sure they are killed, by heating the food to 116–120°C under pressure. The need to destroy heat-resistant spores is also the reason for elaborate sterilisation procedures in hospitals.

The size, shape and position of the spore within the vegetative cell is characteristic of particular species; e.g. in *Bacillus* organisms, the spore is oval and fits within the normal diameter of the cell, but in the slender cells of *Cl. tetani* it forms a terminal bulge which gives the cell its 'drumstick' appearance (Figure 4.12b). Spores are highly refractile and are thus easily recognised under the light microscope (they are bright under phase-contrast). Mature spores are not stained by Gram's or other simple stains, and hence appear as a clear space in a stained cell (Figure 4.12b). Special spore stains are available, using heat or detergent to assist penetration of the wall. Spores are slightly acid-fast, and a modified Ziehl–Neelsen method can be used in differential staining.

Sporulation is a response to conditions of inadequate nutrition. In a well-sporulating culture, e.g. in the stationary phase after exhaustion of nutrients, most of the cells form a spore. The generalised structure of a spore is shown in Figure 4.12a. The central *core* consists of the material necessary for resuming growth later as a vegetative cell, i.e. the bacterial chromosome, ribosomes, enzymes, etc. It contains very little water and the state of dehydration probably accounts for the heat stability of core proteins and nucleic acids, which would otherwise be readily heat-denatured. The core also carries a very high concentration of calcium in the form of its salt with *dipicolinic acid*, a substance rarely found elsewhere in nature and which may constitute 10–15% of spore weight (Figure 4.12c). Dipicolinic acid is formed from diaminopimelic acid (DAP), a precursor of lysine. Calcium dipicolinate may contribute to heat stability in some cases. The

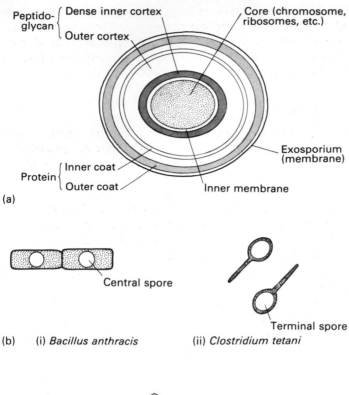

(a)

Peptido-glycan { Dense inner cortex / Outer cortex

Core (chromosome, ribosomes, etc.)

Exosporium (membrane)

Protein { Inner coat / Outer coat

Inner membrane

(b)

Central spore

(i) *Bacillus anthracis*

Terminal spore

(ii) *Clostridium tetani*

(c)

HOOC — N — COOH

core is surrounded by the cell membrane and outside this a thick peptidoglycan wall, the *cortex*. The innermost layer of the cortex is tightly cross-linked, while the outer cortex is more loosely cross-linked than the wall of the parent cell and is rapidly autolysed during germination. The spore is further surrounded by a *coat*, of which 1–3 layers may be seen, made of a tough *keratin-like protein*, rich in cross-linking disulphide bonds; it is these protein layers that are responsible for resistance to chemicals and stains. In some species, a thin lipid membrane, the *exosporium*, is found around the entire surface of the spore. The spore is liberated by disintegration of the parent cell.

Spores have no metabolic activity and remain in a dormant state until *activated* by damage to the coat through heat, acid or an SH compound, or simply as a result of ageing. *Germination* then occurs, in the presence of water and a triggering germination agent, such as a metabolite or inorganic ion. It is a rapid process, completed in $1\frac{1}{2}$–2 hours. The peptidoglycan is broken down by a spore-lytic enzyme and calcium dipicolinate released from the core. The spore loses its refractility and resistance to heat and staining. Germination produces a vegetative cell which, under

Figure 4.12 Bacterial spores. (a) Structural elements of a spore as seen by electron microscopy. (b) Typical appearance of spores (unstained) in stained cells. (c) Dipicolinic acid.

suitable environmental conditions, immediately proceeds to grow and divide. For clostridia, most of which are obligate anaerobes, the conditions include a low oxidation-reduction potential, with exclusion of oxygen, as found in dead or severely injured tissue, or in cooked food.

BACTERIAL TOXINS

We have noted above that production of a toxin is often a major factor in bacterial pathogenicity. A toxin can be defined as a naturally-produced poisonous substance which, in relatively small amounts, either kills cells or adversely affects their function, with harmful consequences for the host. Some, such as the powerful toxins of the tetanus and botulism clostridia, are among the most lethal substances known — 4 kg of botulinum toxin would be sufficient to eliminate the entire population of the world! — while others are less potent. Thus it is possible to distinguish between toxins which are virtually wholly responsible for the course of certain diseases from those which are primarily adjuncts to local bacterial invasion and which, as far as the production of the disease is concerned, may be dispensable. The former group includes the toxins of diphtheria, cholera, tetanus, botulism, and gas gangrene, while among the latter are the cell-damaging products of streptococci and staphylococci.

A basic distinction can be drawn between *exotoxins*, which are often secreted by bacteria as they grow, and *endotoxins*, molecules which are integral components of the cell envelope of Gram-negative bacteria and are released in quantity only on disruption of the organism after death (autolysis). The properties of these two groups are compared in Table 4.3. Exotoxins are *proteins*, whereas endotoxins are complex *lipopolysaccharides*. This basic

Table 4.3 Comparison of exotoxins and endotoxins.

	Exotoxins	Endotoxins
Producing organisms	Gram-positives and Gram-negatives	Gram-negatives; (v. little in Gram-positives)
Release	Often secreted by living organisms	Mainly by autolysis of dead organisms
Nature	Protein	Lipopolysaccharide
Location in microbe	Cytoplasm	Outer membrane of envelope
Effect of heat	Usually labile	Usually stable
Antibody	Antitoxin, neutralising	Anti-O, non-neutralising, but contributes to tolerance
Tolerance*	No	Yes
Activation of macrophages	No	Yes
Toxoid	Yes	No
Activity	Highly specific	Activates many pathways
Toxicity for host	Lethal; can be very powerful poisons	Lethal, but less potent than many exotoxins

*non-immunological

structural divergence leads to other differences, such as susceptibility to inactivation by heat or formaldehyde. Only exotoxins are readily heat-denatured, while formaldehyde converts them into non-toxic derivatives called *toxoids*, but does not affect endotoxins. The importance of toxoids is that they retain the antigens of the toxin, making them invaluable in vaccination against those diseases in which the toxin plays a predominant role. Exotoxins and their toxoids stimulate production of antibodies (*antitoxins*) which neutralise the toxic molecule, usually by preventing it from binding to receptors on target cells; equine or human antitoxins are used in treatment of diseases such as diphtheria and tetanus by passive immunisation. Antibodies are much less effective in neutralisation of endotoxins, as the effective part of the endotoxin molecule is the non-immunogenic lipid. With respect to potency, exotoxins are generally more powerful; a characteristic effect of endotoxins is their ability to cause *fever* (e.g. typhoid).

In the following pages, the structure and mechanism of action of major types of bacterial toxin are described (some toxins not mentioned here can be found in later subsections dealing with individual bacterial genera). In considering their relative significance in the diseases with which they are associated, the following are some key criteria to bear in mind. (1) The level of toxin production *in vivo*; (2) the correlation of toxigenicity with the organism's virulence; (3) the occurrence of sterile lesions at sites distant from those of bacterial multiplication; (4) the ability of the toxin alone to produce disease symptoms when injected; and (5) the ability of antitoxins to prevent the disease.

Exotoxins: mechanisms of action

Exotoxins display a variety of different modes of action, which on the basis of our present knowledge can be divided into three categories: (i) toxins which enter their target cells and exert an intracellular enzymatic action; (ii) toxins which damage cell membranes; and (iii) neurotoxins which interfere with nervous transmission at synapses or neuromuscular junctions. A summary of the properties of exotoxins can be found in Table 4.4.

Exotoxins with intracellular enzymatic action

ADP-RIBOSYLTRANSFERASES

Diphtheria and *cholera* toxins are the prototypes of this group; their actions are well understood in molecular terms and, despite the disparate nature of the diseases, show some basic similarities. Both are essentially enzymes which act inside their target cells. Their toxicity thus involves three stages: (i) *binding* to receptor molecules on the cell membrane; (ii) *entry* into the target cell by transportation across the membrane; and (iii) intracellular *enzymatic action*. Their molecular structure is consequently *bifunctional*—one part of the molecule is specifically involved in the binding reaction, while another is responsible for enzymatic

Table 4.4 Bacterial exotoxins.

Organism	Disease	Toxin	Genetics*	Cellular and other effects	Mechanism of action
Streptococcus pyogenes	Pharyngitis, impetigo, etc.	Streptolysin O		Haemolytic, leucocidic, cardiotoxic	Binds to membrane cholesterol; releases lysosomal enzymes in neutrophils
		Streptolysin S		Haemolytic, leucocidic	Damages membranes; non-antigenic
	Scarlet fever	Erythrogenic toxin	Lysogenised phage	Skin rash; pyrogenic	Hypersensitivity reaction in skin
Streptococcus pneumoniae (pneumococcus)	Pneumonia, bronchitis, etc.	Pneumolysin		Weak haemolysin	Binds to membrane cholesterol; oxygen-labile
Staphylococcus aureus	Pyogenic infections, septicaemia	α-haemolysin (α-toxin)		Lethal vascular smooth muscle spasm; lyses rabbit rbc	Unknown
	Pyogenic infections	β-haemolysin (β-toxin)		Toxic for tissue culture cells and animals; hot-cold lysis (sheep rbc)	Sphingomyelinase C
	ditto	γ-haemolysin (γ-toxin)		Lysis of rabbit rbc	Synergistic action of two protein components
	ditto	δ-haemolysin (δ-toxin)		Lyses rbc of several spp.; also leucocytes and other cells	Surfactant; synergises with α-toxin; v. poor antigen
	ditto	Leucocidin (Panton-Valentine)		Specifically toxic for neutrophils and macrophages	F and S proteins act on cell membrane leading to extracellular release of lysosomal contents
	Food poisoning	Enterotoxins	Lysogenised phage	Vomiting, diarrhoea	Stimulate vomiting centre via vagus nerve (neurotoxic action); do not raise intra-cellular cAMP
	Scalded skin syndrome	Exfoliation	Chromosome or plasmid-coded	Separation of epidermis at the stratum granulosum	Destruction of desmosomes

continued on next page

Table 4.4 *continued*

Organism	Disease	Toxin	Genetics*	Cellular and other effects	Mechanism of action
Vibrio cholerae	Cholera	Cholera enterotoxin		Watery diarrhoea due to hypersecretion of water and electrolytes from intestinal epithelium	Irreversible activation of adenylate cyclase by ADP-ribosylation, causing raised intracellular cAMP
Vibrio parahaemolyticus	Food poisoning	Kanagawa haemolysin		Haemolytic, cytotoxic, cardiotoxic, lethal	
Escherichia coli	Infantile diarrhoea, Traveller's diarrhoea	Heat-labile toxin (LT)	Plasmid-coded	As for cholera toxin	As for cholera toxin
		Stable toxin (ST)	Plasmid-coded	Inhibits uptake of NaCl and water by intestinal epithelium	Activation of guanylate cyclase, causing increased intracellular cGMP
Pseudomonas aeruginosa	Opportunistic infections	Toxin A		Inhibition of protein synthesis	As for diphtheria toxin
		Haemolysin		Toxic for alveolar macrophages	
		Leucocidin		Lyses leucocytes, but not red cells	
		Enterotoxin		Diarrhoea	
Corynebacterium diphtheriae	Diphtheria	Diphtheria toxin	Lysogenised β-phage	Highly lethal for many cells; causes lesions in heart, kidney, nerves, adrenals	Inhibits protein synthesis by ADP-ribosylation of EF-2
Bordetella pertussis	Whooping cough	Pertussis toxin		Lymphocytosis, insulin release, increased sensitivity to histamine	Activation of adenylate cyclase by ADP-ribosylation
Bacillus anthracis	Anthrax	Anthrax toxin			3 components (PA, LF, EF) of which EF is a soluble adenylate cyclase, causing increased cAMP in target cells

Organism	Disease	Toxin	Genetic element*	Effects	Mode of action
Clostridium perfringens	Gas gangrene	α-toxin		Lethal, necrotising, haemolytic, cytotoxic	Phospholipase C; disrupts cell membranes by acting on lecithin and other phospholipids
		θ-toxin		Haemolytic, cytotoxic, lethal	Bind to membrane cholesterol; oxygen-labile
		(Several other minor toxins)			
	Food poisoning	Enterotoxin		Diarrhoea	
Clostridium tetani	Tetanus	Tetanus toxin (tetanospasmin)		Increased muscle tone; severe, generalised muscular spasm (trismus, etc.)	Neurotoxin; acts centrally; increases motor neurone stimulation by preventing release of glycine at inhibitory synapses on anterior horn cells
		Tetanolysin		Haemolysin	Binds membrane cholesterol; oxygen-labile
Clostridium botulinum	Botulism	Botulinum toxins (8)	Lysogenised phage (toxins C,D,E)	Flaccid paralysis, esp. in parasympathetic system and respiratory muscles	Neurotoxin; acts peripherally; inhibits release of acetylcholine from nerve terminals at motor end-plate and synapses

* Chromosomal gene unless stated

activity. In the case of diphtheria toxin, the binding and enzymatic elements are initially part of a single polypeptide chain, while in cholera toxin they are distinct protein subunits bound together. Another common feature is the intracellular reaction which the two toxins catalyse, called *ADP-ribosylation*, i.e. the active part of both toxins is an ADP-ribosyltransferase enzyme. In this reaction, which is shown in Figure 4.13, ADP-ribose is transferred from the cofactor NAD to a specific acceptor protein with an essential cell function.

Figure 4.13 Mechanism of ADP-ribosylation by diphtheria and cholera toxins.
*acceptor proteins: elongation factor 2 (EF2) for diphtheria toxin, adenylate cyclase regulator (G) protein for cholera toxin.

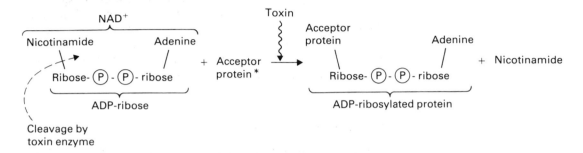

The toxins act on different acceptor proteins, but both acceptors have *GTPase activity* which is blocked after ADP-ribosylation (Figure 4.14). The fact that the end-effects of diphtheria and cholera toxins on their target cells are entirely different is basically a reflection of the different functions of the GTPase proteins involved.

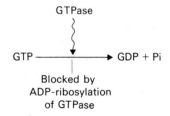

Figure 4.14

Diphtheria toxin

The toxin of *Corynebacterium diphtheriae* is perhaps the most thoroughly studied of all bacterial toxins. Its discovery dates back to 1888, when Roux and Yersin showed that sterile bacteria-free supernatants of *C. diphtheriae* cultures produced all the relevant symptoms of diphtheria in animals. The toxin plays a major role in the disease (p. 572): firstly, its lethal effect on neutrophils and macrophages enables the organisms to establish their local infection in the throat and avoid phagocytosis, and secondly, its dissemination in the bloodstream leads to lesions in several organs with a relatively large blood supply, including the heart, kidney and nervous system, and often to death from heart failure. The organisms remain localised in the throat and are not found in the other lesions. Severe disease is always due to toxigenic strains; non-toxigenic strains produce little more than a mild sore throat with fever. Moreover, diphtheria can be treated in infected

414

individuals by passive immunisation with antitoxin sera, and prevented altogether by active immunisation with the toxoid; the latter is routinely administered to infants as part of the triple vaccine. The efficacy of vaccination with toxoid has made diphtheria a very rare disease today.

Potency

In susceptible species, including man, rabbits and guinea-pigs, diphtheria toxin is lethal at very low doses (50–100 ng per kg). It is also extremely toxic for all cells of these species, so much so that the presence of a *single molecule* of toxin in a cell is sufficient to kill it. Interestingly, rats and mice are resistant, either because their cells lack the receptor molecules for the toxin or because toxin is not transported across the cell membrane. It does not harm prokaryotic cells.

Production and genetics

Diphtheria toxin is produced only by certain (toxigenic) strains of *C. diphtheriae*. A remarkable fact, discovered in 1951, is that toxigenic strains are always *lysogenic*, i.e. they have incorporated into their genomes the DNA information of a bacteriophage, in this case a corynephage called β. Lysogeny (p. 446) is essential for toxin production, and non-toxigenic strains become toxigenic if infected by β phage (*lysogenic conversion*). The process of insertion of the phage genome into that of *C. diphtheriae* is essentially as described on p. 447 for λ phage in *E. coli*. The phage does not replicate in this state (prophage), but some of its information is expressed; the surprise is that this includes the structural gene (*tox*) coding for diphtheria toxin. In other words, the toxin is not a product of the native bacterial genome itself, but is acquired from the phage (Figure 4.15). Such a situation is not unique to diphtheria toxin: lysogenised phages are also responsible for botulinum toxin types C and D, for *Clostridium novyi* α-toxin, and for streptococcal erythrogenic toxin (Table 4.4). The evidence that β phage DNA actually includes the toxin gene—as opposed to, say, a regulator which switches on a bacterial toxin gene—is conclusive. Thus, (a) lysogeny of mutant phages leads to production of defective, non-toxic molecules closely similar in structure to the normal toxin; and (b) pure β phage DNA can be transcribed and translated in a cell-free system *in vitro*, producing diphtheria toxin without any contribution from the *C. diphtheriae* organism. However, the corynebacterium has the ability to regulate the expression of the *tox* gene by producing a *repressor protein*. In the presence of inorganic iron (Fe^{2+}) the repressor binds to the *tox* gene and prevents its transcription. Hence, toxin is only synthesized in quantity when the external supply of Fe^{2+} has fallen to a low level, which in culture is in the late stages of bacterial growth. The repressor is produced by corynebacterial strains irrespective of whether they are toxigenic or not, and is a product of the normal genome. Mutant organisms which lack the repressor molecule produce toxin continuously whatever the Fe^{2+}

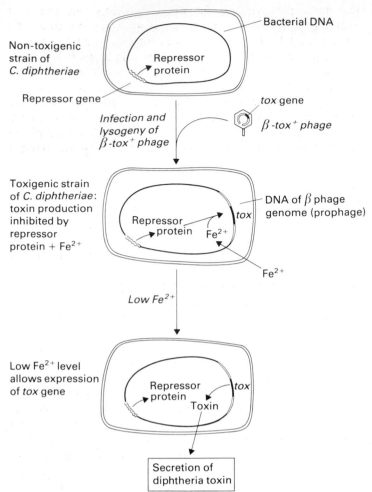

Figure 4.15 Lysogeny of β-phage and synthesis of diphtheria toxin.

Non-toxigenic strain of *C. diphtheriae*

Bacterial DNA

Repressor protein

Repressor gene

tox gene

Infection and lysogeny of β-tox$^+$ phage

β-tox$^+$ phage

Toxigenic strain of *C. diphtheriae*: toxin production inhibited by repressor protein + Fe^{2+}

Repressor protein

tox

Fe^{2+}

DNA of β phage genome (prophage)

Fe^{2+}

Low Fe^{2+}

Low Fe^{2+} level allows expression of *tox* gene

Repressor protein

tox

Toxin

Secretion of diphtheria toxin

concentration, indicating that the repressor and Fe^{2+} act together to regulate the *tox* gene. Figure 4.15 illustrates the details of toxin production.

Mechanism of action

The cytocidal properties of diphtheria toxin are due essentially to its enzymatic action. The mechanism has been studied *in vitro*, both with intact cells and cell-free systems of protein synthesis. On exposure of susceptible cells to toxin, there first occurs a lag period of 60–90 minutes, during which the toxin binds to membrane receptors and enters the cells in an activated state; thereafter, cellular protein synthesis is rapidly inhibited, leading ultimately to the death of the cell. Using cell-free systems, it has been shown that inhibition of protein synthesis depends on the presence of the cofactor NAD and occurs by ADP-ribosylation (Figure 4.13). The enzymatically active part of the toxin transfers ADP-ribose from NAD to a protein called *elongation factor 2* (*EF2*), which is essential for reactions on the ribosome—EF2 is

416

the translocase required for the GTP-driven movement of peptidyl-tRNA from one site to another in the eukaryotic ribosome. ADP-ribosyl-EF2 is unable to perform this function, so translation of messenger RNA is halted. This is the molecular mechanism underlying the damaging effects of diphtheria toxin on body tissues. It explains the potency of the toxin, since its enzymatic activity enables its action to be amplified to the point where a single toxin molecule can kill a cell; selectivity for animal cells can also be accounted for, as prokaryotic cells use a different elongation factor (EFG) which is not affected by diphtheria toxin.

Structure

The native toxin molecule, as released from the bacterial cell, has no enzymatic activity and does not inhibit protein synthesis in cell-free systems. It is a single polypeptide chain of about 60,000 mol.wt, containing two intrachain disulphide bridges as shown in Figure 4.16. In this state it can be regarded as a *proenzyme*, i.e. a precursor of the toxic enzyme which is activated by a proteolytic cleavage reaction. When the native toxin is treated with a protease, followed by reduction of its disulphide bonds with thiol, it is split into two fragments, termed A and B. *Fragment A*, of 21,000 mol.wt, has all the ADP-ribosyltransferase activity and is able to inhibit protein synthesis in cell-free systems (Figure 4.16), but although it is the active part of the molecule, A is unable to act on intact cells because it cannot bind to and cross cell membranes. *Fragment B*, which comprises the remainder of the molecule, is responsible for binding to and entry into target cells. In consists of the carboxyterminal end of the toxin, which binds to cell membrane receptors, and a hydrophobic sequence which probably assists passage across the membrane itself. Thus the diphtheria toxin molecule is bifunctional in structure, with binding and enzymatic regions combined initially in a single

Figure 4.16 Diphtheria toxin: structure and activation.

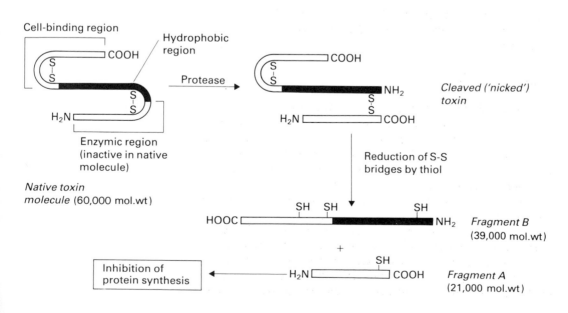

polypeptide chain. (Note that in intact toxin, A is buried on the inside of the molecule and its determinants are not available to antibody.)

This interpretation of the anatomy of the molecule has been confirmed by experiments which can be called 'molecular complementation', using mutant toxins lacking toxic activity. Thus, it is possible to obtain inactive toxins which either lack part of the carboxyterminal B sequence, or have an aberrant A fragment; the former are unable to bind to target cells, while the latter cannot generate active enzyme. As Figure 4.17 shows, such molecules can be mixed and exposed to mild proteolysis and thiol reduction, followed by reoxidation, whereupon active toxin molecules are generated in which both necessary fragments have been recombined. The 'hybrid' molecules have all the activity expected of the toxin, confirming the concept of two functional molecular regions.

Entry into cells and activation

As indicated above, cells susceptible to diphtheria toxin possess membrane receptors to which the molecule binds. The identity of the receptor is unknown, but it seems to be a large protein. The only events in the entry process which are known for certain are that the B region of the toxin binds to the receptor and that the A fragment then crosses the membrane and enters the cell. It has been proposed that activation takes place within the membrane, as illustrated in Figure 4.18. The carboxyterminal (hydrophilic) portion of the B region may be proteolytically separated at the

Figure 4.17 'Molecular complementation' of mutant diphtheria toxins.

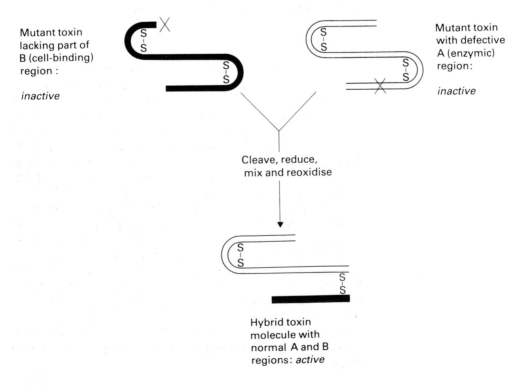

Mutant toxin lacking part of B (cell-binding) region:

inactive

Mutant toxin with defective A (enzymic) region:

inactive

Cleave, reduce, mix and reoxidise

Hybrid toxin molecule with normal A and B regions: *active*

Figure 4.18 Diphtheria toxin: possible mechanism of entry into cells. (a) The cell-binding region of the toxin molecule interacts with a membrane receptor; (b) the hydrophilic C-terminal region of the toxin is removed, allowing the hydrophobic portion to draw the A region into the membrane; (c) within the membrane, the A fragment is split off by proteolytic cleavage and reduction, after which (d) A is released into the cytoplasm. (From Stephen and Pietrowski, 1981)

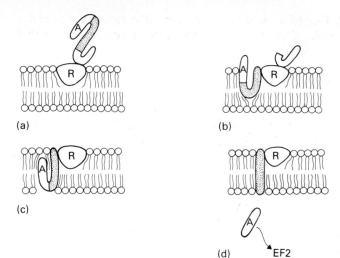

outer surface of the cell, enabling the hydrophobic portion to enter the membrane, taking the A region with it. Inside the membrane, the hydrophobic sequence may interact with lipid and thus span the bilayer, drawing the A region to the inner surface. Membrane-associated proteases could then 'nick' the molecule between the remaining disulphide bridge, allowing reduction by glutathione to release the A fragment into the cell, where it rapidly exerts its protein-inhibitory effect.

Pseudomonas aeruginosa toxin A

There is a fascinatingly close resemblance between diphtheria toxin and one of several toxins produced by the Gram-negative bacillus *Pseudomonas aeruginosa*. This is a prominent and troublesome opportunistic pathogen, harmless in healthy adults but a major cause of infection in hospitals among patients with severe burns or whose immune defences are impaired by immunosuppressive therapy. Pseudomonas toxin A appears to have a very similar production, structure and mode of action to diphtheria toxin. Thus, it is a molecule of 60,000–70,000 mol.wt, the production of which is related to the Fe^{2+} concentration in the organism's surroundings; it is activated by proteolysis and thiol reduction, when it gives rise to a small fragment with ADP-ribosyltransferase activity; finally, it inhibits protein synthesis by modifying EF2 in the same way as diphtheria toxin. However, the two molecules are not identical: they are antigenically distinct (and therefore have differences in amino acid sequence), their receptors on target cells are different, and toxin A can act on mouse cells. Nevertheless, their close structural and functional similarities raise interesting questions of a possible common origin.

Cholera toxin

Although the cholera vibrio was discovered by Koch in 1883, it was not until 1959 that its exotoxin was recognised, though Koch himself had postulated its existence. The toxin is responsible for the massive outpouring of fluid into the gut which characterises cholera, leading to intense watery diarrhoea and the loss of up to 20 litres of water per day; if untreated, there is extreme dehydration, hypovolaemic shock and rapid death (p. 564). The term *enterotoxin* is used for a group of exotoxins, of which cholera toxin is the major example, which are produced by enteric organisms and act on the intestinal mucosa to reverse the normal flow of electrolytes and water, causing diarrhoea. Others discussed below include those of *E. coli*, shigellae, *Staph. aureus* and *Cl. perfringens*. Unlike other enteric pathogens, such as salmonellae and shigellae, *Vibrio cholerae* is not an invasive organism and does not give rise to inflammatory lesions in the intestine. The pathogenesis of cholera is dependent on production of enterotoxin, which acts locally on the epithelium of the small intestine and is not disseminated around the body; its action is primarily one of interference with cellular function. Mutant strains which produce inactive toxins cause no more than a mild diarrhoea in a minority of infected persons.

Assay

The method commonly used to assay enterotoxins was developed by De, the discoverer of cholera toxin, and involves its injection into isolated ligated loops of rabbit ileum (*in vivo*). The toxin causes an accumulation of fluid into the loop (Figure 4.19), an effect also produced by living vibrios. Alternative *in vitro* methods utilise the fact that cholera toxin, for reasons described below, has the same effect on cells as cyclic AMP. Hence, it can be assayed by induction of elongation of cultured Chinese hamster ovary (CHO) cells (which respond to picogram amounts of toxin) and steroidogenesis and shape changes in mouse Y-1 adrenal tumour cells.

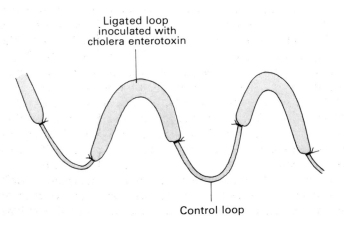

Ligated loop
inoculated with
cholera enterotoxin

Control loop

Figure 4.19 Ligated ileal loop test for cholera (or other) enterotoxin activity. Segments of rabbit ileum are ligated and inoculated with culture filtrates from cholera vibrios or other enterotoxigenic bacteria, intervening loops serving as negative controls. After 24 hours (*in vivo*) the test loops are distended due to accumulation of fluid, while controls remain collapsed.

Figure 4.20 Effects of cholera toxin on epithelial cells of the villi and crypts in the small intestine.
(a) Anti-absorptive effect on villus cells.
(b) Secretory stimulation in crypt cells.

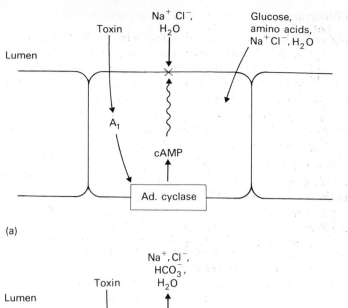

(a)

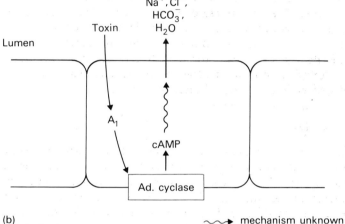

(b)   ∿→ mechanism unknown

Mechanism of action (Figure 4.20)

The basic cause of cholera diarrhoea is an increase in the intracellular level of cyclic AMP in intestinal epithelial cells (enterocytes). Like diphtheria toxin, cholera enterotoxin achieves its effects by ADP-ribosylation: a fragment (A_1) of the toxin can be separated and shown in cell-free systems to be an enzyme with ADP-ribosyltransferase activity. Once it has gained access to the inside of cells lining the villi and crypts of the small intestine, the A_1 fragment causes the transfer of ADP-ribose from NAD to a regulatory protein which is part of the *adenylate cyclase* enzyme complex responsible for intracellular generation of cAMP from ATP. The result is the *irreversible activation* of adenylate cyclase and overproduction of cyclic AMP in the cell. Cyclic AMP in turn (a) inhibits uptake of Na^+ and Cl^- ions by cells lining the villi and (b) stimulates hypersecretion of Cl^- and HCO_3^- ions together with Na^+ by cells in the crypts of Lieberkühn. The uptake of water which normally accompanies NaCl absorption in villus cells is thus blocked, while the secretion of electrolytes from crypt cells causes a concomitant passive outflow of water across the mucosal cells. These events are the basis of the loss of water and electrolytes in cholera diarrhoea.

It is important to note that cholera toxin does not affect the uptake of Na^+ and water which accompanies absorption of *glucose* or amino acids in villus cells. This has made possible oral rehydration with glucose-electrolyte solutions and has greatly simplified therapy of cholera over the last decade by replacing intravenous rehydration in many cases (p. 566).

The effects of cholera toxin on adenylate cyclase are shown in greater detail in Figure 4.21. The enzyme is a complex situated on the inner (basal) surface of the epithelial cell membrane; the toxin must therefore *enter* the cell via the mucosal surface in order to influence the enzyme. Adenylate cyclase has three components: the catalytic protein itself (C), which converts ATP into cyclic AMP; a regulatory protein (G) with GTPase activity, which binds GTP and causes the activity of C to be

Figure 4.21 Molecular mechanism of activation of adenylate cyclase.
(a) Physiological (reversible) activation by hormone binding.
(b) Irreversible activation by cholera toxin.
H, G and C are hormone receptor, GTP-binding regulatory subunit and catalytic subunit respectively of the adenylate cyclase complex.

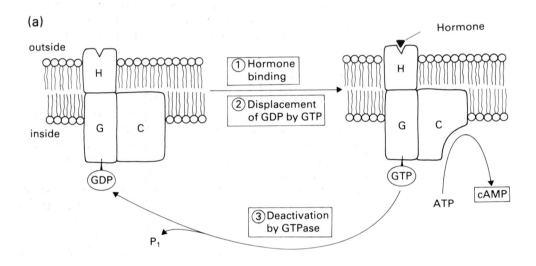

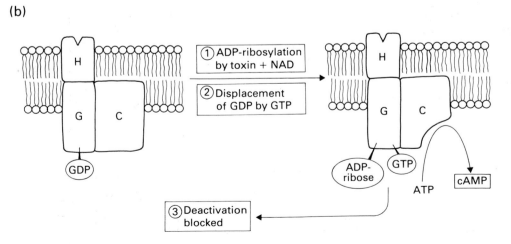

switched 'on' or 'off'; and a membrane receptor (H) responsible for binding a hormone to which the cell is required to respond. (Note that this nomenclature is not yet internationally agreed.) The G protein is associated with both C and H. In the resting (inactive) state of the complex, G carries the nucleoside diphosphate GDP; activation occurs on the substitution of GDP by the triphosphate GTP, and under physiological conditions this is stimulated by reaction of hormone with its receptor H at the outer surface of the cell membrane (Figure 4.21a). Binding of GTP by G evidently results in a conformational change via which G in turn activates the enzymatically active protein C. Subsequent return to the resting state (deactivation) is brought about by the GTPase action of the G protein. The action of the A_1 fragment of cholera toxin is to cause *ADP-ribosylation* of the G protein, the ADP-ribose group becoming covalently linked to a single arginine side-chain. In this state, the G protein can still bind GTP, but cannot exert its GTPase function. Hence, activation of adenylate cyclase is not followed by deactivation, and the enzyme is 'locked' into a permanently active state, with consequent overproduction of cylic AMP (Figure 4.21b).

Structure

Like diphtheria toxin, the molecular structure of cholera toxin is designed to enable binding to the target cell membrane, followed by detachment of the enzymatic fragment and its entry into the cell, the rest of the molecule remaining membrane-bound. Unlike diphtheria toxin, however, there are separate binding (B) and enzymatically active (A) subunits. The structure of the toxin, which has been studied by electron microscopy, is shown in Figure 4.22. Five B subunits form a ring into which the A subunit is partly inserted. The B subunits, each of 11,000 mol.wt, are bound tightly together by non-covalent interactions; A (28,000 mol.wt) is held in place by weaker interactions. The A

Figure 4.22 Structure of the cholera toxin molecule.
(a) Schematic diagram of polypeptide chains (after Holmgren, 1981)
(b) Electron microscope appearance.
(c) Model, showing the A subunit inserted into the ring of B subunits.

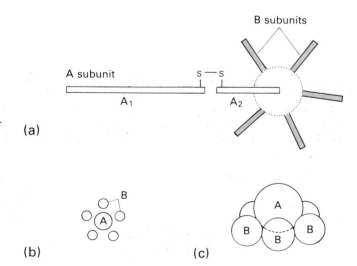

subunit is 'nicked' by bacterial proteases into two fragments A_1 (23,000) and A_2 (5000), which remain linked together by a single disulphide bridge; the active part of the toxin, the A_1 fragment, can thus be released intracellularly by thiol reduction (cf. diphtheria toxin). Experiments in which A and B subunits have been separated by gel filtration under acid conditions, confirm that the B subunits bind to cells but are non-toxic, and that the A subunit is enzymatically active in cell-free systems but is non-toxic for intact cells. Fully active toxin can be reconstituted by reassociating the A and B subunits.

Cell binding and entry

The membrane receptors for cholera toxin are not protein in nature but are composed of a specific *ganglioside*, GM_1, which carries sugar residues to which the toxin B subunits bind. One toxin binding site consists of 5 GM_1 molecules (to pair with 5 B subunits) and there is a direct relation between the amount of GM_1 in the membrane and the number of toxin molecules bound. Interestingly *V. cholerae* organisms produce a neuraminidase which can, by removing N-acetylneuraminic acid residues, convert other gangliosides into GM_1, thereby creating more binding sites for its toxin; for some reason this generation of additional receptors does not occur on intestinal epithelium cells. Cell entry is thought to be via the insertion of the B subunits into the membrane forming a hydrophilic transmembrane channel through which the A subunit can pass into the cytoplasm (Figure 4.23). Thereafter, the disulphide bond joining A_1 and A_2 is probably reduced by glutathione, releasing the active A_1 fragment. Cell binding and entry takes 10–60 minutes, but once inside the cell the action of the toxin is very rapid, with elevation of cyclic AMP production occurring within a minute.

Figure 4.23 Proposed mode of entry of cholera toxin into cells.

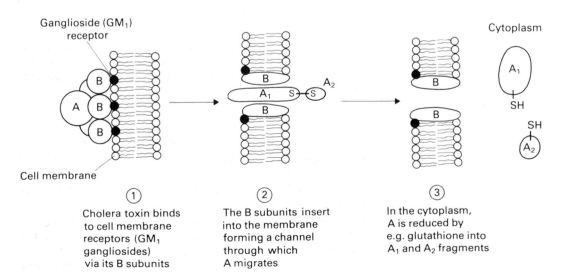

Ganglioside (GM₁) receptor

Cytoplasm

Cell membrane

① Cholera toxin binds to cell membrane receptors (GM₁ gangliosides) via its B subunits

② The B subunits insert into the membrane forming a channel through which A migrates

③ In the cytoplasm, A is reduced by e.g. glutathione into A₁ and A₂ fragments

Implications for vaccination

Immunity against cholera requires the secretion of IgA antibodies into the gut against both the toxin and the organism itself, to neutralise the former and prevent adherence and colonisation by the latter. Such antibodies are present for about three years after natural infection, but have been difficult to stimulate effectively by vaccination. The standard vaccine consists of killed organisms and is administered by parenteral inoculation. Not surprisingly, protection is poor and short-lived (about six months), both because this is an unsatisfactory route for generating the necessary *local* intestinal immunity and because of the lack of antitoxin. A toxoid preparation made by glutaraldehyde inactivation is antigenic but confers no protection against experimental challenge with living bacteria.

Interest currently centres around the development of *oral* cholera vaccines and in this the comprehensive knowledge which now exists about cholera toxin has made it possible to develop a preparation containing the purified B subunit (a 'subunit vaccine'). The B subunit can be readily separated from the A subunit by column chromatography and should be an effective 'toxoid' since it lacks all toxicity, is native rather than denatured by chemical treatment (such as formaldehyde), and stimulates antibodies which neutralise the intact toxin by inhibiting binding to cells. Immunisation with the B subunit protects rabbits against experimental cholera and has recently been used together with killed organisms in human volunteers, in whom the orally administered mixture stimulated secretory IgA responses. However, the protective value of such a vaccine has yet to be evaluated by field trials.

Perhaps the most promising possibility is the isolation, by genetic methods, of mutants of *V. cholerae* which have selectively lost the gene for the A subunit, yet continue to produce the B subunit. Such organisms should be the ideal attenuated strains, since they retain the ability to colonise the gut, and hence to stimulate antivibrio IgA, as well as secreting the inactive toxin which stimulates antitoxin IgA. The first such strain to be developed, called Texas star, is now being evaluated in volunteers. To date it has been found to produce the undesirable side-effect of mild diarrhoea in about 20% of recipients. Ultimately its usefulness will depend on its inability to revert to toxigenicity.

Escherichia coli labile toxin

Certain strains of the normally commensal organism *Escherichia coli* are capable of producing enterotoxins and give rise to acute diarrhoea in man and animals, including severe gastroenteritis in infants and traveller's diarrhoea (p. 548). Two toxins are involved, both of which act by increasing levels of cyclic nucleotides (cyclic AMP or cyclic GMP) in cells of the intestinal epithelium. Of particular interest is the fact that one, known as *heat-labile toxin* (LT) is very similar in structure and activity to cholera toxin. It has the same subunit structure (except for lacking the A_2 fragment), possesses ADP-ribosyltransferase activity and increases intracellular cyclic AMP. Indeed, the similarity extends to antigenic cross-reactivity with cholera toxin and partial amino acid sequence identity, indicating a common genetic origin for the two molecules. An important difference between them is that the gene coding for cholera toxin is part of the chromosome of *V. cholerae*, whereas that for *E. coli* LT is carried extrachromosomally on a *plasmid* (p. 468). The significance of the latter lies in the possible transfer of the LT gene to other Gram-negative organisms by conjugation; this may account for the occasional production of LT by strains of *Salmonella*, *Pseudomonas* and *Yersinia*. (See also *E. coli* stable toxin, p. 433).

Bordetella pertussis toxin

Bordetella pertussis is the causative agent of whooping cough. The role of its toxic products in the disease is far from clear-cut, but one molecule present in culture supernatants, variously known as pertussis toxin, lymphocytosis promoting factor or islet activating protein, has several biological effects and may be central to pathogenesis. For instance, it can induce the lymphocytosis which is a diagnostic feature of whooping cough; it also releases insulin from the pancreatic islets and increases sensitivity to histamine and anaphylaxis. Recently it has been shown that this molecule too activates adenylate cyclase by ADP-ribosylation, though it seems that the subunit of the enzyme complex which is ADP-ribosylated it not the same as that affected by cholera toxin. *Bord. pertussis* also secretes its own soluble cyclase, as discussed below.

BACTERIAL ADENYLATE CYCLASES

ADP-ribosylation of adenylate cyclase is one mechanism for raising intracellular cyclic AMP; another is the secretion by a bacterium of its own adenylate cyclase which, if it can secure entry, may act inside an animal cell. The following examples are known.

Anthrax toxin

Recent studies of the anthrax organism, *Bacillus anthracis*, have revealed that, like a number of others, it secretes a soluble adenylate cyclase; the bacterial enzyme is distinct from that of mammalian cells in its greater heat stability and lack of regulation by GTP. It seems that adenylate cyclase forms part of the complex of three proteins which make up the anthrax toxin. The role of these components has seemed enigmatic and complicated for a long time. They are called *protective antigen* (PA or factor II), *lethal factor* (LF or factor III), and *oedema factor* (EF or factor I). Neither alone has toxicity, but the combination of PA and LF is lethal for rodents, while that of PA and EF produces oedema on injection into the skin; PA itself is a protein which induces immunity to anthrax toxin. It has now been discovered that together PA and EF increase cyclic AMP levels in cultured cells and alter the morphology of Chinese hamster ovary cells (p. 420), while *in vitro* EF is a highly active adenylate cyclase in the presence of *calmodulin*, the calcium-activated regulator protein present in animal cells. It appears that PA is required for the entry of EF into cells, a role analogous to that of the B subunit of cholera toxin, which accounts for the inhibitory effect of anti-PA antibodies. This is the first example of a toxin which increases cyclic AMP in eukaryotic cells as a result of its own intracellular cyclase action rather than by activation of the eukaryotic enzyme. However, the relevance of this novel mechanism to anthrax itself has yet to be clarified, as it is not certain whether EF or LT has the more important part in toxicity *in vivo*.

Bordetella pertussis toxin

It is possible that soluble adenylate cyclase plays a role in the virulence of other bacteria as well. For example, *Bord. pertussis*, one toxin of which was noted above for its ADP-ribosyltransferase activity, also secretes an adenylate cyclase. This enzyme can be taken up by human neutrophils, in which it leads to a marked rise in cyclic AMP; this depresses the antibacterial functions of neutrophils and may thus aid the invasiveness of the organism.

BACTERIOCINS (COLICINS E2 AND E3)

Some bacteria produce exotoxins called *bacteriocins* which are lethal for other bacteria rather than eukaryotic cells. Unlike antibiotics, bacteriocins are proteins which in several respects resemble the toxins discussed above. *Colicins* are the bacteriocins produced by *E. coli* and related enterobacteria; about 40% of the *E. coli* strains isolatable from man and animals are colicinogenic (Col$^+$). Other Gram-negative, as well as Gram-positive, organisms produce similar substances. Two interesting properties of bacteriocins are (i) their lethal action is usually restricted to organisms closely related to the producing strain, and (ii) they may be prevented from acting on the organisms which produce them by an *immunity protein* which inhibits their intracellular action.

Two examples out of a great many are the colicins E2 and E3. They resemble diphtheria toxin in structure and their action on target cells is enzymatic and intracellular; however, they are not ADP-ribosyltransferases, but a DNase (E2) and RNase (E3). *Colicin E3* consists of a complex of two protein subunits tightly bound together; the major chain is similar to diphtheria toxin in having both cell-binding and enzymatic regions, while the minor component is the immunity protein mentioned above (Figure 4.24). Through its association with the main chain, the immunity protein assists in cell binding, but does not enter the target cell. It inhibits the action of colicin *in vitro*, and this is doubtless the basis of its protective action in producer cells, but it is perhaps more appropriate to regard it as an integral part of the secreted

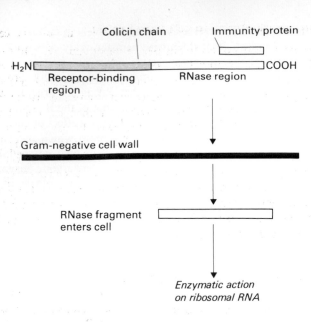

Figure 4.24 Structure and action of colicin E3.

molecule, necessary for cellular entry. Colicin E3, like other colicins, binds to a receptor in the outer membrane of its Gram-negative target cell. The receptors are proteins which generally have some other function, e.g. transport proteins responsible for the uptake of essential metabolites such as vitamin B_{12}, chelated iron, nucleosides, etc. Strains lacking the appropriate receptor cannot be killed by the colicin. It seems that E3, after binding, is split into N-terminal and C-terminal fragments, of which only the latter enters the cell, leaving the immunity protein behind. Its intracellular mode of action as an RNase is to cleave a 50-nucleotide fragment from the 16S ribosomal RNA of intact ribosomes; this reaction prevents the initiation of transcription of mRNA so that protein synthesis soon comes to a halt. *Colicin E2*, which is also a complex of colicin and immunity protein, acts as a DNase.

Like the *E. coli* enterotoxins, colicins and their immunity proteins are coded by genes on plasmids (Col plasmids) which may be transferrable by conjugation to other bacterial strains (see also p. 455); some bacteriocins of Gram-positive bacteria (staphylococcins, streptococcins) are also plasmid-encoded. The significance of bacteriocin production is, in principle, that it gives the organism an advantage when faced with local competition from related species with similar requirements of nutrition and habitat; a Col$^+$ strain of *E. coli*, for example, would derive a selective advantage if it can kill its closely related Col$^-$ competitors. One Col plasmid (Col V) also carries genes for virulence factors which are responsible for the invasiveness of certain pathogenic strains of *E. coli* (p. 469).

Exotoxins which act on cell membranes

There are a variety of exotoxins whose major action is to disrupt cell membranes, ranging from *Clostridium perfringens* α-toxin, which plays a major role in gas gangrene, to the haemolysins and leucocidins of pyogenic cocci, where an important pathogenic role is more questionable. For some, the mechanism of action is well understood—*Cl. perfringens* α-toxin was the first toxin to be shown to have an enzymatic action; for others, however, the details have still to be worked out. Membrane-acting toxins may be directly lytic, through gross membrane damage, or cause membrane fragility which only becomes damaging at low temperatures ('hot-cold lysis'); others induce more subtle permeability changes or activate membrane enzymes. Examples of these modes of action are described below.

ENZYMATIC ACTION ON MEMBRANES

Clostridium perfringens α-toxin

Although *Cl. perfringens* has a wide range of toxic products (p. 580), its α-toxin is the most important, deriving particular significance from its role in gas gangrene, where it is responsible both for local tissue destruction in the infected wound and a severe and often lethal toxaemia. It is lethal on intravenous inoculation into animals, necrotising if injected intradermally, and haemolytic for most species of red cells other than horse and goat. Haemolysis is of the 'hot-cold' variety, in that lysis occurs best if the red cells are treated at 37°C and then cooled. α-toxin is also reponsible for the characteristic ability of sterile culture filtrates of *Cl. perfringens* to cause opalescent turbidity in human serum and extracts of egg yolk. The latter is used in a standard method of identifying the organism called *Nagler's reaction*: when *Cl. perfringens* is grown on nutrient agar into which egg yolk has been incorporated, colonies are surrounded by an opalescent halo, which can be inhibited if anti-α-toxin is also present in the agar. All these properties of α-toxin result from its activity as a *lecithinase* (*phospholipase C*), i.e. an enzyme which acts on the phospholipid lecithin and splits it into phophorylcholine and a diglyceride, as shown in Figure 4.25. While lecithin is the preferred substrate, α-toxin also acts on other phospholipids, as well as sphingomyelin and cephalin. The insolubility of the free diglyceride leads to the turbidogenic reactions with egg yolk (a rich source of lecithin) and serum (due to separation of lipid from lipoproteins). The lethal and necrotising, as well as cytotoxic and haemolytic, properties of α-toxin are due to the fact that lecithin and its other phospholipid substrates are essential components of the membranes of animal cells.

Gas gangrene arises in injured tissue contaminated with *Cl. perfringens* spores, which germinate in conditions of low redox potential (p. 579). Once the organisms are established, the production and diffusion of α-toxin kills more local tissue, especially muscle, as well as destroying leucocytes; the newly

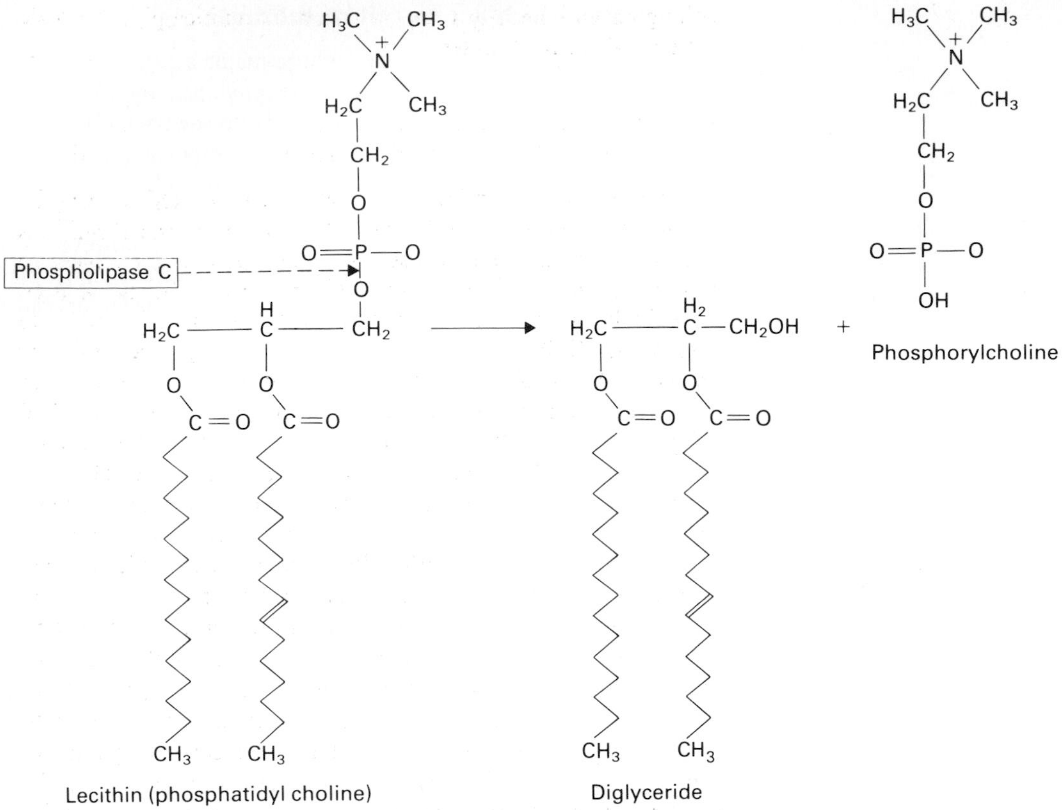

Lecithin (phosphatidyl choline)

Diglyceride

Phosphorylcholine

Figure 4.25 Action of phospholipase C on lecithin.

necrotic area thus prepared can then be freely colonised by the organisms, with further production of toxin and rapid progressive spread of infection until the whole muscle or limb segment is involved. Note that the organisms remain localised for most of the disease, only entering the bloodstream sometimes as a terminal event. Experimental evidence for the role of α-toxin comes from the protective effect of immunity, stimulated by α-toxoids, in sheep with artificially infected gunshot wounds. The immunity was strictly antitoxic rather than antibacterial, as growing organisms could be recovered from the wounds some weeks after infection. Moreover, antitoxin protects animals from an otherwise lethal challenge by *Cl. perfringens*. However, the α-toxin is not the only property of the organism involved in its virulence, and the cumulative effect of its other toxic or aggressive products must also be recognised (p. 580). Thus, in man the protective effect of antitoxin is much less convincing clinically.

Staphylococcus aureus β-haemolysin

This is another example of a 'hot-cold' haemolysin; it is a sphingomyelinase C which splits sphingomyelin into phosphoryl-choline and N-acylsphingosine (i.e. like phospholipase C but with specificity for sphingomyelin). The sensitivity of red cells of different species to β-haemolysin parallels their content of sphingomyelin, namely sheep > human > guinea-pig. It is toxic for animals in large doses.

OXYGEN-LABILE HAEMOLYSINS
(THIOL-ACTIVATED CYTOLYSINS)

Several organisms release cytolytic toxins which can be recognised most easily in the laboratory by their lysis of red cells and which are irreversibly inactivated by oxgen. These molecules possess sulphydryl (-SH) groups which must be in the reduced state for haemolytic activity but which are oxidised in the air to disulphide (S-S) bonds. Reactivation is through reduction by thiols such as glutathione (hence the term 'thiol-activated cytolysins'). Examples are the streptococcal haemolysin called streptolysin O (for 'oxygen labile'), pneumococcal pneumolysin, tetanolysin of *Cl. tetani*, θ-toxin of *Cl. perfringens*, cereolysin of *Bacillus cereus*, and several others. Similarities between these toxins include immunological cross-reactivity, the conditions under which they react with cells, a lethal cardiotoxicity when injected, and irreversible inactivation by cholesterol. They act by binding to cholesterol in cell membranes, followed by aggregation of the toxin-cholesterol complexes, which are visible as arcs or rings in the electron microscope. The structural reorganisation of the membrane involved in forming these aggregates leads to permeability changes and eventual lysis of cells or lysosomes (physical 'holes' in the membrane are not necessary). It is the cytotoxic rather than haemolytic properties of these molecules that gives them a role in the pathogenesis of certain infections, haemolysis simply being useful in identifying the organisms in the laboratory.

Streptolysin O of Streptococcus pyogenes

This is one of the best studied of the oxygen-labile haemolysins. Its contribution to streptococcal infection is exerted locally, through its toxic action on leucocytes which would otherwise attempt to dispose of the organisms by phagocytosis. When added to a suspension of neutrophils, streptolysin O induces the disintegration of *lysosomal granules* (degranulation), with intracellular discharge of their destructive hydrolytic enzymes, leading to rapid death of the cell. A similar toxic action is exerted on macrophages, and streptolysin O also inhibits leucocyte chemotaxis. Through its leucocidic action it enhances the survival of streptococci, though its precise value is difficult to evaluate in view of the variety of other pathogenic devices these organisms use to promote their invasiveness (p. 498). The release of enzymes from killed neutrophils may well also contribute to tissue damage in streptococcal lesions. When injected intravenously into rabbits, guinea-pigs and rodents, the toxin is lethal due to its cardiotoxic action, and it has been suggested that this contributes to heart damage in rheumatic fever (p. 503). Neutralising antibodies to streptolysin O (ASO) appear during the course of infection and a rising titre is useful in diagnosis.

Staphylococcus aureus α-haemolysin

Four distinct haemolysins ($\alpha,\beta,\gamma,\delta$) are produced by *Staph. aureus* of which α-haemolysin is the principal one and responsible for the fatal outcome of staphylococcal septicaemias. α-Haemolysin is lethal when injected, due to induction of spasm in smooth muscle. It is lytic for rabbit red cells, but human red cells are much less sensitive; no specific lipid has been identified as its membrane target molecule and the mechanisms are not well understood.

Staphylococcus aureus (Panton–Valentine) leucocidin

Staph. aureus also produces a separate leucocidin, known as Panton–Valentine (PV) leucocidin, which is specific for neutrophils and macrophages and is not haemolytic. It consists of two separate protein components, designated 'fast' (F) and 'slow' (S) after their relative rates of electrophoretic migration. They undergo a complex and incompletely understood synergistic interaction on leucocyte membranes, the result of which is an alteration in permeability to cations, notably an *influx of Ca^{2+} ions* and resultant efflux of K$^+$. The increase in intracellular Ca^{2+} has important effects which follow its binding to *calmodulin*, the intracellular calcium-binding protein with the role of intermediary in Ca^{2+}-dependent activities, including secretion and activation of certain enzymes. One result is degranulation, with discharge of lysosomal contents to the exterior, and another is calmodulin-mediated activation of membrane enzymes

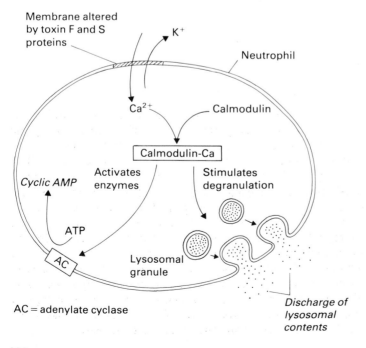

Figure 4.26 Mechanism of action of *Staph. aureus* leucocidin (Panton–Valentine leucocidin).

Membrane altered by toxin F and S proteins

K$^+$

Neutrophil

Ca^{2+}

Calmodulin

Calmodulin-Ca

Cyclic AMP

Activates enzymes

Stimulates degranulation

ATP

AC

Lysosomal granule

Discharge of lysosomal contents

AC = adenylate cyclase

including adenylate cyclase (Figure 4.26). Eventually cell death follows, without physical membrane lysis. As with streptolysin O, staphylococcal leucocidin contributes to the local survival of organisms when faced with phagocytes, though it is again difficult to judge how important it is to the development of lesions. It is one of several products, the effects of which are often *synergistic* rather than simply additive; an example of synergy is provided by α- and δ-haemolysins themselves, a mixture of which produces lysis at lower concentration than either alone. (α-haemolysin damages membranes by detergent-like surfactant properties.)

Streptolysin S of Streptococcus pyogenes

This streptococcal toxin contributes to haemolysis by β-haemolytic organisms and acts on membranes of red cells and leucocytes. Unlike streptolysin O, however, it is stable in oxygen, non-antigenic, and is a small polypeptide of 28 amino acids. 'S' refers to its extractability from intact streptococci with serum—it readily forms a complex with serum albumin and can also associate with other 'carriers' such as RNA. In general, however, it remains cell bound and exerts its toxic effect on leucocytes after the organisms have been phagocytosed. Streptolysin S injures membranes by a mechanism which is not completely understood, but is clearly different from that of its thiol-activated counterpart. Phospholipids seem to be its membrane receptor, as treatment of membranes with phospholipase C prevents toxin binding and free phospholipids or serum lipoproteins inhibit haemolysis. Streptolysin S is lethal for mice and a pathogenic role in human infections is possible. However, it only seems to 'rescue' the occasional organism from within neutrophils, since the majority of phagocytosed streptococci are killed.

TOXIN-INDUCED ACTIVATON OF MEMBRANE ENZYME

Escherichia coli stable toxin

We have previously described *E. coli* labile toxin, which has intracellular ADP-ribosyltransferase activity. Enteropathogenic *E. coli* also secrete an enterotoxin remarkable for its stability to heat, enzymes and acid, and hence known as *stable toxin* (ST). It is a polypeptide of 40–50 amino acids (5000 mol. wt) which is unrelated to LT or cholera toxin. ST acts by increasing cellular cyclic GMP, via activation of guanylate cyclase, but probably does so without entering the cell, by combining with the appropriate *hormone receptor* associated with guanylate cyclase on the plasma membrane. A raised intracellular cyclic GMP level inhibits NaCl transport across the membrane, but has a smaller effect than cyclic AMP on secretion of anions by crypt cells. The ST gene, like that for LT, is plasmid-borne. Enterotoxigenic strains of *E. coli* may produce ST, LT or both; in the last type, the ST and LT genes are carried on the same plasmid.

Exotoxins acting on the nervous system (neurotoxins)

The toxins produced by *Clostridium tetani* and *Cl. botulinum* are the most potent bacterial poisons known, with tetanus toxin only slightly less powerful then botulinum toxin. Both are neurotoxins which act by interfering with the release of neurotransmitter substances, either centrally at synapses in the CNS (tetanus toxin) or peripherally at neuromuscular junctions and parasympathetic synapses (botulinum toxin). Tetanus toxin prevents the release of the inhibitory transmitter *glycine* at motor synapses, leading to overexcitation of motor neurones and hence generalised muscular contraction (*spastic paralysis*); botulinum toxin, in contrast, inhibits release of *acetylcholine* and therefore blocks muscle contraction (*flaccid paralysis*). The evidence suggests that both toxins interfere with the availability or action of calcium ions required for transmitter release. Structurally, the toxins are similar and there is at least a superficial resemblance with diphtheria and cholera toxins. Thus, they are secreted as single polypeptide chains, but their activation involves proteolytic cleavage and reduction of a disulphide bridge; moreover, there are two molecular regions, termed A and B, of which the latter is responsible for binding to cellular receptors, which are membrane *gangliosides*. However, there is little, if any, evidence for an intracellular site of action or for enzymatic activity by the A fragments of the neurotoxins.

There is a single antigenic type of tetanus toxin, but eight of botulinum toxin, secreted by different *C. botulinum* types. A genetic point of interest is that some types of botulinum toxin are coded by bacteriophages and only produced by lysogenic organisms (cf. *C. diphtheriae*); this is not the case for tetanus toxin.

Tetanus toxin (tetanospasmin)

Tetanus (p. 585) results from contamination of a wound by spores of *Cl. tetani*. The spores germinate under anaerobic conditions and toxin is produced inside growing organisms, but only released by autolysis after their death. The symptoms of tetanus are predominantly those of rigidity of voluntary muscles, including characteristic trismus (lockjaw) and violent spasms in the abdomen, back and limbs, with death commonly due to asphyxiation. The organisms themselves remain localised in the wound and the disease is due solely to the toxin; hence the curative effects of antitoxin immunoglobulin and the very successful use of tetanus toxoid in prophylaxis. Thus, where vaccination is practised, tetanus is very uncommon (there are less than 150 cases annually in the USA), though on a worldwide scale it continues to be a major problem with over 250,000 cases annually. In many countries, the toxoid is administered to infants together with diphtheria toxoid as part of the triple vaccine.

Mechanism of action (Figure 4.27).

Tetanus toxin acts centrally rather than locally. Access to the

434

Figure 4.27 Mode of action of tetanus toxin.
(a) Transportation to CNS.
(b) Synaptic events in CNS.

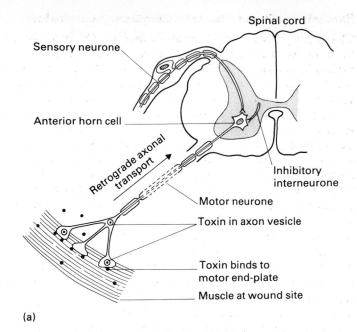

(a)

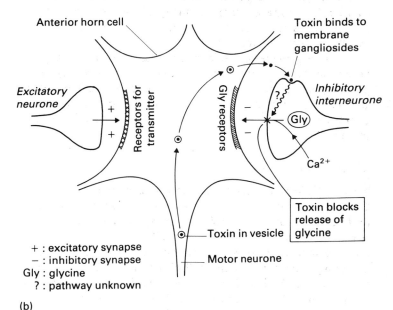

+ : excitatory synapse
− : inhibitory synapse
Gly : glycine
? : pathway unknown

(b)

CNS is by transportation within the axons of motor and sensory nerve fibres, so-called *intra-axonal retrograde transport* (Figure 4.27a). In the area of the wound itself and, following its distribution in the bloodstream, at other sites in the body, toxin molecules bind to ganglioside receptors on motor nerve terminals; pre-incubation of toxin with purified gangliosides GD_2 and GD_{1b} blocks uptake. After binding, the toxin is apparently endocytosed in vesicles and transported in this state within the axoplasm. Evidence for axonal transport includes both immunological detection with antitoxin antibodies and localisation of radio-

435

labelled toxin by autoradiography. On reaching the spinal cord, the toxin emerges and proceeds to interfere with synaptic transmission to anterior horn cells, at first locally but later elsewhere in the spinal cord.

As Figure 4.27b shows, motor neurones normally receive excitatory stimulation, e.g. from sensory neurones or excitatory interneurones, at the same time as inhibitory impulses from inhibitory interneurones. The nature of the excitatory transmitter is not known, but the inhibitory transmitter in the spinal cord is generally glycine. Motor neurone stimulation depends on the outcome of these opposing excitatory and inhibitory influences. A single sensory nerve fibre can form synapses with both types of interneurone, ensuring that the contraction of a particular muscle is accompanied by relaxation of antagonistic muscles. Tetanus toxin acts specifically on the *inhibitory synapses*, preventing the release (rather than either synthesis or action) of glycine from interneurone termini; it has no effect on excitatory transmission. The lack of inhibition leads to over-excitation of motor neurones, which is manifested as increased muscular tone, rigidity and spasm. Such events may be seen as local muscle contraction and twitching around the wound site, but more usually as the generalised form of tetanus, characterised by trismus (lockjaw) and widespread muscular spasms (p. 587).

While it is clear that tetanus toxin acts pre-synaptically, the mechanistic details are less definite. It is widely supposed that there is an intracellular site of action, but there is as yet no firm evidence for this. The toxin may interfere with the release of synaptic vesicles containing glycine by binding to an actomyosin-like protein involved in the release process and inhibiting its calcium-dependent ATPase activity. An effect on cyclic nucleotide metabolism has also been suggested. In any event, the minute amounts of toxin required do indicate that its action is likely to be enzymatic.

Structure

Tetanus toxin is produced as a single polypeptide chain of molecular weight $\sim 150,000$ daltons ('intracellular' or 'progenitor toxin'). The toxicity of this molecule in cell lysates requires proteolytic cleavage, either by bacterial proteases released at the same time, or by added trypsin, to give 'extracellular toxin'. On reduction of a disulphide bond, two polypeptide chains can be obtained from the cleaved toxin, the A and B fragments. Of these, B (100,000 mol.wt) binds to membrane gangliosides and is non-toxic, while A (50,000 mol. wt) is also non-toxic, but required for the activity of the whole molecule. These properties invite comparison with diphtheria toxin but, as there is no proof of an intracellular enzymatic activity by the A fragment of tetanus toxin, it would be premature to suggest that the molecules are strictly analogous.

Botulinum toxin

This is the most poisonous bacterial product known, the lethal dose for man being about 1 μg. Unlike tetanus, botulism is not usually an infectious disease in man, but rather an *intoxication* brought about by the ingestion of toxin *preformed* in food—quite literally a food poisoning (p. 589). Thus the role of toxin in the disease is beyond any possible doubt. (Occasional infection of the gastrointestinal tract with *Cl. botulinum* occurs in infants, with production of toxin *in vivo*.) There are eight antigenically distinct types of botulinum toxin, each produced by a different *Cl. botulinum* type and designated A, B, C_1, C_2, D, E, F and G. Differences exist in the distribution of the toxin types and in the susceptibility to each of different species: human botulism is caused by types A, B, E and F, with A being present in some 60% of cases. The sources of type A toxin can be home-preserved fruit, vegetables or meat, while B is usually acquired from meat and E from uncooked seafood. The spores, which withstand boiling for several hours, germinate in the anaerobic conditions provided by preserved foods. Like tetanus toxin, botulinum toxin is released from the organisms by autolysis. Botulism leads to flaccid paralysis of skeletal and respiratory muscles (especially those innervated by the parasympathetic nervous system) and is very often fatal despite antitoxin treatment, unless the latter is instituted before the onset of clinical symptoms.

Mechanism of action

There are some parallels but also important differences between the actions of botulinum and tetanus toxins. Botulinum toxin is absorbed from the gut, seemingly unaffected by stomach acid or intestinal proteases, possibly even activated by the latter. It is carried in the bloodstream to peripheral neuromuscular junctions where its action is to block release of acetylcholine (ACh) from the nerve terminals at the motor end-plate; since ACh is responsible for transmission of stimuli from nerve to muscle (Figure 2.54) this interference leads to the abolition of muscle tone. Thus, botulinum toxin acts *presynaptically* and, as with tetanus toxin, the first step is binding to membrane gangliosides; this is followed by inhibition of release of ACh vesicles, probably by interference in the supply of Ca^{2+} ions required for ACh release. In an experimental model with isolated synaptosomes, the effect of botulinum toxin could be overcome by an ionophore which allows Ca^{2+} ions to cross membranes freely. Calculations of the number of toxin molecules likely to reach neuromuscular junctions and the number of ACh vesicles and release sites suggest that the mechanism may be a direct consequence of toxin binding rather than an enzymatic effect.

Structure and genetics of production

The eight types of botulinum toxin are distinct both antigenically and in their relative toxicities for different species;

nevertheless, they are all of similar structure and resemble tetanus toxin in having a protein chain of ~ 150,000 mol.wt which is activated by proteolytic cleavage. The neurotoxin is not the only component of the molecule as found in culture fluids, but is complexed with a large haemagglutinin (~ 500,000 mol.wt) which seems to protect the neurotoxin from destruction by acid and proteolysis in the gut. Like diphtheria toxin and streptococcal erythrogenic toxin, production of certain types of botulinum toxin (C, D and E) is dependent on lysogenised bacteriophages (p. 446). Lysogenic strains of *Cl. botulinum* can be 'cured' of their phages by heating the spores to 70°C for 15 minutes, whereupon production of toxin by the vegetative organisms is abolished; cured organisms can then be reinfected with an appropriate phage and will then start producing the toxin coded by that phage. In this way, a type C organism was converted into type D or into *C. novyi* type A (when infected by phage NA_1 which specifies production of α-toxin by that organism). Thus the 'type' of these clostridia is wholly determined by the phage with which they are silently infected.

Endotoxin

In contrast with exotoxins, which are soluble proteins usually secreted by growing organisms, endotoxins are complex cell-associated molecules (lipopolysaccharides, LPS) which form part of the outer membrane of Gram-negative bacteria (p. 394). It is often stated that endotoxin is only released by cell lysis, and while this may indeed be the major source, it is also shed by growing organisms. Although less potent than many exotoxins, endotoxin nevertheless plays a significant part in the pathogenesis of diseases caused by Gram-negative organisms, in particular the characteristic fever of *typhoid*, abortion in animals with *brucellosis*, and the syndrome of *septic shock* which accompanies septicaemia or extensive local infection by various Gram-negative bacteria. The effects of endotoxin are made complicated by the multiplicity of its interactions with the cells and molecular systems of inflammation, immunity and haemostasis. Indeed, it has been exceptionally difficult to distinguish primary effects from secondary changes or trivial responses and this has given rise to a rather confused picture. Note that while the terms lipopolysaccharide and endotoxin are often interchangeable, the latter is generally used in discussing toxicity and the former when referring to structure.

STRUCTURE AND TOXICITY

The Gram-negative cell envelope and structure of LPS have been described on p. 394 (Figure 4.6b, c), and it will be recalled that the outer membrane is a bilayer in which the lipid of the outer layer consists largely of LPS. *Lipid A*, rather than carbohydrate, is the important toxic moiety (toxophore) of LPS. Thus, the toxicity of LPS isolated from rough organisms (mutants which lack the O side-chains) is undiminished. Due to its insolubility, free lipid A itself has only modest biological activity; in the intact molecule the polysaccharide is responsible for solubility, but can be replaced artificially by protein carriers such as BSA. Purified lipid A solubilised in this way or by chemical means has all the toxicity of intact endotoxin.

ASSAY

A sensitive assay for endotoxin is based on the 'gelation' of extracts of blood cells of the horseshoe crab *Limulus polyphemus*; this is sensitive to picogram amounts and is thus useful for detecting small quantities in the circulation. It can also be employed in detection of meningitis due to Gram-negative organisms and for pyrogen screening of solutions to be administered by parenteral inoculation.

TOXIC EFFECTS IN VIVO

The effects of injection of purified endotoxin depend on the dose and route of administration. Intradermal injection of small amounts (0.1-1.0 nanogram) causes an inflammatory response with infiltration of mononuclear cells and, at higher doses, neutrophils. When given intravenously, the most sensitive response is *fever*, the minimum dose required to produce a pyrogenic (febrile) reaction in man being only 1-5 ng per kg. Fever occurs within 90-120 minutes, lasts for several hours and may be accompanied by chills, headache, muscular pain and vomiting. If repeated intravenous injections of endotoxin are given, or if it is infused continuously, a state of *tolerance*—a decline in the febrile response to a particular dose—develops within a few hours, and can be observed during typhoid fever itself. Tolerance lasts for two weeks after contact with endotoxin and is overcome by increasing the dose; it does not occur on injection of endotoxin into the tissues.

As well as inducing fever, endotoxin inoculation causes changes in the level of circulating leucocytes, especially granulocytes; an initial reduction (leucopenia) is followed by increased production from the bone marrow (leucocytosis) within a few hours. There are also important *metabolic changes*, including transient hyperglycaemia followed by marked hypoglycaemia, resulting from the increased uptake of glucose by peripheral tissues and the failure of the liver to make good circulating levels.

High doses of endotoxin induce lethal *shock*, due to hypotension and fall in cardiac output following the release of vasoactive substances such as histamine and kinins and activation of complement, though the nature of the response is species-dependent. Activation of the clotting system also occurs, with *disseminated intravascular coagulation* (p. 444). A much studied experimental model for endotoxin-induced shock is the *Schwartzmann reaction*, which is produced in rabbits when two injections of small amounts of endotoxin are given to the same animal, separated by an interval of 24 hours. The reaction can take one of two forms. (a) The *local* Schwartzmann reaction occurs when the first inoculation of endotoxin is intradermal and the second intravenous: a few hours after the second injection, a haemorrhagic lesion develops at the original inoculation site, with platelet thrombi in venules. (b) The *generalised* Schwartzmann reaction is seen when both injections are intravenous: 24 hours after the second, the animal usually dies of shock, with intravascular coagulation and renal cortical necrosis as characteristic findings. These lesions are most readily produced in rabbits, which have a poorly developed fibrinolytic system.

Endotoxin is also an abortifacient. Its injection into pregnant guinea-pigs, rabbits and rats almost invariably induces abortion, and it underlies the abortion in ungulates which results from infection with *Brucella abortus*.

Altogether, endotoxin poisoning affects many organs, including the liver, kidneys, skeletal muscle, cardiovascular system, gastrointestinal tract and the immune system. In order to understand these complex and widespread reactions, we must first consider what is known of the effects of endotoxin on cells and molecular pathways.

CELLULAR EFFECTS OF ENDOTOXIN

Although endotoxin will kill some cells outright when present at high enough concentrations, its main effects are seen in living cells as alterations of function and metabolic processes. The cell types which are particularly influenced by endotoxin *in vivo* are phagocytes (including granulocytes and macrophages), platelets, B lymphocytes and fibroblasts. The initial event in all cases is binding to cell surface receptors, which may be followed by endocytosis. Although endotoxin reacts non-specifically with membrane phospholipids such as lecithin, the specific receptor has not yet been identified. Interestingly, there are strains of mice which are genetically resistant to the cellular, pyrogenic and lethal effects of endotoxin (e.g. C3H/HeJ), probably because their cells lack the specific receptors.

Kupffer Cells

The liver is a major target organ of intravenously injected endotoxin and is responsible for clearing more than 80% from the circulation in the first hour after inoculation. In the liver, endotoxin is associated both with the phagocytic Kupffer cells and with parenchyma. Like other phagocytes, such as neutrophils, Kupffer cells are induced by endotoxin to synthesize and release small proteins (10,000–20,000 mol.wt) known collectively as *endogenous pyrogen*. These proteins are responsible for the fever which accompanies the presence of endotoxin and which typifies infections by certain Gram-negative organisms (e.g. typhoid fever). The action of endogenous pyrogen may be directly on the thermoregulatory centres of the hypothalamus, but is perhaps more likely to occur via stimulation of prostaglandin synthesis, either locally in the brain or in extraneural tissues, since prostaglandins are probably the final mediators of febrile responses. Thus aspirin and indomethacin suppress induction of fever by endotoxin (p. 37). The reason for believing that Kupffer cells, rather than neutrophils, are the main source of endogenous pyrogen in response to endotoxin is that in the state of tolerance which follows repeated daily injections of a particular dose of endotoxin, Kupffer cells are inhibited in their production of endogenous pyrogen, whereas granulocytes are not affected. This type of tolerance can also be overcome by 'blockading' (saturating) the reticuloendothelial system with agents such as thorium oxide or India ink, presumably because more endotoxin is then available to neutrophils which do not show tolerance. (While the alteration of Kupffer cell responsiveness probably accounts for a rapidly developing but transient tolerance, there is a more prolonged tolerant state which develops after a few days and is more likely due to the presence of antibodies specific for the polysaccharide moieties of endotoxin (anti-O, anti-core). Thus, the latter type of tolerance, but not the former, is transferable with serum.)

Granulocytes

The neutrophil is one of the primary targets for the action of endotoxin, a reaction which has important secondary consequences through the role of this cell in inflammation and tissue damage (see Sections 1 and 2). Neutrophils are a source of endogenous pyrogen and may therefore contribute to fever, though for the reason mentioned above they are thought to be less significant in this respect than Kupffer cells. The most important result of uptake of endotoxin by neutrophils is the release of their lysosomal contents to the outside. As described in Section 1 (p. 18), this leads to the generation of vasoactive mediators of acute inflammation (i) by release of kallikrein, which causes formation of *kinins* such as bradykinin, (ii) by the action of proteases on complement, with production of the anaphylatoxins C3a and C5a, and (iii) via cationic proteins which, like anaphylatoxins, stimulate release of histamine from mast cells. The inflammatory mediators play an important role in the production of septic shock by causing vasodilatation in the peripheral circulation. Moreover, after an initial leucopenia, endotoxin causes a surge of production of granulocytes from the bone marrow, reaching a peak after 12–24 hours. The young granulocytes are a particularly rich source of cationic proteins, the release of which also contributes to the stabilisation of fibrin clots. It must also be remembered that neutrophil enzymes will contribute to tissue damage, as in Type III hypersensitivity. Enzyme release from neutrophils (and macrophages) is inhibited by hydrocortisone, which stabilises lysosomal membranes; this may account for the ability of hydrocortisone to protect against lethal endotoxaemia.

Macrophages

Macrophages are brought to a state of activation by endotoxin, with hyperplasia, greatly increased speed of phagocytosis and increased production of lysosomal enzymes; like granulocytes, they are also induced to shed their enzymes to the outside, which may lead to enzymatic activity in the blood. Macrophage activation may be important in the increased resistance to infection of endotoxin-treated animals. Endotoxin-activated macrophages will kill tumour cells in a non-specific manner (but selective for transformed over normal cells), evidently also by releasing the contents of their lysosomal granules. An inhibitory effect of endotoxin on human cancer has been recognised for many years and is probably mediated by macrophages, since endotoxin itself does not kill tumour cells directly (see also p. 745). An antitumour factor (tumour necrosis factor) is present in the circulation of animals injected with endotoxin and seems to be macrophage-derived.

Platelets

The interaction of endotoxin with platelets is probably involved in the induction of the intravascular coagulation and thrombosis of small blood vessels which are characteristic of septic shock, although the importance of platelet involvement varies in different animal species. Thus, in rabbits, thrombocytopenia prevents the generalised Schwartzmann reaction (though the effect in dogs is much less pronounced). Endotoxin stimulates the *platelet release reaction* with secretion of the platelets' granular contents, leading to aggregation (Figure 4.28), thrombosis and clotting by the processes described in Section 5, as well as to vascular changes of inflammation (p. 38). Note that human platelets exposed to endotoxin *in vitro* do not show the degranulation and aggregation which is so marked with rabbit platelets.

Lymphocytes

The effect of endotoxin on lymphocytes has been particularly useful in studies of *B cell differentiation*. LPS is a selective lymphocyte *mitogen* which causes B cells to divide but has no mitogenic action on T cells. Moreover, it is a *polyclonal activator* of B cells, meaning that as well as dividing, endotoxin-stimulated B cells mature into antibody-secreting cells and produce IgM; the term 'polyclonal' indicates that most of the Ig is the product of diverse B cell clones with no selection of specificity for endotoxin itself. The ability to act as a maturation signal for B cells has made it a widely used experimental agent. B cells of the C3H/HeJ mouse strain do not divide in response to endotoxin stimulation, due to a defect in a gene locus on chromosome 4 (the *LPS* gene) which probably codes for the receptor leading to cell triggering. *In vivo*, endotoxin is an adjuvant, i.e. it increases the level of immune responses, and this may be one reason it enhances resistance to infection (macrophage activation is another). It is also a well-studied thymus-independent antigen, which induces B cells to make *specific* anti-endotoxin IgM in the absence of T cells, e.g. in nude mice (p. 110). The immunological effects of endotoxin are in general more pronounced in the mouse than in man.

Figure 4.28 Interaction of endotoxin (lipopolysaccharide) and rabbit platelets *in vitro* as seen by electron microscopy.
(a) Normal platelets (×10,000).
(b) A few minutes after addition of endotoxin, platelets show characteristic changes in shape and start to degranulate. In this micrograph, 2 strips of endotoxin can be seen between the adherent platelets (×15,000).
(c) Aggregated platelets after longer incubation; many strips of endotoxin are visible (×10,000).
(Courtesy of Dr Audrey Glauert and Dr J.L. Gordon.)

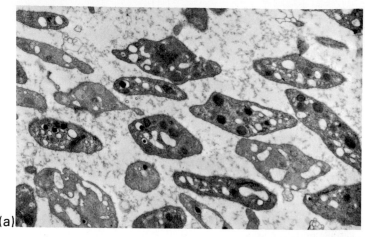
(a)

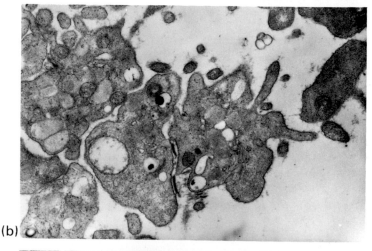
(b)

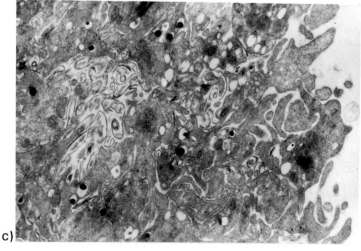
(c)

Endotoxin activates the pathways of inflammation, complement, blood clotting and fibrinolysis (Figure 4.29). The shedding of enzymes by neutrophils is, as we have noted, a starting point for activation of both kinins and complement, and the platelet release reaction provides further enzymes, vasoactive amines and prostaglandins. *Complement* itself can also be activated by endotoxin directly, via the *alternative pathway* (p. 123). During infection by Gram-negative bacteria, this is probably a defence mechanism which may lead to lysis of the organisms or uptake by phagocytes without requiring a specific antibody response. It also generates the anaphylatoxins C3a and C5a, with subsequent release of histamine from mast cells. *Hageman factor*, a central element in the pathways of inflammation (p. 34), coagulation (p. 634) and fibrinolysis (p. 636), is activated by endotoxin, an event which will clearly have far-reaching consequences.

PATHOLOGICAL EFFECTS OF ENDOTOXIN

Fever

We have noted that a pyrogenic response follows intravenous injection of endotoxin, and this is likely to be involved in the fever which is prominent in some diseases caused by Gram-negative bacteria, including typhoid fever, plague, tularaemia and brucellosis.

Disseminated intravascular coagulation (DIC)

The activation of the clotting system by endotoxin leads to

Figure 4.29 Pathways of endotoxin action.

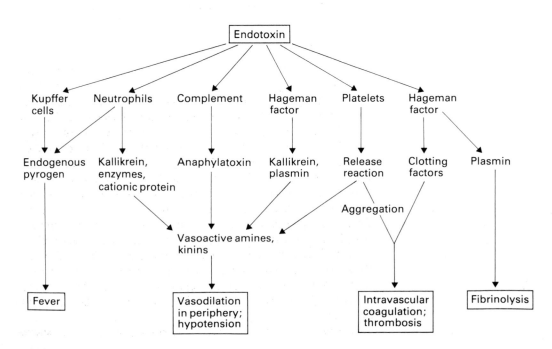

deposition of *fibrin thrombi* in small blood vessels and ischaemic tissue damage to various organs. It is characteristic of septicaemia with Gram-negative bacteria and is part of the syndrome of septic shock, which it greatly aggravates. The effects are generally most severe in the kidneys, due to obstruction of arterioles and glomeruli, with renal tubular injury and typical *cortical necrosis*. The lungs, brain and adrenals are sometimes also affected; e.g. adrenal haemorrhage and acute adrenocortical insufficiency (the *Waterhouse–Friderichsen syndrome*) are severe complications of meningococcal septicaemia (p. 536).

Endotoxin-stimulated mechanisms of clotting in DIC are threefold (Figure 4.29): (i) activation of Hageman factor (Factor XII) and hence the intrinsic clotting cascade (p. 633); (ii) activation of platelets, providing both platelet factor 3 and the conditions for thrombosis (p. 641); and (iii) release from neutrophils of cationic proteins which contribute to stabilisation of fibrin. One of the consequences of DIC, paradoxical at first sight, is a *haemorrhagic state* with profuse bleeding from mucous membranes (e.g. in the gastrointestinal tract) which is the dominant clinical feature of its later stages. The bleeding tendency arises for several reasons: clotting factors and fibrinogen become consumed during intravascular coagulation; platelet levels also fall significantly (thrombocytopenia); and the fibrinolytic enzyme *plasmin* (p. 636), activated by Hageman factor, destroys both fibrin (e.g. in thrombi) and fibrinogen. Fibrin degradation products (FDP) further interfere with clotting.

Another consequence of DIC is that the presence of fibrin strands in small vessels causes fragmentation of red cells as they are 'sieved' through the fibrin mesh, leading to a haemolytic anaemia in which characteristic odd-shaped fragments can be seen in the blood (*microangiopathic haemolytic anaemia*).

Septic shock

This occurs during severe infections with Gram-negative organisms, when bacteria enter the bloodstream in large numbers (bacteraemia, septicaemia, p. 489), or in peritonitis. The organisms commonly involved are *E. coli*, Klebsiella, Proteus, and *Pseudomonas aeruginosa*. It is a complication of gastro-intestinal or urogenital surgery, perforation of the bowel, or infection of burns (where *P. aeruginosa* is a common oppor-tunistic pathogen); immunodeficient or immunosuppressed patients are also at risk. Septic shock develops in about half the patients with bacteraemia due to these organisms. A central feature is *hypotension* (fall in blood pressure) due to decreased peripheral vascular resistance; this in turn is a consequence of the release of vasoactive amines, such as histamine, and kinins through the action of endotoxin on neutrophils, platelets and complement (Figure 4.29). DIC is a further aggravating factor. The mortality is very high, especially in the elderly, death often being due to heart failure.

It is also held that endotoxin contributes to non-septic shock following *haemorrhage*, when its absorption from the alimentary tract occurs.

GENETIC ASPECTS OF PATHOGENICITY

INTRODUCTION

The pathogenetic attributes of bacteria are genetically determined and stably inherited, with variants of greater or lesser degrees of virulence arising through the normal processes of mutation and selection. However, there is also the possibility for a bacterial organism to acquire new inheritable characteristics by taking up genetic material which then becomes added to its own, and it is with the processes and implications of such *gene acquisition* that we are concerned here. The mechanisms include infection by bacteriophages which, instead of multiplying, insert their genome into that of the bacterial cell (*lysogeny*), and the transfer of DNA between bacterial cells by *transformation, transduction* and *conjugation*. These processes may be collectively described as *infectious heredity*. Genetic material thus acquired is of particular interest when it alters or adds to the characteristics of the cell, and especially when it enables an organism to become more virulent. For example, the new genes may code for toxins or bacterial wall structures associated with pathogenicity or may confer resistance to antimicrobial drugs.

Plasmids are vehicles for gene transfer which have received much attention in recent years; they are independent loops of DNA which are not associated with the bacterial chromosome and which may carry virulence or drug-resistance factors as well as other genes. The transfer of plasmid-borne genes by conjugation has created antibiotic-resistant organisms which have been the cause of some major epidemics in recent years and are an increasing medical problem. Plasmids are also central to *recombinant DNA* research and technology ('genetic engineering') on which an exciting new industry, full of potential applications to medicine, has been based.

LYSOGENY

The term lysogeny means the persistence in a bacterial cell of the genetic information of a *bacteriophage* (a virus which infects bacteria), generally by integration of phage DNA into the cell chromosome. Its significance for bacterial pathogenicity lies principally in the introduction of genes coding for *toxins* into otherwise avirulent cells, the most prominent example being the production of diphtheria toxin by strains of *C. diphtheriae* which carry the β corynephage in their chromosomes (p. 415).

Bacteriophages may be either *virulent* or *temperate*. Virulent phages multiply in the cells they infect, which are ultimately killed and from which progeny phage are released by lysis. Temperate phages may also undergo such a replicative (vegetative) cycle, but alternatively their DNA may persist in the cell without production of phage particles (lysogeny). The replicative and lysogenic phases of a temperate phage are illustrated in Figure 4.30. The persistent, but non-infectious, phage DNA is called a *prophage* and the bacterial organism is referred to as *lysogenic*, indicating a tendency to lyse should the prophage become activated. From time to time, a prophage may shift into a replicative state, whereupon it is released from the chromosome and proceeds to reproduce like a virulent phage; such activation is encouraged by low levels of u.v. irradiation or other agents (below). Many bacteria are lysogenic for some or other phage in their natural environment. A small proportion of the organisms of a lysogenic strain usually release progeny phage through spontaneous activation.

Insertion

One of the best studied examples of lysogeny is that of λ phage in *E. coli* strain K12. The process of *insertion* of the λ prophage into the chromosome is shown in Figure 4.31; it proceeds by the circularisation of the linear λ genome, followed by its integration

Figure 4.30 Modes of development of a temperate bacteriophage.

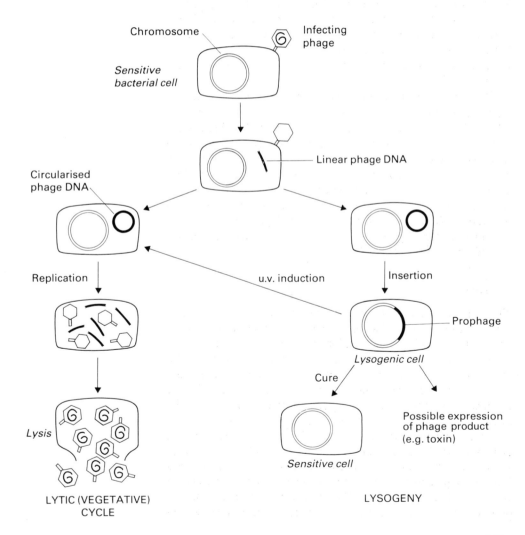

447

at a specific fixed point on the chromosome by a single reciprocal crossover between λ and cell DNA. Essentially the same events occur in insertion of β phage DNA into the *C. diphtheriae* chromosome (Figure 4.15).

Immunity

An important phenomenon associated with the lysogenic state is *immunity* to superinfection: if a lysogenic cell is infected by a phage particle of the same type as the prophage it carries, the cell is protected from lysis through an ability to inhibit productive phage replication. The infecting phage adsorbs to the cell and its DNA enters but fails to replicate. The basis of immunity is the

Figure 4.31 Model for integration of λ phage DNA into bacterial chromosome as prophage.
A, U, h, cl, mi = λ genes or markers
Gal, Bio = bacterial genes
P, P' = λ attachment sites
B, B' = bacterial attachment sites.

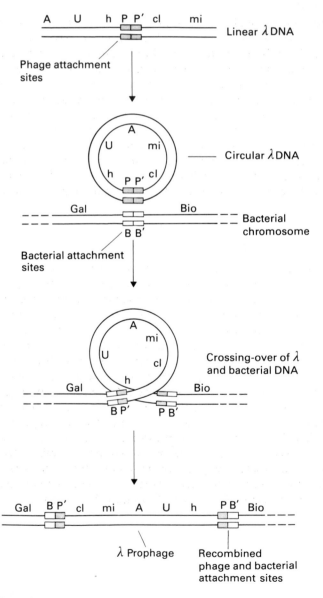

λ Prophage   Recombined phage and bacterial attachment sites

presence in the cell of an inhibitory protein known as the *immunity repressor*, coded by the prophage, which actively and specifically prevents replication by inhibiting transcription of phage DNA. The presence of the repressor is in fact an indispensable feature of lysogeny, as the state can only exist and be maintained through the action of the repressor. Mutations in the phage repressor gene prevent lysogenisation, but allow replication. Thus, mutant phages give rise to clear plaques of complete lysis on sensitive bacteria, whereas the native temperate phages produce turbid plaques (partial lysis). The λ immunity repressor has been isolated and shown to be an acidic oligomeric protein which binds to operator sites on DNA, thus preventing transcription and suppressing the expression of most phage genes.

Reactivation

Reactivation of the phage can, as noted above, occasionally occur spontaneously in rare cells; it does not lead to lysis of neighbouring organisms as they are already immune. Large-scale activation is initiated by procedures which impair the repressor, such as u.v. irradiation in doses too low to damage the phage DNA (u.v. induces a cellular protease which destroys the repressor protein). Other activating agents are X-irradiation, thymine starvation, alkylating agents and some carcinogens. In the normal course of events, activation leads to cell *lysis*; sometimes, however, the prophage can be removed from the chromosome without entering a replicative cycle. Lysogenic bacteria from which a prophage has been removed are said to be *cured*.

Lysogenic conversion

Although most prophages do not alter the characteristics of the bacterial cell, other than inducing immunity to superinfection, a few are responsible for an important virulence property, namely toxin production. In addition to diphtheria toxin, botulinum toxin types C and D, streptococcal erythrogenic toxin (of scarlet fever) and *Cl. novyi* α-toxin are all products of lysogenised phages (Table 4.4). The introduction of a new property such as toxigenicity into a strain via a phage is called lysogenic conversion. Usually the toxin genes are not immediately essential to phage survival, since mutations in them do not affect replication or lysogeny. Nevertheless, they are presumably useful to the phages since they help secure better prospects for growth of their bacterial hosts. The phenomenon of conversion raises the possibility that these genes, though carried by phages, are in fact of cellular origin and have been picked up by the phage at some stage in its (perhaps recent) past (cf. transduction, below).

Gene transfer between bacteria

In the transfer of genetic material between bacteria by transformation, transduction or conjugation, part of the genome of a donor cell is transferred to a recipient cell. The transferred DNA is generally a plasmid or a fragment of the chromosome, though it is possible for long stretches of DNA, or even the entire chromosome, to be transferred by conjugation. The transferred genes may then be inserted into the recipient chromosome by recombination, either being added to the genome or replacing an existing chromosomal gene or, if in plasmid form, remain free in the recipient cytoplasm. There are obvious parallels between processes of DNA transfer between bacteria, especially conjugation, and sexual reproduction of eukaryotic cells though, as will become evident, the analogy is a very partial one.

TRANSFORMATION

Discovery

This was the first phenomenon involving interbacterial gene transfer to be discovered (Griffith, 1928) though its significance as such went unrecognised for several years; it became the means by which molecular genetics was launched when, in 1944, Avery, MacLeod and McCarty showed that the 'transforming principle' was DNA. Griffith's original experiment involved virulent and avirulent forms of pneumococci (*Streptococcus pneumoniae*). The virulence of these organisms depends on the presence of the antiphagocytic bacterial capsule, non-encapsulated forms being harmless (unless they revert to an encapsulated form). Encapsulated organisms form smooth (S) colonies on agar, while the non-encapsulated variants, derived from the former by mutation, grow as rough (R) colonies. (The organisms themselves are also referred to as smooth (S) and rough (R) respectively, p. 401). Another point used in the experiment is that there are several pneumococcal types with distinct capsular polysaccharides recognised by type-specific antisera. Griffith inoculated a mixture of heat-killed S cells of type 1 pneumococci and living R cells of type 2 pneumococci into mice (Figure 4.32). Neither of these organisms alone could harm the animals, but the mixture proved virulent and the mice died. Although this might have been due to reversion of type 2 organisms from R into S (which did in fact also occur), it was possible to demonstrate that the mice carried *living* S forms of the *type 1* pneumococci. The only feasible way these could have arisen was that type 2 R cells had been *transformed* into type 1 S cells by a substance derived from killed type 1 organisms.

Process of DNA transfer

We now know that transformation results from the physical transfer of fragments of naked DNA from one organism to another; in the case of the Griffith experiment, the transferred DNA carried the gene determining presence and type of the

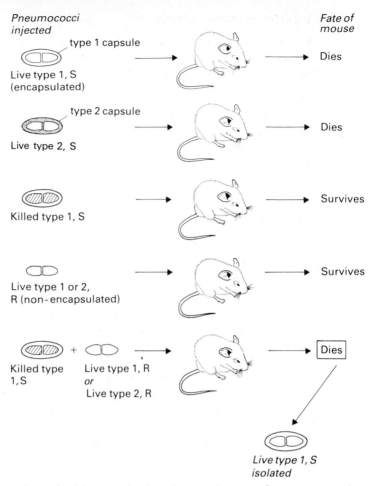

Figure 4.32 Griffith's experiment demonstrating transformation of pneumococci.
S = smooth
R = rough

Pneumococci injected

Fate of mouse

type 1 capsule
Live type 1, S (encapsulated)
Dies

type 2 capsule
Live type 2, S
Dies

Killed type 1, S
Survives

Live type 1 or 2, R (non-encapsulated)
Survives

Killed type 1, S + Live type 1, R or Live type 2, R
Dies

Live type 1, S isolated

polysaccharide capsule, but in practice any fragment may be transferred. DNA released by lysis of dead cells is split into fragments of varying sizes by enzymes or mechanical damage. Pneumococci, and a variety of other organisms, take up double-stranded DNA (including that of distantly related bacterial species) at certain sites in the cell wall; single-stranded DNA does not bind. The presence of adsorption/entry sites determines the *competence* of the cell to take up DNA and depends firstly on a particular stage of the cell cycle—the entry zones seem to be regions of cell wall synthesis—and secondly on a soluble protein called *competence factor* which facilitates the process of uptake and can be found in bacterial culture supernatants. Once adherent to the bacterial membrane, the DNA is cut to an approximately constant length by a membrane endonuclease; *one strand only* is then taken up into the cytoplasm. In order to become inserted into the chromosome, it must find a closely similar (homologous) stretch of DNA with which it first pairs by hybridisation, displacing the chromosomal partner strand and becoming integrated by a double crossover (Figure 4.33a). Thus, transformation can only be efficient between closely related bacteria, generally within a species, because of the requirement for regions of DNA homology.

451

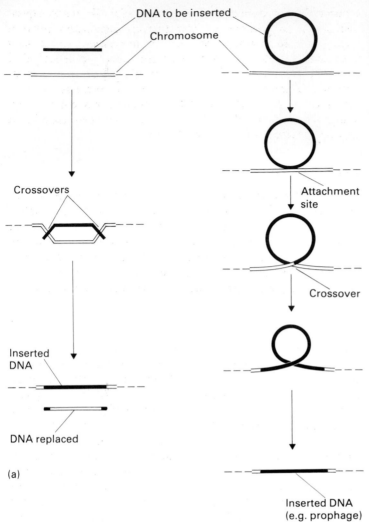

DNA to be inserted

Chromosome

Figure 4.33 Mechanisms of insertion of DNA into a bacterial chromosome.
(a) Integration of linear DNA by double crossover (e.g. transformation, generalised transduction).
(b) Integration of circular DNA by single crossover (e.g. lysogeny, specialised transduction).

Crossovers

Attachment site

Crossover

Inserted DNA

DNA replaced

(a)

Inserted DNA
(e.g. prophage)

(b)

Occurrence

Transformation can occur within several genera besides *Streptococcus*, including *Haemophilus*, *Staphylococcus*, *Neisseria* and *Bacillus*; it does not normally occur with the Gram-negative enteric organisms unless the cell wall is damaged. However, enterics can be induced to take up DNA by brief exposure to $CaCl_2$, a technique used in genetic engineering where it is necessary to introduce recombinant DNA into cells of *E. coli* (p. 474). The term *transfection* is used for this mode of transformation.

Significance

Transformation requires bacterial enzymes specialised for the purpose and must therefore have evolved as a mechanism of gene transfer. Its occurrence in nature is thus very likely and experimentally it is possible to show that transformation between related avirulent strains can lead to increased pathogenicity (complementation). It may therefore have epidemiological importance as a means of quickly generating virulent organisms, but its significance in this respect is difficult to assess. *In vitro*, resistance to antimicrobial drugs, including penicillin, streptomycin, sulphonamides and optochin, has been transferred between pneumococci by transformation.

TRANSDUCTION

In this phenomenon, genes are transferred between bacterial cells by means of a bacteriophage vector. As in transformation, only a small part of the genome can be transferred, generally no more than 1–2%. However, since the DNA transferred is protected by the phage coat, rather than naked as in transformation, transduction is the easier to demonstrate. There are two separate mechanisms, namely generalised and specialised transduction.

Generalised transduction

This occurs as a side-effect of the lytic cycle of a replicating phage. During phage replication, the host genome is enzymatically degraded into small fragments and, provided they are small enough, they may occasionally be incorporated into the phage particle as it assembles, *replacing* the phage nucleic acid (Figure 4.34a). Such particles, which represent only about 0.1% of mature phage progeny, can then transfer the genomic fragment to a recipient bacterium, as they have all the apparatus for infection; they are known as *transducing particles*. After entering the cell, the transduced DNA may be successfully integrated into the recipient's chromosome as in transformation and be replicated with it when the cell divides (*complete transduction*). Often, however, the fragment fails to integrate (or multiply within the cell), and is then carried into only one of the daughter cells on division (*abortive transduction*).

Specialised (restricted) transduction

This is a much more limited phenomenon which occurs during the activation of prophages in lysogenic bacteria. Activation entails excision of the prophage from its site of integration; while this is generally very accurate, it can happen that a chromosomal gene(s) neighbouring the prophage is excised with it, phage gene(s) being lost (deleted) at the same time to compensate for length. The excised phage DNA with its attached bacterial gene may then be replicated and incorporated into phage particles which are subsequently released from the cell on lysis; infection and lysogenisation of a recipient cell then introduces the linked bacterial gene into the recipient chromosome (Figure 4.34b). Since the insertion of prophages only takes place at specific chromosomal sites, this form of transduction can only transfer

(a)

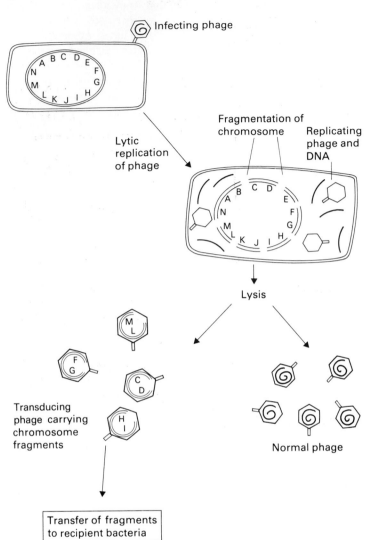

Figure 4.34 Mechanisms of transduction.
(a) Generalised transduction.
(b) *opposite* Specialised transduction, with λ phage as example.

Infecting phage

Lytic replication of phage

Fragmentation of chromosome

Replicating phage and DNA

Lysis

Transducing phage carrying chromosome fragments

Normal phage

Transfer of fragments to recipient bacteria

genes in the immediate vicinity of the insertion points. Thus, in a classic example of specialised transduction by λ phage in *E. coli*, the genes for galactose utilisation (*gal*) or biotin synthesis (*bio*), which adjoin the λ insertion site, are transferred (Figure 4.34b). The transducing phage may be *defective* if the deleted phage genes are necessary for replication; in this case a defective prophage cannot be reactivated from the recipient after lysogeny except in the presence of a coinfecting normal λ particle to act as helper by replacing the missing functions. Specialised transduction has been very useful in bacterial genetic studies.

Like transformation, transduction may have some importance in generating bacterial variants under natural conditions, though its significance in producing strains of increased virulence is unknown.

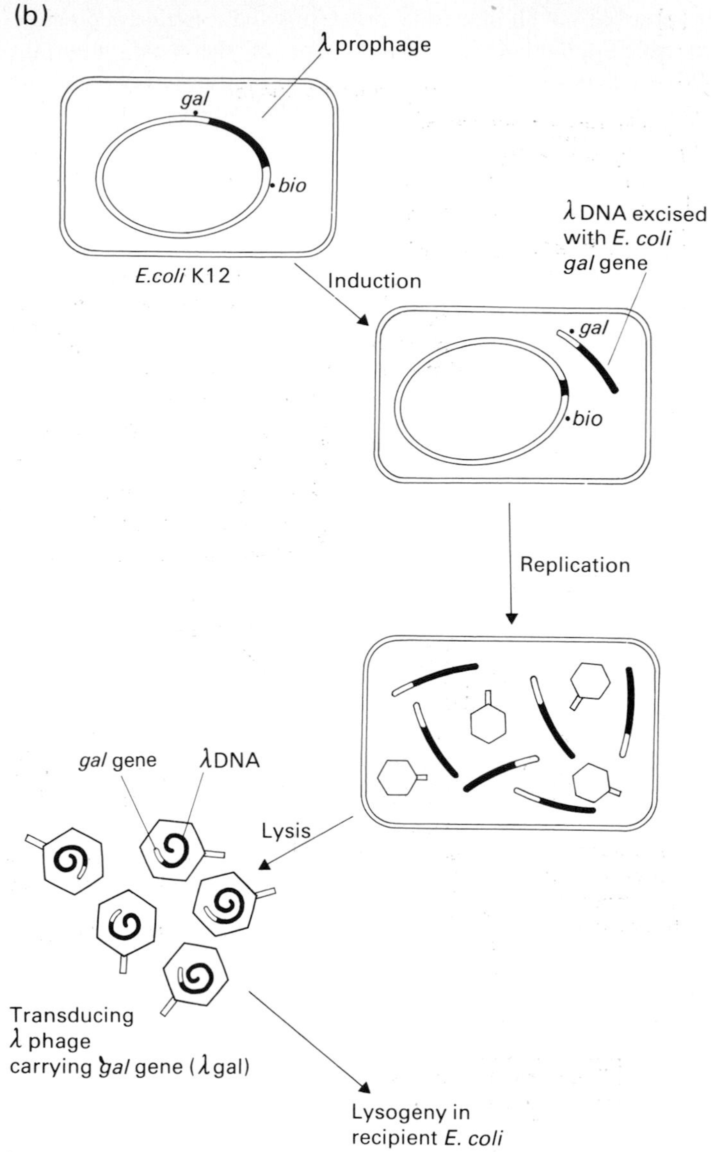

(b)

PLASMIDS

Introduction

Not all bacterial genes are carried chromosomally: some are found instead on separate loops of DNA called plasmids. While plasmid-borne genes are not usually essential to the survival of the organism in its natural environment, they include some which play an important role in bacterial infection, among them genes which enable bacteria to resist the action of antimicrobial drugs such as antibiotics (*resistance* or *R genes*) and others which code for virulence factors including toxins. Plasmids occur in virtually all the classes of bacteria infecting man and animals; they are present in most but not all individual organisms and it is always possible to isolate plasmid-free variants. One of the most important properties of plasmids is their ability to be transferred from one organism to another by the process of *conjugation* (mating) and in this way plasmid-borne genes can be acquired by different species and genera. Thus, plasmids are *extrachromosomal agents of infectious inheritance.*

Antibiotic resistance stands out as a plasmid-borne trait which has become a serious medical problem throughout the world, especially dangerous in epidemics of diseases caused by Gram-negative organisms, such as typhoid fever and bacillary dysentery, as well as being troublesome in infections by opportunistic pathogens in hospitals. Plasmid genes are directly responsible for certain important diseases, including the gastroenteritis caused by enteropathic strains of *E. coli* and staphylococcal impetigo. However, other plasmid genes are of distinct ecological benefit, such as those which enable the bacteria associated with the roots of leguminous plants (*Rhizobium* spp.) to fix nitrogen, or which code for antibiotics (chloramphenicol genes in *Streptomyces*).

Plasmids themselves are responsible for the phenomenon of bacterial conjugation by coding for the necessary structures involved (sex pili). Sometimes during conjugation the bacterial chromosome itself is transferred from one organism to another, and by following the appearance of chromosomally-coded traits in the recipients it is possible to utilise conjugation as a means of mapping bacterial genes; indeed it became invaluable for this purpose in the 1950's and 1960's. More recently, plasmids have assumed a new importance in genetics through their use as vectors in *gene cloning*. By means of certain specialised enzymes, DNA from any source, including man, can be inserted into a plasmid and introduced into bacteria; as the plasmids multiply with the organisms, the 'foreign' genes can thereby be 'grown' in quantity and subsequently isolated in a pure state from individual bacterial clones. This *recombinant DNA* methodology is the basis of genetic engineering, one aim of which is the production of proteins useful to man from bacteria carrying cloned human (or other) genes. Thus plasmids have become vital to the new industry based on biotechnology.

General properties of plasmids

Bacterial plasmids are circular molecules of double-stranded DNA; although RNA plasmids occur in fungi, they are as yet unknown in bacteria. Plasmid size is variable: the smallest, with about 1500 base pairs, only carry the information for one or two small proteins, while the largest are equivalent to nearly 10% of the *E. coli* chromosome and possess many genes. The number of copies of a plasmid in the cell (the copy number) is also very variable, from one to over 100. Small plasmids are present in larger numbers, e.g. those specifying antibiotic resistance are present at about 15 copies per cell, while large ones are found at only one or two per cell. The copy number is an individual property of the plasmid and is not influenced by the bacterial chromosome.

In replication, plasmids utilise the enzymes of the host cell, but are otherwise *autonomous*, i.e. their replication is independent of that of the chromosome and can occur throughout the cell cycle. A useful point is that, unlike the chromosome, they do not require protein synthesis for replication; thus in bacterial cells treated with chloramphenicol, chromosomal replication is inhibited but plasmid replication continues for several hours. In this way, cells containing very large numbers of plasmids (up to 1000 per cell) can be obtained and this is very useful in increasing plasmid yield during isolation from bacterial cultures. The plasmids are obtained by cell lysis, followed by density centrifugation.

The fact that plasmids can have low copy numbers, such as one or two per cell, yet can be present in over 99% of the cells in a culture indicates that they are inherited in a regular fashion, i.e. during bacterial replication there is a mechanism to ensure that each daughter cell receives a copy. However, the details of segregation are not known. Plasmids can also be lost from cells; loss is encouraged by substances called *curing agents*, which include inhibitors of DNA replication such as acridine orange and mitomycin C.

Classification

Several criteria are used in classifying plasmids. One is on the basis of *compatibility*, i.e. whether two different plasmid types can coexist in the same cells over many generations. Two *incompatible* plasmids cannot coexist for reasons concerned with their replication, and after a few rounds of bacterial division one will be lost. Many bacteria contain two or more compatible plasmids. Another criterion is whether the plasmid carries genes required for conjugation. *Conjugative plasmids* code for the structures involved, namely the tubes known as sex pili (below), and thus they can transfer copies of themselves to other bacteria. *Non-conjugative plasmids* do not code for their own transfer, but can nevertheless be 'mobilised' by the presence of a conjugative plasmid. Plasmids can also be classified on the basis of the most important genes they carry. Thus *R* (*resistance*) *plasmids* carry the genes for resistance to antimicrobial agents; *virulence plasmids* code for toxins and adherence proteins involved in bacterial pathogenicity; *Col plasmids* code for colicins (p. 427); and *degradative plasmids* specify various catabolic enzymes.

Conjugation

We have noted above that conjugative plasmids carry the information for bacterial conjugation and can thereby transfer copies of themselves from one organism to another. They are found in most Gram-negative bacteria, but in only three genera of Gram-positive organisms, (*Streptococcus, Clostridium* and *Streptomyces*). The commonest result of conjugation is that the

457

plasmid itself is transferred; however, sometimes a fragment of the chromosome is transferred as well or even, on very rare occasions, the entire chromosome. In this way, following recombination, new combinations of *chromosomal* genes may be formed and new bacterial strains evolve. Some plasmids have a wide host range and can transfer themselves between several groups of Gram-negative bacteria.

The most detailed studies of conjugation have been made with the *E. coli* strain known as K-12. The first plasmid to be discovered was the F plasmid of *E. coli* K-12, 'F' indicating fertility. The presence of F enables a cell to serve as a *donor* of genetic material, i.e. F^+ cells are 'males', while F^- cells act as recipients or 'females'. Thus F was also known as the 'sex factor'. The most obvious feature coded by F (and F-like) plasmids are the specialised, flexible hollow tubes called *sex pili* (F pili) found on the surface of all F^+ cells (Figure 4.35a). They can protrude for a considerable length (up to 20 μm), though most are short (about 2 μm), and 1–3 copies may be present on each cell. They carry receptors for certain bacteriophages, such as MS2, which often specifically cover their surface (Figure 4.52). Sex pili are essential for conjugation and it is thought, though it is not yet certain, that they are conduits through which which DNA passes from the F^+ to the F^- cell. The tip of the sex pilus attaches to a specific receptor present on the surface of F^- cells, this receptor is rendered ineffective on F^+ cells, so that the latter cannot conjugate with themselves or each other. Once donor and recipient cells have made effective contact, the F plasmid begins to replicate; as it does so, a *single* plasmid strand passes to the recipient, probably through the pilus channel (Figure 4.35b). This strand enters the recipient cell, whereupon its complementary strand is synthesized. Thus *both* cells are now F^+ through possession of the F plasmid, so that after conjugation the recipient cell has acquired the information to become a future donor (Figure 4.35c).

On rare occasions, the transfer of F also enables the transfer of chromosomal genes to take place. Although this was the first type of chromosomal transfer to be discovered (by Lederberg and Tatum), its mechanism is not clear. A separate phenomenon is the existence of certain strains of *E. coli* K-12 in which chromosomal transfer is common, called *high frequency recombination* or *Hfr* strains. In these, the F plasmid is no longer free, but has become integrated with the cell chromosome (i.e. covalently attached to the chromosomal DNA) so that when conjugation occurs the chromosome itself undergoes transfer in the same manner as a free F plasmid. (A genetic element such as F which can exist either free or integrated in a chromosome is called an *episome*.) Because its DNA is so long, the chromosome usually breaks before transfer is complete and passage of an entire chromosome is thus rare. By artificially disrupting the process of conjugation of an Hfr strain, the number of chromosomal genes transferred can be restricted. Since, in a given Hfr strain, transfer always begins at the same locus in the genome (the point of attachment of F) and then proceeds at a constant rate, the time required to transfer any particular gene is proportional to its

Figure 4.35 Stages in transfer of F plasmid by conjugation.
(a) Cells before conjugation.
(b) Conjugation.
(c) Cells after conjugation.

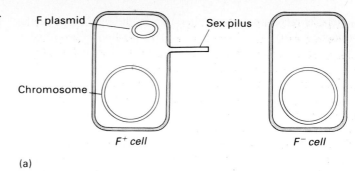

(a)

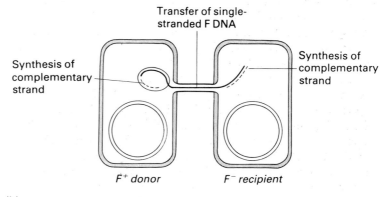

(b)

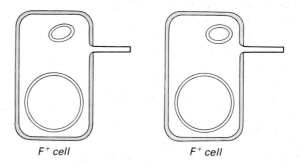

(c)

distance from the starting point (origin) of transfer. This technique of *interrupted mating* can therefore be used to determine the sequence of genes in the *E. coli* chromosome, the position of each gene being deduced from its *time of entry* into a recipient. The *E. coli* chromosome is '100 minutes long', i.e. it takes 100 minutes for the transfer of the entire genome by conjugation. In different Hfr strains, transfer starts at different points on the chromosome, and by comparing results obtained by this method it was first realised that the bacterial chromosome is circular (a fact later confirmed by autoradiography). The successful passage of a gene is recognised by an alteration in the phenotype of the recipient, as it acquires a property which it previously lacked such as an enzyme. The interrupted mating method, first introduced by Jacob and Wollman, has been used to map many of the 680 loci which are now known on the *E. coli* chromosome. The F plasmid can also be employed in other Gram-negative species and the *Salmonella typhimurium* genome has also been mapped in this way.

The F plasmid is unusual in that all the genes it carries are concerned with conjugation. However, it is possible for certain chromosomal genes to become linked to F, the resulting hybrid plasmids being designated F′ (F prime). An F′ plasmid originates in an Hfr strain where, as noted above, F is integrated with the chromosome; F can be excised from the chromosome, at low frequency, and in this process chromosomal genes adjoining F may be excised with it (cf. specialised transduction, in which an activated prophage is excised with a flanking gene, p. 453). F′ plasmids transfer their associated genes at high frequency by conjugation (called F-duction or sexduction) and have been very useful in the transfer and isolation of particular chromosomal genes. Another important property of F and other conjugative plasmids is that they bring about the simultaneous transfer of non-conjugative plasmids in the same cell, i.e. those which cannot mobilise themselves as they do not code for sex pili.

R plasmids and transferable drug resistance

The resistance (R) plasmids carry genes which confer on an organism resistance to antimicrobial drugs, including antibiotics. Drug resistance due to R plasmids has become an ever-increasing problem in recent years, especially where there is heavy reliance on one particular drug to treat a disease. In the 1970's there were major epidemics of typhoid fever and bacillary dysentery in several parts of the world, with thousands of unnecessary deaths, due to the unexpected resistance of the bacteria to the antibiotics in standard use. A particularly menacing phenomenon is the occurrence of *multiple drug resistance*, in which a species becomes resistant to several antimicrobial agents at the same time. R plasmids occur both in Gram-negative and Gram-positive bacteria; although especially prevalent in enterobacteria (*E. coli*, *Shigella*, *Salmonella*), they have by now been found in almost all bacterial species pathogenic for man or animals. Moreover, there are hardly any antimicrobial agents in use for which a corresponding plasmid-borne resistance gene has not been found, and there is the alarming prospect that such genes already exist for drugs which have not yet been discovered or invented. This is possible because resistance genes are *not* mutants, but exist in the cell for some other purpose, antedating the medical use of the drug.

Two particular features of R plasmids make them more important than resistance due to mutation of chromosomal genes, namely (1) their *transmission* between species by conjugation, and

(2) the fact that R genes belong to a special category of genetic elements called *transposons* which can move from one plasmid to another. These properties are responsible for transmissible multiple drug resistance. Of course, drug resistance is sometimes due to mutation of a chromosomal gene followed by selection of the resistant variant by antibiotic treatment, rather than to an R plasmid. This often appears to be the case for sulphonamide resistance in organisms other than enterobacteria, and there are doubtless other examples. However, most resistance genes are plasmid-borne and invariably so in transmissible and multiple drug resistance.

History of antimicrobial drug resistance

Drug-resistant organisms were first recognised a few years after the introduction of chemotherapy with sulphonamides and penicillin, the assumption at that time being that they were resistant variants arising by mutation and selection. Sulphonamides were first introduced in 1935 and were used to great effect in the treatment of gonorrhoea; by the late 1940's, 80–90% of *Nesseria gonorrhoeae* strains were resistant, but fortunately penicillin was by then available. During this period, *N. meningitidis,* enterobacteria and *Strep. pyogenes* also became resistant to sulphonamides. After the introduction of penicillin in the 1940's, resistant strains of *Staph. aureus* developed rapidly and today almost all strains of this organism isolated from hospitals are penicillin-resistant.

The role of plasmids in resistance only became apparent in the late 1950's in connection with an outbreak of bacillary dysentery in Japan, in which some patients failed to respond to one or more of the antibiotics generally effective against *Shigella dysenteriae,* namely sulphonamides, tetracycline, streptomycin and chloramphenicol. By 1960, 10% of all shigella strains showed *multiple resistance* to all four antibiotics, and in time these strains became the majority type of shigellae in Japan. Studies of the resistant organisms showed that the same strain could exist in fully sensitive or multiple-resistant forms, sometimes both even isolable from the same patient; moreover, in patients excreting multiple-resistant shigellae, it was possible to find strains of *E. coli* with multiple resistance to the same group of antibiotics. It was also shown that the resistance genes were transferable from resistant to sensitive organisms by conjugation, thus resembling the F plasmid, and that transfer could occur *in vivo* in the gut. Thus it was suggested that multiple resistance arose initially in *E. coli* and was transferred to shigella during infection by the latter *in vivo*. Multiple-resistant shigellae (*Sh. dysenteriae*) were also responsible for a major pandemic of dysentery in Central America in 1969 and 1970; the disease was unusually severe with high morbidity and mortality. There were over 500,000 cases, and in Guatemala alone 125,000 people died in one year. The proportion of fatalities was exceptionally high because the unexpected resistance to antibiotics confused diagnosis, and physicians treated the disease as amoebiasis; once the organisms were found to be susceptible to ampicillin, mortality rapidly declined. A similar outbreak caused thousands of deaths in Bangladesh in 1973. (*Sh. dysenteriae* causes the severest form of bacillary dysentery, p. 551).

In 1972, there were 14,000 deaths in Mexico during an epidemic of typhoid fever which failed to respond to chloramphenicol, the most effective antibiotic against *Salmonella typhi*. The disease was more severe, more protracted and had a higher rate of complications than usual. Once again, the organisms showed plasmid-borne multiple resistance to strep-tomycin, sulphonamide and tetracycline as well as chloram-phenicol, and it is assumed that this R plasmid was also acquired by *S. typhi* from other enteric organisms in which it was origin-ally formed. (The plasmids implicated in the 1969–70 and 1972 epidemics were genetically distinct, though their occurrence in the same geographical area within a short period of time had suggested that they were the same.) Epidemics of typhoid fever due to chloramphenicol-resistant *S. typhi* have since also occurred in India and other parts of Asia.

Mechanisms of transfer

The transfer of multiple resistance, such as that which occurred in the examples cited above, is due to *conjugative* R plasmids. Like the F plasmid, they code for their own mobility by carrying genes for sex pili, etc., and are called 'F-like'. Only a small fraction (~0.1%) of the cells carrying conjugative R plasmids actually express sex pili and take part in conjugation, as the relevant genes are usually repressed (in contrast with F^+ bacteria where *all* organisms have sex pili). Many R plasmids are *non-conjugative*, and cannot mobilise themselves; nevertheless they too are readily spread by conjugation because they can be mobilised by the presence of a conjugative plasmid. An individual organism may carry more than one R plasmid, some conjugative and others non-conjugative. In Gram-positive organisms, R plasmids are generally non-conjugative; *Staph. aureus*, in which R plasmids are common, does not conjugate at all and its plasmids are transmitted instead by generalised transduction (p. 453), which very possibly occurs naturally between *Staph. aureus* organisms infecting man. It is possible that plasmids from *Staph. aureus*, or other Gram-positives, would be conjugative if introduced into a Gram-negative cell.

R genes as transposons

In addition to transmissibility, a most important feature of R genes is the ability to move from one plasmid to another by a process of *transposition*. This is not restricted by the requirement which accompanies normal recombination, namely that the DNA regions involved be homologous (i.e. very similar in nucleotide sequence). The R genes are parts of mobile genetic elements called *transposons* (transposable elements), meaning that they are associated with nucleotide sequences which enable copies of the R genes to become inserted into the DNA at many different points (one copy being retained at the original site). This ability to acquire new genes or rearrange existing ones by transposition endows R plasmids with great structural flexibility and it can be assumed that the origin of multiple drug resistance is often by accumulation of individual transposons on a single R plasmid. The medical significance is that selection of one R gene results in simultaneous selection of all the other R genes to which it has become linked on the same plasmid; in other words, the use of a single antibiotic can lead to the appearance of organisms with resistance to several other unrelated agents, a prospect with disturbing clinical implications.

Strategies of resistance to antibiotics and other antimicrobials

Four biochemical mechanisms of plasmid-encoded resistance to antimicrobial drugs have been described: (i) production of an enzyme which destroys or inactivates the drug; (ii) blocking entry of the drug into the cell; (iii) alteration of its intracellular target site in such a way that the drug can no longer bind; and (iv) providing an enzyme which bypasses the reaction which the drug normally inhibits. Thus, in many cases resistance depends on a plasmid-coded enzyme, the expression of which may be *inducible* (occuring only in the presence of the drug) or *constitutive* (continuous). Specific examples are described below and summarised in Table 4.5.

(i) *Destruction or inactivation* of the antimicrobial agent is responsible for resistance to penicillins, cephalosporins, chloram-

Table 4.5 Mechanisms of plasmid-coded resistance to antibiotics and other antimicrobial agents.

Agent	Mechanism of resistance
Penicillins	Hydrolysis by β-lactamases (penicillinases)
Cephalosporins	Hydrolysis by β-lactamases
Chloramphenicol	O-acetylation* by chloramphenicol acetyltransferase
Hg^{2+}	Reduction to free Hg
Tetracycline	Inhibition of membrane transport
Aminoglycosides (streptomycin, etc.)	Modification of antibiotic by N-acetylation*, O-phosphorylation* or O-nucleotidylation* leads to blocking of membrane transport system
Macrolides (erythromycin)	Methylation of ribosomal RNA prevents binding of antibiotic to ribosome
Lincomycin	ditto
Sulphonamides	By-pass enzyme: dihydropteroate synthetase which is resistant to sulphonamides
Trimethoprim	By-pass enzyme: dihydrofolate reductase which is resistant to trimethoprim

* O-acetylation, N-acetylation: acetylation of the oxygen atom of a hydroxyl (OH) or nitrogen of an amino (NH_2) group, respectively.

phenicol and mercury compounds. *Penicillins* are inactivated by *β-lactamases* (penicillinases) which hydrolyse their β-lactam ring. Many strains of *Staph. aureus* are now resistant to penicillin G, the first penicillin introduced, though it can still be used against other Gram-positive organisms; *Pseudomonas aeruginosa* is often resistant to ampicillin, the penicillin derivative with a wide spectrum of activity which includes Gram-negative bacteria. Penicillinase-resistant penicillins have been developed, such as methicillin, which is highly effective in severe infections by penicillinase-producing staphylococci, though there is an occasional problem of toxicity. *Cephalosporins* are also destroyed by certain β-lactamases, notably those produced by Gram-negative bacteria, but are not affected by the staphylococcal enzyme. As this implies, there are several types of β-lactamase, the genes for which may either be chromosomal or on R plasmids; being transposons, they have been acquired by many unrelated plasmids and widely distributed. β-Lactamases act extracellularly, so their effectiveness depends on their concentration in the medium into which they are released. They are inducible in Gram-positive bacteria, but expressed constitutively in *E. coli*.

Resistance to *chloramphenicol* occurs by an enzyme which modifies rather than destroys the antibiotic molecule. The enzyme, *chloramphenicol acetyltransferase*, catalyses the O-acetylation of chloramphenicol to produce an inactive acetoxy derivative; the reaction takes place intracellularly and involves acetyl CoA (Figure 4.36). Resistance to *mercuric ions* (Hg^{2+}) is often conferred by plasmid-borne genes. For example, the staphylococci responsible for outbreaks of postsurgical 'suture-line' infections are resistant to the mercury-based disinfectants used to sterilise sutures, and possess plasmids which also confer resistance to compounds of other metals, including arsenic, bismuth, zinc and cadmium. While little is known in most cases about the mechanisms, resistance to mercuric salts is caused by a reductase which reduces Hg^{2+} ions to free mercury; the latter subsequently vapourises.

Figure 4.36 Inactivation of chloramphenicol.

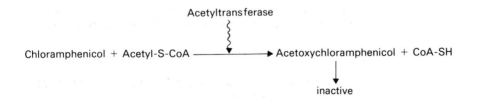

Chloramphenicol + Acetyl-S-CoA ⟶ Acetoxychloramphenicol + CoA-SH

Acetyltransferase

inactive

(ii) *Interference with entry* of the drug and its intracellular accumulation can, in principle, occur whenever there is a specific transport system for the antimicrobial. A well-studied example is that of *tetracycline resistance* in Gram-negative organisms and *Staph. aureus*. Resistance apparently involves the introduction of a protein(s), coded by the R plasmid, into the bacterial membrane; production of the protein is inducible by tetracycline. Resistance to *aminoglycoside* antibiotics, such as streptomycin, spectinomycin, neomycin, kanamycin and gentamicin, also involves interference with transport, but depends on modification of the antibiotics by plasmid-coded modifying enzymes, of which there are a large number. The enzymes cause acetylation, phosphorylation or nucleotidylation of the antibiotic, the result of which is to block the transport mechanism, though the precise details are unclear.

(iii) *Alteration of the intracellular target site* of the drug is only known to occur in one case, namely resistance to the *erythromycin-lincomycin* type antibiotics in streptococci and staphylococci. In these Gram-positives, the plasmid codes for an enzyme (methylase) which transfers methyl groups to two specific adenine residues on 23S RNA molecules in the bacterial ribosome (the large 50S subunit). The antibiotics cannot bind to the modified ribosomes and thus cannot exert their normal mode of action, namely disruption of protein synthesis. Interestingly, Gram-negative organisms, which are in general less sensitive than Gram-positives to macrolides such as erythromycin, have 23S ribosomal RNA which is naturally methylated; so too does the producer organism, *Streptomyces erythreus*, presumably to protect itself from its own product.

(iv) *Enzymatic by-pass.* There are two examples of R plasmids which code for an *enzymatic by-pass* of a reaction which the antimicrobial would normally inhibit; both occur in the folic acid pathway (Figure 4.37). *Sulphonamides* act by competing with para-aminobenzoate (PAB) for the active site of the enzyme *dihydropteroate synthetase*, which condenses PAB with a pteridine to form dihydropteroate, the immediate precursor of folic acid. The R plasmids of Gram-negative bacteria resistant to sulphonamides code for a dihydropteroate synthetase which is not inhibitable by sulphonamide, thus effecting a by-pass (Figure 4.37). It is fascinating that a similar by-pass exists in resistance to *trimethoprim*, a drug which affects the same pathway but at a later stage, namely the reduction of dihydrofolate to tetrahydrofolate by *dihydrofolate reductase*. Once again, there is a plasmid-coded enzyme which in this case is several thousand times less sensitive to trimethoprim than that coded by the bacterial chromosome.

Evolution and selection of R plasmids

A striking feature of these mechanisms is the specificity of each for a particular antimicrobial drug. How and why they have evolved is not easy to answer. It is clear, however, that they are not mutants of existing bacterial enzymes selected for the first time by human use of antimicrobials; rather, the R genes have evolved as a result of selective advantages in the organisms' natural environments and their appearance is by no means a recent event. Thus R plasmids can be isolated from organisms which were stored before the clinical use of antibiotics and from people in isolated parts of the world who had never received antibiotics. Their original role may have been to protect bacteria in

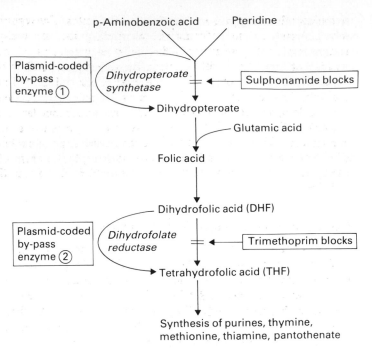

Figure 4.37 Folic acid pathway showing mechanism of resistance to sulphonamide and trimethoprim.

① Resistance to sulphonamide

② Resistance to trimethoprim

soil against antibiotics produced by themselves or other organisms, including fungi, or against traces of toxic heavy metals. For example, we have noted that *Streptomyces erythreus* protects itself from its own product, erythromycin, by a chromosomal gene directing the same mechanism as R-plasmid genes in other organisms; chromosomal genes such as these are likely progenitors of their plasmid counterparts. The speed with which R plasmids appear for newly-introduced antimicrobials is impressive. Resistance to trimethoprim, a synthetic drug with no natural counterpart, was first encountered on plasmids in 1972, only three years after its first clinical use.

Resistant organisms are often in a minority in their natural population and only become dominant as a result of *selection* by the antibiotic, because they survive where sensitive competing organisms are killed. For example, resistant strains of *E. coli* can be demonstrated in over 50% of normal people, but unless an individual is treated with an antibiotic, the proportion of his intestinal organisms showing resistance will usually be low (approximately 0.1%). Once an antibiotic is introduced, the resistant strains pre-existing in the natural flora can be selected. Thus, during oral administration of tetracycline, the predominant strains of *E. coli* in patients' faeces are usually tetracycline-resistant after a few days; on cessation of the antibiotic treatment, resistant organisms apparently compete less well and their numbers usually fall back again after 2–3 weeks, though sometimes they may predominate for several months. The regular use of, and in some countries overindulgence in, orally administered antibiotics means that resistant organisms of the normal intestinal flora will be selected frequently; since their R plasmids are often conjugative, it is hardly surprising to find multiple drug resistance, probably acquired from the existing natural flora, among virulent organisms such as salmonellae and shigellae. The use of antibiotics as growth promoters in animal feed is also a cause of concern due to possible transmission of resistant enterobacteria from animals to man; hence drugs of therapeutic use in man or animals are now prohibited as feedstuff additives.

Current problems associated with R plasmids

Resistant strains of bacteria have become a common, serious problem in hospitals. Since a large proportion of hospital patients receive antibiotics, it is inevitable that drug-resistant organisms will undergo intensive selection. They may be acquired by patients with burns or indwelling urethral catheters, or by those whose ability to combat infection is lowered by their medical condition or the use of immunosuppressive treatment. In other words, drug resistance will complicate infection by *opportunistic pathogens* (p. 478). The latter include organisms in which R plasmids are common, among them Gram-negative bacteria such as *Pseudomonas aeruginosa* and enterobacteria, while *Staph. aureus*, the most important Gram-positive hospital-acquired pathogen, can also often be multiresistant. Patients with burns are particularly vulnerable; *P. aeruginosa* and *Serratia marcescens*, sometimes in combination with *Staph. aureus*, can soon colonise burns and cause bacteraemia. *P. aeruginosa* is often particularly problematic (p. 569), because of its innate resistance to many drugs, which can be compounded by acquisition of an R plasmid. Drug resistant strains of *Salmonella* have been responsible for potentially fatal infections in paediatric units and nurseries in many parts of the world. Since resistance is usually multiple, there can be severe difficulties in treating septicaemia or meningitis due to these organisms. The prophylactic use of antibiotics, the use of broad-spectrum agents or massive doses of any antimicrobial agent entail the risk of secondary infection with resistant bacteria in hospital patients and are therefore to be avoided as far as possible (see also p. 484).

The problem of drug-resistance is also threatening to encroach on conditions which generally respond well to a particular antibiotic. In *gonorrhoea*, for example, where penicillin is the treatment of choice, penicillinase-producing strains of *Neisseria gonorrhoeae* first came to light in 1976, and these strains have now been isolated in more than 15 countries from individuals infected in the Far East or West Africa. A number of cases are identified each year in the UK among people infected abroad. However, the much-feared spread of the resistant strains has not materialised in Europe, probably because the plasmids have proved to be unstable in the absence of continuous selective pressure by antibiotics. In countries such as the Philippines and Singapore, where prophylactic use of oral penicillins is widespread, especially among prostitutes, resistant strains are now very common. The instability of gonococcal R plasmids is extremely fortunate, for otherwise the use of penicillin G and ampicillin for gonorrhoea therapy would come to an end. The plasmid carrying the β-lactamase gene is non-conjugative, but is mobilised by a conjugative plasmid present in about 10% of gonococci.

In *Haemophilus influenzae*, the rise in resistance to ampicillin has become of major concern, since the organism is responsible for serious infections of childhood, such as meningitis and pharyngitis. Chloramphenicol is now often used together with ampicillin in initial treatment, until the antibiotic sensitivity of the organism has been assessed; however, this is by no means a satisfactory situation, as chloramphenicol carries a risk of bone marrow depression and even in rare cases potentially fatal aplastic anaemia.

Virulence plasmids

Some plasmids carry genes whose products are directly involved in bacterial pathogenicity. While they are suspected of occurring in a variety of organisms, the best studied examples are those of virulent strains of *Escherichia coli*.

Enteropathogenic strains of *Escherichia coli*

Although *E. coli* is normally found as a harmless commensal in the large intestine, certain strains are responsible for important diarrhoeal illnesses in man (infantile diarrhoea, traveller's diarrhoea) and domestic animals (piglets, calves, lambs). These strains are *enterotoxigenic*, secreting either the labile toxin (LT), or the stable toxin (ST), or quite often both (p. 548). The toxins are coded by plasmid-borne genes, and in strains producing ST and LT one plasmid may carry both genes. However, the production of enterotoxin is not in itself sufficient to make the organisms pathogenic: to cause disease they must also be able to colonise the small intestine (where most absorption of water occurs). Accordingly, enteropathogenic strains have specialised surface *pili* which enable them to adhere to the wall of the small intestine. These structures are characterised by their antigens and are referred to as *colonisation or adherence factors*. They too are often coded by plasmid-borne genes, but on separate plasmids from those coding for the toxins. Colonisation factor antigens are specific for a particular animal species; thus, antigen K88 is associated with *E. coli* strains causing diarrhoea in piglets, while K99 is present on those which are pathogenic in calves. In man, two antigens (CFAI and CFAII) have been found on *E. coli* responsible for diarrhoea (p. 548). The pili bind to specific receptors on intestinal epithelial cells and it is interesting that the receptors for K88 are similar to the GM_1 gangliosides which bind LT and cholera toxin.

In order to cause intestinal disease, a strain of *E. coli* must possess toxin *and* adherence factor plasmids. It has been possible to prove this by exploiting the transmissibility of the plasmids to construct a set of *E. coli* strains differing only in the presence or absence of the virulence plasmids. From the ability of the organisms to cause diarrhoea in piglets, it was evident that pathogenicity was not conferred by either toxin or adherence factor plasmids alone, while together they were sufficient to convert a harmless strain into an enteropathogenic one. Since the K88 adherence antigen is essential for pathogenicity, it has been possible to use it as a vaccine in piglets, where diarrhoea, being a major cause of death, is of considerable economic importance. Sows are immunised with a K88 antigen preparation and transfer protective IgA antibodies to their offspring via colostrum during the first feeds (all maternal antibody is acquired by this route in piglets, there being no placental transfer). Maternal anti-K88 retained in the small intestine of the newborn is effective in protecting against diarrhoea.

Invasive strains of *Escherichia coli*

While the enterotoxigenic strains are non-invasive, other strains of *E. coli* cause generalised, non-intestinal infections in man and animals. Unlike the enteropathogenic strains, these are opportunistic and in man they are the major agents of urinary tract infections, as well as being found in septicaemias, peritonitis and meningitis; they are also an important cause of death among calves and chickens. These organisms possess several distinctive virulence factors, the genes for some of which are carried on plasmids. One virulence plasmid is known as *Col V*, because it also codes for the antibacterial protein *colicin V* (below). Strains carrying the Col V plasmid are thirty times more lethal for chickens than cured strains (i.e. from which the plasmid has been lost) and reintroduction of the plasmid by conjugation restores virulence. One of the genes on Col V confers resistance to complement-mediated killing, thus enhancing survival of the organisms in blood and other body fluids. Another codes for a novel iron-uptake system which is also important for pathogenicity. All bacteria require iron for growth, but in nature iron is present as high molecular weight aggregates while *in vivo* it is complexed to iron-binding proteins such as transferrin and therefore inaccessible. Bacteria can overcome this problem by producing specialised iron-binding agents called *siderophores* (e.g. enterochelin of *E. coli* and *Salmonella typhi*). The Col V plasmid codes for such a siderophore (hydroxamate) which chelates ferric iron and can remove it from transferrin, subsequently transporting it into the bacterial cell. The combined abilities to scavenge iron and resist the antibacterial effects of serum are vital plasmid-coded factors in the invasiveness of opportunistic *E. coli* strains.

Bacteriocin plasmids

The properties of some bacteriocins have been described on p. 427. They are toxins which kill strains of bacteria closely related to the organism secreting the bacteriocin. The *colicins* of *E. coli* and related enterobacteria are coded by genes on *Col plasmids*, which also carry the genes for the immunity proteins responsible for protecting the bacterial cell from the toxicity of its own products. We have noted above that one such plasmid, Col V, carries genes for *E. coli* virulence factors as well as for colicin V. Col V is also a conjugative plasmid and codes for F-like pili which enable conjugation to occur (some other Col plasmids are non-conjugative). An individual Col plasmid can carry genes for more than one colicin, and may also carry R genes.

Possession of a bacteriocin plasmid presumably confers an advantage on a strain in competing with related organisms in the same environment. This also ensures the survival of the plasmid: any organisms which lose the plasmid become susceptible to Col^+ cells and are hence replaced. Nor can competing organisms easily become bacteriocin-resistant, as the bacteriocin receptors are usually required for uptake of essential metabolites. The degree to which these plasmids are helpful to bacteria is difficult to assess, but the fact that nearly half the *E. coli* strains of man and animals are Col^+ is an indication of their importance. Since Col V carries genes both for a colicin and for virulence, it is possible that this is one case where the ability to produce a bacteriocin may also be relevant to the organism's pathogenicity for man or animals.

Plasmids and genetic engineering

The term 'genetic engineering' refers to the technique by which DNA segments of any origin—eukaryotic, prokaryotic or viral—can be introduced into bacterial cells and by which they can be homogeneously multiplied or 'cloned' (Figure 4.38). Plasmids are a key element in the method through their use as *vectors* or vehicles on which the foreign DNA is carried: by a series of specialised enzymatic steps, a gene of interest is physically integrated with a plasmid, and the resulting recombinant plasmid (*recombinant DNA*) is then induced to enter bacterial cells such as *E. coli*. As the recipient organisms grow, the foreign DNA is replicated and can ultimately be recovered in quantity and pure form (*gene cloning*). While genetic engineering has brought about a revolution in modern genetic research, perhaps its most dramatic practical application is in the intro-duction of genes from animal cells into bacteria in order for the latter to express the products of the genes and essentially become microbial 'factories' making molecules useful to man. To date such molecules include hormones (growth hormone and insulin), interferons, and antigens of viral or parasitic pathogens for use in vaccines; but the potential scope of the technique, coupled with industrial-scale manufacture, is immense.

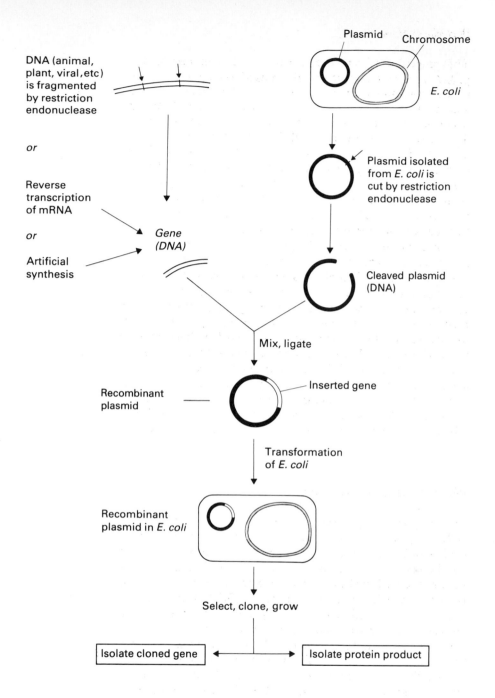

DNA (animal, plant, viral, etc) is fragmented by restriction endonuclease

or

Reverse transcription of mRNA

or

Artificial synthesis

Gene (DNA)

Plasmid   Chromosome

E. coli

Plasmid isolated from *E. coli* is cut by restriction endonuclease

Cleaved plasmid (DNA)

Mix, ligate

Recombinant plasmid

Inserted gene

Transformation of *E. coli*

Recombinant plasmid in *E. coli*

Select, clone, grow

Isolate cloned gene   Isolate protein product

Figure 4.38 Principle of genetic engineering.

Outline of method

The isolation and cloning of a particular gene in bacteria using plasmids involves the following steps (Figure 4.38). (i) Preparation of the plasmid and of the foreign DNA to be incorporated into it (the 'insert'). The latter may be a fragment of chromosomal DNA produced by enzymatic action, or a DNA sequence copied from specific messenger RNA (complementary or cDNA), or chemically synthesized. (ii) Insertion of the foreign

DNA into the plasmid. This is usually accomplished with a specific enzyme known as a *restriction endonuclease* which breaks the plasmid at a single point, thus converting it from a DNA loop into a linear molecule. The ends of the foreign DNA insert are joined to the ends of the plasmid by another enzyme (a *ligase*) to re-form a circular molecule in which plasmid and foreign DNA have been recombined (hence the widely used term *recombinant DNA*). (iii) Introduction of the recombinant plasmid into bacteria by *transformation*. (iv) Isolation and identification of clones of bacteria carrying the foreign DNA; only a small fraction of the recipient cells will carry the DNA of interest. (v) Growth of those clones in bulk and purification either of the foreign gene or of its protein product. Some details of these procedures are now described.

Restriction endonucleases

These bacterial enzymes are indispensable tools in genetic engineering, used both to prepare and recover DNA inserts and to open plasmids at specific single points. They are obtained from a variety of bacterial species, whose own DNA is protected from their action. The enzymes are given abbreviated names indicative of their origin, such as *Eco*Rl (from *E. coli* where it is coded by an R plasmid), *Hind*III (from *Haemophilus influenzae* serotype d), and so forth. Over 100 restriction endonucleases are known, each acting on DNA at very specific points through recognition of particular nucleotide sequences. In most cases, the DNA site recognised by the enzyme is symmetrical and is called *palindromic*; this is illustrated by the site at which *Eco*Rl, one of the most commonly used endonucleases, attacks DNA (Figure 4.39). Its action leaves two tails of unpaired nucleotides called 'sticky ends', which will pair with each other again under appropriate conditions. A given DNA molecule is always cut at the same point(s) by a particular enzyme, and for a small plasmid it is usually possible to find several restriction endonucleases which will make a *single* cut at a known site to open the loop.

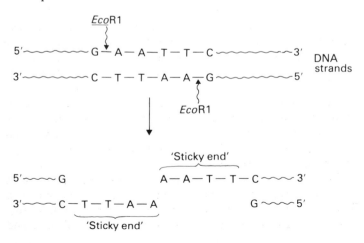

Figure 4.39 Site of action of restriction endonuclease *Eco*Rl.

472

Plasmids as vectors

The plasmids into which foreign DNA is inserted usually have two particularly useful properties. One is that they continue to multiply in bacteria treated with chloramphenicol, which inhibits replication of the bacterial chromosome (p. 457); the plasmids are thus increased in number and easily isolated from cultures stopped by chloramphenicol. Secondly, they are derived from R plasmids and hence carry certain *antibiotic-resistance* genes; this property is exploited when it comes to identifying the bacterial clones carrying recombinant plasmids. For example, a widely used plasmid, denoted pBR322, has genes for ampicillin and tetracycline resistance (Figure 4.40). Insertion of a foreign DNA segment into the tetracycline resistance gene leads to loss of resistance to this antibiotic, but ampicillin resistance remains. Thus, at a later stage, bacteria which have received the recombinant plasmid can be identified because they will be resistant only to ampicillin.

When treated with an appropriate restriction endonuclease, a plasmid such as pBR322 can, as we have noted, be opened at a single specific point, leaving free sticky ends (Figure 4.40a). If the DNA insert has been obtained using the same enzyme, it will have identical sticky ends. Thus, by mixing together the opened plasmid with the fragment, the two will join at their free ends by complementary base-pairing and their union can be made permanent by forming covalent bonds using a DNA ligase. By adjusting the proportions of plasmid to insert, the tendency of the plasmid to recircularise itself can be minimised and the chances of recombination with the DNA insert favoured.

Reverse transcription

We have noted that a major use of genetic engineering is to obtain bacteria in which eukaryotic genes are functionally expressed. However, in their chromosomal form such genes differ structurally from prokaryotic genes and could not be translated in a bacterial cell. The major difference is that eukaryotic genes are often *split*, i.e. the nucleotide sequence coding for the gene product is not continuous but is interrupted by non-coding sequences or *introns* (Figure 4.40b). After the gene DNA has been transcribed into mRNA in the eukaryotic nucleus, introns are removed by enzymatic *splicing*, leaving a continuous coding sequence which is translated into protein on ribosomes. Bacteria lack the necessary splicing enzymes (splicases) and therefore cannot translate many eukaryotic genes in their native form. To overcome this problem, the spliced mRNA transcript of the eukaryotic gene is obtained from the eukaryotic cytoplasm and converted back into a DNA copy lacking introns by use of the enzyme *reverse transcriptase* (p. 781). It is this complementary DNA copy, or *cDNA*, which in double-stranded form is introduced into the bacterial plasmid for cloning, as shown in Figure 4.40b. In order to insert it into the plasmid, free complementary (sticky) ends are created on both plasmid and

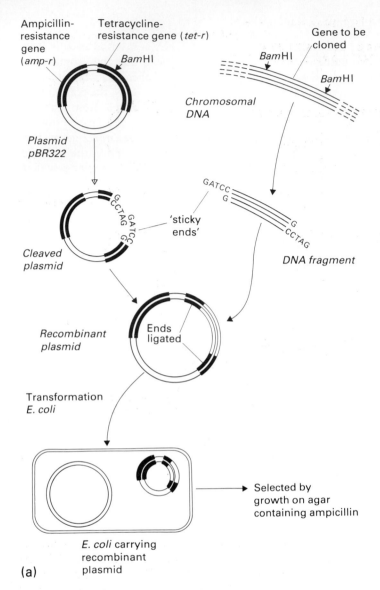

Figure 4.40 Recombinant-DNA techniques for gene cloning with plasmid pBR322.
(a) Using a restriction endonuclease to prepare the DNA insert.
(b) *opposite* Using DNA copied from messenger RNA of a 'split' eukaryotic gene.
*Bam*HI, *Pst*I: restriction endonucleases

Figure labels:
Ampicillin-resistance gene (*amp-r*)
Tetracycline-resistance gene (*tet-r*)
*Bam*HI
Gene to be cloned
*Bam*HI
*Bam*HI
Chromosomal DNA
Plasmid pBR322
'sticky ends'
Cleaved plasmid
DNA fragment
Recombinant plasmid
Ends ligated
Transformation E. coli
Selected by growth on agar containing ampicillin
E. coli carrying recombinant plasmid
(a)

cDNA using enzymes called terminal transferases; ligation can then proceed as described above.

Transformation

Transformation is used to introduce recombinant plasmids into bacterial host cells, usually *E. coli*. To induce the latter to take up a plasmid, the cells are treated with $CaCl_2$, whereupon they bind and absorb externally added DNA, as described on p. 452 (transfection).

Detection of recombinant bacteria

The problem remains of identifying bacteria which have taken up the recombinant plasmid. Initial detection of such cells is

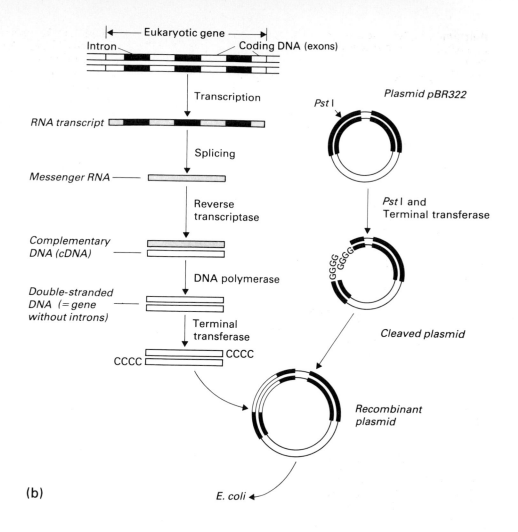

Intron — Eukaryotic gene — Coding DNA (exons)

Transcription

RNA transcript

Splicing

Messenger RNA

Reverse transcriptase

Complementary DNA (cDNA)

DNA polymerase

Double-stranded DNA (= gene without introns)

Terminal transferase

CCCC   CCCC

Pst I   Plasmid pBR322

Pst I and Terminal transferase

GGGG GGGG

Cleaved plasmid

Recombinant plasmid

E. coli

(b)

relatively straightforward, as they will have acquired antibiotic resistance by virtue of the R genes present on the plasmid. In the case illustrated in Figure 4.40a of a pBR322 plasmid in which DNA has been integrated into the *tet-r* (tetracycline-resistance) gene, the bacteria sought will have acquired resistance to ampicillin but not tetracycline; by making replica agar plates containing one or the other antibiotic, colonies with single resistance can be identified. The next step is to discover which of these clones has received the gene of interest and this may be a more complicated procedure. To detect a mammalian gene, for example, in a bacterial cell, it is possible to search either for the gene DNA itself or for its protein product. To identify the DNA requires *hybridisation* with a complementary nucleic acid 'probe', such as the appropriate radiolabelled mRNA transcript; alternatively, the cloned DNA may inhibit translation of specific mRNA in a cell-free translation system. If a sufficient amount of protein is successfully translated from the gene in the bacterial host cells, it can be detected by *radioimmunoassay* using specific antibodies.

Isolation of active protein

When a eukaryotic gene is inserted into a plasmid, it is often flanked on either side by parts of a plasmid gene, such as the *tet-r* gene in Figure 4.40a. Consequently, the bacterially translated product will be a hybrid molecule in which the eukaryotic protein is fused at the ends to parts of the plasmid-coded protein, and in order to isolate a biologically active product it is necessary to cleave off enzymatically the bacterial contribution. For example, when the gene for rat insulin was cloned in *E. coli*, it was inserted into the penicillinase gene on pBR322 (as in Figure 4.40b); recombinant bacteria synthesized a molecule which was part-penicillinase, part-insulin, from which the penicillinase polypeptide sequences were removed with trypsin.

Practical applications

In principle, any protein useful in human or veterinary medicine could be made by these methods, but interest has naturally centered on those which are in short supply or difficult to obtain from natural sources. Into this category come hormones and clotting factors, for use in replacement therapy, and interferon. Industrial-scale production is easily possible and in many parts of the world new industrial and research companies are springing up to exploit the commercial potential of these and similar products. Successes to date include the large-scale production of human growth hormone, insulin, and all three types (α,β,γ) of human interferon. Recombinant *E. coli* carrying such genes can be grown in fermenters of huge capacity and the product subsequently extracted.

Until now, the source of *human growth hormone* (HGH) has been cadaver pituitaries and there has been scarcely enough available to treat children suffering from growth hormone deficiency; there are about 100 new cases annually in the UK and 60,000 pituitaries must be processed each year to meet the worldwide demand. Human growth hormone from *E. coli* carrying the HGH gene is now available and clinical trials with the bacterially synthesized product are in progress. Trials are also being carried out with *human insulin* similarly produced from 'engineered' *E. coli*. In this case, synthetic genes for the separate A and B chains of insulin were inserted into plasmids and thence into *E. coli*; the organisms synthesizing each chain are grown separately and the chains then extracted and chemically linked to create the human insulin molecule. Its advantages over the insulin currently obtained from ox and pig pancreas will firstly be its cheapness, and secondly it will avoid the possibility of anti-insulin antibodies which are sometimes made by diabetics.

Interferons (p. 246) are a particularly good example of substances which may only become available for large-scale clinical trials (e.g. for cancer therapy) and eventual clinical use through successful production in recombinant bacteria. The isolation of interferons has been simplified by another breakthrough in biotechnology, namely monoclonal antibodies (p.

100). Monoclonal anti-interferon can be used to separate interferon very efficiently from unwanted bacterial proteins; the antibody is insolubilised by conjugation to cellulose beads and specifically binds interferon present in bacterial supernatants or extracts. Subsequently, pure interferon can be easily eluted from the beads (Figure 2.16).

Genetic engineering methods are not only being used for animal genes and proteins, but are also being applied in the production of pure components of pathogenic microorganisms for use as *vaccines*. It is often the case that antibodies directed against an antigen on the surface of a virus, bacterium or parasite will provide immunity against reinfection, e.g. by preventing adherence to a target cell or mucous surface, etc. Such antigens can, if isolated, be useful vaccines. If they are identifiable proteins, there is every possibility that their genes can be isolated and cloned in *E. coli* (or other cells) and the antigens thereby obtained in pure form and in quantity. In this way vaccines could be developed without the usual necessity of growing the microbe in culture, which is sometimes very difficult or hazardous. Purified protein vaccines also avoid problems which sometimes accompany the use of whole living or inactivated organisms in vaccines, such as the reversion of attenuated strains to virulence or incomplete inactivation of a virus; they also have the advantage that a high dose of the specifically protective antigen can be given, increasing the chances of an effective immune response.

Three examples where such vaccine proteins are in the process of development from recombinant bacteria are hepatitis B virus (the agent of serum hepatitis, p. 358), foot and mouth disease virus, and *Plasmodium falciparum*, the malarial parasite. *Hepatitis B virus* has been impossible to grow in culture, but a vaccine has been prepared from the surface antigen (HBsAg) present in carrier serum (p. 363); recently the HbsAg gene has been cloned in *E. coli* and the HBs protein synthesized by the organisms. This may in time become the source of HBsAg for vaccines, free of contaminating human serum protein or lipid. For *foot and mouth disease*, the problem is not one of growing the virus, but rather lies in the preparation of sufficient killed virus to meet vaccine demand and in the multiplicity of viral types. It remains one of the world's most serious animal diseases and the vaccine requirement is huge. Methods which could increase the yield would therefore be very welcome. Recently, the gene of the virus coat protein, responsible for the protective antibody response, has been introduced on a plasmid into bacteria and the yield of viral antigen promises to exceed that obtained from the mammalian cell cultures currently used to grow the whole virus. Immunisation against *malaria* presents a complicated problem because of the complex life cycle of the parasite and the difficulty of growing it in culture, so that as yet no vaccine is available. *Plasmodium* is thus a prime target for the development of a vaccine by genetic engineering and at the time of writing, work in this direction is in progress. We can anticipate that in the next few years the list of vaccines obtained through these modern genetic methods will be considerably extended.

OPPORTUNISTIC PATHOGENS

Primary pathogens are those which have the ability to cause disease in the normal body; such organisms possess, in varying degree, the virulence attributes of toxigenicity and invasiveness described above. *Secondary* or *opportunistic pathogens* are organisms which take advantage of a localised or generalised defect in the antimicrobial defences of a host to cause disease. Where defence mechanisms, in the broadest sense of that term, are defective, the host is described as 'compromised' and appreciation of the underlying conditions which enable opportunistic infections to occur is particularly important (below). The fact that an organism is opportunistic under suitable conditions does not preclude primary pathogenicity; e.g. *Streptococcus pyogenes* and *Strep. pneumoniae* are primary pathogens which also frequently cause disease in compromised hosts. However, there are many opportunistic organisms which

Table 4.6 Opportunistic bacterial pathogens.

Organism	Predisposing conditions and examples of opportunistic infections
Staphylococcus aureus	Injury to the skin (infection of wounds, suture lines, burns) Infectious diseases (bronchopneumonia following influenza, measles, whooping cough) Lung diseases (pneumonitis, without septicaemia, in cystic fibrosis; pneumonitis with septicaemia in other chronic lung disease) Diabetes mellitus (septicaemia) Heroin addicts (acute endocarditis) Newborns (skin infection, conjunctivitis, bronchopneumonia, osteomyelitis) Childbirth (puerperal sepsis) Neutrophil defects (chronic granulomatous disease) Hypogammaglobulinaemia, immunosuppression
Staphylococcus epidermidis	Intravenous cannulation (septicaemia) Cardiac surgery (endocarditis) Urinary tract anomalies (cystitis) Neutrophil defects (chronic granulomatous disease) Immunosuppression (septicaemia)
Streptococcus pyogenes	Injury to the skin (infection of wounds, burns, incisions) Infectious disease (pneumonia following influenza, measles, rubella, chickenpox, whooping cough) Childbirth (puerperal sepsis) Cancers of head, neck, gastrointestinal tract (septicaemia) Immunosuppression, hypogammaglobulinaemia (septicaemia, systemic infection)
Streptococcus agalactiae	Diabetes mellitus (pyelonephritis, pneumonia, arthritis) Newborn (septicaemia, meningitis, pneumonia)
Streptococcus viridans	Damaged heart valves (subacute bacterial endocarditis)

478

Table 4.6 *continued*

Organism	Predisposing conditions and examples of opportunistic infections
Streptococcus pneumoniae	Infectious disease (pneumonia following influenza, whooping cough, pulmonary tuberculosis) Congestive heart failure (pneumonia) Diabetes mellitus (pneumonia) Anaesthesia, alcoholism (pneumonia) Sickle cell anaemia (septicaemia, meningitis, pneumonia, osteomyelitis) Hypogammaglobulinaemia, incl. multiple myeloma and chronic lymphocytic leukaemia (pneumonia, septicaemia)
Escherichia coli	Urinary tract obstruction, incl. pregnancy; catheterisation, cystoscopy (urinary tract infections) Cirrhosis (peritonitis) Newborns (meningitis, gastroenteritis)
Klebsiella spp. (*K. pneumoniae,* etc.)	Frequent infections in hospitals, e.g. intensive care units Chronic lung disease (pneumonia) Diabetes mellitus (pneumonia) Urinary tract obstruction or instrumentation (cystitis)
Serratia marcescens	Common infections in hospitals, e.g. intensive care and chronic disease units Urinary tract instrumentation and anomalies (urinary tract infections) Injury to skin (infections of wounds and burns) Heroin addicts (endocarditis) Neutrophil defects (chronic granulomatous disease)
Proteus spp. (*P. mirabilis,* etc.)	Urinary tract infections
Enterobacter cloacae	Urinary tract infections
Salmonella spp. (*S. cholerae-suis* etc.)	Defective cell-mediated immunity, immuno-suppression (salmonellosis and septicaemia in leukaemia, Hodgkin's disease, treated solid tumours, kidney graft recipients, systemic lupus erythematosus, sarcoidosis) Haemolysis (osteomyelitis, pneumonitis, septicaemia in sickle cell disease and other haemoglobinopathies, malaria, bartonellosis) Neutrophil defects (septicaemia in chronic granulomatous disease) Newborn (septicaemia, meningitis) Elderly (septicaemia)
Haemophilus spp. (*H. influenzae,* etc.)	Sickle cell disease, agammaglobulinaemia (septicaemia, meningitis in children) Cranial trauma, diabetes mellitus, alcoholism (meningitis) Respiratory infections or chronic lung disease (pneumonia)

Table 4.6 *continued*

Organism	Predisposing conditions and examples of opportunistic infections
Pseudomonas aeruginosa	Injury to skin (infection of burns and wounds, leading to septicamia, pneumonitis) Cystic fibrosis (pneumonia without septicaemia) Eye surgery or injury (corneal infection) Urinary tract catheterisation or irrigation (urinary tract infections, septicaemia) Heroin abuse (endocarditis) Newborns (enterocolitis, meningitis, etc.) Immunosuppression, acute myeloblastic leukaemia (pneumonitis, septicaemia)
Clostridium perfringens	Deep wounds with muscle necrosis and infection by facultative bacteria (anaerobic cellulitis, gas gangrene) Abortion (uterine infection, septic abortion, septicaemia) Childbirth (puerperal sepsis) Surgery on biliary or gastrointestinal tract (septicaemia)
Clostridium tetani	Wounds and burns with necrosis and/or presence of facultative bacteria (tetanus) Infection of umbilical stump (tetanus neonatorum)
Mycobacterium tuberculosis	Diabetes mellitus, silicosis, malnutrition, chronic alcoholism (exogenous infection, exacerbation of existing tuberculosis, reactivation of latent lesions) Defective cell-mediated immunity in Hodgkin's disease, immunosuppression, cancer chemotherapy and inherited T cell defects (as above with disseminated infection, miliary tuberculosis; disseminated infection after BCG vaccine)
Atypical mycobacteria (*M. kansasii*, *M. fortuitum*)	Cancer and cancer chemotherapy, immuno-suppression (pulmonary disease, occasionally disseminated)
Listeria monocytogenes	Newborn (meningitis, septicaemia) Cirrhosis, diabetes mellitus (meningitis, septicaemia) Hodgkin's disease, immunosuppression for transplantation (meningitis, septicaemia)

rarely, if ever, cause disease in the normal body, but do so when host defences are reduced; they include *Staphylococcus aureus* and members of the normal flora such as faecal and viridans streptococci, *Escherichia coli*, *Bacteroides* spp., and *Staph. epidermidis*, as well as exogenously acquired organisms such as *Pseudomonas aeruginosa* and clostridia. Thus, the state of host resistance often has a determining effect on whether an infection can occur and what its outcome will be; the terms 'non-pathogenic' and 'avirulent' are readily seen to be applicable only in reference to a *normal* host, since in the compromised body many otherwise harmless microbes may cause severe, even life-threatening disease. It should be noted that, while this section is concerned with bacteria, opportunistic pathogens are also found among viruses and fungi, where the same general principles apply (e.g. pp. 151, 271).

Conditions for opportunistic bacterial infection

The phrase 'reduced host defence' encompasses a wide variety of conditions, from local damage to, or reduced effectiveness of, the barriers to infection of the skin and alimentary, respiratory and urinary tracts, to generalised deficiencies in phagocytic cells or the immune system. Some of these are summarised below and in Table 4.6, while others can be found in the descriptions of specific genera.

BREAKDOWN OF LOCAL TISSUE BARRIERS AND OTHER MECHANISMS

Skin

The skin is a major barrier to infection and its damage by surgical or traumatic wounding can be followed by infection with *Staph. aureus*, *Strep. pyogenes*, Gram-negative bacilli (*E. coli*, *P. aeruginosa*, *Klebsiella* spp., *Serratia marcescens*) and anaerobes (*Clostridium perfringens*, *Cl. tetani*). Similarly, burns destroy the skin's effectiveness as a defensive barrier. Gram-negative rods such as *Pseudomonas* and *Serratia*, as well as pyogenic cocci (*Staph. aureus*, β-haemolytic streptococci) cause burn infections which may lead to dangerous septicaemia. Intravenous catheterisation also breaches the skin defences and can lead to infection and septicaemia.

Gastrointestinal tract

The gastrointestinal tract is protected to a large extent by stomach acidity; increased susceptibility to infection by *Salmonella* spp. or *Vibrio cholerae* occurs in achlorhydria (absence of HCl from the gastric juice), e.g. in atrophic gastritis or following surgical removal of part of the stomach (gastrectomy). In such patients, the small intestine, which normally has a sparse microflora, is densely colonised by bacteria, often leading to diarrhoeal diseases.

Lower respiratory tract

The lower respiratory tract is physically protected by its mucus coating in which organisms become trapped; the mucus is swept upwards from the respiratory tree by *ciliary action* to be either coughed and expectorated or swallowed, the latter event exposing the organisms to the sterilising conditions of the stomach. Damage to the ciliated epithelium, especially by influenza, predisposes the patient to secondary pneumonia due to bacteria which may already be carried in the upper respiratory tract (*Strep. pneumoniae*, *Strep. pyogenes*, *Staph. aureus*, *Haemophilus influenzae*). Cystic fibrosis, in which mucociliary clearance and phagocytosis in the lung are depressed by the viscosity of the mucus, is often complicated by infection with *Staph. aureus* or *P. aeruginosa*. Other chronic lung diseases, including chronic bronchitis, bronchiectasis and emphysema, in which there is depression of pulmonary clearance and normal respiratory function, are also complicated by secondary pneumonia. Manipulations of the respiratory tract (tracheostomy, aspiration, use of contaminated respirators) can be hazardous as they bypass or overwhelm normal respiratory defences.

Urinary tract

The urinary tract (ureter, bladder, urethra) is protected by the flow of urine which ensures that infecting organisms are regularly washed out. Opportunistic infection occurs when excretion of urine is impaired by congenital anomalies, acquired obstruction (e.g. due to pregnancy, enlargement of the prostate or calculi), paralytic disease affecting bladder function, or manipulations such as catheterisation or cystoscopy. *E. coli* is the commonest organism involved; other enterobacteria (*Klebsiella*, *Proteus*, *Enterobacter*, etc.) and *P. aeruginosa* are also Gram-negative opportunists in these conditions. Streptococci (especially enterococci), *Staph. aureus* and *Staph. epidermidis* also cause opportunistic infections of the urinary tract.

Heart valves

Heart valves, either congenitally malformed or damaged by rheumatic fever or syphilis, can be colonised by bacteria of normally low virulence, such as viridans streptococci; the organisms are protected from blood-borne host defences by small thrombi which form on the lesions and by the relative avascularity of the valves. Colonisation of the valves leads to the serious condition of *subacute bacterial endocarditis*. This provides a further example of endogenous opportunistic infection (i.e. by organisms already present in the body), as the viridans streptococci are commensals in the mouth which enter the bloodstream normally harmlessly during dental extractions, vigorous chewing or brushing of the teeth. A small proportion (2–4%) of prosthetic heart valves become infected in a similar way, usually more than two months after surgery (early endocarditis is more likely to be due to organisms acquired during the operation).

GENERALISED DEFICIENCIES IN INFLAMMATORY AND IMMUNE RESPONSES

Defects in phagocytosis, antibody production, complement or cell-mediated immunity all predispose to opportunistic infection; such defects may be primary (inherited) or secondary to neoplasia (leukaemias, Hodgkin's disease) or the immunosuppressive and cytotoxic drugs used in cancer therapy and transplantation. The types of organisms which appear as opportunists in such conditions reflect the importance of the affected defence process in combating those organisms.

Neutrophils

Inherited defects in the bactericidal function of neutrophils occur in chronic granulomatous disease and glucose-6-phosphate dehydrogenase deficiency. As described on p. 24, they lead to infection by catalase-positive bacteria, with adenitis, pneumonia, osteomyelitis and septicaemia. In the Chédiak-Higashi syndrome (p. 25) a defect in the number, chemotaxis and phagocytic activity of neutrophils leads to upper respiratory tract infections, pneumonia, abscesses and skin infections by pyogenic cocci and Gram-negative bacilli. The 'lazy leucocyte syndrome' and 'Job's syndrome' are rare defects in neutrophil chemotaxis associated with infection by pyogenic cocci. The neoplastic neutrophils in leukaemia do not function normally.

Neutropenia (agranulocytosis) is a reduction in the number of peripheral blood neutrophils (and other granulocytes) which may be an inherited disorder or acquired through drug toxicity or irradiation. Many of the chemotherapeutic drugs used in cancer treatment lead to neutropenia by reducing production (proliferation) of granulocytes in the bone marrow, while certain other drugs cause excessive destruction of mature granulocytes, also within the bone marrow. Stomatitis (infection within the mouth) and other infections occur due to *Staph. aureus* or a range of Gram-negative rods (*E. coli, Pseudomonas, Klebsiella, Proteus*). Neutrophil function is also depressed in sickle cell anaemia and other haemoglobinopathies, renal failure, diabetes mellitus and malnutrition, all of which are frequently complicated by opportunistic bacterial infections of the urinary and respiratory tracts and the skin, and by septicaemia.

Antibody production

Primary B cell deficiencies such as Bruton type agammaglobulinaemia (p. 78) lead to infection with extracellular pyogenic organisms for which antibody-mediated defence (opsonisation, lysis) is crucial, including streptococci, *Staph. aureus*, *Neisseria meningitidis*, *Haemophilus influenzae* and *P. aeruginosa*. Recurrent pneumonia, upper respiratory tract infections, skin infections, meningitis and septicaemia are common. Secondary defects in antibody production occur in lymphoproliferative disorders such as chronic lymphocytic leukaemia, multiple myeloma and lymphosarcoma, with infections due to a similar range of organisms. Cytotoxic drugs used in cancer therapy kill B cells (among others) and hence also lead to similar opportunistic infections.

Complement deficiencies

Complement deficiencies affect the bactericidal function of serum antibody (classical pathway) and normal serum (alternative pathway) as well as the opsonising activity of IgM. The consequences are described on p. 123.

T cell defects

T cell defects, such as thymic hypoplasia or aplasia (DiGeorge's syndrome) and the Nézelof syndrome lead to a reduction in cell-mediated immunity and T cell help for antibody production. In T cell deficiency, opportunistic infections are principally those due to intracellular parasites (*Mycobacterium, Listeria, Brucella, Nocardia, Salmonella*) for which lymphokine-mediated activation of macrophages is the normal mechanism of recovery. Hodgkin's disease provides an example of secondary deficiency in CMI; patients with Hodgkin's disease treated with immunosuppressive agents also suffer infection by opsonin-requiring bacteria such as *Staph. aureus* and *P. aeruginosa*.

Combined T and B cell defects

Combined T and B cell defects as in severe combined immunodeficiency, the Wiskott–Aldrich syndrome and ataxia telangiectasia, have a predictable tendency to infections by many types of organism.

Use of cytotoxic drugs, irradiation, etc.

The use of cytotoxic drugs, irradiation, steroids and similar agents during the therapy of cancer, after transplantation or in treatment of systemic lupus erythematosus, etc., carries the hazards of secondary infection as a result of suppression of part or all of the body's immune defence and phagocytic systems. Cytotoxic agents affect B cells more than T, reduce leucocyte numbers and damage mucous membranes; irradiation additionally affects phagocytosis; corticosteroids damage T cells more than B and suppress neutrophil activity. Almost any organism may cause infections in these circumstances. In transplant patients, pneumonia is seen mainly after renal, cardiac and liver grafting, and septicaemia after bone marrow, liver and renal transplantation.

ANTIMICROBIAL DRUGS

The use of antimicrobial drugs, including antibiotics, can encourage opportunistic infection by altering the normal flora of the skin, mucous membranes and gastrointestinal tract, reducing the numbers of competing commensal organisms which normally help to prevent colonisation by pathogens; in consequence, resistant organisms are selected. The latter may be variants of common pathogens with plasmid-borne resistance genes, such as penicillin-resistant staphylococci, or bacteria with a high degree of natural resistance to antimicrobial agents, such as *P. aeruginosa*. The use of excessive doses of antibiotics, especially those with a broad spectrum of action, is especially liable to result in super-infection, usually after 4–5 days of treatment. It may seem paradoxical at first that the wider the antimicrobial spectrum, the greater the danger of opportunistic infection. Endogenous Gram-negative rods and resistant strains of *Staph. aureus* are prominent.

484

Normal neonates are often at risk of opportunistic infection because of the relative immaturity and incompetence of their defensive processes, including specific immune responses, phagocytosis and complement. This is particularly the case for babies born prematurely and with a low birth weight, who are about five times more likely to develop serious infections than full-term babies of normal weight. Bacterial infection (neonatal sepsis) is responsible for 10–20% of all neonatal deaths. Important agents are *E. coli*, the enteropathogenic strains of which cause infantile gastroenteritis with severe diarrhoea and dehydration (p. 548), and the group B β-haemolytic streptococcus *Strep. agalactiae* (p. 507), which has become one of the commonest causes of neonatal disease (pneumonia, meningitis, septicaemia). *Staph. aureus* is also a common cause of infection among newborns. Neonatal infection is more likely to occur if the baby is deprived of maternal IgA antibodies in colostrum and milk, or if infected with organisms to which the mother has no immunity. Normally, infants receive organisms and corresponding antibodies from the mother, but this balanced situation may be upset in hospitals.

NOSOCOMIAL (HOSPITAL-ACQUIRED) INFECTIONS

Many of the conditions predisposing to opportunistic infection exist in hospital patients, so it is hardly surprising that such infections are common in the hospital environment. They occur in approximately 5% of all patients admitted, but this figure can be much higher depending on the type of hospital or ward. The vast majority involve the urinary tract, respiratory tract and surgical wounds and arise either from endogenous flora or are transmitted from other patients, hospital personnel or equipment. A particular problem is that the widespread use of antibiotics in hospitals has led to a prevalence of resistant organisms which are readily acquired by patients soon after admission and which may subsequently cause disease, e.g. in the postoperative period or on treatment with antibiotics, immunosuppressive drugs, etc.

The organisms involved in nosocomial infections include *Staph. aureus*, *P. aeruginosa*, and enterobacteria such as *E. coli*, *Klebsiella pneumoniae*, *Serratia marcescens* and *Proteus mirabilis*, all of which may possess multiple resistance to antibiotics. Approximately 40% of such infections are due to enterobacteria: *E. coli* is the predominant nosocomial pathogen, accounting for about 20% of all infections and septicaemias, while *Klebsiella* is the main cause of lower respiratory tract infections. *Staph. aureus* and *E. coli* between them account for about 30% of all wound infections. Note that infections which become clinically apparent in hospitals are not necessarily acquired there, but are often due to pre-existing natural flora which become invasive as a result of hospital treatment.

SOURCES AND TRANSMISSION OF
BACTERIAL INFECTION

Diseases due to primary pathogens are (by definition) the result of *exogenous* infection, i.e. acquired from a source outside the patient's own body, such as another patient or a healthy carrier. Secondary (opportunistic) infection may also be exogenous but can equally well be *endogenous*, arising from the patient himself; in endogenous infection, an organism which had hitherto been carried harmlessly somewhere in the body is transferred to another body site at which it gives rise to disease.

SOURCES OF EXOGENOUS INFECTION

(Note that the term 'source' implies a growth habitat for the organism rather than simply a vehicle for its transmission).

Humans

Infected humans, often with subclinical or untreated infection, are the exclusive sources of diseases such as diphtheria, whooping cough, pulmonary tuberculosis, leprosy, cholera, typhoid fever, bacillary dysentery, syphilis and gonorrhoea. *Healthy carriers* are often important sources of infection; they are individuals who are infected with pathogenic organisms but show no typical clinical signs or symptoms of the illness (subclinical or inapparent infection). They are nevertheless able to disseminate the organisms and are all the more dangerous for being unrecognised. Sometimes, carriers are *convalescent* individuals who continue to harbour and shed organisms for weeks or months despite the disappearance of their clinical symptoms. Diseases often acquired from healthy carriers include gonorrhoea, diphtheria, bacillary dysentery and typhoid fever. Where asymptomatic carriers are frequent, control of a disease becomes difficult as it requires identification and treatment of carriers as well as patients and in some cases (e.g. streptococci) this is an impracticable task.

Animals

Some of the bacteria causing disease in man have animal hosts. Infectious diseases which primarily affect animals but are transferrable, under appropriate circumstances, to man are called *zoonoses*. Man is generally a 'dead end' host as far as further transmission is concerned, and spread to other persons or back to animals is usually rare. Examples include bovine-type tuberculosis, salmonella food poisoning, brucellosis, anthrax and bubonic plague. Organisms such as clostridia are harmless commensals in the intestines of many animals (including man), but potentially pathogenic if introduced into a wound. Transmission of infection from animal to man can take place by a variety of means, including direct contact, contamination of soil or water, or ingestion of contaminated meat or dairy products. Milk is a vehicle for the spread of several organisms, including tubercle bacilli, staphylococci, streptococci and salmonellae, but milk-borne infection is effectively controlled by pasteurisation.

Soil

The soil is a great source of organisms, most of which grow there as non-pathogenic saprophytes. Some are indigenous, while others derive from excreta or animal cadavers. Human pathogens among soil organisms include *Clostridium tetani* (the tetanus bacillus) and *Cl. perfringens* (gas gangrene), which cause disease after infecting wounds; they enter the soil in human and animal faeces. *Bacillus anthracis* is deposited in the soil from the bodies of animals which have died from anthrax, and may then be acquired by man through the skin or mucous membranes. *Clostridium* and *Bacillus* species can survive in soil for long periods through production of resistant spores. Diseases acquired from the soil are not transmitted from person to person by direct contact.

Water

Both salt and fresh water contain bacteria, but the presence of pathogenic species is usually the result of contamination by human or animal excreta (below). However, water is a natural habitat for *Cl. botulinum* and *Vibrio parahaemolyticus*, which can give rise to food poisoning via contamination of seafood. It is also a vehicle for transmission, rather than a natural habitat for, typhoid and cholera organisms, as described below.

Food

Bacteria multiplying in food are a cause of food poisoning, which should be distinguished from 'food-borne infections' where food serves solely as a vehicle for transmission. The term 'food poisoning' is generally used in reference to acute gastroenteritis, usually manifested as abdominal cramps, vomiting and diarrhoea, all of relatively brief duration; it is not applied to major enteric diseases such as the enteric fevers, cholera or bacillary dysentery, even though these may also be transmitted in food. (Botulism is an exception in that it is often described as a food poisoning—which, of course, it is literally—although its effects are neurological rather than intestinal.) Food poisoning may result from the release of enterotoxins into the food, with no requirement for bacteria to infect the body; *Staph. aureus* food poisoning is the commonest example of this *toxic* type of gastroenteritis. In contrast, food poisoning by *Cl. perfringens*, salmonellae and *V. parahaemolyticus* is *infective*: the organisms multiply in and may invade the small intestine. In these cases, extensive multiplication in the food is necessary since a large infecting dose is required. For clostridia, the heat resistance of the spores enables them to survive most cooking procedures, including boiling, and in fact heat induces the germination of *Cl. perfringens* spores. Other organisms contaminate food eaten raw (e.g. *V. parahaemolyticus*) or are introduced after cooking, in both cases multiplying rapidly in food kept warm.

With the exception of infections transmitted across the placenta, all infectious diseases begin at a body surface, either the skin or the mucous membranes of the respiratory, alimentary and urogenital tracts and conjunctiva.

Skin

When intact, the skin is a remarkably efficient physical barrier to bacterial invasion; in addition, fatty acids and skin pH have an antibacterial effect. However, a burn, wound or even a minor abrasion remove the barrier and facilitate infection, which can be acquired from hands, clothing or other articles, from airborne dust or droplets, or from the soil (see opportunistic infection, above).

Respiratory infections

Respiratory infections can be transmitted either by *contact* with an infected individual or object or by *inhalation* of infected dust particles or droplets. Bacteria in respiratory secretions may find their way into the environment by transfer to the hands, clothing, bedding and objects such as handkerchiefs, cups, cutlery or other household articles (fomites), all of which act as vehicles of infection. Transmission can then take place by contact with the infected person or the contaminated vehicle, organisms being transferred to the recipient's nose or mouth, e.g. via the fingers. Alternatively, dust particles (dried secretions) carrying bacteria may be liberated into the air from the skin, clothing, bedding, handkerchiefs and other objects, to be inhaled directly into the respiratory tract of the new host. For many pathogens, dust is the main vehicle for airborne spread and most respiratory organisms can remain alive for some time if protected from direct sunlight (e.g. streptococci, staphylococci, tubercle bacilli, diphtheria bacilli). However, for those organisms which are susceptible to drying, such as the meningococcus, pneumococcus and whooping cough bacillus, spread in moist droplets is important. This is also true for *Strep. pyogenes*, which remains viable on drying but loses its pathogenicity. Respiratory droplets are expelled during talking, coughing and sneezing, but hardly at all during normal breathing. A sneeze may create a million droplets, varying in size from 10 μm to 2 mm in diameter. Large droplets fall to the ground in a few seconds and are probably not inhaled, whereas smaller ones (< 100 μm) evaporate rapidly in the air, producing *droplet nuclei*, minute residues which remain airborne like dust particles and settle only very slowly. They may be carried in the air for several hours. However, in general, secretion droplets seem to be less important than dust particles in transmission by inhalation. Airborne spread occurs in the relatively close vicinity of the source, i.e. mainly in the same room. Spread to other rooms in a building is generally slight, while the bactericidal effects of ultraviolet radiation, ozone and desiccation mean that the outdoor air rarely contains pathogens.

Faecal-oral routes

Faecal-oral routes of transmission are responsible for major gastrointestinal infections such as typhoid, cholera and bacillary dysentery, the organisms being discharged from the body in faeces and entering by ingestion. Spread may be by hands which become contaminated during cleansing at toilet, followed by transfer of organisms to door handles, taps, towels, etc., from which they can be acquired by a recipient and carried on his hands to the mouth; this is a typical course of events in bacillary dysentery. Faecally-contaminated *water* is often the vehicle for transmission of typhoid fever and cholera. *Food* can be contaminated by flies which have been in contact with faeces, or after handling by carriers; typhoid fever and bacillary dysentery are often food-borne.

Sexual transmission

This is the principal means of spread of certain organisms which are very easily killed by drying and other conditions outside the body, such as *Treponema pallidum* (syphilis) and *Neisseria gonorrhoeae* (gonorrhoea). Many other organisms can be spread by this means, however.

Transplacental transmission

The placenta is a barrier to most bacteria, making transplacental transmission of infection relatively uncommon. The classic example is congenital syphilis which is acquired *in utero* either by direct passage of treponemes from the maternal to the foetal circulation or via a lesion in the placenta from which organisms in large numbers may infect the foetus.

PRESENCE OF BACTERIA IN THE BLOOD

Bacteria often enter the bloodstream, though the numbers are usually too low for them to be observed directly in blood films and culture of the blood is required for their detection. The following are intended as introductory definitions of the relevant terms, further illustrations being provided later in the section.

Bacteraemia is the presence of living bacteria in the circulating blood. As usually used, the term implies that small numbers of organisms are present transiently in the bloodstream with no immediate clinical effects; they are either rapidly killed by antibody and complement or removed by the littoral (sinus-lining) macrophages of the liver, spleen and bone marrow. Bacteraemia by organisms of low pathogenicity resident in the normal flora commonly occurs harmlessly in normal persons, e.g. viridans streptococci often enter the blood with no untoward effect during eating, brushing the teeth or dental extraction. However, bacteraemia may also serve to disseminate organisms to various sites during the development of certain diseases, including typhoid fever, syphilis and tuberculosis, or lead to opportunistic infection where there is an underlying predisposition (e.g. subacute bacterial endocarditis due to viridans streptococci colonising abnormal heart valves).

Septicaemia is the presence of large numbers of bacteria in the bloodstream, in which they multiply. It is thus a severe form of bacteraemia and may involve the rapid multiplication of highly pathogenic organisms such as pyogenic cocci, or of invading opportunists in the compromised host. It occurs when the organisms have overwhelmed host defences and always has serious clinical consequences, leading either to rapid death or the development of foci of infection in various parts of the body. Gram-negative septicaemias are a frequent cause of death following opportunistic infection in compromised patients (Table 4.6).

Pyaemia is invasion of the bloodstream by pyogenic organisms carried on infected emboli (p. 647). It is caused by the disintegration of infected thrombi, such as those which develop in veins (thrombophlebitis) in the neighbourhood of septic foci. Where the emboli become impacted, they give rise to multiple suppurative foci in various tissues (pyaemic abscesses). A striking example occurs in staphylococcal osteomyelitis (p. 526), in which *Staph. aureus* infection of the bone marrow leads to thrombosis in the sinusoids, initiated by the organisms' production of the enzyme coagulase. The thrombi are then softened by neutrophil enzymes released during suppuration, and pyaemia leads to formation of multiple abscesses in the lungs, kidneys and elsewhere.

BACTERIAL FAMILIES AND GENERA

The remainder of this section describes specific bacterial genera of medical importance, with particular emphasis on factors determining their pathogenicity and the processes involved in the diseases for which they are responsible. A classification of these organisms can be found in Table 4.7.

STREPTOCOCCUS

The streptococci are Gram-positive cocci, some of which are pyogenic (pus-inducing) and responsible for a wide variety of important human and animal diseases, while others are harmless commensals. Their natural habitat in man is the upper respiratory tract, which they colonise a few hours after birth and from which they can almost always be obtained by a throat swab; they form part of the normal flora of the nose, throat and mouth, though species are also found in the gut and on the skin. In general, those present in healthy individuals are organsims of low intrinsic pathogenicity (viridans streptococci) which in the mouth are responsible for tooth decay; however, up to 10% of normal people are also carriers of the pathogenic streptococcus (*Streptococcus pyogenes*), the agent of acute suppurative diseases such as pharyngitis, tonsillitis, scarlet fever, erysipelas and impetigo. The main feature of the pathogenicity of this organism is *invasiveness*: it has the ability to remain extracellular and resist phagocytosis, both by means of external structures and by secreted locally-acting toxins and enzymes. As important,

Table 4.7 Classification of selected bacteria of medical importance.

Genus	Morphology and other characteristics	Species	Diseases include
A. Gram-positive organisms			
Streptococcus	Cocci; cells in chains or pairs; non-motile; facultative anaerobes; catalase negative; α-haemolytic, β-haemolytic and non-haemolytic groups	*Streptococcus pyogenes*	Pharyngitis, tonsillitis, scarlet fever, erysipelas, impetigo, rheumatic fever, acute glomerulo-nephritis
		Streptococcus agalactiae	Neonatal sepsis and meningitis
		Streptococcus viridans	Subacute endocarditis
		Streptococcus mutans	Dental caries, gingivitis, periodontitis
		Streptococcus pneumoniae	Lobar pneumonia, bronchopneumonia, empyema, meningitis, pericarditis
Staphylococcus	Cocci; cells in grape-like clusters; non-motile; facultative anaerobes; catalase positive; haemolytic; coagulase positive	*Staphylococcus aureus*	Skin pustules, boils and carbuncles, impetigo, infections of wounds and burns, breast abscess, whitlow, osteomyelitis, bronchopneumonia, septicaemia, acute endocarditis, food poisoning, scalded skin syndrome
	coagulase negative	*Staphylococcus epidermidis*	Cystitis, endocarditis, septicaemia, chronic granulomatous disease
Corynebacterium	Bacilli; club-shaped, beaded; palisades and angular clusters; non-motile; aerobes or facultative anaerobes	*Corynebacterium diphtheriae*	Diphtheria

continued on p. 492

Table 4.7 *continued*

Genus	Species	Morphology and other characteristics	Diseases include
Clostridium	*Clostridium perfringens*	Bacilli; spore-forming, motile with peritrichous flagella (excl. *Cl. perfringens*); obligate anaerobes; many exotoxins	Gas gangrene, food poisoning, enteritis necroticans
	Clostridium septicum		Gas gangrene
	Clostridium novyi		Gas gangrene
	Clostridium tetani		Tetanus, tetanus neonatorum
	Clostridium botulinum		Botulism
Bacillus	*Bacillus anthracis*	Bacilli; spore-forming; grow as chains; most motile with peritrichous flagella (excl. *B. anthracis*); aerobic	Anthrax
Mycobacterium	*Mycobacterium tuberculosis*	Bacilli; acid-fast; obligate aerobes; non-motile	Tuberculosis
	Mycobacterium bovis		Tuberculosis
	Mycobacterium leprae		Leprosy
B. Gram-negative organisms			
Neisseria	*Neisseria meningitidis*	Cocci; cells in pairs; non-motile; aerobic; oxidase positive	Meningococcal meningitis, septicaemia
	Neisseria gonorrhoeae		Gonorrhoea
Klebsiella	*Klebsiella pneumoniae*	Bacilli; non-motile; encapsulated; facultative anaerobes; ferment lactose	Pneumonia, urinary tract infections, wound infections, septicaemia, meningitis (all are opportunistic infections) (Table 4.6)
Proteus	*Proteus mirabilis*	Bacilli; motile with peritrichous flagella; urease positive	Urinary tract and other opportunistic infections (Table 4.6)
Escherichia	*Escherichia coli*	Bacilli; motile with peritrichous flagella; facultative anaerobes; ferment lactose; O, K, H antigens	Diarrhoea in newborns, travellers' diarrhoea; urinary tract infections, neonatal meningitis, other opportunistic infections (Table 4.6)

Genus	Characteristics	Species	Disease
Shigella	Bacilli; non-motile; lactose negative; O antigens	*Shigella dysenteriae* (also *Sh. flexneri*, *Sh. boyii* and *Sh. sonnei*)	Bacillary dysentery
Salmonella	Bacilli; motile with peritrichous flagella; lactose negative; H_2S positive; O, Vi, H antigens	*Salmonella typhi*	Typhoid fever
		Salmonella paratyphi	Paratyphoid fever
		Salmonella typhimurium	Gastroenteritis (food poisoning)
		Salmonella cholerae-suis	Septicaemia
Pseudomonas	Bacilli; motile with polar flagella	*Pseudomonas aeruginosa*	Several opportunistic infections (wounds, burns, lung, eye, urinary tract, septicaemia; Table 4.6)
Vibrio	Curved rods; motile with single polar flagellum	*Vibrio cholerae*	Cholera
		Vibrio parahaemolyticus	Food poisoning
Treponema	Spirochaetes; slender, flexible helices; motile; non-flagellate; axial fibrils; obligate anaerobes; slow growth	*Treponema pallidum*	Syphilis
		Treponema pertenue	Yaws
		Treponema carateum	Pinta

however, are the nonsuppurative complications which may follow untreated streptococcal disease, principally rheumatic fever and glomerulonephritis, both of which are immunological in origin and results of hypersensitivity.

CLASSIFICATION (Figure 4.41)

Streptococci are classified according to their ability to produce *haemolysis*: α and β groups are haemolytic organisms, while γ are non-haemolytic, properties evident from their growth on blood agar plates. Colonies of *β-haemolytic streptococci* on blood agar are surrounded by a broad, clear, almost colourless zone of complete haemolysis in which no surviving red cells are visible by microscopic examination. This is the result of production of the haemolysins called streptolysin O and streptolysin S, both of which give rise to complete haemolysis. The β-haemolytic organisms include *Strep. pyogenes*, the principal streptococcal species pathogenic in man. *α-Haemolytic streptococci* produce a narrow zone of partial (incomplete) haemolysis around the colony when grown aerobically, with a greenish discolouration due to an insoluble reduction product of haemoglobin. They are known as viridans streptococci (Lat. *viridis*, green) and include several species, usually of low pathogenicity (*Strep. salvarius*, *Strep. mutans*, *Strep. sanguis*, etc.), but also *Strep. pneumoniae* (the pneumococcus, p. 510). The non-haemolytic *γ-streptococci* include faecal organisms (*Strep. faecalis*) which are always present as intestinal commensals (also called *enterococci*); they sometimes occur as opportunistic pathogens.

β-Haemolytic streptococci are further subdivided by immunological criteria. In the early 1930's, Rebecca Lancefield discovered that streptococci could be grouped according to the antigens of an extractable carbohydrate present in the cell wall ('C' carbohydrate). The usual method for extraction is by boiling organisms for ten minutes in dilute HCl, followed by neutralisation and centrifugation, whereupon the supernatant contains

Figure 4.41 Classification of streptococci.

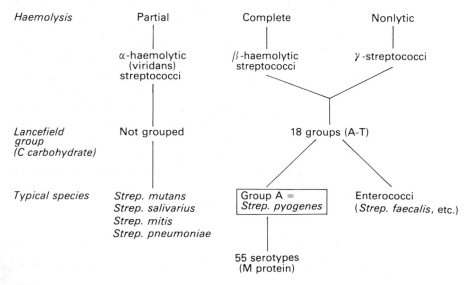

Haemolysis	Partial	Complete	Nonlytic
	α-haemolytic (viridans) streptococci	β-haemolytic streptococci	γ-streptococci
Lancefield group (C carbohydrate)	Not grouped	18 groups (A-T)	
Typical species	Strep. mutans Strep. salvarius Strep. mitis Strep. pneumoniae	Group A = Strep. pyogenes	Enterococci (Strep. faecalis, etc.)
		55 serotypes (M protein)	

the carbohydrate. Antisera were raised against C carbohydrate in rabbits and with them, by means of precipitin tests (p. 125), Lancefield defined 13 groups, denoted A–O (now 18 groups, A–T). The Lancefield groups have different habitats and distributions among animal species: streptococci responsible for human disease are mostly *Group A*, though occasionally organisms in other groups (B,C,D,G) are involved. Some groups are associated with particular animal hosts (Groups B in cattle, E in swine, L and M in dogs). Lancefield groups include all β-haemolytic and γ-streptococci (Group N), but viridans streptococci and *Strep. pneumoniae* are not 'groupable' (Figure 4.41).

Although Group A β-haemolytic streptococci are a *single species* (*Strep. pyogenes*), they are further subdivided into *types* on the basis of the antigens of the *M protein* in the cell wall. The original typing method of Griffiths was by bacterial agglutination using rabbit antisera, though precipitation of extracted M protein is now preferred as it avoids confusion with other antigens. More than 55 immunological types (serotypes) of Group A organisms have been identified according to their M antigens and designated numerically. Some individual serotypes are associated with a particular disease, a good example being the *nephritogenic* strains (e.g. types 12 and 49), which lead to glomerulonephritis. Serotype determination is an important aspect of epidemiology of streptococcal infections.

MORPHOLOGY AND GROWTH

Streptococci are non-motile, spherical or oval cells, $1\,\mu m$ in diameter, which characteristically grow in chains of varying length (Figure 4.2a) as a result of division in a single plane and non-separation of daughter cells. (*In vivo*, the chains tend to be shorter than in culture, or simply pairs). Cells are linked by wall material which has not been cleaved by the normal enzymatic processes and, in fluid culture, formation of long chains is encouraged by antibodies to cell wall antigens. They require a complex growth medium including at least 15 amino acids, all B vitamins and some purines and pyrimidines. In practice they are grown in beef infusion media containing 5% blood or serum. They are *facultative anaerobes* (i.e. can grow in the presence or absence of oxygen), but since they are unable to synthesize haem their respiration is always anaerobic. Thus, all streptococci are lactic acid bacteria, deriving their energy requirement from fermentation of sugars. Their aerobic growth is limited by the bactericidal effects of H_2O_2, which they produce as a result of the oxidation of NADH and NADPH but cannot destroy as they are catalase-negative (catalase is a haem-containing enzyme). In media containing blood, red cells are a source of catalase. (See also p. 24, chronic granulomatous disease.)

STRUCTURE (Figure 4.42).

Structural components of streptococci are not only important in

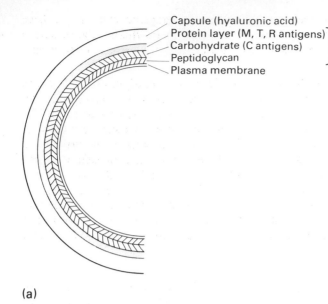

Capsule (hyaluronic acid)
Protein layer (M, T, R antigens)
Carbohydrate (C antigens) } Cell wall
Peptidoglycan
Plasma membrane

(a)

Figure 4.42
(a) Diagrammatic section.
(b) Electron micrograph of thin section of Group A streptococcus, showing fimbriae (f) of M protein.
(c) Electron micrograph of M⁻ strain; note absence of fimbriae. (From McCarty, M. (1971) The streptococcal cell wall. *Harvey Lectures Series* **65**, p. 73)

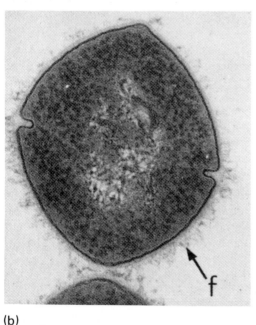

(b)

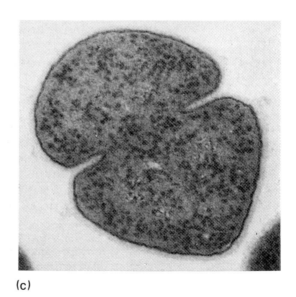

(c)

classification, but by endowing the organisms with antiphagocytic properties, they are also central to their pathogenicity.

Capsule. During periods of active (logarithmic) growth, *Strep. pyogenes* strains often possess a capsule of *hyaluronic acid*, which tends to be lost when rapid division ceases. Hyaluronic acid is a mucopolysaccharide composed of repeating units of glucuronic acid and N-acetylglucosamine which is chemically and antigenically indistinguishable from the same component of normal connective tissue (p. 666, 850). Thus the streptococcal capsule is *non-antigenic* (i.e. does not stimulate antibody production); this might be a powerful and dangerous adaptation were it not for the fact that other surface molecules are antigenic and, as we have noted, the capsule tends to be lost. Nevertheless, the capsule is antiphagocytic and thus contributes to the organisms' survival.

M protein is the antiphagocytic component of the cell wall, and as already noted, shows considerable variation between strains, the basis of typing of streptococci. M protein is present as hairlike fimbriae on the cell surface which appear as a surface 'fuzziness' in thin sections under the electron microscope (Figure 4.42b); fimbriae are absent from M⁻ mutants which present a smooth appearance (Figure 4.42c). The M protein is the target of the antibody response which is required for opsonisation; only anti-M antibodies are protective and immunity is therefore type-specific. Given that there are at least 55 M-types, there is little likelihood of an individual becoming immune to Group A streptococcal infection.

R and T proteins are also antigenic wall constituents, but neither seems to have a bearing on virulence. There are two antigenically distinct R proteins and several T proteins, the strain distribution of which is not related to M.

Group carbohydrate. The C carbohydrate makes up about 10% of the dry weight of the cell and in Group A organisms is composed of 60% rhamnose and 30% N-acetylglucosamine. It is covalently attached to the underlying rigid wall peptidoglycan. The variability of its sugar composition gives rise to the different antigens which are the basis of Lancefield groups.

The *peptidoglycan* is similar to that of other Gram-positive bacteria (p. 388). Interestingly, it produces some of the reactions usually associated with endotoxin of Gram-negative organisms, such as fever, dermal and cardiac necrosis, lysis of red cells and platelets and non-specific enhancement of resistance to infection.

Glycerol teichoic acids are associated with peptidoglycan and contribute about 1% of the dry weight of the cells.

CELL SURFACE AND VIRULENCE

The antiphagocytic properties of streptococci are essential for their pathogenicity, as once phagocytosed by neutrophils they are usually quickly killed. Both the capsule and M protein are involved, as demonstrated using variants lacking one or the other or both. In experimental animals (mice, rats), strains with both capsule and M protein are the most virulent, while absence of either leads to intermediate virulence and strains lacking both are the least virulent. Moreover, in these experiments virulence was inversely correlated with the degree of phagocytosis occurring early after infection; the extent of phagocytosis of non-encapsulated/M⁻ organisms is about 20 times that of encapsulated/M⁺ cells. The capsule and M protein can also be removed artificially by enzymatic treatment with hyaluronidase and trypsin respectively; by selective removal, it was found that the M protein makes a slightly greater antiphagocytic contribution than the capsule, but that to prevent phagocytosis effectively, the combined action of both is required.

EXTRACELLULAR PRODUCTS

A considerable number of soluble products are released from Group A β-haemolytic streptococci, among them toxins (streptolysins S and O, erythrogenic toxin) and enzymes (hyaluronidase, DNase, proteinase, etc.), some of which are probably involved as local adjuncts to pathogenicity (Figure 4.43). Immunoelectrophoresis of streptococcal culture supernatants reveals at least 20 products, of which several have yet to be identified.

Toxins

Streptolysins O and S act on cell membranes and are responsible for β-haemolysis around streptococcal colonies on blood agar plates. Their mechanism of action has already been described (p. 431, 433). The significance of streptolysin O in invasiveness is principally as a leucocidin which kills neutrophils by stimulating the *intracellular* release of their lysosomal contents; it also suppresses chemotaxis. The cardiotoxic properties of streptolysin O may be involved in rheumatic fever. Streptolysin S is also antichemotactic and leucotoxic and is probably the more significant of the two; it is largely cell-bound and will kill phagocytes which have made contact with or engulfed *Strep. pyogenes*.

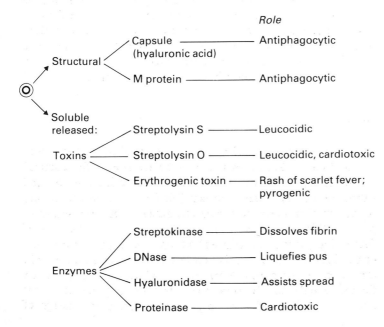

Figure 4.43 Structural components and soluble products involved in virulence of *Streptococcus pyogenes*.

However, as we have already noted, the majority of phagocytosed organisms are rapidly killed, so after engulfment streptolysin S at best only allows a few organisms to escape. The death of neutrophils in foci of infection, accelerated by streptolysins, contributes to local tissue damage by release of enzymes (p. 25). The *antistreptolysin test*, for antibodies against streptolysin O, is widely used in diagnostic laboratories as an indicator of streptococcal infection. Streptolysin S is one of the few toxins which are non-antigenic, due to its small size (p. 433).

Erythrogenic toxin is responsible for the rash of *scarlet fever*, an acute pharyngitis caused by toxigenic strains of *Strep. pyogenes*, generally in children. It provides an example of toxin production by lysogenic organisms (p. 446, Table 4.4). The toxin exists in three antigenically distinct forms, A, B and C, and is a small protein released as a complex with hyaluronic acid, which acts as carrier. Apart from the skin rash, its toxic manifestations include pyrogenicity, low lethality and myocardial necrosis. Its most remarkable property is an ability to intensify the action of other toxins, including endotoxin and streptolysin O, a form of synergistic interaction. Thus, rabbits become thousands of times more sensitive than normal to endotoxin in the presence of erythrogenic toxin; anaphylactic responses to antigens are also enhanced. The mechanism of these interesting phenomena is unknown. It has been proposed recently that in some individuals the rash of scarlet fever may be a hypersensitivity reaction against toxin localised in the skin, rather than the direct effect of erythrogenic toxin on blood vessels.

In individuals not previously exposed, injection of erythrogenic toxin into the skin leads to a localised erythema after 8–12 hours, becoming maximal after about 24 hours; this is known as the *Dick test* and a positive reaction indicates susceptibility to scarlet fever. On recovery from the disease, the presence of circulating antitoxin causes the Dick test to be negative; similarly, injection of antitoxin into the skin of a child with scarlet fever blanches the rash around the injection site (*Schultz–Charlton test*), a reaction which can be of value in distinguishing scarlet fever from similar skin rashes.

Enzymes

Hyaluronidase is produced by certain strains of *Strep. pyogenes* in culture (types 4, 22) and is thought to be more generally produced *in vivo*. It attacks the hyaluronic acid of connective tissue ground substance and may well be responsible for the impressive ability of the organism to spread through mammalian tissues ('cellulitis', p. 501). Thus, hyaluronidase is also called *spreading factor*. Interestingly it is also produced by *Staph. aureus*, which typically causes localised lesions. It is noteworthy that hyaluronidase will also attack the organism's own capsule, which may be the reason for the capsular loss by streptococci in stationary (non-dividing) cultures. The fact that an organism produces the means of destroying one of its own virulence structures seems surprising, but the M protein will maintain the antiphagocytic properties of the cell even if its capsule is lost.

Streptokinase catalyses activation of plasminogen into plasmin, which in turn dissolves fibrin clots (p. 636). It occurs in two forms (A and B) in different strains of *Strep. pyogenes*. It is usually suggested that the enzyme plays a role in assisting bacterial spread by lysis of fibrin barriers formed from inflammatory exudate, though antistreptokinase antibodies do not appear to affect the invasiveness of the organisms. The latter finding underlines the multiplicity of invasive mechanisms employed by virulent streptococci. Delayed-type hypersensitivity to streptokinase (SK) and streptodornase (SD, below) develops during the course of streptococcal infections.

DNase (streptodornase). Four distinct types of DNase (A–D) have been isolated from streptococcal cultures. The enzyme is an effective means of thinning out the viscous pus which forms in abscesses around pyogenic cocci following the disintegration of neutrophils; DNase thus increases the mobility of the bacteria in pus. In fact, preparations of streptokinase and streptodornase have been used therapeutically to liquefy purulent exudates in pneumococcal empyema. DNase does not enter cells and is therefore not leucotoxic.

NADase. Some strains of *Strep. pyogenes* produce an enzyme which removes the nicotinamide from NAD. Although especially associated with nephritogenic strains, such as type 12, there is no other evidence to link it with glomerulonephritis.

Proteinase. This enzyme has the interesting property of destroying M protein (cf. hyaluronidase); it is only released between pH 5.5 and 6.5, but this may occur in the environment of an abscess as the pH falls due to production of lactic acid by organisms and cells. It is cardiotoxic on intravenous injection into animals, producing necrotic myocardial lesions; a possible role in rheumatic fever is a matter for conjecture.

SUMMARY OF VIRULENCE ATTRIBUTES

The significance of each individual product of pathogenic strep-tococci may be open to question, but cumulatively they contribute to the success of the organisms in their *extracellular* life style (Figure 4.43). We have noted elsewhere that these organisms must avoid phagocytosis in order to survive and that they have therefore become endowed with the structural means to remain outside neutrophils (antiphagocytic capsule and M protein) as well as producing the leucocidic streptolysins. The fact that one of these (streptolysin S) is non-antigenic means that immunity to the pathogenic products of *Strep. pyogenes* is never complete.

Their enzymatic products seem chiefly effective in maintaining the freedom of the organisms in the face of local obstacles, such as natural tissue barriers (hyaluronidase) or other impediments to their movement resulting either directly or indirectly from the acute inflammatory response (streptokinase, DNase). It seems that a certain degree of 'overkill' is necessary in the interests of the organisms' survival.

DISEASES DUE TO GROUP A β-HAEMOLYTIC STREPTOCOCCI

Strep. pyogenes is responsible for a prodigious variety of seemingly unrelated diseases. We can distinguish three types of host–parasite relationship with pathogenic streptococci. (1) Asymptomatic infection, or carrier state, in which the organisms are present in the upper respiratory tract with no sign of inflammation; some carriers may be convalescent after an acute sore throat. (2) Acute diseases, which are often suppurative, due to streptococcal invasion of a tissue. (3) Non-suppurative sequels of an immunological origin involving hypersensitivity mechanisms. *Strep. pyogenes* is a *primary pathogen* in pharyngitis and tonsillitis, where no predisposing factor is evident. All other streptococcal infections are *secondary* or *opportunistic*, predisposing conditions including trauma (skin infections), childbirth (puerperal sepsis) and influenza (pneumonia). Streptococci typically produce spreading lesions with inflammation of the soft or supporting tissues, called *cellulitis*; abscesses tend to occur later than in the more localised infections of *Staph. aureus*. An important clinical point is the speed with which *Strep. pyogenes* can kill; e.g. puerperal sepsis and pneumonia can both kill within 12 hours of the illness being recognised.

Transmission of infection

Streptococcal throat infections are acquired principally by the respiratory route, especially from droplets released from individuals with acute disease or harbouring organisms asymptomatically (carriers). Experimental studies show that streptococci in dry form on dust or fomites (contaminated articles) are far less infectious than in moist secretions. Nasal, pharyngeal and salivary secretions are the sources of droplets carrying streptococci and all may be involved in an acute infection such as pharyngitis or sinusitis. Nasal shedding is particularly important, either from individuals with acute sinusitis or from *nasal carriers*. The latter shed about a hundred times more organisms than pharyngeal carriers and, while they are less common, are regarded as a major source of infection. Throat and saliva carriers, on the other hand, are a more persistent reservoir, since 10% of children harbour *Strep. pyogenes* in the throat at any one time and this figure rises during outbreaks. Other dangerous sources are patients with otitis media, vulvovaginitis or infected skin lesions, the last especially in tropical climates.

Pharyngitis and tonsillitis are the most familiar manifestations of suppurative streptococcal disease, with sore throat, inflamed oedematous (beefy red) pharynx, tonsillar exudate, peritonsillar abscesses and fever. (Note that viral infections are a more common source of sore throat than streptococci.) However, this degree of inflammation only occurs in about 20% of those infected, in whom it can be extremely severe; the remainder experience fever or sore throat alone, or non-specific symptoms such as headache, nausea, etc., or are entirely symptomless. The acutely infected throat is a source of spread to cervical lymph nodes (lymphadenitis), nasal sinuses (sinusitis), the middle ear (otitis media), the mastoid process (mastoiditis) and occasionally from the sinuses or middle ear to the meninges (meningitis). Spread to the lower respiratory tract, with streptococcal bronchopneumonia, occurs as a *secondary (opportunistic) complication* of respiratory viral infections such as influenza or measles.

Scarlet fever used to be a common, virulent childhood disease complicating pharyngitis or tonsillitis, but is now rather rare thanks to prompt antibiotic intervention. It is caused by strains of *Strep. pyogenes* which produce erythrogenic toxin (p. 499), resulting in a diffuse pink-red skin rash. The development of antitoxin prevents recurrence of the rash, but provides no resistance to reinfection with other toxigenic strains, since immunity is directed against the organism and is therefore type-specific (anti-M). (See also Dick test, p. 499).

Puerperal sepsis or child-bed fever was at one time a dreaded complication of child birth and abortion, with multiplication of *Strep. pyogenes* (or other pathogens) in the uterus and subsequent spread as pelvic cellulitis, peritonitis or septicaemia; it still occurs occasionally. Before 1935 and the introduction of sulphonamides a fatal outcome was very common, but today severe illness or death from puerperal sepsis is rare in civilised countries. It occupies an important place in medical history, and is particularly associated with the names of Ignaz Semmelweis and Oliver Wendell Holmes. Semmelweiss, a Hungarian physician working in Vienna in the first half of the nineteenth century, showed that the disease was contagious and that the major source of infection was from the contaminated hands and clothing of doctors and students attending the birth straight after dissecting cadavers; it was far less common among women attended only by midwives. Through promoting simple measures of cleanliness and washing hands in antiseptic solutions, he eventually succeeded in reducing puerperal sepsis from a disease affecting up to 25% of all women after childbirth to one seen in less than 1%, but only at the expense of great personal unpopularity among the medical profession. Holmes also propounded the infection theory of puerperal sepsis over 40 years before the first isolation (from the vaginal discharge of a woman with fatal sepsis) of the causative streptococci by Pasteur in 1879.

Skin infections. Strep. pyogenes is responsible for two diseases of the skin, namely erysipelas and impetigo. *Erysipelas* is a spreading infection of the dermis (*cellulitis*), mostly affecting the face (bilaterally), an arm or a leg. The infected area is raised, red, tender and well demarcated. An allergic reaction to streptococcal products, such as SK and SD, may be involved. *Impetigo*, in contrast, is a *pyoderma*, a vesiculopustular infection seen mostly in young children. The lesions are purulent vesicles or ulcers which can occur on normal skin or may be secondary to other skin infections, dermatitis or insect bites. It is more common in warm (or tropical) climates, where it may be followed by glomerulo-nephritis (but not rheumatic fever).

Wounds and burns can become infected by *Strep. pyogenes*. Its introduction into a small wound can lead to a cellulitis of local tissues (e.g. septic finger), lymphadenitis or even fatal septicaemia. In the past, septicaemia from infected wounds sometimes occurred in surgeons and pathologists who had handled tissue infected by streptococci.

Non-suppurative sequels of Streptococcus pyogenes infections

Rheumatic fever

Before the use of antibiotics, rheumatic fever was a common complication of *Strep. pyogenes* throat infections, occurring primarily in children and young adults between two and four weeks after pharyngitis. If the latter is untreated, rheumatic fever follows in 0.1–3% of children, depending on the severity of the infection. The prompt (within five days after infection) and thorough use of penicillin, as well as improvements in social conditions, have made it a relatively rare disease in developed countries, but it remains common in parts of Africa and India. As the name suggests, an obvious symptom is *arthritis*, usually of the ankles, knees, elbows or wrists, which are often painful, tender and swollen. However, its great importance is as a cause of *pancarditis* (inflammation affecting endocardium, myocardium and pericardium), which in the acute stage seriously affects myocardial function and has the unfortunate long-term con-sequence of damage to the heart valves. Rheumatic fever has a marked tendency to recur and with each recurrence the de-formities of the valves become more severe. Other sites affected are the brain, giving rise to involuntary movements known as *chorea*; subcutaneous tissues over the bony prominences of the arms and legs where *nodules* may develop transiently; and the skin, where a rash known as *erythema marginatum* may occur. Lesions, apart from those of the heart, resolve.

During acute rheumatic fever, carditis occurs in about half the patients with arthritis. One manifestation is *fibrinous pericarditis*, fibrin being deposited from inflammatory exudation onto the surface of the pericardium; fibrin is subsequently organised and may cause fibrous adhesions. In the myocardium, there are characteristic foci known as *Aschoff bodies*, small granulomas consisting of inconspicuous accumulations of macrophages, lymphocytes and some multinucleate cells (Aschoff giant cells) around eosinophilic hyaline material derived from collagen fibres (note the resemblance with other chronic inflammatory lesions, p. 59). There is little other sign of myocardial damage and the fact that acute rheumatic fever may end in fatal heart failure is a result of functional disturbance in the myocardium, though this aspect is not fully explained. The endocardium is also affected.

On the *heart valves*, the lesions are small *vegetations* consisting of platelet thrombi on which fibrin is subsequently deposited; they gradually become organised into fibrous tissue and it is this healing process which has the most important *long-term* effects, unlike the arthritic and other manifestations of rheumatic fever, which do not lead to permanent disability. Valvular damage worsens with the recurrences to which patients are particularly prone. Fibrosis leads to thickening, fusion of the margins and distortion of valve cusps, resulting eventually in *stenosis* (narrowing), usually of the mitral and aortic valves—rheumatic fever is the major cause of mitral stenosis. In addition, thickening and retraction of the cusps and shortening of chordae tendineae prevents valves from closing efficiently (*incompetence*). The consequences of valvular stenosis are seen in adults rather than children, as it takes years for development of enough fibrosis of the mitral and aortic valves to cause obstruction: a reduction of about 30% in the mitral or aortic orifices is required for the condition to be clinically significant. Chronic rheumatic heart disease leads to heart failure, thrombosis in the atrium due to fibrillation, angina pectoris, arrhythmias and infective endocarditis (p. 508). Interestingly, it is quite possible for rheumatic heart disease to develop from *subclinical* rather than acute rheumatic fever; evidently the disease can proceed for many years without overt manifestation until the valvular deficiencies finally become noticeable.

The processes underlying rheumatic fever are almost certainly to a large degree immunological, though several aspects remain unexplained. We have noted that it follows some 2–4 weeks after infection of the throat by *Strep. pyogenes* and that it does not occur if penicillin is administered promptly. Moreover, the organisms themselves are *not* present in the lesions in the heart, joints, or elsewhere, and if penicillin is given *after* recovery from the sore throat it does not arrest the development of rheumatic fever. The time lag is presumably required for the development of an immune response against streptococcal antigens. Patients with rheumatic fever develop unusually high levels of antibodies to streptococcal products, including streptolysin O (the ASO titre is used diagnostically), secreted enzymes and cell wall proteins. Arthritis probably results from deposition of *antigen-antibody complexes* in joints (p. 160). It is often held that the basic cause of myocardial and valvular damage is a direct action of antibodies made against streptococcal antigens but cross-reacting significantly with cardiac components. Such cross-reactions have been demonstrated between the group A carbohydrate and the structural glycoproteins on heart valves, and between an M-associated antigen and cardiac muscle. The cross-reacting antibodies are thus *autoantibodies*, and the mechanism of their formation has been suggested on p. 192. It is plausible that their binding to heart antigens could damage heart muscle cells, inducing functional disturbances, or initiate inflammation or thrombosis (this last perhaps by interaction between antibody on valves and platelet Fc receptors). Indeed, deposits of Ig and complement can be found in the heart and blood vessel walls in chronic rheumatic heart disease and are especially plentiful in fatal cases of acute disease. On the other hand, antibodies are not present in the Aschoff bodies, which rather resemble sites of cell-mediated hypersensitivity, with lymphocytes perhaps reacting against cardiac muscle (sarcolemmal) antigens and attracting macrophages to the site. A similar explanation may apply to the subcutaneous nodules which are larger than, but histologically similar to, Aschoff bodies in the heart.

However, these findings are not the whole explanation for cardiac damage in rheumatic fever. For example, pericarditis, the most obvious inflammation, is so far unexplained, as cross-reaction with pericardium has not been found; and the myocardium itself, supposedly a target of antibody attack, does not suffer much inflammatory damage (in fact the muscle fibres look normal after rheumatic heart failure.) Another unexplained fact is that rheumatic fever does not follow streptococcal skin infections which nevertheless stimulate antibody production leading to glomerulonephritis (p. 506). There may well be non-immunological contributing factors, such as the cardiotoxic properties of certain streptococcal products, notably streptolysin O and protease. An immune causation would be consistent with the common recurrence of rheumatic fever, through restimulation of the secondary antibody response, though the interval between reinfection and cardiac damage is not shortened (see below). Note that neither initiation nor recurrence of rheumatic fever is dependent on any particular serotype of *Strep. pyogenes* (cf. glomerulonephritis), so that the antigens involved must be shared by many streptococcal serotypes; however, here too there is an inconsistency with the immunological hypothesis, because rheumatic fever can also follow reinfection by strains which seem to lack the cross-reactive antigens. Also, there is no convincing evidence that second attacks of rheumatic fever occur more quickly after infection than first attacks; a more rapid, secondary response is the hallmark of an allergic disease.

In order to prevent recurrences, people who have suffered rheumatic fever are maintained continuously on penicillin as a prophylactic measure and it is often suggested that this be continued for life. (To date, *Strep. pyogenes* is one of the few bacteria which have not developed resistance to penicillin.) It is especially important to administer antibiotics during dental treatment in order to avoid the dangerous possibility of subacute bacterial endocarditis in individuals with damaged heart valves (p. 508).

Acute glomerulonephritis

This is another complication of *Strep. pyogenes* infection involving a hypersensitivity reaction, this time affecting the kidney. Thus there is a delay of 1–4 weeks after acute streptococcal disease before renal damage becomes apparent, the time taken to induce primary antibody formation. Unlike rheumatic fever, however, the initial infection can be either in the throat (pharyngitis) or the skin (impetigo), and in warm climates the latter is more likely to be the case. Moreover, only certain serotypes of *Strep. pyogenes* (so-called *nephrito-genic strains*), are associated with acute glomerulonephritis, most commonly type 12 in throat infections and type 49 in impetigo. As a result, second attacks are very rare because the antibody (anti-M) response also provides serotype-specific immunity (cf. rheumatic fever, where recurrences are common because the antigens involved are shared by many serotypes, while immunity is type-specific.) Post-streptococcal glomerulonephritis occurs particularly in children and young adults, the vast majority (85–95%) of whom recover completely after a week or two. The condition tends to persist for a longer time in adults and fewer make a complete recovery. The acute clinical features are those of oedema, due to proteinuria or water retention, dark urine containing blood, oliguria (less than 500ml of urine passed daily) and hypertension. Sometimes death occurs in the acute stage from the effects of hypertension (acute heart failure), while in others the disease may become progressive, culminating in death from hypertension and renal failure within two years.

As in the lesions of rheumatic fever, there is no evidence for streptococcal invasion of the kidney. Rather, the cause of renal damage is the deposition of antigen-antibody complexes in glomerular capillary walls in the diffuse, irregular, granular ('lumpy-bumpy') distribution typical of Type III hypersensitivity (p. 162). An autoimmune reaction against basement membrane as a result of cross-reaction with a streptococcal antigen has been suggested, along the lines of rheumatic fever, but the granular localisation of the complexes seems to rule this out (p. 139), moreover, early in the disease, streptococcal antigen has been demonstrated in the kidney lesion, indicating that this is an immune complex disease. The processes involved, with activation of complement, influx of neutrophils and release of tissue-damaging enzymes, have been described elsewhere (p. 162). Immunofluorescent staining for IgG and complement presents a picture of the glomerulus which is simliar to that in Figure 2.28b, and serum C3 levels are depressed as complement is deposited. The nature of the streptococcal antigen is unknown, but in all likelihood it is a type-specific component such as M protein or another protein. However, it is not known why only certain strains are nephritogenic, while other serotypes, and indeed other bacteria, are not.

Treatment of Streptococcus pyogenes infections

Strep. pyogenes is susceptible to several antimicrobials, penicillin being the agent of first choice. Penicillin-resistant strains have fortunately not appeared (cf. staphylococci), though resistance to sulphonamides and tetracyclines is common. Therapy with penicillin is continued for up to ten days in cases of acute pharyngitis in order to eliminate the organism entirely from the throat and reduce to a minimum the risk of non-suppurative complications. In people who have suffered rheumatic fever, the continuous prophylactic use of penicillin prevents recurrences. The organism frequently reappears when penicillin is discontinued. Vaccination is not practicable because of the large number of serotypes.

GROUP B β-HAEMOLYTIC STREPTOCOCCI

Although Group A organisms are the predominant pathogenic streptococci in man, those of other groups (B, C, D, G) are occasionally involved. Group B infections by the organisms known as *Strep. agalactiae* are of particular significance in the newborn and, together with *E. coli*, are now the commonest cause of invasive bacterial disease during the first 4–6 weeks of life (neonatal sepsis, neonatal meningitis). In the first few days after birth, Group B infection is seen as pneumonia and septicaemia (early onset disease), while in slightly older babies (over ten days) it causes meningitis (late onset disease). It appears that the early infection is acquired during birth, since *Strep. agalactiae* is present in the normal vaginal flora of about 25% of all women and is even more common in pregnancy. The later infection, on the other hand, is acquired after birth and the mother does not seem to be its source. Mortality in neonatal *Strep. agalactiae* infections is high, especially where maternal antibody is lacking, and accounts for about 1–2 deaths per 1000 neonates.

In the past, the bovine strain of *Strep. agalactiae* was an important cause of mastitis in cows, a disease which is a considerable problem in the dairy industry. Penicillin therapy has greatly reduced this cause of bovine mastitis, which is now more commonly due to *Staph. aureus* (p. 528) or *E. coli*.

DISEASES DUE TO α-HAEMOLYTIC STREPTOCOCCI

These organisms, known collectively as *viridans streptococci*, are generally commensals of very low pathogenicity which are universal inhabitants of the human upper respiratory tract and mouth. They are not groupable by Lancefield carbohydrate. Their low intrinsic virulence derives from an absence of antiphagocytic properties—they are non-capsulate, do not possess M protein and do not produce leucocidic toxins—and they therefore cause disease only in conditions where acute inflammation is minimised and they are not endangered by phagocytes. However, they are associated with one life-threatening infection, a serious disease of the heart known as *subacute bacterial endocarditis*, while in the mouth they are a major cause of tooth decay and periodontal disease.

This is an infection of the endocardium, the lining membrane of the heart, affecting in particular the heart valves. *Strep. viridans* species are often the causative organisms, but sometimes *Strep. faecalis*, *E. coli*, fungi and some other organisms of low intrinsic pathogenicity are responsible. The term 'chronic' would describe its course more accurately than 'subacute'. It occurs principally in individuals whose heart valves are congenitally deformed or have been damaged by rheumatic fever, or who have been treated surgically for these conditions; normal valves are rarely attacked. It used to be seen mostly in children and young adults with chronic rheumatic heart disease, but as acute rheumatic fever is now much less common, older age groups have become the most affected.

Endocarditis is often initiated by entry of *Strep. viridans* from the mouth into the bloodstream, which frequently follows dental treatment such as extraction, but may also be caused simply by vigorous chewing or brushing, especially in those with loose teeth. The streptococcal *bacteraemia* is transient and in normal persons quite harmless, organisms being removed by littoral macrophages in the liver, spleen and bone marrow. However, the organisms can be trapped at sites of existing endocardial damage, usually in a tiny fibrin clot. On the heart valves (mitral, aortic or both, in post-rheumatic cases), they become enmeshed in a thrombus composed of fibrin, platelets and red cells, to form *vegetations*. Within vegetations, bacterial colonies can grow protected from the bloodstream by the thrombus; the initial avascularity of the valves accounts for the poor acute inflammatory response and hence the survival of these otherwise vulnerable organisms. The vegetations are friable (crumble easily) and fragments are carried away in the bloodstream in the form of emboli, which impact in the brain, intestines, kidney or spleen, where infarction results (p. 649). Note that the emboli rarely cause foci of infection in these organs, possibly because once in the bloodstream the bacteria are exposed to neutrophils and high titres of circulating antibody. A characteristic complicaton is glomerulonephritis, with haematuria as a useful diagnostic symptom; this is probably due to immune complexes and may result in renal failure.

If untreated, endocarditis is invariably fatal, as a result either of heart failure or embolism, but antibiotic therapy has reduced mortality to about 20%. It is obviously important that individuals at risk (those with valvular anomalies) be given penicillin as a prophylactic measure before dental treatment and also before operations on the urinary tract, a source of bacteraemia by endocarditis-causing organisms such as *E. coli*. (*Strep. viridans* can be resistant to penicillin, so in patients with congenital or rheumatic heart disease on long-term penicillin, erythromycin is used in dental prophylaxis.)

Dental disease

Viridans streptococci such as *Strep. mutans* and *Strep. sanguis*, as

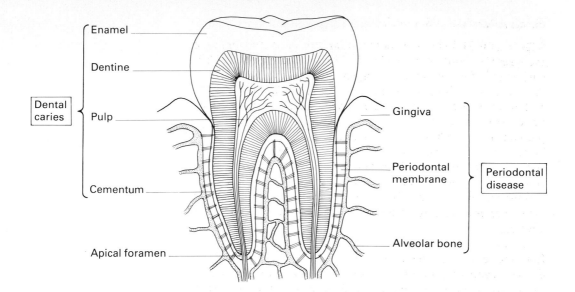

Figure 4.44 Cross-section of a molar, showing sites of dental disease caused by streptococci and other organisms.

well as the non-haemolytic *Strep. faecalis*, are among the oral bacteria responsible for dental caries and periodontal disease. As indicated in Figure 4.44, *caries* usually affects the enamel surface of the tooth, which is progressively destroyed until the dentine is exposed forming a cavity, with the accompanying pain of toothache. *Periodontal disease* refers to inflammation or degeneration of surrounding tissues, especially the gums (*gingivitis*) and ultimately the bone supporting the tooth (*periodontitis*). The initial, reversible phase of all these conditions is the accumulation of *dental plaque* on the surface of the teeth, a familiar soft whitish material consisting of polysaccharide (dextran), salivary glycoproteins and entrapped bacteria. *Strep. mutans*, one of the normal bacterial inhabitants of the mouth, produces an extracellular enzyme, dextransucrase, which converts sucrose into dextran and releases fructose (Figure 4.45). By adhering to the tooth, plaque brings the bacteria into intimate contact with the enamel surface; damage is then done by the local production of lactic acid, resulting from anaerobic respiration by the streptococci and other acidogenic microbes such as *Lactobacillus acidophilus*. Moreover, plaque prevents acid from diffusing away and also prevents its neutralisation by saliva.

Experimentally, it can be shown that intake of sucrose-rich food encourages caries and that germ-free animals remain caries-free until infected with acid-producing streptococci. Intake of sugary, sticky foods and sweets is certainly a very important contributor to tooth decay in man; the presence of sugar in the

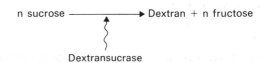

Figure 4.45 Action of dextransucrase.

mouth causes the pH at the dental surface to fall from 7 to 5 within a few minutes.

Caries can begin on the smooth surfaces of the sides of the teeth, but is particularly likely to occur where plaque can become immobilised for long periods, namely in the fissures of the biting surfaces of molars and premolars and in the areas between teeth. It may also start at the neck (exposed root) of the tooth in the cementum, especially where the gums have receded in the elderly. The enamel consists of crystals of calcium apatite (calcium phosphate and hydroxide) in an organic matrix, and is susceptible to gradual dissolution by lactic acid. The incorporation of fluoride (as fluorapatite) leads to acid resistance. Once the enamel has been penetrated, caries of the dentine is more rapidly destructive because of the latter's lower inorganic (mineral) content. Ultimately the pulp itself becomes acutely inflamed (*pulpitis*) and exudate accumulates in the pulp chamber; acute pulpitis is a particularly painful form of toothache.

The accumulation of plaque at the margins of the teeth and gums is the cause of chronic inflammation of the periodontal tissues. In *gingivitis*, the gums are inflamed and bleed easily; inflammation is a result both of damage by the action of bacterial products (toxins and enzymes) and of immune responses against them. In *periodontitis*, the gingiva gradually retract towards the root apex and lose their attachment to the teeth. Bacterial growth continues in the pockets between gum and tooth, and the supporting bone then begins to be destroyed, loosening the teeth. Acute infection, in the form of periodontal abscesses in the pockets, can be superimposed on this chronic process and leads to pain.

Among the measures which can be taken to avoid bacterial dental disease are careful removal of plaque from tooth surfaces by regular brushing and from areas between teeth with dental floss; avoidance of sweet sticky foods, especially as snacks between meals; incorporation of fluoride into the developing enamel via consumption of fluoridated water or fluoride tablets (about 1 mg fluoride per day is optimal); and application to formed teeth of fluoride compounds during cleaning of teeth or as a mouthrinse. The possibility of vaccination with *Strep. mutans* is being explored, and appears to be effective in non-human primates.

STREPTOCOCCUS PNEUMONIAE, THE PNEUMOCOCCUS

The pneumococci are pyogenic organisms closely related to streptococci, with which they are usually grouped, and the most appropriate generic name for the species is probably *Streptococcus pneumoniae* (the term *Diplococcus pneumoniae* has also been widely used, in reference to their characteristic growth as pairs of cocci). As the name suggests, pneumococci are associated with diseases of the lung and are the principal agents of lobar pneumonia; they also cause bronchopneumonia. Before the use of antibiotics, both diseases were major causes of death, and pneumococcal bronchopneumonia is still a common and serious illness, especially in the elderly, though nowadays it is much less often fatal. The organisms are resident in the throats of many healthy people where they act as an endogenous source of *secondary* (opportunistic) infection of the respiratory tract. In terms of mechanism, the pneumococci provide an example of organisms whose virulence is predominantly invasive in character, with minimal demonstrable toxigenicity. They have played a central role in the development of microbiology, both in understanding the relationship between bacterial structure and pathogenicity and, through the phenomenon of transformation, in ushering in the modern era of molecular genetics.

MORPHOLOGY, GROWTH, CLASSIFICATION

The pneumococci are Gram-positive cocci, about 1 μm in diameter, typically found as pairs of lancet-shaped cells joined by their broad ends, though they can also form short chains (hence streptococci). They are usually encapsulated and over 80 serological types are distinguishable on the basis of capsular antigens (below). They resemble viridans streptococci in their nasopharyngeal habitat and also form α-haemolytic colonies when grown aerobically on blood agar. (Under anaerobic conditions, colonies are surrounded by a zone of β-haemolysis, due to the oxygen-labile haemolysin, pneumolysin.) However, pneumococci can be differentiated by their capsule, their solubility in bile, ability to metabolise inulin, sensitivity to optochin and (in most cases) virulence for mice. Like other streptococci, they are facultative anaerobes which produce lactic acid even when growing in the air. On blood agar plates, encapsulated pneumococci grow as glistening *smooth* colonies, surrounded by a zone of partial haemolysis, while non-encapsulated variants form granular *rough* colonies; this is an important distinction as rough organisms are avirulent. During their growth in culture, pneumococci tend to *autolyse* and become Gram-negative; the centre of the colony collapses and stationary (post-log phase) cultures clarify. Autolysis is due to production of an enzyme (amidase), normally required during division, which destroys the cell wall by splitting the tetrapeptide from the muramic acid in peptidoglycan (p. 390). 'Bile solubility' occurs through activation of this enzyme by surface acting agents, including bile salts and sodium deoxycholate.

STRUCTURE

Capsule

The capsule is the most important structural feature of pneumococci, at least as far as pathogenicity is concerned, as it is wholly responsible for virulence and immunity. The capsule consists of *polysaccharide* which is both antigenic and chemically distinct from the hyaluronic acid of other streptococci (p. 401, Figure 4.9). The capsule forms a hydrophilic, acidic, antiphagocytic gel on the surface of the organism. Variation in the capsular polysaccharide as recognised by specific antisera has led to the identification of over 80 pneumococcal serotypes (i.e. it is the type-specific antigen). The reaction of type-specific antibody with its appropriate antigen leads to a characteristic reaction of capsular swelling, the *quellung reaction*, which is useful in *typing* and identification of pneumococci. In this reaction, the definition of the capsule is increased so that it can be seen more readily by light microscopy (Figure 4.46). Pneumococci can also be typed by agglutination. Through its antiphagocytic nature, the capsule enables the organism to survive *in vivo* and is essential to virulence (below). Capsular size varies with type; type 3 organisms, which are often associated with disease, have particularly large capsules.

Smooth and rough forms. Encapsulated pneumococci are known as smooth (S) because of the appearance of their colonies on agar, while variants which lack the capsule are rough (R) and grow as granular colonies. Loss of the ability to form a capsule is a result of mutation in an S organism, and R mutants can be selected by growing S organisms in the presence of antiserum to the capsular polysaccharide. Since they are unable to resist phagocytosis, R organisms are totally avirulent. Thus, if a mixture of R and S forms is injected into a mouse, only S organisms can be recovered from the dead animal, R cells having been phagocytosed and destroyed. For this reason, passage through mice is a conventional method of maintaining the virulence of cultured pneumococci, a necessary procedure since R mutants may outgrow S organisms during culture.

(a)

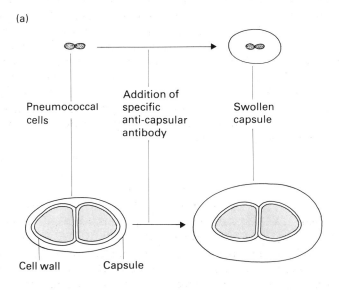

Cell wall   Capsule

(b)

Pneumococcal cells

Addition of specific anti-capsular antibody

Swollen capsule

Figure 4.46 Pneumococci and the quelling reaction of capsular swelling.
(a) By light microscopy, e.g. stained with methylene blue.
(b) From electron micrographs.

Cell wall carbohydrate

Pneumococci possess a species-specific carbohydrate designated *C polysaccharide* (C substance) which is analogous to, but structurally distinct from, the group-specific carbohydrate of haemolytic streptococci. It contains galactosamine-6-phosphate and phosphorylcholine, as well as minor sugar components. The *C-reactive protein* (CRP), which is present in the blood during the acute phase of many bacterial infections, including pneumonia and other inflammatory diseases, was discovered by its ability to precipitate pneumococcal C polysaccharide (see p. 42). CRP binds to the phosphorylcholine component of C polysaccharide.

Cell wall proteins

These include *M antigens* similar to those of Group A β-haemolytic streptococci and which are also type-specific. Anti-M sera only agglutinate R pneumococci, since in S organisms the antigens are hidden by the capsule. However, unlike pathogenic streptococci, pneumococci do not derive virulence properties from their M proteins, as the latter are not antiphagocytic in this species; nor are anti-M antibodies protective. *R antigens* are other proteins present in the wall, also apparently not involved in virulence.

EXTRACELLULAR PRODUCTS

Extracellular products of *Strep. pneumoniae* include the weak haemolytic toxin, *pneumolysin*, which is related both in structure and action to other oxygen-labile haemolysins such as streptolysin O, tetanolysin and *Clostridium perfringens* θ-toxin (p. 431). A toxic *neuraminidase* is also secreted, and another toxin which is released on autolysis produces dermal and internal haemorrhages when injected into rabbits. However, there is no evidence that any of these products are important in the pathogenesis of pneumococcal infections. On the other hand, soluble capsular polysaccharide material is shed by the organisms as they grow and, although non-toxic, it will bind to and block opsonising anticapsular antibodies and hence can inhibit phagocytosis.

CAPSULE AND PATHOGENICITY

The capsule is the vital pathogenic factor in pneumococcal infections, enabling invasion to occur by resistance to phagocytosis. Thus (i) only encapsulated (S) organisms are able to establish an infection in man or animals, while their non-encapsulated, but otherwise identical, R mutants are non-pathogenic; (ii) in some organisms, such as type 3 pneumococci, virulence can be related to capsular size, variants with smaller capsules being less virulent than the fully encapsulated parent form; and (iii) anticapsular antibodies, either actively stimulated by immunisation with purified capsular polysaccharide or injected passively, are protective. Neutrophils are able to phagocytose encapsulated pneumococci to a certain extent by surface phagocytosis (p. 17), and this occurs in the lung during lobar pneumonia, but they are much less effective where the organisms are suspended in exudate or mucus. Thus the excessive mucus secretion during viral infection of the upper respiratory tract and its aspiration into the lower respiratory tract is one factor encouraging pneumococcal lung disease. Phagocytosis readily occurs in the presence of *opsonising anticapsular antibodies*, and this causes the sudden disappearance of organisms from the lung at the 'crisis' of lobar pneumonia. The shedding of soluble capsular polysaccharide by growing organisms, noted above, helps them to avoid opsonisation, as the free antigenic polysaccharide blocks the incoming antibodies before they can bind to the organisms.

PNEUMOCOCCAL DISEASE

Pneumonia is an acute inflammation of the lung characterised by the presence of purulent exudate in the alveolar spaces leading to consolidation (firmness caused by the presence of exudate extending the alveoli). In *lobar pneumonia*, the exudate spreads rapidly through the alveoli to involve an entire lobe, which becomes consolidated, while in *bronchopneumonia* only the alveoli contiguous with the terminal and respiratory bronchioles are affected and there are numerous discrete foci of acute inflammation and consolidation around the terminal bronchioles. Pneumococci produce both lobar pneumonia and bronchopneumonia, while in the upper respiratory tract they are a cause of sinusitis and otitis media in children and may spread from the latter to the subarachnoid space to cause meningitis. However, although pathogenic, they are present asymptomatically in the nasopharynx of as many as 50% of healthy persons at any one time, and can be found in oral and nasal secretions. Healthy carriers are the principal source of spread of the organisms, but patients with, or convalescent from, pneumonia are also a source of infection. Pneumococci are relatively resistant to drying and can be transmitted as air-borne infections on dust derived from dried secretions, as well as in moist droplets; they are also acquired by contact with contaminated articles. Pneumococcal disease is characterised by an acute inflammatory response, often suppurative in the lung in bronchopneumonia, paranasal sinuses (sinusitis), middle ear (otitis media) and meninges (meningitis). Pneumococcal meningitis can be a particularly rapid killer.

Not all the 80-odd different pneumococcal types are equally virulent in man. *Type 3* has the highest fatality rate and is generally well represented among the types causing lobar pneumonia; together, types 1, 2 and 3 are responsible for 70% of all cases, other virulent serotypes being 4, 5, 7, 8, 12 and 14, the last particularly common in children. These virulent pneumococci are often acquired *exogenously* from active cases or convalescent patients and can give rise directly to primary lobar pneumonia in hitherto healthy persons, mostly between the ages of 30 and 50 but seen in all groups (except infants below one year). The less virulent (low grade) types are usually an *endogenous* source of disease, i.e. the organisms have been carried as commensals in the throat for some time and only become pathogenic as secondary (opportunistic) invaders after primary viral respiratory diseases such as influenza and the common cold. They lead to bronchopneumonia, especially in individuals with low resistance, usually the very young and the elderly: 70% of deaths due to bronchopneumonia occur in the over-65 age group and 10% in young children. Additional factors which predispose to bronchopneumonia are alcoholism, malnutrition and exposure to cold, all of which further reduce resistance. That the last of these is particularly important is shown by the prevalence of bronchopneumonia among infants and old people at the coldest times of winter; atmospheric pollution in the form of fog is an additional hazard at that time of year. However, a hard and fast distinction between the origins of lobar and bronchopneumonia is not always possible. Thus, lobar pneumonia is encountered in vagrants and alcoholics exposed to cold, and it is often difficult to be sure that an infection which appears to be primary is not the consequence of an unrecognised initiating cause. Also, bronchopneumonia is more frequently due to exogenous infection by organisms other than pneumococci, such as *Staph. aureus, Strep. pyogenes* and *Klebsiella pneumoniae.*

Lobar pneumonia

Since the introduction of antibiotics, the full course of lobar pneumonia has become a clinical rarity in developed countries, but is still common in those parts of the world where the standard of medical care is poor. The process begins with inhalation of virulent pneumococci into lung, or aspiration of thin mucus containing pneumococci during an upper respiratory tract viral infection such as the common cold. The disease progresses in four stages, though all parts of the lobe may not be at the same stage at the same time (Figure 4.47). It presents a classic picture of an acute inflammatory response followed by resolution.

The multiplication of pneumococci in the lung initiates the first stage (duration 1–2 days) in which alveolar capillaries are dilated and engorged with red cells, capillary walls are lined with marginating neutrophils and protein-rich exudate pours into the alveoli. The speed with which this occurs suggests IgE-mediated hypersensitivity, as it is difficult to explain by toxic action of the organisms themselves. Pneumococci are plentiful and multiply freely. The exudate spreads very rapidly to adjacent alveoli through the interconnecting pores of Kohn and alveolar ducts, and soon fills the entire lobe, which becomes heavy, dark red and firm, and sharply demarcated from the neighbouring lobe(s). Organisms are present in the blood during the early stages (bacteraemia) and this can lead to extrapulmonary complications such as suppurative meningitis or infective endocarditis.

The second stage (2nd–4th day of illness) is called *red hepatisation* because the lobe is red, solid and feels like liver. The

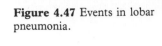

Figure 4.47 Events in lobar pneumonia.

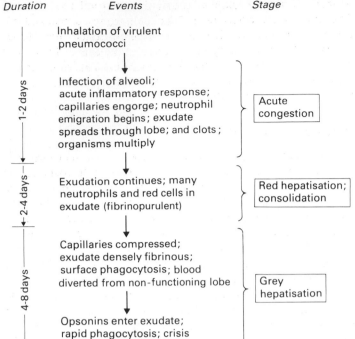

exudate now contains a fine network of fibrin, large numbers of neutrophils which have emigrated from the capillaries by diapedesis, and many extravasated red cells. The lobe, which is airless, is firm, heavy and swollen and described as *consolidated*.

The third stage (4th–8th day) is *grey hepatisation* in which the blood flow is reduced and the exudate is clearly fibrinous, the fibrin forming a dense ('inspissated') network at the surface of which phagocytosis of bacteria by neutrophils can take place. Capillaries are compressed by the distended alveoli and the alveolar space is packed with neutrophils, many of which are dead and disintegrating (pus). During this stage, anticapsular antibodies enter the exudate in sufficient quantity to assist the process of phagocytosis by opsonisation; destruction of pneumococci is now rapid and the fever, which at the onset of disease has risen rapidly, now falls precipitately (*crisis*). Those who die of lobar pneumonia usually do so at this stage, with incipient abscess formation.

The final stage is one of *resolution* in which macrophages replace neutrophils in the alveoli, engulf any remaining pneumococci and take up the cellular debris of the exudate. Fibrin is dissolved by fibrinolysin, and the liquefied exudate drained off via the lymphatics and alveolar capillaries. It takes from one to three weeks for the lobe to return to normal, and it is common for some residual fibrin to be converted into fibrous pleural adhesions, which are of little consequence. In a small proportion of cases (less than 5%), resolution fails to occur and the alveoli become organised by the laying down of fibrous tissue; a fibrosed zone is leathery and non-functional.

Acute bronchopneumonia

Here the causative pneumococci are the less virulent serotypes which have established a commensal existence in the nasopharynx and only invade the lower respiratory tract as opportunistic pathogens secondarily to predisposing conditions in the host. Thus the infection is endogenous in origin and occurs in a state of lowered host resistance. As noted above, it is most often seen in infants or in the elderly, and in the latter may be a terminal event in cancer, stroke and uraemia. Acute respiratory infection such as influenza, measles and whooping cough, or chronic conditions such as chronic bronchitis and cystic fibrosis, all predispose to bronchopneumonia, as do chilling, excess alcohol, morphine and volatile anaesthetics. All these conditions, by damaging the epithelium or affecting the secretion of mucus, interfere with the primary defence mechanism of the lower respiratory tract, namely the mucus blanket which traps inhaled organisms and is carried to the pharynx to be swallowed or expectorated. Alcohol, morphine and anaesthetics also depress the cough reflex which may encourage the inhalation of organisms in the upper respiratory tract, proliferation of which, together with excessive mucus secretion, is often a complication of the common cold. Finally, pulmonary oedema fluid provides an excellent culture medium for pneumococci (and other organisms) and an oedematous lung is much more susceptible than a dry one; hence conditions such as cardiac failure or pulmonary stasis during prolonged bed rest also encourage development of bronchopneumonia.

In contrast with lobar pneumonia, the pneumococci in bronchopneumonia establish discrete foci of infection around terminal bronchioles in several lobes. They do not cause a rapid outpouring of exudate; instead, each small infected area, of about 1 cm diameter, shows consolidation and microscopically consists of inflamed bronchioles full of pus and adjoining alveoli which contain fibrinous exudate and large numbers of neutrophils. If the organisms can be removed by phagocytosis at this stage, recovery is more gradual than in lobar pneumonia and fever subsides in step-like fashion ('lysis') rather than by crisis. On the other hand, inflammation may continue, so that focal areas enlarge and coalesce, and in time large areas of the lobe may be involved. Bronchopneumonia is often prolonged and resolution inadequate and *repair* converts fibrin into fibrous tissue. Thus *chronic inflammation* supervenes in which lung tissue is progressively destroyed and fibrosed. The destruction of the muscular and elastic tissue of bronchi and replacement by fibrous tissue leads to bronchial dilatation, due to stretching of this tissue;

this is a condition known as *bronchiectasis*, which in turn predisposes to further attacks of infection including bronchopneumonia.

Vaccination

The capsular polysaccharides of pneumococci are immunogenic and are safe, effective vaccines. Because immunity is *type-specific*, it is necessary to make a mixture of the polysaccharides of virulent strains occurring most frequently in the locality (about ten in practice) to ensure wide cover. Although they are not in general use at present in the UK, such multiple vaccines could potentially be of value in protecting the elderly and the susceptible young from the risk of pneumococcal pneumonia and bacteraemia; they are used for this purpose in the USA.

STAPHYLOCOCCUS

The staphylococci include two species which commonly infect man and domestic animals. The major pathogenic species is *Staphylococcus aureus* (*Staph. pyogenes*), while *Staph. epidermidis* (*Staph. albus*) is a very widespread, non-pathogenic commensal. They are Gram-positive cocci and *Staph. aureus* is characteristically *pyogenic*. Their natural habitat in man is principally the skin and nose, and most familiar manifestations of *Staph. aureus* infection are minor skin abscesses (pustules, boils) arising in infected hair follicles or sebaceous glands. However, it is also the cause of a variety of more serious suppurative conditions, in many of which it is an *opportunistic pathogen*; in this role it causes infection where natural tissue barriers have been breached or where host resistance is either underdeveloped, suppressed by therapeutic agents or compromised by chronic debilitating disease. In such circumstances, *Staph. aureus* gives rise to wound infections, puerperal sepsis, bronchopneumonia, osteomyelitis, meningitis and endocarditis; not surprisingly it is a common pathogen in hospital-acquired infection. *Staph. aureus* often enters the bloodstream and staphylococcal septicaemia can be fatal. In pyogenic infections, the organism is primarily *invasive* and possesses a variety of mechanisms for avoiding or surviving phagocytosis. However, there are also important *toxins* and two diseases in which toxigenicity is the major factor are staphylococcal food poisoning and a skin condition with the exotic name of staphylococcal scalded skin syndrome.

MORPHOLOGY, GROWTH, ETC.

The characteristic microscopic appearance of staphylococci is as grape-like clusters of cells (Gk. *staphule*, bunch of grapes); when chains appear they are rarely more than four cells long (Fig. 4.2c). Agar colonies of most *Staph. aureus* strains are golden-yellow in colour due to carotenoid pigments (Lat. *aureus*, golden), though there is wide variation from white or cream to orange; *Staph. epidermidis*, on the other hand, usually forms white colonies (hence the alternative name of *Staph. albus*). Both species are facultative anaerobes; unlike streptococci, their growth is not retarded by oxygen because they produce *catalase*, the enzyme which destroys H_2O_2. During its growth, *Staph. aureus* releases a variety of soluble products (toxins, enzymes) which are not found in the non-pathogenic species. The one which is most consistently associated with virulence is *coagulase*, an enzyme which causes clotting of plasma: coagulase-positive staphylococci are, by definition, *Staph. aureus*. Coagulase is detected by adding a loopful of a colony from an agar plate or a drop of a young broth culture to 0.5 ml citrated rabbit plasma and incubating at 37°C; clotting occurs within a few minutes. *Staph. aureus* also has the ability to grow in a high salt concentration, e.g. in broth containing 10% NaCl, which inhibits the growth of most other organisms, and this is useful in selectively detecting its presence in faeces or food.

Among the non-spore-forming bacteria, staphylococci are some of the most resistant to adverse environmental conditions. They can survive in dry conditions for many weeks (e.g. in dried crusts of pus) and some strains resist heating to 60°C for 30 minutes. However, they do not generally grow outside the body, except sometimes in meat, milk and dirty water. *Staph. aureus* may resist disinfectants such as phenol and mercuric chloride, resistance to the latter being due to a plasmid-borne R gene (p. 464), it can be killed by basic dyes such as gentian violet.

CLASSIFICATION

As with other pyogenic cocci, *Staph. aureus* is a species which can be further divided into a large number of *types*. However, although serological methods can be used (i.e. typing via specific cell surface antigens using agglutination with appropriate antisera) they present technical problems and a more widely used method is *phage typing*, which depends on susceptibility to specific bacteriophages rather than on cell surface variation (Figure 4.48). A panel of 20–24 (numbered) phages is used in typing, the phages being divided into four groups according to their host range (Fig. 4.48a); each group contains a combination of phages which differ serologically and morphologically. A strain of *Staph. aureus* is typed by testing each phage for ability to lyse the organism in question. In practice this is a simple procedure in which a drop of a suspension of each phage is placed on a separate area of a lawn of the organism on an agar plate; circumscribed zones of lysis become visible after a few hours incubation (Fig. 4.48b). The organism can thereby be assigned to one of the phage groups and the combination of phages which lyse that strain becomes its individual designation. Thus a strain in phage group III might be identified as 47/53/75/77, indicating that it can be lysed by those four particular phages of that group.

The reason for the type-specific patterns of lysis is not an absence of phage receptor in the bacterial wall, but is due to the immunity to lysis associated with lysogeny (p. 448). Virtually all strains of *Stap. aureus* are lysogenic, i.e. carry phage DNA in non-

Group	Phage number						
I	29	52	52A	79	80		
II	3A	3C	55	71			
III	6	42E	47	53	54	75	77
	83A	84	85				
IV	42D						
Unassigned	81	94	95	96			

(a)

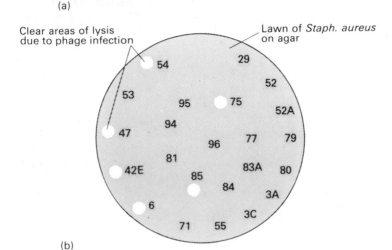

(b)

Figure 4.48 Phage typing of a strain of *Staphylococcus aureus*.
(a) Lytic groups of staphylococcal typing phages.
(b) Appearance of a phage-typing plate.

replicating form as a prophage incorporated into chromosomal DNA or as a plasmid; the presence of a prophage in the organism causes it to resist lysis on external infection by that phage.

Staphylococcus aureus

STRUCTURE, PRODUCTS AND PATHOGENICITY

As with other pyogenic cocci, local invasiveness is the principal feature of the pathogenicity of *Staph. aureus* leading to suppuration. Several contributing factors enable it to avoid or survive phagocytosis but, unlike streptococci or pneumococci, it is not possible to pinpoint a specific attribute as being of overwhelming importance. *Staph. aureus* strains do not generally possess structural antiphagocytic components akin to the capsule and M protein of *Strep. pyogenes*, for example. Rather, their invasiveness depends on a combination of properties which include (i) an ability, ascribed to the cell wall, to resist intra-cellular killing after uptake by neutrophils and macrophages; (ii) production of toxins with a lethal effect on phagocytes; and (iii) release of enzymes including coagulase, which forms a fibrin barrier against neutrophils, and others which may assist in the organisms' spread. There is a variety of staphylococcal toxins, some of which promote extracellular survival in localised lesions, while others have a more decisive role in disease. Thus staphylo-coccal food poisoning is wholly due to ingestion of *enterotoxins* preformed in food, the dermatological lesions of the scalded skin syndrome are due to a toxin called *exfoliatin*, and the fatal outcome of septicaemia is ascribed to α-toxin. The virulence factors of *Staph. aureus* are summarised in Table 4.8 and detailed below.

Structural surface components

Capsule. Only rare strains of *Staph. aureus* possess an antiphagocytic carbohydrate capsule, but when present the capsule does increase virulence. Two of those analysed consist of hexosaminouronic acid.

Protein A is found on the surface of the cell wall of *Staph. aureus* and is specific for the species. It has a remarkable ability to bind the Fc region of immunoglobulins (mainly IgG) of practically all mammalian species. Protein A binds (and precipitates) IgG, a property utilised in immunological laboratories to remove antibody or antigen–antibody complexes from solution. The free molecule inhibits opsonisation by competing with neutrophil Fc receptors for the Fc portion of opsonising IgG antibody (and cell bound protein A probably behaves similarly). Thus protein A released from the organism's surface could be an important factor in helping *Staph. aureus* to frustrate the action of phagocytes in acute inflammatory exudate. After reacting with IgG, protein A activates complement.

Table 4.8 Virulence factors of *Staphylococcus aureus*.

Virulence factor	Possible role
(a) *Structural*	
Capsule (rare strains only)	Antiphagocytic
Cell wall (component unknown)	Resists destruction in neutrophils
Protein A (also released)	Inhibits opsonisation by binding Fc of IgG; activates complement
(b) *Soluble*	
(i) *Toxins*	
Leucocidin	Kills neutrophils and macrophages
α-Haemolysin (α-toxin)	Leucocidic; responsible for death in septicaemia (smooth muscle spasm)
δ-Haemolysin (δ-toxin)	Leucocidic; synergistic interaction with α-toxin
Enterotoxin	Responsible for food poisoning
Exfoliation	Responsible for scalded skin syndrome
(ii) *Enzymes*	
Coagulase	Forms fibrin barrier which impedes approach of neutrophils and phagocytosis
Staphylokinase	Dissolves fibrin by activating plasmin; may assist spread
Hyaluronidase	May assist spread by breaking down connective tissue
Lipase	Promotes development of boils in hair follicles and sebaceous glands

Bound coagulase (clumping factor). *Staph. aureus* cells are rapidly clumped in the presence of a trace of plasma, due to the action of surface-bound coagulase (the enzyme also released in free form, below). The clumping reaction may be due to cross-linking by fibrinogen rather than production of fibrin.

Species-specific carbohydrate antigens of the staphylococcal wall are teichoic acids. In addition, there are several type-specific antigens detectable by agglutination tests with antisera, but the chemical nature of most is undefined.

We have noted above that virulent staphylococci are resistant to intracellular killing by phagocytes; they may survive within phagocytic vacuoles for long periods. It is not known which wall component (peptidoglycan, carbohydrate, protein or other) confers the ability to resist the enzymes and oxidative mechanisms of neutrophils and macrophages. However, killing proceeds quite efficiently once the organisms have been coated by antibody and complement, though there may still be some survivors.

Enzymes

Coagulase causes plasma to clot by activating a protein called coagulase-reacting factor, which is probably prothrombin itself; thus thrombin is formed and converts fibrinogen to fibrin (p. 632). Clotting of exudate is thought to aid survival either by walling off lesions, thereby preventing the approach of neutrophils, or by coating the organisms themselves in fibrin to reduce phagocytosis (though ultimately this does not seem to prevent engulfment). In view of this seemingly modest role, it is perhaps surprising that production of coagulase corresponds so closely with pathogenicity; indeed, as already noted, it is the 'marker' property for the species and by definition is never present in *Staph. epidermidis*.

Staphylokinase. In view of the above, it is paradoxical that *Staph. aureus* produces an enzyme which leads to dissolution of fibrin, via activation of plasminogen (cf. streptokinase, p. 500). A role in spreading is possible (but see below).

Hyaluronidase is produced by *Staph. aureus* strains and, as with the streptococcal enzyme, may serve as a 'spreading factor'. However, this is not likely to be of great importance as staphylococcal lesions are typically localised and in general show less tendency then streptococcal infection to spread through a tissue; moreover, strains lacking hyaluronidase (or staphylokinase, for that matter) show no diminution of virulence in experimental infections.

Lipases and esterases are useful to staphylococci growing on the skin, enabling them to metabolise sebaceous secretions; the common staphylococcal skin lesion is an abscess arising in a hair follicle or sebaceous gland.

Staph. aureus strains can produce a range of toxins, including four haemolysins, a specific leucocidin, enterotoxins and the epidermolytic agent exfoliatin. Individual strains produce one or more haemolysins, which are responsible for the zone of complete lysis surrounding *Staph. aureus* colonies on agar containing blood of an appropriate species. (At 37°C, lysis on rabbit blood agar is due to α or δ haemolysins for reasons explained below.) Although easily demonstrated as haemolysins *in vitro*, during an infection these toxins probably damage other cells.

α-Haemolysin (*α-toxin*) is the major haemolytic toxin of human strains of *Staph. aureus* (see also p. 432). Rabbit red cells are the most sensitive to lysis and human red cells are not affected. It was first isolated in 1929, following a notorious tragedy in Bundaberg, Australia, when 16 out of 21 children inoculated with the contents of a vial of diphtheria toxin-antitoxin mixture (then used in immunisation) became acutely ill and 12 died of staphylococcal septicaemia and toxaemia. The vial was subsequently shown to be contaminated by *Staph. aureus*. The α-toxin seems to be responsible for death in such cases. While it acts as a haemolysin and leucocidin, lethality is due to pharmacological effects on vascular smooth muscle, in which it induces spasm. In localised infections, its main role is probably that of a leucocidin. Its mode of action on cell membranes is controversial, but may involve enzymatic activity on membrane proteins, leading to lysis.

β-Haemolysin (*β-toxin*) causes lysis of red cells through its enzymatic action as a *sphingomyelinase C* (p. 430). Being a 'hot-cold' haemolysin, it is only revealed by incubating blood-toxin mixtures or blood agar plates carrying *Staph. aureus* cultures, first at 37°C, then overnight in the refrigerator. It occurs mainly in strains of animal rather than human origin and is toxic in large doses.

γ-Haemolysin (*γ-toxin*) is also lytic, principally for rabbit red cells. It consists of two separate proteins, neither of which is toxic in its own right, but which in combination have lytic activity, a phenomenon described as *synergy*. The details of its action on the red cell membrane are unknown, but it is inhibited by sulphated polymers such as agar and so does not contribute to lysis on blood agar plates. A leucocyte-damaging action has been claimed.

δ-Haemolysin (*δ-toxin*) is produced by most human strains of *Staph. aureus* and acts on the red cells of several species, as well as on leucocytes and other cells. Its action on membranes resembles that of surfactants, such as detergents, which accounts for its wide range. Perhaps its main significance as a factor in pathogenicity derives from its synergistic interaction with α-toxin; thus low concentrations of α- and δ-toxins, each well below the lytic threshold, will cause lysis if mixed together, providing mutual enhancement of their membrane-damaging effects. Another feature which may be relevant in the course of disease is that, like streptolysin S, it is a small molecule (5000 mol.wt peptide) and therefore a very weak antigen, and this may partly explain the apparent ineffectiveness of immunity to *Staph. aureus* and *Staph. aureus* vaccines.

Panton–Valentine (PV) leucocidin is specifically toxic to phagocytes and is non-haemolytic. As described earlier (p. 432), the toxin causes discharge of lysosomal contents into the medium and activation of membrane enzymes (protein kinases, adenylate and guanylate cyclases) with cell death following, perhaps as a result of raised intracellular cyclic AMP. These effects are due to the action of the toxin on the plasma membrane, causing an influx of Ca^{2+} ions into the cell; in calcium-free medium, degranulation does not occur. Raised intracellular Ca^{2+} activates membrane enzymes via calmodulin, the calcium-activated regulator protein (Figure 4.26).

Enterotoxins. Staph. aureus is a major cause of food poisoning due to the production of enterotoxins, of which six antigenically distinct types have been recognised (A, B, C_1, C_2, D, E). About half the strains of *Staph. aureus* can produce an enterotoxin. Like botulism, staphylococcal food poisoning is an *intoxication* which follows ingestion of toxin formed by the organisms in contaminated food; it is not necessary for intestinal infection to occur. The enterotoxins are remarkably heat-resistant proteins, which can withstand boiling for 30 minutes and can therefore persist in *cooked* food even though the organisms themselves have been killed. Within a few hours of ingestion, vomiting and diarrhoea occur, but the mechanimsm is apparently different from that of the enterotoxins of Gram-negative bacteria such as *V. cholerae* and *E. coli*. Thus, staphylococcal enterotoxin will induce vomiting if injected intravenously in monkeys, by acting as a neurotoxin directly on the vomiting centre of the brain. After ingestion, stimulation of the vomiting centre can occur via the vagus nerve which innervates abdominal viscera. The basis of the diarrhoea is not clear, in particular whether or not there is an intracellular effect on adenylate cyclase. Enterotoxin B is involved in staphylococcal *enterocolitis*, a rare and often fatal infection complicating abdominal surgery.

Exfoliatin, or epidermolytic toxin, is the agent of a group of exfoliative skin diseases known collectively as the *staphylococcal scalded skin syndrome* from the characteristic peeling of large areas of epidermis which leaves the skin looking as if it had been scalded (see p. 525). The syndrome principally affects newborn babies and is caused by staphylococci of phage group II; however, the organisms are often not found in the skin lesions themselves, but at distant sites, indicating involvement of a toxin. It has been shown that a soluble product of group II *Staph. aureus* will produce a very similar condition in newborn mice and that the experimental disease is prevented by specific antitoxin. The toxic product is now known as exfoliatin and it is produced by about

5% of all *Staph. aureus* organisms isolated from humans. The toxin exists in two forms, one coded chromosomally, the other plasmid-coded. Its action leads to physical detachment of the outermost layer of the skin as a result of destruction of the intercellular connections (desmosomes) between cells of the stratum granulosum.

DISEASES DUE TO *STAPHYLOCOCCUS AUREUS*

Like other pyogenic cocci, *Staph. aureus* is often carried by healthy individuals, predominantly in the nose and on certain moist areas of the skin: some 30–50% of normal adults carry the organism in the anterior nares (nostrils) and 10–20% have *Staph. aureus* on perineal skin. In fact, the organisms colonise the nose, skin and umbilicus of newborn babies within the first few days of life, by infection from the mother, nurse or environment. The strains carried by healthy people are virulent and commonly give rise to minor, superficial disease. More serious, deep-seated staphylococcal diseases are rare in comparison, but *Staph. aureus* has the tendency to invade as an *opportunistic pathogen* wherever the resistance of a tissue or host is compromised, and hence is the cause of a wide variety of different conditions. Their common feature is *suppuration* and the typical lesion is the *abscess*, the development of which has been described in Section 1. Abscess formation will not be further discussed here except to say that microscopically the pus contains neutrophils and staphylococci, the latter often within the phagocytes but resisting destruction. Compared with β-haemolytic streptococci, *Staph. aureus* produces a more rapid development of suppuration and its lesions are more localised, with less tendency to spread, perhaps due to the action of coagulase. Staphylococci often invade the bloodstream from a local focus of infection such as in the skin; *bacteraemia* can lead to suppurative infection of bone (osteomyelitis) or lungs, from where further bacteraemia causes abscesses in the liver, kidneys, brain, etc. *Pyaemia* occurs when staphylococci are carried on infected emboli (p. 490). *Septicaemia* itself (with toxaemia) is a further, potentially fatal complication.

Skin infections

These often take the form of small abscesses (pustules) or inflammatory nodules developing in hair follicles (folliculitis). *Boils* (furuncles) are acute tender nodules on various areas of the skin (neck, face, buttocks, breasts, fingers, etc.) which are larger and have a central necrotic core which discharges purulent exudate. A cluster of boils, with deep suppuration, is called a *carbuncle*; they are often found on the nape of the neck, are slow to heal and form a large scar. Carbuncles are more common where there is underlying predisposing disease such as diabetes mellitus.

The *scalded skin syndrome* has been noted above as being due to infection by toxigenic strains producing exfoliatin. Its generalised exfoliative form occurs in newborns, sometimes as epidemics in nurseries. It starts as a localised crusted lesion around the mouth, but within 48 hours large areas of the skin become displaced and wrinkle and peel off at the slightest pressure (desquamation), leaving the baby with a moist, red, glistening surface as if burned. The disease progresses rapidly and may be fatal, but because only the most superficial layers of the epidermis are affected, massive fluid loss does not occur and secondary infection of the exposed area is avoided, so that recovery is usual. (*Bullous impetigo* is a more localised form of exfoliation, with fluid-filled bullae (large blisters) in the nappy area, around the mouth and on the trunk.) Scalded skin syndrome occurs sporadically in older children and adults and is known as *toxic epidermal necrosis* (TEN), but this is more often due to hypersensitivity to a drug than to *Staph. aureus* infection. The occurrence of staphylococcal skin disease in neonates is one form of opportunistic pathogenicity, the newborn being particularly susceptible as a result of its immunological immaturity and the relative slowness with which it responds to primary infections. Maternally acquired antibodies are of course present and act as opsonins, but evidently do not always provide sufficient protection. Other staphylococcal infections of babies are noted below.

Wounds and burns

These often become infected by *Staph. aureus*, an example of opportunistic infection following penetration or removal of a natural defensive barrier, viz. the skin. Both accidental and surgical wounds can be affected, the latter usually through infection acquired in the operating theatre itself or subsequently on the ward. Contamination of a suture by only a small number of staphylococci (less than 100 cells) is capable of leading to a *stitch abscess*, and staphylococci associated with such a 'foreign body' are much more likely to cause a suppurative lesion than the same number of organisms inoculated into the skin. Epidemics of such suture-line abscesses have been caused by *Staph. aureus* strains resistant to mercury-based antiseptics used to sterilise sutures (p. 464). The effects of infection by *Staph. aureus* on a wound or burn range from a delay in healing to bacteraemic spread and possibly fatal septicaemia, the latter being a common cause of death in severely burned patients. A problem with staphylococcal wound infections acquired in hospitals is the multiple resistance of the infecting strains to antibiotics (p. 467).

Osteomyelitis

Spread of staphylococci in the bloodstream from a local lesion can cause infection of the bone marrow (osteomyelitis) and of different sites in the bone itself (osteitis, periosteitis). Osteomyelitis of this type occurs paricularly in childhood, the inital infection being in the skin or middle ear. There is also a risk (at all ages) of bacterial contamination of a compound fracture or of direct spread of an infection to bone from an adjacent tissue (e.g. from an apical tooth abscess to the jaw); however, haematogenous spread is the commonest route. Unless treated promptly, staphylococcal bone infection leads to extensive suppuration in the marrow and then extension through the metaphysis to form subperiosteal abscesses; these may spread along much of the shaft of the bone or burst through the periosteum, infecting adjacent muscular tissues. Thrombosis in bone marrow sinusoids is initiated by the production of coagulase by the organisms, which causes clotting in the vessels. The thrombi are then softened by enzymes present during suppuration and small fragments, infected with *Staph. aureus*, are carried away in the bloodstream as emboli. This condition is *pyaemia* (lit. pus in the blood) and trapping of infected emboli in the lungs, kidneys and myocardium leads to multiple abscesses in these tissues. Thrombosis also leads to bone necrosis and in extreme cases a large part of the diaphysis (shaft) may die and become separated from the living bone as a 'sequestrum'. A new tube of bone, known as an involucrum, then forms around the dead bone from the periosteum; but pus may continue to be produced inside the involucrum and drain to the surface through small openings in it, eventually discharging at the skin as a sinus.

If acute osteomyelitis fails to heal completely, the disease may become chronic, with repeated appearance of abscesses over a long period. However, the advanced stages of staphylococcal osteomyelitis and its complications are rarely seen today in developed countries, due to the use of antimicrobial therapy, but they are still common in tropical countries where treatment in likely to be delayed.

Bronchopneumonia

Staphylococcal pneumonia is another example of opportunistic infection, usually being a secondary complication of an acute viral respiratory disease such as influenza, or chronic respiratory illness such as cystic fibrosis (p. 829). Influenza, measles and whooping cough all predispose to opportunistic invasion of the lung by *Staph. aureus* for reasons discussed in connection with pneumococci. Both in young children and adults, the pneumonia may be acute and rapidly lethal. Alternatively, in older children and adults, areas of consolidation form which develop into pulmonary abscesses; these may rupture into the pleural cavity where the presence of purulent exudate is known as *empyema*. Another predisposing cause of staphylococcal pneumonia is inadequate host immune defence, either as a result of the use of immunosuppressive drugs in transplantation or of cytotoxic agents in cancer therapy, or due to primary immunodeficiency diseases affecting antibody production (hypogammaglobulinaemia, agammaglobulinaemia, etc.). These will be recognised as general causes of opportunistic infection (p. 482, Table 4.6).

Food poisoning

As already mentioned (p. 524) many strains of *Staph. aureus* produce enterotoxins and the introduction of toxigenic organisms into food is a common source of food poisoning. Food handlers, who may be healthy carriers or have staphylococcal skin lesions, may contaminate food such as meats and meat products, pastries, custards and salad dressings, all of which are common vehicles for staphylococci. The effects of staphylococcal food poisoning are due to enterotoxins released in the food and begin within 1–6 hours of ingestion as vomiting, nausea, cramps and diarrhoea. They are short-lived, however, and recovery within 24 hours is usual.

Bovine mastitis

Bovine mastitis, inflammation of the udder, is a serious economic problem in the dairy industry: the combined annual loss through reduction in milk yield, discarding of antibiotic-contaminated milk, veterinary fees and loss of animals through culling is estimated at £100 million in the UK alone. *Staph. aureus* and *E. coli* are the major causes today (see also *Strep. agalactiae*, p. 507). Acute mastitis during the first few weeks of lactation is particularly critical as it can prevent attainment of peak milk yield or prevent milk production altogether in the infected quarter; it may necessitate culling the animal as it becomes unprofitable to keep it. Defence against bacterial infection in the mammary gland relies, as elsewhere, on phagocytosis by neutrophils brought to the site of infection by an acute inflammatory response. Often this ensures that disease is mild or the infection subclinical. During acute mastitis itself, especially in mid or late lactation, the response is quite obvious, with a swollen udder and discoloured milk, but with the rapid destruction of bacteria the udder soon returns to normal. One problem during early lactation is that the inflammatory resonse in the udder may be suppressed, allowing multiplication of organisms to occur unchecked; toxin production may then lead to severe gangrenous damage to the udder and even generalised, fatal toxaemia. Moreover, the lack of tell-tale inflammation makes diagnosis difficult. The reasons for lack of inflammatory response in such cases are as yet unknown. Infected milk from cows with mastitis can be a source of food poisoning in man.

It is common for staphylococcal infections in the udder to become chronic; after apparent recovery from acute mastitis, a persistent subclinical infection remains which may flare up again from time to time in an acute form. Such chronic infections are refractory to antibiotics, not through inherent resistance of the organisms but because the staphylococci can persist within neutrophil lysosomal vacuoles; although antibiotics can penetrate the neutrophil, most fail to kill there, either because of the acidic environment or the dormant state of the organisms. Rifampicin is one antibiotic which will kill *Staph. aureus* inside neutrophil vacuoles, but resistance to it often appears. Thus at present chronic staphylococcal mastitis remains an intractable problem.

We have noted that *Staph. aureus* is carried harmlessly by a sizeable proportion of healthy people, especially in the nostrils and on moist areas of the skin. For this reason, the development of a lesion is often the result of *endogenous* infection, e.g. by transfer of organisms on the fingers from the nose to a hair follicle or perhaps to a surgical or accidental wound. Alternatively, infections may be acquired from an *exogenous* human or animal source. These sources of cross-infection fall into two categories. (a) Individuals with suppurating, but not necessarily large, skin lesions, e.g. doctors and nurses with pustules on the hands, can transfer infection to their patients by contact. Larger abscesses or infected wounds and burns are sources of large numbers of staphylococci in pus and exudate. Patients with bronchopneumonia discharge organisms in sputum. (b) Healthy carriers, some of whom are 'shedders' and liberate organisms as plentifully as patients with actual lesions; carriers are especially common among hospital staff. Similarly, animals can be a source of infection for man, and the example of food poisoning via contaminated milk has been cited above.

Among possible mechanisms of spread, both direct contact and airborne transmission are common. Touch is an effective route, e.g. via the hand of a nasal carrier who has picked his nose or of a nurse who has handled a patient or an infected baby. Contaminated dust particles can be liberated from handkerchiefs carrying dried sputum or nasal secretion, from surgical dressings of infected wounds on which pus or exudate has dried and powdered, and from the skin, clothing and bedding of patients and carriers, etc. Droplet infection, e.g. from the nose by sneezing or from patients with bronchpneumonia, is probably less frequent than the other routes.

Suitable conditions for the transmission of *Staph. aureus* and for the establishment of infection exist in hospitals: doctors, nursing staff and patients are all sources and vehicles of organisms and there are many potential recipients for opportunistic infection. The latter include newborn babies and their mothers, patients with surgical wounds, and others with lowered resistance due to debilitating disease or immunosuppressive therapy. Thus it is hardly surprising that sporadic *Staph. aureus* infections and even epidemics are common. Infection of newborn babies provides a good example. Babies are born free of bacterial colonisation, but in hospital nurseries they acquire infection at the umbilical stump, usually from a nurse or the mother, and the skin and nose are soon colonised thereafter. Minor staphylococcal skin infections and conjunctivities are common in babies, with a few developing bullous impetigo, osteomyelitis or bronchopneumonia. A baby may in turn transfer infection from its nose to the milk ducts of the nursing mother, frequently a cause of breast abscesses which develop a few weeks after delivery. Interestingly, infection of newborns with pathogenic *Staph. aureus* can be prevented by colonising them deliberately with a strain of low virulence (502A) applied to the nostrils and umbilicus, a method known as *bacterial interference*. Competition for carriage sites by the avirulent strain very effectively prevents virulent organisms from establishing themselves and in American trials this has been shown to prevent outbreaks of staphylococcal disease in nurseries.

Another example of nosocomial (hospital-acquired) staphylococcal infection is sepsis of surgical wounds. Contamination has been known to occur via small punctures in surgeons' gloves through which drops of sweat carrying organisms can pass, from nasal carriers in attendance in operating theatres, contaminated sutures, or subsequently on the ward from a nurse or the patient himself. Patients with open wounds or burns are particularly susceptible.

An important problem is that the strains of *Staph. aureus* which are common in nosocomial infections are often *resistant* to several antibiotics, including penicillin, the agent most widely used in the past in staphylococcal infections. The historical development of antibiotic resistance and its genetic basis have been described previously (p. 461). Staphylococcal resistance genes are plasmid-borne and transmitted by generalised transduction. In treating a staphylococcal infection, it is therefore essential to establish the drug-sensitivity of the strain isolated from the patient. Until this is known, it is usual to commence treatment with a penicillinase-resistant penicillin, such as methicillin or cloxacillin, or with cephalosporins, to which most strains are susceptible.

Staphylococcus epidermidis

By definition, this is the species of coagulase-negative staphylococci; it lacks the other virulence factors of *Staph. aureus* as well and is therefore never a primary pathogen. It is universally present as a harmless commensal colonising the entire surface of the skin (cf. *Staph. aureus*), the nostrils, mouth, external ear and urethral meatus. However, it is a potential opportunist, in which role it occasionally appears as the agent of endocarditis after cardiac surgery and of cystitis (inflammation of the bladder) where there is an abnormality of the urinary tract. Opportunistic invasion by *Staph. epidermidis* (and others) occurs in chronic granulomatous disease where phagocytic mechanisms are defective (as described on p. 24) and may be a cause of septicaemia in immunosuppressed and immunodeficient patients.

NEISSERIA

The neisseriae are Gram-negative pyogenic cocci which include two pathogenic species responsible for serious but quite different diseases: *Neisseria meningitidis* (the meningococcus) is the most frequent cause of *epidemic bacterial meningitis*, while *Neisseria gonorrhoeae* (the gonococcus) is the agent of the major sexually-transmitted disease, *gonorrhoea*. While modern therapeutics and vaccination have made epidemics of meninogococcal meningitis uncommon in many countries, gonorrhoea is all too prevalent; around 60,000 cases of gonorrhoea are reported in the UK annually, while in the USA it is currently at veritable epidemic proportions and is the most prevalent communicable human disease in that country. Like the other pyogenic cocci, neisseriae are invasive organisms which cause suppuration as a result of their interaction with neutrophils during the acute inflammatory response. Gonococci are specially equipped to invade the urogenital tract through possession of surface pili which serve as adhesion structures. In addition, neisseriae share with other Gram-negative organisms the presence of lipopolysaccharide *endotoxin* in the cell wall, which makes an important contribution to their virulence. They do not secrete haemolysins or other exotoxins. Non-pathogenic species (*N. sicca, N. flava*) are common commensals in the upper respiratory tract.

MORPHOLOGY, GROWTH, ETC.

The organisms are non-motile cocci, generally found in pairs; they are slightly smaller than the Gram-positive diplococci, and the opposed surfaces may be concave so that individual cells are bean-shaped (Figure 4.2d). Pathogenic neisseriae are difficult to grow in culture because of their susceptibility to toxic fatty acids and trace metals in peptone and agar; however, blood prevents the action of the toxic substances and good growth occurs on 'chocolate blood agar' (blood agar after heating to 80°C for 10 minutes), especially under 5–10% CO_2. They are essentially aerobic organisms and are *oxidase positive* (possess cytochrome c). The latter property, which is useful in localising colonies of neisseriae in a heavily mixed culture as from a vaginal swab, can be demonstrated by oxidation of dimethyl- or tetramethyl-p-phenylenediamine. Oxidase-positive colonies sprayed with these compounds first turn pink, then rapidly develop a dark purplish-black colour; non-pathogenic neisseriae also react, but more slowly. The non-pathogenic species are easier to grow and will multiply at 22°C on simple media, whereas the pathogens do not grow well below 37°C and not at all at 22°C.

Neisseriae are particularly sensitive to adverse physical and chemical conditions, and the fact that the gonococcus is so easily killed by drying, cold and exposure to air means that it cannot survive outside the body, hence the requirement for intimate sexual or other wet contact for its spread.

STRUCTURE, SECRETED PRODUCTS AND PATHOGENICITY

The invasiveness of neisseriae depends on the properties of their outer surface (Figure 4.49); neither meningococci nor gonococci produce an exotoxin, nor is there the range of secreted enzymes which contribute to the survival and spread of pathogenic Gram-positive cocci. The cell wall resembles that of other Gram-negative organisms, with a thin layer of peptidoglycan and an outer membrane containing LPS (Figures 4.6 and 4.49b). The wall may be surrounded by a capsule and have filamentous pili.

Figure 4.49
(a) Gonococcus as seen under the electron microscope.
(b) Generalised outer structure of neisseriae.

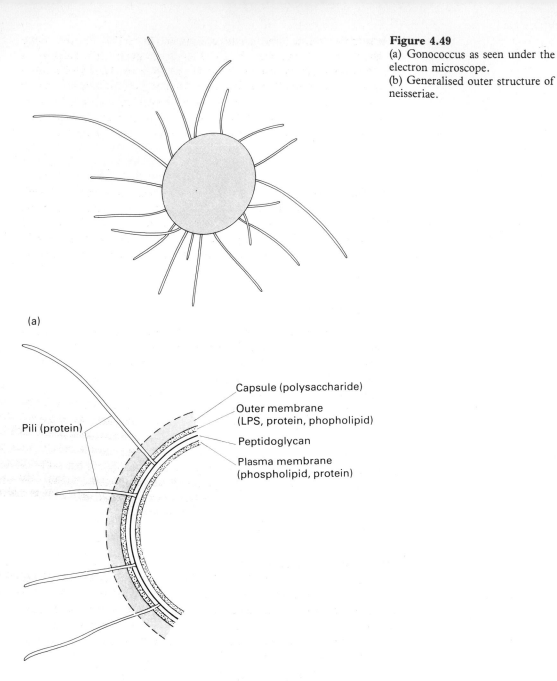

(a)

(b)

Capsule (polysaccharide)
Outer membrane
(LPS, protein, phopholipid)
Peptidoglycan
Plasma membrane
(phospholipid, protein)
Pili (protein)

Capsule

Most meningococci possess a polysaccharide capsule which is antiphagocytic and plays an important part in virulence by assisting extracellular suvival. Thus, non-encapsulated strains are relatively avirulent in mice and anticapsular antibodies are protective. The capsular polysaccharide is the *group-specific antigen* of meningococci (below) and undergoes a quellung

532

reaction with appropriate antiserum (p. 512). In the three pathogenic groups (A, B, C), the polysaccharide is a polymer of N-acetylmannosamine phosphate (group A) or N-acetylneuraminic acid (groups B and C). Some virulent gonococci have recently also been shown to possess a polysaccharide capsule, both by quellung and electron microscopy of organisms treated with antisera; its nature and properties are under investigation.

Proteins

The outer membrane of meningococci contains antigenic proteins; organisms of group A share common protein antigens, while in group B several serotypes are distinguishable. Some of the proteins have antiphagocytic properties, so that certain (group B) serotypes are particularly associated with disease (e.g. serotype 2).

Pili (fimbriae)

Meningococci and gonococci both possess these fine filamentous projections, which for the latter are essential for pathogenicity (see also p. 538). Only gonococci with pili are able to *adhere* to epithilial cells of the genito-urinary tract and thus avoid being washed out of the urethra by urine; non-piliated forms do not adhere and, as studies in male volunteers have shown, do not cause genito-urinary disease. In addition, gonococcal pili, which have no binding affinity for neutrophils, are antiphagocytic. Antibodies to pili prevent adherence to cells *in vitro* as well as being opsonising. The pili of meningococci may also facilitate binding to cell surfaces, but no specific role has been proposed for them.

Endotoxin

Endotoxin (LPS) is present in the outer membrane of neisseriae and is likely to be important in the inflammatory lesions of both meningitis and gonorrhoea. The haemorrhagic manifestation of meningococcal septicaemia and its sometimes rapidly fatal outcome are also due to endotoxin (p. 445). Electron microscopy shows the release of endotoxin in 'blebs' from the surface of the organisms.

IgA protease

This is an enzyme released by several bacteria which cleaves the secreted and serum forms of IgA. It is highly specific for human IgA (and only the IgA_1 subclass) and makes a single cut in the 'hinge' region of the heavy chain leading to detachment of Fc. While this should leave the antibody binding sites intact, after action of IgA protease the IgA molecule is apparently functionally defective. All strains of the gonococcus and meningococcus produce this enzyme, which may serve an important role in their pathogenicity by destroying the activity of locally produced IgA in genital secretions (gonococcus) and the nasopharynx (meningococcus and gonococcus). IgA protease may account for the very poor immunity to reinfection by the gonococcus.

INVASIVENESS AND IMMUNITY

As with other pyogenic cocci, the invasiveness of neisseriae depends on their ability to avoid phagocytosis and/or phagocytic destruction. Microscopic examination of neisserial pus, such as the cerebrospinal fluid in meningitis or urethral discharge in gonorrhoea, characteristically shows that some neutrophils carry large numbers of diplococci. Thus in some neutrophils at least, the organisms apparently survive and multiply. Often, however, it seems that they are killed in phagocytes, whence the importance of antiphagocytic structures such as the capsule and pili to virulence. Antibodies against these structures may act as opsonins to enhance phagocytosis; they are also *bactericidal* and, like other Gram-negative cells, neisseriae can be killed by antibody and complement. The importance of the latter in defence can be judged from the frequency of gonococcal and meningococcal infections in the rare patients with deficiencies of the late components of complement (C5-9). Gonococci are also susceptible to the bactericidal action of normal human serum, via endotoxin-induced activation of complement (p. 123).

MENINGOCOCCAL MENINGITIS

This is the main epidemic form of meningitis and is also called epidemic cerebrospinal meningitis, cerebrospinal fever and spotted fever. During the last century and up to the Second World War, epidemics of meningitis were greatly feared, due to the speed of onset of the disease, its rapidly fatal course in some of those infected, and high mortality ($\sim 50\%$). Those most at risk were, and still are, young children and military recruits (below). The situation changed radically with the introduction of sulphonamides in 1941; not only did they prove a highly effective treatment for the disease itself, but were also used prophylactically, eliminating carriage and preventing epidemics, especially in the crowded conditions of military barracks. The world-wide emergence of sulphonamide-resistant meningococci after 1963 meant that prophylaxis was no longer possible (penicillin, to which the organisms are sensitive, fails for unknown reasons to eliminate the carrier state) and led to the introduction of vaccines for groups at risk. Epidemics may be uncommon today in many countries, but they are still a danger elsewhere; a good example was the large urban epidemic in Sao Paulo, Brazil, which reached a peak in the summer of 1974 when 13,000 cases occurred in two months. Meningococcal meningitis is also seen as occasional sporadic (endemic) cases, at about one per 50,000 population per annum in the UK and USA.

Nine serogroups of meningococci are known (A, B, C, D, W-135, X, Y, Z and 29-E), of which group A contains the strains responsible for most of the epidemics in the past; groups B and C

534

are generally endemic strains, but C has been a cause of epidemics (e.g. Brazil, above). Those most at risk are generally children under the age of 5 years and the highest incidence is in infants between 3 and 12 months of age (maternal antibodies protect the baby during the first three months of life). However, all ages may be affected, and epidemic outbreaks occur in young adults brought together in semi-closed groups, such as military recruits, refugees, etc. Large epidemics occurred among the troops in training during the early years of both world wars and localised outbreaks continue to occur in military camps from time to time.

The pathogenesis of meningococcal disease is outlined in Figure 4.50. *N. meningitidis* can usually be found in the nasopharynx of healthy carriers, generally 5–10% of the normal population, though in military camps this figure can be much higher and may exceed 90%. The carrier state can last for a few days to several weeks, and in general the individual makes an antibody response which leads to immunity and prevents development of meningitis. Thus a large proportion of the adult population is immune to common strains and during epidemics the overwhelming majority of cases are in individuals who did not possess antibodies at its outbreak. Transmission is by the respiratory route via droplet infection. Three stages in the development of the disease are recognised. Initial infection occurs in the nasopharynx and is frequently asymptomatic; if it proceeds no further, the individual is a temporary carrier. In a small proportion, the organisms invade the bloodstream, from which they can be cultured at this stage (*meningococcaemia*); although its severity varies, this is a true *septicaemia*, with multiplication of bacteria in the blood. A rash frequently develops and in severe cases there are haemorrhagic spots in the skin (petechiae) which gave rise to the old name of 'spotted fever'. Septicaemia may be so severe that death occurs in a few hours, with or without

Figure 4.50 Pathogenesis of meningococcal meningitis.

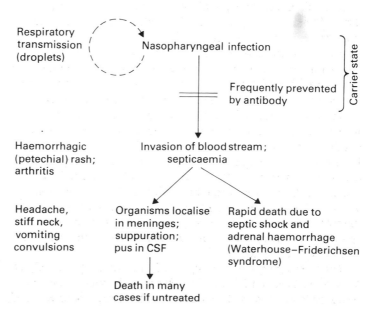

meningitis, due to septic shock and the effects of the *Waterhouse–Friderichsen syndrome*. The latter is an acute adrenocortical insufficiency associated with gross adrenal haemorrhage. The role of *endotoxin* in producing haemorrhage and shock has been described on p. 445, and there is little doubt that endotoxin is primarily responsible for the manifestations of meningococcal septicaemia.

In general, meningococcaemia is less severe but leads to meningitis, known as *leptomeningitis* to indicate that it affects the pia mater and arachnoid mater rather than the dura mater. The reasons for the preferential localisation of the organisms in the meninges are obscure. They enter the subarachnoid space and are widely distributed by the movement of cerebrospinal fluid (CSF) within it, CSF constituting a good culture medium. The whole of the pia-arachnoid system is inflamed and exudate, frequently purulent, fills the subarachnoid space around the brain and spinal cord, and often the ventricles of the brain and the spinal canal as well. The CSF can be sampled by lumbar puncture (insertion of a hollow needle into the subarachnoid space of the lumbar spine), and during the early stages of infection it contains large numbers of neutrophils and Gram-negative diplococci; the latter are both free in the pus and inside some of the phagocytes. The characteristic early symptoms of meningitis are fever, with vomiting and severe headache, the latter due to the increased pressure of the CSF. Irritation of spinal nerves causes a stiff neck, and in small children the head and spine may be drawn backward like a bow; infants show bulging fontanelles. In the brain, increased pressure of fluid occurs when the pus becomes thick and blocks the passages between the ventricles and the spaces in the spinal meninges; this can lead to fatal internal *hydrocephalus* (abnormal increase of CSF in the ventricles) unless relieved. The organisms are prevented by the pia mater from invading the tissue of the brain and spinal cord itself and neurological complications after recovery are not common.

Sulphonamides were formerly used in treatment of meningococcal disease, but the prevalence of resistant strains means that penicillin is now the agent of choice. Early use of antibiotics reduces the mortality to below 10%; otherwise the risk of death is high. Immunity is mediated by opsonising and bactericidal anticapsular antibodies and purified capsular polysaccharides of Groups A and C are effective vaccines. They have been used in many countries for the control of epidemics, especially among the military, though routine vaccination of civilians is not practised. However, Group C vaccines are not very effective in infants under the age of two years, in whom the peak incidence occurs.

GONORRHOEA

Gonorrhoea is a sexually-transmitted disease of world-wide prevalence and may well be the commonest communicable disease in the world today: in 1968, the WHO estimated the incidence at 150 million cases. It is also one of the oldest of all diseases, having apparently existed since prehistoric times, and was well known in the ancient world. In recent years it has grown to epidemic proportions in some countries, with over a million cases reported annually in the USA; this probably represents only about a third of the total in that country, where it is now the most frequent notifiable infection. In the UK, the situation is rather less dramatic; there was a steady decline in gonorrhoea in the early 1950's following the success of antibiotic treatment, but a more than threefold increase then occurred, from the low point of about 18,000 reported cases in 1954 to over 60,000 annually in the early 1970's.

Several reasons can be found for this current high prevalence of gonorrhoea, some social, others biomedical. Among the former are: (i) the increase in and acceptance of promiscuity in our permissive society, together with the shift in contraceptive practice from the condom to the pill and intrauterine devices; (ii) a lesser fear of infection due to the safety-net of antibiotic therapy; (iii) the widespread lack of sex education; and (iv) increased personal mobility, including rapid air travel. Biomedical reasons include: (i) the high infectivity rate of the disease; (ii) the fact that women, and to a lesser extent passive male homosexuals, may be asymptomatic carriers; (iii) the short incubation period, which makes it difficult to break the chain of infection; and (iv) the emergence in some places of antibiotic-resistant strains of *N. gonorrhoeae*.

There are at least 16 antigenically distinct strains of *N. gonorrhoeae*, which differ in their outer membrane proteins. However, there is no satisfactory system of classification. Each strain can exist in five colonial *types* (T1–5), according to its appearance on translucent agar. Types 1 and 2 are small, well-demarcated colonies formed by virulent organisms, whereas the larger and more diffuse colony types 3, 4 and 5 are avirulent; microscopic examination shows that only type 1 and 2 organisms possess pili. Pili tend to be lost during culture on laboratory media, so that a strain which forms type 1 and 2 colonies when first isolated, gradually becomes 3, 4 or 5 after repeated subculture. A new method for strain-typing which is now widely used is *auxotyping*, in which strains are classified by their requirements for specific nutrients in defined media. More than 30 auxotypes have been identified and, unlike colony form, this is a stable characteristic. Some auxotypes have recognisable pathogenic features and increased virulence. For example, virulent strains requiring arginine, hypoxanthine and uracil for their growth (Arg^-, Hyx^-, Ura^-)—nutrients not normally required by isolates from genito-urinary disease—are resistant to the bactericidal action of antibody and complement. They cause an unusual severe disseminated bacteraemic gonorrhoea with arthritis in females, are more likely to give rise to asymptomatic urethritis in males, and are very sensitive to penicillin and tetracycline.

The sensitivity of gonococci to conditions outside the body (drying, heat, soap and water) means that intimate contact is necessary for transmission. While this is usually during *coitus*, infection of the eye is possible by hand-to-eye contact, or can be acquired in the eye of the newborn as the baby passes through the birth canal of an infected mother (*ophthalmia neonatorum*); the latter leads to blindness if not treated promptly. Under natural conditions, the organism is restricted to man and studies of the pathogenesis of gonorrhoea have been delayed by lack of a suitable animal model; many studies have been carried out on human male volunteers and infection has now also been transmitted experimentally to chimpanzees. These studies have confirmed that the possession of pili is the most important virulence attribute of gonococci; pili enable the organisms to adhere to the epithelial cells of the genito-urinary tract and so avoid being washed away in the urinary stream. After adherence, gonococci enter epithelial cells by phagocytosis and multiply intracellularly; lysis of infected cells releases organisms into the subepithelial tissue spaces, where they stimulate an acute inflammatory reaction, leading to suppuration and the characteristic discharge of pus from the urethra or cervix. About 50% of women having coitus with an infected male will become infected, while the risk for a man having intercourse with an infected woman is about 25–50%.

In *males* the infection is almost always clinically apparent, *acute urethritis* developing after an incubation period of 2–10 days (mean 8 days). This begins in the anterior urethra; after damage by gonococci, the mucous membrane becomes heavily infiltrated by neutrophils which collect as pus in the urethral lumen, and this emerges as the yellowish-green urethral discharge. Because of the inflammation, urination is accompanied by a burning pain and becomes frequent and urgent. Having penetrated into the underlying submucosa, the gonococci spread freely parallel to the surface, both in tissue spaces and lymphatics, and if treatment is not successful they infect the posterior urethra and prostate gland. A *chronic* infection there can lead to urethral stricture (narrowing) which in turn predisposes to periurethral abscess; should this perforate the perineum or scrotum, a fistula results. The organisms may also descend from the posterior urethra to the vas deferens and epididymis, which becomes inflamed; if bilateral, epididymitis may cause sterility.

Females acquire the infection during coitus directly from the male discharge; the organisms invade the cervix (the primary site of infection), urethra and para-urethral glands, and the ducts of Bartholin's glands. An important point is that the symptoms may be trivial or non-existent. Thus, in about two-thirds of women, gonorrhoeal infection is *asymptomatic* and unsuspected until it arises in a male contact, who may sometimes reinfect the source of his own infection! Since infected women may be carriers for weeks or months, they represent one of the major problems in control of the disease. Where female infection is clinically apparent, the cervix is inflamed and discharges pus. Although many women recover spontaneously, spread of gonococci can occur, in acute or chronic fashion, via the uterus (endometritis) to involve the Fallopian tubes (salpingitis) and then even into the pelvic peritoneum (peritonitis). These inflammations are accompanied by fever and severe abdominal pain akin to appendicitis. Healing in the Fallopian tubes can lead to fibrotic occlusion and *sterility*.

In both sexes, gonorrhoea may affect the rectum (proctitis); in females, organisms often spread to the anus from the copious vaginal discharge, while in male homosexuals the rectum can be the site of primary infection. Gonococcal pharyngitis due to orogenital contact is also recognised. *Arthritis* is a rare complication today, found mainly in females, in whom it may occur without genital symptoms. A solitary joint in an upper limb becomes acutely inflamed, swollen and tender, and pus in the synovial fluid may contain gonococci indicating bacteraemic infection of the joint, though an allergic (immune complex) reaction may also be involved. The acute purulent conjunctivitis of newborns (ophthalmia neonatorum), acquired during birth if organisms are present in the birth canal, is greatly reduced by the routine use of silver nitrate eye drops (1% solution) which are bactericidal for gonococci. In young (prepubertal) girls, vulvovaginitis may be due to gonococcal infection; it is now rare and associated either with contaminated bedding, towels, etc., or occasionally with sexual offences.

Immunity to gonococci after recovery from gonorrhoea is unfortunately poor or non-existent and reinfection commonly leads to a fresh attack. In the USA, 40% of infected patients return within 12 months and it is not unusual for an individual to acquire 20 or more separate infections. (Boswell, the biographer of Dr Johnson, boasted of 12!) In principle, one would expect that IgA (and other) antibodies in urogenital secretions might provide protective immunity by blocking attachment of gonococci to epithelial cells. Indeed, such antibodies can be detected in genital (e.g. vaginal) secretions of patients with gonorrhoea and their blocking activity tends to be specific for the infecting serotype. There is also evidence that women who fail to make a local IgA response to gonococci are more likely to develop salpingitis. Yet local immunity is clearly inadequate in preventing reinfection. The recurrence of gonorrhoea may be due to the short-lived nature of the local IgA response, to the ability of gonococci to produce IgA protease, or to reinfection by a different serotype (of which there are many). Vaccines are not available, but could be based in the future on purified pili protein.

Treatment is with penicillin, which replaced sulphonamides in 1943. (Before the introduction of antimicrobial therapy, patients essentially had to cure themselves and complications were common.) Penicillin-resistant strains are an increasing problem in some parts of the world. As described on p. 467, this may be due to the presence of R plasmids carrying the gene for penicillinase and their transmission by conjugation. Such strains appeared suddenly in 1976 and are completely resistant to penicillin and ampicillin, with serious implications for the control of gonorrhoea. First isolated in the USA, there have been cases in a number of countries, including outbreaks in England (Liverpool); in general, they originate in the Far East. Resistance due to mutation rather than R plasmids is also recognised and accounts for the more gradual decrease in susceptibility to penicillin that has been found in clinical practice. Three genetic loci are involved, one of which (*pen* A) is specific for penicillin, while the others (*pen* B, *ery*) are non-specific and are also involved in resistance to tetracyclines and chloramphenicol. Resistant strains bind less penicillin than sensitive strains. (Resistance of this type can be overcome by increasing the dose of the antibiotic.)

Control of this very widespread disease depends to a large extent on the tracing and treatment of contacts of patients. The fact that infection in women is often asymptomatic is a major problem, as illustrated by the results of a mass screen of some 9 million women in the USA in the 1970's, when about 4% were found to be carriers. Annual screening in the USA has significantly reduced the reservoir of carriers and contributed to a small downturn in the incidence of gonorrhoea since 1975. Individuals can protect themselves by the use of the condom, but most effectively by restricting the number of their sexual partners to one.

ENTEROBACTERIACEAE

This is a large family of related Gram-negative facultative bacilli (rods) that inhabit the large intestine of man and animals: together with the vibrios, they are often loosely called the enteric bacilli or simply 'enterics'. They make up some 5% of the normal gut flora (the majority of the latter being obligate anaerobes such as *Bacteroides* and not part of this family). The commonest representative of the enterobacteriaceae in aerobic stool cultures is *Escherichia coli*, and the term 'coliform' is sometimes used in reference to it and related normal members of the intestinal tract. Altogether the family comprises 12 genera (Figure 4.51).

While most are harmless commensals under normal circumstances, some genera include the primary agents of major intestinal diseases, such as typhoid fever (*Salmonella typhi*), bacillary dysentery (*Shigella* spp.) and infantile diarrhoea (enteropathic *E. coli*), as well as milder forms of gastroenteritis. Diarrhoeas due to enterobacteria (as well as viruses and protozoa) are merely an inconvenience to adults in developed countries, but can be crippling and life-threatening in the very young and old, as well as in the undernourished populations of

Figure 4.51 Enterobacteriaceae.

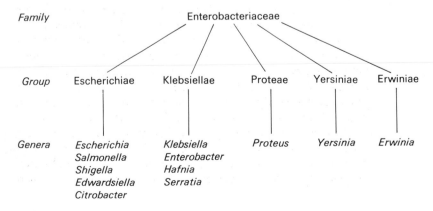

540

some parts of the Third World. In addition, there are many examples where enteric commensals, lacking the ability to cause intestinal disease, give rise to *opportunistic infection* in other body sites; *E. coli*, for example, is a particularly frequent pathogen in the urinary tract. Their tendency to invade tissues and hosts where resistance has been lowered in various ways has made them responsible for many *nosocomial* (hospital acquired) infections, such as wound infections, secondary pneumonias, meningitis and septicaemia, a problem made more serious by the frequent occurrence in them of multiple resistance to antibiotics.

E. coli itself is the most minutely studied organism in all microbiology and the numerous references to it in other parts of this book make clear its importance to biochemistry, genetics and molecular biology in the last few decades.

MORPHOLOGY, GROWTH, ETC.

The enterobacteria are relatively small, non-spore-forming rods (3 μm × 0.5 μm). Most are motile, possessing peritrichous flagella (i.e. distributed around the cell) as in Figures 4.2g, 4.10, *Shigella* and *Klebsiella* are the non-motile genera. In motile species, flagella vary in number from a few, as in *E. coli*, to several hundred per cell in *Proteus*. The organisms grow well on simple media and are facultative anaerobes (i.e. can live in the presence or absence of oxygen) which ferment glucose with production of acid, reduce nitrates to nitrites, and are oxidase-negative. The ability to resist bile salts is characteristic and selective media such as McConkey's, which incorporates bile salts, are useful in distinguishing the enteric bacilli from the bile-sensitive Gram-positive organisms in faecal cultures.

Fermentation of different sugars, etc. is used to identify different genera, especially in separating pathogenic from non-pathogenic species. Many of the organisms which are normally commensal, such as *Escherichia*, *Citrobacter*, *Klebsiella* and *Enterobacter*, ferment *lactose* to acid (lactose-positive), while the major pathogens, *Salmonella* and *Shigella*, are unable to utilise lactose (lactose-negative); these groups can be distinguished on solid media containing lactose and an acid-base indicator, such as McConkey's agar, on which lactose-positive organisms give rise to coloured colonies due to formation of acid and lactose-negative colonies remain colourless. Lactose is a disaccharide of glucose and galactose, into which it is hydrolysed intracellularly by β-galactosidase; its rapid uptake into bacterial cells requires a specific membrane transport protein, galactoside permease. Thus, only organisms possessing the permease and β-galactosidase can ferment lactose promptly. Some enterics lack the permease and utilise lactose slowly, but such organisms can be recognised with ortho-nitrophenyl-β-galactoside (ONPG), which does not require the permease and is hydrolysed by β-galactosidase to give bright yellow ortho-nitrophenol. (Shigellae and salmonellae lack both permease and β-galactosidase.) The genes for lactose utilisation make up the *lac* operon, one of the classic genetic models studied in *E. coli*.

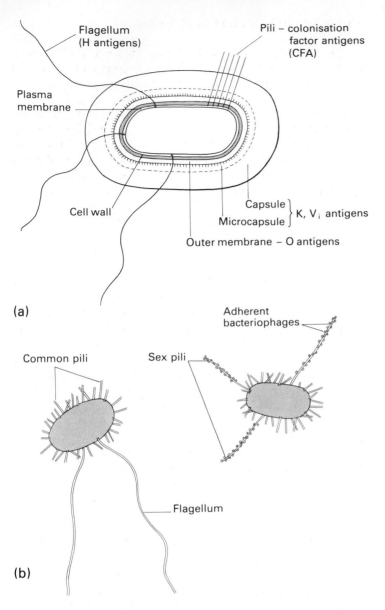

(a)

(b)

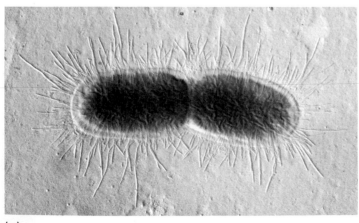

(c)

Figure 4.52 Enterobacteria.
(a) Outer structures and
corresponding antigens.
(b) Cells of *E. coli* drawn after
electron micrographs.
(c) Electron micrograph of
salmonella showing surface pili.
Shadowed preparation, x20,000
(Courtesy of Dr P.D. Walker.)

While the major genera of the family can be identified using fermentation and other tests, further subdivision into species and types often depends on identification of *surface antigens* using specific antisera. There are three categories of antigen, each related to a particular surface structure, as shown in Figure 4.52a, namely: (i) the *O* or *somatic antigens*, carried on the LPS molecules in the outer membrane; (ii) the *K antigens* associated with the capsule; and (iii) the *H antigens* present on flagella. Within a genus or species, there may be many O, K or H antigens, so that by serological tests such as agglutination (or staining with fluorescent antibody) many different *serotypes* of each genus may be recognised. The surface antigens of *E. coli, Klebsiella, Salmonella* and *Shigella* are particularly diverse and identification of serotypes is an important part of epidemiological studies.

The *O (somatic) antigens* are carried on the polysaccharide side chains of the LPS molecules and derive their great diversity from different sugar residues and glycosidic linkages in the chains (p. 395). In *E. coli*, over 150 O antigens have been found, and 64 in *Salmonella*. Loss of O antigens sometimes occurs on growth in culture and is accompanied by a change from smooth to rough colonial form; rough organisms lack the endotoxin side chains and are less virulent than their smooth counterparts. Agglutination by anti-O antibodies may be inhibited by the presence of flagella or a capsule, in which case the latter must be destroyed first by boiling the organisms for two hours. The detection of anti-O (and anti-H) antibodies in patients' sera is used diagnostically in typhoid fever (the *Widal test*, p. 135) when a titre rising over 4–7 days during the second week of the disease is an indication of *Salmonella* infection.

Capsular (K) antigens are polysaccharides which also exist in a variety of antigenically distinct forms—90 K antigens for *E. coli* and 72 for *Klebsiella* are known; the latter can be typed by a capsular quellung reaction similar to that used for pneumococci. The capsule of *Salmonella typhi* and *S. paratyphi*-C is known as the *Vi antigen* because of its association with virulence.

Flagellar (H) antigens are determinants on flagellin (the flagellar protein) and the extensive variation which can occur is due to (minor) alterations in amino acid sequence; a large number of H antigens are known for *E. coli* and salmonellae. Many species of *Salmonella* possess two distinct flagellar antigens, called phase 1 and phase 2, which differ markedly from one another: the phase 1 antigens are restricted to one or a few species (types), while those of phase 2 are shared by many (i.e. phase 1 antigens are the more specific, while phase 2 are widely distributed). A given cell expresses only one H antigen phase at a time, and the two phases correspond to *two different flagellin molecules*. As an individual cell replicates, the flagellar phase can switch from 1 to 2, or vice versa, at a fixed frequency ($10^{-3}/10^{-5}$ per cell per generation), a phenomenon known as *phase variation*. This occurs because there are two flagellin genes, *H1* and *H2*, coding for phase 1 and phase 2 flagellin respectively, and only one gene is expressed at a time. The state of the H2 gene ('on' or 'off') determines the bacterial phase: when H2 is expressed (on) it causes synthesis of H2 flagellin and at the same time a repressor of the H1 gene, so that the latter is expressed only when H2 is switched off.

STRUCTURE, PRODUCTS AND PATHOGENICITY

The pathogenic enterobacteria have virulence attributes which may be structural or secreted products; in some the main pathogenic mechanism is invasiveness, while in others toxins are paramount.

Capsules and phagocytosis

The importance of the capsule varies among the different genera. For *Klebsiella pneumoniae*, an important agent of secondary bacterial pneumonia, the capsule is often large and serves to prevent phagocytosis as it does in pneumococci; thus, non-encapsulated (R) strains are avirulent. For *Salmonella typhi*, the capsule or Vi antigen is thin in comparison (a microcapsule) and its precise role in pathogenicity is still unclear. Studies in human volunteers show that Vi-positive strains are clearly more virulent than those lacking Vi. The functions usually attributed to it are: (i) to inhibit phagocytosis; (ii) to protect *S. typhi* from intra-cellular destruction in phagocytic cells of the reticuloendothelial system (the organisms are often found multiplying in macro-phages in the lesions of typhoid fever); and (iii) to prevent the lytic action of antibody and complement. The capsule of *E. coli* is also thin and seems to have similar properties.

Pili and adhesion

Enteropathogenic strains of *E. coli*, which cause gastroenteritis in infants and newborn animals and 'traveller's diarrhoea', must adhere to the small intestine to cause diarrhoea. They do this by means of surface pili which are identified by specific antigens: K88 and K99 are the pilial antigens on strains infecting piglets and calves respectively, CFAI and CFAII are those of strains which are pathogenic in man. Their role in pathogenicity is described on p. 468.

Endotoxin

The outer membrane of all these organisms contains endotoxin, an important factor in the pathogenesis of invasive disease (e.g. typhoid fever) and in septicaemia caused by the enteric bacilli. The mechanisms of endotoxin action are described at length elsewhere (p. 438), including its causative role in *septic shock* which frequently develops in septicaemia and is associated with a high mortality. While cell bound, the polysaccharide side chains of LPS perform some of the functions of a capsule, viz. inhibition of phagocytosis and resistance to complement-mediated lysis. Thus the loss of O antigens, which occurs on subculturing, gives rise to rough variants which are less virulent than the smooth, O-positive cells.

Enterotoxins and intestinal disease

Enterotoxins (toxins which act on the intestine) are responsible for the production of diarrhoea in *E. coli* gastroenteritis and may be involved in bacillary dysentery (shigellosis) and *Salmonella* gastroenteritis. The action of the heat-labile and stable enterotoxins of *E. coli* (LT, ST) on the small intestine is described on p. 425, 433, and their genetic coding on plasmids on p. 468. Both LT and ST raise intracellular cyclic nucleotide levels in intestinal epithelial cells, leading to secretion of water and salts into the lumen of the intestine and hence to production of watery diarrhoea.

An enterotoxin is also produced by pathogenic shigellae (*Sh. dysenteriae, Sh. flexneri, Sh. sonnei*), but its role in dysentery is less clear than that of cholera and *E. coli* toxins in watery diarrhoea. Unlike those diseases, in bacillary dysentery there are *inflammatory* lesions throughout the colon and frequently in the lower ileum; shigellae are primarily *invasive*—loss of invasiveness means loss of their virulence—whereas cholera vibrios and enteropathogenic *E. coli* are primarily toxigenic. Nevertheless, watery diarrhoea is not uncommon in dysentery, suggesting the action of an enterotoxin causing secretion of water. As long ago as 1903, a *neurotoxin* was demonstrated in culture filtrates of *Sh. dysenteriae*, which caused limb paralysis and death in experimental animals and inflammatory lesions in the rabbit large intestine. A role in human dysentery was subsequently discounted, however, until the 1970's, when it was found that *Sh. dysenteriae* (type 1) culture filtrates caused accumulation of fluid in rabbit ileal loops, i.e. secretion of water into the small intestine (cf. cholera enterotoxin, p. 420). The toxin also causes inflammatory changes in the jejunal mucosa similar to those produced by whole organisms. Moreover, purification of shigella enterotoxin showed that the same molecule possessed neurotoxic activity and was cytotoxic for cultured human cells such as HeLa cells. Its action and structure are apparently different from cholera enterotoxin in that it does not stimulate adenylate cyclase nor cross-react immunologically; its mechanism of action in producing diarrhoea is unknown, but it inhibits protein synthesis in HeLa cells and mammalian cell extracts. Although the properties of shigella toxin point to an involvement in dysentery, this is not borne out by volunteer studies designed to assess the relative importance of invasiveness and toxigenicity in the disease. Thus (a) strains of *Sh. dysenteriae* which are non-invasive but toxigenic are harmless, and conversely (b) lack of toxin production does not prevent an invasive strain from causing dysentery in just as severe a form as that of toxigenic strains. Thus the relevance of enterotoxin is as yet unproven.

There have also been reports of an enterotoxin produced by

Salmonella typhimurium, a major agent of gastroenteritis; this molecule resembles cholera toxin and *E. coli* LT in producing elongation of Chinese hamster ovary cells, and it can be neutralised by antibodies to cholera toxin. It may well have been acquired by transfer of the LT plasmid from *E. coli*. In general, however, exotoxins are not known to be involved in *Salmonella* enteric disease. Enteropathogenic strains of *Klebsiella pneumoniae* and *Enterobacter cloacae* also produce LT.

DISEASES DUE TO ENTEROBACTERIACEAE

In general terms there are two main routes whereby this family of organisms causes clinical disease (Figure 4.53).

(i) *Intestinal infections* by primary pathogens, organisms endowed with the virulence necessary to cause disease in healthy individuals, notably *Salmonella*, *Shigella*, and the enteropathogenic strains of *E. coli*. Pathogenic processes which are essentially *invasive*, as in *Salmonella* and *Shigella* infection, can be differentiated from those in which *toxin production* is the central event, as in the cholera-like *E. coli* diarrhoeas. This in turn leads to marked differences in the clinical nature and course of these diseases.

(ii) *Extraintestinal infections* by organisms which under normal circumstances are harmless enteric commensals but act as secondary or opportunistic pathogens where natural defence mechanisms have been damaged or suppressed. This group includes organisms of several genera (*E. coli*, *Klebsiella*, *Proteus*, *Serratia*, *Enterobacter*, etc.) and the sites of clinically apparent pyogenic infection are the urinary tract, lungs, wounds, meninges and the

Figure 4.53 Routes of production of disease by Enterobacteriaceae.

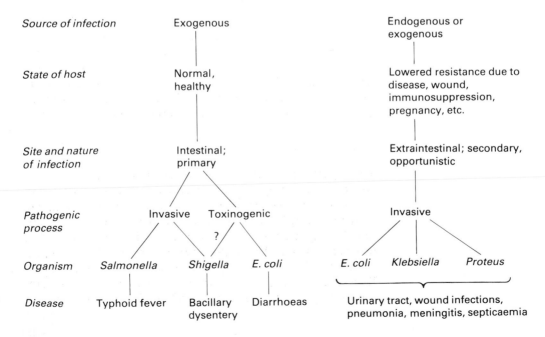

bloodstream. Although there are differences in epidemiology, severity and frequency, these diverse genera give rise to essentially similar clinical conditions. Pathogenesis is that of *invasion* of the compromised host or tissue and exotoxins do not play a prominent role.

Finally, we may note that many Gram-negative bacilli tend to cause bacteraemia or septicaemia, regardless of the initial site of infection. This can be a very serious clinical state and, where *E. coli*, *Proteus* and *Klebsiella* are involved, often leads to death as a result of septic shock (p. 445).

Escherichia coli

Infection by *E. coli* can be manifested in three possible ways, depending on the strain of the organism and the status of the host. (1) It is the major *aerobic* species in the large intestine where it is a life-long commensal following infection (by ingestion) in the first few days after birth. (2) Outside the intestinal tract it occurs as an opportunistic pathogen, and is a major cause of urinary tract infections, wound infections, meningitis, peritonitis and septicaemia. At special risk are infants and those debilitated by immunosuppressive therapy. Many of these infections are pyogenic. They may be acquired endogenously, from the patient's own intestinal flora, or exogenously. (3) Enteropathogenic strains of *E. coli* are primary intestinal pathogens which cause gastroenteritis in the form of diarrhoeas in infants, in adults during journeys abroad, and in newborn domestic animals. These strains are acquired exogenously (e.g. from contaminated food) and carry plasmids which give them the ability to colonise the small intestine and produce enterotoxins.

PROPERTIES OF THE ORGANISM

Most of these have been described above. *E. coli* is usually motile and ferments lactose with gas production; some strains cause β-haemolysis on blood agar. It does not grow outside the human or animal body, but is often present in the soil due to faecal contamination. The presence of *E. coli* in water indicates recent contamination by human or animal faeces, so that tests for its growth are routine in public health laboratories.

CLASSIFICATION

The organisms possess LPS in the outer membrane, a narrow polysaccharide capsule and flagella, and are typed by the corresponding O, K and H antigens. The K antigens are divided into 3 groups (L, A, B) on the basis of their physical behaviour. The capsule may prevent agglutination by anti-O sera and is then removed by boiling before O-serotyping. At least 160 O antigens, 90 capsular K antigens and 50 H antigens have been described. Each serotype is given a numerical designation in the form O type: K type: H type, such as 111:58(B4):2, an enteropathogenic strain.

The factors imparting virulence to the enteropathogenic strains have been described elsewhere. In summary, they comprise the presence of *adherence structures* (pili) which enable them to colonise the surface of the intestinal mucosa, together with production of *enterotoxins* (LT and ST). Pili and toxins are coded by genes on transmissible plasmids. The antigens known as K88 and K99 are present on those adherence pili responsible for colonisation of the small intestine of piglets and calves respectively; similar antigens on pili of strains causing human diarrhoeal disease are called *colonisation factor antigens* CFAI and CFAII. Strains bearing these specialised pili usually also produce ST and LT, so identification of CFA pili is presumptive evidence of an enterotoxigenic strain. CFA antigens can be detected by agglutination of the organisms with specific anti-CFA sera and by a characteristic type of haemagglutination. All *E. coli* strains agglutinate human and guinea-pig red cells by means of common pili and this is usually inhibitable by mannose, while strains with CFA pili produce agglutination of human or bovine red cells which is *mannose-resistant*.

The K1 capsular antigen confers virulence on certain *E. coli* strains involved in neonatal meningitis by increasing resistance to phagocytosis. The majority of strains from urinary tract infections, peritonitis, meningitis and septicaemia possess particular virulence properties which are less common among the normal faecal flora. Some of these are determined by genes carried on plasmids such as Col V; the nature of these factors has been described on p. 469.

ACUTE GASTROENTERITIS

Acute gastroenteritis due to *E. coli* is characterised by a cholera-like outpouring of fluid into the small intestine, leading to massive fluid loss, acute dehydration, acidosis and hypovolaemic shock; as in cholera there is little or no evidence of inflammation in the intestinal mucosa, due to the non-invasive character of the infection. Outbreaks of gastroenteritis in infants, often under 18 months, occur in nurseries and paediatric units—*infantile* or *nursery diarrhoea*—and are especially common among the under-nourished in developing countries. The diarrhoea leads to severe, life-threatening dehydration. Several *E. coli* serotypes have been found, particularly in epidemics, the most frequent in the past being those carrying O antigens 26, 55 and 111; however, nowadays the association with particular serotypes is less regular, probably due to the transmission of the virulence plasmids to other strains. The infection is probably transmitted to infants by inadequately sterilised feeding bottles, teats or feeds, and is more likely to occur in bottle-fed than in breast-fed babies. Thus breast-feeding is the best preventative measure, as well as providing protective maternal IgA antibodies. Treatment essentially consists of replacement of lost fluid and electrolytes (oral or intra-venous rehydration) together with antibiotics. Enteropathogenic strains of *E. coli* cause *traveller's diarrhoea* in persons of all ages newly arrived in a foreign country, especially those travelling from temperate to tropical countries where there may be more opportunity for infection.

It is also possible for certain invasive, non-toxigenic strains to cause diarrhoeal disease which originates in the large intestine rather than the small intestine; this is a *bacillary dysentery* resembling that of shigellosis, with blood and mucus in the stools in addition to diarrhoea. It occurs in infants and young children among crowded impoverished populations and is less common in Europe and the USA than the watery diarrhoea syndrome. These enteroinvasive strains of *E. coli* can be detected by the *Sereny test* in which a drop of culture placed in the eye of a guinea-pig causes keratoconjunctivitis.

URINARY TRACT INFECTIONS

As an extraintestinal, opportunistic pathogen, *E. coli* is responsible for over 80% of urinary tract infections, most of which occur in women. They are encouraged by certain well recognised predisposing conditions, including urethral *catheterisation* or other instrumentation; *obstruction* of the urinary tract with urinary stasis; and *pregnancy*, in which stasis occurs because of the hormonally-produced relaxation of urinary tract muscles and, in later stages, the pressure of the enlarged uterus. The importance of urinary stasis is that it allows *E. coli* to grow in the stagnant urine retained in the bladder, causing inflammation (*cystitis*). While the bladder is the principal site of infection, the organisms can also ascend the ureters to infect the renal pelvis and calyces and the tissue of the kidney itself (*pyelonephritis*).

In the urinary tract in normal circumstances, organisms such as *E. coli*, *Proteus* and Gram-positive cocci are mostly found on the mucosa of the distal part of the urethra, from where they are washed out by the urinary stream; the rest of the tract is relatively free of bacteria. *Bacteriuria* (presence of bacteria in the urine) is common and normal, but when it exceeds 100,000 organisms per ml, urinary tract infection is indicated. Significant bacteriuria may be asymptomatic and as such is seen in some 5% of pregnant women, in whom it is often followed by cystitis; it also occurs in a small proportion of young children, as a prelude to chronic pyelonephritis. Where urinary obstruction occurs due to stricture, calculi or neurogenic disturbance of bladder control, cystitis is likely to be prolonged and reflux of urine into the ureters is encouraged. Bacteria can then ascend the ureters to the kidneys to cause *acute pyelonephritis* with acute inflammation, suppuration and extensive destruction of cortical tissue, especially tubules but sparing glomeruli. In contrast, *chronic pyelonephritis* is in many cases not preceded by clinically apparent bladder infection, though the organisms reach the kidneys by the same route. When severe, the chronic disease is characterised by extensive *scarring* of kidney tissue with destruction of parenchyma, and is an important cause of renal failure. Chronic pyelonephritis also often leads to hypertension which can be of the malignant variety (p. 673).

OTHER INFECTIONS

E. coli is an important cause of meningitis among newborns, infection being acquired from the mother during birth. This disease has a high mortality and survivors may show neurological abnormalities. Wound infections are a further example of *E. coli* as an opportunist. It is also the commonest organism in Gram-negative septicaemia leading to septic shock (p. 445), especially in cancer patients being treated with corticosteroids or other immuno-suppressive drugs; septicaemia can also follow gastrointestinal or genito-urinary surgery. The strains involved in septicaemia are often endowed with resistance to lysis by antibody and comple-ment by genes on the Col V plasmid (p. 469). Needless to say, *E. coli* is one of the most important agents of hospital-acquired disease.

Shigella

The characteristic feature of dysentery is diarrhoea with blood, mucus and pus in the stools; it can be caused by bacterial or protozoal infection and results from inflammation of the mucosal lining of the colon. Bacillary dysentery has been recorded as a common serious disease since biblical times and has been played a role in military history by incapacitating the soldiers of entire armies. Epidemics of severe dysentery still occur in tropical countries and reached huge proportions in Central America in 1969–70 and Bangladesh in 1973; these recent epidemics were compounded by the antibiotic resistance of the organisms and led to thousands of deaths. Such severe outbreaks are due to *Shigella dysenteriae*, a species now rather infrequently encountered in Europe and North America, where most cases are relatively mild and often due to *Sh. sonnei*.

CHARACTERISTICS AND CLASSIFICATION

There are four species of shigella, all of which cause dysentery, namely *Sh. dysenteriae*, *Sh. flexneri*, *Sh. boydii* and *Sh. sonnei*, in descending order of severity. They are similar in morphology and structure to the other enterobacteria, and like salmonellae they do not ferment lactose (*Sh. sonnei* utilises lactose slowly). Shigellae can be distinguished from salmonellae by the following: (1) they are non-flagellate and hence non-motile, (2) they do not produce gas during fermentation of carbohydrate (except for some types of *Sh. flexneri*), (3) they do not produce H_2S, and (4) some species, particularly *Sh. dysenteriae*, produce indole. Shigellae are classified by their O antigens into four groups (A, B, C, D) corresponding to the four species, and then into a relatively small number of serotypes (ten of *Sh. dysenteriae*, only one of *Sh. sonnei*). As the organisms are non-flagellate, there are no H antigens, while capsular K antigens are significant only in so far as they interfere with O-typing; boiling the suspension removes the capsule and prevents this interference. Plasmids carrying antibiotic-resistance genes are widespread among shigellae and can be acquired from other enterics by conjugation (p. 460).

PATHOGENESIS OF BACILLARY DYSENTERY

In contrast with *Vibrio cholerae* and enterotoxic *E. coli*, the important feature of shigella infections (shigelloses) is the *invasiveness* of the organisms; non-invasive strains are non-pathogenic. Although an enterotoxin is produced in culture by *Sh. dysenteriae* type 1 and other species, its importance in the disease process is suspected but not proven, as discussed on p. 545. (The fact that early in the disease the faeces are watery suggests the action of enterotoxin in the small intestine before the colon is invaded.) Infection and lesions occur throughout the colon and often the terminal ileum; moreover, the lesions are *inflammatory*, with mucosal ulceration and suppurative exudate containing large numbers of neutrophils (cf. *V. cholerae* and *E. coli* infections which permeate the small intestine and do not cause inflammation). On the other hand, shigellae are less invasive than virulent salmonellae and rarely spread beyond the intestinal submucosa; bacteraemia and invasion of other organs is therefore very uncommon.

The organisms are acquired by ingestion, the infecting dose required being very small indeed—in volunteer studies, 200 cells of *Sh. dysenteriae* could cause disease in 25% of individuals (ID_{25}), in comparison with 10^6–10^7 *E. coli* organisms and 10^5 *Salmonella typhi*. In the large intestine, they adhere to mucosal epithelial cells which they then enter by phagocytosis and in which they multiply. Ultimately the infected cells are killed (perhaps through endotoxin action) and the organisms spread to adjacent cells and invade the lamina propria; however, the infection is limited to the mucosa and submucosa of the intestine. Pyogenic inflammation occurs in the mucosa, with sloughing of the epithelium and ulceration. In the case of infection with *Sh. dysenteriae*, these events lead to a severe illness with abdominal pain, prostration and fever, and the passage of fresh blood, pus and mucus in the stools. Dehydration is the most important consequence and may be fatal, especially in children less than two years old or debilitated adults. Intravenous fluid and electrolyte replacement are needed, together with antibiotic therapy; this form of dysentery can have a high mortality in children in tropical epidemics, especially when complicated by multiple drug resistance. In contrast, illness due to *Sh. sonnei*, the common species in W. Europe and N. America, is much less incapacitating, with relatively mild abdominal discomfort and passage of some loose stools. Mild forms of dysentery are self-limiting and do not require treatment.

TRANSMISSION

Since shigellae only infect man and other primates, patients and carriers are the sources of organisms; asymptomatic infection is common and carriers are important in spreading the disease. Infection is by the faecal-oral route, via 'fingers, faeces, food and flies'. Because so few organisms are required, an infective dose can be picked up on the hands from toilets, door handles, washbasin taps, hand towels, and other objects contaminated by patients or carriers, and the organisms transferred to the mouth and ingested. In countries with good sanitation, shigellosis occurs mainly in young children whose toilet habits at primary school usually leave something to be desired, particularly in the matter of washing the hands. Food and eating utensils can also be contaminated by carriers, while in countries where sewage disposal is inadequate, flies can transfer organisms mechanically from faeces to food. Water supplies contaminated by sewage have been responsible for large-scale outbreaks.

IMMUNITY

Immunity to shigellae evidently depends on production of IgA into the gut; during infection antibodies are made (locally) both against the organisms and enterotoxin. Where the organisms are endemic, immunity is widespread, probably from inapparent infection, but can be overcome by a high infecting dose. Oral vaccines of promise are being developed in the form of living strains which have lost the ability to invade the epithelium. Competition from the normal gut flora evidently plays a role in natural resistance to infection: germ-free animals are especially sensitive to shigella but become resistant if their intestinal tract is infected with *E. coli*. As with other enteropathogens, control of dysentery in the community depends on good personal hygiene, proper sewage disposal and chlorination of water.

Salmonella

This is a large, diverse genus of over 1800 'species' (more precisely serotypes) which infect both man and animals. They are invasive enteric organisms and in man cause three distinct types of disease (salmonelloses). (1) The most severe infections are the *enteric fevers* of which the prototype is typhoid fever (*Salmonella typhi*); this is a generalised bacteraemic (septicaemic) disease lasting several weeks. (2) The salmonellosis most frequently encountered in Europe and the USA is *food poisoning* (acute gastroenteritis), often due to *S. typhimurium* or *S. enteritidis*, with vomiting, diarrhoea and abdominal pain, with a brief self-limiting course and restricted to the intestinal tract. (3) Occasionally, *septicaemia* leading to focal suppurative lesions in extraintestinal tissues occurs without major intestinal involvement and is caused by *S. cholerae-suis*, especially as an opportunistic infection where there is underlying disease or reduced host defence.

CHARACTERISTICS AND CLASSIFICATION

Salmonellae are motile (flagellated) Gram-negative bacilli which do not ferment lactose. With the notable exception of *S. typhi*, they produce gas from glucose fermentation and H_2S from thiosulphate (cf. shigellae). They are capable of tolerating high concentrations of bile and *S. typhi* regularly infects the gall bladder; bile resistance is used in the design of selective growth media. However, they are sensitive to acid, including normal stomach fluid (pH 3.5). The principal antigens are the somatic O antigens of LPS and the flagellar H antigens, the latter usually exisiting in two phases as described on p. 543. In addition, *S. typhi* and *S. paratyphi B* possess a narrow glycoplipid capsule which carries the Vi (virulence) antigen; this microcapsule inhibits agglutination by anti-O sera and can also be detected by anti-Vi sera.

Classification in the *Kaufmann–White scheme* makes use of the O and H antigens. Major (strongly-reacting) O antigens are used to divide salmonellae into groups which are designated alphabetically (and numerically after Z); there are minor (weaker) O antigens which may be shared between groups. Each species (serotype) is defined further by its H antigens, phase 1 (originally lower case letters) and phase 2 (originally numbered). Thus, to identify a particular isolate the group is first identified by anti-O sera and the species then determined with anti-H. According to the traditional scheme, each serotype is given the status of a species, of which over 1800 have now been described. Thus, *S. typhimurium* belongs to Group B and is designated 4,12:i:1,2 (O antigens 4 (major) and 12 (minor): phase 1 H antigen i: phase 2 antigens 1 and 2), while *S. typhi* is Group D and identified as 9,12,Vi:d: − (i.e. no phase 2 flagella). More recent practice (in the USA) is to use only three species designations, *S. typhi*, *S. cholerae-suis* and *S. enteritidis*; the first two are each a single serotype, while *S. enteritidis* contains all the other types, each referred to by name (e.g. *S. enteriditis* sero typhimurium is *S. typhimurium* of the Kauffmann–White scheme).

Phage-typing has become important for the salmonellae causing enteric fevers: there are 90 phage types of *S. typhi*, 50 of *S. paratyphi B* and 6 of *S. paratyphi A*. The fact that all patients infected from a common source yield the same phage type is of great value in tracing the origin of an outbreak, especially where there is a symptomless carrier.

Most salmonellae infect many animal species as well as man, but some have particular preferred hosts. An important example of this is *S. typhi* itself which *only* infects man; thus the source of typhoid fever is always a human carrier or patient (*S. paratyphi A* and *C* are similarly restricted to man). A few species preferentially infect certain animals, such as *S. cholerae-suis* in pigs, though this species is a pathogen in man and other animals as well.

DETERMINANTS OF PATHOGENICITY

Salmonellae are invasive pathogens. Like the shigellae, the first stage in their invasion of the intestinal wall depends on adherence to epithelial cells, followed by uptake by phagocytosis; the bacterial component responsible for adherence is unknown. Subsequent cellular damage is probably caused by endotoxin, which is also responsible for other clinical aspects of typhoid fever, such as the pyrexia itself (p. 439) and inflammation in various organs. *S. typhi* and the paratyphoid organisms are the most invasive and spread to the local and regional lymph nodes and thence to many internal organs to which they are carried by the bloodstream. Their most important attribute is the ability to survive and multiply inside phagocytic cells, notably macrophages; resistance to destruction is apparently provided by the capsule, as variants lacking the Vi antigen are non-invasive. This *intracellular* existence means that, as in the case of infection by mycobacteria and brucellae, cell-mediated immunity involving sensitised T cells and macrophage activation plays an important role in recovery; cell-mediated *hypersensitivity* is involved in the later lesions.

The salmonellae which remain localised to the intestinal mucosa and cause gastroenteritis lack the capsular Vi antigen. It is possible that enterotoxins are involved in causing diarrhoea. Thus, a relatively heat-stable enterotoxin has been found in *S. enteritidis* which stimulates fluid accumulation in rabbit ileal loops (p. 420); it also seems that *S. typhimurium* may produce an enterotoxin closely related to LT of *E. coli* and cholera toxin. However, the role of these products in salmonellosis is not yet clear and there are alternative explanations for the production of diarrhoea (p. 559).

TYPHOID AND PARATYPHOID FEVERS

The enteric fevers, as these diseases are called, are uncommon today in countries with a high standard of public health and adequate sewage disposal, where water supplies are unpolluted and milk is pasteurised. In Britain, enteric fevers are now rare and most recorded cases are imported, especially from the Indian subcontinent, while in the USA the annual incidence is below 400 cases. Paratyphoid fevers resemble typhoid, but are milder and have a shorter incubation period; they are due to *S. paratyphi* types A, B or C.

Pathogenesis of typhoid fever is shown schematically in Figure 4.54. The infection is acquired from contaminated food or water, particularly the latter, and since *S. typhi* is restricted to man, all cases originate from another patient or carrier. Compared with shigellae, a large number of organisms are required to initiate disease, 10^5 being the ID_{25} and 10^7 the ID_{50} (the numbers of organisms required to produce disease in 25% and 50% of individuals respectively). Many organisms are killed by gastric acidity, but those which enter the small intestine adhere to epithelial cells, which then engulf them. They multiply in and pass through these cells and invade the lamina propria and submucosa, where they are found in neutrophils and macrophages. The salmonellae are then carried in the lymphatics to the

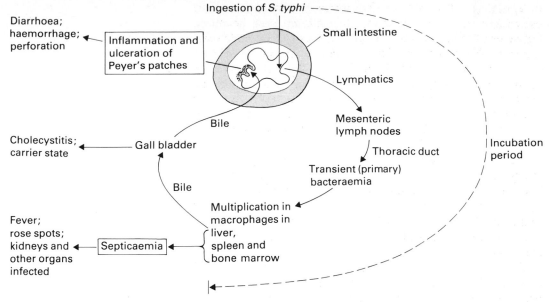

Diarrhoea;
haemorrhage;
perforation

Inflammation and
ulceration of
Peyer's patches

Ingestion of *S. typhi*

Small intestine

Lymphatics

Bile

Mesenteric
lymph nodes

Thoracic duct

Incubation
period

Cholecystitis;
carrier state

Gall bladder

Bile

Transient (primary)
bacteraemia

Fever;
rose spots;
kidneys and
other organs
infected

Septicaemia

Multiplication in
macrophages in
liver,
spleen and
bone marrow

Figure 4.54 Pathogenesis of
typhoid fever.

mesenteric lymph nodes where multiplication within macrophages takes place—as already noted, they are resistant to intracellular killing by normal macrophages. After release, they are drained via the thoracic duct into the bloodstream, in which they are disseminated but do not multiply significantly (primary transient *bacteraemia*). The organisms are rapidly removed from the blood by the littoral macrophages of the reticulendothelial system lining the sinusoids of the liver, spleen and bone marrow, and proceed to multiply intracellularly until the macrophages are killed. *S. typhi* organisms are now released in large numbers into the blood. This is the secondary bacteraemia, in fact *septicaemia*, which marks the onset of serious clinical illness. During its first week, the typical symptoms are the progressive, stepwise increase in temperature, epistaxis, headache, abdominal tenderness, and constipation rather than diarrhoea; organisms can be cultured from the blood at this stage.

From the liver, *S. typhi* is carried into the gallbladder, multiplying freely in the bile; sometimes the wall of the gallbladder itself becomes inflamed (*cholecystitis*). The flow of bile into the small intestine leads to *reinfection* of the intestinal tract, the organisms now localising particularly in the lymphoid tissue of Peyer's patches in the distal ileum and causing inflammation, necrosis and ulceration (*typhoid ulcers*). Thus during the second week of illness, together with sustained fever of 40°C (104°F), diarrhoea occurs with typical 'pea-soup' stools; organisms are present in the faeces. It is noteworthy that the major cell types in the ulcerated Peyer's patches are macrophages, the number of lymphocytes being reduced, and with very few neutrophils: the intestinal lesions are probably the sites of a cell-mediated immune response to *S. typhi* initiated by T cells sensitised during the incubation period. Activation of macrophages by lymphokines leads to intracellular destruction of salmonellae, but the release of inflammatory lymphokines causes the tissue damage and ulceration (cell-mediated or Type IV hypersensitivity, p. 163). Haemorrhage may occur from the ulcers during the third week or, more seriously, there may be perforation of the small intestine with generalised peritonitis, the commonest cause of death in typhoid fever. In uncomplicated cases, however, the ulcers heal, the fever falls by *lysis* (i.e. gradually) and the patient recovers rapidly during the fourth and fifth weeks.

Figure 4.55 shows the time-course of appearance of salmonella organisms in the blood, faeces and urine during typhoid, and of serum antibodies, all of which are valuable aids to diagnosis. (It is noteworthy that none of these is positive in all cases.) *S. typhi* can be cultured from the blood during the first week of fever and thereafter appears in the faeces. Bacteria in the blood are cleared by antibody—like other Gram-negative organisms, *S. typhi* are killed by anti-O antibodies and complement—and a rising anti-O (and anti-H) titre in the blood during the second and third weeks is a diagnostic test for typhoid (Widal test, p. 135). Before this occurs, however, septicaemia has distributed the organisms widely: infection of the kidneys leads to the presence of organisms in the urine in 20% of patients (bacilluria); bacteria in the skin account for the rose-coloured spots which appear on the abdomen and chest in about 10% of cases; and possible complications include endocarditis, bronchopneumonia, meningitis, periosteitis and arthritis. Infection of the bone marrow leads to suppression of granulocyte production, so that instead of the leucocytosis which usually accompanies acute bacterial infections, the white cell count is typically somewhat depressed ($<4 \times 10^6$ per ml; *leucopenia*) due to the decrease in neutrophils. Circulating endotoxin is responsible both for fever and for lesions in the heart, liver and kidneys.

In most cases the *S. typhi* bacilli are completely eliminated during the process of recovery. However, a small proportion of

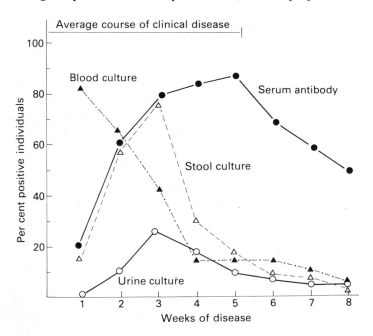

Figure 4.55 Typhoid fever: frequency among patients of positive blood, stool, and urine cultures and of antibody in serum.

patients, (2–5%) recover from the clinical disease but continue to harbour the organisms as a chronic infection in the gall bladder (some may suffer from cholecystitis) and less often in the urinary tract. These individuals are *carriers* who continue to excrete the organisms in faeces (or urine) for long periods of time and are a most important source of outbreaks of typhoid fever; about half of these remain carriers for less than a year while the rest are *chronic carriers* in whom infection may be lifelong. The chronic carrier state is more common in typhoid than paratyphoid.

Treatment of enteric fevers is generally with chloramphenicol, which produces rapid recovery but has little effect on carriers. Most of the latter can be cured by cholecystectomy (removal of the gallbladder) or ampicillin.

Transmission and epidemiology. Typhoid and paratyphoid organisms are acquired either from patients or carriers, via a faecal–oral route (water, food, hands, eating utensils, etc.). Infected water, contaminated by human faeces, is the main vehicle in typhoid, while paratyphoid tends to be carried primarily in food; both may be transmitted in infected milk or dairy products such as ice cream, as well as in other foods. Typhoid fever was not unusual in Britain in the days before purification and chlorination of water supplies, with about 9000 deaths annually during the 1870's; this number had fallen to less than 1000 in 1917 and in the decade 1962–71 there were only 26 deaths. Milk is a major source of infection in countries where pasteurisation is not practised. Food may be contaminated indirectly via flies, a particular hazard in the tropics. An infective dose may develop from subsequent multiplication. Chronic carriers (and ambulant patients) are the chief sources of the organisms, and are especially dangerous when handling food or employed in dairies or water works. The most notorious example is undoubtedly that of 'Typhoid Mary' (Mary Mallon) who was a typhoid carrier employed as a cook in New York between 1901 and 1914, during which period she caused over 1300 cases of typhoid fever. An example of a large food-borne outbreak occurred in Aberdeen in 1964. A 6 lb can of imported corned beef had been contaminated through the use of unchlorinated river water during the process following sterilisation of the can, and some organisms had evidently entered through unsealed joints; 515 cases of typhoid resulted. Shellfish grown in contaminated river estuaries are responsible for occasional cases.

The enteric fevers are of world-wide prevalence and their incidence depends on the efficiency of sanitation and steps taken to prevent contamination of food and water supplies. In the UK the vast majority of the 200 or so cases of typhoid reported annually are imported, either from the Indian subcontinent (60–70%), the Middle East, North Africa, or European countries bordering the Mediterranean (Spain and Italy). There are about 100 cases of paratyphoid each year, also imported, two-thirds of which are paratyphoid A and the remainder B. In Europe, the largest numbers of cases of typhoid and paratyphoid occur in Italy

(10,000), Spain (2000–3000), Portugal (1000) and Yugoslavia (2000) (1970 figures). Epidemics can be made more severe by antibiotic-resistant strains of *S. typhi*, which caused a large number of deaths in Mexico in 1972 (p. 462).

Prevention depends on purification of drinking water, pasteurisation of milk, banning chronic carriers from food-handling and isolation of patients. An acetone-killed vaccine, given subcutaneously, is used to protect exposed individuals during epidemics, and has replaced the use of the formaldehyde-inactivated triple typhoid vaccine (TAB—typhoid plus paratyphoid A and B organisms). Attenuated vaccines are useless, as the antigens against which protection is needed are lost.

FOOD POISONING (GASTROENTERITIS)

Salmonellae are one of the three principal causes of bacterial food poisoning in Europe and the USA, the others being *Clostridium perfringens* (p. 583) and *Staph. aureus* (p. 527). While the latter two are due to production of toxins into the food, salmonella food poisoning is an acute intestinal infection. It is also by far the commonest of the three: although only a fraction of the cases of salmonella food poisoning are notified, the estimate of 2 million annually in the USA is often quoted. In contrast with the enteric salmonellae, which are spread by human patients or carriers, the principal reservoir for the food poisoning species are the animals themselves, principally chickens, turkeys, pigs and cows.

Pathogenesis. Several salmonella species are able to produce food poisoning, principal among them *S. typhimurium*, *S. agona* (in the UK), *S. enteritidis*, *S. heidelberg*, *S. newport*, etc. The infective dose required is very high (10^8 bacilli or more), so the organisms must multiply extensively in the food before it is ingested. All species invade the intestinal mucosa, being taken up by epithelial cells in the manner described for *S. typhi*, but, unlike the latter, the infection is usually confined to the intestine and organisms reaching extraintestinal sites are phagocytosed and killed. This can be attributed to their lack of Vi antigen, and consequent inability to resist macrophage killing. Occasionally, however, septicaemia and focal infection in different tissues occurs (below).

In response to local damage, an acute inflammatory response occurs in the ileum and caecum, sometimes with ulceration, and leads to diarrhoea, abdominal pain, vomiting and fever; diarrhoea is the main feature and varies from the slight to the violent. These symptoms usually occur about 12–24 hours after ingestion of the contaminated food. The stools, which may contain neutrophils, mucus and blood, are often watery, and dehydration and electrolyte imbalance can be serious in the very young or the elderly. Three key events are responsible for the diarrhoea, namely: (i) invasion of the intestinal mucosa, (ii) a local acute inflammatory response, and (iii) secretion of fluid and electrolytes

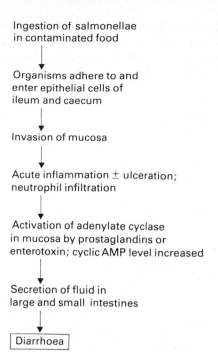

Figure 4.56 Pathogenesis of salmonella food poisoning.

Ingestion of salmonellae
in contaminated food

↓

Organisms adhere to and
enter epithelial cells of
ileum and caecum

↓

Invasion of mucosa

↓

Acute inflammation ± ulceration;
neutrophil infiltration

↓

Activation of adenylate cyclase
in mucosa by prostaglandins or
enterotoxin; cyclic AMP level increased

↓

Secretion of fluid in
large and small intestines

↓

Diarrhoea

following activation of mucosal adenylate cyclase (Figure 4.56). Thus, only invasive salmonellae are associated with gastro-enteritis, and suppression of the inflammatory response prevents secretion of water into the intestine. The activation of adenylate cyclase is very reminiscent of the action of cholera toxin and *E. coli* LT, but the role of a similar enterotoxin in salmonella diarrhoea is not established (p. 554). Instead, it has been suggested that intestinal ulcers or other sites of inflammation release or cause production of *prostaglandins*, which are known to be powerful activators of adenylate cyclase. The resulting rise in cyclic AMP would then induce secretion of water and electrolytes as described elsewhere (p. 421).

In most cases, gastroenteritis lasts for 2–5 days and is self-limiting; in uncomplicated infection, antibiotics are not used as they do not shorten the illness, but rather prolong faecal excretion of organisms and may select resistant strains. Following recovery, individuals may continue to excrete salmonellae for several weeks and act as a source of infection. However, a chronic carrier state lasting over a year is much less common (~ 0.1%) than for *S. typhi* (~ 3%).

Transmission. These salmonelloses are *zoonoses* (i.e. the major route of transmission is from animals to man) and the animal reservoir is enormous: besides the domestic species regularly utilised as food by man, many other wild and domestic animals harbour infection—for example, rats and mice commonly carry salmonellae and may contaminate food with their faeces. The fact that *S. typhimurium* is a primary pathogen in a wide variety of animals has led to it being the commonest food poisoning organism in Europe and the USA. The organisms usually cause a typhoid-like disease in their natural animal hosts, but almost always only a localised gastroenteritis in man. The main vehicles of transmission to man are poultry and meat which have been inadequately cooked or refrigerated. Contaminated poultry (chicken, ducks, turkeys) and poultry products are the largest single source in the UK and USA; salmonellae are also often present in egg products, especially those imported, such as dried or frozen whole egg and frozen egg whites, huge quantities of which are used in the bakery trade. In England and Wales, liquid egg is now pasteurised to destroy salmonellae, by a method similar to that used for milk. Salmonellae may be introduced into meat in abattoirs, since cross-contamination of healthy animal carcasses can occur from intestinal contents of an infected animal killed at the same time, with subsequent multiplication. Efforts are being made to reduce salmonellosis in livestock and poultry by improving conditions on farms, animal transporters and abattoirs. In Denmark, all animal feeds are heat-treated to kill salmonellae before distribution and this has significantly reduced infection. In the USA, pet turtles were a major cause of human salmonellosis in the early 1970's, causing an estimated 300,000 cases annually. As a result, many states now ban the sale of turtles or require that they be certified as salmonella-free.

Note that the infection of food is not in itself sufficient to cause salmonella food poisoning: the food must be moist and stored under conditions promoting bacterial growth (24 hours in a warm area or several days in a cool larder) and not subjected to thorough cooking. The latter is especially easy with chilled solid food through which heat may take a considerable time to penetrate. An important precaution is that raw food, which may be contaminated, should never have contact with cooked food, a situation which is very likely to occur in domestic refrigerators.

SEPTICAEMIAS

Salmonellae may cause septicaemia with or without evidence of gastrointestinal infection, from where it presumably originates, and the organisms may not be isolable from faeces. *S. cholerae-suis* can cause prolonged septicaemia with foci of suppuration in several organs including the biliary tract, kidneys, heart, spleen, joints and meninges. It is a common cause of osteomyelitis in children with sickle-cell anaemia (p. 863) or Gaucher's disease (p. 856). As its name implies, *S. cholerae-suis* is often acquired from contaminated pork. Other salmonellae which cause septi-caemia are *S. paratyphi C* and recently *S. napoli*. *S. typhimurium*, which normally causes food poisoning, may rarely cause septi-caemia. Septicaemia due to salmonellae is rare in the UK.

VIBRIO

Vibrio cholerae is the agent of cholera, one of the major tropical diseases and historically among the most feared. Endemic for centuries in the Indian subcontinent and today widespread in S.E. Asia and Africa, it is estimated that in India alone the death toll through cholera in this century exceeds 20 million. In the past, cholera was by no means confined to the tropics, but spread throughout the world where conditions of poverty, overcrowding and bad sanitation allowed; the infection is transmitted, like typhoid, principally in faecally-contaminated water. During the course of one such epidemic in Egypt in 1883 the German bacteriologist Robert Koch was the first to isolate the causative agent, which he termed the 'Kommabacillus' from its slightly curved microscopic appearance. Other vibrios are associated with *food poisoning*, particularly in Japan where they are acquired from raw or undercooked seafood (*V. parahaemolyticus*), or occasionally with wound infection and fatal septicaemia (*V. vulnificus*).

Vibrio cholerae

HISTORY AND NATURE OF CHOLERA

Since 1817 there have been seven great pandemics of cholera, spreading from the endemic areas in the delta of the Ganges and lower Bengal, to China, the Philippines and Japan in the east and Africa, Russia, Europe and North America in the west. In the nineteenth century, the infection reached Europe on several occasions by overland routes, sometimes carried by pilgrims returning from Mecca. It was spread to the USA in the late 1860's, while in England it decimated the populations of overcrowded towns and cities. In the 1890's, European Russia was mostly affected, while in the early part of this century another great pandemic spread from India to China and the Philippines and thence to Europe by 1908–10. During the 1950's, cholera was confined to its traditional endemic area, the Bengal region of India and Bangladesh, but in 1961 the most recent pandemic occurred due to a strain of *V. cholerae* known as the *El Tor biotype*, distinguishable from the 'classical' cholera vibrio but causing the same disease. This pandemic originated in Indonesia, spreading extensively in the Far East, then through Indo-China and Thailand to India, West Pakistan, the Middle East and many African countries. By 1970–71, it was reported in over 40 countries in Africa and Asia; it even reached Europe (Portugal, Spain, France), N. America and Japan, though limited by good sanitation in these countries. Several cases were reported in Texas in 1981.

Clinically, cholera is an acute, life-threatening illness with uncontrollable watery diarrhoea and vomiting, in which an untreated patient rapidly loses huge amounts of water and electrolytes; during epidemics, 50% of patients may die through the effects of dehydration (hypovolaemic shock). Man is the only host and transmission is by water or food contaminated with faeces of infected individuals. The cholera vibrio, unlike shigellae and salmonellae, does not invade the intestine, but merely colonises its surface; diarrhoea is due solely to production of the powerful cholera enterotoxin, which stimulates the intestinal epithelium to secrete water and electrolytes (p. 420).

Vibrios are short, Gram-negative, highly motile rods, characteristically 'comma-shaped' on initial isolation (they revert to straight forms on repeated laboratory subculture). Their motility is due to a single, thick, polar flagellum (Figure 4.2h). They are facultative anaerobes which grow rapidly in simple media. Vibrios are extremely sensitive to acid pH (<pH6) and grow best at pH7; however, they tolerate alkaline conditions which kill enterobacteria, a property utilised in selective media. The organisms are oxidase-positive (cf. enterobacteria), ferment sucrose and mannose, but not arabinose, and produce acid but not gas. Outside the human body, *V. cholerae* dies in fresh water and is killed by chlorination, but survives for several days in water that is slightly dirty or polluted.

Vibrios causing epidemic cholera can be divided into two *biotypes* (i.e. on the basis of biochemical rather than serological differences) known as *classical* and *El Tor*. The classical type was the one isolated by Koch and responsible for most occurrences of cholera until 1961. The El Tor biotype was first isolated in 1900 at a quarantine station of that name in Sinai from pilgrims bound for Mecca, and differed from classical *V. cholerae* in producing a haemolysin for goat and sheep red cells. At that time, El Tor organisms were not associated with disease, but in 1961 they suddenly became the dominant choleragenic type in Hong Kong and over the next few years spread worldwide as described above, displacing the classical biotype in India and elsewhere. Most El Tor species are now no longer haemolytic, but there are other differentiative tests; for example, only El Tor has a cell-associated haemagglutinin for chicken red cells, inhibitable by mannose and readily detected in a rapid slide test, and most El Tor strains are resistant to polymyxin and phage IV, to which the classical strains are sensitive. While both biotypes cause an identical disease, El Tor is rather less virulent, due to lower production of enterotoxin, and gives rise to a large number of asymptomatic (subclinical) infections.

Serological classification of *V. cholerae* is much simpler than most other Gram-negative bacteria. Somatic O antigens divide vibrios into six groups, of which the cholera organisms are group 1. Each biotype exists in two major serotypes, called Inaba and Ogawa, identified by O antigens called A, B and C: Inaba is A,B and Ogawa A,C. There is a third rare serotype, Hikojima, which is A,B,C (Figure 4.57). The organisms share common flagellar

Figure 4.57 Classification of *Vibrio cholerae.*

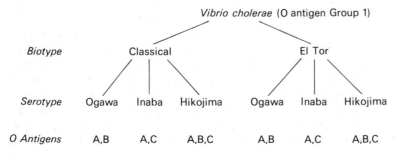

antigens. Vibrios that are biochemically similar to the epidemic strains of *V. cholerae* but do not agglutinate in O-group 1 antiserum have been referred to in the past as *non-agglutinable vibrios* (NAGs) or as *non-cholera vibrios* (NCVs). The former term is something of a misnomer, as they are agglutinated by antisera directed specifically against them. They are best referred to as non-O group 1 (non-O 1) *V. cholerae*. They have caused outbreaks and sporadic cases of gastrointestinal illness, far less severe than true cholera, and occasionally extraintestinal disease, generally by production of an enterotoxin very similar to cholera toxin itself. These strains are widely distributed in Europe, Asia and the USA in sewage, contaminated water, estuaries, seafood and animals.

STRUCTURAL AND SOLUBLE DETERMINANTS OF VIBRIO PATHOGENICITY

The major factor determining the pathogenicity of *V. cholerae* is its production of *enterotoxin* (p. 420); atypical O Group 1 organisms which lack the toxin genes have been isolated and are non-enteropathogenic. *V. parahaemolyticus*, which gives rise to cholera-like watery diarrhoea, produces a heat-stable haemolysin (*Kanagawa haemolysin*) which is associated with pathogenicity, all food poisoning strains being haemolysin positive. In high doses, the isolated haemolysin is cytotoxic, cardiotoxic and lethal, and produces degenerative changes in the intestinal mucosa. In order to cause disease, *V. cholerae* must adhere to the small intestine, but the bacterial molecules involved in adherence have not been defined: no pili or surface structures other than the flagellum are visible by electron microscopy. *Motility* may well be important in helping the organisms to penetrate intestinal mucus, as non-motile varieties do not succeed in attaching to the epithelium; enzymes such as *neuraminidase* and *proteinases* which degrade mucus are also produced to this end (*V. cholerae* neuraminidase is the 'receptor destroying enzyme' for influenza-virus, p. 320).

CHOLERA

Pathogenesis

Cholera is a secretory, non-inflammatory diarrhoeal illness in which cholera vibrios stimulate profuse watery diarrhoea by means of their enterotoxin (choleragen). The secretory nature of the diarrhoea is demonstrable experimentally *in vivo* in rabbit isolated ileal loops inoculated either with the vibrios themselves or with the enterotoxin, as described on p. 420. Unlike shigellae and salmonellae, cholera vibrios are not invasive and do not enter or destroy the intestinal epithelium; hence there is no pus or blood in the stool as in dysentery, nor any indication of acute inflammation in the mucosa. The diarrhoea fluid is not an inflammatory exudate and has a low protein content. The mechanism of action of cholera toxin is described elsewhere (p. 421). Diarrhoea occurs when the water-absorptive capacity of the large intestine is exceeded. Normally, of the 8–10 litres of water which enter the gut each day in the form of ingested liquid and alimentary secretions, 90% is absorbed in the small intestine and less than a litre passes into the caecum. Passage through the caecum, colon and rectum removes all but the remaining 100 ml or so which remains in the faeces daily, but 4–5 litres could probably be absorbed in the large intestine if necessary. This capacity is greatly exceeded in cholera, where the volume of fluid lost may be more than 20 litres in a single day (though usually much less).

In order to colonise the small intestine, cholera vibrios must first negotiate the stomach, and as we have already noted they are acid sensitive. The infective dose in healthy American volunteers has been found to be very large, with up to 10^{11} vibrios having little effect when ingested in water, the vast majority being killed in the stomach. Neutralisation of gastric acidity with bicarbonate reduces the number of organisms required by several orders of magnitude to about 10^4. While the stomach is an important and efficient barrier to vibrios present in water, organisms entering with food are relatively protected and more likely to be infective. Moreover, individuals who are naturally hypochlorhydric are the most liable to contract cholera.

Once in the small intestine, the organisms adhere to the brush border (microvilli) of epithelial cells (Figure 4.58); the nature of the intestinal receptors for vibrios has not been defined. Enterotoxin production follows rapidly and the incubation period is usually less than 3 days and may be as short as 24 hours. Hypersecretion by enterocytes of sodium, potassium, chloride and bicarbonate ions, with accompanying water, leads to the voluminous, isotonic diarrhoea. The faeces are watery and pale, with flakes of mucus floating in them, resembling the fluid of boiled rice ('rice-water' stools). They contain up to 10^8 organisms per ml, so a patient may shed up to 2×10^{12} vibrios daily; hence diarrhoea is the organism's means of ensuring its own distribution. The diarrhoea is accompanied by vomiting, but there is no pain, nausea or fever. The faeces contain the same Na^+ concentration as serum, but twice the HCO_3^- and five times the K^+; thus metabolic acidosis and hypokalaemia develop. Severe water and electrolyte depletion lead to intense thirst, oliguria (decreased urinary output), painful muscular cramps, weakness, and a shrunken appearance with sunken eyes and wrinkled skin.

Massive fluid and electrolyte loss has several systemic consequences: the fall in blood volume, and consequently in cardiac output and blood pressure, leads to a condition of *hypovolaemic shock*; the blood proteins and cells become more concentrated, with increased blood viscosity (haemoconcentration); urine may cease altogether (anuria) with renal failure and uraemia; acidosis and severe K^+ depletion lead to circulatory collapse and stupor. In untreated cases, death occurs in a few days, or the patient recovers within a similar period (3–6 days). In untreated outbreaks or epidemics there is often a greater than 50% mortality, but this is reduced to less than 1% by prompt and adequate replacement of water and electrolytes.

564

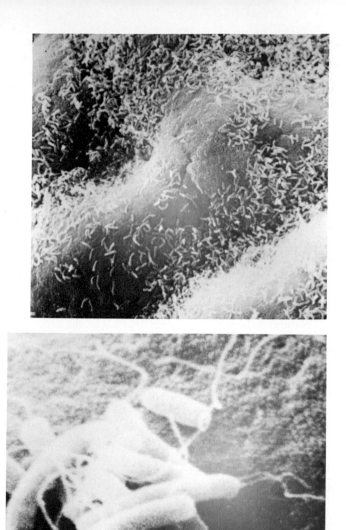

(a)

(b)

Figure 4.58 Colonisation of the
intestinal surface by *Vibrio
cholerae* in experimental rabbit
ileal loops.
(a) Scanning electron microscopy
showing vibrios adhering to the
epithelial surface (× 3000).
(b) Higher magnification of
vibrios close to the tips of
microvilli. Each cell has a single
polar flagellum.
(c) Transmission electron
micrograph of vibrios adhering to
the tips of microvilli.
(From Nelson, Clements and
Finkelstein (1976) *Infect.
Immunol.*, **14**, 527.)

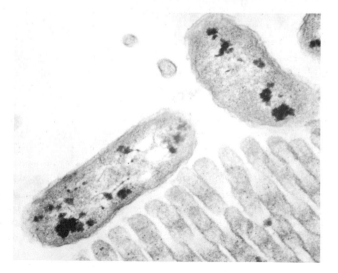

(c)

Treatment

Until recently this consisted of intravenous replacement of an amount of fluid and electrolytes equivalent to that lost, the patient's fluid loss being measured in graduated buckets underneath an appropriate hole in the hospital bed. However, absorption of fluids through the gut can occur efficiently in the presence of *glucose* (p. 422) and current practice is therefore oral administration of solutions containing NaCl, KCl, NaHCO$_3$ and glucose. Almost all cholera patents can be maintained in this way until they recover and the WHO and UNICEF distribute packets of the salts and glucose to be made up in water as required. Prompt and adequate fluid replacement is life-saving in almost all cases. Tetracyclines are adjuncts to this treatment but are not a substitute for fluid/electrolyte replacement, which is essential; the antibiotics are useful as they shorten the period of diarrhoea. Pharmacological agents which suppress cholera diarrhoea, notably chlorpromazine and nicotinic acid, may become useful in treatment.

Natural recovery from cholera depends on the development of antibodies (IgA) against the organisms and the enterotoxin, and the regeneration of normal intestinal epithelium (convalescent patients may continue to excrete vibrios for a time). Immunity, which lasts at least three years, follows recovery and is due to intestinal IgA, which prevents binding both of organisms and toxin to the mucosa. Because intestinal immunity is effective and long-term, most of the patients during outbreaks in areas of endemic infection are children, whereas in epidemics in newly-infected regions cholera most frequently affects adults.

It is important to note that infection with *V. cholerae* does not necessarily lead to cholera—indeed, the El Tor biotype establishes a large number of asymptomatic infections which may outnumber clinical cases by from 10:1 to 100:1, a much higher ratio than in classical cholera infections. *Symptomless carriers* excrete organisms in their faeces and are an important element in the rapid spread of the El Tor strains; the carrier state induces immunity. Factors such as stomach pH, the size of the infecting dose, its volume and whether it is ingested in food, are all significant in determining whether illness will occur and if so its severity. Although rare, a long-term carrier state may be established, with vibrios surviving in the gallbladder (cf. typhoid bacilli). A classical case was 'cholera Dolores' in the Philippines, who harboured vibrios for 12 years (1962–73); however unlike Typhoid Mary, she did not act as a source of dissemination.

Diagnosis

Diagnosis can be quickly achieved by direct bright or dark-field microscopic examination of the liquid stool for rapidly moving bacteria. Addition of a drop of specific anti-*V. cholerae* O group I serum inhibits motility. The presence of *V. cholerae* in stools or rectal swabs can also be confirmed by immunofluorescent staining with anti-O serum.

Transmission

As with typhoid fever, man is the only host of the cholera vibrio and transmission is therefore by ingestion of water or food contaminated by faeces of patients or carriers. Water is the main vehicle and infection usually occurs by drinking; cholera is therefore basically a disease of poor sanitation. Spread also occurs via contaminated milk, cold cooked foods, vegetables sprinkled with water, and uncooked fruit, or directly from faeces and vomit. The vibrios survive for a few days in water, but do not multiply, so constant reinfection from patents or carriers must occur. Obviously the introduction of safe drinking water, through adequate sewage treatment and water purification, would go a considerable way towards controlling the disease, but this is only a long-term prospect in the underdeveloped parts of the world in which it is endemic or likely to be epidemic. (In London in 1854, John Snow halted an epidemic merely by removing the handle of the Broad Street pump—a contaminated water supply—a demonstration, if one were needed, that an advanced theoretical knowledge may be quite unnecessary in preventing a disease.)

Vaccination

Vaccination may provide the best short-term prospect of cholera control. However, the traditional vaccine of killed organisms administered parenterally gives little protection to individuals who have never been exposed to cholera, though it does restimulate existing immunity. Similarly, injection of a cholera toxoid has been shown in controlled studies to be an ineffective means of vaccination. Efforts to produce an oral vaccine using live avirulent variants have been described on p. 425.

Vibrio parahaemolyticus

This organism was first recognised as a cause of food-borne diarrhoeal illness in Japan in the early 1950's and in recent years has become an important agent of *food poisoning* in many parts of the world, including the UK and USA; in Japan itself, *V. parahaemolyticus* is responsible for about 50% of all such cases. It is a marine organism, common in estuaries, which resembles *V. cholerae* in most respects, but with an additional growth requirement of 2% NaCl (a halophytic or salt-loving organism). Under appropriate conditions, it grows extremely rapidly with a generation time of only 9–15 minutes, an important factor in production of gastroenteritis. It is transmitted exclusively in seafood, primarily that eaten raw or inadequately cooked; it is therefore not surprising that it is such a hazard in Japan, where raw fish is a national dish.

The clinical syndrome generally occurs some 15 hours after ingestion, as an explosive, watery, cholera-like diarrhoea, free of blood or mucus, with abdominal cramps, vomiting and fever. However, a shigella-like dysenteric disease due to this organism has also been reported in Japan, Australia and India, and it seems that it has a greater invasive tendency than *V. cholerae*. Despite intensive study, the pathogenic mechanisms are not known. There is as yet very little evidence for a cholera-like enterotoxin; thus *V. parahaemolyticus* produces inflammation rather than outpouring of fluid in the rabbit ileal loop, and culture filtrates do not induce morphological changes or steroidogenesis in Y-1 adrenal cells (p. 420). However, it has been reported that a labile factor produced a reaction in Chinese hamster ovary cells similar to that of cholera toxin. As noted on p. 563, only strains producing the Kanagawa haemolysin are enteropathogenic, though the mechanism responsible for this relationship is also unknown.

Food poisoning due to *V. parahaemolyticus* is predominantly a summertime disease, reflecting the prevalence of the organisms and the opportunity for rapid multiplication in non-refrigerated food. Two simple measures reduce its incidence, namely adequate refrigeration of seafood eaten raw (growth of the organisms being inhibited below 15°C) and adequate cooking (since they are destroyed at 65°C).

PSEUDOMONAS

This is a large genus of over 140 species, naturally inhabiting soil and water; while the majority are non-pathogenic in man or animals, *Pseudomonas aeruginosa* (*P. pyocanea*) is one of the most important and versatile *opportunistic pathogens* of man. While it seldom causes disease in healthy individuals, *P. aeruginosa* is a major cause of infection under conditions of impaired host or tissue resistance and is often acquired in hospitals. Indeed, some 20% of nosocomial infections may be due to this organism and it is a common cause of Gram-negative septicaemias, which have a particularly high mortality. It is included here to illustrate the many varieties of opportunistic infection.

MORPHOLOGY, GROWTH, ETC.

P. aeruginosa is an ubiquitous free-living organism, very often found in moist environments. It is a motile Gram-negative rod, usually with a single polar flagellum (occasional strains have two or three flagella). The cell wall resembles that of enterobacteria and contains endotoxin, though of a less toxic nature than in other Gram-negative bacilli. The organisms are often surrounded by a type-specific polysaccharide slime layer which is antiphagocytic, and strains isolated from clinical infections usually possess pili, which may also be antiphagocytic as well as promoting adherence to cell surfaces. In terms of growth requirements, it is a particularly adaptable species which can utilise over 80 different organic compounds and can use ammonia as nitrogen source. Energy is derived solely from *aerobic*, non-fermentative respiration and they are the only Gram-negative bacilli to give a rapid oxidase reaction (cf. neisseriae). Colonies are greenish-blue due to characteristic production of pigments, including *pyocyanin* (a blue-green phenazine pigment) and *fluorescein*; the latter shows green fluorescence, with the result that colonies of *P. aeruginosa* and wounds infected with the organism fluoresce under u.v. light. One of the pigments functions in iron uptake by the organisms. All strains are haemolytic on blood agar plates. There are several typing systems—serology, phage-sensitivity, and the specificity of the bactericidal action of pseudomonas bacteriocins called pyocins; 105 pyocin types of *P. aeruginosa* are now recognised.

An important property of *P. aeruginosa* is its innate resistance to salts, dyes, chemical disinfectants, antiseptics, hexachlorophene soaps and many of the commonly used antibiotics; it even multiplies in dilute disinfectants. This resistance together with nutritional versatility explains its ubiquitous distribution in hospitals: when provided with adequate moisture it can survive in respirators and humidifiers and on medical instruments, bedpans, taps, floors, baths and mops, as well as being constantly introduced from the outside on fruit, vegetables, cut flowers and plants. Among the agents which kill it are phenolic disinfectants, boiling water and complete dessication. Due to its resistance, *P. aeruginosa* often becomes dominant as a commensal and in lesions when other organisms are suppressed by antimicrobial treatment; it was therefore selected in hospitals with the introduction of broad-spectrum antibiotics. Antibiotic resistance of the species is at least partly due to transferable R plasmids.

STRUCTURE, PRODUCTS AND PATHOGENICITY

The pathogenicity of *P. aeruginosa* derives both from its invasive properties and its toxigenicity. It is an extracellular organism and, like the pyogenic cocci, its invasiveness depends on antiphago-cytic devices to prevent uptake by neutrophils. The properties of the slime polysaccharide and surface pili have already been mentioned. Large amounts of extracellular polysaccharide are produced by strains which cause chronic lung infection in children with cystic fibrosis, for whom *P. aeruginosa* is a major hazard. Strains causing pulmonary infection also produce a glycolipid haemolysin which is toxic for alveolar macrophages. A second haemolysin, a *phospholipase C*, may contribute to invasiveness in the lung by destroying pulmonary surfactant and attacking lung tissue. A few strains secrete a thermolabile *leucocidin* which kills neutrophils and lymphocytes without being haemolytic; this is highly toxic in mice, but is unlikely to be a major factor as it is only produced by some 5% of isolates.

Having secured its extracellular survival, *P. aeruginosa* produces at least three other exotoxins (A, B and C) of which *toxin A* is the most potent and best studied. Its molecular action is to inhibit protein synthesis and we have noted elsewhere its striking similarity to diphtheria toxin (p. 419). It is toxic to animals and cultured cells, and under experimental conditions in mice its main action seems to be on the liver, causing cellular swelling, fatty change and necrosis; it does not affect neutrophil phagocytosis, nor does it cause skin necrosis. The lethal dose for a mouse is about 0.2 μg. Its part in human disease is not well defined, but the fact that most patients who survive *P. aeruginosa* septicaemia have elevated levels of antibodies to toxin A, or are infected with strains which produce little or no toxin A *in vitro*, suggests a significant pathogenic role. Moreover, mutant strains deficient in toxin A are less virulent in several animal models than their toxin-producing counterparts. An *enterotoxin* has been discovered recently in connection with diarrhoea due to intestinal infection by *P. aeruginosa*. *Endotoxin* is important in septic shock, often the outcome of pseudomonas septicaemia.

Many strains of *P. aeruginosa* produce extracellular *proteases*, at least one of which can digest the elastin component of connective tissue; they may assist in tissue invasion and probably contribute to the tissue destruction which accompanies infections in the skin, eye and lung. Thus, in animals, injection of proteases into the relevant local sites induces haemorrhagic lesions in the skin, corneal destruction and lung damage. Other adjuncts to the invasiveness of this organism are products which prevent the growth of competing bacteria, including the pyocyanin pigment and pyocins.

While *P. aeruginosa* possesses a range of attributes which are relevant to its potential pathogenicity, they are evidently not sufficient to overcome the defensive barriers and mechanisms of a healthy body. As is the case for other extracellular organisms, host resistance, once natural barriers have been traversed, depends on phagocytosis by neutrophils in conjunction with opsonising antibodies. Thus it is not too surprising that clinical conditions which prejudice the efficiency of phagocytosis, such as reduction in the numbers of circulating neutrophils (neutropenia) and deficiencies in antibody production, predispose to infection by *P. aeruginosa*. Conversely, impaired cell-mediated responses, as in Hodgkin's disease and inherited thymic deficiencies, do not generally lead to susceptibility.

OPPORTUNISTIC INFECTIONS BY *P. AERUGINOSA*

The organism causes a wide variety of diseases affecting almost any tissue or body site. They are a catalogue of opportunistic infection, following destruction or circumvention of normal tissue barriers, reduced tissue resistance or generalised deficiency in host immunity. As already noted, *P. aeruginosa* is most commonly pathogenic in hospitalised patients, for obvious reasons. Although it is present as a commensal in the stools of about 10% of healthy individuals and sporadically on the skin, the incidence of silent infection (carrier rate) rises sharply to around 30% within 72 hours of admission to hospital and up to 40% of all hospital in-patients are infected during their stay at some time or other. Spread may be airborne, but patient-to-patient transmission via the hands of hospital personnel is probably more significant in a hospital unit; contaminated instruments, catheters, respirators and even soap are vehicles for transmission. Infections may be localised in burns or wounds, in the eye, urinary tract or lungs, or may invade the bloodstream, causing a dangerous septicaemia. The latter occurs especially in older or debilitated patients, or those treated with immunosuppressive drugs, etc. The mortality associated with septicaemia can be as high as 80%, with death often due to septic shock (p. 445). While most *P. aeruginosa* infections arise from exogenous sources, some may be endogenous. The following are representative examples.

(i) Infection of burns and other wounds by *P. aeruginosa* is particularly common and up to 30% of infections in burn units are due to this organism; septicaemia often follows.

(ii) Urinary tract infections occur through introduction of the organisms on infected catheters or in irrigating solutions.

(iii) The lungs of patients with *cystic fibrosis* are often chronically infected with *P. aeruginosa*, which has replaced *Staph. aureus* as the major pathogen in such cases. Chronic bronchitis, bronchiectasis (p. 518) and pneumonia result and may be ultimately fatal. The organisms grow in the thick respiratory mucus secretions. Interestingly, the patients have high levels of circulating antibodies which, though unable to clear the organisms from the lungs, prevent them from invading the bloodstream and causing septicaemia. The strains involved secrete large amounts of extracellular slime polysaccharide which inhibits phagocytosis; they form mucoid colonies on agar due to slime production.

(iv) Pneumonia due to *P. aeruginosa* is also common in patients receiving mechanical ventilation, the source of infection being contamination of the respirators; the apparatus must be carefully monitored and cleaned to avoid this problem. Pneumonia also often leads to septicaemia. Infection of tracheostomy wounds, sometimes spreading to the lungs, is an important problem in intensive care units.

(v) Severe corneal infections, which may result in loss of the eye, follow eye surgery (postoperative ophthalmitis) or injury. Infection may be due to contaminated eye drops or contact lenses. As noted above, corneal damage is a result of protease production by *P. aeruginosa*.

(vi) Middle ear infections due to *P. aeruginosa* have been troublesome in divers engaged in oil explorations in the North Sea.

(vii) Due to their immunological immaturity, babies are targets of opportunistic infection and sporadic cases or larger outbreaks of infection with *P. aeruginosa* occur among newborns and young infants in maternity units and paediatric wards.

(viii) Children with primary (inherited) immunodeficiency involving B cells, such as Bruton-type agammaglobulinaemia, are very susceptible to infection with extracellular pathogens including *P. aeruginosa* (pneumonia and septicaemia).

(ix) The deficiencies in host defence which occur in cancer patients, either due to the disease itself or to therapeutic measures, predispose to septicaemic infection with *P. aeruginosa*.

Mortality is highest in severely neutropenic patients. Neutropenia (diminished production of granulocytes in the bone marrow) occurs particularly in acute leukaemia, myeloma and secondary bone marrow tumours. Irradiation, antimetabolites and other cytotoxic agents used in cancer therapy also cause neutropenia or even agranulocytosis (no circulating granulocytes). Suppression of antibody responses also occurs through the use of these agents and corticosteroids, and in patients with lymphoid neoplasms.

Treatment

Treatment is rendered difficult by the resistance of *P. aeruginosa* to most antimicrobial agents. A combination of an aminoglycoside antibiotic such as gentamicin, together with carbenicillin (a penicillin) is often used to treat severe, life-threatening infections, e.g. in patients with leucopenia. Vaccines are being developed and this is especially important in view of the high mortality associated with septicaemia in burns victims. In trials with a heptavalent vaccine preparation (Pseudogen), mortality was reduced from 15% to 3%. The vaccine has also been used to raise human antibodies (hyperimmune gamma globulin) for use in passive immunisation, and clinical trials suggest that the latter is valuable in treating immunosuppressed patients and others suffering from pseudomonas infection. Passive immunisation may be used alone or in conjunction with vaccination. As yet, however, these methods are not in general use.

CORYNEBACTERIUM

Until the end of the Second World War, *diphtheria* was one of the major life-threatening epidemic diseases of childhood and was prevalent throughout the world; it was common in Europe and the USA and exacted a heavy toll of death. During the war itself, the annual incidence in mainland Europe was estimated at 600,000 cases, with total deaths at 150,000, many of them in Germany (in the UK during this period, deaths fell from 2,390 in 1941 to 584 in 1945). The 1950's saw a dramatic downturn in the incidence of diphtheria: the number of cases fell to a low level and deaths became a rarity in most developed countries. In 1976, just two cases were notified in England and 128 in the USA (though outbreaks still occur in many countries). This near disappearance of a once common disease was solely the result of widespread immunisation (with toxoid) which became routine for all infants after the war. Its great effectiveness is due to the fact that antibodies against diphtheria toxin provide complete protection from the disease. Diphtheria is the prototype of an illness caused by a powerful toxin. The organism, *Corynebacterium diphtheriae*, settles in the throat where it establishes a local infection and secretes its potent exotoxin; the latter is absorbed by the lymphatics and distributed by the bloodstream, causing lesions in organs with a high blood supply and thus often death through heart failure. The action of diphtheria toxin is described on p. 414.

Diphtheria occupies an important place in the history of bacteriology and immunology. Following the discovery of the toxin by Roux and Yersin in 1888, von Behring and Kitasato showed that the serum of animals injected with sublethal doses of diphtheria or tetanus toxins contained agents—antitoxins—which specifically neutralised the toxins and protected animals against them. This was one of the first clear demonstrations of antibody formation. The therapeutic value of antitoxin was quickly recognised by Ehrlich and on Christmas night, 1891, a diphtheria patient was successfully treated for the first time by *passive immunisation*, which to this day remains the only effective treatment for the disease. Subsequently, it was discovered (Ramon, 1923) that diphtheria toxin could be inactivated by formaldehyde yet retain its antigenicity, opening the way to *active immunisation* against diptheria and tetanus with the respective toxoids.

Corynebacteria, though not acid-fast, are structurally related to the mycobacteria and nocardiae (the CMN group); all three genera have mycolic acids and arabinogalactan in their cell walls (p. 397) and the peptidoglycan contains meso-diaminopimelic acid (meso-DAP). *C. diphtheriae* is the only major human pathogen among the corynebacteria; *C. ulcerans* causes localised ulcerations in the throat and some other species are throat commensals. *C. ovis*, *C. pyogenes*, *C. renale*, etc., cause suppurative lesions in domestic animals.

MORPHOLOGY, GROWTH, IDENTIFICATION

C. diphtheriae is a Gram-positive rod which is non-motile, non-sporing and non-capsulate. In stained smears, the cells characteristically appear as parallel rows (palisades) or sharply angled pairs (V, L) which are likened to Chinese characters and caused by a snapping movement which occurs on cell division (Figure 4.2e). Although uniform in shape when grown on nutritionally complete media, organisms cultured on suboptimal media, such as Loeffler's coagulated serum medium used in primary isolation from patients, are pleomorphic with granular, uneven staining. The typical forms are *club-shaped* (Gk, *koryne*, club), beaded or barred. The beads are metachromatic granules (Babes–Ernst granules), consisting of intracellular deposits of polyphosphates, which stain reddish with methylene blue or toluidine blue.

The organisms are facultative anaerobes growing best aerobically. In addition to Loeffler's medium, media containing *tellurite salts*, which depress the growth of Gram-negative organisms, are used in their identification; on tellurite agar, the colonies have a grey or black colour due to intracellular precipitation of free tellurium. Three types of colony are recognisable, corresponding to the three biotypes of *C. diphtheriae*, namely *gravis*, *intermedius* and *mitis*; to a certain extent they can be correlated with the severity of the disease, gravis being the most virulent and mitis the least, determined by the amount of toxin each produces. However, there is no constant relationship between colonial morphology and clinical severity. Serotypes, bacteriophage types and bacteriocin types can be distinguished within each biotype.

Only strains of *C. diphtheriae* which produce diphtheria toxin are virulent; demonstrating the toxigenicity of an isolate is therefore an important part of diagnosis. Both *in vitro* and *in vivo* tests for this are used. The former involves immunoprecipitation in gel between toxin and horse antitoxin antibody (Elek test) as illustrated in Figure 4.59. Heavy inocula of the organisms under test are streaked across the surface of agar medium on a Petri dish, and a strip of filter paper soaked in specific horse antitoxin is placed across the plate at right angles to the streaks. (The antiserum is preabsorbed with corynebacterial non-toxin proteins to ensure specificity for toxin.) The plates are incubated and, if the organisms produce toxin, a line of precipitation (toxin–antitoxin) forms at an angle of 45° to the streak; its identity can be confirmed by using a reference toxigenic strain (Park Williams no. 8, PW8) as a neighbouring streak—the precipitin lines from the two inocula should meet and form a continous arch. The particular appearance of the precipitin line occurs because the toxin (antigen) diffuses into the gel at right angles to the streaked inoculum and meets the antitoxin diffusing similarly at right angles to the filter paper; the precipitate forms at optimal proportions, and since precipitates with horse antisera characteristically dissolve in antibody excess, the line starts at a certain distance from the filter paper (see also p. 128).

Figure 4.59 Elek gel diffusion test for detection of toxin-producing *Corynebacterium diphtheriae*.
PW8 = Park Williams no. 8 strain

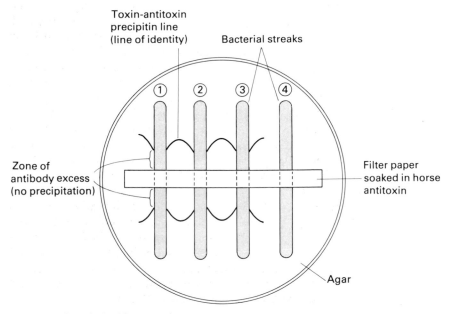

Toxin-antitoxin
precipitin line
(line of identity)   Bacterial streaks

Zone of
antibody excess
(no precipitation)

Filter paper
soaked in horse
antitoxin

Agar

Streaks in this example:
① PW8 – toxigenic *C.diphtheriae* reference strain
② Test strain – toxigenic
③ PW8
④ Test strain – non-toxigenic

Toxigenic organisms can also be identified by *in vivo* inoculation into the skin of a guinea-pig or rabbit, and antitoxin is again used. A small amount (0.2 ml) of a 48-hour broth culture of the isolated organisms is injected subcutaneously into a test site on the shaved skin, followed after 5 hours by intraperitoneal or intravenous injection of horse antitoxin; 30 minutes later, a second 0.2 ml aliquot of the culture is injected into another area of skin on the same animal (the control site). The presence of circulating antitoxin can neutralise the second inoculum but is too late to affect the first; thus, if the organisms are toxigenic *C. diphtheriae*, a necrotic ulcerated area appears at the test site after 48–72 hours, while the control site merely develops a pinkish nodule which does not ulcerate.

As noted elsewhere, diphtheria toxin is only produced when the organisms grow under conditions of low iron (Fe^{2+}) concentration. The PW8 strain, which has been used for many years for commercial production of toxin, has a particular ability to grow well in media containing very low levels of iron, when toxin may account for about 5% of bacterial protein. PW8 has the unusual capacity to increase its mass five-fold after depletion of exogenous iron.

STRUCTURE, PRODUCTS AND PATHOGENICITY

The exotoxin is the major factor in the pathogenicity of *C. diphtheriae* and accounts for essentially all the major manifestations of diphtheria. Its structure, genetics of production and mode of action are described exensively on p. 414. It also assists the organism in colonising the pharyngeal mucous membrane by killing phagocytes and tissue cells, but since both toxigenic and avirulent non-toxigenic strains are able to infect the throat, the toxin is evidently not the only factor in local invasion. Two corynebacterial structural components involved are *K antigens*, heat-labile proteins found near the surface of the cell wall, and *cord factor*. The latter is a toxic surface glycolipid composed of characteristic mycolic acids (cornemycolic and corynemycolenic acids) esterified to trehalose (see p. 399). Like that of mycobacteria, the cord factor of corynebacteria inactivates the membranes of mammalian mitochondria. However, the exact contributions of the K antigens and cord factor to invasiveness are not well defined.

In addition, *C. diphtheriae* produces enzymes which help it to utilise mucous secretion, namely neuraminidase and N-acetyl-neuraminate lyase. The former removes NANA (N-acetyl-neuraminic acid) residues from glycoproteins in mucus and on cell surfaces, while the lyase degrades release NANA to pyruvate and N-acteylmannosamine; pyruvate is a ready energy source and hence actively stimulates corynebacterial growth.

PATHOGENESIS OF DIPHTHERIA

Man is the only natural host of *C. diphtheriae* and hence infection is acquired from a patient or carrier, usually by the respiratory route via contaminated airborne droplets or dust. In the days before immunisation, the incidence was highest in the 5–14 year age group (65% of cases), with 20% of cases in children under 4 and 15% over 15 years. Infants are protected for the first 3–6 months by maternal IgG. Diphtheria is normally an infection of the upper respiratory tract, with organisms colonising the mucous membranes of the tonsils and oropharynx, and sometimes extending to the larynx and trachea; cutaneous diphtheria occurs quite commonly in tropical countries as a secondary infection in wounds, open sores or abrasions. The incubation period (1–4 days) is one of the shortest of any bacterial disease. *C. diphtheriae* grows on the epithelial surface and produces its toxin which kills mucosal cells, initiating an inflammatory reaction and a fibrinous and cellular exudation. The exudate clots and adheres tightly to the underlying tissues, forming the so-called 'false membrane' (pseudomembrane), a thick-textured layer, greyish to black in colour, with a characteristic and unforgettable smell (Gk. *diphtheria*, membrane). The membrane consists of fibrin, leucocytes, necrotic epithelium and bacteria; it can be removed only with difficulty, revealing a raw, bleeding surface. It may spread upwards from the pharynx into the nasal passages (nasopharyngeal diphtheria) or downward into the larynx and trachea (laryngeal diphtheria). The nasopharyngeal form is associated with severe toxaemia, and the laryngeal with mechanical obstruction of the airway (croup) and danger of suffocation, necessitating a life-saving tracheotomy. Typically, the cervical lymph nodes swell enormously and, together wih tissue oedema, give the classic 'bullneck' appearance.

The organisms themselves remain in the membrane and epithelium and rarely if ever penetrate the deeper tissues. From their local site, they secrete diphtheria toxin which is carried into the cervical lymph nodes (to cause the bullneck) and then passes to the blood (toxaemia) and causes lesions in a number of organs, the most serious being in heart muscle, the nervous system, kidneys and adrenals. Heart failure is the commonest cause of death, the myocardium showing fatty degeneration; myocardial damage is reversible, however, and if the patient survives recovery is usually complete. The fatality rate in untreated cases is about 20%, being highest for gravis infections. Persons recovered from diphtheria may become carriers, harbouring organisms in the nose or throat for weeks or months.

TREATMENT: PASSIVE IMMUNISATION

Recovery is brought about by development of antitoxin (and antibacterial immunity) and, as we have noted, administration of antitoxin is the sole effective treatment (passive immunisation). Antitoxin neutralises free toxin by preventing it from binding to cells; antibodies cannot 'rescue' cells to which toxin has already bound, so that speedy treatment is essential. Antitoxin is completely effective if given promptly after clinical onset, but if delayed for more than four days is without benefit. Thus, if there is the slightest suspicion of diphtheria, antitoxin must be given immediately. Diagnosis is therefore clinical, and isolation of the organism and demonstration of toxin production are only retrospective confirmation. Diphtheria antitoxin for passive immunisation is raised in horses and serum sickness is therefore a common allergic complication, seen in about 10% of cases (p. 161); anaphylaxis is rare. Serum sickness could be avoided if human antitoxin were available. Antibiotic therapy is useful, but is not a substitute for antitoxin.

PREVENTION: ACTIVE IMMUNISATION

Since 1923, diphtheria *toxoid* has been used in active immunisation (before that date a toxin–antitoxin mixture was used). It is made by treating toxin with 0.3% formaldehyde, which causes cross-linking of lysine and tyrosine residues via methylene bridges. Toxoid does not bind to cell receptors, possesses no ADP-ribosylating activity and cannot be cleaved into A and B fragments; it is thus completely harmless. However, it retains sufficient antigenicity to make an excellent immunising agent, especially in the form of an alum precipitate in which it is normally administered. (alum has an adjuvent effect). Infants receive diphtheria toxoid in combination with tetanus toxoid and pertussis vaccine during the second month of life, followed by several boosters, including one at school entry. The immunising mixture is 'balanced' in terms of dosage of the three components, to avoid a phenomenon of mutual immunological inhibition called 'antigenic competition'.

While national immunisation programmes have been successful in reducing the occurrence of diphtheria to a low level in Western Europe and the USA, there is a constant danger of an outbreak of disease among non-immune groups. One of the effects of immunisation has been to reduce the carrier rate and hence the opportunity for immunity to be induced or reinforced by natural subclinical infection. As a result, an increasing number of adults are without protective immunity and a smaller proportion of newborns receive maternal antitoxin. It is vital to achieve complete cover of the infant population, as the occasional outbreaks show (San Antonio 1970; Montreal 1974; Würzburg 1975; Seattle 1972–5; Bonn, 1976; Lusaka, 1977).

During each outbreak, the immune status of individuals in the community must be assessed and the classical method employed is the *Schick test*, which assesses the presence of circulating antitoxin. It is performed by injecting a standard small amount of purified toxin into the skin of the forearm; in a non-immune individual (or one with a very low titre of circulating antibody), this causes a local inflammatory reaction which becomes maximal within 4–7 days and fades gradually, leaving a brownish pigmentation. A negative reaction indicates immunity to normal conditions of exposure while a positive reaction means an absence of immunity (Table 4.9). However, it is possible for a false-positive reaction to occur as a result of delayed hypersensitivity to the toxin or other proteins, the so-called *pseudo-Schick* reaction. Therefore a control is essential, either in

Table 4.9 Interpretation of the Schick test.

| Individual | Result at each site: | |
	Test	Control
Non-immune/non-allergic	Postive	Negative
Immune/non-allergic	Negative	Negative
Immune/allergic	Pseudopositive	Pseudopositive
Non-immune/allergic	Positive, prolonged	Pseudopositive

Test = toxin
Control = heated toxin or toxoid

the form of toxin which has been inactivated by heating to 60°C for 30 minutes, or in the form of toxoid (in which case it is called the Moloney test); the control is injected into the other forearm. The allergic pseudoreaction, a short-lived erythema, is the result of prior infection with corynebacteria or immunisation with toxoid. An allergic individual who is also immune gives an erythematous (pseudopositive) response which peaks at 24–36 hours and then fades and disappears completely within the next 72 hours; the reaction in the test and control arms is the same. One who is allergic but has little or no circulating antitoxin gives the pseudopositive reaction in the control arm, but a prolonged combined positive reaction in the test arm. Such individuals are immunised very cautiously as a full immunising dose would cause severe local and general reactions (in fact, the Schick test alone is often sufficient to restimulate immune levels of antibody). The Schick test has revealed that between 1 and 2% of the human population cannot produce detectable antitoxin in response to immunising doses of toxoid, and thus remain permanently at risk.

It should be possible to achieve the worldwide eradication of diphtheria by immunisation and, as we have noted, the disease is a rarity in countries where immunisation is practised. However, it remains prevalent in other parts of the world.

CLOSTRIDIUM

Clostridia are Gram-positive, spore-forming anaerobes which include organisms responsible for three life-threatening human diseases: gas gangrene (*Clostridium perfringens* and others), tetanus (*Cl. tetani*) and botulism (*Cl. botulinum*). They are widely distributed in nature both in the soil and as commensals in the intestines of man and animals. Most are saprophytic and play an important role in putrefaction of dead animal and plant matter; the decomposition of animal and human corpses is to a large extent due to organisms such as *Cl. perfringens* which enter the bloodstream and tissues around the time of death.

The pathogenic properties of clostridia are determined by a combination of three attributes. (i) Most species are *obligate anaerobes*, growing only in the almost total absence of oxygen, though a few are aerotolerant and will grow slowly in air at atmospheric pressure. True anaerobes will only grow in an environment which is in a chemically reduced state, i.e. one of low oxidation-reduction (redox) potential; in practice this means both the absence of oxygen and the presence of reducing agents. Molecular oxygen may in fact be lethal for such organisms, probably because they lack enzymes such as superoxide dismutase and catalase which would enable them to dipose of superoxide anions (O_2^-) and hydrogen peroxide, both of which are formed by reaction of oxygen with reduced cofactors and are cytotoxic (see p. 21). As a result, clostridia cause disease only where conditions of low redox potential, including oxygen deficiency, can be met, such as in wounds where the blood supply has been impaired and tissue killed (gas gangrene, tetanus) or after anaerobic growth in food (food poisoning, botulism). (ii) Clostridia form *endospores* which are able to resist adverse physical conditions (including oxygen); the spores survive for long periods in soil, in which they can enter wounds, and resist drying, antiseptics and often heating (p. 407). The last point is important in food poisoning, since normal conditions of cooking may not destroy the spores of *Cl. perfringens* and *Cl. botulinum*. (iii) Powerful *exotoxins* are produced by several species and are central to the pathogenesis of clostridial disease, including the α-toxin of *Cl. perfringens* and neurotoxins of *Cl. tetani* and *Cl. botulinum*. In gas gangrene, α-toxin assists the organisms in spreading through infected tissue and then causes lethal toxaemia, while the clinical effects of tetanus and botulism are entirely due to their neurotoxins. The organisms in gas gangrene are intensely invasive, though generally confined to the local tissue, while botulism is an intoxication in which they need not enter the body at all.

Clostridia often infect wounds and in taking advantage of damaged tissue will be recognised as typical *opportunistic pathogens* (p. 478). Even if they can secure entry, they fail to invade healthy oxygenated tissues (with a normal redox potential) and their spores and vegetative cells can be rapidly disposed of by phagocytes. They only successfully colonise tissues damaged by trauma, ischaemia or other circumstances which, by killing tissue and lowering redox potential, create the conditions necessary for their germination and anaerobic growth.

The major clostridial diseases do not occur as epidemics — there is no person-to-person spread—but are nevertheless important causes of mortality under appropriate circumstances. Thus gas gangrene has historically been responsible for many deaths among wounded soldiers and tetanus is still a leading cause of death in some underdeveloped tropical parts of the world.

Clostridium perfringens

This is the species principally associated with the necrotising, massively damaging infection of wounds known as *gas gangrene* (clostridial myonecrosis). Other species associated with the same condition are *Cl. novyi* and *Cl. septicum*. *Cl. perfringens* (formerly known as *Cl. welchii*) is classified into five types (A, B, C, D and E), each distinguishable by the particular combination of exotoxins it produces (below). *Type A* is the major pathogen in man and is responsible for gas gangrene and food poisoning; the other types are mainly animal pathogens, except for some type C species which cause a more severe variety of food poisoning in man (enteritis necroticans), especially in New Guinea where it is called 'pig-bel'. Type A organisms are also very widespread commensals in the intestinal tracts of animals, while their spores are ubiquitous in soil, dust and air as well as often present on the human skin.

MORPHOLOGY, GROWTH, ETC.

Cl. perfringens is a relatively large, plump Gram-positive rod (1 μm × 2–4 μm) with rounded ends (Figure 4.2i); it is capsulate and non-motile, in which respects it differs from most other clostridia, which are generally non-capsulate and peritrichously flagellated. Spores are formed under natural conditions in the intestines. Although anaerobic, *Cl. perfringens* is more aerotolerant than most anaerobes and will survive and grow under low O_2 tension. It grows rapidly at 37°C and even more so at 45°C, at which temperature the generation time is as brief as ten minutes (a fact relevant to its multiplication in warmed food). Large amounts of gas (CO_2 and H_2) are produced during fermentation.

Three aids which are useful in identification of *Cl. perfringens* are a characteristic pattern of haemolysis on blood agar plates, production of opalescent precipitation in human serum or media containing egg yolk, and 'stormy' fermentation of milk media. (i) On blood agar plates, its colonies are typically surrounded by a double zone of haemolysis, an immediate narrow region of complete lysis and a wider one of incomplete haemolysis. The former is due to *θ-toxin*, the latter to *α-toxin*. (ii) As described on p. 429, α-toxin is a *phospholipase C* and acts on phospholipid (lecithin) in serum and egg yolk to release free diglyceride which precipitates in the form of a dense opalescence. This is known as *Nagler's reaction* and is inhibitable by antitoxin. *Cl. perfringens* can be identified by streaking on both sides of an egg yolk agar plate, one half of which has been covered with anti-α-toxin; opalescence occurs only on the untreated half. (iii) In milk media (though rarely used today) *Cl. perfringens* ferments lactose and produces both sufficient acid to cause a 'clot' or precipitate of casein, as well as a large volume of gas which tears the clot apart—the so-called stormy fermentation or stormy clot reaction.

TOXINS, ENZYMES AND PATHOGENICITY

Between them, the five types of *Cl. perfringens* produce four major exotoxins, given Greek designations α, β, ϵ, ι, and eight minor antigens, some of which are toxins and others enzymes—γ, δ, η, θ, k, λ, μ, ν. Of the major toxins, type A organisms produce only α-toxin; this has a powerful cytotoxic action, disrupting the phospholipids of cell membranes and mitochondria. α-toxin is the organism's principal virulence factor, both in local invasiveness and production of necrosis during gas gangrene, and probably in the subsequent generalised toxaemia and death. θ-toxin is haemolytic for horse, ox, sheep and rabbit red cells and is one of the group of oxygen-labile haemolysins described on p. 431; it is also a cytotoxic molecule which probably contributes to cell damage in wound infections. Other products are enzymes which assist in the invasiveness of type A organisms, namely a collagenase (k toxin) and hyaluronidase (μ toxin) which destroy connective tissue, and a DNase (ν toxin).

Food poisoning strains of type A organisms produce an *enterotoxin* which is responsible for diarrhoea; it is a structural protein of the spore and is in fact released during sporulation (spore formation) in the course of intestinal infection. It has been purified and is a heat-labile molecule of 35,000 mol.wt. Like the enterotoxins of cholera and *E. coli*, it reverses the net flow of Na^+, Cl^- and water across the epithelial cells, from absorption to secretion, and causes fluid accumulation in the ligated rabbit ileal loop. However, its action is not via raised intracellular cyclic AMP, but seems to be at the cell membrane; electron microscopy shows that morphological changes occur within a few minutes in epithelial cells of the villi in rat and rabbit intestine exposed to the toxin, and it seems that the structure and function of the membrane eventually breaks down. In cultured cells, the toxin inhibits energy production and protein and nucleic acid synthesis. The cell membrane action of *Cl. perfringens* enterotoxin is unique among bacterial products causing diarrhoea. The more severe enteric disease caused by *Cl. perfringens* type C is due to the β-toxin, which is instrumental in damaging the mucosa and causing intestinal necrosis.

PATHOGENESIS OF GAS GANGRENE

Gangrene is a rather inconsistently used clinical term for a visibly necrotic area of tissue in the living body, which may putrefy as a result of invasion and digestion by bacteria. The gangrenous area is in continuity with adjacent living tissue and becomes dark coloured (almost black) and foul smelling due to volatile products; gas may be produced, resulting in a crackling sound when the area is pressed. The organisms responsible for putrefaction are often anaerobic saprophytes, such as clostridia, which cannot invade living tissues. We can distinguish (a) *primary gangrene*, a continuous process of invasion in which tissue is killed by the action of bacterial toxins, followed by invasion of the newly necrotic area by the organisms, and (b) *secondary gangrene*, in which necrosis is due to ischaemia (loss of blood supply) and the dead tissue is then subjected to putrefaction by bacteria.

Gas gangrene is a primary gangrene: there must be an initial focus of dead tissue, as in a wound, in which growth of the anaerobic organisms can commence, but thereafter the destruction of the tissue is due to their toxic action and invasion. It is classically associated with severe traumatic injuries to muscle, involving laceration, crushing and vascular damage; the wound is infected by spores or vegetative cells of *Cl. perfringens* and related species, typically from soil during warfare or accidental injury, but also from the skin, faeces or clothing. The spores germinate and vegetative cells grow provided the appropriate tissue conditions of reduced oxygen tension and low oxidation-reduction potential prevail, usually where the normal blood supply is impaired through crushing or severing of arteries and where tissue is devitalised or necrotic. Blood clots, foreign bodies and infection with pyogenic facultative anaerobes all help to create suitable anaerobic conditions. Because of these restricting conditions, the incidence of gas gangrene is low compared with the frequency with which clostridia are found in wounds.

Once the organisms germinate and grow, they produce α-toxin which kills muscle fibres in surrounding healthy tissue (*myonecrosis*) and enzymes which destroy connective tissue. The organisms can then follow into the area which their products have rendered necrotic, where they ferment the muscle carbohydrate with production of lactic acid and the characteristic gas (mostly H_2 and CO_2). A whole area of muscle is invaded very rapidly, though the organisms show no tendency to bacteraemic spread except as a terminal event. Oedema fluid and gas increase tissue pressure and thus impair the local circulation, providing further opportunity for the organisms to spread. Thus the picture is one of progressive, massive muscular damage with organisms moving in behind their destructive toxins and spreading along tissue planes until a whole muscle group or limb segment is involved. During this time the skin darkens and becomes black, and the tissue is 'crepitant' (creaking) and may burst open due to the pressure of fluid and gas. Where large muscle masses are involved, there is severe shock and prostration.

The entry of α-toxin (and θ-toxin) into the bloodstream causes acute haemolysis, haemoglobinuria and renal failure; the severe toxaemia (which may also be due to toxic products of dead tissue) affects all internal organs and, when untreated, leads to rapid death from peripheral vascular collapse. Post-mortem examination shows clostridia in many tissues but, as noted above, their spread in the bloodstream is purely a terminal event.

Besides infecting massive wounds, *Cl. perfringens* was a common cause of infection of the uterus following abortions carried out illegally by non-medical practitioners before legalised abortions became generally available. The source of infection in such cases is often endogenous, from faecally-contaminated skin. After causing necrosis of the uterine muscle, the organisms may invade the bloodstream (septicaemia) with intravascular haemolysis, renal failure and often death. Another mode of infection, leading to gas gangrene, is intramuscular injection of adrenaline contaminated with clostridial spores; the local ischaemia caused by adrenaline-induced vasoconstriction can allow the organisms to grow.

Cl. perfringens is also involved in wound infections of lesser severity than gas gangrene. In *anaerobic cellulitis*, the organisms infect tissue which is already dead as a result of ischaemia or trauma, but do not kill healthy intact muscle; toxaemia, if any, is slight. In *simple wound contamination*, pathogenic clostridia can be isolated from the wound but do not lead to pathological events.

Treatment

Gas gangrene has a high mortality (15–30%) and extensive surgery and amputation are often necessary as infected and necrotic tissue must be surgically removed. Antibiotics (such as penicillin) and passive immunisation with antitoxin are of doubtful value. However, if available, hyperbaric oxygen treatment can limit the degree of surgery required and avoid amputation. The patient is placed in a special pressurised chamber and breathes pure oxygen at 3 atmospheres pressure for 1–2 hours daily over 5–7 days. In many cases the improved oxygenation of the infected tissues halts the spread of the organisms, both by direct toxicity and by raising tissue redox potential.

The most important thing is to *prevent* gas gangrene by thorough cleansing of wounds, removing non-viable tissue, and giving prophylactic antibiotics.

Epidemiology

In the past, the battlefield was the principal setting for gas gangrene, where the contamination of massive wounds by infected soil, clothing or metal fragments was common. It was prevalent in the 1914–18 war but less so in 1939–45. The prompt evacuation of the wounded and adequate medical treatment have greatly reduced its occurrence and it was not often seen, for instance, among US casualties in Vietnam. In civilian life, gas gangrene can follow agricultural accidents—contaminating organisms are prevalent in manured and cultivated soil—traffic accidents, gunshot wounds, compound fractures, complication of surgery (even operating theatres may harbour clostridia and their spores), and in septic abortion.

FOOD POISONING

Food poisoning due to *Cl. perfringens* was first described in 1945 and since then has become increasingly common: in the period 1973–75, there were 6500 cases in England and Wales in 150 outbreaks, most originating in canteens in schools, hospitals and institutions. It takes the form of acute abdominal pain and diarrhoea some 8–24 hours after eating contaminated food, but vomiting is uncommon; symptoms last for about a day and recovery is complete. Compared with other forms of food poisoning, it is generally mild. The contaminated food is very often meat (roasts, poultry, stews) that has been pre-cooked and either eaten cold or subsequently reheated and held warm for several hours. The factors which have made it so common today are: (i) the frequent occurrence of food poisoning strains of *Cl. perfringens* in the environment and in human faeces; (ii) the heat resistance of the spores, which can withstand boiling for one hour; and (iii) the rapid growth of the organisms in meat or other food held at 40–50°C. The organisms are type A *Cl. perfringens*, which differ from the classical gas gangrene strains in the heat resistance of their spores and in being non-haemolytic.

Food poisoning by *Cl. perfringens* requires the ingestion of large numbers of viable organisms which have multiplied in the infected food. Contamination of raw meat by clostridial spores is commonplace, whether during slaughter, through handling in the kitchen or by exposure to flies and dust. The spores not only survive the cooking procedure, but are induced to germinate by heating, after which the vegetative bacterial cells multiply rapidly in the meat as it cools or on subsequent storage or inadequate reheating. Ingestion of 10^8–10^9 viable bacteria is needed, but it has been shown experimentally that this number is easily attained in a meal if 200,000 cells or spores are incubated in freshly cooked lamb and gravy and allowed to stand at 40–50°C for three hours. In the small intestine, the organisms sporulate and in so doing release enterotoxin, the properties of which are described above (p. 581).

ENTERITIS NECROTICANS

This is a more severe food poisoning caused by type C organisms. Diarrhoea and abdominal pain are intense, there may be intestinal bleeding, and the illness may be fatal. As in type A food poisoning, it is caused by strains with heat-resistant spores. Major outbreaks have occurred in New Guinea, the vehicle being contaminated and inadequately cooked pork eaten during pig feasting. This disease, called locally 'pig-bel', has a mortality of 30–40%. The organisms produce a powerful toxin (β-toxin) which destroys the intestinal mucosa.

Clostridium tetani

Like gas gangrene, *tetanus* is the consequence of contamination of a wound by clostridial spores, in this case of *Cl. tetani*, followed by growth of the organisms under anaerobic conditions and production of a powerful exotoxin. However, in contrast with *Cl. perfringens* α-toxin, tetanus toxin does not enable the organisms to damage and invade the tissue: it is a *neurotoxin* which is carried in the fibres of peripheral nerves to the CNS, where its effects lead to localised or widespread muscular spasm. Since these often affect the jaw (*trismus*), tetanus has the informal name of *lockjaw*. It is a disease of high mortality and in some more primitive areas of the world is still a major cause of death; the worldwide incidence is some 300,000 cases per year. However, it is a comparative rarity in well-developed countries today as a result of the complete protection provided by active immunisation with tetanus toxoid. Like *Cl. perfringens*, the tetanus bacilli are intestinal commensals in many animals and form hardy spores which are commonly present in manure and soil.

MORPHOLOGY, GROWTH, ETC.

Cl. tetani is a straight, slender rod, longer and thinner than other pathogenic clostridia, 3–8 μm in length and 0.2–0.5 μm wide. It is Gram-positive, but Gram-negative forms are common in

584

smears made from wounds. It forms a prominent, terminal, spherical spore which, being of considerably greater diameter than the vegetative cell, gives the organisms their typical 'drumstick' appearance (Figure 4.2i, 4.12b). *Cl. tetani* is highly motile with numerous peritrichous flagella; this motility causes colonies to 'swarm' on agar plates. Like most other clostridia, it is an *obligate anaerobe*. The resistance of the spores varies, but they often survive boiling for 20 minutes, as well as various disinfectants. Serologically, ten different *Cl. tetani* types can be distinguished on the basis of flagellar antigens; however, a point of great practical importance is that a single antigenic type of neurotoxin is produced by all pathogenic strains. It is not known what structural components (if any) enable the tetanus organisms to survive in infected tissue. The horse and man are the species most susceptible to tetanus.

TOXINS

All the clinical features of tetanus derive from the action of tetanus neurotoxin (*tetanospasmin*), which is second only to botulinum toxin in potency (the minimum lethal dose for a 20 g mouse is about 30 pg, or 3×10^{-11} g). Its nature and mode of action have been discussed on p. 434. Inoculation of the toxin into mice or guinea-pigs leads to the typical signs of tetanus, with death occurring in 1–2 days. Lethality for mice and their protection by specific antitoxin are used in the identification of organisms cultured from wounds. Another toxic product, *tetanolysin*, is an oxygen-labile haemolysin (p. 431) but no great significance is attached to its production.

PATHOGENESIS OF TETANUS (Figure 4.60)

Spores of *Cl. tetani* are widely distributed in the soil and are also present on dirty clothing and dust; thus, in the days before active immunisation, tetanus, like gas gangrene, was seen particularly in war casualties with deep lacerated wounds into which soil particles had entered. In civilian life, agricultural wounds and road accidents can also be readily contaminated; however, many wounds leading to tetanus have been of the simple puncture variety—nails, splinters, thorns, etc., and recently through contaminated syringe needles used by drug addicts in 'skin-popping'. Thus, tetanus can occur without any history of recent injury. Tetanus can also develop in the newborn (*tetanus neonatorum*) as a result of infection of the umbilical stump, either through use of non-sterile instruments or subsequent insanitary conditions, such as the bizarre habit of applying dung to the stump as a dressing, which is practised in some primitive communities. Neonatal tetanus is a significant cause of mortality of newborns in some developing countries, but can be largely prevented by ensuring that all pregnant women are immunised and hence provide adequate passive immunity to their offspring via the placenta.

Though wounds may be contaminated quite regularly,

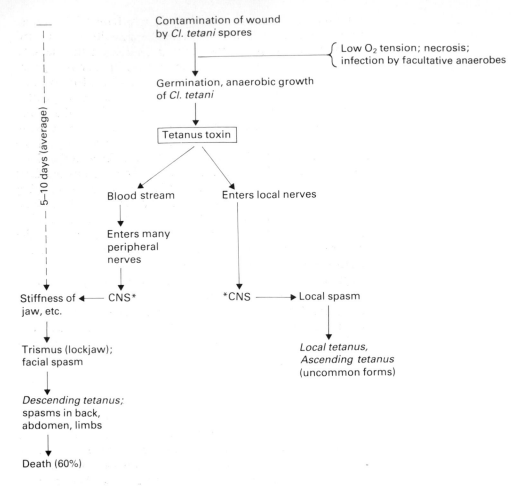

Contamination of wound
by *Cl. tetani* spores

{ Low O$_2$ tension; necrosis;
infection by facultative anaerobes

Germination, anaerobic growth
of *Cl. tetani*

Tetanus toxin

Blood stream   Enters local nerves

Enters many
peripheral
nerves

5–10 days (average)

Stiffness of ◄── CNS*   *CNS ──► Local spasm
jaw, etc.

Trismus (lockjaw);   *Local tetanus,*
facial spasm   *Ascending tetanus*
                                      (uncommon forms)

Descending tetanus;
spasms in back,
abdomen, limbs

Death (60%)

tetanus is an unusual outcome in non-immunised persons because of the rather stringent conditions required for germination of the spores and growth of the bacilli. The oxygen tension in the tissue must be reduced and there is usually also tissue necrosis resulting from the wound and the presence of facultative anaerobes, which will assist in removing oxygen and then continue to grow anaerobically. The importance of tissue necrosis is demonstrable experimentally—mice injected intramuscularly with heavy doses of tetanus spores fail to develop disease unless necrotising chemicals, such as CaCl$_2$ or lactic acid, are injected at the same time. When the oxidation-reduction potential of the tissue is lowered sufficiently for the spores to germinate, the organisms proceed to grow locally in the wound, but do not spread into adjacent tissue or enter the bloodstream.

Tetanus toxin is produced locally and, as related elsewhere, initially enters local motor nerves by adhering to the nerve terminals of the motor end-plate; it is then taken up in vesicles and transported intra-axonally to the CNS. In itself, this leads to *local tetanus*, with spasms in the muscles around the wounds, which can be reproduced by local injection of small doses of toxin in animals. Thereafter, spread of the toxin up the spinal cord produces *ascending tetanus* as an extension of the local form.

Figure 4.60 Pathogenesis of tetanus.
*see also Figure 4.27

However, local tetanus is a relatively rare form of the disease occurring in individuals with partial immunity or very few organisms; it may persist for weeks or months and then subside. The classic and much more common form of tetanus is generalised and is caused by entry of the toxin from the local site into the bloodstream and its *toxaemic* dissemination, duplicated experimentally by intravenous inoculation of toxin. Entry into the CNS is nevertheless still *via nerve fibres*, the toxin being adsorbed at motor end-plates in the general musculature of the body. Muscles with the shortest neuronal distance to the CNS, namely those of the head and neck, are therefore affected first; thus the earliest symptom is often *stiffness of the jaw*, developing later into spasm of the masseter muscles (trismus, lockjaw) with a descending progression to the trunk and limbs (*descending tetanus*). The disease increases in severity, producing the characteristic grin of *risus sardonicus* through spasm of the facial muscles, and then more generalised convulsions. Spasms are often triggered by insignificant stimuli such as a footstep or flash of light, and although brief in duration can be frequent and exhausting. The patient usually remains mentally clear and aware of his condition throughout. Death frequently results after a few weeks, but in those who recover there are no permanent disabilities.

IMMUNITY

Clinical tetanus itself does *not* lead to immunity, either because the amount of toxin produced in the course of the disease is below the immunogenic level or because it is rapidly bound by nervous tissue. *Passive immunisation* with antitoxin is used in treatment, human antibodies being employed wherever possible to avoid serum sickness. Tetanus is very efficiently prevented by *active immunisation* with tetanus toxoid, which is now routine for all babies and infants in developed countries and administered as part of the triple vaccine (p. 166). The effects are nowhere seen more dramatically than in wartime. During the Second World War, there were only 12 cases of tetanus out of 2.7 million immunised soldiers admitted to hospital for wounds and injuries, while in the British action at Dunkirk there were seven cases out of 16,000 wounded—and all in men who had refused to be immunised. After the standard immunising course, immunity can be maintained by a single booster every ten years. Boosters are also given when a previously immunised individual has a serious wound (those not previously immunised being given prophylactic antitoxin). In countries where immunisation is practised efficiently, the annual incidence of tetanus is about one per million population, but in underdeveloped tropical countries the incidence is high and tetanus is among the leading causes of death.

Clostridium botulinum

Botulism is a rare but usually fatal type of food poisoning caused by ingestion of botulinum toxin, the most poisonous of all bacterial products. Botulism is almost always an *intoxication* rather than an infection, so naturally all the clinical effects relate solely to the toxin. The recently recognised *infant botulism* is one of the rare instances where the disease results from release of toxin by *Cl. botulinum in vivo*, growing within the intestinal tract of babies; very rarely the organisms infect wounds. In general, the toxin is formed in food after the anaerobic germination of contaminating *Cl. botulinum* spores; the latter have an exceptional degree of heat resistance which enables them to survive cooking procedures, and most outbreaks in Europe and the USA are thus due to home-preserved food which has not been heated to a high enough temperature before storage. The intestinal effects of botulinum toxin are insignificant compared with its action on the nervous system; it produces paralysis by blocking transmission at neuromuscular junctions and, after a rapid course, death occurs through respiratory or cardiac failure. In addition to its occasional occurrence in man, botulism is economically very important in some parts of the world, including the USA, where it causes the deaths of thousands of animals and birds each year. This may occur from drinking alkaline swamp water, as happened in the Norfolk Broads in 1976.

MORPHOLOGY, CLASSIFICATION, ETC.

Cl. botulinum is a straight or slightly curved Gram-positive bacillus, with peritrichous flagella providing motility; the spores are oval and subterminal. It is strictly anaerobic. The resistance of the spores to adverse conditions is remarkable; they are among the most heat-resistant of all spores, capable of surviving for hours at 100°C. They are usually killed in a few minutes by moist heat at 121°C and in canning factories food in cans is autoclaved at 116°C for 10 minutes or 121°C for 3 minutes (depending on the food) to ensure destruction of the spores.

Although it is convenient from the medical point of view to think of *Cl. botulinum* as a single species, it is in fact a heterogeneous group of organisms which are brought together because they produce a pharmacologically similar toxin rather than because of close serological or genetic relationships. There are eight antigenically distinct types of botulinum toxin and hence eight corresponding *Cl. botulinum* types, designated A, B, C_1, C_2, D, E, F and G. All the toxin types have the same pharmacological action. The toxins affect different species, a selectivity which is partly related to their abilities to pass through the intestinal wall of different hosts: humans are susceptible to A, B, E and F, while C and D occur solely in animals and birds, and G is so rare that its species-specificity is unknown. The toxins of *Cl. botulinum* types C and D are coded by lysogenised phages carried by the organism (cf. diphtheria toxin); thus toxigenicity is lost if the organism is 'cured' of its phage, and organism types C and D can be interconverted by the appropriate specific phages. Type C organisms can even be transformed into a different species, *Cl. novyi*, by curing them of the botulinum phage and reinfecting with the phage that codes for *Cl. novyi* α-toxin.

Cl. botulinum is found naturally in the sediments of lakes and rivers, in soil both cultivated and virgin, and in the intestinal tracts of birds, fishes and mammals.

PATHOGENESIS OF BOTULISM

Botulism in man is caused by toxin types A, B and E (F affects man but is very rare); in the USA, type A accounts for about 60% of cases, B for 30% and E for 10%. Type A botulinum toxin is not only the most poisonous of all toxins, but the most poisonous substance known: the minimum lethal dose for a 20 g mouse is about 5×10^{-12} g (5 pg) and for an average man is of the order of 10^{-8} g. (Another way of looking at this is that 50 people could be killed by the amount of toxin accommodated on a pin-head!) After ingestion of food containing botulinum toxin, there may be early gastrointestinal efects, including nausea, pain, vomiting and diarrhoea or sometimes constipation. A fraction of the toxin consumed is absorbed from the small intestine, thence into lymphatics and the bloodstream. It exerts its effects on the *peripheral* nervous system: at neuromuscular junctions it binds to presynaptic nerve terminals and, by blocking acetylcholine release, inhibits transmission of nerve impulses from motor nerve to muscle fibre, as described on p. 437. Cholinergic transmission at synaptic ganglia is also inhibited. The result is *flaccid paralysis*. The major effects occur in the parasympathetic nervous system: involvement of cranial nerves leads to the classical presenting symptoms of diplopia (double vision), dysphagia (difficulty in swallowing) and dysphonia (difficulty in speaking). The pupils are dilated and the tongue is very dry as saliva production ceases; urinary retention is another symptom. There are no sensory abnormalities. As the disease progresses, the muscles of the neck and respiratory system become weak and death is due to sudden respiratory paralysis or heart failure. Mortality is about 20–40% and is highest for type A toxin, followed by type E and then type B; this seems to reflect the strength of binding of each to human neural tissue. Treatment is by passive immunisation with polyvalent horse antitoxin.

EPIDEMIOLOGY

Human botulism has a restricted geographical distribution and is found primarily in the northern hemisphere between 30 and 65 degrees latitude. Most outbreaks occur in seven countries, namely the USA, Canada, Germany, France, Poland, Japan and Russia, in all of which countries it is rather rare. Thus, in the USA in 1978 there were 58 reported cases of food-borne botulism. In the UK there have been only a handful of incidents since the Loch Maree outbreak in 1922, when eight people died after eating contaminated duck paté. One of the most recent was in 1978 when four elderly people in Birmingham were poisoned by tinned North American salmon and two subsequently died; type E *Cl. botulinum* was isolated from the salmon.

Botulism was originally described in connection with food poisoning via contaminated sausages (Lat. *botulus*, sausage), but meat is now a rare source of the organisms. Canning factories employ rigorous sterilisation procedures, but there have been occasional incidents, like the one just noted, involving canned salmon, tuna fish or vichyssoise soup. However, most cases can be traced to home-preserved meat and vegetables; since the spores survive boiling for many hours, food for preservation must be raised to a higher temperature (116–120°C) in a pressure cooker. The toxin itself is heat-sensitive, so as an additional precaution before consumption, home-preserved food should be boiled for one minute or heated at 80°C for five minutes to destroy any toxin present. Acid fruits are safely preserved through heating at 100°C since *Cl. botulinum* cannot grow at low pH.

In contrast with its scarcity in man, botulism is an important cause of paralytic disease in animals, with considerable economic implications. Examples include grass or fodder sickness of horses, limberneck in chickens and lamziekte of cattle. Type C toxin is the cause of extensive epidemics among aquatic and shore birds in the USA, South America, Australia and South Africa, and it is the major natural cause of death of ducks in the western USA. The ducks are poisoned when they feed on fly larvae infected with *Cl. botulinum*; their carcasses are in turn fed upon by larvae, which then poison more ducks and so on. Type C is also the cause of botulism in chickens. Interestingly, carrion-feeding birds such as vultures are resistant to botulinum toxin; the mechanism of resistance is unknown.

INFANT BOTULISM

Infant botulism is an infection of the intestinal tract by *Cl. botulinum*. It is restricted to infants, perhaps because competing intestinal flora are less well established. All reported cases have recovered, but it has been suggested as one cause of the sudden infant death syndrome (cot death).

MYCOBACTERIUM

Mycobacteria are responsible for two of the world's major diseases, *tuberculosis* and *leprosy*, which together currently affect some 30 million people, mostly in tropical countries. Two species of 'tubercle bacilli' cause tuberculosis in man, namely *Mycobacterium tuberculosis* and *M. bovis* (the human and bovine types respectively), while leprosy is due to *M. leprae*. Tuberculosis was formerly one of the great agencies of death throughout the world, but over the last 40 years has become very much less common in Europe, North America and the rest of the developed world. Nevertheless, in countries with poor standards of living and health care it remains very prevalent, and on a global scale it is still the most important infectious disease (an estimated 15–20 million cases) and the leading killing infection (1–2 million deaths annually). Similarly, leprosy is a rarity in developed, temperate countries, but affects some 15 million people in the tropics in Africa, Asia and parts of South America.

Mycobacteria have several unusual properties both from the bacteriological and pathological points of view, all of which derive from the unique chemical composition of the cell wall. The latter is unlike that of either Gram-positive or Gram-negative organisms; it is waxy, very hydrophobic and has an extremely high lipid content—up to 60% of the dry weight of the wall is lipid, much of it in the form of esterified *mycolic acids* (see p. 397). This has several important consequences. (i) The most familiar result is the staining property of mycobacteria: they are not easily stained, but once they have taken up dyes such as carbolfuchsin, they resist decolourisation with acid-alcohol and are hence known as *acid-fast* organisms. (ii) The hydrophobicity of the wall limits the rate at which nutrients in solution can enter the cell and as a result they are among the slowest growing of all bacteria (while the leprosy bacillus has yet to be cultivated on artificial media at all). (iii) The wall resists degradation by lysosomal enzymes of phagocytes so that the pathogenic mycobacteria characteristically survive and grow *intracellularly* in macrophages; indeed, for *M. leprae*, growth only occurs intracellularly. Moreover, even when the organisms have been killed by activated macrophages, cell wall elements may persist for some time and provide prolonged antigenic stimulation. (iv) The cell wall has an important effect on the immune system which is summed up in the term *adjuvanticity*. This is the ability to stimulate both antibody and cell-mediated immune responses to a higher level than would otherwise be attained. The cell-mediated response is a particularly important factor in the pathogenesis of tuberculosis and leprosy, where *hypersensitivity* is an essential element. Protective immunity also depends on the CMI response, with activation of macrophages by T-cell lymphokines. (v) As a result of points (iii) and (iv), mycobacteria give rise to *chronic granulomatous infections*, in which the host immune response is often responsible for the nature and course of the disease. Many of the immunological and cellular events involved in mycobacterial infection have been described in detail in Sections 1 and 2 (p. 59, 163).

Mycobacteria have been important in the history of microbiology, *M. leprae* being the first pathogenic organism to be seen and described in a human disease (Hansen, 1874). *M. tuberculosis* was first isolated in 1882 by Robert Koch who transmitted tuberculosis experimentally to guinea-pigs and rabbits and showed that it obeyed the criteria now known as *Koch's postulates*; these had been established by Koch for anthrax some years before and came to be regarded as essential in proving the microbial causation of a disease. They are (in summary) (a) that the organism must always be associated with the clinical disease; (b) that it be isolated from a case and grown in a series of pure cultures; (c) that a late pure culture reproduce the disease in a susceptible animal; and (d) that the organism be subsequently reisolated from the latter. (Ironically, these conditions cannot be satisfied for *M. leprae*, as this organism cannot be grown in culture.)

MORPHOLOGY, STAINING, ETC.

M. tuberculosis is a slender, straight or slightly curved bacillus, 1–4 μm in length, which is non-motile, non-encapsulated and does not form spores (Figure 4.2j). While the cells do not readily take up the Gram-stain, the genus is generally considered to be Gram-positive. The *Ziehl-Neelsen stain* is routinely used for mycobacteria and is designed to demonstrate their acid-fast property. In this method, a smear of the organisms is covered with carbolfuchsin and heated in steam to facilitate penetration of the dye; thereafter, the stained smear is washed in acid-alcohol (3% HCl, 95% ethanol) and counterstained with methylene blue. Only mycobacteria, being acid-fast, retain the red carbolfuchsin after this treatment and appear as brilliant red rods against a deep blue background; all other organisms lose the red dye and stain blue. Acid-fastness is due to the high hydrophobicity of the cell wall which prevents the release of carbolfuchsin trapped inside the cell; evidently the impenetrability of the wall is greater after staining as a result of complexing of the dye to mycolic acids. Stained organisms often have a beaded or granular appearance due to deposits of polyphosphate and unstained vacuoles.

M. tuberculosis is an *obligate aerobe*, the growth of which is hampered by even a small reduction in oxygen tension. The very hydrophobic nature of its wall is responsible for its characteristic growth properties. Thus, it grows very slowly and even under optimal culture conditions divides only every 18–24 hours. On solid media, enriched by serum or egg yolk, colonies take many days or even several weeks to develop and are dry and tightly matted with a wrinkled surface. On liquid medium, if undisturbed, the organisms grow at the surface (like a layer of fat) in the form of a wrinkled skin or pellicle, and are only dispersed into a regular suspension by incorporation of a detergent such as Tween 80.

Another consequence of the waxy wall is the high degree of resistance of the organisms to drying, which is important in their usual method of transmission in the air. A practical consideration is that they remain alive in dried sputum for up to 6–8 months and during this period can be distributed in the air in dust. They are also resistant to chemical disinfectants. However, mycobacteria are readily killed by moist heat, a fact used to advantage in *pasteurisation*, which is designed to kill *M. bovis* in milk. Pasteurisation involves heating to 63°C for 30 minutes or to 72°C for 20 seconds; while this does not produce sterilisation, it is sufficient to kill mycobacteria and has been instrumental in eliminating milk-borne tuberculosis, which in Britain formerly accounted for 5–10% of all cases and 25% of tuberculosis in children. Mycobacteria are also very susceptible to ultraviolet light and are killed by direct sunlight in two hours, though organisms in sputum are killed rather more slowly; thus the long-term survival to which they are otherwise suited depends on protection from daylight.

While man is the principal host of *M. tuberculosis*, other animals may be readily infected, either naturally or artificially. Guinea-pigs are highly susceptible and have been widely used experimentally. Guinea-pig inoculation was employed as a sensitive diagnostic test where tubercle bacilli cannot be detected in specimens by direct microscopic examination, but modern culture methods are just as sensitive.

CELL WALL AND PATHOGENICITY

Neither exotoxins nor endotoxins are produced by *M. tuberculosis* and pathogenicity is in very large measure, if not entirely, dependent on the chemical nature of the cell wall. As noted above, components of the wall (a) confer on the organisms the ability to resist intracellular destruction, at least in normal macrophages, (b) act as a persistent antigenic stimulus and (c) interact with the immune system to stimulate a very active cell-mediated response. Details of the chemistry of the mycobacterial wall can be found on p. 397 (Figure 4.8), and it will be recalled that most of the lipid is in the form of characteristic high molecular weight branched-chain fatty acids called *mycolic acids*. They occur in glycolipids, both free and linked to peptidoglycan. In virulent strains, one of the forms in which mycolic acids are present is as the dimycolyl ester of trehalose, the so-called *cord factor* (Figure 4.8c). Cord factor is responsible for growth of virulent strains in culture as *serpentine cords*, a result of close parallel arrangement of bacilli; attenuated and avirulent forms grow in a random pattern and do not possess cord factor in their walls. Not only does cord factor correlate with virulence, but it also possesses toxic properties similar to those of the viable organisms themselves. Thus, intravenous injection of cord factor into mice gives rise to granulomas which are indistinguishable from tubercles caused by *M. tuberculosis* infection, while intraperitoneal injection of cord factor dissolved in oil leads to wasting and death. Intracellularly, cord factor inhibits oxidative respiration by disrupting mitochondria. Its activity is potentiated by closely related sulphatides (sulpholipids, p. 399) located in the periphery of the wall. Suphatides inhibit an essential part of the phagocytic process, namely the fusion of phagosomes with lysosomes (p. 19) and this may be one mechanism whereby mycobacteria survive intracellularly in macrophages.

The wall component responsible for the immunostimulating properties of mycobacteria (adjuvanticity) has been intensively studied. At first it was also thought to involve mycolic acids, as chloroform extraction of mycobacterial walls yielded a fraction called *wax D*, containing mycolic acid linked to arabinogalactan and peptidoglycan (Figure 4.8b), which possessed all the adjuvant activity of whole organisms. As described on p. 400, chemical structures much smaller than wax D and free of mycolic acid retain all the ability to stimulate the immune response. The minimal fragment with adjuvanticity is in fact very small indeed, a conjugate of N-acetylmuramic acid and two amino acids, L-alanine and D-*iso*-glutamine, known as *muramyl dipeptide* or

MDP (Figure 4.8d). This structure is part of the peptidoglycan and is also present in the wall of other organisms, which raises the unanswered question of why few bacteria have the powerful adjuvant properties of mycobacteria. One can envisage that components such as the capsule or outer membrane prevent contact between the peptidoglycan of many organisms and lymphoid cell surfaces; in fact the isolated peptidoglycan of practically all Gram-positive and Gram-negative species is immunostimulatory. MDP is able to replace whole killed *M. tuberculosis* in Freund's complete adjuvant (p. 80), in which form it stimulates antibody formation and delayed hypersensitivity to protein antigens. Injection of a synthetic MDP into guinea-pigs leads to development of massive granulomas indistinguishable from those of tuberculosis. MDP does not stimulate lymphocytes directly and has no mitogenic effect on T cells. Its primary target of action is the macrophage, with T cells being stimulated subsequently, either through an effect on antigen presentation (p. 114) or by soluble macrophage products (monokines).

TUBERCULIN AND THE TUBERCULIN TEST

When tubercle bacilli are grown in broth culture and the organisms subsequently filtered off, the culture fluid contains a mixture of mycobacterial proteins which stimulate a delayed hypersensitivity reaction in the skin of individuals sensitised to *M. tuberculosis* through natural infection or vaccination. The protein mixture is called *tuberculin* and the skin reaction is the *tuberculin test*, which plays a valuable role in the diagnosis and control of tuberculosis (details of the mechanism of the reaction are described on p. 163). Koch's original preparation of tuberculin (heat-sterilised culture filtrates concentrated to one-tenth volume) is known as Old Tuberculin (OT), but a semipurified preparation called PPD (purified protein derivative) is now in standard use in the tuberculin test. PPD is a mixture of low molecular weight tuberculoproteins and polypeptides.

The significance of the tuberculin test is that, in a non-vaccinated population (e.g. the USA), a positive reaction in an individual indicates current or previous infection with tubercle bacilli, not necessarily accompanied by symptoms of disease. Conversely, a negative test in a person in good physical condition shows that there has been no infection—past or present—by tubercle bacilli or other mycobacteria. Apart from its epidemiological significance, the tuberculin test is also helpful in tracing contacts of infectious cases and as a post-vaccination check on the effectiveness of BCG vaccination. A positive test in a healthy person without current mycobacterial infection indicates increased resistance to externally acquired tuberculosis. Where BCG vaccination is widely practised, the test loses its usefulness as an indicator of natural infection, as all vaccinated persons are tuberculin-positive; for this reason, large scale vaccination is not carried out in some countries where the incidence of tuberculosis is low, including the USA.

The standard form of the tuberculin test, and one which

enables a quantitative assessment of response to be made, is called the *Mantoux test* (introduced by Mantoux in 1908). 0.1 ml of a preparation of PPD, containing 5 tuberculin units, is injected intracutaneously and the injection site examined 48–72 hours later. A positive reaction consists of an area of oedema or induration (hardness) 5 mm or more in diameter and a wider zone of erythema (reddening); reactions of less than 5 mm are doubtful or negative. In an alternative form now in common use, known as the *Heaf test*, tuberculin is applied with a multiple puncture apparatus giving six intradermal injections; despite certain advantages of speed and reproducibility, the Heaf test is less easily standardised than the Mantoux test.

Some individuals, especially Negroes and those with skin, eye or glandular infection, are extremely sensitive to PPD and suffer large necrotic reactions to the standard Mantoux test. On the other hand, the reaction is commonly suppressed during measles infection as a result of viral infection of lymphocytes (p. 341). In some patients with very severe tuberculosis, the tuberculin test may also be negative, supposedly due to a blocking effect of the large amount of tuberculoprotein released from lesions.

The tuberculin reaction occurs because of the specific sensitivity, in the form of T cell reactivity, which develops to mycobacterial products during the course of infection. It is interesting that only a small fraction of the material injected in the test remains at the site of injection, 95% diffusing away during the first 24 hours. However, some tuberculin remains fixed to cells in the skin for a long period. The cellular events involved and the histological appearance of the site of a positive reaction are described on p. 163.

The regular tuberculin testing of herds of cattle and the slaughter of all positive animals has led to a great reduction in tuberculosis in cows, formerly an important source of human infection. Pasteurisation of milk prevents any residual bovine infections from reaching man.

EPIDEMIOLOGY OF TUBERCULOSIS

In developed countries there has been a very rapid decline in the incidence and mortality of tuberculosis over the last 30 years. However, the disease remains very common in countries such as India and Pakistan, where 1–2% of the population suffer from active tuberculosis against a constant background of poverty, dirt, poor hygiene, malnutrition, overcrowding and overpopulation. In England and Wales in 1925 there were about 60,000 notifications of respiratory tuberculosis, which fell slowly to about 45,000 by 1950; but in 1971 there were only 11,000 cases and in 1976 fewer than 8,000, which only 1100 deaths. A similar decline has occurred in Western Europe and the USA; in the USA, about 30,000 new cases are recognised each year, with about 3,000 deaths, but few of these are new infections. Tuberculosis as a result of new infection is now rare in developed countries. Forty years ago, morbidity and mortality due to tuberculosis were highest in young children and young adults, the most susceptible groups, and relatively low in the elderly. Today the situation is the reverse, with few cases among the young and the highest incidence in older people, especially elderly, impoverished men living alone in city slums, often alcoholic and undernourished. In the past, mortality (overall) was approximately equal among males and females (with a preponderance of females among young adults); today, most deaths from respiratory tuberculosis occur in men over 55 years of age, generally through *reactivation* of latent disease. In the UK in the 1970's, tuberculosis was much commoner among immigrants than among the native born: in 1971, 32% of all cases were in immigrants who at that time constituted about 5% of the population.

A number of factors have contributed to the successful reduction in tuberculosis in the developed world: the efficient detection of infectious cases with mass miniature diagnostic radiography; isolation of infectious cases in sanatoria; effective treatment and prophylaxis by antimicrobial drugs, such as isoniazid and streptomycin, and by surgery (removal of infected organs); protective vaccination with BCG; and a rising standard of living with less poverty, overcrowding, etc. Milk-borne tuberculosis has been eliminated, as described above. Recently there has been concern in England over the occurrence of severe tuberculosis in badgers, since mycobacteria may be transmitted from them to cattle by contamination of pastures.

Genetic factors, both familial and racial, are very important in determining whether infection with *M. tuberculosis* will lead to clinical disease. Some families are more susceptible to tuberculosis than others; Jewish families, for example, often show an increased resistance to the disease, though not to infection (see also p. 864). Among racial groups, American Negroes, American Indians and Eskimos have more severe forms of tuberculosis than the White man; in studies in the US army between 1922 and 1936, the morbidity due to tuberculosis was the same among White and Black soldiers, but the mortality was four times higher among the Negroes. Because these groups were not exposed to tuberculosis until the last 200–300 years, there has presumably been less selection of resistance genes in them than among Europeans. Experimentally, rabbits have been bred for high or low resistance to tuberculous infection.

PATHOGENESIS OF TUBERCULOSIS

Tuberculosis is most commonly a disease of the *lung*, both because it is usually transmitted by inhalation and because the lung provides a good environment for the multiplication of the aerobic organisms. Lesions often also occur in draining lymph nodes and, when the organisms are distributed by bacteraemia, scattered lesions are found in many other organs, including the liver, kidneys, spleen, meninges and brain. Ingestion of *M. bovis* in infected milk leads to infection of the tonsils or intestines. In adults, tuberculosis is usually a *chronic* disease, which often leads to death after a variable, prolonged course, while in children (or adults infected for the first time) it can be acute and rapidly fatal.

In endemic areas, disease in children is common, with a very high risk of mortality in those under three years. In adults, certain conditions predispose to the development of tuberculosis, including chronic alcoholism, other chronic lung disease (e.g. silicosis), diabetes mellitus and corticosteroid therapy.

M. tuberculosis is a highly infectious organism and man is very susceptible; tuberculous disease, however, is relatively rare as infection is usually clinically asymptomatic. However, there are no healthy carriers; i.e. individuals who spread infection always have lesions. Infection is transmitted very effectively via the respiratory route, mostly from 'open' cases of pulmonary tuberculosis (i.e. discharging tubercle bacilli from the lung) who expectorate organisms in sputum or expel them in droplets during coughing or speaking. Bacilli are acquired either in moist droplets or more often dried dust particles, and it will be recalled that mycobacteria are able to resist drying conditions for many months.

The essential feature of the pathogenesis of tuberculosis is the involvement of the host cell-mediated immune response which, besides providing the means of recovery, is responsible for the form and development of lesions through hypersensitivity. The basic lesion, the tubercle, is the classic example of a *granuloma*, a chronic inflammatory focus arising, in this instance, through an immunological process. The cellular and molecular events involved have been described in Section 1, which should be consulted for an account of the origin and development of tubercles. The following is confined to a brief review of the gross events in human infection.

Two patterns of the disease are distinguished according to whether the infection is acquired for the first time (*primary tuberculosis*) or as a result of reinfection or reactivation of a dormant lesion (*reinfection* or *post-primary tuberculosis*). In areas where infection is common, primary tuberculosis occurs in infants and children, and is also called the 'childhood type'; it either heals or is rapidly fatal. The reinfection pattern of disease affects adults, who probably have a certain degree of immunity as a result of childhood exposure but evidently insufficient to dispose of the organisms quickly; the disease then takes a chronic course (the 'adult type'). In communities where tuberculosis is uncommon, primary infection may occasionally occur in adults. One of the key differences between primary and reinfection disease is in the spread of organisms from the original site of infection to lymph nodes. *Lymph node infection* is the rule in individuals exposed for the first time; it enables the organisms to multiply and then become further disseminated via lymphatics and the bloodstream before the development of a cell-mediated immune response. In contrast, the lesions of reinfection (chronic) tuberculosis remain localised in the lung, often developing into large cavities, with little or no lymph node involvement.

Primary tuberculosis. A primary lesion develops at the point of entry, usually the lung, but in the tonsils or intestine in cases of ingestion. Initially the organisms are taken up by neutrophils, but within a short time macrophages enter the area and take up, but do not kill, the mycobacteria. This early accumulation of macrophages occurs without involvement of lymphocytes and essentially resembles a foreign body reaction. Development of a true tubercle, with epithelioid cells, giant cells, and lymphocytes, takes place over the next 2–3 weeks (p. 59). In the lung, the primary lesion, which is single, 1–2 cm in diameter, and found in the midzone, is termed the *Ghon focus*; is shows the caseation characteristic of tubercles and gradually enlarges. The organisms spread to the local hilar lymph nodes (tracheobronchial, mediastinal) in which tubercles form, the nodes becoming converted into large caseous masses. The combination of the Ghon focus and caseous lymph nodes is called the *Ghon complex* (after the Prague pathologist, Anton Ghon).

The Ghon complex generally heals, either by fibrosis or calcification; in the latter case it is readily identified by chest X-ray. Sometimes, however, the outcome is less favourable, the possibilities being (a) progression in the lung to *tuberculous bronchopneumonia*, with lesions around the terminal bronchi in both lungs, development of lung cavities and a rapidly fatal course, or (b) widespread dissemination of the bacilli in the bloodstream (*generalised miliary tuberculosis*). The latter occurs when caseation in the primary complex extends into the wall of an adjacent vein and caseous material containing large numbers of bacilli enters the circulation. Many small lesions, 1–2 mm in diameter, called *miliary tubercles*, are then found in several organs, especially in the lungs, where they are most plentiful, the liver, spleen, kidneys, meninges and brain; there is no cavitation in the lungs nor bacilli in the sputum, and organisms in the lesions are scanty. In such untreated cases, death occurs after about a month from tuberculous meningitis. Bacteraemic spread is usually a complication of primary childhood disease, but can occur during reinfection disease in adults treated with corticosteroids or other immunosuppressive drugs.

Reinfection or chronic tuberculosis is almost always a disease of the lungs and occurs when there is some immunity due to prior infection or BCG vaccination. While it may result from exogenous infection due to inhaled organisms, it may equally well be a *reactivation* of a dormant primary lesion under circumstances such as malnutrition, alcoholism or severe illness. The initial lesion occurs in the well-ventilated apical region of one lung, usually the right, and the infection does not spread to the hilar lymph nodes, but develops locally as a cluster of tubercles which enlarge, caseate and merge into larger lesions. Progression is slow, due to the existing state of partial immunity. Cavities eventually form by liquefaction and discharge into a bronchus, enlarging until much of the upper lobe is a single large cavity with a necrotic lining and a fibrous wall. The discharge of a tuberculous lesion into a bronchus can distribute bacilli via the air passages throughout the lungs, leading to acute tuberculous bronchopneumonia and rapid death (galloping consumption). Adults with open lesions of this type are the main sources of spread of the disease, the tubercle bacilli proliferating in the aerobic lining of the cavity and discharging into the bronchus.

TREATMENT

The availability of effective chemotherapy for tuberculosis was a major factor in the dramatic reduction of the disease which occurred in developed countries after the Second World War. The drug almost always used in treatment is isoniazid (isonicotinic acid hydrazide, INH), the other 'first-line' agents being rifampicin, streptomycin and ethambutol. Streptomycin, which was the primary agent from 1945 to 1951, has the disadvantages of toxicity (damage to the 8th cranial nerve) and inability to kill intracellular mycobacteria; INH, introduced in 1951, and rifampicin both lack toxicity and are effective against organisms sequestered in macrophages. INH interferes with mycolic acid synthesis and is a specific antimycobacterial agent. Drug-resistant mutants are common, and to avoid their selection two or more antimicrobials are used together. For complete effectiveness, treatment must be continued for at least a year and often up to two years, because of the inactive state of the organisms in lesions. An open case becomes almost non-infectious after a few weeks' treatment.

Drug treatment greatly reduces the dense fibrosis and calcification which normally accompanies 'natural' recovery. When organisms are killed by antimicrobials, resolution largely replaces repair, with absorption of necrotic and caseous material and minimal fibrosis. Early lesions disappear completely, but cavities formed during chronic disease persist, lined by a thin layer of fibrous tissue overlaid with epithelium. Because of the safety of modern anaesthetics, surgery is important in removing parts of diseased organs, under the cover of antibiotics. This rapidly eliminates the source of infection.

VACCINATION

Active immunisation against tuberculosis is carried out with the living attenuated strain of *M. bovis*, known after its French discoverers as *Bacille Calmette et Guérin* (BCG). It was produced by attenuation of the bovine mycobacterium by several hundred subcultures on unfavourable (bile-containing) media, and has remained avirulent since its discovery. Killed vaccines give no protection. Since its introduction in 1924, BCG has been given to an estimated 250 million people. In countries where tuberculosis is common and early protection important, BCG is given to babies during the first month after birth; in the UK and other countries with a low level of infection, it is administered to tuberculin-negative schoolchildren between the ages of 11 and 13. Controlled trials, especially that carried out by the Medical Research Council in England, have demonstrated the high degree of protection provided by BCG. Over 50,000 children in the 14–15 year age group were included in the MRC trial, which began in 1952, and were followed up for 15 years; those who were tuberculin-negative at the start of the trial were either vaccinated or left as non-vaccinated controls. The results showed a better than 80% protection in the vaccinated group following a single BCG injection; a comparable degree of protection was given by the vole bacillus (fully virulent for voles). BCG was not accepted in the USA when it might have been useful and today prevalence is too low to justify its widespread use there.

The undesirable effect of mass vaccination, especially when performed at an early age, is that it eliminates the usefulness of the tuberculin test as an indicator of natural infection in the community, since all who receive BCG become tuberculin-positive. This is avoided to a certain extent in the UK by delaying vaccination to older children who are skin-tested first. In the USA, where mass vaccination is not employed, BCG is given only to those groups who might be at special risk, including hospital staff, who are often exposed to infection, and naval and other military personnel confined to crowded quarters. In these circumstances, the tuberculin test has the significant diagnostic usefulness described on p. 594.

Mycobacterium leprae

Leprosy is a chronic, highly disfiguring disease of the skin and peripheral nerves which has been known—and feared—since antiquity; today it is still very prevalent in the tropics, where there are millions of infected people. Although the leprosy bacillus, *M. leprae*, was discovered in 1874 and was in fact the first bacterial pathogen to be described, less is known about it than most other organisms because of the failure to grow it in culture. However, it clearly has many of the properties of *M. tuberculosis*, including a highly waxy, impervious cell wall, acid-fastness, slow growth and the ability to stimulate a strong immune response. The form of the immune response is crucial to the pathogenesis of the disease and shows wide host variation.

PREVALENCE OF LEPROSY

During the Middle Ages leprosy was widespread in Europe, where it persisted, especially in Northern countries, into the nineteenth century; in Britain it continued to exist in northern Scottish islands during the eighteenth century, the last patient there dying on Papa Stour in 1798. Leprosy was still present in Norway in the second half of the last century and it was there that Amauer Hansen discovered the organism in biopsies of patients. Today it is not a numerically important disease in the Western world: about 300 cases are known in Britain, all imported from tropical countries, while in the USA there are about 2000 existing cases and about 150 new ones each year, mostly from three states where leprosy is still endemic, namely California, Texas and Hawaii. The major areas in the world where it is common are in the tropics—Central Africa, South and South East Asia (Southern China and India), Central and South America. In some parts of Africa, up to 10% of the population is infected. The prevalence of leprosy worldwide is estimated at about 15 million persons, with 100,000 new cases registered annually.

A CLINICAL AND IMMUNOLOGICAL SPECTRUM

Despite the obvious clinical differences between leprosy and tuberculosis, there are many parallels in the pathogenic processes involved. Both are chronic diseases in which the basic lesions are *granulomas*—accumulations of macrophages at foci of infection—the form of which is determined by the nature of the *host immune response*. In this respect, leprosy presents an additional complexity which is much less obvious in tuberculosis, namely a wide range of intensity in the cell-mediated immune response among different individuals and a corresponding range of clinical forms of the disease. At one extreme are patients who, as in tuberculosis, develop a highly active cell-mediated response and hence a state of immunity to the organisms and hypersensitivity to their products. They have *tuberculoid* leprosy, a relatively benign form, so called because of the histological resemblance of the skin lesions to tubercles (i.e. with epithelioid macrophages, lymphocytes and few organisms), and indeed the lesions arise through a similar mechanism of cell-mediated hypersensitivity. At the other extreme are individuals who show a complete absence of cell-mediated responsiveness to *M. leprae* and a total inability to deal with the organisms. This is the *lepromatous* form of leprosy, which is much more severe and represents a state of specific unresponsiveness in the cell-mediated arm of the immune response to *M. leprae*, reflected in the lack of lymphocytes in the skin lesions and accumulation of unaltered macrophages containing many bacilli. Instead of CMI, there is an intense antibody response in these patients. Thus, clinically and immunologically, leprosy is a *spectrum* of possible conditions, with intermediate forms (borderline or dimorphous leprosy) between the polar extremes; the greater the degree of cell-mediated immune response, the more the condition becomes tuberculoid (Figure 4.61). In short, the course of leprosy is determined as much by the nature and degree of the host response to infection as by the pathogenic qualities of the organism.

Figure 4.61 The leprosy spectrum.

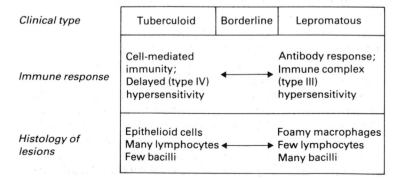

Clinical type	Tuberculoid	Borderline	Lepromatous
Immune response	Cell-mediated immunity; Delayed (type IV) hypersensitivity	⟷	Antibody response; Immune complex (type III) hypersensitivity
Histology of lesions	Epithelioid cells Many lymphocytes Few bacilli	⟷	Foamy macrophages Few lymphocytes Many bacilli

MORPHOLOGY AND GROWTH

M. leprae organisms are acid-fast rods identified by Ziehl-Neelsen staining. Recently it has been found that the acid-fastness of *M. leprae* is lost after pyridine extraction, while that of *M. tuberculosis* and other mycobacteria is unaffected, and pyridine extraction has become a routine diagnostic aid. *M. leprae* is an *obligate intracellular parasite* and in lepromatous lesions is seen packed in cigar-like array in macrophages known as *lepra cells*. The rods have a granular, beaded appearance when stained, which becomes more noticeable in organisms from patients undergoing chemotherapy; the proportion of solid staining to beaded rods (the 'morphological index') is an indicator of viability. Despite many well-controlled attempts, *M. leprae* has never been grown *in vitro*, either in culture media or in various human cell types, and this has obviously limited studies of the organism. It can be grown in two animal species—the mouse and the nine-banded armadillo. Besides providing a model for the pathogenesis of leprosy (below), infection of the mouse footpad is a sensitive, if slow, means of detecting bacilli and confirming a doubtful diagnosis. The infection in the armadillo, a disseminated form of leprosy, has also been widely used as an experimental model.

The growth of the organisms is even slower than that of other mycobacteria, with a mean generation time of 12 days in the mouse footpad. One important feature is the striking temperature dependency of their growth, which occurs much more rapidly at 30°C than 37°C; this doubtless accounts for their localisation in the cooler regions of the body (skin; peripheral nerves; mucous membranes of the mouth, nose, pharynx and larynx; eye; testes), with only infrequent invasion of internal organs. Man is the only natural host.

FACTORS IN PATHOGENICITY

The cell wall resembles that of *M. tuberculosis* in structure, but there is less information on the chemical correlates of pathogenicity. Nevertheless, it is clear that the two most important factors are (i) ability to resist intracellular destruction in macrophages, in which the organisms proceed to grow, and (ii) stimulation of a vigorous immune response. The latter may be either a strong cell-mediated (T cell) response leading to destruction of the organisms (immunity) and concomitant tissue damage (Type IV hypersensitivity), or an exceptionally high antibody (B cell) response with hypergammaglobulinaemia, auto-antibody formation and manifestations of immune complex disease. The nature of response depends on the host, in whom it is genetically determined. (In principle, the exaggerated CMI and antibody responses could both arise through activation of T cells, with hyperstimulation of CMI effector T cells in the former and helper T cells for antibody formation in the latter.)

LEPROMIN TEST

This skin test is analogous to the tuberculin test and is positive in individuals developing a cell-mediated immune response to *M. leprae*. Since the organisms cannot be grown in culture, lepromin is prepared somewhat differently from tuberculin, namely by grinding lepromatous tissue in saline, filtering off the debris and autoclaving the supernatant. Intact bacilli are present in the final preparation. In the test, a small amount of lepromin is injected intracutaneously. Two types of reaction occur—an early or *Fernandez reaction*, which resembles the tuberculin reaction and peaks at about 48 hours, and a late or *Mitsuda reaction*, developing after 7 days and reaching a peak after 3–4 weeks; the Mitsuda reaction is an allergic granuloma stimulated by the presence of persistent intact (dead) organisms. Both reactions reflect the state of sensitivity to *M. leprae* antigens brought about by existing or previous infection. Patients with the tuberculoid form of leprosy are lepromin-positive, but those with lepromatous disease are lepromin-negative, in accord with the inability of the latter to make a CMI response. The fact that lepromatous patients are often tuberculin-positive indicates that their unresponsiveness to *M. leprae* is specific for the antigens of this organism. Some of the antigens in lepromin evidently cross-react with those of tubercle bacilli, as a positive lepromin reaction occurs in healthy people immunised with BCG in countries where there is no leprosy, and in patients with tuberculosis.

PATHOGENESIS OF LEPROSY

As man is the only natural host of the leprosy bacillus and there are no healthy carriers, infection is acquired solely from patients. Although one of the first diseases to be recognised as infectious, leprosy is not highly contagious and in fact attempts at experimental infection have nearly always failed. Prolonged, close contact with a patient who is shedding bacilli in large numbers— in practice usually a lepromatous case—is required, organisms entering the body either through skin abrasions or via the respiratory tract in droplets or dust. The incubation period is variable, but usually very long, of the order of 2–4 years. The organisms localise in the skin in macrophages and also characteristically in Schwann cells of peripheral nerves. The clinical outcome of infection depends on the strength of the individual's cell-mediated (T cell) response to *M. leprae* antigens. This is illustrated by experimental infection in the mouse. In a normal mouse, leprosy bacilli cause a localised 'tuberculoid-like' lesion when injected into the footpads, and even if administered intravenously the lesions are restricted to the nose and front feet. However, if the animal's T cell response is eliminated by neonatal thymectomy or antilymphocytic serum, a generalised infection occurs and the lesions are 'lepromatous'.

For the sake of simplicity, we will concentrate on the polar forms, but it should be borne in mind that there is a spectrum of disease and some patients will be intermediate or 'borderline' between the tuberculoid and lepromatous forms (Figure 4.61). Moreover, the clinical state can be 'shifted' by chemotherapeutic agents which can move a patient from lepromatous towards tuber-

Table 4.10 Comparison of the tuberculoid and lepromatous forms of leprosy.

Feature	Tuberculoid	Lepromatous
Skin lesions:		
Numbers	1–3	Very many
Symmetry	Asymmetrical	Symmetrical
Anaesthesia	Marked, rapid	None or late
Histology of lesions:		
Granuloma cell	Epithelioid	Foamy macrophages
Lymphocytes	Many	Few or absent
Dermal nerves	Destroyed	Normal
M. leprae bacilli	Few or none	Plentiful, intracellular
Lymph nodes:		
Paracortical areas	Immunoblasts	Foamy macrophages
Germinal centres	Normal	Hypertrophied
Lepromin test	Strongly positive	Negative
ENL*	Absent	Common
Infectivity	−	+
Autoantibodies	−	+
CMI	+	−
Hypersensitivity	Type IV	Type III

*ENL: erythema nodosum leprosum

culoid by lowering the number of organisms. The polar forms are compared in Table 4.10.

Tuberculoid leprosy is relatively benign with well-defined, sharply demarcated skin lesions, which are large (several centimetres in diameter), hypopigmented, few in number (1–3) and asymmetric. The area of the lesion is *anaesthetic*, loss of sensation being caused by obliteration of cutaneous nerve twigs and swelling of the larger superficial nerves (e.g. the ulnar nerve may be palpated above the elbow). Anaesthesia leads to deformities such as 'claw hand' and 'claw toe', often accompanied by wounds and secondary infection. The cellular picture is that of an immunological granuloma and closely resembles a young tubercle, with Langhans giant cells, epithelioid cells and dense lymphocytic infiltration, but without necrosis or caseation. It is often impossible to detect any viable organisms in the tissue. The lesion is clearly the site of an intense T cell reaction in which macrophages have accumulated and, after activation by lymphokines, have successfully destroyed the intracellular organisms. In the process, nerves are damaged and the anaesthetic lesion develops as a result of cell-mediated hypersensitivity. An antibody response to *M. leprae* also occurs, but is modest in size.

Lepromatous leprosy is the most severe and disfiguring form of leprosy. The skin lesions are small, but very numerous, bilaterally-distributed macules, papules and nodules. They commonly affect the face, the skin of which becomes thickened and folded, with lesions especially on the nose and earlobes;

eyebrows and eyelashes are lost as the typical 'leonine facies' (lion-like countenance) develops. Lesions also occur on the oral, nasal and respiratory mucosa, with marked vocal changes when the larynx is affected, in the eye, where blindness may ensue, and in the testis, where orchitis leads to testicular atrophy. In the later stages of the disease, paralysis occurs, and death is due to respiratory obstruction, renal failure or secondary infection.

The lesions of lepromatous leprosy are also granulomas, but unlike those of tuberculoid cases there is *no lymphocytic involvement*. The majority cell population consists of macrophages known as *lepra cells*, which are infected with massive numbers of growing bacilli; the macrophages have a unique foamy appearance due to the accumulation of mycobacterial lipid. Up to 10^7 organisms may be present per gram of infected tissue. Here there is lack of T cell sensitisation and, in consequence, an inability to activate macrophages to a state in which they can kill the growing organisms. Nerves are also infected and large numbers of bacilli can be found in Schwann cells but, despite extensive superficial nerve involvement, anaesthesia does not occur. Lepromatous patients have a continuous bacteraemia and shed large numbers of bacilli in nasal secretions (the source of infection).

In contrast with the absence of CMI, there is vigorous antibody production in lepromatous leprosy. (The term 'split tolerance' is sometimes used to describe such a state of unresponsiveness affecting only one of the limbs of the immune system.) Polyclonal hypergammaglobulinaemia is often present. While some of the Ig is directed against *M. leprae* antigens, autoantibodies are often also present, including rheumatoid factor (anti-IgG), antinuclear factor (anti-DNA), antithyroglobulin, antitesticular antibody and Wassermann antibody (anticardiolipin). This points to an abnormality or breakdown in the regulation of B cell activity by suppressor T cells, in line with the absence of lymphokine-releasing and other T cells involved in CMI.

The high level of antibody can lead to *immune complex (Type III) hypersensitivity* in lepromatous patients if a large amount of antigen enters the circulation; this is indeed what often happens during the first year of sulphone chemotherapy for leprosy. Complexes deposit in the skin where they cause characteristic acute inflammatory nodules with large numbers of neutrophils and fibrinoid necrosis of dermal vessels; these lesions are called *erythema nodosum leprosum* (ENL). They resemble an Arthus reaction (p. 163) and can be shown to contain antibody, mycobacterial antigen and complement. Immune complexes may also cause arthritis and glomerulonephritis. Amyloid disease (p. 66) is another complication.

When the organisms are killed during drug treatment, it may become evident that individuals with lepromatous leprosy are, after all, capable of mounting a cell-mediated response. As this happens, the patient makes a transition across the disease spectrum to a more tuberculoid state, with vigorous cell-mediated hypersensitivity in the tissues where antigen remains and a severe peripheral neuritis. Such an event is called a *reversal reaction*.

The question of why an individual fails to make the T cell response to *M. leprae* and develops the lepromatous disease is not readily answerable. There are several complexities. For example, the deficiency seems to be specific for *M. leprae* antigens, as we have already noted, yet there is also evidence for more general unresponsiveness; thus lepromatous patients may fail to become sensitised by chemical skin-sensitising agents such as dinitro-chlorobenzene, and may even accept skin allografts. There is also the indication (above) that some degree of CMI can develop in lepromatous patients once the antigenic load is reduced, demonstrating that T cell unresponsiveness is not an absolute state. Genetic factors are important in determining the level and type of response to *M. leprae*, and genes linked to the HLA-D region appear to be involved (p. 169).

TREATMENT

Drugs are available which kill the leprosy bacillus, the most widely used being sulphones, especially *dapsone* (4,4'-diamino-diphenylsulphone). This halts the progress of the disease, but must be continued for a very long period — 3–5 years for tuberculoid patients, a lifetime in lepromatous cases. Side effects, caused by immune complex hypersensitivity or reversal reactions, have been noted above. *Rifampicin* is a more effective alternative, but its use is limited by greater cost.

VACCINATION

There is a high degree of antigenic cross-reaction between *M. tuberculosis*, *M. bovis* and *M. leprae*, as evidenced by the positive lepromin reactions in people infected with *M. tuberculosis* or vaccinated with BCG. There is also support from some (but not all) field trials for a protective effect of BCG on leprosy, and the use of BCG for the active immunisation of children in endemic areas has been recommended. Its effectiveness will only become apparent in future years.

SPIROCHAETACEAE: TREPONEMA

The spirochaetes are a family of organisms of unique appearance—slender, flexible, helical cells, relatively long (up to 20 μm) and actively motile though non-flagellate. Three genera cause human disease, namely *Treponema* (syphilis, yaws, pinta), *Borrelia* (relapsing fever) and *Leptospira* (leptospirosis); here we will be concerned mainly with treponemes and syphilis. The pathogenic species of Treponema are *T. pallidum* (syphilis), *T. pertenue* (yaws) and *T. carateum* (pinta), and all cause epidemic diseases of great importance in many parts of the world. Syphilis is the most serious of the sexually-transmitted (venereal) diseases and is of worldwide occurrence; yaws is an important tropical disease found in Africa, India and South America; and pinta occurs in tropical areas of Central and South America. They are all complex, chronic diseases which share common features, notably a very prolonged course which may last for over 30 years, distinct acute clinical stages with intervening asymptomatic periods and, except for the tertiary stage of syphilis, a non-fatal outcome. The pathogenic processes in these diseases are not completely understood and several important questions remain to be answered.

Treponema pallidum

MORPHOLOGY, GROWTH, ETC.

The organism is a delicate, narrow, flexuous helix ('corkscrew-shaped'), 6–15 μm in length and 0.1–0.2 μm wide (Figure 4.2k). *T. pallidum* has 4–14 tightly wound coils or 'waves' (in two dimensions), at regular intervals of 1 μm along most of its length, tapering towards the ends. The organisms are so thin that the living cells are difficult to resolve by normal transmitted-light microscopy and ordinary bacterial stains, but can be viewed with the dark-ground microscope, in which they appear as bright spirals against a dark background. They can also be visualised after silver staining, the diameter of the cells being increased by a silver precipitate on the surface; silver impregnation can be used to demonstrate them in tissues such as aorta and brain. They have characteristic motility, either rotating about the longitudinal axis in corkscrew-like fashion, or with a slower undulation or a sluggish forward and backward spring-like motion. They often bend to a right angle or more without losing the regular spiral form (Figure 4.2k).

T. pallidum is usually considered an obligate anaerobe, though recent evidence suggests it is really micro-aerophilic, surviving best at low (1–5%) oxygen tension. Despite many efforts, it has yet to be grown in culture; the cells remain alive for several days in anaerobic media, but do not divide. They are therefore propagated in animals, usually in the rabbit testis, where the rate of growth is very slow (the generation time is about 30 hours); the Nichols strain, used in diagnostic syphilis tests, has been maintained in this way for many years. Division is by transverse binary fission. Non-pathogenic treponemes, such as the Reiter strain, can be grown in culture; this organism is a distant relation of *T. pallidum*.

SENSITIVITY

T. pallidum is highly sensitive to conditions outside the body; it is rapidly killed by drying, mild heat (42°C), cold, exposure to oxygen, and most disinfectants. Hence transmission depends on direct personal contact or transplacental infection.

STRUCTURE

In addition to their distinctive morphology, the surface structure of spirochaetes presents some unique features, as illustrated in

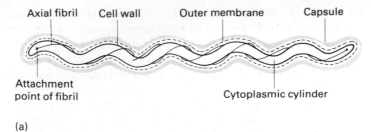

Axial fibril   Cell wall   Outer membrane   Capsule

Attachment point of fibril

Cytoplasmic cylinder

(a)

Figure 4.62 Structure of *Treponema pallidum*.
(a) Schematic diagram of main features (only 2 axial fibrils shown; helix has up to 14 coils).
(b) (i) Schematic longitudinal section.
    (ii) Transverse section as seen in electron microscope.
(c) Mode of attachment of *T. pallidum* to cell surfaces, as seen by scanning electron microscopy.

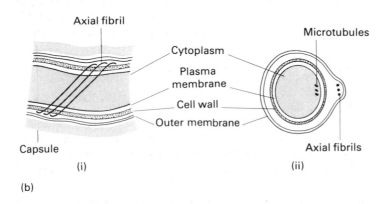

Axial fibril

Microtubules

Cytoplasm

Plasma membrane

Cell wall

Outer membrane

Capsule

(i)

Axial fibrils

(ii)

(b)

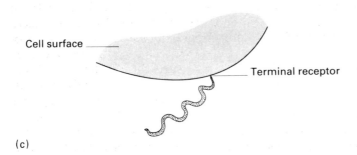

Cell surface

Terminal receptor

(c)

Figure 4.62. The cytoplasmic cylinder is enclosed by the plasma membrane and a closely fitting peptidoglycan cell wall, which is responsible for the helical shape; outside this is a second membrane, the outer envelope or sheath. To this extent they resemble Gram-negative bacteria, but the outer membrane does not contain lipopolysaccharide. Between the cell wall and the outer membrane are found one or more *axial fibrils* (axial filaments) which are much like flagella except that, instead of projecting from the surface, they are wound tightly around the cylinder and are covered by the outer membrane. Axial fibrils are attached by a 'disc' at each end of the cell and run more than half its length; thus the fibrils from opposite ends overlap in the midregion of the organism. The number of axial fibrils varies among different species, with a minimum of one pair; in *T. pallidum* there are six in all, three inserted at each end. They are assumed to be involved in motility, though this has not been unequivocally established. A cross-section shows that within the cytoplasm are 6–8 tubules, or body fibrils, which also arise at each end and wind around the cylinder to the midpoint.

The existence of a capsule has been established by electron microscopy; that of *T. pallidum* is composed of acidic mucopolysaccharide (glycosaminoglycan) containing N-acetyl-glucosamine and N-acetylgalactosamine, and is thus similar to the hyaluronic acid and chondroitin sulphate components of connective tissue. The organism also possesses a *mucopolysaccharidase* enzyme which can digest the latter molecules, perhaps to provide the sugars required for its own capsular synthesis. The proportion of *T. pallidum* cells with a detectable capsule varies from 50% to 90% of freshly isolated organisms.

TREPONEMAL ANTIGENS AND SYPHILITIC ANTIBODIES

Analysis of the antigenic surface molecules of *T. pallidum* has been hampered by the inability to grow the organism in culture. One membrane component of particular interest is the phospholipid known as *cardiolipin* (diphosphatidylglycerol), the antigen which stimulates the diagnostic *Wassermann antibodies* (anticardiolipin) found in syphilitic serum (p. 194). It is well known that cardiolipin is present in normal mammalian tissues, where it forms part of the mitochondrial membrane, so that anticardiolipin is an *autoantibody*. Until recently it was assumed that the antibody was probably made in response to cardiolipin released from tissues damaged during the course of the disease, and indeed its non-specific presence in other chronic conditions (malaria, leprosy, SLE) supports this view. However, it has now been demonstrated that cardiolipin exists in the treponemal cell membrane, making it equally if not more likely that the Wassermann antibody is a direct response to the organism. Free cardiolipin itself is non-immunogenic, but the bacterium would serve as the carrier for an antibody response. Anticardiolipin antibodies do not bind to the intact organisms, but other antibodies present in the serum during syphilis do react with *T. pallidum* and are used in the specific confirmatory tests for the disease (p. 618).

Certain group-specific antigens are shared by all treponemes, including the non-pathogenic Reiter strain. Antitreponemal sera absorbed with Reiter organisms become specific for the virulent treponemal species (*T. pallidum*, *T. pertenue* and *T. carateum*), but no species-specific antigen for *T. pallidum* has been found and the three organisms appear to be antigenically identical. Nor is it known which antigen is responsible for the immunity which develops during syphilis.

DETERMINANTS OF PATHOGENICITY

The particular properties of *T. pallidum* which underlie its virulence are incompletely understood. It is not a toxigenic organism: no exotoxins have been identified, nor does the cell wall contain endotoxin. Indeed, in early lesions the organisms multiply to considerable numbers without producing gross tissue damage. Most of the organisms in a lesion are extracellular, and are probably killed if taken up by phagocytes; nevertheless, a small number evidently can survive intracellularly in macrophages and in non-phagocytic cells (endothelial cells, fibroblasts), and this may explain the persistence in the body of *T. pallidum* during the long asymptomatic periods which characterise the full course of syphilis (below). *Invasiveness* is the key property and is probably dependent on the mucopolysaccharide capsule which is believed to be antiphagocytic; it also protects the organisms from bactericidal attack by antibody and complement and accounts for the non-reactivity of freshly-isolated organisms in serological tests. The capsular material is water-soluble and is continuously being shed (dissolved) and resynthesized; in solution it could block opsonising antibodies or sensitised T cells and thereby contribute further to the survival of *T. pallidum* during the primary and secondary stages of syphilis (cf. shedding of capsular material by pneumococci).

The organisms also carry a mucopolysaccharidase enzyme which digests the hyaluronic acid and chondroitin sulphate components of connective tissue ground substance. Two functions for this enzyme have been proposed: (i) as a receptor enabling the organisms to adhere to cell surfaces and to connective tissue, and (ii) to break down ground substance to provide the constituent sugars for the synthesis of the organism's own capsule. As far as adherence is concerned, it is known that *T. pallidum* will attach to the surface of many different cells in culture, probably binding to membrane sugar residues; electron microscopy of bound organisms shows that binding occurs by the tapered end only (Figure 4.62c) and it has been suggested that this outer tip may be the location of the mucopolysaccharidase acting as a receptor. The organisms probably attach in this way to the inside of blood vessels before invading perivascular tissues. In its enzymatic role, the mucopolysaccharidase causes the destruction of ground substance and may contribute to invasiveness as well as to the pathological changes in and around blood vessels that are characteristic of syphilitic lesions. The known inability of some treponemes to synthesize N-acetylglucosamine (not yet confirmed for *T. pallidum*) would be a rationale for the localisation of organisms in connective tissue around blood vessels, where ground substance polymers could provide a source of the sugars for capsular biosynthesis.

HISTORY AND EPIDEMIOLOGY OF SYPHILIS

Syphilis has been known in Europe for a little less than 500 years —a short time when compared with some diseases—and there is no evidence that it existed in ancient times. It was not described until it first appeared in Europe at the end of the fifteenth century; popular belief has it that the disease was imported in 1493 by Columbus's sailors returning from their discovery of the

West Indies, but this may be apocryphal. An epidemic certainly broke out among the French soldiers at the siege of Naples in 1494 and thereafter syphilis spread all over Europe and was probably exported to the Far East by Vasco da Gama's sailors. It was extremely virulent for about 60 years, subsequently becoming milder; the late consequences remained serious however, and until recent times were among the main causes of admission to mental hospitals.

The worldwide incidence of the disease became enormous and has remained so; in 1970 there were an estimated 50 million cases of early syphilis in the world. After the Second World War, the widespread use of penicillin led to a rapid decline in its incidence in developed countries, but the trend was reversed in the early 1960's, especially in the USA. Today, syphilis is a much less common sexually-transmitted disease than gonorrhoea. In England and Wales, the number of new cases fell rapidly from a peak of 24,000 in 1947, and since 1965 has been around 2000 annually, with little tendency to increase, at a time when gonorrhoea is reaching epidemic proportions (p. 536). One reason

Figure 4.63 Pathogenesis of syphilis.
? : uncertain

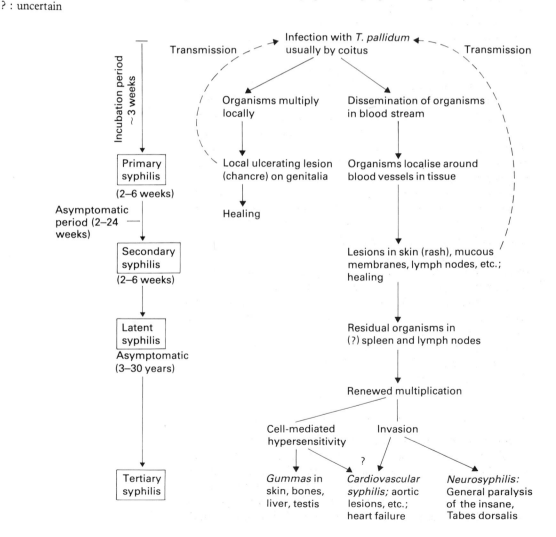

611

is that asymptomatic female carriers, of major importance in the spread of gonorrhoea, are far less frequent in syphilis. In the USA there has been a significant increase from the low point in 1958 and there are now about 30,000 reported cases of primary and secondary syphilis annually (the true number of cases may be considerably higher), the greatest incidence (45 per 100,000 population) being in the 20–24 year age group. Male homosexuals account for many cases in cities.

PATHOGENESIS OF SYPHILIS   (Figure 4.63)

Syphilis is a chronic granulomatous disease, the full course of which is extremely prolonged (the lesions of the final stage may be delayed for up to 30 years after initial infection). There are three well-defined stages—primary, secondary and tertiary— separated by asymptomatic periods of varying lengths. After an incubation period of 3–4 weeks, an acute localised *primary lesion* appears which heals in 2–6 weeks and is followed by an asymptomatic phase lasting 2–3 months. Then follows the acute *secondary stage*, with generalised lesions, which again heal in 2–6 weeks. This stage is succeeded by a *latent period* of several years' duration, during which time there are no clinical manifestations, but which in a minority of patients leads to the most serious form of the disease, *tertiary syphilis* with cardiovascular and neurological involvement. This relapsing course is the result of the ability of *T. pallidum* organisms to survive in the body for many years, emerging to multiply and produce the secondary and tertiary stages when 'circumstances', such as perhaps a reduced immune response, permit. While the host response to *T. pallidum* leads to healing, it does not eliminate the organisms completely, some of which go into 'hiding' in an unknown way in the clinically silent periods.

Although the histological appearance of syphilitic lesions is well known, the processes involved are not easy to explain and there are several unanswered questions in connection with this fascinating disease. Among them are the following: Why does the active host immune response fail to eliminate the organisms after the primary lesions or the secondary stage? How does such a seemingly delicate organism manage to escape destruction for such long periods of time? What becomes of it during the silent periods of the disease? And what factors cause it to re-emerge from its hiding place in the secondary and tertiary stages? Man is the only natural host for *T. pallidum* and, in the past, experimental inoculation with living organisms has been performed in volunteers to study events such as immunity. The best animal model is the rabbit, in which primary and secondary syphilis, but not the later stages, can be reproduced.

Syphilis is normally acquired by direct contact, the organisms being too sensitive to drying to survive for long periods outside the body; infection usually occurs during sexual intercourse, though occasionally by kissing or other close bodily contact. A person having coitus with an infected partner has about a 10% likelihood of acquiring the disease. It has been known for syphilis to be transmitted by blood transfusion, especially when fresh blood is used, as the organisms are disseminated in the bloodstream before the primary lesion appears. However, storage of blood at 5°C for 72–96 hours leads to the disappearance of *T. pallidum*. Congenital infection is described on p. 616. When sexually transmitted, *T. pallidum* enters the body either through a minute break or abrasion in the penile skin or intact mucous membranes in females (labia, vagina, cervix) or male homosexuals (rectum); these are also the sites at which the primary lesion eventually appears. While some of the infecting organisms attach to the local subepithelial tissue at the point of entry, others are rapidly carried away in lymphatics and the bloodstream. Organisms distributed in this early *bacteraemia* adhere to the inner walls of capillaries in many tissues and apparently pass between endothelial cells into the perivascular areas. Thus, syphilis is a generalised infection *from the outset*, though disseminated lesions do not appear until the secondary stage.

After an incubation period of 2–3 weeks, the single primary lesion appears, the *primary sore* or *chancre*, usually on the external genitals at the initial site of infection; it is a small, hard, painless nodule, dull red in colour, which forms an ulcer about 1 cm in diameter, with a clean, firm base. The local lymph nodes enlarge and become hard and rubbery. The chancre, which persists for some weeks, is a *highly infective* lesion, containing many living treponemes identifiable in the serous exudate by dark-ground microscopy. Histologically, there is a dense cellular infiltration, the typical cells involved both here and in later lesions being lymphocytes and plasma cells, with some macrophages and giant cells. Thus the lesion is not an acute inflammatory response to treponemal tissue damage, but rather the site of an *antitreponemal immune reaction*. T and B lymphocytes are both present: the T cells and macrophages represent a cell-mediated response to the organisms, while the B cells, and especially the plasma cells, are engaged in local Ig production, though it is not known why plasma cells are so well represented. A characteristic feature of this and other syphilitic lesions is the involvement of blood vessels. Thus infiltrating lymphocytes lie mainly around arterioles and capillaries (*perivascular cuffing, periarteritis*) while, within the vessels, endothelial cells swell and proliferate (*endarteritis*). When the lumen of the vessels is reduced to such an extent that blood flow ceases, the condition is called *endarteritis obliterans*, and this leads to necrosis distal to the block and the ulceration of the chancre. As the organisms are removed, the lymphocytes and other cells gradually disappear and the chancre heals with slight scarring. There then follows a clinically silent period of 2–24 weeks.

The immunological processes which eliminate *T. pallidum* from the chancre do not prevent the organisms from multiplying slowly at the sites to which they were distributed at the outset of the infection. In the *secondary stage* of syphilis, these sites now become apparent as lesions in the skin and mucous membranes (*mucocutaneous rash*). The skin rash, which may be macular, papular or pustular, often occurs first on the palms of the hands and soles of the feet, eventually spreading elsewhere with multiple symmetrical lesions. In the moist regions of the skin, such as membranes of the external female genitalia or around the anus, raised papules occur called *condylomata lata*, while on the mouth and tonsils moist patches or papules break down to give '*snail-track ulcers*'. Like the chancre, these lesions contain many organisms and all are highly infective; they also show a similar histological appearance, with invasion by lymphocytes, prominent plasma cells and some macrophages, accompanied by vascular changes. Lesions may also occur elsewhere (meninges, bones, eyes, liver), some being due to deposition of *immune complexes* composed of antitreponemal antibody and treponemal antigen. Such complexes are found in the glomerular basement membrane of the kidney, where they give rise to glomerulonephritis as part of a *nephrotic syndrome*; they also affect the joints (arthritis, arthralgia). Host immune defence leads to healing of the lesions of secondary syphilis after a few weeks, though they sometimes recur up to three times. Once the secondary lesions have healed, the individual is no longer a danger to others (except to a foetus).

The host is by now solidly immune and for many patients the disease is at an end; in others it enters a prolonged quiescent phase with no clinical manifestations, the *latent period*, which generally lasts for several years. In these individuals, some organisms remain in the body, sequestered especially in the spleen and lymph nodes and presumably intracellular. In experimental syphilis in rabbits, there is a similar state of latent infection after recovery from the secondary stage. In both rabbit and man, this asymptomatic infection can be terminated with penicillin, proving that viable, growing organisms must be present. For reasons which are not entirely clear, but are thought to involve a decline in antitreponemal immunity, the treponemes emerge from their latent state after a number of years and give rise to *tertiary syphilis*, which can affect almost any tissue and may be fatal. Tertiary syphilis can take three forms: benign tertiary syphilis, cardiovascular syphilis and neurosyphilis.

(i) *Benign tertiary syphilis*, which develops after 3–10 years, is characterised by large granulomas called *gummas*. A gumma contains a central area of necrosis, surrounded by lymphocytes, plasma cells, giant cells and epithelioid cells, with an outer region of fibrous tissue; the infiltrating cells are again found around blood vessels which become occluded by endarteritis. The zone of *gummatous necrosis* is firm and rubbery and the structural outline of the dead cells is preserved, without the tendency to caseation seen in tuberculous lesions. Gummas, which are found particularly in the liver, testis or bone, are very destructive, due to the ischaemia resulting from endarteritis obliterans. They contain *very few organisms* and are interpreted as being a cell-mediated hypersensitivity reaction to a depot of treponemal antigen, i.e. of essentially similar origin to the granulomas of tuberculosis. Gummas are generally not lethal, hence the epithet 'benign'.

(ii) *Cardiovascular syphilis* affects the aorta and aortic valves and usually takes at least 10 and up to 40 years to appear. The condition is caused by obliterative endarteritis of the vasa vasorum, which results in degeneration of the media and replacement of elastic lamellae and muscle by fibrous tissue. The fibrous tissue stretches, resulting in *aneurysmal dilatation* of the wall (p. 47). This damage to the media is associated with atherosclerotic thickening of the intima (p. 650), often with a characteristic focal lymphocytic/plasma cell infiltration in the adventitia. Serious clinical effects occur when the aortic valve dilates, with separation of the valve cusps; the aortic valvular incompetence can eventually lead to left ventricular failure and death.

(iii) *Neurosyphilis* may affect the meninges at any stage and result in nerve palsies, damage to the spinal cord, or cerebral infarction (p. 649) (*meningo-vascular syphilis*). Direct damage to the brain may also occur, associated with the presence of abundant organisms and atrophy of the white matter. This leads to the classical *general paralysis of the insane* (general paresis), which was frequently encountered in mental hospitals, but is now uncommon; among its more extreme manifestations are temper tantrums, frequent weeping, depression and delusions of grandeur. *Tabes dorsalis* (locomotor ataxia) is a degeneration of the posterior column and roots of the spinal cord; there are numerous symptoms, including intense stabbing pains at irregular intervals in the legs (lightning pains), unsteadiness of gait, loss of bladder sensation (with consequences for the urinary tract), impotence and blindness. The pathogenic mechanism is unknown.

THE IMMUNE RESPONSE IN SYPHILIS

The chronic nature of the disease and the persistence of organisms over very long periods of time is not due to lack of an immune response against *T. pallidum*; indeed, the constant finding of lymphocytes and plasma cells in the lesions indicates a continuous response on the part of T and B cells. Cell-mediated and antibody responses to treponemal antigens both develop; the antibodies are used in the serological tests for syphilis and are detailed below. The fact that more than 50% of untreated patients do not progress clinically beyond the primary stage shows that immunity develops and can be successful. Although its induction is a rather slow process, patients are immune to reinfection after healing of the primary lesion, though this may not prevent them from harbouring treponemes for many years and passing through further stages of the disease. Antibodies alone are not responsible for immunity, as shown by the inability to prevent syphilis in rabbits by passive transfer of immune serum (though the lesions do become less severe); as noted above, the capsule probably helps to protect the organism against the lytic and opsonising effects of antibody. The existence of CMI is demonstrable *in vivo* by delayed hypersensitivity to treponemal antigens in secondary, latent and tertiary syphilis, and *in vitro* by stimulation of patients' lymphocytes to transform into blast cells and divide after exposure to treponemal antigens, with release of lymphokines such as macrophage migration inhibition factor (MIF). However, the role of CMI in immunity and recovery is unclear, and transfer of sensitised lymphocytes (T cells) provides only partial protection in rabbits. Immunity seems to require both antibody and CMI responses acting in concert. As far as contribution to tissue damage is concerned, we have already noted that the gumma is a cell-mediated reaction to treponemal antigens, in which very few, if any, viable organisms are present, as in all late lesions except general paresis.

There is some evidence for *immunosuppression* during syphilis, and one hypothesis is that this permits the multiplication of, and tissue invasion by, *T. pallidum* during the secondary stage in the face of immune processes designed to kill it. Although this is controversial, it seems that some interference with immune mechanisms is probably involved at the onset of the secondary and tertiary stages. For example, the incidence of disseminated lesions in rabbits, similar to the secondary stage in man, is much higher in animals treated with immunosuppressive agents. Moreover, an immunosuppressive factor has been found in the blood of syphilitic patients and rabbits which interferes with T cell responses to treponemal antigens. This factor may be the capsular mucopolysaccharide, as it is claimed that it can be destroyed by treatment of syphilitic serum with hyaluronidase. However, although the theory is attractive, the relevance of immunological perturbations of this type to the progress of syphilis requires further study.

CONGENITAL SYPHILIS

This is a result of infection of the foetus *in utero*; treponemes present in the circulation of a pregnant woman cross the placenta during the second trimester and infect many foetal organs. Thus, infection is prenatal and the mother always has the disease, though not necessarily clinical symptoms. The effects on the foetus depend on the number of transmitted organisms and this is determined in turn by the stage of the mother's disease. At the primary stage, treponemes will be plentiful in her circulation and the foetus may receive an overwhelming infection leading to its death *in utero* (stillbirth). If the mother's disease is at the secondary or latent stage, the baby survives but is likely to have congenital syphilis, either apparent at birth or becoming apparent by two years (*early congenital syphilis*) or thereafter (*late congenital syphilis*). In practice, one third of pregnant women with untreated syphilis produce healthy children, one third have babies with congenital syphilis, and the remainder end in stillbirth or abortion.

In early congenital syphilis, there is no primary lesion as the infection is blood-borne, and the symptoms are those of the secondary stage. Organisms abound in lesions in the skin and mucous membranes of the nose, mouth, throat and larynx; 'snuffles' follows destruction of nasal bones; the liver and spleen are enlarged; and abnormalities of the long bones develop. Alternatively, the disease may only become clinically apparent some years later, and the lesions are then typical of the tertiary stage, with gummas and neurosyphilis. Many children with late congenital syphilis have dental 'stigmata' in the form of maldeveloped permanent teeth—characteristically peg-shaped incisors (Hutchinson's teeth) and dome-shaped molars (Mulberry molars). Three common manifestations make up *Hutchinson's triad*: interstitial keratitis (corneal inflammation), deafness (due to 8th nerve involvement) and Hutchinson's teeth. The determining factors in the development of early versus late disease are probably the stage of the disease in the mother, the number of organisms infecting the foetus, the age of the foetus at which infection occurs, and the extent to which it is able to make an immune response (maternal IgG antibodies will also cross the placenta, but evidently do not prevent infection).

Congenital syphilis only occurs when the mother's disease is not diagnosed and treated during pregnancy; where routine antenatal diagnostic tests for syphilis are carried out, congenital syphilis is relatively rare. Nevertheless, despite widespread antenatal programmes, there have been some 400–500 cases annually in the USA in recent years (10–20 in the UK). Once a woman has been adequately treated, future pregnancies are safe.

TREATMENT

Syphilis can be cured by penicillin, the drug of choice since 1943; fortunately, resistant strains of *T. pallidum* have not emerged. All clinical stages, including latency and congenital syphilis, can be treated successfully with penicillin, indicating the presence of viable organisms throughout the disease. A few hours after starting antibiotic treatment, especially in early syphilis, there may be a *Jarisch-Herxheimer reaction*, a temporary exacerbation of lesions such as the chancre or secondary rash, accompanied by headache, fever, malaise and aching bones. The reaction usually subsides within 24 hours and has no serious consequences but, rather, indicates effective therapy. It seems to be an Arthus-type reaction in the lesions caused by complexes of antibody with the treponemal antigen released from killed organisms. If penicillin is given early in the primary stage of the disease, immunity fails to develop and the patient remains susceptible to further infection; if treatment is delayed, immunity is permanent.

DIAGNOSTIC SEROLOGICAL TESTS FOR SYPHILIS

The antibodies present in the blood during syphilis are very valuable diagnostic aids. Two types of test are employed, namely (a) those which detect antibodies against cardiolipin, of which the Wassermann reaction is the classic example, and (b) those which detect antibodies reacting with the treponemal organisms themselves.

Anticardiolipin tests (also known as 'standard tests for syphilis' or

STS). In 1906, Wassermann discovered that the serum of syphilitics reacted with an antigen present in extracts of liver from human foetuses which had died of congenital syphilis; the antigen was subsequently found in normal liver extracts and indeed in many mammalian tissues, and was identified as the phospholipid *diphosphatidylglycerol* (*cardiolipin*). The preparation in current use is an extract of beef heart mixed with lecithin and cholesterol. (Heart muscle is rich in mitochondria, which contain cardiolipin in their membranes.) The original *Wassermann reaction* employed complement fixation as the assay, as described on p. 136; however, flocculation (precipitation) tests have become more widely used, particularly the Venereal Disease Research Laboratory (VDRL) test, which is rapid, reliable and simple to perform. In the VDRL test, cardiolipin antigen is mixed with the patient's serum on a slide for 4 minutes and then examined under the low power of the microscope for flocculation. By making serial dilutions of the test serum, the strength of reaction can be expressed as an end-point; a prozone (inhibition by antibody excess) may occur with strongly positive sera.

The drawback of anticardiolipin tests is their relative lack of specificity for syphilis, leading to biological (i.e. not simply due to technical error) *false-positive reactions* with sera from individuals who are either healthy or have some quite unrelated disease. Thus, 1% of normal adults have anticardiolipin antibodies; infections such as pneumonia, hepatitis and malaria, cause a transient false-positive reaction, while chronic conditions such as systemic lupus erythematosus, rheumatoid arthritis and leprosy give reactions which persist for many months. It is assumed that anticardiolipin is made in these diseases because cardiolipin is frequently released or revealed through tissue damage, followed by an autoimmune response which seems to occur quite readily (p. 193). As we have already noted, cardiolipin is also one of the membrane lipids of *T. pallidum* and this may be the source of antigenic stimulation in syphilis itself.

Antitreponemal tests. In order to confirm a diagnosis of syphilis by serology, it is necessary to rule out a false-positive reaction by turning to a specific test using *T. pallidum* as the antigen; anti-treponemal tests are therefore used as a follow-up to a positive Wassermann or VDRL test.

(i) In the *Treponema pallidum immobilisation* (*TPI*) *test* the presence of serum antibodies which can inhibit the motility of *T. pallidum* is detected; the organisms are killed by the bactericidal action of the antibodies and complement and thus stop moving. Living organisms are incubated with the serum and guinea-pig complement for 18 hours at 35°C, followed by examination using dark-field microscopy. However, the TPI test is technically complicated as well as expensive to perform, and therefore is not in routine use.

(ii) *The fluorescent treponemal antibody* (*FTA*) *tests* are indirect immunofluorescence tests (p. 137). The test serum is allowed to react with a film of *T. pallidum* (Nichols strain) fixed on a slide; antitreponemal antibodies bind to the organisms and are detected by addition of fluorescent antihuman Ig followed by darkground microscopy in u.v. light. The FTA test is made more specific for *T. pallidum* if antibodies to group-specific treponemal antigens are first removed by absorption with the Reiter treponemes (the FTA-ABS test).

(iii) The *Treponema pallidum haemagglutination (TPHA) test* is an indirect (passive) haemagglutination test (p. 135) using red cells to which treponemal antigens have been coupled. The antigens are obtained from sonicated organisms and the coupling occurs by treating the red cells with tannic acid, whereupon they will absorb protein to their surface. The test serum is titrated and a drop of antigen-coated red cells added to each dilution; a positive reaction is seen as haemagglutination and the titre can be determined. The test has the advantages of simplicity and sensitivity and can be automated to deal with large numbers of serum samples. It is therefore an ideal screening test for syphilis and other treponematoses.

The serological tests are positive through all the stages of untreated disease, persistent organisms providing a constant stimulus to antibody production. After clearance of the organisms by penicillin, antibody production eventually ceases and Wassermann antibodies are generally undetectable after 3–6 months, though antitreponemal tests remain positive for a longer period.

CONTROL OF SPREAD

Control of spread of syphilis is difficult and involves tracing all known sexual contacts and treating them with penicillin. In women especially, the early lesion may go unnoticed; a single promiscuous person may transmit organisms to many sexual partners. Since immunity develops during the course of the disease, vaccination against syphilis should be possible. However, inactivated organisms fail to induce immunity in rabbits, presumably because of the labile nature of the protective antigens (as yet unidentified). There are no living, attenuated strains of *T. pallidum*.

FURTHER READING

General

Christie A.B. (1980) *Infectious Diseases: Epidemiology and Clinical Practice*, 3rd edition. Churchill Livingstone.

Davis B.D., Dulbecco R., Eisen H.N. & Ginsburg H.S. (1980) *Microbiology*, 3rd edn. Harper and Row.

Duguid J.P., Marmion B.P. & Swain R.H. (eds.) (1978) *Mackie and McCartney's Medical Microbiology* Volume 1: Microbial Infections, 13th edn. Churchill Livingstone.

Gillies R.R. & Dodds T.C. (1973) *Bacteriology Illustrated*, 3rd edn. Churchill Livingstone.

Joklik W.K., Willett H.P. & Amos D.B. (eds.) (1980) *Zinsser, Microbiology* 17th edn. Appleton Century Crofts.

Milgrom F. & Flanagan T.D. (1982) *Medical Microbiology*. Churchill Livingstone.

Mims C.A. (1982) *The Pathogenesis of Infectious Disease*, 2nd edn. Academic Press.

Turk D.C. & Porter I.A. (1978) *A Short Textbook of Medical Microbiology*, 4th edn. Hodder and Stoughton.

Volk W.A. (1978) *Essentials of Medical Microbiology*. J.B. Lippincott.

Specific topics

Adam A., Petit J.F., Lefrancier P. & Lederer E. (1981) Muramyl peptides: chemical structure, biological activity and mechanism of action. *Molec. Cell. Biochem.*, **41**, 27.

Bradley S.G. (1979) Cellular and molecular mechanisms of bacterial endotoxins. *Ann. Revs. Microbiol.*, **35**, 67.

Bullock W.E. (1978) Leprosy: A model of immunological perturbation in chronic infection. *J. Infect. Dis.*, **137**, 341.

Davies J. & Smith D.I. (1978) Plasmid-determined resistance to antimicrobial agents. *Ann. Revs. Microbiol.*, **32**, 469.

Ellwood D.C., Melling J. & Rutter I. (eds.) (1979) *Adhesion of Microorganisms to Surfaces*. Academic Press.

Elwell L.P. & Shipley P.L. (1980) Plasmid-mediated factors associated with virulence of bacteria to animals. *Ann. Revs. Microbiol.*, **34**, 465.

Field M. (1979) Modes of action of enterotoxins from *Vibrio cholerae* and *Escherichia coli*. *Revs. Infect. Dis.*, **1**, 918.

Fitzgerald T.J. (1981) Pathogenesis and immunology of *Treponema pallidum*. *Ann. Revs. Microbiol.*, **35**, 29.

Formal S.B. & Hornick R.B. (1978) Invasive *Escherichia coli*. *J. Infect. Dis.*, **137**. 641.

Gilbert W. & Villa-Komaroff L. (1980) Useful proteins from recombinant bacteria. *Scientific American*, **242**, 68.

Hardy K. (1981) *Bacterial Plasmids*. Aspects of Microbiology series, no. 4. Nelson.

Holmgren J. (1981) Actions of cholera toxin and the prevention and treatment of cholera. *Nature*, **292**, 413.

Honda T. & Finkelstein R.A. (1979) Selection and characterisation of a novel *Vibrio cholerae* mutant lacking the A (ADP-ribosylating) portion of the cholera enterotoxin. *Proc. Nat. Acad. Sci. USA*, **76**, 2052.

Inouye M. (1979) *Bacterial Outer Membranes: Biogenesis and Function*. Wiley.

Johnson R.C. (1977) The spirochaetes. *Ann. Revs. Microbiol.*, **31**, 89.

Lai C.Y. (1980) The chemistry and biology of cholera toxin. *CRC Crit. Rev. Biochem.*, **9**, 171.

Mäkelä P.H. & Stocker B.A.D. (1981) Genetics of the bacterial surface. *Symp. Soc. Gen. Microbiol.*, **31**, 219.

Mass W.K. (1981) Genetics of bacterial virulence. *Symp. Soc. Gen. Microbiol.*, **31**, 341.

McGhee J.R. & Michelek S.M. (1981) Immunobiology of dental caries: microbial aspects and local immunity. *Ann. Revs. Microbiol.*, **35**, 595.

McNabb P. & Tomasi T.B. (1981) Host defense mechanisms at mucosal surfaces. *Ann. Revs. Microbiol.*, **35**, 477.

Novick R.P. (1980) Plasmids. *Scientific American*, **243**, 76.

Ouchterlony O. & Holmgren J. (eds.) (1980) *Cholera and Related Diarrhoeas: Molecular Aspects of a Global Health Problem*. 43rd Nobel Symposium. S. Karger, Basel.

Pappenheimer A.M. (1982) Diphtheria: studies on the biology of an infectious disease. *Harvey Lectures*, series 76, 45.

Parker M.T. (ed.) (1979) *Pathogenic Streptococci: Streptococcal Disease in Man and Animals*. Reedbooks.

Parry W.H. (1979) *Communicable Diseases*, 3rd edn. Hodder and Stoughton.

Robins-Browne R.M. (1980) Enterotoxins and disease. *South African J. Sci.*, **76**, 352.

Rogers H.J., Perkins H.R. & Ward J.B. (1980) *Microbial Cell Walls and Membranes*. Chapman and Hall.

Schofield C.B.S. (1979) *Sexually Transmitted Diseases*, 3rd edn. Churchill Livingstone.

Stephen J. & Pietrowski R.A. (1981) *Bacterial Toxins*. Aspects of Microbiology Series. Nelson.

von Graevenitz A. (1977) The role of opportunistic bacteria in human disease. *Ann. Revs. Microbiol.*, **31**, 447.

SECTION 5   THE CIRCULATION

Introduction

This section deals with pathological changes in the circulation, disorders which together account for about half the human mortality in the developed parts of the world. The major components of cardiovascular disease, namely *atherosclerosis, hypertension* and their sequels, are peculiarly human conditions, encountered only infrequently among other species, even other primates. They are also primarily diseases of the 'civilised' nations and are rare among so-called 'primitive' peoples. The high mortality with which they are associated derives mainly from complications of atherosclerosis, such as *coronary thrombosis*. Both atherosclerosis itself and thrombosis result in large measure from deviations of normal processes involved in repair of blood vessels and cessation of bleeding (*haemostasis*), brought about by abnormal conditions in the circulation. Specialised blood cells, the *platelets*, play a central role both in the normal and pathological events. Their activities and specific disorders are discussed in the opening part of this section, together with the *blood clotting* system. The processes involved in thrombosis and atherosclerosis and their sequels (*embolism, ischaemia, infarction*) are then described. The later part of the section deals with the origins of hypertension, a disease affecting a significant proportion of Western populations and one which is important to the development of other cardiovascular disorders. The section concludes with an account of *oedema*, the abnormal accumulation of fluid in tissues, which is one of the important results of circulatory disease.

THE PLATELETS

Platelets are of major importance in haemostasis and thrombosis, both of which begin with their adherence on and around the surface of damaged blood vessels. Platelets play two distinct haemostatic roles in the circulation. The first is to prevent leakage of red cells from blood vessels in areas of minor endothelial damage. Such 'wear and tear', with shedding of endothelial cells, can frequently occur under the normal haemodynamic stress forces of the circulation; at points where endothelial cells have been lost, platelets adhere to the basement membrane to re-establish the integrity of the wall and avoid loss of red cells (Figure 5.9). In due course the endothelium grows back over the damaged area. Their second role is to arrest haemorrhage after vascular injury. Their importance in these processes is indicated respectively by the *purpura* (bleeding into skin) and increased bleeding time in patients with severe *thrombocytopenia* (platelet deficiency). Platelet mechanisms in haemostasis are more 'primitive' than blood clotting and in lower animals in which a clotting system is lacking, cells which are the equivalents of platelets, called amoebocytes, form solid aggregates at the sites of vascular injury. In their normal state in circulating blood, platelets are convex discs, $2-5$ μ in diameter, and are the smallest blood elements; they number $200,000-400,000$ per cubic millimetre. They are formed in a highly unusual way by the disintegration of enormous precursor giant cells in the bone marrow called *megakaryocytes*. These cells develop a polyploid nucleus with up to thirty-two times the normal chromosome number before delicate processes form in the cytoplasm, which then breaks up into tiny fragments. Each fragment becomes a platelet and 3,000–4,000 are produced by each megakaryocyte. The life-span of platelets in the blood is about 10 days.

Structure of platelets

Figure 5.1 shows some details of platelet structure. Within a smooth membrane, they contain mitochondria, electron-dense granules and a system of microtubules running just beneath the membrane. There is no nucleus, few ribosomes and no endoplasmic reticulum. The granules, which contain substances important to the functioning of platelets, are of two types. The α granules are essentially lysosomes, containing enzymes such as acid hydrolases and cathepsins, as well as cationic substances which increase vascular permeability. The other type of granule, the dense body, is of higher electron density and contains calcium, ADP and the vasoactive amine 5-hydroxytryptamine (5-HT or serotonin), which has properties similar to histamine. Associated with the platelet membrane is a phospholipid called *platelet factor 3*, an essential component of the blood clotting system (p. 635). Platelets are thus equipped, through their granular and membrane components, both to play a major role in clotting and haemostasis, and also to provide mediators of acute inflammation (Section 1). About 15–20% of the total platelet protein is actomyosin, which may be responsible for many of the characteristic reactions of platelets (below) including the release reaction, aggregation, shape changes and contraction of blood clots. *Thrombosthenin* is another term for this platelet contractile protein.

Figure 5.2 Platelet reactions in haemostasis.

Reactions of platelets

The characteristic reactions of platelets take place when, due to a break in the vascular endothelium or damage to the vessel, the platelets come into contact with connective tissue in the vessel wall or surrounding tissues. These reactions are (i) *adhesion* to foreign surfaces, (ii) the *platelet release reaction*, in which 5-HT and ADP are released from platelet granules, leading to (iii) *aggregation* to form tightly-packed platelet masses, and (iv) interaction with the blood clotting system by platelet clotting factors (Figure 5.2). These reactions serve to arrest bleeding at sites of vascular damage, but also initiate the process of thrombosis. Adhesion and aggregation are also accompanied by characteristic changes of shape including swelling and formation of pseudopodia.

1 *Platelet adhesion* is initiated by contact with many surfaces including, most importantly, connective tissue fibres, especially collagen, and also by glass, metal and some tissue cells. Adhesion

Figure 5.1 Platelet
ultrastructure.

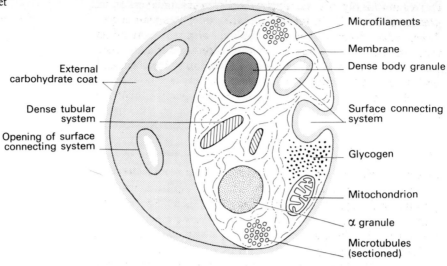

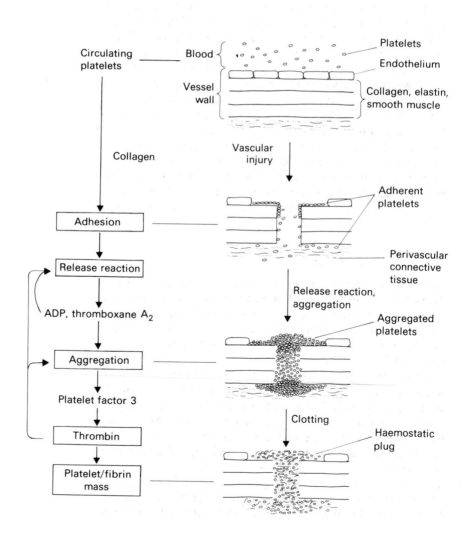

is a very rapid process, occurring with a few seconds of surface contact. Clearly the normal endothelial surface does not provoke platelet adhesion; when, however, the endothelium is damaged or lost, sub-endothelial collagen is revealed and the adhesion to it of platelets is the first step in endothelial repair, haemostasis and thrombosis. The specificity of platelet adhesion is shown in the electron micrographs of Figure 5.3. It is not known why platelets adhere to collagen. One theory is that an enzyme on the platelet membrane which can bind to sugars (glycosyltransferase) forms a complex with sugar residues on collagen (galactosyl hydroxylysine groups). Similar models, involving glycosyltransferases specific for different sugars, have been used as general mechanisms to explain the adhesion of cells to each other in tissues (p. 711, Figure 6.6).

2 Adhesion to collagen initiates the *platelet release reaction*, with the liberation of ADP, 5-HT and various other constituents. The

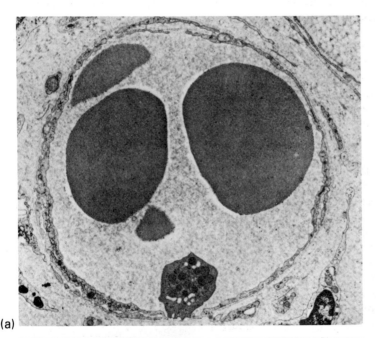

(a)

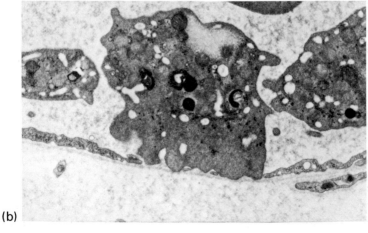

(b)

Figure 5.3 Platelet adhesion.
(a) Transverse section through a capillary in which a platelet has filled a small gap between two endothelial cells by adhering to exposed subendothelium.
(b) Higher magnification of a platelet similarly adhering to basement membrane exposed between two endothelial cells.
(Courtesy of Dr H.R. Baumgartner.)

importance of the ADP is that it is a very effective agent in causing platelet aggregation, which thus rapidly follows adhesion. ADP itself causes further ADP release, so it is easy to envisage the chain reaction which leads to formation of tightly-packed platelet aggregates (Figure 5.2). In addition to collagen and ADP, *thrombin* is a third important stimulator of the release reaction. As will be further discussed, this is another example of *positive feedback*, since activation of the clotting enzyme thrombin is one of the end results of these platelet reactions. In common with other cellular secretory reactions, the release reaction is controlled by the levels of cyclic AMP in the platelet. In this case a fall in cyclic AMP triggers release, while an increase is inhibitory. Both thrombin and collagen (but not ADP) directly inhibit adenylate cyclase, the enzyme in the platelet membrane which produces cyclic AMP from AMP, and hence cause the fall in cyclic AMP levels. Calcium is also involved in the release reaction and it is likely that the fall in cyclic AMP causes the release into the cytoplasm of calcium stored inside platelets; this event is the direct trigger for the release of the contents of the dense granules (ADP, 5HT), which are then shed to the outside. A fall in cyclic AMP levels can also be produced by certain prostaglandin derivatives called *thromboxanes* which thereby trigger the release reaction. The role of these molecules in platelet reactions is now recognised as being of great importance and is described further below.

3 The *aggregation of platelets* by ADP can take place in two stages. If ADP or thrombin in low concentrations are added to platelets, a reversible aggregation is produced, in the absence of the release reaction; *in vivo*, this reversible aggregation may be produced by low amounts of ADP shed from damaged red cells or tissues. In the presence of higher amounts of ADP or thrombin, the release reaction takes place and then aggregation becomes irreversible. Collagen induces irreversible aggregation because it induces the release reaction. The permanent aggregation which follows the release reaction is partly due to endogenous ADP which is shed from the platelet granules. In addition, prostaglandins and thromboxanes are produced by platelets; the latter are particularly potent aggregator substances and cause irreversible aggregation. *Aspirin* inhibits both the platelet release reaction and permanent aggregation because it prevents synthesis of thromboxanes and prostaglandins. A characteristic feature of aggregation is that platelets change in shape from discs to irregular spheres. The function of aggregation is to build up a platelet mass, the *haemostatic plug*, capable of arresting bleeding from cut vessels. As with other features of platelet physiology, the precise mechanism whereby ADP and thromboxanes aggregate platelets is still elusive. It is probable that ADP interacts with actomyosin at the platelet surface and that this is one stage in rendering the platelets sticky, leading to aggregation. Extracellular calcium is required for aggregation. (Platelet aggregation is shown in Figure 5.9c.)

4 The platelet aggregates which form under the influence of ADP and thromboxanes are not in themselves strong enough to be permanent and now require *fibrin* deposition to give

mechanical strength. For this, the interaction between platelet aggregates and the blood clotting system is vital. The role of platelets in blood clotting is described at length in the following pages. In brief, the process of aggregation makes available the phospholipid platelet factor 3, which is not released but rather revealed on the platelet surface where it is required for the activation of thrombin from prothrombin. Thrombin is the enzyme which causes fibrin formation, and in this way platelet masses stabilised by fibrin are formed. As already noted, thrombin also leads to further platelet aggregation and stimulates the release reaction. Platelets also release a protein called *platelet factor 4* which promotes clotting by neutralising the action of heparin (p. 635). The formation of platelet/fibrin masses is the central event in haemostasis and thrombosis.

Platelets and prostaglandins

The prostaglandins are hormone-like molecules which are present in almost all tissues and which can produce a variety of important pharmacological effects; their structure and role in acute inflammation have been described in Section 1. In recent years it has become clear that prostaglandins and the closely related molecules thromboxanes play a central role in the reactions of platelets and can mediate aggregation and the release reaction. Indeed, the production of these molecules is probably the common pathway through which agents such as collagen, ADP and thrombin affect platelets. The starting point of prostaglandin metabolism is the precursor fatty acid *arachidonic acid*, and it is likely that the diverse aggregating agents all cause the generation of arachidonic acid (through the initiation of the hydrolysis of membrane phospholipid by phospholipases); this is a necessary step, since prostaglandins are not stored in cells, but synthesized as and when required. Arachidonic acid is then converted by an enzyme, cyclo-oxygenase, into an unstable intermediate called a prostaglandin (PG) *cyclic endoperoxide*. The latter is the precursor of prostaglandins and thromboxanes (Figure 5.4). The cyclo-oxygenase enzyme is inhibited by aspirin, which thus blocks the synthesis of PG endoperoxide and the production of prostaglandins and thromboxanes; this explains the well-known inhibition of platelet aggregation and the release reaction by aspirin. In platelets the PG endoperoxides are converted into the highly unstable thromboxane known as *thromboxane A_2* or *TxA_2*, by thromboxane synthetase. TxA_2 is the major mediator of platelet reactions, causing irreversible aggregation as well as initiating the release reaction; in the latter, ADP is made available and this leads to aggregation and further production of TxA_2 by the same pathway (Figure 5.4). The instability of TxA_2 makes its continued synthesis in this cyclic manner essential. Endoperoxides are also converted into prostaglandins E_1 and E_2 mentioned in Section 1 in connection with inflammation; the effects of PGE_1 and PGE_2 on platelet aggregation are, however, insignificant compared with the powerful action of TxA_2. As already noted, TxA_2 is very unstable, with a half-life of about 30

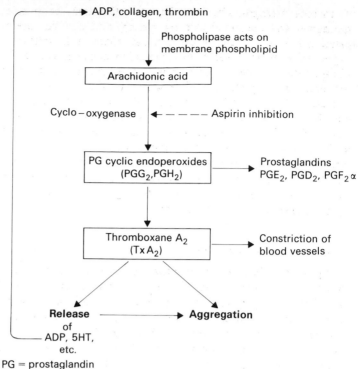

Figure 5.4 Thromboxane A_2 in platelet reactions.

ADP, collagen, thrombin

Phospholipase acts on membrane phospholipid

Arachidonic acid

Cyclo – oxygenase ◀ ─ ─ ─ ─ Aspirin inhibition

PG cyclic endoperoxides (PGG$_2$,PGH$_2$) → Prostaglandins PGE$_2$, PGD$_2$, PGF$_2\alpha$

Thromboxane A$_2$ (TxA$_2$) → Constriction of blood vessels

Release → Aggregation
of
ADP, 5HT,
etc.

PG = prostaglandin

seconds; it is rapidly converted to a stable, but inactive molecule, thromboxane B_2. Besides aggregating platelets, TxA_2 is a powerful agent of arterial constriction which is important in the arrest of bleeding. Thus, it is clear that TxA_2 has a crucial role in the processes of blood clotting, haemostasis and thrombosis.

Obviously, it is important that the synthesis and activity of a potent agent such as TxA_2 be subject to controls and one such control mechanism has been discovered. It has been found that the walls of blood vessels do not convert PG endoperoxide into TxA_2; instead they transform endoperoxide by a different pathway into an unstable prostaglandin called *prostacyclin* or PGI_2. This molecule is an antagonist of TxA_2: it inhibits platelet aggregation and relaxes arterial muscle. It is very likely that the balance between TxA_2 from platelets and PGI_2 from the vessel wall is a crucial factor in the control of haemostasis. The level of spontaneous production of PGI_2 by normal endothelium is extremely low and insufficient to influence platelets. However, once endothelium has been damaged, PGI_2 is readily produced and becomes an important protective mechanism; indeed the sensitivity of PGI_2 release in response to even the mildest trauma has made its role *in vivo* difficult to study, since procedures such as insertion of a syringe needle into a vessel cause a significant rise in local PGI_2 levels. Two antithrombotic roles for PGI_2 seem likely. In haemostasis, the release of PGI_2 by traumatised endothelium around the site of a wound will restrict the development of the platelet/fibrin mass and prevent its propagation as a thrombus into the lumen. Secondly, in minor damage to endothelium, the release of PGI_2 may prevent platelet aggregation leading to thrombosis. (Note that adhesion is not inhibited by PGI_2, so that the process of endothelial repair would not be affected.)

Recent understanding of the role of PGs in platelet reactions have possible clinical implications. For example, agents which prevent TxA_2 production may lower the incidence of thrombosis. Aspirin is one such agent but, disappointingly, a large scale clinical trial recently completed in the USA showed a slight *increase* in deaths due to coronary thrombosis in patients with ischaemic heart disease given daily aspirin, over untreated controls. Other smaller trials showed a small (10–20%) reduction in mortality with aspirin. The fact that aspirin will inhibit both TxA_2 and PGI_2 synthesis may explain the marginal nature of the results of these trials (see also p. 671). An important property of PGI_2 is its ability to *disaggregate* platelets, which may prove to have clinical applicability for conditions where platelet thrombi are involved (coronary thrombosis, stroke, etc.). Like its thromboxane counterpart, PGI_2 has a very short half-life (2–3 minutes) and stable analogues for therapeutic use are being sought. PGI_2 has already been used successfully in therapy of ischaemic lower limb disease, where it increases the blood flow through arteries narrowed by atherosclerosis.

BLOOD CLOTTING

The appearance of fibrin is the last stage in the complex series of reactions which make up blood clotting or coagulation. The clotting sequence is another example of a biological amplification mechanism whereby a small stimulus is enabled to produce a major biological effect. Thus clotting involves a *cascade* type of reaction in which enzyme intermediates normally present in the blood as inactive proenzymes are activated by one another in sequence. Complement activation and kinin formation are other instances of this principle which have been described in Section 1.

The final events in the clotting sequence have been known since the turn of the century (Morawitz, 1905). They are the activation of the enzyme *thrombin* from its plasma precursor *prothrombin*, and the subsequent action of thrombin on plasma *fibrinogen* to produce *fibrin*. Calcium ions are required for this reaction. It is immediately apparent that there must be some additional agent involved to activate prothrombin, and this has traditionally been termed *thromboplastin*:

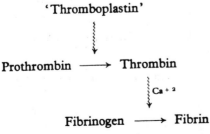

Thromboplastin is unfortunately a rather vague term and one which is almost rendered obsolete by our more detailed present knowledge of events. It is not a single substance and is best thought of as 'the plasma activity capable of converting pro-thrombin into thrombin'.

Since clotting involves a complex series of interactions, an internationally agreed reference system for the substances involved has been devised. Those derived from the plasma are termed *factors* and denoted by Roman numerals from I to XIII, with the activated forms indicated by the suffix 'a' and subsequently inactivated forms by the suffix 'i'. Factor I refers to fibrinogen, factor II to prothrombin, factor III to thromboplastin and factor IV to calcium. Factor VI is no longer used. The remaining eight plasma factors are enzymes or enzyme cofactors involved in coagulation. Substances from platelets are termed *platelet factors* and designated with Arabic numerals from 1 to 5, the most important being platelet factors 3 and 4. Less well defined agents from tissues are at present simply called *tissue factors*.

Two pathways are known for the generation of 'thromboplastin activity' for the ultimate activation of prothrombin (Figure 5.5). In the *extrinsic* system, damaged tissue contributes a tissue factor and a phospholipid which together generate and catalyse the action of thromboplastin; in the *intrinsic* system, on the other hand, all the elements involved derive from plasma precursors and platelets. While the extrinsic system is triggered by tissue damage, the intrinsic system is initiated by contact of the blood

Figure 5.5 Pathways of blood clotting.

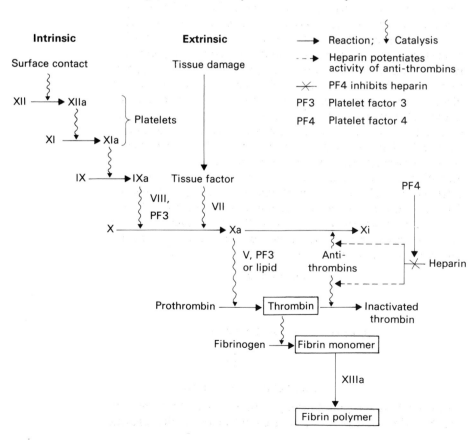

with a foreign surface such as glass or, *in vivo*, connective tissue collagen and is by far the more important physiological clotting mechanism.

The central event for both pathways is the activation of plasma factor X to produce factor Xa, an esterase which in association with phospholipid and factor V catalyses prothrombin conversion:

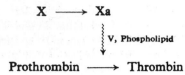

In the extrinsic system, the phospholipid is tissue derived; in the intrinsic system it is the platelet factor 3. The difference between the two systems is essentially in the means of activating factor X (Figure 5.5). Extrinsic clotting has as its starting point the release of two factors from damaged tissue: one tissue factor is an active protein or lipoprotein which converts X into Xa, in the presence of plasma factor VII; the other tissue factor is the phospholipid referred to above. Hence 'tissue thromboplastin' consists of these two tissue-derived factors and plasma factors Xa, VII and V. Brain extract is a particularly rich source of the tissue factors and is used as such in various laboratory tests. That blood will clot without these tissue factors has been known since Lister's demonstration of contact activation in 1863. Its physiological importance can be inferred from *haemophilia* where there is a failure of the blood to clot on contact with glass, yet normal clotting occurs on addition of normal or haemophilic tissue extracts. The latter observation indicates a defect which lies outside the tissue-activated system. The intrinsic pathway for prothrombin activation is shown in Figure 5.5, and it involves several enzymatic steps leading up to activation of factor X. First, surface contact causes the activation of factor XII, Hageman factor, which will be familiar from Section 1 for its key role in generation of acute inflammation (Figure 1.13). Platelets are also involved in the contact activation steps. Activated Hageman factor, XIIa, activates factor XI and XIa activates factor IX in turn. Factor IXa then forms a complex with factor VIII, platelet factor 3 and calcium ions, and the complex catalyses the important activation of factor X to Xa. Factor Xa, factor V and platelet factor 3 (phospholipid) constitute 'plasma thromboplastin', the intrinsic prothrombin activator.

The final stages in clotting are then common to both systems. Thrombin is formed by activation of prothrombin and is a protease which acts on fibrinogen. The latter is normally solubilised by its high negative charge due to glutamic acid residues; thrombin splits off from fibrinogen two peptide fragments, which contain the charged residues, to produce fibrin monomer. Fibrin monomers polymerise readily to form molecular aggregates which, however, are easily disrupted. The fibrin network is stabilised by plasma factor XIII which creates covalent bonds between the aggregates to give a firm gel.

It is clear from the above that platelets make a vital contribution to intrinsic clotting. Platelet adhesion and aggregation, triggered initially by surface contact, makes available the phospholipid platelet factor 3, probably as a result of a change affecting the platelet surface membrane. Platelets adsorb other clotting factors to their surface and it is on or around the platelet membrane that thrombin is formed. The important feedback relationship which exists between thrombin and platelets has already been noted (p. 629), in which thrombin itself causes the aggregation of platelets and hence further appearance of platelet factor 3 (Figure 5.6). This mutual enhancement effect is important in development of platelet haemostatic plugs and thrombi. Thrombin also potentiates the activity of factors V and VIII.

Figure 5.6 Positive feedback of thrombin on platelet aggregation.

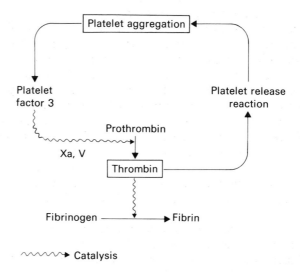

Control of clotting

Clearly it is important that blood clotting be controlled so that propagation of the clot into the circulation does not occur at the site of haemorrhage. Indeed clotting activity tends to disappear a few minutes after fibrin formation. This inhibition is accomplished by plasma *antithrombins*—glycoproteins present in the α_2-globulin fraction which inactivate thrombin—and *heparin*, which inhibits the action of thrombin on fibrinogen, probably by potentiating the activity of antithrombins (Figure 5.5). Heparin, frequently used in the laboratory as an anticoagulant, is a widely distributed sulphated mucopolysaccharide found in the granules of mast cells. It is noteworthy that platelets contain a heparin-neutralising substance, platelet factor 4. Heparin may be administered therapeutically in acute thrombo-embolic disease. Anticoagulant therapy is also frequently employed in the long-term treatment of venous thrombosis and this takes advantage of the fact that some clotting factors are dependent on vitamin K for their synthesis by the liver, notably prothrombin and factors VII, IX and X. Vitamin K antagonists, such as the coumarin and indandione derivatives, reduce the levels of these factors and hence the extent of any tendency towards clotting.

Fibrinolysis

Once formed, fibrin can be solubilised by fibrinolysis, principally through the action of the enzyme *plasmin*, present as its pro-enzyme plasminogen in the blood. The formation of plasmin has already been discussed in the context of acute inflammation (Section 1) and it will be recalled that plasminogen activation is catalysed by active Hageman factor. Thus Hageman factor, once activated, initiates both the appearance of fibrin and the means of its dissolution (fibrinolysis). In addition, activators of plasminogen are produced by the endothelium of small vessels and the fibrinolytic activity of the blood is to a large extent due to the release of these activators (Figure 5.7). The absence of post-mortem clots which is noticeable after sudden death, shock or asphyxia, is due to plasmin activity following release of the activators from endothelium, which is promoted by exercise, adrenaline, injury and stress. Plasmin can also be activated by streptokinase, an enzyme found in culture filtrates of β-haemolytic streptococci, and urokinase, a similar enzyme present in human urine. The activation of plasminogen and activity of plasmin itself are controlled by various inhibitors, as indicated in Figure 5.7. Human plasmin, activated by streptokinase, is used in therapy as an adjunct to anticoagulants, and may be administered in attempts to dissolve newly formed thrombi.

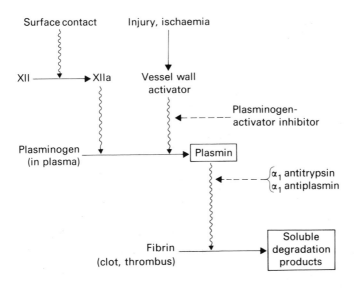

Figure 5.7 The fibrinolytic system.

The sequence of events which act to stop haemorrhage when a blood vessel is injured, haemostasis, can now be summarised (Figure 5.8). Within seconds after injury, platelets adhere to the collagen exposed by the disruption of the endothelium. The subsequent synthesis of thromboxane TxA_2 and rapid release of platelet ADP, together with ADP derived from damaged tissue, cause platelet aggregation; this in turn promotes further TxA_2 production and ADP release and continued aggregation (p. 630). A platelet mass, the haemostatic plug, is thus quickly formed to fill the opening and in small vessels this is sufficient to stop blood flow in 2–3 minutes. 5-HT released from platelets is also important in causing local vasoconstriction. At the same time, the intrinsic clotting system is activated by contact of factor XII with exposed collagen and, of lesser importance, the release of tissue clotting factors contributes by the extrinsic activation of thrombin. (Note that factor XIIa also activates an inflammatory response in the area of damage, as well as the fibrinolytic system). Platelet factor 3, made available by platelet aggregation, enables thrombin and fibrin to form rapidly round the platelets and thrombin itself causes further platelet aggregation. The otherwise fragile platelet mass is gradually stabilised and strengthened by fibrin deposition and becomes a more effective plug. After 24 hours, the plug is composed largely of fibrin, with platelets still visible but more widely spaced. The retraction of the clot is brought about by the contraction of platelet thrombosthenin. Subsequently, in the course of healing, the fibrin clot is dissolved by plasmin.

Figure 5.8 Events in haemostasis.

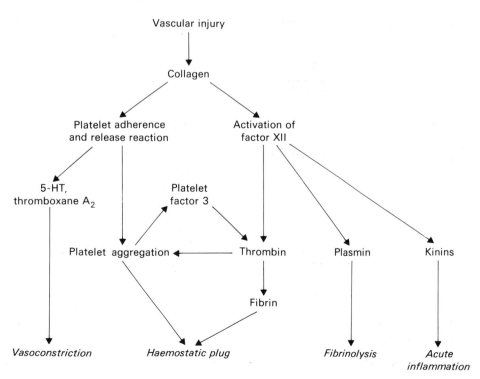

637

Bleeding disorders

Efficient haemostasis involves vasoconstriction, platelet aggregation and blood clotting and it is to be expected that deficiencies in these last two processes would lead to bleeding disorders. Haemorrhagic diseases do indeed occur either as a result of platelet abnormalities, as in *thrombocytopenic purpura*, or defects in the clotting mechanism, as in *haemophilia*. Several types of test are used to discover the cause of abnormal haemostasis. One important test is the *bleeding time*, which is the time taken for a small skin puncture to stop bleeding and is essentially a measure of the ability of platelets to aggregate and form a plug. Thus bleeding time is prolonged in platelet deficiencies or disorders, but is normal in haemophilia. Deficiencies of plasma clotting factors, such as occur in the latter, are revealed by a variety of *in vitro* clotting tests which can discriminate between deficiencies of the intrinsic and extrinsic systems.

Thrombocytopenia is a decrease in the number of platelets and causes an increased tendency to bleed. In severe cases, bleeding into the skin and mucous membranes occurs, characteristically as small petechial haemorrhages ('petechial' meaning less than 2 mm in diameter). This condition is known as *purpura*. The bleeding time is prolonged, due to the inability to form an adequate platelet plug, but the clotting time of the blood measured *in vitro* is normal because only small numbers of platelets are required to catalyse coagulation. In *primary* thrombocytopenic purpura, an autoimmune mechanism seems to be responsible for platelet destruction. Antiplatelet antibodies are found in many patients, and the antibody-coated platelets are destroyed in the spleen. For this reason splenectomy has a beneficial effect in most cases. *Secondary* thrombocytopenia may follow the administration of certain drugs, such as 'Sedormid', quinidine and sulphonamides, which initiate a Type II hypersensitivity reaction (p. 160). The drug, or one of its metabolised products, becomes attached to platelets and acts as a hapten. An antibody response against the drug thus results in the coating of platelets with anti-drug antibody and their subsequent complement-mediated destruction. Other drugs, including cytotoxic agents used in cancer therapy, produce thrombocytopenia by direct depression of platelet production in the bone marrow. Other conditions affecting the bone marrow, such as leukaemias, aplastic anaemia, X-irradiation or severe infection, also give rise to thrombocytopenic purpura.

The excessive bleeding and purpura of thrombocytopenia emphasize the chief functions of platelets, namely in haemostasis and in the repair of minor endothelial damage which might otherwise lead to haemorrhage. In the latter process of endothelial repair, platelet and fibrin deposition on a damaged vascular wall quickly ensures the integrity of the wall and rapid re-endothelialisation then follows over the platelet layer (Figure 5.9a,b).

Besides the gross deficiency in platelet number of thrombocytopenia, bleeding disorders can also be a result of abnormalities of the vital platelet reactions of adherence, release and aggregation

(Table 5.1). Examples of defective platelet function, with normal platelet levels, are seen in *von Willebrand's disease* and the *Bernard-Soulier syndrome*, where the platelets fail to adhere to collagen; in *thrombasthenia*, where adherence is normal and release occurs but aggregation is defective; and in *aspirin-induced defects*, where both release and irreversible aggregation fail to occur. *Von Willebrand's disease* is related to haemophilia, because they both involve deficiency of the plasma clotting factor VIII (antihaemophilic globulin). In von Willebrand's disease, however, both bleeding time and coagulation are prolonged, whereas in haemophilia the bleeding time is normal and only the clotting time is abnormally protracted. Note too that von Willebrand's disease is inherited as an autosomal dominant, in contrast with haemophilia, which is an X-linked recessive (Section 7), indicating that different proteins are defective in the two disorders. In von Willebrand's disease platelet adherence to subendothelial collagen is impaired, but aggregation on the few adherent platelets is normal. The adherence defect is not in the platelets themselves, but in a plasma factor required for platelet adherence. The factor involved is called *von Willebrand factor*; it seems to be involved with factor VIII in such a way that deficiency of von Willebrand factor leads to reduction in factor VIII activity as well. It is possible that the two form a macromolecular complex in which von Willebrand factor plays an essential role in the coagulative activity of factor VIII.

The other platelet anomalies are inherent in the platelets themselves. In the rare *Bernard-Soulier (giant-platelet) syndrome*, platelets do not adhere to collagen even in the presence of normal amounts of factor VIII. *Aspirin*, as noted on p. 629, inhibits both the platelet release reaction and the irreversible aggregation induced by collagen, thrombin and ADP, while the reversible aggregation produced by ADP can still occur. Aspirin can thus produce mild haemostatic defects in normal subjects, which can last for several days after ingestion. Indeed, one 300 mg aspirin tablet is sufficient to produce detectable changes in platelet aggregation. The action of aspirin is to suppress synthesis of prostaglandins and thromboxanes from arachidonic acid by inhibition of the enzyme cyclo-oxygenase (Figure 5.4); the thromboxanes are required both for the release reaction and for permanent aggregation (p. 630). One case has been discovered of an inherited absence of the cyclo-oxygenase enzyme, which produces the same deficiencies as those induced by aspirin.

Table 5.1 Platelet disorders

Disorder	Cause
Thrombocytopenia	Deficiency in platelet numbers
Von Willebrand's disease	Defective adherence to collagen
Bernard-Soulier syndrome	Defective adherence to collagen
Thrombasthenia	Defective aggregation
Aspirin-induced defect	Defective release reaction and aggregation by collagen
Storage pool disease	Defective release reaction and aggregation by collagen

A deficiency of ADP in granules can also occur, and this too leads to defective aggregation, because ADP both participates directly in aggregation as well as stimulating synthesis of thromboxane TxA_2 (Figure 5.4). In this 'storage pool' disease, the number of dense bodies is much reduced and the basic defect probably lies in the formation of these granules which are the store of ADP, serotonin and calcium.

Haemophilia is caused by an inherited deficiency in a plasma blood-clotting factor, factor VIII (antihaemophilic globulin). It is a sex-linked recessive condition, occurring only in males (Section 7). Deficiencies of other clotting factors are known, such as *Christmas disease* (lack of factor IX), which are inherited as autosomal, recessive traits. (Factor VIII deficiency is sometimes referred to as haemophilia A, and factor IX deficiency as haemophilia B. The clinical symptoms are the same for both.) Characteristic in haemophilia is the tendency for serious, even fatal bleeding to occur from minor wounds or incisions (e.g. dental extractions). Spontaneous bleeding into the joints (haemarthrosis) and soft tissues, as well as from the natural orifices, is common. Changes in the joints as a result of haemorrhage lead to crippling deformity in many instances. However, in contrast to platelet inadequacy, purpura is uncommon. The severity of bleeding in haemophilia emphasizes the importance of the intrinsic clotting mechanism in haemostasis; clotting of haemophilic blood with tissue thromboplastin can be shown to occur normally *in vitro*. It is interesting that the rare deficiency of factor XII (Hageman factor) is not associated with clinical abnormalities, especially in view of the important role this factor is believed to play in initiation of intrinsic clotting and inflammation. Some observations suggest that platelets contain substances that can bypass the requirement for factors XII and XI in initiation of clotting, which may explain why the patients with factor XII deficiency do not bleed.

THROMBOSIS

Definitions and terminology

Thrombosis is the formation of a solid mass, a *thrombus*, in the lumen of a blood vessel or in the heart from the constituents of the blood during life. Thrombi may occur anywhere in the circulation, although they are relatively uncommon in capillaries. They are always attached at one or more points to the vessel wall. A *mural* thrombus is attached to the wall at one side but does not occlude the vessel. It may develop into an *occluding* thrombus, which fills the lumen of the vessel and obstructs blood flow. In veins, once occlusion has occurred, the thrombus is often *propagated* by clotting in the stagnant blood proximal to the occlusion. A mural thrombus is *pale* due to its large platelet and fibrin component; a propagating thrombus is *red* in its early stages because of its content of red blood cells. Most thrombi are *mixed* in appearance, with pale platelet and red clot components.

Thrombus formation

As in haemostasis, the interaction of platelets and the clotting mechanism is involved in thrombosis. Essentially, a thrombus is formed by the accumulation of platelets on the damaged or inflamed wall of a blood vessel or heart valve and the stabilisation of the platelet mass by a fibrin clot. As noted above, this process is constantly occurring for the repair of minor endothelial damage (Figure 5.9a,b). It does not normally lead to thrombosis because of the rapid dissipation of blood clotting components in the blood stream and efficient growth of new endothelium contiguous with the intima as the platelet aggregate is dissolved. It is only when conditions in the circulation allow the build-up of a certain local thromboplastin concentration or encourage excessive platelet aggregation that a thrombus can develop (Figure 5.9c). The form of the thrombus is then determined by the type of vessel and the local conditions of flow. In veins, for example, where sluggish blood flow is often a major contributing factor in thrombosis, the lumen of the vessel may become blocked over a considerable length by a long red thrombus, composed mainly of a 'tail' of clotted blood. Closer examination will show this structure to be anchored at its point of origin to the vessel wall by a pale 'head', which may show characteristic surface markings known as the *lines of Zahn*. The head is composed of platelets and fibrin and is formed first; the tail is a result of clotting in the stagnant column of blood formed after the occlusion of the vein by the platelet/fibrin mass. A thrombus of this type is distinguished from the more gelatinous post-mortem clot by its dry, granular appearance and its attachment, by the head, to the vessel wall. In the rapid-flowing arterial system, thrombi are pale, firm, compact structures composed mainly of platelets and some fibrin. If they occlude the vessel they are short, without an obvious head and tail. Here they are commonly associated with atherosclerosis (p. 654). In the heart, thrombi form on the wall of the left ventricle after myocardial infarction, or on the valves after inflammatory damage, where they are called *vegetations*.

The accumulation of platelets on vessel walls has been studied experimentally for over a century, since the observations of Zahn in 1875 on the effects of injury to vessels in frog mesentery, and there is no doubt that this is the first step in thrombus formation (Figure 5.9a). The multiple factors which contribute further to the pathogenesis of thrombosis can be largely interpreted by their part in encouraging platelet adhesion and aggregation. These factors are summarised in the classical hypothesis of Virchow (1856) and are known as *Virchow's triad*. They are (i) changes in the vessel wall, (ii) changes in the local pattern of blood flow, and (iii) changes in the constituents of the blood. Virchow's triad remains a most useful guide to the aetiology of thrombosis.

(i) *Changes in the vessel wall* will encourage the adhesion of platelets if they reveal subendothelial collagen. Experimentally, damage to the wall by crushing or chemical irritation will induce thrombosis and so will the introduction of a foreign surface such

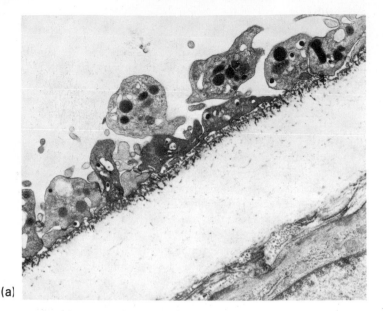

(a)

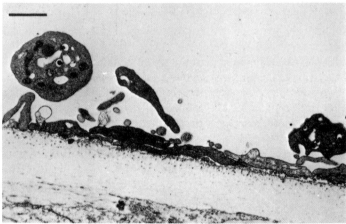

(b)

Figure 5.9 Interaction of platelets with subendothelium. (a) Electron micrograph of platelets adhering to the subendothelial surface of rabbit aorta *in vivo* 10 minutes after removal of the endothelium. (Endothelium was stripped off using a balloon catheter, p. 657) Platelets change shape and spread out as a continuous layer; they still contain some α granules and dense body granules. (b) 30 minutes later, the platelets are even more flattened and have degranulated. This picture is a prelude to endothelial repair. (c) Electron micrograph of a section through a platelet thrombus formed *in vivo* 10 minutes after removal of the endothelium from a rabbit iliac artery. Note the interdigitation of the platelets and typical changes in shape. Platelets nearest to the subendothelial surface have degranulated, while those more peripheral still contain most of their granules. (From Baumgartner, H.R. & Muggli, R. (1976) in Gordon, J.R. (ed.) *Platelets in Biology and Pathology*. North Holland.)

as a suture passed through the vessel. The loss of endothelium is probably important in thrombosis in diseased arteries, for example in atherosclerosis, where surface damage or ulceration can bring the blood into direct contact with the intima. Similarly, inflammation in veins leads to endothelial loss or damage and predisposes to thrombosis (*thrombophlebitis*). However, in the more common thrombosis of the veins encouraged by venous stasis (*phlebothrombosis*), gross endothelial changes may be difficult to demonstrate, though more subtle damage may very likely be caused, for example, by mechanical effects of prolonged immobilisation in bed or by anoxia from venous stasis. Platelet adhesion requires a break in the continuity of the endothelium, though platelets can take advantage of very small intercellular gaps (Figure 5.3). However it must be acknowledged that the presence of venous damage as initiator of thrombosis is often uncertain and it seems that in areas of static blood flow in valve pockets, platelet release and aggregation probably occur without initial binding to

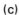

(c)

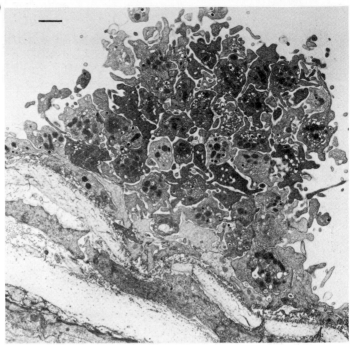

collagen. Young platelets are especially likely to be hyperactive in this respect. Moreover, endothelial damage, where present, is not sufficient in itself to allow the formation of an occluding thrombus, and platelet aggregates will soon be dispersed if other circulatory factors do not operate.

(ii) *Changes in the local pattern of blood flow* are especially important here and are of two main types, namely *turbulence* (whirling, eddying) and *stasis*. Both of these changes will encourage platelets to leave their normal axial flow and make contact with the vessel wall. Eddy currents are important in the fast-flowing arterial system, where platelet aggregates would otherwise be swept rapidly away. Eddying in arteries results from atherosclerosis and encourages platelet contact with the damaged or irregular vessel wall and hence aggregation. Eddying also occurs at sites of branching of arteries. In the venous system, on the other hand, a very slow blood flow allows platelets to simply fall out of the axial stream. Stasis in veins also has the important effect of allowing plasma clotting factors to accumulate in sufficient concentration for clotting to occur. It is easy to understand why venous thrombosis is such a common hazard for patients confined to bed for long periods, especially with cardiac disease or after abdominal surgery; heart failure, shallow breathing and lack of muscular activity in the legs all greatly impair venous return and lead to venous stasis.

(iii) *Changes in the composition of the blood* which are significant and encourage thrombosis, include an increase in the platelet number and in their tendency to adhere to foreign surfaces. A rise in the platelet count follows tissue injury such as parturition, major surgery and myocardial infarction and is correlated with a tendency to thrombosis about 7–10 days afterwards. Adhesiveness too is higher in the postoperative and *postpartum* period and also in hyperlipidaemia. Any increased tendency of the blood to coagulate would be expected to predispose to thrombosis. Likewise, a decrease in fibrinolytic activity would also encourage the stabilisation of thrombi by fibrin. It is noteworthy in this respect that a decreased content of activators of fibrinolysis in vessel walls and a defective release of such activators has been found in patients with recurrent venous thrombosis. For these reasons, anticoagulants (p. 635) are useful in treatment of thrombosis in which the clotting component is most significant, namely deep venous thrombosis, and hence also in pulmonary embolism (p. 647). The value of anticoagulant therapy in arterial thrombosis (e.g. coronary artery disease, cerebrovascular disease), where the platelet component predominates, is much less convincing.

Process of thrombosis

In contrast with a simple clot or a haemostatic plug, the thrombus possesses a certain architecture which is the result of its method of formation in the flowing bloodstream. The process of thrombosis can be divided into several stages (Figure 5.10).
1   Initial damage to the vessel wall, which may be quite trivial in extent, triggers platelet adhesion; aggregation follows by release of ADP and thromboxanes, as already described, and leads to a white (primary) platelet thrombus. Its growth is encouraged by factors mentioned above such as eddying or stasis. However, the granular platelet aggregate is fragile and to remain must be stabilised by fibrin, in the same way as a platelet plug.

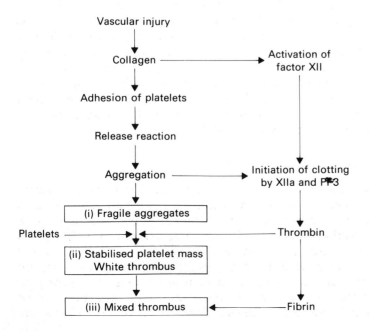

Figure 5.10 Events in thrombosis.

2   Thrombin formation is activated by factor XIIa and platelet factor 3, first in pockets within the platelet mass where clotting factors are protected from natural inhibitors such as the antithrombins. Fibrin forms most rapidly in veins where stasis allows clotting components to accumulate.

3   Thrombin and fibrin promote further platelet aggregation and deposition which now occurs in the form of pale layers across the stream. In this way a platelet framework is built up which is often likened to coral (*coralline thrombus*). In the spaces of this structure there is stasis and fibrin clot can form, trapping leucocytes and red cells in it. Thus, on section, a thrombus shows branches of fused platelets alternating with fibrin clot. The term *mixed thrombus* indicates its composition at this stage. The lines of Zahn are formed by the retraction of fibrin, which leaves elevated platelet ridges at the free surface.

4   As the coralline thrombus grows, the vessel becomes gradually occluded and in veins resultant stasis leads to a larger clot component so that the later additions are red. Eventually, the lumen is completely blocked by an *occluding thrombus*. When this occurs in an artery supplying a vital organ such as the heart or brain, serious and often fatal consequences follow immediately. An essential difference between arterial and venous thrombi should be noted at this point. For arterial thrombi, the major component is the closely packed platelet mass interspersed with fibrin strands and leucocytes, whereas for venous thrombi the platelet component is relatively minor and the main bulk is composed of fibrin and red cells.

5   In veins it is common for the stationary column of blood beyond the thrombus to coagulate, i.e. proximal to the occlusion; this process is the same as *in vitro* clotting and should be distinguished from thrombosis which occurs only in flowing blood. The blood usually clots up to the next venous junction, where it may act as the stimulus for further platelet deposition and growth of a second thrombus. In this way *propagation* along the vein occurs, with anchorage at each venous junction. Alternatively, if there is sufficient stasis after the first occlusion, the blood may clot rapidly along a considerable length of the vein to form a single strand anchored only at the base. In this case there is considerable danger of the propagated clot breaking to release a section of the tail as an *embolus* which will impact in the lungs (pulmonary embolism, p. 647).

Thrombosis in veins

Deep venous thrombosis is an especially important complication following major surgery. This is termed *phlebothrombosis* and as already noted is caused mainly by venous stasis, in contrast with *thrombophlebitis* in which an inflamed venous wall initiates thrombosis. It is in order to avoid phlebothrombosis and possible pulmonary embolism that patients are encouraged to leave bed and take some exercise as soon as possible after surgery or parturition, since venous return depends to a large extent on muscular activity in the legs. The deep veins of the calf are a common starting point for the thrombus. Phlebothrombosis is surprisingly free of painful symptoms and the first indication may well be pulmonary embolism. In contrast, thrombophlebitis is a very painful condition in which thrombosis is initiated by inflammation of the vein wall. Here stasis does not occur, since the inflammation rather increases blood flow, and so there is little likelihood of propagation. The thrombus is firmly attached and does not embolise unless the inflammation is of bacterial origin. Then invasion by pyogenic organisms may cause the disintegration of the thrombus and the dissemination of tiny infected emboli (*pyaemia*, p. 490). Thrombophlebitis, however, can be sterile and indeed may be induced deliberately in treatment of varicose veins by injection of 'sclerosing solutions' (sodium morrhuate or sodium tetradecyl sulphate) into small varicose branches after surgical removal of the main affected veins.

Thrombosis in arteries

Thrombosis in arteries is rather less common than in veins because of the rapid removal of clotting factors in the blood stream. Nevertheless, its occurrence is of great importance, being closely associated with atherosclerosis of which it is the most serious complication, and it is described in that connection on page 668. Where there is a gross local dilatation (an aneurysm) of the heart, aorta or other artery, stagnation and eddying of blood often leads to some thrombosis.

Fate of thrombi

Old thrombi become pale and brownish as the trapped red cells lyse and diffuse away and haemosiderin is stored in macrophages. The changes which may occur in thrombi can be summarised as resolution, organisation or embolism (below). Removal of a thrombus by *resolution* or lysis occurs partly as a result of activation of the fibrinolytic system (plasmin, p. 636) and partly by autolytic enzymes released from degrading trapped leucocytes. Venous endothelium contains a plasminogen activator which may be important here, and therapeutically thrombolysis is encouraged by administration of streptokinase-activated human plasmin. Alternatively, *organisation*, the conversion of fibrin into vascular connective tissue, may occur and involves a process essentially similar to that described in Section 1 for healing tissues. A special feature of organisation in thrombi is *recanalisation* in which new vascular channels develop through the body of an occluding thrombus, to form literally a new artery or vein within the original vessel. In this way blood flow can in time be restored through an occluding thrombus. Simple retraction of thrombi with a large clot component can also create a new channel to re-establish flow. Mural thrombi become covered with endothelium within a few days and gradually become organised; they are an important cause of intimal thickening. In arteries, mural thrombi form on atherosclerotic lesions and contribute greatly to the narrowing of the arteries which is the main feature of the disease. The role of mural thrombi in the possible aetiology of atherosclerosis is discussed on page 668.

EMBOLISM

Embolism is one of the most important features of the pathology of thrombosis. The term is defined as the tranportation of undissolved material in the bloodstream and its impaction somewhere in the circulation. The material transported is the *embolus*. While thrombi are the commonest source of emboli, other examples include tumour cells and tumour fragments, as part of the process of metastasis (p. 735), and also fat droplets and gas bubbles. The most frequently encountered emboli are fragments of—or entire—thrombi which have become detached. They may arise from the long propagated thrombi of phlebothrombosis, in which case they become impacted in the pulmonary circulation; on the arterial side, emboli can be derived from mural thrombi formed on atherosclerotic lesions, or may arise in the heart as detached vegetations. Although emboli can thus originate from thrombi anywhere in the circulation, they impact only where trapped by the progressive narrowing of the lumen of the vessels in which they are carried; hence emboli impact only in the arterial circulation.

The most important example of embolism is seen in the pulmonary circulation, *pulmonary embolism*. This occurs when the long strand of clotted blood which has propagated in the veins of the leg following thrombosis becomes fragile and breaks, perhaps as a result of a sudden movement. The detached clot can be as much as 40–50 cm in length. It is carried into the heart and through the right ventricle and impacts in the main branches of the pulmonary artery or at the bifurcation of the pulmonary trunk. In such cases, death understandably follows in a few minutes. However, the cause of death is not always immediately obvious, especially when only one branch of the pulmonary artery is blocked. In this case, release of 5-hydroxytryptamine from the embolus may cause secondary spasm in the lung vessels. It is important to be aware of the differences in appearance between a massive pulmonary embolus and a post-mortem clot. The former is dry, granular, friable and tightly coiled by impaction into the pulmonary vessels; the latter is moist, gelatinous and elastic and more loosely inserted in the vessel. The embolus is paler and browner than the clot in which the trapped red cells are dark purplish red. Furthermore, the shape of the embolus, when unfolded, corresponds to the lumen of the leg veins, whereas that of the clot resembles the pulmonary tree in which it forms. Not all pulmonary emboli have serious effects or are even noticed during life; small emboli occur frequently and many are only detected at autopsy.

In the systemic circulation, emboli may arise from thrombi in the heart and aorta; they will impact in and occlude arteries in organs such as the brain, kidney and spleen. Embolism of the coronary arteries is rare because of the flow pattern around the aortic valve cusps. Arterial obstruction by thrombosis or embolism reduces the local tissue blood supply. This condition is called *ischaemia* (below).

ISCHAEMIA AND INFARCTION

Thrombosis, embolism and atherosclerosis are the major causes of local ischaemia, which is defined as a state of inadequate blood supply to an area of tissue. The chief effect is to damage the tissue as a result of hypoxia (oxygen lack). It should be noted that ischaemia can be sudden or develop gradually and that a vessel may be completely or partially occluded. The seriousness of the outcome depends on the sensitivity of the tissue to hypoxia, the degree of ischaemia and the ability of the tissue cells to regenerate if conditions improve. Particular attention must be paid here to the vital organs, the brain and the heart, in neither of which can functional cells be regenerated or replaced, other than by non-functional connective tissue. The brain is particularly sensitive to a reduction in its oxygen supply, so much so that following cardiac arrest, consciousness is lost after a few seconds and irreparable brain damage is done after a matter of 3–4 minutes. Death is inevitable if the brain is deprived of oxygen for more than about 8 minutes. Less extensive cerebral ischaemia following thrombosis or embolism is damaging but not necessarily fatal. In the heart, sudden occlusion of a coronary artery by a thrombus causes the ischaemic muscle to become hyperexcitable and death may result suddenly from ventricular fibrillation. If the occlusion develops more slowly by the gradual thickening of the coronary arteries, partial ischaemia results in which muscle fibres die gradually and are replaced by the more resistant fibrous tissue (*replacement fibrosis*). Since cardiac muscle cannot regenerate, even subsequent improvements in blood supply cannot reverse this situation.

Clearly the effects of thrombosis and embolism also depend largely on the degree of ischaemia produced and this is a variable factor governed by the type of vessel affected, the size of the occlusion and the extent to which a local collateral circulation is able to maintain the blood supply. The latter point is particularly critical: if there is a good collateral supply, ischaemia may be avoided altogether. In veins, where cross-anastomoses are common, obstruction of small vessels is without serious consequences. On the arterial side, however, many of the distributing arteries are functionally, if not always anatomically, 'end-arteries' with no effective anastomoses. This applies to the central artery of the retina and many cerebral vessels. In the normal heart a potential collateral circulation between the branches of the coronary arteries exists, but this is normally incapable of preventing ischaemia after sudden occlusion of a coronary artery. However, gradual occlusion of the coronary vessels (such as occurs in atherosclerosis with mural thrombosis) stimulates a collateral circulation to develop with actual increase in length and circumference of anastomosing vessels. This is often of crucial importance in determining the degree of ischaemia, and hence the fate of the heart and the patient if occluding thrombosis should subsequently occur.

A certain degree of ischaemia may be mild enough to go unnoticed in resting tissue but lead to insufficient oxygen supply for exertion or exercise. This is again well illustrated in the ischaemic heart. The characteristic thoracic pain known as *angina pectoris* is caused by a temporary inability of the coronary arteries to supply sufficient oxygenated blood called for by exertion or emotional stress, even though the supply is sufficient for the heart during rest or more moderate activity. The anginal pain is probably caused by substances such as potassium ions and lactic acid released by the ischaemic muscle.

Besides interfering with the function of an organ, ischaemia leads to cell death of varying degree. Where there is no collateral supply, occlusion of an artery leads to the death of all the cells supplied by it causing a necrotic area of tissue to form, the shape of which roughly corresponds to the distribution of the particular artery. This process is called *infarction* and the circumscribed necrotic area is an *infarct*. Infarcts are usually cone shaped, with the base of the cone towards the periphery of the organ. Colour changes in an infarct indicate their stage of development. At first they are *red*, due to dilatation of the blood vessels; as the dead cells in the tissue swell, blood is forced out again and the infarct becomes *pale*, unless there is bleeding into the necrotic tissue as happens in the lung and sometimes the brain and heart. The usual fate of an infarct is its organisation into fibrous scar tissue. This is again well illustrated in the heart following infarction of the wall of the left ventricle. *Myocardial infarction* is caused by the ischaemia following coronary thrombosis and/or atherosclerosis. If immediate ventricular fibrillation does not cause death, the infarct develops and is in due course replaced by fibrous tissue. If the scar replaces most of the thickness of the myocardium, this portion of the wall may be stretched due to the action of the heart to form a non-contractile sac known as an *aneurysm*. Within the aneurysm, thrombosis may occur due to eddying, and it may even rupture with fatal haemorrhage. In the brain, an infarct often becomes soft and creamy; *cerebral infarction* is caused by cerebral artery thrombosis, embolism from the heart or as a complication of atherosclerosis. *Pulmonary infarction* is rare, even if a main pulmonary artery is occluded, because the lung has a low metabolic rate, double circulation and direct access to oxygen. Infarcts occur only if the lungs are congested through heart failure or mitral stenosis; an embolus from the leg veins then results in bleeding into the affected cone of tissue, thus cutting off the oxygen in the inspired air.

A noteworthy point is the release by recently infarcted tissue of enzymes such as creatine phosphokinase, transaminases and lactic dehydrogenase. Measurements of activity of such enzymes in serum can thus be useful in diagnosis of myocardial and other infarctions.

ATHEROSCLEROSIS

Atherosclerosis and its sequels are the major causes of death in the developed world today. At the turn of the century, this statement would have been made of the acute infectious diseases, but with their eradication and the resulting longevity of the population, cardiovascular diseases have emerged as the most important factor in human mortality. At present about 50% of all deaths in the UK are attributable to cardiovascular disease, compared with 16% for cancer, the next commonest cause of death, and of that 50% the large majority of deaths are the result of the effects of atherosclerosis.

Definitions

The general term for conditions in which arteries are thickened and hardened is *arteriosclerosis*; as such it includes atherosclerosis and also *arteriolosclerosis* (thickening of arterioles associated with benign hypertension) and *Mönckeberg's medial sclerosis*. *Atherosclerosis* is a disease of the large and medium-sized arteries, in which the intima of the arterial wall is thickened by the development of fibrous tissue and the accumulation of lipid. (Greek, athere—gruel or porridge; sclerosis—hardening). The term *atheroma* is frequently used to describe the lesions of atherosclerosis especially those in which extracellular lipid is particularly evident.

Atherosclerosis affects the elastic arteries, including the aorta, and the larger distributing or muscular arteries. Clinical disease most often results from lesions in the aorta and arteries supplying the heart, brain and lower limbs. These lesions may cause *ischaemia* or lead to *haemorrhage*. The narrowing of the arterial lumen has particularly serious consequences for the circulation to the heart and brain; the ischaemia brought about by the gradual occlusion of the coronary and cerebral vessels is compounded by *thrombosis* leading to sudden occlusion, the most serious sequel of atherosclerosis. In order to appreciate how these events come about, the structure of the arterial wall in health and disease must first be described.

The normal artery wall

The wall of a normal artery consists of three distinct layers, namely *intima*, *media* and *adventitia* (Figure 5.11). The *intima*, which lies immediately beneath the single layer of endothelium, is the region of greatest interest in the present context, because this is where the lesions of atherosclerosis develop. It consists of an extracellular connective tissue matrix in which are found a small number of smooth muscle cells. It is normal for the intima to be very thin at birth and in children and to increase gradually in thickness with age, with further deposition of connective tissue and a parallel increase in the number of smooth muscle cells. The absence of fibroblasts from the intima is especially noteworthy; intimal smooth muscle cells themselves are able to produce the collagen, elastin fibres and mucopolysaccharides which make up the connective tissue and which elsewhere would be produced by fibroblasts. Since fibrosis contributes a major part of the thickening of the intima in atherosclerosis, it is important to note

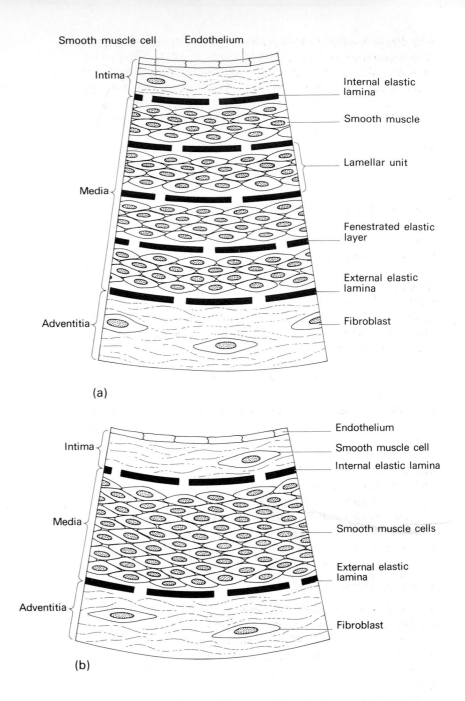

Smooth muscle cell   Endothelium

Intima

Internal elastic lamina

Smooth muscle

Media

Lamellar unit

Fenestrated elastic layer

External elastic lamina

Adventitia

Fibroblast

(a)

Endothelium

Intima

Smooth muscle cell

Internal elastic lamina

Media

Smooth muscle cells

External elastic lamina

Adventitia

Fibroblast

(b)

Figure 5.11 Structure of the normal artery wall.
(a) Elastic artery.
(b) Muscular artery.

that it is also a part of the normal development of the intima, probably a response to the continual stress of blood flow under pressure.* Exaggerated intimal thickening occurs in areas of special stress, such as branch points and around the ostia of blood vessels, where thickened intimal 'pads' or 'cushions' soon appear. It is therefore not surprising that such locations are also the sites where the pathological changes of atherosclerosis are seen first. The intima is separated from the media by a sheet of elastic fibres, the internal elastic lamina. The *media* is the muscular layer of the wall. In elastic arteries, such as the aorta, the media is composed of lamellar units, each consisting of a layer of elastic fibres and a layer of smooth muscle cells; in muscular arteries, the media consists wholly of smooth muscle cells (Figure 5.11). In large arteries the small blood vessels known as *vasa vasorum* penetrate a little way into the media from the outside of the artery, but the inner part of the media as well as the intima are devoid of capillary and lymphatic supply. Naturally, the blood in the lumen of the artery itself supplies nutrients, by diffusion, to the inner part of the vessel wall. Nevertheless, the fact that this region is avascular may be significant in some of the pathological changes of atherosclerosis (p. 668). The *adventitia* is the outermost layer, made up of connective tissue, and is the only layer to contain fibroblasts.

Lesions of atherosclerosis

The typical lesions are local, nodular changes in the intima of the arterial wall; their focal nature distinguishes atherosclerosis from diffuse intimal thickening which occurs in man with increasing age and which is exacerbated by hypertension. Three principal types of lesion are recognised, namely the *fatty streak, fibrous plaque* and *complicated lesion.* The fibrous plaque is the most characteristic feature of developing atherosclerosis, while the complicated lesion is an advanced stage which derives from the fibrous plaque. The fatty streak, on the other hand, is an early stage and the question of whether streaks can develop into plaques is controversial.

(i) *Fatty streaks* and dots are superficial fatty patches, yellow in colour, which are only slightly raised and do not cause narrowing of the lumen or clinical symptoms. Their colour is due to the deposited lipid (cholesterol and cholesteryl oleate) which is intracellular, contained in 'foam cells', lipid-laden smooth muscle cells. Streaks are very common at all ages, including childhood, and in all races and environmental conditions. 30–50% of the aortic surface at the age of 25 may be covered by fatty streaks. Thus, dots and streaks are the earliest and most universal of the fatty changes in the intima. However, it is by no means certain that they develop into plaques. Another lesion, a small area of intimal oedema called the *gelatinous lesion*, is more likely to be a precursor of the fibrous plaque.

(ii) *Fibrous plaques* are raised greyish-yellow areas of intimal thickening which protrude into the lumen of the artery. Histologically, the plaque consists of a superficial accumulation of smooth muscle cells and fibrous connective tissue (collagen, elastin, mucopolysaccharide) lying under the intima. The cells are loaded with lipid (again cholesterol and its esters) which now also lies extracellularly in the connective tissue. Beneath this fibrous layer lies a larger deposit of free extracellular lipid and cell debris (Figure 5.12). The porridge-like appearance of this deposited fat gives atherosclerosis its name. The fibrous connective tissue of

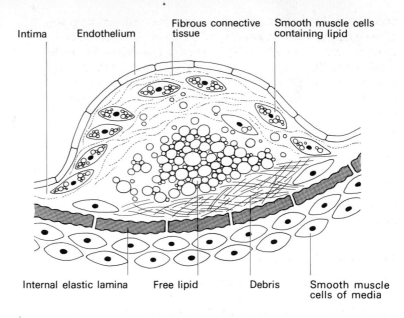

Figure 5.12 Section through fibrous plaque.

Intima   Endothelium   Fibrous connective tissue   Smooth muscle cells containing lipid

Internal elastic lamina   Free lipid   Debris   Smooth muscle cells of media

the plaques is produced by the smooth muscle cells, rather than fibroblasts (which are not found in plaques); the lipid is derived from the plasma. An *atheroma* is a plaque in which there is an amorphous necrotic mass containing much extracellular lipid lying beneath a fibrous cap. The media underlying the fibrous plaque or atheroma is thinned, thus partially accommodating the extra tissue.

(iii) *Complicated lesions* derive from the raised plaques as they become haemorrhagic, ulcerated, calcified (a distinctive feature), or the site of thrombosis. The complicated lesion is the cause of occlusion of the artery.

DISTRIBUTION OF THE LESIONS

The raised lesions show local preferences in their early distribution for certain sites in the arterial tree and occur frequently at points of branching, at bends and where arteries are relatively immobilised. For example, the bifurcation of the aorta and the entrances to the branches of the aorta (intercostals and coronaries) are sites which are commonly affected first. The occurrence of more severe atheroma in the proximal rather than the distal segments of the coronaries may be because they are especially twisted. The local sites first affected are often points of particular haemodynamic stress, which both damages the endothelium and stimulates fibrosis.

Consequences of atherosclerosis

The development and complication of the fibrous plaque are responsible for the consequences of atherosclerosis, outlined in

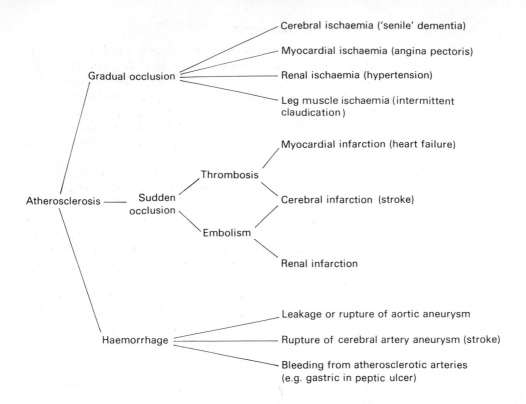

Atherosclerosis

- Gradual occlusion
  - Cerebral ischaemia ('senile' dementia)
  - Myocardial ischaemia (angina pectoris)
  - Renal ischaemia (hypertension)
  - Leg muscle ischaemia (intermittent claudication)
- Sudden occlusion
  - Thrombosis
    - Myocardial infarction (heart failure)
    - Cerebral infarction (stroke)
  - Embolism
    - Renal infarction
- Haemorrhage
  - Leakage or rupture of aortic aneurysm
  - Rupture of cerebral artery aneurysm (stroke)
  - Bleeding from atherosclerotic arteries (e.g. gastric in peptic ulcer)

Figure 5.13. The continuing narrowing of the lumen of the vital coronary and cerebral blood vessels results in ischaemia or infarction of the heart muscle and the brain. The most important complicating factor is thrombosis, caused by the disturbance of blood flow over, and the reaction of platelets with, the roughened and in later stages ulcerated arterial surface. An occluding thrombus may be immediately fatal for obvious reasons. Moreover, mural thrombi are a most important cause of the growth of the plaques themselves. Thrombi forming on the surface of fibrous plaques become organised into fibrous tissue and may become covered by endothelium, thus enlarging the underlying plaque and further narrowing the lumen of the vessel. This process of *encrustation* of mural thrombi is very significant in causing the occlusive effects of atherosclerosis and is discussed further below. In the advanced lesions there is also calcification, ulceration and damage to the underlying elastic lamina and the media. In consequence there is weakening of the arterial wall, possibly aneurysmal dilatation, and a tendency to rupture and haemorrhage. Of course, the clinical consequences of atherosclerosis are dependent on other factors besides the presence of raised and advanced lesions, some of which have been described in previous paragraphs on thrombosis and ischaemia. Indeed, the majority of middle-aged men have lesions of atherosclerosis without ischaemic heart disease; but the presence of this silent condition is almost always the cause of the mortality and morbidity of coronary disease, due to coronary thrombosis and subsequent myocardial infarction.

Figure 5.13 Consequences of atherosclerosis.

Outline of pathogenesis

Atherosclerosis is a very complex disease to which many factors contribute. Moreover, some of these serve to augment the development of the fibrous plaque and complicated lesion rather than to initiate their appearance. It is helpful, therefore, to outline a current synthesis of the processes involved in atherogenesis as a preliminary to the evidence implicating different factors in its pathogenesis. Three main processes can be distinguished (Figure 5.14).

1 *Injury to the endothelium* is probably the initial event in atherosclerosis. Damage will reveal subendothelial collagen and lead to accumulation of platelets on the wall, with their characteristic responses of adhesion, release, aggregation and activation of blood clotting. One of the recent advances in understanding the role of platelets in atherosclerosis is the finding that they release a factor which promotes the division of smooth muscle cells and production of fibrous connective tissue.

2 *Infiltration of lipid* from the plasma will follow endothelial damage, as a result of the increased permeability of the endothelium. Once deposited, cholesterol itself is toxic and irritating; it causes necrosis and stimulates further smooth muscle proliferation and fibrosis around the lipid deposit. Hence through endothelial injury and lipid infiltration, the key features of the fibrous plaque will develop, namely smooth muscle proliferation, fibrosis and deposition of lipid.

Figure 5.14 Pathogenesis of atherosclerosis.

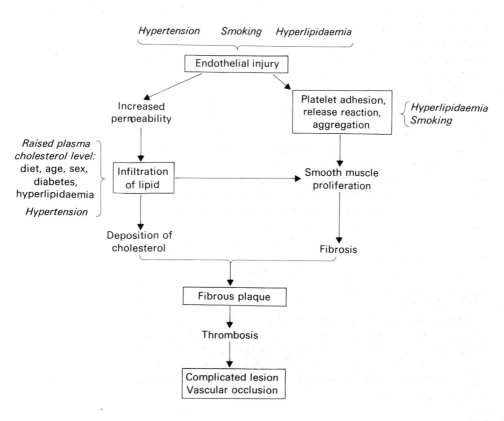

3 The fibrous plaque grows by *thrombosis*, in which mural thrombi form on the altered arterial surface, then become organised into fibrous tissue and ultimately incorporated into the plaque. Calcification of the lesion follows later.

Risk factors such as hypertension, raised plasma cholesterol levels, smoking, stress, diabetes mellitus, etc., are involved when they contribute to these principal events (Figure 5.14). Some of these factors may explain why atherosclerosis is such a peculiarly human disease, advanced lesions resembling those of man hardly ever being seen in other mammals, including the primates.

The endothelium and endothelial injury

The earliest stages in atherosclerosis are damage to the endothelium and an increase in its permeability, leading to platelet deposition and the entry of harmful lipids into the intima (Figure 5.15). The normal endothelium forms a tight barrier which prevents the entry of macromolecules, including lipoproteins (the transport form of most lipids, including cholesterol, p. 660), from the blood into the arterial wall. The endothelial cells are locked together by closed interdigitating junctions, and are more tightly associated than in capillaries and venules of the

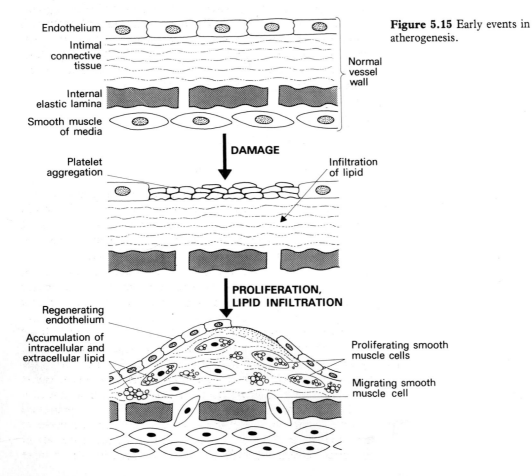

Endothelium
Intimal connective tissue
Internal elastic lamina
Smooth muscle of media

Normal vessel wall

DAMAGE

Platelet aggregation
Infiltration of lipid

PROLIFERATION, LIPID INFILTRATION

Regenerating endothelium
Accumulation of intracellular and extracellular lipid
Proliferating smooth muscle cells
Migrating smooth muscle cell

Figure 5.15 Early events in atherogenesis.

microcirculation (Section 1). Consequently, the arterial endothelium is a more effective permeability barrier and thereby serves to prevent the loss of lipoproteins and other large molecules from the circulation before the blood reaches the tissues. A limited passage of macromolecules occurs across the arterial endothelium in vacuoles after pinocytosis by endothelial cells.

Endothelial injury leads to formation of gaps between cells, exactly as in the microcirculation during acute inflammation (Section 1) or, if violent, to detachment of endothelial cells from the wall. The effects of damage can be studied experimentally by injuring an area of endothelium by means of a balloon catheter (an inflatable rubber tube inserted into the artery which strips off endothelial cells). The immediate result is the increased permeability of the damaged area to macromolecules, including lipoproteins, and the adherence of platelets to the exposed surface. A few days later, smooth muscle cells invade the area, migrating into the intima from the media through fenestrae in the internal elastic lamina, proliferate and begin to form connective tissue collagen and elastic fibres. An important finding is that these subsequent changes do not occur in the presence of platelet inhibitors or in thrombocytopenic animals (p. 658).

Under normal circumstances, endothelial damage occurs particularly at sites which are exposed to *haemodynamic stress*, such as the entrance regions to vessels, bifurcations and branch points ('flow dividers'), and the flow of lipid across the endothelium is always increased at such points. These are among the arterial sites which are particularly prone to atherosclerosis, and there is little doubt that the effect of mechanical stress on the endothelium contributes to the local distribution of lesions.

RISK FACTORS CONTRIBUTING TO
ENDOTHELIAL DAMAGE

Hypertension

An important role for arterial blood pressure in atherosclerosis is immediately indicated by the exclusive occurrence of lesions in the arterial, i.e. high pressure, system and their absence on the venous side. Moreover, hypertension is one of the most important factors predisposing to atherosclerosis and ischaemic heart disease, and some blood vessels, such as the pulmonary arteries, only show lesions in cases of hypertension. One of the reasons for this association is the effect of hypertension on the endothelium; when severe, it opens endothelial junctions by causing the cells to contract away from each other. This increases the permeability of the endothelium and hence infiltration of lipid. This effect of hypertension may in fact be caused by angiotensin itself, the circulating level of which is often increased in hypertensive patients (p. 676). Besides raising the blood pressure, angiotensin has been shown to increase arterial permeability by opening up endothelial junctions. Hypertension also increases turbulence at flow dividers in the arterial sytem, and hence the frequency of collisions between platelets and damaged endothelium at these points. It is noteworthy that normal human blood pressure is higher than in other species, as well as other primates; this is likely to be one of the reasons that atherosclerosis is very common in man, yet rare in the other primates, including the anthropoid apes.

Hyperlipidaemia

The central role of the blood cholesterol level in the development of atherosclerosis is discussed at length below. It can generally be attributed to the increased rate of entry of lipid into the intima when the cholesterol level is raised. However, it has recently been shown that hypercholesterolaemia can itself lead to endothelial injury, with actual loss of endothelial cells, and hence also initiate the influx of cholesterol into the intima as well as the adhesion of platelets to the exposed connective tissue.

Smoking and hypoxia

Smoking promotes atherosclerosis, probably through the increased carbon monoxide level in the blood. A high circulating CO level will produce hypoxia of the endothelium and open the intercellular junctions.

Antigen–antibody complexes

When antigen–antibody complexes form in the circulation they can deposit on the endothelium and cause the death of endothelial cells, probably through complement activation. This can promote atherogenesis in animals which already have high circulating lipid levels.

Role of platelets in atherosclerosis

The adhesion of platelets to the arterial wall after endothelial injury is one of the important initiating steps in atherosclerosis (Figure 5.15); in this respect there is a strong parallel between this process and thrombosis (p. 644) which, it will be recalled, also starts by platelets adhering to revealed collagen. Following experimental injury to the endothelium, the response of the arterial wall consists of the migration of smooth muscle cells into the intima where they proliferate and produce collagen fibrils, elastic fibres and mucopolysaccharides (glycosaminoglycans). The intima increases in thickness as a result of this activity. An important observation implicating platelets in these events is that the intimal response does not occur in animals in which platelet function has been suppressed, either by inhibitors such as dipyridamole or by antiplatelet serum. This provides good experimental evidence that platelets are required for the characteristic proliferation of smooth muscle in the intimal response to vascular injury. The adhesion of platelets is followed by the release of serotonin, ADP and lysosomal enzymes from platelet granules and some of these may further increase the permeability of endothelium around the damaged area. Moreover, it has been discovered that platelets release a macromolecular factor which promotes the proliferation of smooth muscle cells in culture. In fact, platelets are not the only source of this mitogenic factor, which can also be produced by monocytes or macrophages (which may be present in lesions) and by endothelial cells themselves. It seems likely that this factor is an important trigger of the response of smooth muscle cells in the intima following endothelial damage; its action is augmented by plasma lipoproteins, containing cholesterol, which will infiltrate into the intima at this time as a result of removal of the endothelial barrier. It is envisaged that under favourable circumstances, endothelial cells grow back over the damaged area and restore the integrity of the endothelium, whereupon growth of smooth muscle cells ceases. The thickening of the intima is reversible, and the initial lesion will normally regress *unless* repeated damage to the same area occurs. In the latter situation, the lesion can develop into a fibrous plaque.

Certain additional factors encourage platelet aggregation, including a raised blood lipid level, a condition which is itself the result of a variety of contributing elements (p. 661, Figure 5.14). Hyperlipidaemia both increases the agglutinability of platelets as well as inhibiting fibrinolysis, hence raising the thrombotic tendency of the blood. In such circumstances, if platelet aggregates form spontaneously on normal endothelium they might cause endothelial damage and perhaps themselves initiate the cycle of events leading to atherosclerosis.

Platelets not only play a central role in the initiation of the lesions, but are also vital to their further development by thrombosis (p. 668).

Cholesterol and atherosclerosis

Of all the components of atherosclerosis, greatest attention in the past has been given to cholesterol, being the principal component of the lesion which leads to narrowing of the lumen. It is certainly true that high plasma cholesterol levels encourage the development of lesions; what is more debatable is whether cholesterol is itself an initiating factor. Recent findings that raised plasma lipids can (a) damage arterial endothelium and increase permeability, (b) promote smooth muscle proliferation and (c) enhance platelet aggregation, all indicate that cholesterol can indeed contribute to the initiation as well as the development of fibrous plaques.

The classical view of the involvement of cholesterol in arterial lesions derived from the insight of the great nineteenth century pathologist Virchow. The *infiltration theory* which he put forward for atherosclerosis was that mechanical forces injure the intima and allow lipid from the plasma to infiltrate under arterial pressure; the lipid in the intima could itself act as an irritant and stimulate chronic inflammatory changes, the result of which would be intimal fibrosis. In this way, two features of the raised lesions, namely lipid accumulation and fibrosis, could be accounted for. This hypothesis greatly contributed to the contemporary view that atherosclerosis is a response of the arterial wall to injury and is supported by more recent knowledge on the properties of cholesterol, its transportation in the blood and its irritant qualities, as well as by the evidence, some of it described below, that plasma cholesterol levels directly determine the development of lesions.

TRANSPORTATION OF CHOLESTEROL IN THE BLOOD

Cholesterol, like other lipids, is almost completely insoluble in aqueous media and does not exist free in the plasma. It is solubilised for transportation by forming soluble complexes with carrier proteins, the complex being called a *lipoprotein*. Other fats, such as phospholipids and triglycerides, are also transported as lipoprotein complexes, and triglycerides are also carried in particulate form as chylomicra. The lipoproteins are separable into four classes on the basis of their density, namely high, low and very low density lipoproteins and chylomicra; electrophoretically they can be separated as α, β and pre-β lipoproteins, which correspond to the high, low and very low density classes respectively (Table 5.2). Lipoproteins are very large complexes in which the carrier proteins (apoproteins) perform a detergent-like role in solubilising the lipid. Non-polar lipids, such as triglycerides and cholesteryl esters, are found in the centre of such complexes, while the polar cholesterol and phospholipids together with the apoproteins form an outer shell (Figure 5.16). Most of the cholesterol is transported as low density lipoprotein (LDL) and it is with the properties of this complex that we shall be particularly concerned. The cholesterol is mainly in the form of its ester with linoleic acid and it is important to note that the cholesterol in fibrous plaques is also largely cholesterol linoleate. This is obviously consistent with a plasma origin for the lipid in atherosclerosis. However, in fatty streaks, the cholesteryl ester is mainly with oleic acid, which suggests that fatty streaks and fibrous plaques may have different origins.

The normal fasting concentration range of low density lipoprotein in man is 400–600 mg/100 ml plasma and of cholesterol is 150–280 mg/100 ml plasma, and these are higher than the levels in most other animals, including other primates. This correlates with the low occurrence of atherosclerosis and ischaemic heart disease in species other than man; man may

Table 5.2 Plasma lipoproteins

Class	Mobility	Density (g/cc)	Major lipid component	Major apoprotein
Chylomicra		<0.950	Triglyceride	Apo–A,B,C
Very low density lipoproteins (VLDL)	Pre-β	0.950–1.006	Triglyceride	Apo–B,C,E
Low density lipoproteins (LDL)	β	1.006–1.063	Cholesterol	Apo–B
High density lipoproteins (HDL)	α	1.063–1.210	Phospholipid, cholesterol	Apo–A

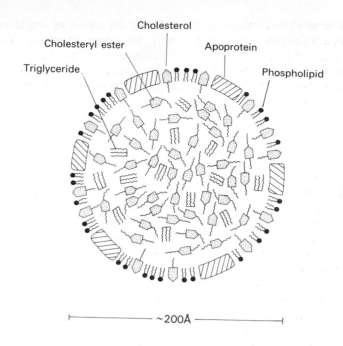

Figure 5.16 Diagrammatic structure of low density lipoprotein (LDL).

Cholesterol

Cholesteryl ester

Triglyceride

Apoprotein

Phospholipid

~200Å

therefore be naturally predisposed by his cholesterol level to arterial disease. (In this connection, it has already been noted that man is naturally hypertensive in so far as human blood pressure is higher than that of other primates; the importance of hypertension in atherosclerosis is not less than that of plasma lipid levels.) The levels of both LDL and HDL are relevant to atheroma. Thus, national surveys have shown a strong positive correlation in the population between a higher than average level of plasma LDL-cholesterol and ischaemic heart disease. In contrast, there is an *inverse* correlation between the level of cholesterol carried as HDL and ischaemic heart disease—the risk decreases with higher HDL-cholesterol levels. The protective effect of HDL is obviously of great interest; the mechanism is uncertain, but the evidence favours a 'reverse cholesterol transport' hypothesis, in which HDL mobilises cholesterol from the intima into the blood.

VARIABILITY OF HUMAN BLOOD CHOLESTEROL
LEVEL: DIET, AGE, SEX, PERSONAL HABITS

There are many reasons for implicating the level of cholesterol in the blood as a major cause of atherosclerosis, one of which is the incidence of the disease within and between populations. Although the fatty streak is a universally distributed lesion, the occurrence of fibrous plaques, complicated lesions and ischaemic heart disease is considerably higher in the affluent societies of the world than it is where living standards are low. For example, in the USA, Negroes have the same incidence of atherosclerosis as Whites in the same area, which is much higher than in the Jamaican or African Negro populations. Ethnic differences play relatively little part in such variations, the causes of which are environmental and mainly reflect differences in *diet*. Frugal dietary habits, whether enforced during wartime or voluntary, as in certain religious orders or vegetarians, lead to a reduced level of atherosclerosis and its consequences. In all cases, the effect of dietary restriction is to lower the level of lipoproteins circulating in the blood. The important dietary component involved, however, is not necessarily cholesterol itself or even the total lipid content. Rather, the type of fat in the diet, particularly the proportions of saturated and unsaturated fat, determines the concentration of plasma cholesterol. Thus, a diet rich in saturated animal fats, such as butter, eggs, beef fat, etc., maintains the plasma cholesterol at a higher level than one containing instead unsaturated fats or oils of fish or vegetable origin. Poorer communities consume less saturated fat than rich ones and this is one of the main factors determining the lower incidence of atherosclerosis in the less affluent populations of the world. However, lipid is not the only dietary component which can affect plasma cholesterol levels; carbohydrate intake also makes an important contribution. It is significant, for example, that certain primitive populations such as the Masai and other nomadic tribes, as well as Eskimos, consume a high level of animal fats but very little carbohydrate, and that their incidence of atherosclerosis and abnormal blood lipid levels is extremely low. Restriction of carbohydrate in the Western diet may be as important to the prevention of atherosclerosis as the limitation of saturated animal fats. Interestingly, alcohol consumption can protect against arterial disease by increasing plasma HDL-cholesterol, and patients with alcoholic liver disease rarely have atheroma.

Within a given population, atherosclerosis shows strong correlations with *age* and *sex*, increasing steadily with age after the third decade and being more common in young men than young women. In women, there is quite a rapid increase in atherosclerosis after the menopause, and in the over-50 age group there is little difference between the sexes. These trends can again be correlated with plasma cholesterol levels, which increase with age and are higher in young males. The sex difference is hormonally determined; oestrogens depress the level of plasma cholesterol. Oestrogens may also have a direct effect on the arteries by stabilising lysosomal membranes and limiting release of lysosomal enzymes into the cells and tissues. Thus women are to a degree protected from atherosclerosis during their reproductive life. It is noteworthy that oral contraceptives reverse the depressive effect of oestrogen and increase cholesterol levels; the long-term results of this increase have yet to be observed.

Among other personal habits which may affect atherosclerosis and coronary disease, cigarette smoking stands out as increasing both, though a direct effect of smoking on cholesterol levels is difficult to prove. Exercise, on the other hand, has a beneficial influence, which seems to be exerted via a rise in the level of plasma HDL-cholesterol. Running 12 miles per week can increase plasma HDL-cholesterol by up to 30%, while running 24 miles per week leads to increases of 50% or more.

The most striking examples of correlations between the severity of coronary disease in individuals and their cholesterol levels are the cases of *inherited hyperlipidaemias*. These are conditions in which, because of an inherited metabolic disorder, blood lipid levels are considerably higher than the normal range. Those hyperlipidaemias in which the cholesterol level is markedly increased, such as *familial hypercholesterolaemia*, are closely associated with severe atherosclerosis occurring at an early age, including among children (juvenile ischaemic heart disease). Hypercholesterolaemia may be secondary to other conditions, such as hypothyroidism and diabetes, in which there is also increased arterial disease as a result. However, other hyperlipidaemias in which the triglyceride level, but not the cholesterol level, is markedly raised are *not* associated with atherosclerosis. Experimentally, hypercholesterolaemia can be induced in many species by feeding large amounts of cholesterol, although this is difficult in some such as the rat and dog. One of the findings is the focal loss of approximately 7% of the endothelial surface from arterial walls. Thus, chronic hypercholesterolaemia can directly lead to endothelial injury with both gap formation and loss of endothelial cells, initiating the adherence of platelets and the increased permeability of the wall to cholesterol.

Recently, a cellular defect involved in familial hypercholesterolaemia has been discovered. Normal fibroblasts and certain other cells, including arterial smooth muscle cells, have receptors for low density lipoproteins (LDL), the chief plasma transport form of cholesterol. After binding to these surface receptors, the lipoproteins are internalised and digested in the cell by lysosomal enzymes to release cholesterol, which is used for membrane synthesis. The accumulation of cholesterol in the cell inhibits both the synthesis of cholesterol by the cell and also the formation of the LDL receptor itself. In hypercholesterolaemia, the receptor is absent from the cell surface, presumably because of a defect in the gene coding for the receptor molecule. As a result, LDL carrying cholesterol is not removed from the bloodstream by tissue cells and, moreover, cellular synthesis of cholesterol is not suppressed, despite the high circulating cholesterol level. The plasma cholesterol level thus rises to very high levels which may exceed 800 mg per 100 ml, about four times the normal value, in individuals homozygous for the defective gene (i.e. possessing two copies of it). Heterozygotes are also affected, though less severely (Section 7). As already noted, severe forms of hypercholesterolaemia are accompanied by cardiovascular disease in young people.

EXPERIMENTAL EVIDENCE ON THE ROLE OF CHOLESTEROL

The theory that circulating cholesterol is a key factor in the development of lesions has classically been supported by a large body of evidence which in summary shows that (i) the lipid which accumulates in atherosclerotic lesions is derived directly from the plasma, (ii) cholesterol is an irritative agent and can stimulate proliferative and fibrous changes in the intima and (iii) the plasma levels of cholesterol and low density lipoprotein have a determining effect on the disease. These conclusions are supported both by animal experiments and by the foregoing clinical evidence. Animal experiments usually involve the effect on atherosclerosis of raising blood cholesterol levels by means of different diets. These experiments have a long history, dating back to early studies in rabbits by Ignatowski (1908) and Anitschkow (1913) who showed that the feeding of cholesterol caused the development of nodular fatty thickening in the intima of the aorta. The rabbit has been the animal of choice for most of the feeding experiments because, being herbivorous, its cholesterol levels are normally very low but are very easily increased by cholesterol feeding. Indeed it is possible to increase plasma cholesterol concentrations in the rabbit to 10,000 mg/100 ml (cf. normal rabbit level of 100 mg/100 ml.) Needless to say, the rabbit does not normally show signs of atherosclerosis in the aorta. By means of suitable diets containing cholesterol and animal fats, it takes a few months of elevated cholesterol levels ($\sim$ 500 mg/100 ml) to produce lesions in the rabbit aorta and its branches which resemble, in some degree, those in man, i.e. there is localised intimal thickening with accumulation of lipid and overgrowth of fibrous tissue. In fact, the fibrous component is very small unless special techniques are employed, such as alternation of a high fat diet with periods of a normal one. What happens in this case is presumably that, during periods of normal diet, there is a slowing of lipid accumulation and an enhanced fibrogenic response to the fatty lesions. The lipid is frequently contained intracellularly in foam cells and is superficial. Raised plaques are preceded in appearance by fatty streaks which form after a few weeks. In these experiments the degree and duration of the raised plasma cholesterol level correlates with the severity of the lesions, and the lipid in the aorta derives from the plasma.

Experiments such as these in the rabbit are open to the objection that they do not necessarily bear on the situation in man. The rabbit is a herbivore and especially sensitive to cholesterol; cholesterol levels attained in some experiments are clearly excessive, beyond anything which might be found naturally even in man. Indeed, the striking observation is precisely that the blood cholesterol levels have to be raised to very high levels to produce visible plaques. This confirms that the normal undamaged endothelium is a highly efficient barrier to the entry of lipid. However, if feeding of cholesterol to rabbits is combined with experimental damage to the endothelium, plaques appear at the sites of injury after only two weeks and at cholesterol levels of only 150 mg/100 ml. Similar effects have been found in rats, which are normally very resistant to induction of atherosclerosis by feeding cholesterol, as well as in primates. Experimental hyperlipidaemia on its own must be regarded as inefficient at producing lesions, while hyperlipidaemia combined with endothelial damage is highly effective, producing lesions which both develop more rapidly and are more severe. By the same token, experimental damage to the endothelium in the absence of hypercholesterolaemia leads to intimal thickening which is reversed when the endothelium is repaired. If cholesterol levels are raised, however, lesions do not regress, but grow into lipid-rich fibrous plaques. Once again, the interdependence of hyperlipidaemia and endothelial damage in the pathogenesis of lesions is evident. It is relevant to recall at this point that prolonged exposure to excessive cholesterol levels can itself be a cause of endothelial damage, as noted on page 658. In an animal which more closely resembles man, namely the Rhesus monkey, raising the plasma cholesterol to levels which might be encountered in humans (250–600 mg/100 ml), has produced lesions which resemble those in man and, if continued for very long periods (over 3 years), has led to occlusion of the coronary arteries and myocardial infarction.

REGRESSION OF CHOLESTEROL-INDUCED LESIONS

Both clinical and experimental evidence suggest a primary role for cholesterol in the pathogenesis of atherosclerosis. Not surprisingly, there is considerable interest in whether reduction of plasma cholesterol levels can lead to regression of existing atherosclerotic lesions in man. The evidence cited above of the effect of severe dietary restriction during wartime suggests that it may. Experimental lesions induced in primates by cholesterol feeding are apparently reversible and regress when the diet returns to low fat. In man, in addition to dietary regulation, drugs have been used to reduce cholesterol levels, but their effect both on blood lipid and incidence of heart disease has been found to be marginal in clinical trials. Surgical intervention can also be used to reduce absorption of cholesterol from the gut (the partial ileal bypass operation), and this lowers blood cholesterol levels by between 30% and 60%. Some improvement in the condition of coronary arteries in patients has been noted following this operation. Thus, some regression of established lesions seems to be possible, particularly for those which have not progressed to the complicated stage, providing reduction of blood cholesterol is sufficiently great; in practice this may mean levels of around 200 mg per 100 ml which can be achieved by vigorous treatment. However, even after loss of lipid from lesions, a fibrous scar, possibly with calcification, may remain and it is most unlikely that this will ever be resolved. Nevertheless, the calibre of the lumen of the vessel may be beneficially increased. It is unlikely that complicated, i.e. calcified and ulcerated, lesions ever regress; nor can severe damage to the arterial wall (medial degeneration, ruptured internal elastic lamina) be reversed.

FATE OF LOW DENSITY LIPOPROTEIN IN THE INTIMA

In the fibrous plaque, cholesterol is found both as extracellular deposits and intracellularly within smooth muscle cells ('foam cells'). Figure 5.17 indicates the pathways by which lipid can

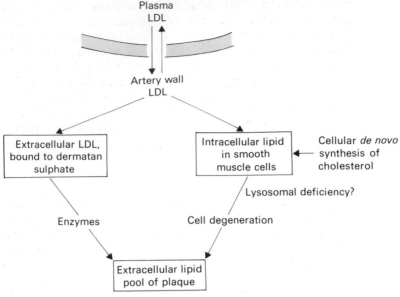

Plasma
LDL

Artery wall
LDL

Extracellular LDL,
bound to dermatan
sulphate

Intracellular lipid
in smooth
muscle cells

Cellular *de novo*
synthesis of
cholesterol

Lysosomal deficiency?

Enzymes

Cell degeneration

Extracellular lipid
pool of plaque

Figure 5.17 Routes of deposition
of lipid in the intima.

LDL = low density lipoprotein

accumulate in the intima, having penetrated the endothelium. These are (i) trapping of LDL by certain connective tissue constituents (mucopolysaccharides) and (ii) uptake by smooth muscle cells and subsequent release when the cells die.

Trapping by mucopolysaccharides

Having entered the intima as a result of increased endothelial permeability, LDL can be selectively trapped as a result of 'sieving' by and interaction with intimal connective tissues, especially mucopolysaccharides (glycosaminoglycans). These molecules are a major constituent of the intercellular matrix and include hyaluronic acid, haparan sulphate, chondroitin sulphate and dermatan sulphate. In structure, they are long, unbranched chain molecules which form a molecular network in the matrix. The effect of this network is first to slow up the rate of diffusion through the intima of large molecules such as LDL, acting in short as a 'molecular sieve'. Secondly, they are negatively charged, because of their carboxyl and sulphate groups, and can therefore bind proteins by ionic interaction. In particular, LDL, but not HDL, binds well to dermatan sulphate; the reaction can be demonstrated as precipitation on mixing solutions of LDL and the mucopolysaccharide in the presence of calcium ions. The selectivity of the reaction is significant, since it is the LDL which is retained by the intima. In fibrous plaques, the connective tissue matrix is produced by the proliferating smooth muscle cells. It is very interesting that, in culture, these cells produce 60–80% dermatan sulphate, 10–20% chondroitin sulphate and less than 5% hyaluronic acid. This contrasts markedly with dermal fibro-

666

blasts, which produce about 60% hyaluronic acid, 10–20% chondroitin sulphate and only 10% dermatan sulphate. The high proportion of dermatan sulphate produced in human aortas is particularly striking in the light of the particular affinity of this molecule for LDL. Once bound in the intima, LDL is dissociated, probably by enzymatic action, to release cholesterol and its esters. Since cholesterol stimulates growth of smooth muscle cells and production of connective tissue, a cycle of events can ensue in which cholesterol deposition promotes production of dermatan sulphate which in turn progressively traps more LDL, and so on.

Uptake by smooth muscle cells

LDL binds to the surface of smooth muscle cells at specific LDL receptors and is then endocytosed in vesicles, which eventually become incorporated into lysosomes. (Bulk phase uptake of extracellular fluid may also occur, of course, and with it uptake of entrapped lipoprotein.) The lysosomal enzymes include proteases, which destroy the protein part of the LDL to release cholesterol and cholesteryl ester, and a hydrolase which acts on the esters to free cholesterol. The latter reaction is essential both for the passage of cholesterol out of the lysosome for cellular excretion and for its utilisation in membrane synthesis. A recent hypothesis suggests that, if there is an excessively large uptake of LDL, lysosomal hydrolase may be inadequate to deal with the influx, and an accumulation of cholesteryl esters in the lysosomes could occur. It has been found that the number of lysosomes in intimal smooth muscle cells increases during experimental atherogenesis (hypertension plus hypercholesterolaemia) and that they are the intracellular sites of lipid accumulation. In due course, the excessive concentration of cholesteryl ester in the cell could result in cell death and the release of lipid contents, which could then contribute to the extracellular lipid pool. It is interesting to draw a parallel here with the lysosomal storage diseases (see Section 7), in which certain substrates accumulate in lysosomes because of an inherited deficiency in a degradative enzyme. For example, in the Hurler syndrome, a mucopolysaccharide storage disease, dermatan sulphate accumulates in fibroblast lysosomes due to their deficiency of the enzyme L-iduronidase (p. 851). The dermatan sulphate is released into the circulation when these cells die and accumulates *inter alia* in smooth muscle cells in the walls of blood vessels. It is particularly noteworthy in this context that this results in smooth muscle proliferation, the subendothelial thickening of artery walls and, since the coronary arteries may be affected, eventual myocardial ischaemia and infarction. It is possible that an analogous situation exists in the developing fibrous plaque in atheroma and that accumulation of cholesteryl esters is partly a result of insufficiency of lysosomal hydrolase in the smooth muscle cell.

The free cholesterol and cholesteryl esters deposited extracellularly are virtually unable to diffuse through the intima unless resolubilised by protein or other lipotropic agents. Nor is the intima supplied with the lymphatics or capillaries via which lipid could be removed. Even in large arteries where the vessels of the vasa vasorum partially penetrate the media from the adventitia, there is an avascular gap between the endothelium and the outer part of the wall across which molecules must diffuse before they can be drained off by lymphatics. There is also no significant catabolism of cholesterol by the arterial wall; the liver and some endocrine organs are able to degrade cholesterol to water soluble cholic acids, but other tissues lack this capacity. Hence a pool of insoluble cholesterol and cholesteryl linoleate accumulates in the intima and frequently crystallises. We have noted elsewhere that the protective effect of HDL may be due to solubilisation of cholesterol from the vessel wall and its removal into the blood, accounting for the fact that a high plasma HDL-cholesterol level correlates with a reduced risk of heart disease.

Further development of lesions: atherosclerosis and thrombosis

The similarity between initial stages in atherosclerosis and thrombosis is evident, since both begin by adherence of platelets to collagen following endothelial damage. Normally, in the absence of gross architectural changes in the vessel wall, thrombosis does not occur in arteries because of the rapid dispersal of clotting factors in the bloodstream. The development of the fibrous plaque protruding into the lumen disturbs the normal blood flow and leads to eddying which encourages platelet deposition on the raised arterial surface. However, the surface of the fibrous plaque is covered by endothelium and in order for a thrombus to form on it some damage to the surface is again necessary. The surface of the atheroma breaks easily and the plentiful collagen below is probably frequently exposed. Platelets then deposit on the fractured surface, encouraged by the haemodynamic factors such as eddying, and a mural thrombus forms over the fibrous plaque (Figure 5.18). The thrombus becomes overgrown by endothelium and then follows one of the fates of thrombi, namely organisation, with transformation into fibrous tissue (p. 646). Thus, in effect, a new fibrous layer is added to the fibrous plaque, which now protrudes further into the arterial lumen. The organising thrombus also acquires lipid by infiltration from the plasma. The growth of plaques by incorporation and organisation of mural thrombi is called *encrustation*; a repetition of the process will lead to progressive narrowing of the artery. In this way, the coronary and cerebral arteries gradually become occluded (Figure 5.18). In fact, encrustation was one of the oldest theories for the origin of atherosclerosis, originally proposed by the German pathologist Rokitansky in 1852; it was revived by Duguid in 1948 on the basis of accumulating histological evidence which showed that the lesions on the arterial wall developed by repeated mural thrombosis. While encrustation is responsible for the growth of lesions, they are not usually initiated by thrombosis, since the organising thrombi are always found on existing fibrous plaques and never on normal arterial wall.

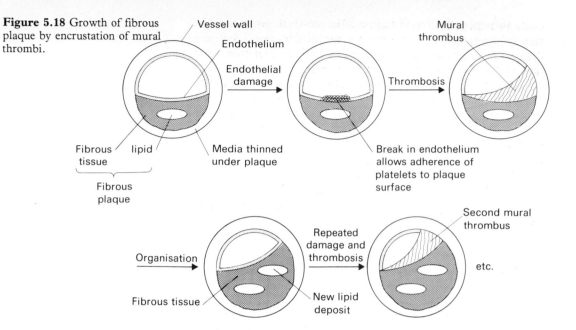

Figure 5.18 Growth of fibrous plaque by encrustation of mural thrombi.

Vessel wall

Endothelium

Endothelial damage

Fibrous tissue   lipid

Media thinned under plaque

Fibrous plaque

Mural thrombus

Thrombosis

Break in endothelium allows adherence of platelets to plaque surface

Organisation

Repeated damage and thrombosis

Second mural thrombus

etc.

Fibrous tissue

New lipid deposit

Modern theories of the pathogenesis of atherosclerosis

RESPONSE TO INJURY HYPOTHESIS

Contemporary understanding of the processes of atherosclerosis is founded largely on the classical theories of Virchow (arterial injury and infiltration of lipid) and Rokitansky (encrustation of mural thrombi) as refined by current experimental and clinical evidence. The response to injury hypothesis in its present form integrates these themes, as shown in Figures 5.14 and 5.15. Any hypothesis has to account for the key features of the fibrous plaque, namely smooth muscle proliferation, formation of fibrous connective tissue and accumulation of lipid, as well as explaining the growth of the plaque to occlusion of the vessel. In this theory, the first event is endothelial injury caused by mechanical stress, hypertension, hyperlipidaemia and other risk factors noted on page 655. Once the endothelium has been injured or removed, two consequences follow: (i) the barrier properties of the endothelium are lost at that point, so that lipids and other macromolecules can enter the vessel wall from the plasma, and (ii) platelets adhere to revealed collagen, release their granular contents and aggregate. These events lead to the local influx and division of smooth muscle cells, their production of the fibrous and matrix elements of connective tissue, and the accumulation of insoluble cholesterol and its derivatives. Mitogenic platelet factors and lipoproteins both contribute to smooth muscle cell proliferation and production of connective tissue. Thus a small lesion forms, which will soon be covered again by re-endothelialisation; providing the injury and response are both of limited size and duration, the process of thickening can probably be reversed and the area return to its normal appearance. The platelet and intimal response can then be regarded as a normal means of repairing minor endothelial damage. A fibrous plaque will only develop at the site if the injury is continuous or repetitive, which at certain points it inevitably will be, and if other risk factors encourage its formation. Among the latter, hypertension and a high circulating LDL-cholesterol level play the major role in causing the normal transient process of repair to become chronic and develop into atherosclerosis. Continuous injury and infiltration of lipid will stimulate the processes of smooth muscle proliferation and repair to the stage where they become irreversible and lead to clinical consequences. Once the lesion has reached a size and condition where a mural thrombus is likely to develop on top of it, it will grow by encrustation and in time occlude the lumen of narrow arteries (Figure 5.18).

The response to injury hypothesis serves to integrate the results of endothelial damage, platelet involvement and raised plasma cholesterol. It emphasizes the view that clinically important atherosclerosis is the result of normal repair mechanisms functioning in an altered environment (high cholesterol, hypertension). However, it is not the only hypothesis, and the following is a radically different alternative approach.

THE MONOCLONAL HYPOTHESIS: ATHEROSCLEROSIS AS BENIGN TUMOUR

A new theory of atherosclerosis has been suggested by some unexpected observations on the nature of the proliferating cells in the fibrous plaques. It has been emphasized above that, rather than typical fibroblasts, these are mainly smooth muscle cells, which have the ability to produce the collagen which makes up the stroma of the plaque. It has been suggested by E. Benditt that these cells are abnormal and that an atherosclerotic plaque is in fact a benign smooth muscle neoplastic tumour producing collagen. The evidence for this is the finding that in many plaques the proliferating cells are apparently *monoclonal* in origin, i.e. they are all descendents of a single cell and represent a single clone. This has been ascertained by using the fact that in females one of the X chromosomes in each somatic cell is randomly inactivated (the Lyon hypothesis, p. 819). Therefore, each cell will contain the products of the genes of only one of the two X chromosomes. One X-linked gene product is the enzyme glucose-6-phosphate dehydrogenase, and this occurs in two allelic forms (A and B) in Negroes. Therefore, in a heterozygous (i.e. A/B) female Negro, individual cells will produce either the A form of the enzyme or the B form, but never both, since one X chromosome is always inactivated. The normal intima in such women can be shown to be a mosaic of both cell types, and even very small areas of intima contain both forms of the enzyme. The same is expected of normal repair tissue. However, when quite large areas of atherosclerotic plaques were examined they were found to contain either the A form or the B form of the enzyme, but rarely both. This strongly suggests that the cells proliferating in the plaque are not a random collection of cells, but have all derived from a single cell, for only in this case would they all produce the same enzyme form. Hence the smooth muscle cells in the plaque seem to make up a single clone and in this way resemble a tumour, which also originates from a single cell (p. 729), rather than the mixed cell population expected in repair tissue. If the plaque really does represent a benign tumour of smooth muscle cells, one could speculate that the initiating agent is a lipid-soluble mutagen or virus associated with cholesterol, and that many of the factors invoked in atherogenesis, such as mechanical stress and hypertension, act as promotors in the sense of encouraging neoplastic growth (p. 766). While at the moment these are purely speculative suggestions, the discovery of the monoclonal origin of the plaques must be a challenge to the more conventional views of atherogenesis.

Prevention of atherosclerosis and thrombosis

What therapeutic and prophylactic uses can be made of the growing understanding of the mechanisms involved in atheroma and thrombosis? In the first place, there is strong evidence to support the beneficial effects of a restricted intake of dietary animal fats, regular exercise and abstinence from smoking. Secondly, there is the possible use of drugs to regulate blood lipids or prevent the thrombotic action of platelets, with the object of preventing ischaemic heart disease or its progression in those most at risk. The effectiveness of such agents can only be judged from properly conducted clinical trials. These can be either of 'primary prevention', in persons with no history of heart disease, or 'secondary prevention', in patients who have already suffered myocardial infarction. Both types of clinical trial have been used to test the benefits of drugs which lower the concentration of plasma cholesterol, including clofibrate, colestipol, cholestyramine and gemfibrozil. For example, in the primary prevention trial with clofibrate completed by the WHO in 1978, a reduction in serum cholesterol of 10% was accompanied by a fall of 25% in non-fatal myocardial infarction, while the incidence of fatal coronary thrombosis was not reduced. There was, however, a disturbing increase of about 25% in non-cardiovascular mortality (e.g. due to cancers). As far as secondary prevention is concerned, no effect of lipid-lowering drugs on morbidity or mortality has been found; thus, control of plasma cholesterol seems largely irrelevant to the prognosis once the disease has already progressed to the stage of myocardial infarction.

There have been several trials, mostly of the secondary prevention type, of antithrombotic agents, such as anticoagulants and antiplatelet drugs. Anticoagulant drugs produce a modest decrease in mortality of about 20%. With the increased understanding of the role of prostaglandins in platelet reactions, there has been great interest in the potential usefulness of antiplatelet agents such as aspirin, dipyridamole and sulphinpyrazone. Aspirin has received the most attention, with six clinical trials, the largest being the aspirin—myocardial infarction study

(AMIS) recently completed in the USA. In this trial, 2267 patients received 1000 mg aspirin daily, while 2251 acted as controls. Disappointingly, there were 245 deaths in the aspirin-treated group during the period of the trial, compared with only 219 in the untreated controls. All the other (smaller scale) trials have pointed to a 10–20% reduction in mortality through the use of aspirin. The problem seems to be that aspirin prevents the potentially beneficial as well as the thrombotic effects of prostaglandins, by inhibiting synthesis both of thromboxanes and prostacyclin (p. 630). The ideal dosage of aspirin would be one which selectively inhibited TxA_2 production and left PGI_2 synthesis unaffected, and this may be true at about 30–50 mg daily; however, such low doses have not yet been used in clinical trials. Specific inhibitors of thromboxane synthetase would perhaps be the ideal agents for preventing thrombosis.

HYPERTENSION

Definitions

Hypertension, or excessively raised arterial blood pressure, is a very common chronic condition, which affects as much as 5% of Western populations as a whole and which makes an important contribution to human mortality. However, despite the frequency of the condition, it is difficult to state precisely how high the arterial pressure must be to constitute hypertension. Arterial pressure, like characteristics such as individual height or weight, shows a continuous variation in the population, and it is not easy to draw a firm dividing line between the normal and the pathological (Figure 5.19). The most satisfactory definition of hypertension is probably in terms of the benefits which are conferred on the patient by therapeutic reduction of blood pressure

Figure 5.19 Hypertension in males and females.
Frequency distribution of diastolic pressure in males and females between the ages of 40 and 49 in a London sample (modified from Pickering, 1974). While the diastolic pressure is higher on the average in females, the definition of hypertension is also higher. The stippled area above 110 mm Hg shows patients known to be at risk; those in the ruled area are also likely to benefit from hypotensive therapy.

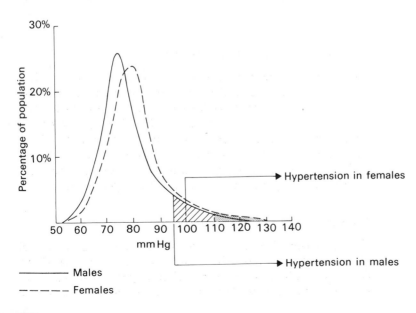

672

(hypotensive therapy). Using this criterion, it can be said that individuals showing a diastolic pressure of 95–100 mm Hg or more will benefit from a lowering of arterial pressure and are therefore hypertensive. There is a significant sex effect here, for although females in the middle age range and older tend to have higher arterial pressures than males of the same age group, they show less susceptibility to its adverse effects. Hence the definition of what constitutes hypertension is at a rather higher level for women ($\sim$ 100 mm Hg) than for men ($\sim$ 95 mm Hg) (Figure 5.19). Treatment becomes essential for either sex if the diastolic pressure rises above 110 mm Hg. In general, both systolic and diastolic pressure are raised in hypertension, but the diastolic pressure is the better guide to its severity. (There are some conditions in which only the systolic pressure is raised—systolic hypertension—generally a result of increased stroke output from the left ventricle. Systolic hypertension is not further discussed here.)

Age dependence

The normal values of systolic and diastolic pressure generally lie in the range of 90–140 mm Hg and 60–90 mm Hg respectively, depending on age and sex. Arterial pressure in our society increases with age, so it is not surprising that hypertensive disease becomes more frequent in middle and higher age groups. This statement is not true of all populations, however. In particular, primitive peoples who have been studied, such as the nomadic tribes of Kenya, have been found not to show the age-dependent increase in arterial pressure which is so characteristic of 'civilised' societies. When members of such primitive groups enter Western civilisation their blood pressures take on the same pattern of gradual increase as that of the community they join. These observations raise several interesting possible reasons for the increase in arterial pressure, such as diet or the stress of our way of life.

Secondary and essential hypertension

In a small proportion of cases ($\sim$ 10%) hypertension is a manifestation of another identifiable disease, most commonly of the kidney and urinary tract (nephritis, chronic pyelonephritis), and occasionally of an endocrine disorder (Cushing's syndrome, Conn's syndrome, phaeochromocytoma) or coarctation of the aorta. This is called *secondary hypertension*. However, in the vast majority there is no readily identifiable cause or associated disorder and they are said to have *essential hypertension*.

Malignant and benign hypertension

The pathological effects which result from raised arterial pressure, whether it is primary or secondary, take one of two courses depending on the severity of the hypertension. *Malignant hypertension* is rapidly progressive to a fatal termination with a diastolic pressure often above 130 mm Hg and rising. Death occurs in a majority of untreated cases within a year of diagnosis, either from uraemia, left ventricular failure or cerebral haemorrhage. Failing vision progressing to blindness is a characteristic feature. Only about 5% of hypertensive patients develop this form, which can occur at any age and is commonest around 40. The most frequently encountered form of hypertension has a much more stable course and is called *benign hypertension*; this is especially common in the middle aged and elderly with essential hypertension. Here the clinical effects are due to the gradual development of cardiovascular disease, particularly atherosclerosis, which is accelerated by hypertension. Retinal changes are unusual and renal function is generally good.

Consequences of hypertension

The greater the degree of hypertension, the more severe are its clinical effects, regardless of the underlying causes of the raised pressure. The consequences of hypertension fall into two groups, namely (a) degenerative changes in arteries and arterioles, including atherosclerosis, fibrinoid necrosis, hyalinisation and aneurysmal dilatation, and (b) hypertrophy of the arteries and of the heart, the latter due to the work load.

Atherosclerosis. Hypertension is an important risk factor in the development of fibrous plaques and complicated lesions. By increasing haemodynamic stress on the arterial wall, raised pressure causes endothelial damage and hence increased permeability to lipid and platelet adhesion. Via its acceleration of atherosclerosis, hypertension leads to ischaemic heart disease and myocardial and cerebral infarction, these being the main long-term effects of benign hypertension.

Hyaline thickening is a change frequently seen in arterioles in benign hypertension, especially in the afferent arterioles of the renal glomeruli. The wall of the vessel takes on a homogeneous, 'glassy' (hyaline), pink appearance (on staining with haematoxylin and eosin), with a loss of its underlying structural detail. The hyaline material is an acellular mass formed from fibrin or collagen fibres. The lumen of the affected vessels is narrowed. While hyaline thickening is a consequence of hypertension, it may also lead to further hypertension by reducing the blood flow through the renal arterioles. The kidney responds to reduced flow by releasing renin, an enzyme which catalyses formation of the pressor substance angiotensin and hence raises arterial pressure. (These events are described more fully on p. 676.)

Medial hypertrophy is an increase in thickness of the media by extra growth of smooth muscle in response to raised pressure. This is a widespread change in benign hypertension, which is likely to raise peripheral resistance (p. 675) and thereby contribute to the maintenance of raised pressure in essential hypertension.

Fibrinoid necrosis of small arteries and arterioles is the characteristic vascular lesion of malignant hypertension. An intense exudation of plasma takes place into the wall due to fragmentation of muscle fibres; inflammatory changes occur, neutrophils and red cells are found in the necrotic wall and fibrin is deposited. Haemorrhage may occur or the vessel may thrombose, or repair may lead to extreme fibrous thickening of the intima. Fibrinoid necrosis is responsible for the serious consequences of untreated malignant hypertension, in particular ischaemia and destruction of the kidney with renal failure, the typical ischaemic retinal changes which can lead to blindness (neuroretinopathy), and cerebral haemorrhage. The vascular changes can be arrested if the arterial pressure is reduced by suitable drug therapy.

Aneurysms. A further consequence of severe hypertension is that the media of the small arteries of the brain gives way and a dilatation or *microaneurysm* is formed. The rupture of an aneurysm results in cerebral haemorrhage, a common cause of death in both malignant and benign hypertension. The term *stroke* refers to the sudden and persistent interruption of cerebral function which can be caused by haemorrhage, thrombosis or embolism. There is a close association between the occurrence of strokes due to cerebral haemorrhage and severely raised arterial pressure (greater than 170/110 mm Hg), and hypotensive therapy is more effective in preventing strokes than it is in myocardial infarction.

Effects on the heart. In addition to the arterial changes, severe hypertension has a direct effect on the heart. The increased load on the heart caused by a raised arterial pressure leads to an increase in size of cardiac muscle fibres and hence in the size of the heart itself (*cardiac hypertrophy*). The greater the degree of hypertension, the more the heart is enlarged. When hypertension is very severe, the heart may be unable to maintain its output and enters into heart failure (left ventricular failure). This can be fatal at the first or any subsequent attack and is most likely to occur in malignant hypertension, because of the rapidity with which the pressure increases.

Hypertension and the regulation of blood pressure

The level of the mean arterial pressure is determined by two factors, namely *cardiac output* and *peripheral resistance*:

mean arterial pressure = cardiac output × peripheral resistance

Peripheral resistance is created mainly by the small arteries and arterioles with lesser contributions from the capillaries and small venules. In most cases of hypertension, cardiac output is normal and the raised arterial pressure is due to the increase in peripheral resistance, brought about by the decreased diameter of these blood vessels. There are also cases where an increase in blood volume, and hence cardiac output, is the underlying cause of hypertension. Physiological regulation of arterial pressure takes place largely through adjustments in peripheral resistance, and this is achieved both via the nervous system as well as hormonal mediators. Disturbances of these regulatory processes lead to hypertension.

Arterial baroreceptor reflexes

The baroreceptors are stretch receptors situated under the adventitia of large elastic arteries at points where the wall is particularly thin and where the smooth muscle of the media is replaced by elastic tissue, e.g. the carotid sinus and under the arch of the aorta. When arterial pressure rises, the frequency of firing of nerve impulses from the stretch receptors also increases, signalling the pressure change to the medullary centres in the brain. The pressor areas are inhibited, leading to dilatation of peripheral blood vessels and decrease in resistance. At the same time the heart is slowed through stimulation of the vagal cardio-inhibitory centre. If arterial pressure is raised for a long time, the sensitivity of the stretch receptors is decreased, and in chronic hypertension they are effectively reset at a higher pressure level. A similar decreased sensitivity occurs with age and contributes to the rise in blood pressure with ageing. Atherosclerotic lesions in these areas also decrease the sensitivity of the baroreceptors.

Adrenaline (epinephrine) and noradrenaline (norepinephrine)

Both these vasoactive amines exert a pressor action, through constriction of arterioles (noradrenaline being the neurotransmitter of the nerve terminals of the sympathetic system). Their secretion from the adrenal medulla increases the arterial pressure during stress, excitement, exercise and asphyxia. *Phaeochromocytoma* is a tumour of the chromaffin cells of the adrenal medulla, the cells which secrete adrenaline and noradrenaline. The tumours secrete excessive amounts, particularly of noradrenaline, and hence lead to secondary hypertension.

The renin-angiotensin-aldosterone system

The association between kidney disease and hypertension is well known, and was reproduced experimentally in the classic experiments of Goldblatt (1934). He showed that hypertension could be induced in the dog by constriction of the renal arteries, i.e. reduction of blood flow through the kidney. Clinical hypertension is seen in chronic pyelonephritis, chronic glomerulonephritis, stenosis of the renal artery and polycystic disease. When blood flow through the kidney is reduced, either due to a fall in blood pressure or renal disease, the kidney responds by releasing the proteolytic enzyme *renin* from cells in the walls of the afferent arterioles in the juxta-glomerular complex. Renin catalyses the splitting of angiotensinogen, an α_2-globulin in the plasma, and releases a decapeptide called *angiotensin I*. This is further converted to *angiotensin II*, an octapeptide, by a plasma converting enzyme; angiotensin II is a highly active pressor substance, causing arteriolar constriction and also stimulating the release of noradrenaline from sympathetic nerve endings and the adrenal medulla. Angiotensin II is converted to a hexapeptide, *angiotensin III*, and finally degraded by angiotensinase to amino acids and small peptides. The release of renin and angiotensins forms the basis of hypertension secondary to renal disease (Figure 5.20). Angiotensins II and III inhibit the release of renin in a negative feedback loop.

Renin and angiotensin are also closely involved in the regulation of body sodium and water content. A fall in plasma sodium level or in plasma volume, as in sodium deprivation, dehydration or blood loss, also stimulates the release of renin and production of angiotensins. The latter, and in particular angiotensin III, cause the secretion of *aldosterone* by the zona glomerulosa of the adrenal cortex, and this hormone increases the readsorption of sodium from the distal tubules. Water is retained with sodium, but potassium is lost in exchange. If the production of aldosterone is excessive, there will be pathological over-retention of sodium and water and an expansion of the blood volume. This can also raise the arterial pressure, through the increase in cardiac output. Such events are seen in the hypertension which accompanies *Conn's syndrome* (primary aldosteronism), where a tumour (adenoma) of the adrenal cortex secretes a high level of aldosterone. The renin level is low in this form of hypertension, which is caused mainly by the excessive plasma volume rather than by peripheral resistance. In kidney disease, as we have noted above, renin is

Figure 5.20 The renin-angiotensin-aldosterone system in the regulation of arterial pressure.

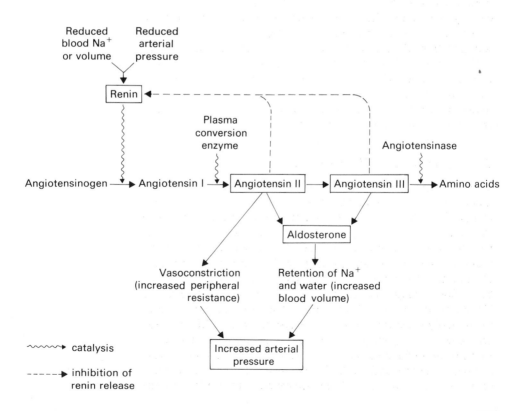

produced in excess from the juxta-glomerular apparatus; this in turn leads to a condition of secondary aldosteronism with sodium and water retention. Hence renal hypertension is the result of both increased peripheral resistance (due to angiotensin) and increased blood volume (due to aldosterone), as illustrated in Figure 5.20. Later on, changes in blood vessels, such as intimal thickening or fibrinoid necrosis, lead to a permanent rise in peripheral resistance and arterial pressure.

The kallikrein-kinin-prostaglandin system

Besides its ability to increase arterial pressure by releasing renin, the kidney also exerts a counterbalancing antihypertensive effect to antagonise the activities of the angiotensins and aldosterone. The renin-angiotensin system is opposed in the kidney by the kallikrein-kinin system which acts in conjunction with a prostaglandin (PGE_2) to produce intra-renal vasodilatation and increased excretion of sodium and water. The kallikrein-kinin system therefore leads to *lower* arterial pressure, while the renin-angiotensin system raises it. The ramifications of the effects of kallikrein, kinins and prostaglandins on salt and water balance and on blood pressure are complex and still being worked out. Their relevance to hypertension has been indicated by the finding that some patients with essential hypertension excrete less kallikrein in their urine than normal. Urinary kallikrein reflects the production of this enzyme in the kidney, so these observations suggest that a reduced secretion of renal kallikrein may be involved in the development of hypertension.

Kallikrein will be familiar from Section 1 as the plasma enzyme which produces bradykinin from a plasma precursor, bradykininogen; bradykinin is an important mediator of acute inflammation, causing vasodilatation, increased vascular permeability and pain. In the kidney, a related kinin, kallidin (lysyl-bradykinin) is also produced, a decapeptide with the same properties as bradykinin itself. Kallikrein is stored in the kidney in its precursor form, prekallikrein, probably in the juxta-glomerular apparatus, the same location as renin. The chief stimuli to kallikrein release are an increase in blood volume or arterial pressure and, significantly, both angiotensin and aldosterone. Kinins will then be formed by the action of kallikrein on kininogen. The kinins dilate renal blood vessels and thereby increase the flow of blood through the kidney; one result of this may be to curtail the release of renin and hence prevent an excessive rise in arterial pressure. Secondly, kinins increase the excretion of water, though their effect on sodium excretion is variable. This will counter the tendency to hypertension due to an increased blood volume, as in aldosteronism. Indeed, aldosterone itself is a potent stimulator of the kallikrein-kinin system, and Conn's syndrome (primary aldosteronism) is one instance where the hypertension is accompanied by a rise in urinary kallikrein, in contrast to the fall in essential hypertension. The main role of the kallikrein-kinin system is thus to protect the kidney from the vasoconstrictive effects of angiotensin and to balance the effects of angiotensins and aldosterone on arterial pressure and blood volume (Figure 5.21).

The vasodilatation and increased water excretion which are the main results of renal kinin activity are amplified and mediated by prostaglandins (Figure 5.21). The main prostaglandin in the kidney is PGE_2, and it is known to be produced in response to angiotensin. It appears that renal production of PGE_2 is dependent on bradykinin and kallidin; these activate the enzyme phospholipase, which in turn catalyses production of arachidonic acid, the prostaglandin precursor (Figure 5.22, see also p. 34). PGE_2 enhances the vasodilatation brought about by bradykinin, besides causing vasodilatation in its own right; it is responsible for about 30% of the renal vasodilatation produced by kinins. Moreover, the kinin-stimulated excretion of water is mediated by PGE_2. The control of production of PGE_2 may be achieved by channelling prostaglandin synthesis into another end-product, $PGF_{2\alpha}$ rather than PGE_2; $PGF_{2\alpha}$ lacks the effects of PGE_2 on vasodilatation and excretion. The proportions of these prostaglandins which are produced may be regulated by kinins themselves (Figure 5.22). Another important point for the control of the system is that both kinins and prostaglandins are rapidly inactivated, the former by kininases, and will thus only exert an effect locally within the kidney itself. However, although bradykinin and PGE_2 are unlikely to be released from the kidney to act as circulating hormones, PGE_2 can be produced by the walls of some arteries in response to angiotensin, noradrenaline and sympathetic stimulation and can counter the vasoconstrictive action of these stimuli in certain parts of the circulation. Prostaglandins are therefore likely to be of widespread importance in the regulation of blood pressure.

Figure 5.21 The kallikrein-kinin-prostaglandin system in the regulation of arterial pressure.

The pathological significance of the kallikrein-kinin-prostaglandin system is that, since it is in large measure responsible for the antihypertensive action of the kidney, a defect in it could lead

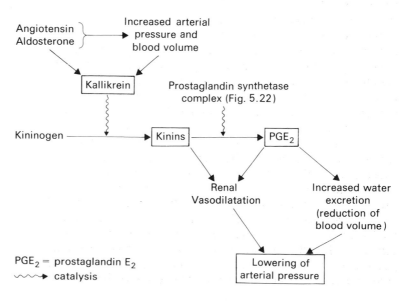

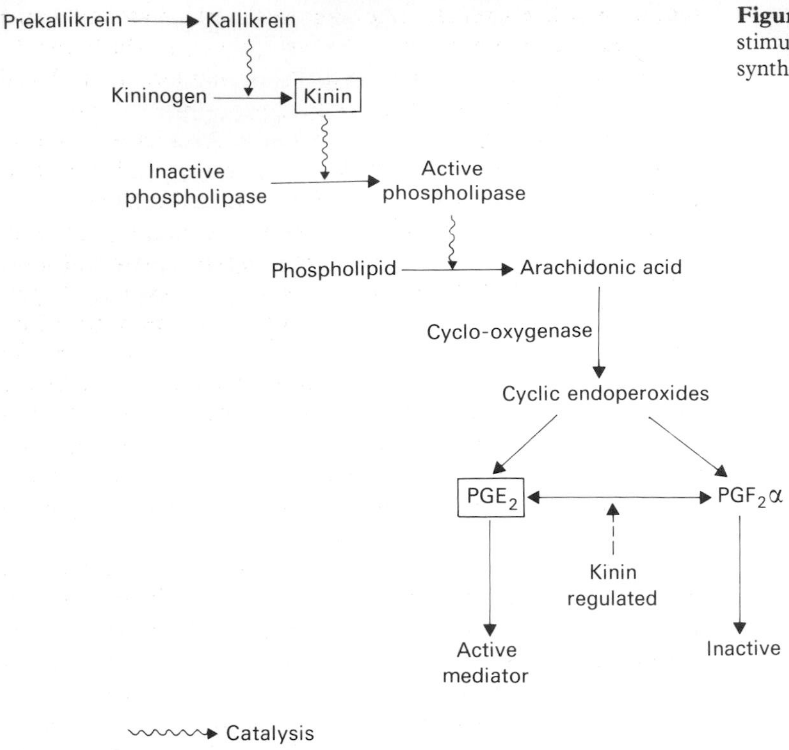

Prekallikrein ⟶ Kallikrein

Kininogen ⟶ | Kinin |

Inactive phospholipase ⟶ Active phospholipase

Phospholipid ⟶ Arachidonic acid

Cyclo-oxygenase

Cyclic endoperoxides

| PGE_2 | ⟷ | $PGF_2\alpha$

Kinin regulated

Active mediator   Inactive

∿∿∿⟶ Catalysis

Figure 5.22 Pathway of stimulation of prostaglandin synthesis by kinin.

to hypertension. The urinary kallikrein concentration reflects the level of production of the enzyme by the kidney and has been found to be reduced by about 50% in patients with moderate to severe essential hypertension compared with normal controls. Furthermore, an inhibitor of prostaglandin synthesis, indomethacin, can raise the blood pressure experimentally in the anaesthetised dog and rabbit (though there is no evidence that aspirin, another inhibitor, raises arterial pressure in man). Hence it is possible that a deficiency in the kallikrein-kinin system plays a part in the development of hypertension by decreasing the production of PGE_2 and hence reducing the antihypertensive effect of the kidney. Moreover, a low renal kallikrein activity could be an inherited characteristic which may be important in the genetic predisposition to hypertension (below).

Aetiology of hypertension

It is often easy to understand the development of secondary hypertension, especially where there is a demonstrable excess in the circulation of active substances, as in phaeochromocytoma (adrenaline, noradrenaline), Conn's syndrome (aldosterone) or Cushing's syndrome (cortisol). However, the basis of essential hypertension remains difficult to explain satisfactorily, especially since there are several possible different pathways by which arterial pressure could be permanently raised. Serum levels of renin, vasoactive amines, aldosterone and cortisol are sometimes increased, but there are no consistent changes which can be demonstrated in all or most patients. The renin level in the blood of hypertensive patients has been studied carefully and while about 15% have high plasma renin levels, 25% have low renin activity, while the remaining 60% have normal renin levels. This heterogeneity among patients is relevant to the progress of the disease and its treatment. Thus, patients with high plasma renin have the highest risk of cardiovascular disease, stroke and renal failure, while this tendency is reversed with low-renin hypertension. In the former group, hypertension is the result of increased peripheral resistance and treatment is often successful with propanolol, a β-adrenergic blocking agent which blocks adrenaline-like affects on the heart and blood vessels and interferes with renin production. The low-renin group of patients, on the other hand, have an expanded plasma volume and respond well to diuretics, such as the aldosterone antagonist spironolactone.

There is an inherited component in hypertensive disease, as shown by the increased tendency to hypertension in close relatives of hypertensive patients. However, the inheritance is generally multifactorial, with contributions from several genes as well as from environmental factors. A possible genetic determination of renal kallikrein levels has already been mentioned (p. 680). According to Pickering, an individual's tendency to have a raised arterial pressure is inherited, but the rate of rise of arterial pressure with age is determined by the environment. Blood pressure is constantly being affected by external factors and is increased by stress, fear, anger, pain, exercise, coitus, etc. It could be envisaged that if environmental stimuli such as these are repeated over a long period of time, gradual structural changes in the arteries and arterioles may develop; particular emphasis has been laid on hypertrophy of the media in this respect. Such changes, which also include intimal thickening (fibrosis), result in permanent narrowing of the vessels, increase in peripheral resistance and hence raised arterial pressure. The development of hyaline thickening of the renal arterioles could lead to renin release and high-renin hypertension. For hypertensive patients with a normal or low renin but a raised blood volume, a decreased capacity of the kidney to excrete sodium or an increased aldosterone or reduced kallikrein level are possible underlying causes of increased arterial pressure.

OEDEMA

Oedema is the excessive accumulation of fluid in tissues leading to swelling. It may be a *local* event resulting from an inbalance in factors which govern the amount of fluid in a particular tissue; or it may be *generalised* (widespread) and involve an abnormal retention of water in the body as a whole and a resultant increase in body weight. Renal function plays an important role in the development of generalised oedema.

Terminology

Special terms are used for oedema in body cavities, namely *ascites* for oedema in the peritoneal cavity, *hydrothorax* in the pleural cavity and *hydropericardium* in the pericardial cavity. Generalised oedema is called *anasarca*. Oedema in tissues can be recognised by 'pitting'—when an oedematous area is pressed firmly for a few moments an indentation or pit forms which is slow to disappear, hence the term *pitting oedema*.

Formation of oedema

One example of oedema, namely *inflammatory exudation*, has already been described (Section 1) and it will be recalled that the factors which determine the exchange of fluid between the blood and the tissues are described by Starling's hypothesis (Figure 5.23 and p. 5). These factors include (a) the difference in hydrostatic pressure between the blood and the interstitial fluid, which tends to force fluid from the blood into the tissue, and (b) the osmotic pressure exerted by the plasma proteins, which draws fluid back from the tissues into the blood. Of these opposing forces, the hydrostatic pressure is in excess at the arteriolar end of tissue capillary circulation, while at the venous end, where the hydrostatic pressure in the vessels is lower, the plasma osmotic pressure is the greater force. Hence a balance is set up between the blood and the tissue which determines the normal amount of extracellular fluid. An exact equilibrium between these forces does not exist, however, and the lymphatics have the important role of draining off excess fluid in the tissue as it forms. The local tissue tension also tends to resist excess fluid accumulation and, while the pressure involved is low (3–4 mm Hg), it does play an important part in determining the areas in which oedema is particularly likely to occur. Thus, areas where tissue pressure is normally low such as the eyelids, external genitalia, ankles and over the sacrum, may be the first to show subcutaneous oedema.

Figure 5.23 Factors involved in development of oedema.
* Normal values ∿ 32 mm Hg at arterial end, ∿ 12 mm Hg at venous end (in skin at heart level).
† Normal value ∿ 25 mm Hg.

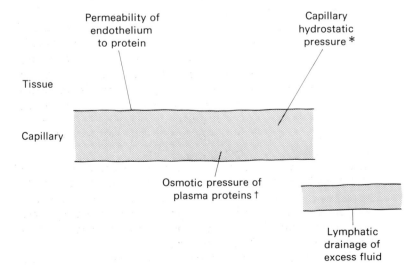

It is immediately apparent that any of the following events could disturb the tissue fluid balance and cause oedema (Figure 5.23).

1 An increase in the permeability of the capillary endothelium. The endothelium normally behaves as a semipermeable membrane, allowing water and low molecular weight solutes to pass through, but preventing molecules larger than a molecular weight of about 10,000 from leaving the plasma. This leads to the importance of plasma proteins in exerting their osmotic force across the capillary wall. If the endothelium becomes permeable to protein, the osmotic pressures of the plasma proteins and of the tissue fluid are equalised and there is therefore no tendency for fluid to return to the circulation. Permeability is increased under the influence of inflammatory mediators in acute inflammation (Section 1) and immediate type hypersensitivity (p. 153). It is also increased by hypoxia of the vessel wall, an important factor in pulmonary oedema (p. 685). The oedema fluid which forms as a result of increased permeability is a protein-rich *exudate* of essentially the same composition as plasma.

2 An increased venous and hence capillary hydrostatic pressure will reduce the effectiveness of the osmotic pressure of the plasma proteins. As a result excess fluid will collect in the tissue despite normal vascular permeability; such an oedema fluid is termed a *transudate*. Postural oedema, which forms in the ankles, feet and legs on standing for long periods is an example, and venous obstruction due to thrombophlebitis or in pregnancy has the same effect. Cirrhosis of the liver leads to ascites due in part to increased pressure in the portal veins as a result of fibrosis in the liver.

3 Lymphatic obstruction prevents drainage of tissue fluid and as a result a transudate accumulates. A well known example is the extensive swelling of the legs and external genitalia known as *elephantiasis* which occurs in the tropical disease filariasis. This is caused by the parasitic nematode worms *Wuchereria bancrofti* which live in the lymphatics of the groin and block them when they die. Much of the oedema is in fact caused by secondary infection and inflammation, with subsequent fibrosis and induration.

4 A fall in plasma protein level reduces the osmotic pressure of the blood and may, therefore, result in a generalised oedema. It can be due to the excessive loss of protein associated with kidney disease, as in the heavy proteinuria of the nephrotic syndrome; to reduced protein synthesis by the liver in cirrhosis; or to inadequate dietary protein intake, which plays a role in *famine or nutritional oedema*. In the latter, prolonged starvation or malnutrition causes oedema of the legs, ankles and feet and sometimes ascites. However, the plasma protein levels are not necessarily the main component in famine oedema, since studies on volunteers have shown that oedema can occur in starvation without a fall in plasma protein level. An important factor is the loss of compact tissue, mainly body fat, and its replacement by loose connective tissue. This exerts a lower tissue tension and as a result takes up more fluid than normal.

5 The overall regulation of total body water, especially the

degree to which the kidneys retain sodium chloride and water, plays an important part in most generalised oedema.

Generalised oedema: cardiac oedema

Oedema is thus clearly multifactorial. Although the principles expressed in the Starling theory provide a satisfyingly logical explanation in many cases, it is important to remember that the causes of oedema are frequently complex and sometimes quite speculative. This is especially true of the generalised oedemas, of which the most important example is the oedema of congestive heart failure, *cardiac oedema*. This ensues when the heart fails as a whole, i.e. there is combined left- and right-sided failure. In this situation there is a general retention of fluid in the body, indicated by an increase in body weight and caused by the retention of sodium and water by the kidney. The distribution of the oedema is influenced by gravity—pitting oedema of the ankles and legs if the patient is ambulatory, of the sacral and genital areas if recumbent. Familiar though the condition is, it has been interpreted in different ways. According to one of the classical views of heart failure, cardiac oedema can be thought of as resulting from increased venous back-pressure, due to failure of the heart to deal with the normal venous inflow. The alternative classical hypothesis is that of forward-failure, in which there is insufficient blood supply to the tissues as a result of poor cardiac output; oedema would then result from stagnant hypoxia of the vascular endothelium. Neither of these approaches provides a convincing or complete explanation. The back-pressure theory attributes tissue oedema to the rise in central venous pressure; as a consequence there should be a fall in plasma volume, followed by compensatory retention of salt and water by the kidneys. The actual events, however, seem to be almost a reversal of this picture. There is usually an increase, rather than a decrease, in plasma volume on heart failure, and although there is a rise in venous pressure the extent of the oedema is not always related to it. However, while increased central venous pressure must play some part in the oedema, stagnant hypoxia in the capillaries probably does not, since the oedema fluid is a typical low-protein transudate with no indication of increased vascular permeability.

The failing of these hypotheses is that they underestimate the important role of renal function in generalised oedema via its regulation of blood volume. In congestive heart failure, the kidneys retain more sodium and as a result more water than normal. This is principally the result of renal vasoconstriction, which occurs in congestive heart failure as a result of sympathetic stimulation and which reduces the renal blood flow and glomerular filtration rate. The kidneys respond by releasing renin from the juxta-glomerular apparatus, production of angiotensin and aldosterone occurs (p. 676) and the latter causes heightened readsorption of sodium from the distal tubules. The fall in glomerular filtration rate also allows a more complete readsorption of sodium than normal. Hence under these conditions of reduced renal blood flow, increased retention of sodium occurs and, since sodium cannot be retained without water, of water also. The effectiveness of a reduced sodium intake, in the form of a salt-free diet, and of diuretics in preventing oedema in heart failure, support the view that the retention of sodium and water is the major factor predisposing to cardiac oedema. The resulting increase in the extracellular fluid compartment creates the circumstances favourable for oedema, which can then be precipitated locally by other conditions, such as increased venous pressure.

Not surprisingly, kidney disease itself is also associated with generalised oedema (*renal oedema*). In acute glomerulonephritis, there is fluid retention and a raised blood volume, while in the nephrotic syndrome the main factor is the characteristic massive proteinuria, which results in a lowered plasma osmotic pressure.

Pulmonary oedema

While congestive heart failure causes generalised oedema, left ventricular failure is particularly associated with *pulmonary oedema*, which is frequently rapidly fatal. In an acute paroxysmal attack, the lungs fill with a pink, frothy fluid which, spreading rapidly even up to the nose and mouth, may asphyxiate the patient in a matter of minutes. Pulmonary oedema is not necessarily fatal, however, and if the acute stage is survived, pulmonary lymphatics rapidly drain away the excess fluid. Alternatively it may run a more prolonged course, lasting for some hours or even days, and the protein-rich oedema fluid may then become infected and lead to bronchopneumonia. The rapid development and spread of oedema in the lungs is caused by certain features peculiar to the pulmonary capillaries and lung structure. The key features are (a) that the endothelium of the lung capillaries normally receives its oxygen directly from the alveolar air and not from the venous blood, and (b) that the alveoli are usually kept 'dry' because the plasma osmotic pressure is at all points in the lungs greater than the capillary hydrostatic pressure. As soon as fluid begins to accumulate in the alveoli, for whatever initial reason, the capillaries become hypoxic and their permeability to protein increases; a vicious circle is rapidly established in which the more fluid collects the more permeable the capillaries become. Since there is no tissue pressure to resist its advance, the oedema spreads rapidly through the lung via the interalveolar pores and the alveolar ducts. What is the immediate initiating cause of formation of the oedema? In left ventricular failure it is largely the increased back-pressure in the pulmonary circulation which results when the left ventricle fails to expel all the blood it receives—the raised pulmonary capillary pressure causes the initial transudation and the vicious circle commences. Adrenaline has a potentiating effect by diverting blood volume from the systemic to the pulmonary circulation as a result of systemic vasoconstriction. The fear and anxiety which inevitably occur during an attack of pulmonary oedema thus encourage its continuation. Neurogenic factors are certainly important, as shown by the favourable effects of general cerebral depressants such as morphine and anaesthetics. It should be noted that pulmonary oedema is a *local* redistribution of fluid which occurs before the generalised fluid retention of heart failure.

Apart from left ventricular failure, the most important practical cause of pulmonary oedema is failure to expand part of the lung, as may occur in the bed-ridden. It is also an important complication of influenza. Pulmonary oedema predisposes to lung infection with bacteria, a complication which contributed to the millions of fatalities in the great influenza pandemic of 1918 (p. 324).

FURTHER READING

General

Hardisty R.M. & Weatherall D.J. (1982) *Blood and its Disorders*, 2nd edn. Blackwell Scientific Publications.
Hughes-Jones N.C. (1979) *Lecture Notes on Haematology*, 3rd. edn. Blackwell Scientific Publications.

Specific topics

Atherogenesis. *Annals N.Y. Acad. Sci.* (1976), **275**.
Barnett H.J.M., Hirsch J. & Mustard J.F. (1982) *Acetylsalicylic acid: new uses for an old drug*. Raven Press.
Benditt E.P. & Benditt J.M. (1973) Evidence for a monoclonal origin of human atherosclerotic plaques. *Proc. Nat. Acad. Sci.* **70**, 1753.
Brown M.S., Kovanen P.T. & Goldstein J.L. (1981) Regulation of plasma cholesterol by lipoprotein receptors. *Science*, **212**, 628.
Dawber T.R. (1980) *The Framingham Study: The Epidemiology of Atherosclerosis*. Harvard University Press.
Duguid J.B. (1976) *The Dynamics of Atherosclerosis*. Aberdeen University Press.
Gordon J.L. (ed.) (1976) *Platelets in Biology and Pathology*. North Holland.
Gordon J.L. (ed.) (1981) *Platelets in Biology and Pathology–2*. Elsevier/North Holland.
Gotto A.M.Jr. & Paoletti R. (eds.) *Atherosclerosis Reviews*, vols 1–11.
Gotto A.M.Jr., *et al.* (1977) *Atherosclerosis*. A Scope publication, The Upjohn Company.
Gresham G.A. (1976) Primate atherosclerosis. *Monographs on Atherosclerosis*, vol. 7.
Gresham G.A. (1980) *Reversing Atherosclerosis*. Charles C. Thomas.
Haemostasis. *British Medical Bulletin* (1977), **33**, no. 3.
Hallam J., Goldman L. & Fryers G.R. (eds.) (1981). *Aspirin symposium 1980*. Royal Society of Medicine and Academic Press.
Hirsch J. & Brain E.A. (1979) *Haemostasis and Thrombosis. A Conceptual Approach*. Churchill Livingstone.
Kinins, renal function and blood pressure regulation. *Federation Proceedings* (1976), **35**, no. 2.
Mollison P.L. (1983) *Blood Transfusion in Clinical Medicine*, 7th edn. Blackwell Scientific Publications.
Pickering G (1974) *Hypertension: Causes, Consequences and Management*, 2nd edn. Churchill Livingstone.
Ross R.R. & Glomset J.A. (1976) *The pathogenesis of atherosclerosis. New Engl. J. Med.*, **269**, 396, 420.
Swales J.D. (1979) *Clinical Hypertension*. Chapman and Hall.

Thomson J.M. (1980) *Blood Coagulation and Haemostasis: A Practical Guide*. Churchill Livingstone.

Thrombosis. *British Medical Bulletin* (1978), **34**, no. 2.

Weiss H.J. (1975) *Platelet physiology and abnormalities of platelet function*. *New Engl. J. Med.*, **293**, 531, 580.

Introduction

Neoplasia (lit. new growth) is a disorder of cell proliferation which, in its malignant form (*cancer*), is second only to cardiovascular disease as a cause of human mortality. Since neoplastic change can arise in the cells of most tissues, neoplasia assumes a great diversity of clinical forms. However, all neoplastic cells share the fundamental aberration of *loss of growth control*. One of the major tasks of medical research is to discover the causes of this cellular abnormality. In this section, we shall be concerned principally with present understanding of the cellular nature of neoplasia, with its known causes as revealed both by epidemiology and experiment, and with the possible pathways to neoplastic change. Some of the theories of neoplasia are discussed, though at present no single theory provides a wholly satisfactory explanation for this most complex of disorders.

Definitions

A *neoplasm* or new growth is the result of an irreversible and inheritable change in a somatic cell or cells leading to their uncontrolled proliferation. This often results in a swelling or *tumour* and although all neoplasms do not result in a tumour (and all swellings are not neoplasms), 'tumour' is commonly used as a synonym for 'neoplasm'. The growth of a neoplasm, while it may be checked by factors such as the need for an adequate blood supply or by attack from the host immune system, is not affected by the regulatory processes which determine the size of normal tissues. A tumour is thus fundamentally different from other examples of pathological proliferation, such as granulomatous inflammation, wound healing or hyperplasia (p. 695), which are all limited by tissue regulatory mechanisms. There are two main groups of neoplasms, divided according to their behavioural characteristics, namely benign and malignant. A *benign neoplasm* is one which remains localised and does not invade the tissue in which it grows or spread through the host; it does not normally cause serious damage to the host, except as a result of a critical positioning or function. In contrast, a *malignant neoplasm* invades and destroys host tissue and spreads throughout the body; it is invariably fatal if unchecked by removal or treatment. The terms *cancer* and *malignancy* are commonly used as synonyms for malignant neoplasm.

CLASSIFICATION OF NEOPLASMS

It is usual to classify neoplasms (i) according to the cell type from which they originate, with a major subdivision into those derived from epithelial tissue and those from connective tissue (mesenchyme), and (ii) according to biological behaviour, that is whether they are benign or malignant. Such a classification is given in Table 6.1. Note that the suffix '-oma' is used to indicate a tumour (it is also used for some non-neoplastic swellings, such as granuloma or haematoma) while the tissue or cell of origin appears as a prefix.

691

Table 6.1. Simple classification of neoplasms.

Tissue of origin	Behaviour	
	Benign	Malignant
Epithelium		Carcinoma
1 Squamous	Squamous cell papilloma	Squamous cell carcinoma
2 Basal cell	Basal cell papilloma	Basal cell carcinoma
3 Transitional	Transitional cell papilloma	Transitional cell carcinoma
4 Glandular	Adenoma	Adenocarcinoma
	Cystadenoma	Cystadenocarcinoma
Pigment cells (melanocytes)	Naevus cell naevus (benign melanoma)	Malignant melanoma
Neural tissue		
1 Nerve sheath	Neurilemmoma	Neurofibrosarcoma
2 Glial tissue	Glioma	Malignant glioma
3 Nerve cells		Neuroblastoma
Connective tissue		Sarcoma
1 Fibrous	Fibroma	Fibrosarcoma
2 Fatty	Lipoma	Liposarcoma
3 Cartilage	Chondroma	Chondrosarcoma
4 Bone	Osteoma	Osteosarcoma
5 Muscle	Myoma	Myosarcoma
(a) Smooth muscle	Leiomyoma	Leiomyosarcoma
(b) Striated muscle	Rhabdomyoma	Rhabdomyosarcoma
6 Vessels	Angioma	Angiosarcoma
(a) Blood	Haemangioma	Haemangiosarcoma
(b) Lymphatic	Lymphangioma	Lymphangiosarcoma
7 Meninges	Meningioma	Malignant meningioma
Lymphoreticular and haematopoietic tissue		
1 Lymphoreticular		Malignant lymphoma
		Lymphocytic leukaemia
		Plasmacytoma (multiple myeloma)
		Reticulum cell sarcoma
		Hodgkin's disease
2 Haematopoietic (bone marrow)		Granulocytic leukaemia
		Monocytic leukaemia
Embryonic tissue		
Multipotential cells in ovary, testis or embryonic rests.	Benign teratoma, dermoid	Malignant teratoma, teratocarcinoma
Trophoblast	Hydatid mole	Choriocarcinoma

1 Benign tumours originating from squamous, transitional or basal cell types of epithelium are called *papillomas*, while those from glandular epithelium are termed *adenomas*. Pedunculated papillomas and adenomas are loosely referred to as *polyps*, a term applied to any pedunculated mass attached to a surface, not necessarily neoplastic. Malignant epithelial tumours are called *carcinomas* and for surface epithelium are classified as squamous cell, basal cell and transitional cell carcinomas. Those derived from glandular epithelium are called adenocarcinomas.

2 Benign growths of connective tissue are named according to cell type, e.g. fibroma, lipoma, osteoma, and so on. Malignancies of connective tissue origin are termed *sarcomas*, thus fibrosarcoma, liposarcoma, osteosarcoma, and so on. The sarcomas of the tissues producing white blood cells are classified separately because of their distinctive biological behaviour, in particular the occurrence of abnormal leucocytes in the blood in large numbers. The latter condition is *leukaemia* and is divided into *granulocytic, monocytic* and *lymphocytic* according to the groups of cells involved (Table 6.1). Although the connective tissues exceed epithelium in mass by about five-fold, carcinomas are about ten times more frequent than sarcomas.

3 Some tumours are composed of more than one histological cell type and are described as *mixed*. Some of these arise in immature embryonal tissues in infants and are highly malignant, such as nephroblastoma of the kidney (Wilms' tumour) which consists of both sarcomatous and tubular structures and may contain bone, cartilage and striated muscle fibres. The most extreme examples of mixed tumours are the *teratomas*, which arise in multipotential cells (i.e. cells which can differentiate into a variety of tissues), mainly in the gonads. Ovarian teratomas (also known as *dermoids*) are common and are usually benign and cystic, while testicular teratomas tend to be malignant and solid. Teratomas contain a great variety of tissues in haphazard arrangement, including cartilage, bone, epidermis, glandular epithelium, hair, teeth and even representation of liver, kidney, nervous and haematopoietic tissue. The development of teratomas from germ cells can be likened to parthenogenesis.

4 *Hamartoma* is a term used for tumour-like malformations which are not truly neoplastic, but in which there is a relative overgrowth of part of a tissue with a disorderly structural arrangement. Common examples are of vascular origin, also called haemangiomas, which include the *vascular naevus* of the skin (a red or purple mole or birthmark). This consists of a closely packed arrangement of capillaries containing blood. The naevus is usually small, but can sometimes form large, flat, red-blue areas on the face or upper part of the body called 'port-wine stains'. Vascular naevi are present at birth and grow with the body, but unlike a true neoplasm growth is coordinated with the rest of the tissue and usually stops after childhood. Another common hamartoma is the familiar *pigmented naevus* or benign melanoma, which varies in colour from brown to black. This type of birthmark consists of clusters of melanocytes containing the black pigment melanin. Unlike the vascular naevus, the pigmented

naevus has a slight tendency towards malignant change, and increased size or pigmentation of such a mole in an adult may indicate this (malignant melanoma arises *de novo* in most cases).

Benign and malignant tumours

Some of the important differences between benign and malignant tumours are summarised in Table 6.2. Benign tumours are slow growing (few mitoses) and, while they expand in size, they do not invade or destroy the tissue in which they grow. As a result, they are often sharply demarcated and, with the exception of papillomas, are usually encapsulated within a wall of connective tissue. Benign tumours are 'organised', in that the architecture of the parent tissue is largely retained in the tumour, and the tumour cells resemble those of the tissue of origin, i.e. are well differentiated.

In contrast, malignant tumours grow rapidly and invasively, with destruction of neighbouring tissue, often developing the claw-like extensions which gave rise to the term 'cancer' (Lat. crab). Hence malignancies have an irregular shape with ill-defined borders, due to their invasion of surrounding tissue. Unlike the normal tissue, the cells of malignant tumours are an extremely heterogeneous population in terms of their morphology, nuclear size and staining properties (*pleomorphism*). The type of cell may also vary from one part of the tumour to another, as may the type and degree of differentiation. Numerous mitoses are evident, but these are frequently abnormal, with chromosome breaks or dispersal; the chromosome numbers in individual cells show marked variation. The nucleus occupies an abnormally large part of the cell. The cytoplasm of malignant cells is more basophilic than normal because of its increased RNA content. The degree of differentiation or specialisation of malignant tumours varies, but they are generally less organised and

Table 6.2. Comparison of benign and malignant neoplasms.

Benign	Malignant
Loss of growth control	Loss of growth control
Loss of feedback regulation by cell products	Loss of feedback regulation by cell products (if any)
Normal regulation of motility	Loss of regulation of motility
Mostly slow growth	Frequently rapid growth
Growth expansive, non-invasive, non-destructive	Growth invasive and destructive
Few mitoses	Many mitoses
Well differentiated; normal cells; resembles architecture of host tissue	Poorly differentiated; pleomorphic; abnormal cells; does not resemble tissue of origin
No metastases	Metastases
Rarely fatal; clinical consequences through over-secretion of hormones, or mechanical blockage or pressure	Invariably fatal if untreated; clinical consequences through destruction of tissues, anaemia, haemorrhage, secondary infection, etc.

differentiated than the normal tissue, and the extent to which the tumour has dedifferentiated parallels its malignancy and rate of cell division.

The most important characteristic of malignancy is the ability to *metastasise*, i.e. for tumour cells to be carried in the lymphatics or the blood to other tissues and there establish further (secondary) growths of the tumour. Metastasis is the most dangerous feature of cancer and in most cases the one responsible for its fatal consequences. The possible harmful effects of benign tumours should not be overlooked, however. Serious mechanical blockages can be caused by histologically benign tumours growing in the respiratory, gastrointestinal or urinary tracts, and a 'benign' brain tumour carries obvious dangers. Adenomas of endocrine glands cause serious disturbances by excessive production of hormones, such as tumours of the adrenal medulla which produce adrenaline and noradrenaline (phaeochromocytoma, p. 676), or of the adrenal cortex which secrete steroid hormones (Conn's syndrome, p. 677, Cushing's syndrome, adrenogenital syndrome, p. 848). However, benign tumours *never* metastasise; they are therefore rarely fatal and generally curable by surgical removal. The structures of some representative neoplasms are shown in Figure 6.1.

Carcinoma *in situ*

From the point of view of cancer treatment, it is especially important that there exists a recognisable pre-invasive stage for certain malignancies. The carcinoma *in situ* is such a lesion, in which the histology and cytology are those of a carcinoma, yet no invasion of neighbouring tissue has taken place and the basement membrane is still intact. This lesion occurs in the uterine cervix, epidermis, lung, prostate and breast. In the *uterine cervix* it may persist for some years before ultimately becoming invasive. Thus, it is practicable to screen for carcinoma *in situ* and take advantage of the delayed invasiveness by prompt treatment. The taking of a cervical smear should be part of the routine physical examination for every woman. Papanicolaou (1942) introduced this exfoliative cytology for diagnosis of cancer of mucous membranes, cells being removed by scraping the membrane and examined, after staining, for abnormal cytology ('Pap smear' test). Carcinoma cells are recognised by their irregular size, increased basophilic staining of the cytoplasm, pronounced nuclear polymorphism, increase in the ratio of size of nucleus to cytoplasm and numerous, sometimes atypical mitoses. If discovered at the carcinoma *in situ* stage, cervical cancer is cured by surgical removal, such as simple hysterectomy.

Neoplasia and hyperplasia

It is useful to compare the unrestricted growth of tumour cells with another pathological cellular overgrowth, *hyperplasia*. This often occurs when a tissue has been damaged and regeneration is

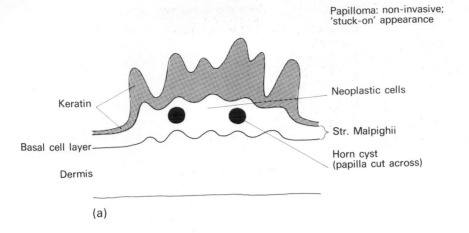

Papilloma: non-invasive; 'stuck-on' appearance

Keratin

Neoplastic cells

Basal cell layer

Str. Malpighii

Dermis

Horn cyst (papilla cut across)

(a)

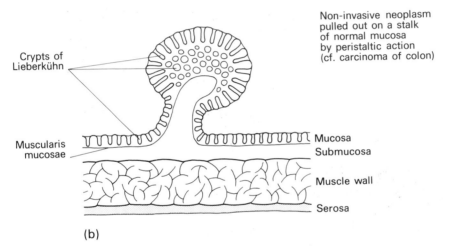

Crypts of Lieberkühn

Non-invasive neoplasm pulled out on a stalk of normal mucosa by peristaltic action (cf. carcinoma of colon)

Muscularis mucosae

Mucosa
Submucosa

Muscle wall

Serosa

(b)

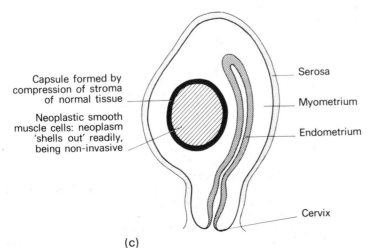

Capsule formed by compression of stroma of normal tissue

Neoplastic smooth muscle cells: neoplasm 'shells out' readily, being non-invasive

Serosa

Myometrium

Endometrium

Cervix

(c)

Figure 6.1 *and on facing page.* Some benign and malignant neoplasms.
Benign
(a) Basal cell papilloma of the skin.
(b) Adenomatous polyp of the intestine.
(c) Leiomyoma of the uterus.
Malignant
(d) Carcinoma of the skin.
(e) Carcinoma of the breast. The carcinoma-bearing breast is smaller than that on the other side although it contains a tumour.
(f) Carcinoma of the colon without fibrotic stromal reaction.
(g) Carcinoma of the colon with fibrotic stromal reaction (different scale).

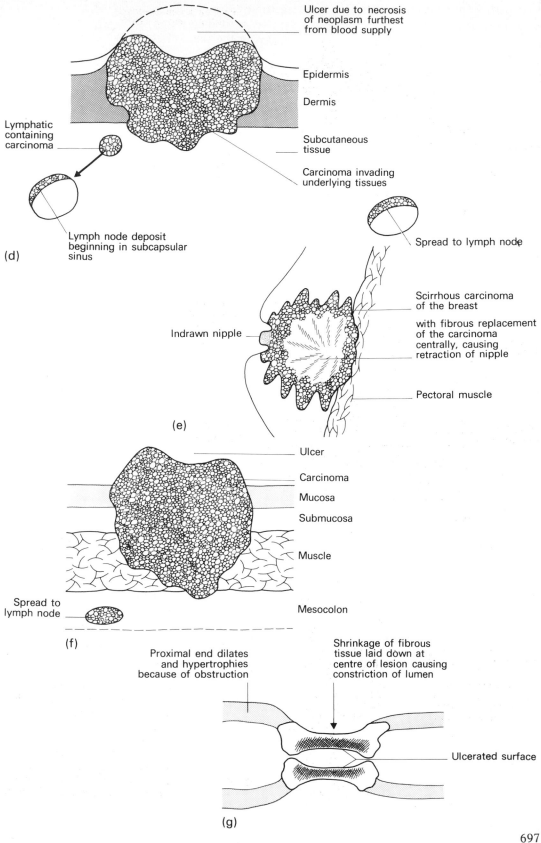

(d)

Ulcer due to necrosis of neoplasm furthest from blood supply

Epidermis

Dermis

Subcutaneous tissue

Carcinoma invading underlying tissues

Lymphatic containing carcinoma

Lymph node deposit beginning in subcapsular sinus

(e)

Spread to lymph node

Scirrhous carcinoma of the breast

with fibrous replacement of the carcinoma centrally, causing retraction of nipple

Indrawn nipple

Pectoral muscle

(f)

Ulcer

Carcinoma

Mucosa

Submucosa

Muscle

Mesocolon

Spread to lymph node

(g)

Proximal end dilates and hypertrophies because of obstruction

Shrinkage of fibrous tissue laid down at centre of lesion causing constriction of lumen

Ulcerated surface

stimulated in order to replace lost cells. If the regenerative process overshoots and the mass of the tissue is increased beyond its normal level, hyperplasia results. This can be seen in the skin epithelium, e.g. during wound healing or as the familiar thickening which follows persistent mechanical stimulation. Hyperplasia is also caused by prolonged, excessive hormonal stimulation; thus, increased secretion of pituitary adrenocortico-trophic hormone (ACTH) causes both an increased production of adrenal cortical hormones and stimulates cell proliferation in the cortex which becomes enlarged. The essential differences between these instances of hyperplasia and neoplastic growth are that hyperplasia is a reversible proliferation which ceases when the stimulus to it is removed, and that although hyperplastic proliferation is greater than the normal it is still strictly under control. In contrast, neoplastic proliferation is a permanent feature of the abnormal tumour cells and is essentially unlimited—in certain situations the size of a tumour may even come to exceed that of the normal animal!

EPIDEMIOLOGY OF CANCER

Statistical measurements of the frequency of cancer within and between populations are an important part of the study of the disease and have produced much information on its possible causes. The two measures of frequency most commonly employed are mortality and incidence. *Mortality* is the annual rate of death attributed to cancer, while *incidence* is the frequency of new cases arising in the population. As a cause of death, cancer is second only to heart disease in the developed world and moreover is showing an increasing incidence. To some extent this is due to the longevity enjoyed by the population in a period when fatal infectious diseases have been largely eradicated and to more refined diagnostic procedures now in use. Even when these points are taken into account, however, some cancers, such as cancer of the lung, show real increases. The rising frequency of cancer is presumably the result of our increased exposure to carcinogenic (cancer-causing) agents.

Within a population, the incidence of cancer varies widely with age, sex, site of origin and various environmental factors. The latter in particular provide valuable information on the aetiology of cancer. Further, there are sometimes wide variations when different populations are compared and this geographical dependence of certain cancers is similarly indicative of important causative factors in the environment.

Age

For most cancers, incidence in the population increases with age. Some, however, show peculiarly high incidence in childhood, notably acute leukaemia and tumours of the central nervous system. For this reason, the overall incidence of cancer is higher in the first five years of life than in the next two five-year periods. In the very aged, the chance of developing certain tumours approaches 100%, for example for carcinoma of the prostate in men, with a similar though rather less extreme situation for cancer of the stomach and lung in men and cancer of the breast in women.

Sex

Overall incidence

In childhood and over 60 years of age, males are more affected than females; between 30 and 60 years the overall incidence is generally higher in females, because of the rise in cervical and breast cancer during this period. However, mortality is higher in males in most age groups, because of their higher frequency of cancers of low curability (lung, stomach); the common cancers of women (breast, cervix) are more readily cured.

Sex and site of origin

The frequencies of some malignancies differ markedly in the two sexes. Thus cancers of the lung and oesophagus are considerably more frequent in males. For lung cancer, the ratio of males to females affected can be as high as 10:1. Stomach cancer and leukaemias are also more common in men, though rather less strikingly so. On the other hand, cancer of the breast, reproductive organs and thyroid are more often found in women. Other tumours are of equal occurrence in both sexes.

Environmental factors

A variety of factors in the environment influence the incidence of certain cancers, and some specific examples are described in detail later (p. 750). We can define the following broad categories of environmental influence.

Personal habits

One of the most important examples of an environmental contribution to cancer is the association of *lung cancer* with cigarette smoking. In several large-scale studies, the mortality from lung cancer has been shown to be over ten times greater in smokers than non-smokers and to be proportional to the number of cigarettes smoked and the number of years over which smoking has been practised. Smoking also leads to increased mortality from cancers of the larynx, oral cavity, oesophagus and bladder. (For further details, see p. 707.) Similarly, air pollution may account for the greater incidence of lung tumours among city dwellers than in the country. Sexual experience influences the incidence of certain cancers. *Cervical cancer* is associated with early sexual relations, an early age of marriage and frequent births, though with respect to the last point it seems that coitus rather than pregnancy is the important factor. Cervical cancer shows its lowest incidence among nuns, virgins and Jewish women. Among the Jews, the practice of circumcision may be one factor responsible for the low frequency of cervical cancer. *Breast cancer* shows the reverse correlation with sexual experience in that it is less frequent among multiparae than women without children. (A possible basis for the protective effect of pregnancy on breast cancer is described on p. 728.) Circumcision soon after birth is responsible for the low incidence of carcinoma of the penis among Jews. When carried out later in life, as at puberty in Moslems, circumcision has a very much smaller effect.

Diet

Differences in the incidence of cancers of the alimentary tract (oesophagus, stomach, colon) may be related to dietary components such as salt level, smoked foods and alcohol. Some pronounced geographical variations in frequencies of these tumours (p. 701) are likely to be the result of different dietary habits in different parts of the world. The association of stomach cancer with low economic status is also likely to be due to dietary factors.

Occupation

There are many examples of cancers which are hazards of particular occupations. The sites most frequently affected are the skin, respiratory tract and bladder, i.e. either the surface with which the cancer-inducing agent first makes contact (skin, respiratory epithelium) or that exposed to its active metabolites in urine (bladder). Among the early examples of occupational cancers were the classical observation of cancer of the scrotum in chimney sweep boys by Percival Pott in 1775, shale-oil cancer in workers in mineral oil distilleries, and the mule-spinner's cancer among workers in the Lancashire spinning mills where mineral oil was used. These are all examples of skin cancers produced by contact with polycyclic aromatic hydrocarbons, such as benzpyrene, during the course of work. *Bladder cancer* was a hazard of the early aniline- and azo-dye industries and is caused by aromatic amines (e.g. β-naphthylamine) and related substances. They are also responsible for bladder cancer among workers in the rubber industry and those involved in the manufacture of rubber-coated electric cables.

Occupational cancers can be caused by irradiation as well as by chemical carcinogens, illustrative examples being the skin cancer of the early radiologists, lung cancer among uranium miners and the 'dial-painter's' osteosarcoma. This last instance occurred in the 1920's when girls employed in painting watch-dials with luminous paint containing radium ingested the element by sucking the tips of their brushes. The radium was deposited selectively in bone where it gave rise to osteosarcomas.

A large proportion of today's occupational cancers are due to *asbestos*, a fact which has given rise to a great deal of public concern. Asbestos workers are at much greater risk of developing carcinoma of the lung (lung cancer) or malignant mesothelioma of the pleura than the rest of the population; among workers dying of asbestosis, lung cancer is present in a high proportion

(20–50%) and malignant mesothelioma in about 10%. (The incidence of mesotheliomas is increasing steeply and it seems that all are connected with asbestos inhalation.) Asbestos encompasses a variety of naturally occurring fibrous silicates of diverse physical and chemical nature. Thus, different types of asbestos vary considerably in the length, diameter and shape of the fibres, their resistance to acid, content of iron and magnesium, and so on, as well as in their carcinogenicity. It was established in South Africa in the 1950's that the development of mesotheliomas of the pleura and peritoneal cavity was closely associated with exposure to the dust of 'blue asbestos' (crocidolite). Tumours developed some years after first exposure and the total intake of the dust was in some cases quite trivial. Moreover, in addition to the workers, people living in the vicinity of crocidolite mines were found to be at risk, making asbestos an environmental as well as an occupational hazard. However, crocidolite only accounts for about 5% of world asbestos production; most is another type known as 'white asbestos' (chrysotile) which is much less dangerous. Nevertheless, excess exposure to all forms of asbestos can lead to asbestosis and carcinoma of the lung. It seems that the risk associated with different types of the material depends primarily on the physical properties of the fibre, because penetration of the lung is determined by its diameter and shape; thus, the thin, straight fibres of crocidolite penetrate more efficiently to the distal subpleural portion of the lung than the curly fibres of chrysotile. An important aspect of the asbestos problem is that cigarette smoking greatly increases the risk of developing asbestos-associated lung cancer (p. 755). Public pressure is now leading to a reduction in asbestos levels in industry, schools and homes. Discouraging smoking is also clearly an important step which, if effective, would be of particular benefit to workers in the asbestos industry, as well as to the population at large.

In principle, occupational cancers are wholly preventable, but in practice, workers will continue to be affected so long as society demands the products of the industries concerned.

Geographical distribution

While some cancers show fairly uniform distributions around the world, there are some striking examples of tumours which are seen frequently in some countries yet are rare in others. Geographical variations seem to reflect differences in environmental rather than racial or genetic factors, for immigrant populations usually assume the pattern of cancer incidence of their adopted countries. Thus by studying these variations it should be possible to identify and perhaps eliminate some environmental causes of cancer. Figure 6.2 illustrates the different mortalities of cancers in a few selected countries.

Good examples of international variation are found in the frequencies of *stomach* and *breast cancer* in Japan and the United States. Stomach cancer is at its highest level in Japan (mortality ∼ 50 per 100,000 population) and lowest among American Whites (∼ 7 per 100,000); exactly the reverse is true of breast

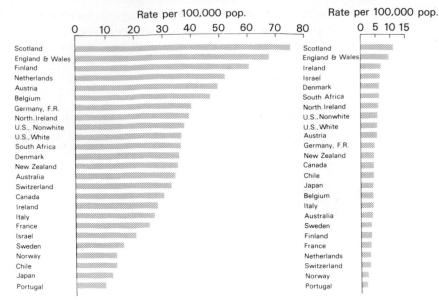

(a)

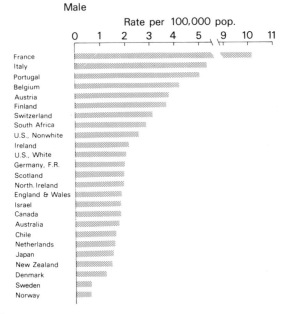

(b)

Figure 6.2 *and on pp. 703–706.*
Death rates for malignant
neoplasms of different sites in
various countries, 1964–5 (from
Clinical Oncology, UICC, 1978).
(a) Lung, bronchus and trachea.
(b) Larynx (rate in females
< 1/100,000 in all countries).

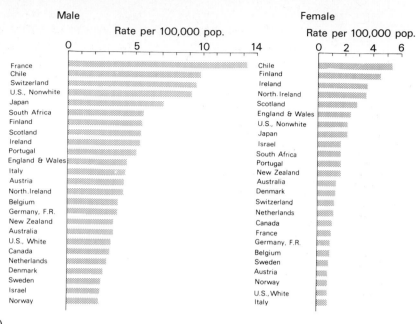

(c)

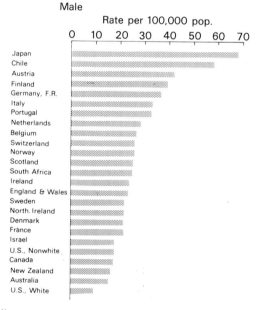

(d)

Figure 6.2 *continued.*
(c) Oesophagus.
(d) Stomach (female rate about
half male rate in most countries).

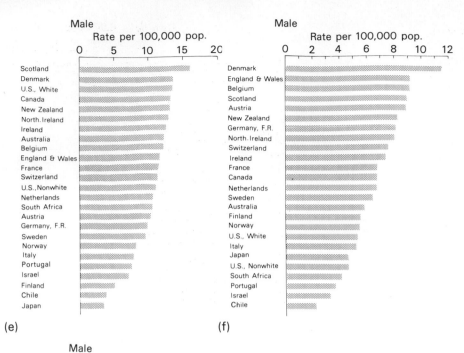

(e)

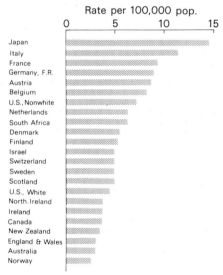

(f)

(g)

Figure 6.2 *continued.*
(e) Intestine excluding rectum (female rate similar to male).
(f) Rectum (female rate about half male rate).
(g) Liver (female rate a little lower).

Figure 6.2 *continued.*
(h) Uterus.
(i) Breast (females).

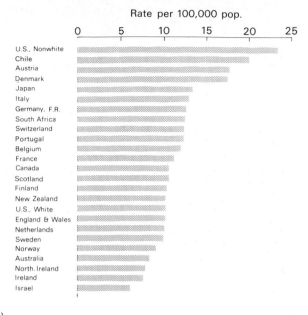

(h)

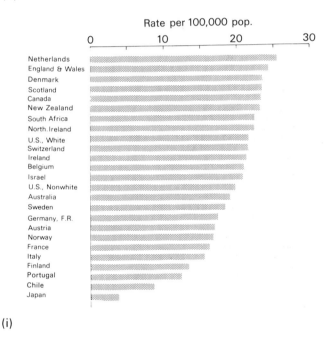

(i)

cancer, which is 5–6 times more frequent among American women than Japanese. The reasons for these differences are speculative, but in the case of stomach cancer the markedly different diets of the two countries are very probably involved. When Japanese settle in the United States, the frequency patterns of these malignancies in their descendents resemble those in the local American population. In Europe, stomach and breast cancer are about equally frequent and in many countries are the commonest cancers. It is interesting that stomach cancer is declining significantly in Europe, but this decline is not seen in

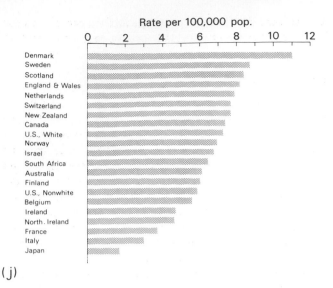

Rate per 100,000 pop.

Figure 6.2 *continued.*
(j) Ovary, Fallopian tube and broad ligament.

(j)

Japan. A further example of geographic variation is provided by *cancer of the colon*, which is common in Western Europe, North America and New Zealand, but several times less frequent in Africa and Japan. Again, dietary factors are probably involved and a high intake of meat or a low intake of cereals seem to be associated with high incidence of cancer of the colon. It is difficult to decide which is the more relevant factor, since the two usually go together. *Cancer of the oesophagus* also shows remarkable epidemiological features. It is very common in parts of the Soviet Union (mortality of ~ 60 per 100,000 among males in Turkmenistan), in parts of South and Central America (~ 17 per 100,000 in Puerto Rico) and France (~ 14 per 100,000). The mortality in male American Whites is only 3 per 100,000 and is even lower in females. Intake of alcohol, hot drinks or spices have been suggested as causative factors. In certain parts of Africa, an unusually high level of *liver cancer* occurs, due in part to contamination of food with toxins produced by a fungus, *Aspergillus flavus* (see *aflatoxins*, p. 760). For *lung cancer*, the highest mortality rates occur in Western Europe, especially the UK, Finland, Austria, Holland and Belgium; in the UK it carries the highest mortality of any cancer. In contrast, lung cancer is a much less frequent cause of death in Japan, Portugal, Chile, Norway and Sweden. An example of a tumour which is restricted by climatic boundaries is *Burkitt's lymphoma*, a tumour of the jaw found in children in Africa and South America. In Africa it is limited to areas with an average temperature of 16°C or over and a rainfall of over 508 mm. It shows a similar distribution to that of endemic malaria, and malarial infection seems to be the predisposing factor (p. 792). Identification of environmental factors which underlie geographical differences in tumour incidence offers one of the best hopes for the control of cancer.

There is no doubt that the single most important contribution of epidemiological data to the field of cancer in recent years has been to reveal the link between smoking and lung cancer, and this provides an excellent illustration of how such data can be applied.

Smoking and cancer of the lung

The results of exhaustive epidemiological studies since 1950 have amply demonstrated the causal association between cigarette smoking and lung cancer. The main lines of evidence are as follows. In initial retrospective studies, in which the smoking habits of known lung cancer patients were ascertained and compared with control groups, it was shown that the proportion of patients who were non-smokers was extremely small ($\sim 1\%$), while more than half had been heavy smokers over a number of years. Prospective studies, in which populations were first characterised in terms of tobacco usage and the appearance of lung cancer then followed for a number of years, were even more conclusive. The risk of developing lung cancer was up to 30 times greater in smokers than non-smokers, and was proportional to the number of cigarettes smoked and the duration of the smoking habit. By giving up smoking, the risk could be very much reduced. The mortality in different age groups at various smoking levels is shown in Table 6.3. The risks involved in pipe or cigar smoking were very much less than from cigarettes and only about twice that of non-smokers. Cigar and pipe smokers, however, do run a considerably higher than average risk of cancer of the lip or oral cavity.

Other aspects of the epidemiology of lung cancer could also be correlated with cigarette smoking. (a) Lung cancer has increased dramatically in incidence in the last 50 years and this can be wholly correlated with increased cigarette consumption. In the UK the death rate for males in the 65–75 age group rose from 36 per 100,000 in 1935 to 650 per 100,000 in 1973. (b) Because of the long latency in the development of lung cancer, the mortality rates in any particular period correlate most closely with the *per capita* consumption of cigarettes 20 years previously. This is particularly well illustrated by the upward trend of lung cancer in women which began in the 1960's and has continued at a faster rate of increase than lung cancer in males. In the UK it was unusual for women to smoke before about 1920, and the main increase in women smoking began in the 1940's. After a lag of 20

Table 6.3 Smoking and death rates from lung cancer (per 100,000 population). Source: Kahn (1966) *The Dorn Study of Smoking and Mortality.* (Nat. Cancer Inst. Monogr. 19.)

	Age group	
Amount smoked	55–64 years	65–74 years
Nil	10	30
Cigarettes per day		
1–9	70	135
10–20	123	265
21–39	205	432
39+	338	696
Cigars only	20	49
Pipe only	24	54

years, lung cancer began to rise rapidly in women, as shown in Figure 6.3. (c) Male mortality from lung cancer has always been much higher than female in all countries (the ratio is about 7:1 in the UK), but in recent years the ratio has started to fall as female mortality has increased. Once again, these features can be accounted for by reference to the smoking habits of the sexes in the last 50 years, as Figure 6.3 shows.

The incidence of lung cancer varies around the world, having its highest incidence in the UK where it carries a higher mortality than any other tumour. It is interesting that for comparable numbers of cigarettes smoked, mortality is significantly higher in the UK than in the USA or South Africa. At first sight, this runs counter to the hypothesis that smoking is the main causative factor, but it may be that the variations can be accounted for by differences in the types of tobacco used in the past in the manufacture of cigarettes in different countries. Cigarette smoke contains, among other substances, radioactive polonium ^{210}Po, and it has been suggested that mortality variations in these countries are proportional to the amount of this element in different tobaccos. There is now a tendency to smoke cigarettes of lower cancer risk, namely filter cigarettes and those with a low tar yield. What influence this has on mortality will only be seen in several years' time.

The association between smoking and cancer is thus very strong and is most probably the result of the carcinogenic substances in tobacco tar. The latter contains several chemical carcinogens, such as polycyclic hydrocarbons, aromatic amines and nitrosamines, as well as radioactive elements, though the mechanism whereby smoking leads to cancer has not been precisely established because of the lack of an ideal animal model. However, while about 10% of heavy cigarette smokers die of lung cancer, others survive to an advanced age without developing the disease. Cigarette smoking may not of itself be a sufficient cause of lung cancer in the absence of some other predisposing

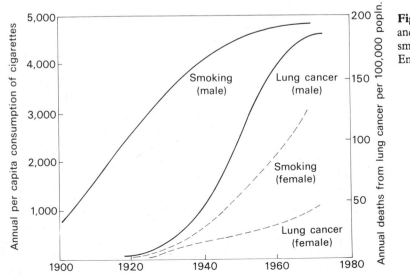

Figure 6.3 Cigarette smoking and lung cancer. Trends in smoking and lung cancer in England and Wales since 1900.

influence in the individual. A genetic influence is one possibility and there is evidence both for a familial incidence of lung cancer which is independent of cigarette smoking, as well as an inherited tendency to become a smoker or non-smoker. There is also some experimental evidence that the basis of genetic susceptibility lies in the inherited ability to produce an enzyme, *aryl hydrocarbon hydroxylase*, which activates polycyclic hydrocarbons in the lung and converts them into carcinogens. Only producers of this enzyme would be able to metabolise the hydrocarbons, which seems to be essential for the expression of their cancer-causing property (p. 754). However, at present the evidence that the level of this enzyme really determines susceptibility in man is inconclusive. It would obviously be a great advantage in prevention of the disease to be able to identify individuals most at risk by means of an enzyme test or other biochemical characteristic.

CHARACTERISTICS OF NEOPLASTIC CELLS

1. NEOPLASIA AND GROWTH REGULATION

As we have noted, the growth of tumour cells is free of the controls which regulate the division of normal tissue cells and which ensure that new cells only arise as and when required. Besides the generalised influence of circulating hormones such as somatotrophin, gonadotrophin and oestrogen, there are two important local means of regulating cell division in normal tissues. One is the inhibition of division by direct membrane contact between cells, so-called *contact inhibition* of mitosis. The second is the production of growth regulatory substances, specific for each particular tissue; most attention has been given to soluble inhibitors of cell division called *chalones*, though stimulatory substances are probably also produced. Neoplastic cells have escaped from both the soluble and membrane methods of control, and it is of key importance to discover how this escape occurs. First, we must describe the phases of the replicative cycle of a normal cell.

The cell cycle

This is the interval between one mitosis and the next occurring in one or both daughter cells. The cycle is divided into four phases of which mitosis itself is one, denoted M (Figure 6.4). The replication of cell DNA takes place before mitosis, in a discrete period of the interphase called the synthetic or S phase. After mitosis and before the S phase is a presynthetic 'gap' termed G_1, while following S comes a postsynthetic or premitotic gap, G_2 (Figure 6.4). The biochemical changes necessary for DNA synthesis occur in G_1, while those required for mitosis occur in G_2. G_1 and S are the longest phases of the cell cycle: G_1 varies in duration from a few hours to several days, while S lasts for about 10–20 hours in human cells. M is short, about 1–2 hours, while G_2 is a little longer, 1–4 hours. Note that in G_2 the cell has twice

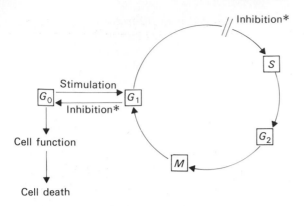

Figure 6.4 The cell cycle.
*indicates points of action of
soluble or contact inhibition.

the normal diploid DNA content, DNA having been replicated in
the S phase. Cells which cease division and temporarily leave the
cell cycle are said to be in a resting or G_0 phase. Resting cells can
re-enter the replicative cycle on appropriate stimulation or by
relaxation of tissue inhibitory mechanisms. Some cells, however,
permanently lose the ability to divide, such as mature
erythrocytes or polymorphonuclear leucocytes. Inhibition of
division by chalones or membrane contact will either arrest the
cell in G_1 or cause it to leave the cycle and become a resting (G_0)
cell. Arrest in the G_2 phase is unusual.

Contact inhibition and membranes of normal and neoplastic cells

When normal cells such as fibroblasts are grown in a culture dish,
they multiply and migrate over the surface of the vessel up to the
point where they form a continuous single layer (a monolayer),
(Figure 6.5a). Both division and migration then stop, a phenomenon known as contact inhibition or density-dependent growth
control. In contrast, the growth of tumour cells does not cease at
the monolayer stage, but the cells continue to divide and migrate
over each other until they have piled up several layers deep in
disorganised array (Figure 6.5b). Clearly, normal cells respond to
the fact that they are in a crowded environment, but tumour cells
have lost the ability either to transmit or receive such information, resulting in the relentless growth of tumours in body
tissues. Inhibition of movement and mitosis are distinct
phenomena, and loss of inhibition of mitosis shows the best
correlation with malignancy. One can also readily see that loss of
inhibition of movement will contribute to the invasive character
of malignant cells *in vivo*.

The control of normal cell growth depends on *cellular interactions*, which in turn involve the *surface membranes* of the interacting cells. There is considerable evidence to suggest that the
altered growth behaviour of tumour cells can be related to
changes in the cell membrane. Three stages in interactions
between cells in growth control can be distinguished, namely
(a) recognition by cells of which of their neighbours they should or

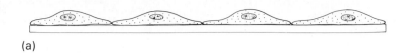

Figure 6.5 Growth patterns of normal and neoplastic cells.
(a) Normal cells grow to a confluent monolayer.
(b) Multilayering of neoplastic cells.

(a)

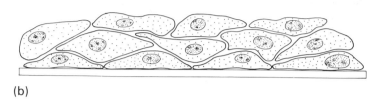

(b)

should not associate with, followed by (b) adherence of cells to each other with formation of mechanical and permeable connections and (c) the transmission of regulatory signals from cell to cell and the effect of those signals on division, movement, metabolism, etc. In principle, the escape from normal growth control could involve a breakdown at any of these stages.

Recognition

Present understanding of how differentiated tissue cells recognise each other is limited and somewhat speculative. That such recognition does exist can be shown by the selective way in which cells of different origins reassociate if mixed together in culture. For example, if cultures of embryonic liver and kidney cells are thoroughly mixed, the two types of cell will eventually segregate themselves, liver with liver and kidney with kidney, and in some cases even organise themselves into characteristic structures such as kidney tubules. While recognition processes must involve the cell surface, the details are as yet obscure. One hypothesis to which particular attention has been given is that sugar-binding enzymes called *glycosyltransferases* are present in the cell membrane and recognise sugar residues on glycoproteins in the membranes of adjacent cells (Figure 6.6). These enzymes normally function inside the cell where they add specific sugars to proteins in the synthesis of glycoproteins. They are highly specific both for the sugar being added and the 'receptor' to which it is being attached (in practice another sugar or amino acid). According to the hypothesis, the specificity with which cells recognise each other is achieved by a particular combination of membrane enzyme and surface sugar residues. There is a certain amount of evidence to suggest that glycosyltransferases may be present on the surfaces of at least some cells. In one experimental model of cell recognition, the localisation of lymphocytes in lymph nodes, a role for surface sugars can be demonstrated. When lymphocytes are injected into an experimental animal they 'home' to the lymph node, where they are evidently recognised as 'belonging'. If, however, the lymphocytes are treated with

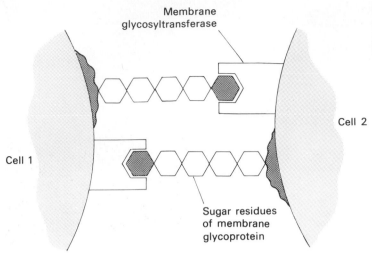

Membrane
glycosyltransferase

Cell 2

Cell 1

Sugar residues
of membrane
glycoprotein

Figure 6.6 Hypothesis of cellular interaction via glycosyltransferases (after Roseman).

enzymes which strip off their surface sugars, the cells are no longer recognised by the node, but continue to float around in the circulation. For tumour cells, a reduced efficiency of these surface interactions could be envisaged as a result of a specific change in the molecules involved (enzyme and oligosaccharide substrate) or by more general alteration in the cell membrane which would reduce cell–cell adhesiveness.

Adhesion

Adhesion involves the formation of physical connections between cells, of which several types are known (Figure 6.7). *Desmosomes* are junctions of a purely mechanical nature holding cells together, seen primarily between epithelial cells. Under the electron microscope they appear as electron-dense material bridging the intercellular gap (about 200 Å). They are composed of a fibrous protein and can be digested away by trypsin, allowing cells to

Figure 6.7 Intercellular connections.
(a) The desmosome.
(b) The tight junction.
(c) The gap junction.
For each, (i) is a diagrammatic representation and (ii) an electron micrograph of a thin section (x 200,000).
(Electron micrographs by courtesy of Dr F.B.P. Wooding.)

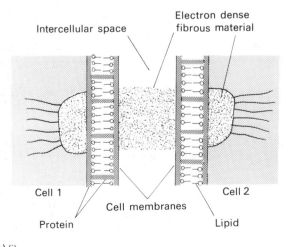

Intercellular space

Electron dense
fibrous material

Cell 1

Cell 2

Cell membranes

Protein

Lipid

(a) (i)

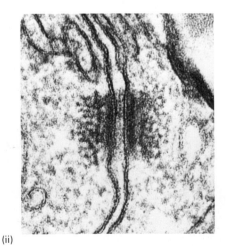

(ii)

712

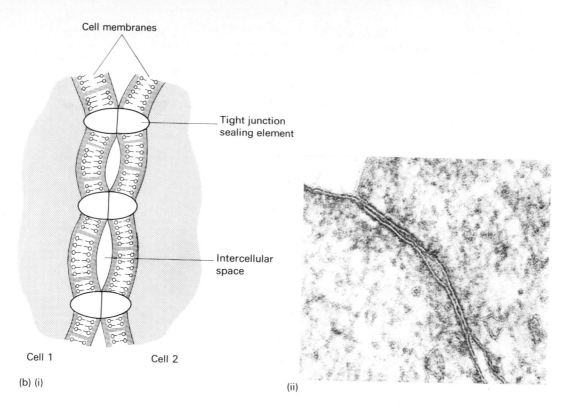

Cell membranes

Tight junction
sealing element

Intercellular
space

Cell 1   Cell 2

(b) (i)

(ii)

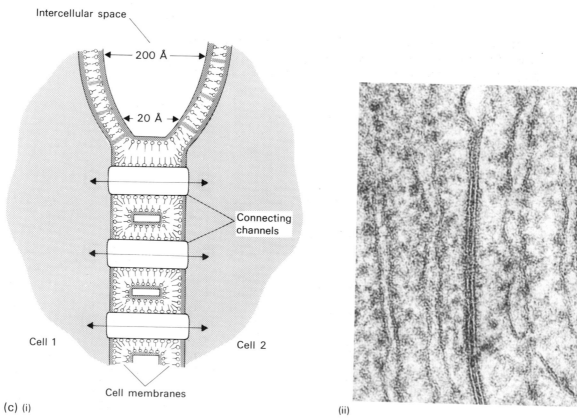

Intercellular space

← 200 Å →

← 20 Å →

Connecting
channels

Cell 1   Cell 2

Cell membranes

(c) (i)

(ii)

separate. A quite different type of intercellular connection, with physiological rather than mechanical significance, is the *tight junction*, an area of very close connection which actually involves fusion of the two cell membranes. The intercellular space is therefore occluded (Figure 6.7b). Tight junctions form impermeable barriers and are prominent in areas where a sharp physical separation is required. For instance, they are in evidence in the endothelial lining of cerebral blood vessels where they help to create the blood-brain barrier.

A third type of junction which may have considerable significance for intercellular communication is the *gap junction*, which differs from the others in that it allows a physical connection between the cytoplasm of adjoining cells (Figure 6.7c). It consists of an array of channels or pores passing through the cell membrane, across a decreased intercellular gap (about 20 Å wide) and through the membrane of the adjacent cell. The pores have a diameter of about 15 Å and allow the passage of low molecular weight material between the cells. The permeability range is up to molecular weights of about 1000 and would thus encompass steroid hormones, metabolites, vitamins, cyclic nucleotides, but of course exclude proteins or nucleic acids. Permeability channels between cells were first discovered by an unexpectedly low electrical resistance between tissue cells, and subsequently confirmed by demonstration of physical intercellular transfer of fluorescent dyes or radiolabelled markers; e.g. when fluorescein is introduced into a single cell, its neighbours soon become fluorescent (Figure 6.8a). The channels are widespread in tissues including the epithelia of the liver, kidney, skin, bladder, thyroid, etc; indeed the only tissues in which they have not been found are skeletal muscle and the nervous system. A particularly interesting feature of gap junctions is that they are not permanent functional entities in the plasma membrane; they form when cells make contact and disappear when cells are separated, the membrane then returning to its impermeable state. The coupling channels take about 10 minutes to form after contact between two cell membranes and can appear at any point after adhesion has brought the membranes into intimate proximity. Clearly, permeability channels could have great significance for the regulation of growth and differentiation. The implication is that there is a common internal milieu for a large community of cells, even entire organs, through which regulators or signalling molecules could rapidly diffuse.

Of all the forms of intercellular connection, the gap junction may have direct relevance to contact inhibition of growth and its loss in neoplasia. It has been found that some tumour cells show a defect in the formation of intercellular channels and that this correlates with the loss of density-dependent growth control. Several cancer cell lines grown *in vitro* have been shown to be 'uncoupled', in that they will not form junctions with each other or permit passage of fluorescein, labelled nucleotides or small ions (Figure 6.8b). However, the junction defect is not found in all cancer cells, so evidence has been sought that, when present, it is

Figure 6.8 Demonstration of permeability channels between normal, but not neoplastic, cells.
(a) Normal cells (and hybrids of normal and neoplastic cells) form gap junctions which permit passage of fluorescent marker between cells.
(b) Neoplastic cells do not form permeability channels and fluorescent dye remains localised in cell into which it is introduced.

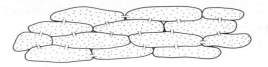

<table>
<tr><td>⊥
⊤ Gap junction</td><td>Fluorescent dye
(introduced into one cell)</td></tr>
</table>

(a)

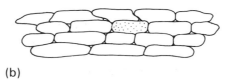

(b)

directly related to the growth abnormality. Such evidence has been found by the technique of *cell hybridisation* (see also p. 730). When tumour cells are fused with normal cells, hybrid cells are produced which frequently show a normal growth pattern with contact inhibition and are no longer malignant (p. 732). The 'normal-growth' hybrids form coupling (gap) junctions, even if the tumour cell is of the uncoupled type. Furthermore, the hybrid cells tend to lose some of their chromosomes and in so doing often revert to the 'uncontrolled-growth' (neoplastic) state; when such revertant cells are grown in culture they are found to have lost the ability to make gap junctions in addition to losing contact inhibition. Evidently, normal cells can provide tumour cells with the genetic information which simultaneously corrects their growth behaviour and re-establishes junction formation, so that the hybrid cell is normal in both these respects. When the information is lost, through chromosome shedding, both characteristics revert to those of the neoplastic cell. Hence there is an indication that contact inhibition requires the formation of permeable channels and that an inability of cells to communicate in this way is an important part of the neoplastic change leading to abnormal growth.

Signals

The details of the signals involved in regulating cell division in contact inhibition are also only incompletely understood. It is likely that cyclic nucleotides function as intracellular messengers in the control of mitosis as they do for so many other cellular events. Thus, mitosis is associated with a fall in the cyclic AMP level in the cell and a rise in cyclic GMP. Moreover, the cyclic AMP level of tumour cells is only about half that of normal cells, and addition of cyclic AMP to their culture medium can cause tumour cells to revert to a normal morphology and growth pattern. A possible link between a lowering of cyclic AMP and changes in the cell membrane is discussed below.

Membrane changes in neoplasia

The cell surface clearly plays a major role in regulating cell division and there is ample evidence for changes in cell membranes associated with neoplasia and with the loss of contact inhibition. One is an increase in the net negative charge of tumour cells, and there is evidence that the more malignant and invasive the cell the greater the increase in charge. All mammalian cell surfaces are negatively charged under physiological conditions. The increased negativity of tumour cells is due to N-acetylneuraminic (sialic) acid residues in cell surface glycoproteins and can be reduced by treating the cells with neuraminidase. It is interesting that injections of neuraminidase-treated malignant cells into animals cause fewer tumours than inocula of untreated cells. In a simplistic way, one could envisage that the greater electrostatic repulsion between highly charged cells would tend to keep them apart and hence reduce adhesiveness and contact inhibition, though this is unlikely to be the whole explanation.

Another change involving the surface glycoproteins of tumour cells has been detected using sugar-binding proteins called *lectins*. These molecules are found in extracts of a variety of plants and invertebrates and are recognised by their ability to agglutinate red blood cells. Each lectin has a highly specific binding site for a particular sugar. The agglutination reaction takes place because lectins are divalent molecules which can cross-link cells after binding to surface sugars, similar to haemagglutination by antibody. The connection between lectins and tumours is that a number of lectins selectively agglutinate tumour cells, but not their normal counterparts (Figure 6.9a, b). For example a lectin called wheat germ agglutinin (WGA) has been shown to aggregate almost every tumour cell type grown *in vitro*, regardless of how the tumour arose (i.e. spontaneously or by chemical agent, virus or irradiation). Lectins will agglutinate a few normal cell types, notably erythrocytes and lymphocytes, but in general the correlation between lectin-agglutination and neoplasia is very strong. This is also shown by isolating from tumour cells grown *in vitro* (tumour lines), occasional cells which have spontaneously reverted to a normal state. These revertant cells grow normally, show contact inhibition of mitosis and, significantly, are no longer agglutinable by WGA. The sugar involved in the tumour cell agglutination phenomenon is N-acetylglucosamine, particularly its dimer, di-N-acetylchitobiose, for which WGA has a specific binding site. An interesting application of this knowledge is an experimental attempt to protect mice from the lethal effects of a transplanted tumour (a myeloma) by preimmunising them

Figure 6.9 Effects of lectins on normal and neoplastic cells.
(a) Normal cells grow to monolayer in culture and are not agglutinated by lectin.
(b) Neoplastic cells grow as multilayers and are agglutinated by lectin.
(c) Normal cells after trypsin treatment enter further replication and are lectin-agglutinable.
(d) Neoplastic cells treated with monovalent (non-agglutinating) lectin grow to monolayer.

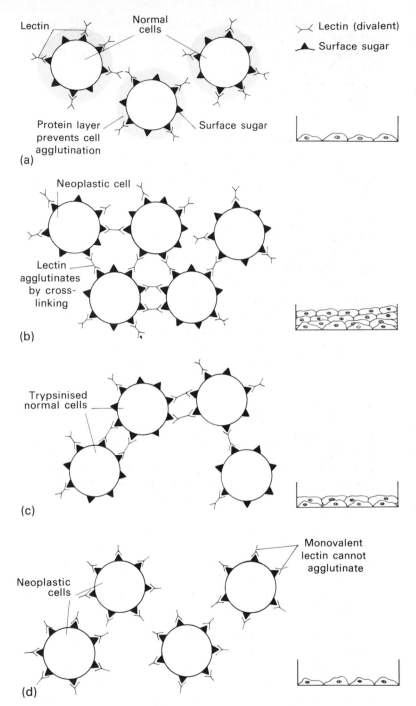

with the N-acetylglucosamine dimer bound to a protein carrier. Indeed, under certain conditions the animals were protected by this procedure.

One can envisage two possible reasons for the enhanced agglutinability of tumour cells. One is that the neoplastic change is accompanied by increased production of glycoproteins carrying

717

N-acetylglucosamine and that these are therefore present in larger amount at the cell surface. This seems not to be the case, because normal and tumour cell surfaces have comparable amounts of N-acetylglucosamine. Moreover, experiments with radioactively labelled lectins show that the same amount of lectin binds to the normal and the neoplastic cell. The second explanation is that some other surface component of normal cells prevents their agglutination after lectin binding. This possibility has been confirmed by treating normal cells with minute amounts of trypsin to remove an outer layer of protein from the cell surface without destroying the cell. After trypsinisation, normal cells do indeed become agglutinable by WGA and, interestingly, they temporarily lose contact inhibition and divide like tumour cells (Figure 6.9c). (The loss of inhibition lasts only for one generation, because the cells soon replace the lost surface protein layer.) The stimulation of growth by protease treatment suggested a converse experiment, notably to try to inhibit the growth of tumour cells by covering the surface agglutination sites (N-acetylglucosamine residues). This can be achieved by treating tumour cells with the sugar-binding lectin, provided the lectin is first made monovalent by enzymatic treatment. This is essential because normal divalent lectin will cause agglutination, whereas monovalent lectin can only bind to the cell surface but cannot agglutinate (Figure 6.9d). When monovalent lectin was added to cultured tumour cells, contact inhibition was successfully restored, i.e. the cells grew to a monolayer and then stopped. This effect was reversible: when lectin was removed from the cell surface by addition of an excess of free N-acetylglucosamine, growth recommenced.

Taken together these observations indicate that the loss of certain cell surface proteins causes both the agglutination of tumour cells by lectins and their loss of contact inhibition. This has led to a suggestion that endogenous proteolytic enzymes could bring about the membrane changes of tumour cells, e.g. enzymes released from cell lysosomes. It is known that an extracellular release of lysosomal enzymes occurs during mitosis, and it has also been shown that low doses of protease inhibitors can restore contact inhibition to growing tumour cells. Several neoplastic cell lines possess higher levels of lysosomal enzymes than normal and release proteases into their environment (see also p. 724).

There is thus good reason to associate membrane changes of neoplastic cells, possibly produced by enzymatic action, with the loss of contact inhibition and perpetual growth of tumour cells. It is noteworthy that similar changes in cell membranes, with ag-glutinability by lectins, can be observed during brief periods of the *normal* cell cycle, and they may be part of a membrane 'signal' to the interior of the cell to enter the S phase of the cycle and replicate DNA before mitosis. The link between the membrane change and cell division may be provided by alterations in the intracellular levels of cyclic AMP and cyclic GMP. We have already noted that the cyclic AMP level of tumour cells is significantly lower than that of normal cells and that cyclic AMP can restore a normal growth behaviour to neoplastic cells in culture. Trypsinisation of contact-inhibited cells also causes a fall

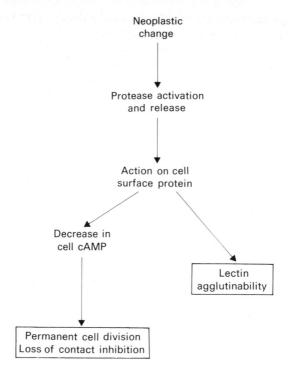

Figure 6.10 Possible role of proteolytic enzymes in producing membrane alterations of neoplastic cells.
(cAMP = cyclic AMP)

in cyclic AMP, as well as the cell division and lectin agglutinability noted above, and addition of cyclic AMP to trypsinised cells prevents their extra round of division. Thus, it is possible to link a permanent intracellular protease activation with membrane changes and decreased cyclic AMP levels in a speculative scheme, showing how lectin agglutinability and loss of contact inhibition might result (Figure 6.10).

Chalones

The observations on contact inhibition *in vitro* and its loss by neoplastic cells have suggested that the growth of a tissue is regulated by interactions taking place at the cell membrane and that when these reach a critical level, cells capable of division receive a signal which arrests the cell cycle and prevents mitosis. This homeostatic mechanism has at some point broken down in the tumour cell, probably at the membrane level. However, this type of regulation by cell contact may not be the only means of setting the rate of division of tissue cells. There is evidence for the existence of soluble substances which can act as local, tissue-specific inhibitors of replication; the term 'chalone' is used to describe these molecules. The principle of their mode of action is simple: they are produced by differentiated tissue cells to provide *negative feedback inhibition* of the proliferative cells in the tissue or organ (Figure 6.11). Hence, the greater the number of cells in the tissue, the more chalone will be produced and the greater the suppression of division. The size of a tissue could then be regulated by the rate of production of chalone and the sensitivity

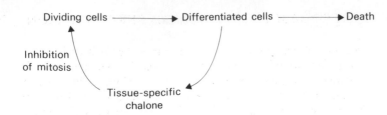

Figure 6.11 Regulation of tissue mass by negative feedback.

of divising cells to its inhibitory effect. There may well also be locally-produced stimulatory molecules which encourage division (growth factors), in addition to stimulatory tissue-specific hormones produced elsewhere (e.g. TSH for the thyroid gland, ACTH for the adrenal cortex, etc.). No doubt physiological regulation depends on a balance between these opposing influences of stimulation and inhibition. Evidence for the existence of chalones is described in Section 1 (p. 54).

If chalones are important in the feedback regulation of growth, it appears that tumour cells have escaped their effect, either through lacking the ability to produce the necessary chalones or through an insensitivity to their action (e.g. loss of a chalone receptor from the cell membrane). In general, it seems that tumours can produce the chalones of their tissue of origin and can also respond to them, but have become less sensitive than normal tissue to chalone suppression of cell division. In short, tumour cells have a reduced receiving efficiency for the chalone signal. This has led to attempts to treat cancers experimentally by a 'chalone therapy', i.e. with tissue extracts. Only occasional successes have been reported—in at least one documented case due to bacterial contamination of the extract—and in general such extracts have not provided much reason to believe that they will be of clinical usefulness.

At the present time, the importance of chalones in growth regulation, and hence of the loss of responsiveness to chalones in neoplasia, is rather uncertain. In part this is due to the failure to obtain the molecules in pure form and to characterise precisely their mechanism of action at a molecular level. Therefore, while there is no disputing the existence of cybernetic and homeostatic mechanisms of growth control in tissues, the important question of which ones are directly relevant to the unregulated growth of neoplastic cells cannot yet be answered satisfactorily. For example, *in vitro* contact inhibition does not appear to depend on soluble mediators, yet its loss is clearly closely related to tumour growth *in vivo*. It is difficult with present methods to assess what level of contribution is made by the additional insensitivity of tumour cells to chalone regulation. Equally, it may well be that the loss of both regulatory effects have one and the same origin, namely alterations either in the cell surface itself or in the means whereby inhibitory signals are transmitted from the surface to the nucleus. Clarification of the derangements of the neoplastic cell will have to await a proper understanding of the molecular basis of normal growth regulation.

2. NEOPLASIA AND CELL DIFFERENTIATION

An important aspect of tumours and tumour cells is their degree of differentiation, i.e. the extent to which they resemble, in structure and function, their tissue of origin. The state of differentiation of a normal tissue is recognised from the characteristic morphology of its cells, from their organisation or architectural arrangement in the tissue, and from specific cell products. At the genetic level, differentiation involves the restriction of the expression of the cell's genetic information. Thus, both liver cells and kidney cells possess the same genome and the identical nuclear content of DNA; the difference between them lies in which genes are active and which repressed in the differentiated state. In general, benign tumours are highly differentiated: they resemble their tissues of origin both in cytological appearance and structure, and continue to synthesize the characteristic products of their normal counterparts, such as hormones, keratin, etc. Thus, while normal control of cell division has been lost, the pattern of gene repression characteristic of the particular tissue has been maintained.

Cancers, on the other hand, show wide variation in their degree of differentiation and are often less differentiated or organised than the normal tissue. In extreme cases, there is complete lack of differentiation or *anaplasia* and the tissue origin may not be at all obvious from histology. Frequently, the more malignant the tumour, the less its degree of differentiation, and correspondingly the worse the prognosis. Hence, evidence of differentiation is an important criterion used in estimating the degree of malignancy, i.e. in *grading* cancers. However, it would be wrong to generalise, as has sometimes been done in the past, that loss of differentiated characteristics (dedifferentiation) is an inevitable attribute of all malignancies, since many examples are known of cancers which retain a differentiated state. The continued production of immunoglobulin by B cell tumours (myelomas) and of hormones by cancers of endocrine glands make this point. So too does the highly organised structure of some malignant tumours, such as the well differentiated squamous cell carcinomas of the skin which produce considerable keratin (laid down as epithelial 'pearls'), or adenocarcinomas which can show a typical glandular cell arrangement. Nevertheless, in their more malignant forms, the squamous cell carcinomas can be anaplastic and fail to produce keratin, and adenocarcinomas form sheets of loosely attached cells rather than a glandular structure.

Changes in the normal pattern of genetic expression in malignant cells are frequently indicated by the loss of expected cell products, due to gene repression, or the appearance of new ones by derepression of normally silent genes. Some examples of the latter are described below and include the inappropriate production of hormones and, perhaps most significantly, the re-expression of foetal or embryonic proteins. These changes indicate that the cancer cell is one which has embarked on an abnormal pathway of differentiation, in which the normal pattern of active and inactive genes is altered (though as we have noted, the degree of such change is variable). In at least some cases there may be a reversion to a quasi-embryonic cell type. Consideration of the changes in cell differentiation which can accompany malignancy leads to the theory that cancer is due to a derangement in the *expression* of the genetic material of the cell, in contrast to the 'mutation theory' which proposes alterations of the structure of the DNA itself (see p. 768).

Metaplasia

While a change in state of differentiation is often seen in neoplasia, normal cells also have the ability to undergo a certain degree of altered differentiation. Metaplasia is the term for a change from one type of differentiated tissue to another normal differentiated type. It can be distinguished from neoplasia in that it does not involve excess proliferation, the cells remain well differentiated and it is reversible. In metaplasia, the scope for alteration is limited and cells remain true to their origins; thus one type of epithelium may change into another type of epithelium, but never into connective tissue. A common example is *squamous metaplasia*, a change to a stratified squamous type of epithelium from either transitional (bladder), simple columnar (gall bladder) or pseudo-stratified columnar epithelia (bronchi). The squamous cell carcinoma of the lung, one of the common varieties of lung cancer, probably arises in areas of bronchial epithelium which have undergone squamous metaplasia. Epithelial metaplasia is a response to chronic damage (inflammation, mechanical irritation, etc.) and in the lung is commonly seen as a consequence of cigarette smoking and in chronic bronchitis. It can also result from vitamin A deficiency.

Biochemical abnormalities of neoplastic cells

The alteration of the normal state of differentiation which accompanies neoplasia is seen as much in changes in the biochemistry of tumour cells as in their ability to become organised into recognisable tissue structures. Abnormalities occur in cell respiration, in the levels of enzymes characteristic of particular tissues and most strikingly in cell products. This last involves the inappropriate production of proteins not normally synthesized by the tumour's tissue of origin, such as the secretion of hormones by tumours of non-endocrine tissue, or the re-expression of molecules which are normally only found during foetal development. The detection of tumour-associated proteins such as these has considerable potential for early cancer diagnosis. All these changes are a result of shift in the normal pattern of gene expression, by repression of some genes and derepression of others.

Respiration

Many malignant cells show a characteristic alteration of their energy metabolism in which they exhibit an unusually high rate of glycolysis under aerobic as well as anaerobic conditions. In glycolysis, glucose is broken down to pyruvate, with production of ATP and the reduced cofactor NADH. Under aerobic conditions, pyruvate enters the Krebs cycle in mitochondria and NADH is oxidised via mitochondrial oxidative phosphorylation to NAD, with further production of ATP. When oxygen is lacking, mitochondrial respiration is reduced or eliminated and glycolysis becomes an important source of energy. Under these circumstances, NADH is reoxidised by alternative means to allow the recycling of NAD, essential because NAD is in limited supply. This is achieved by lactic dehydrogenase, which uses NADH to reduce pyruvic acid to lactic acid, the end-product which diffuses out of the cell in anaerobic glycolysis. However, glycolysis is a very inefficient means of producing ATP from glucose and in normal cells the presence of oxygen inhibits the use of the glycolytic pathway beyond what is required to provide the pyruvate substrate for mitochondrial respiration; this inhibition of glycolysis by oxygen is known as the *Pasteur effect*. Malignant cells do not show the normal Pasteur effect, but instead a high rate of glycolysis and lactic acid production continue even in the presence of adequate oxygen. This feature was discovered by Warburg who believed it to be fundamental to the nature of neoplasia. It is certainly true that the growth rate of cancer cells can frequently be correlated with glycolysis, with a more malignant cell showing a higher rate of aerobic glycolysis than a less malignant cell of similar origin. However, this may be a result of selection of cells capable of rapid growth under the anaerobic conditions which prevail in many tumours with a sluggish blood supply, rather than a basic cause of cancer as Warburg postulated.

Enzymes

Alterations in the intracellular enzyme levels of the normal cell are another common biochemical change in malignancy. Detailed studies with hepatomas have shown that deviations from the normal can be found in a great many pathways of metabolism. In malignant tumours from different sources there is a tendency for the varied enzyme patterns of the differentiated cell types of origin to converge to a common pattern, a biochemical parallel to the morphological changes towards anaplasia. Thus highly malignant, undifferentiated cells of diverse tissue origins may show closer resemblance to each other than to the normal cells from which they have arisen (biochemical convergence). The following are a few specific examples of changes in enzyme levels.
1 The neoplastic granulocytes found in the blood in *chronic myeloid (granulocytic) leukaemia* (CML) show a characteristic deficiency of the enzyme *alkaline phosphatase*, normally found in granulocyte lysosomes. It has been suggested that the deficiency is associated with the presence of the Philadelphia chromosome abnormality which these cells carry (p. 729).
2 Cells of *acute lymphocytic leukaemia* (ALL), unlike normal

tissues, lack an enzyme required for the synthesis of the amino acid asparagine, and are therefore dependent on an exogenous source of asparagine. This is provided by the liver, which releases asparagine into the blood. The enzyme defect in the malignant cells has been exploited in a therapeutic procedure for ALL using administration of another enzyme, *L-asparaginase*. The latter rapidly lowers the plasma asparagine level, which should in principle arrest the growth of ALL cells. While asparaginase therapy is successful in mice, it is less so in man, although it produces remissions in ALL patients, because leukaemic cells eventually reappear which are able to synthesize their own asparagine and are therefore resistant to plasma asparagine depletion.

3 Carcinoma of the *prostate* is associated with an increase in the plasma of *acid phosphatase* released from the cancer. This has some use as a diagnostic procedure.

4 Another enzyme found at raised levels in serum of cancer patients is *carcinoplacental alkaline phosphatase* (CAP). This enzyme is produced by the normal placenta and is therefore also found in pregnancy sera, but is not otherwise present in the blood. About 12% of a variety of tumours produce this enzyme, which is also known as the Regan isoenzyme after the patient in whom it was first discovered. It is of interest as one of several instances of placental products which are re-expressed in tumours, others including placental hormones. Once again, detection of CAP may in time become of diagnostic usefulness.

5 The levels of *lysosomal enzymes* are raised in many tumour cells, and it has been suggested that their release assists in the invasion of host tissue by cancer cells. In particular, release of *collagenases and hyaluronidases*, to digest connective tissue and ground substance, has been implicated in the invasiveness of certain cancers; for example, collagenase activity has been correlated with invasiveness for human breast cancers (see also p. 735.)

Hormones

A variety of tumours synthesize and release hormones which are not produced by the normal cells of their tissue of origin, a phenomenon called inappropriate or *ectopic* hormone production (Table 6.4). This is a good example of the more general ability of tumour cells to synthesize proteins not normally found in their tissues of origin; other instances include inappropriate enzymes, such as CAP mentioned above, and foetal proteins (p. 726). Hormone production is the most dramatic because of its association with clinical syndromes. The ectopic production of hormones by non-endocrine tumours should be distinguished from over-production of hormones by tumours of endocrinal or placental origin, which merely secrete in excess their expected products. Examples of the latter are also shown in Table 6.4. In this group, hormone production is not inappropriate, at least in type, and so it is not an indication of abnormal differentiation in the tumour cell.

Table 6.4 Production of hormones by tumours.

Tissue	Tumour	Product	Clinical features
Hormones appropriate to the tumour's tissue of origin			
Adrenal cortex	Adenoma, carcinoma	Cortisol Aldosterone Androgens	Cushing's syndrome Conn's syndrome Adrenogenital syndrome
Adrenal medulla	Phaeochromocytoma	Adrenaline, noradrenaline	Hypertension
Pancreatic islet cell	Adenoma	Insulin	Hyperinsulinism, hypoglycaemia
Enterochromaffin cells	Carcinoid tumours	Serotonin	Carcinoid syndrome
Placental tissue	Choriocarcinoma, hydatiform mole	Gonadotrophin	
Inappropriate (ectopic) hormone production by non-endocrine tumours			
Lung	Oat cell carcinoma	ACTH* ADH*	Cushing's syndrome Inappropriate antidiuresis, hyponatraemia
	Squamous cell carcinoma	PTH*	Hypercalcaemia
Kidney	Adenocarcinoma	PTH	Hypercalcaemia
Liver	Hepatoma, hepatoblastoma	Gonadotrophin	Precocious puberty, gynaecomastia
Lung	Oat cell carcinoma	Gonadotrophin	Gynaecomastia

* ACTH : adrenocorticotrophic hormone
  ADH : antidiuretic hormone
  PTH : parathyroid hormone

725

The commonest example of ectopic hormone production is the secretion of *adrenocorticotrophic hormone* (ACTH) by lung cancer cells. Clinically-apparent ACTH production is found in about 10% of all lung cancer patients, and ACTH can be detected intracellularly in a higher proportion ($\sim 30\%$). The oat cell carcinomas of the lung and bronchial carcinoids are the tumours most often associated with ACTH. The clinical effect is manifested as *Cushing's syndrome*, due to overproduction of cortisol by the adrenal cortex in response to high circulating ACTH, with its typical features of rounded 'moon' facial appearance, truncal obesity and purple abdominal striae. In middle-aged and elderly patients with lung cancer, the severity of hypercortisolism is often so great that death occurs before all the classical symptoms of Cushing's syndrome are seen. Oat cell carcinomas are also a source of *antidiuretic hormone* (ADH, vasopressin) as well as the other pituitary peptides oxytocin and neurophysin. ADH secretion leads to excessive retention of water and overexcretion of sodium, with a resultant *hyponatraemia* (lowered blood sodium level). When severe, this produces a syndrome of *water intoxication* with lethargy, weakness, and eventually fits and coma. Squamous cell carcinoma of the lung and adenocarcinoma of the kidney may produce *parathyroid hormone* (PTH), with consequent mobilisation of calcium from the bones and hence *hypercalcaemia* (elevated blood calcium). This in turn leads to secondary renal damage.

The ectopic production of hormones can best be regarded as a result of derepression in the tumour cell of genes which are not expressed in normal counterpart cells. If this is so, it might be expected that any tumour showing abnormal differentiation would be able to produce a hormone, but this is not the case. There is clearly a restriction in the types of tumours which will produce particular hormones. Thus ACTH production is mostly seen in lung cancer and never associated with breast cancer, while PTH and ADH secretion are similarly restricted to the cancers mentioned above. The explanation for these restrictions is not known. Nevertheless the derepression theory is the most likely explanation for ectopic hormonal secretion, and one which emphasizes the similarity with inappropriate production of other proteins by tumours.

Foetal or embryonic proteins

Another example of gene derepression as an indicator of altered differentiation in neoplasia is the re-expression by malignant cells of proteins normally found only in embryonic tissue. Some examples are given in Table 6.5. These proteins, some of which are tissue specific, are found in foetal tissues but disappear after birth and are not usually detectable in the adult. Their reappearance in tumours is taken to indicate a process of reversion or dedifferentiation in neoplasia to a more primitive cell type. The phenomenon is widespread and, as well as being found in several human tumours, embryonic proteins also appear on the surface of cancer cells induced experimentally in animals by carcinogenic chemicals or viruses.

726

Table 6.5 Foetal products of cancer cells.

Product	Cancer	% positive serum tests
Carcinoembryonic antigen (CEA)	Colon	77
	Pancreas	92
	Stomach	61
	Lung	76
	Breast	47
	Bone	88
	Neuroblastoma	88
	(Normals	3)
Alpha-fetoprotein (AFP)	Liver	89
	Testicular teratoma	86
	Pancreas	22
	Stomach	25
	(Normals	0)
Foetal sulphoglycoprotein antigen (FSA)	Stomach	90*
Alpha$_2$H-ferroprotein	Teratomas & others in children	80
	(Normal children	10)
Gamma-fetoprotein	Various tumours	75
Leukaemia-associated antigens (LAA)	Various leukaemias	35

*detected in gastric juice.
Data from S. O. Freedman, in *Scientific Foundations of Oncology*, ed. T. Symington and R. L. Carter (Heinemann, 1976).

Carcinoembryonic antigen (CEA) is one of the best known of such re-expressed foetal products. It was discovered by its antigenic properties when extracts of human colonic cancer tissue were injected into rabbits; after absorption with normal colonic tissue, the rabbit antisera still contained an antibody which reacted both with the cancer tissue and the gut tissue of the normal embryo. The antigen recognised by this antibody was called CEA. It is a glycoprotein found on the cell membrane of embryonic gut cells and is also shed into surrounding body fluids, but is only found very occasionally in normal adult plasma. By means of a sensitive radioimmunoassay, significant amounts of CEA are detectable in the plasma of 70-80% of patients with colorectal cancer. It is not unique to the digestive system cancers, however, and is also found in lung and breast cancer, as well as some chronic inflammatory conditions such as chronic bronchitis. Normal colon, liver, lung and breast tissue do contain a little CEA, at about 1/40–1/10,000 of the level of the concentration in colonic cancer, suggesting that the CEA gene is not completely repressed in adult cells. Detection of serum CEA is a useful diagnostic aid for certain cancers where early detection is otherwise difficult (rectum, colon, lung, pancreas). Its major clinical use at present is in monitoring a course of treatment for these cancers.

Another example is provided by *alpha-fetoprotein* (AFP), which is found in the blood of patients with liver cancer (hepatoma), testicular teratoma or viral hepatitis. AFP is a normal liver product in the foetus, but is present in only trace amounts by a few weeks after birth. In almost all cases of liver carcinoma, AFP reappears in the blood. Viral infection of the liver also sometimes causes production of AFP especially in children, at rather lower levels than in cancer. AFP is also found in some other non-neoplastic childhood conditions, especially the rare *ataxia telangiectasia*, an inherited disease involving immune deficiency, cerebellar ataxia and cutaneous telangiectasia (p. 775). Other recently discovered instances of derepressed embryonic products include the Regan isoenzyme (p. 724) found in 12% of patients with various malignancies; fetal sulphoglycoprotein antigen, which has been demonstrated in the gastric juice of 90% of cases of stomach cancer; an antigen common to embryonic and leukaemic leucocytes; and the blood-group precursor substances I,i. Besides their theoretical interest, all these products may in time find diagnostic application as reasonably specific indicators of the existence of cancer.

Another interesting aspect of the derepressed foetal proteins is that when present at the cell surface they behave as tumour-specific antigens and can become targets of attack by cells of the immune system (p. 739). Thus mice can be protected against cancers induced with chemical carcinogens or viruses by pre-immunisation with foetal cells. Apparently, the induced cancer cells share antigens with the foetus which are no longer present in the adult. When the adult is actively immunised against foetal cells, it therefore gains immunity to the cancer cell as well. Medawar has suggested that this could underlie the influence of parity on breast cancer in women. The risk of breast cancer decreases with the number of children a woman has borne, perhaps because she has become immunised against foetal antigens during her pregnancies. The age of the mother at the birth of her first child is a determining factor in this relative resistance, in that the younger the mother the greater the degree of protection. This could be because the neoplastic process in the breast also begins early in reproductive life and the immunological response must therefore be established as soon as possible to be of benefit.

3. NEOPLASIA AND CELL GENETICS

The preceding pages have described some of the abnormalities of growth and differentiation found in neoplastic cells. When a tumour cell divides, it gives rise to daughter cells which carry the same aberrations, i.e. the neoplastic change is *inheritable*. The simplest explanation is that neoplasia is the result of a permanent change in a cell's genetic material, and indeed this has been implicit in much of what has been discussed above on the subject of abnormal gene expression in tumour cells. The basis of this genetic change has been sought first in the gross chromosomal abnormalities which are a common feature of malignancy. However, it has become clear that cells of different cancers show very variable chromosomal changes and in general it has not been possible to detect chromosomal alterations common even to cancers of the same histological type. To search for the more subtle genetic changes which underlie malignancy, the technique of cell fusion has been employed and has yielded particularly exciting results.

Chromosomes of neoplastic cells

The chromosomes of malignant cells are frequently abnormal in two respects. First, there is often a deviation from the normal diploid number (46 in man) and secondly, abnormalities in the structure or shape of individual chromosomes. Such visible changes obviously represent enormous changes in nuclear DNA and it is easy to envisage that they could be connected causally with the neoplastic state. Moreover, many of the agents which are able to cause cancer experimentally, such as chemical carcinogens, ionising radiation and viruses, interact with DNA and produce visible changes in chromosomes such as breaks, gaps, fragmentation, rearrangement, formation of rings, etc. Thus it was hoped that studying the chromosomal changes of specific cancers would reveal common patterns associated with malignancy. However, this search has been disappointing; the diversity of karyotypes found in cancer cells is such that any common pattern has been impossible to discern. The one exception occurs in *chronic myeloid leukaemia* (CML), where the cells almost always share a specific chromosomal lesion called the Philadelphia chromosome (below). Despite this lack of uniformity when different cancers are compared, the cells within an individual tumour show the same abnormalities and most possess the same chromosome number and karyotypic pattern. This is because a tumour grows as a *clone* of cells, i.e. all the cells in a growth are descendents of a single cell in which the neoplastic abnormality first arose, so that they all inherit the same abnormal chromosomes.

In contrast with the considerable variation in chromosome number seen in malignancies, the chromosome count of benign tumours is nearly always the normal 46. A significant deviation from 46 in a benign tumour may therefore be an indication of malignant change. In cancer cells, the number is often near to, but not exactly 46, with a few chromosomes missing or in excess. Some cancers have considerably higher numbers, due to doubling of the normal set (tetraploidy), though in such cases the number is frequently rather in the range of 70–80 rather than the precise 92, due to loss of chromosomes from tetraploid cells.

As we have noted, in addition to an unusual chromosome number, the karyotype of each malignant tumour may have its own individual pattern and often includes distinctive 'marker' chromosomes, with recognisable structural abnormalities, carried by the majority of cells in the tumour. The sole example of a chromosome alteration which is specific for a particular type of cancer is the *Philadelphia chromosome* of CML, which is found in the neoplastic granulocytes of all patients with this disease. It is interesting that this characterises a condition which in many ways is more like a benign tumour than a malignant one. The

Philadelphia chromosome is a fragment of a normal chromosome 22 from which the long arm has been lost. However, the missing part of 22 is still present in the cell, attached to chromosome 9. This is, therefore, an example of a *translocation* between 22 and 9 rather than a deletion (see p. 817); as a result there may in fact be no change in the total genetic material of the cell.

The large number of tumours with apparently normal diploid karyotypes, shows that a cell can be neoplastic without deviating detectably in its content of DNA. In short, gross changes in the amount of DNA in the cell are probably not a necessary condition for malignancy; indeed they may in some instances be a result rather than a cause of neoplasia. This suggests that many of the genetic changes responsible for cancer are below the level of resolution of morphology or number of chromosomes and that more subtle methods will be required to detect them. One such is the use of banding techniques in which each individual chromosome can be identified by a characteristic pattern of bands, revealed by staining with Giemsa stain (G-banding) or a fluorochrome such as quinacrine mustard (Q-banding) (Figure 7.2). Changes in the banding pattern of a specific chromosome might identify a particular chromosomal region responsible for neoplastic change. Another important advance in identifying the chromosomes involved in neoplasia is somatic cell hybridisation.

Cell hybridisation and malignancy

The technique of cell fusion or hybridisation is being applied to a large number of biological problems, including the nature of genetic changes in cancer. The method involves the fusion of different cells to give a *cell hybrid*, i.e. a cell which possesses the chromosomal complement of both parent cells (Figure 6.12). The cells fused can be from different tissues of the same animal or from different species. The agents used to induce fusion include inactivated viruses, of which Sendai virus is the best known, or chemical agents such as polyethylene glycol. A hybrid formed by fusion of two diploid cells is at first tetraploid; with time, however, there is a marked tendency for chromosomes to be lost and for hybrid cells to achieve stability at a chromosome number between diploid and tetraploid. Thus, while the hybrid finally retains some chromosomes of both parents, it does not necessarily possess all of them, even in single copies. An important application of the phenomenon of chromosome loss is in *gene mapping*, because it provides a means of associating directly the presence or absence of certain cell characteristics with the retention or loss of particular chromosomes, i.e. of observing segregation.

When applied to cancer, hybridisation can provide answers to problems such as whether malignancy is a dominant or recessive trait, and on which chromosomes the genes responsible for the malignant state are located. The first of these questions concerns the nature of the genetic change which leads to cancer. If the malignant change is *dominant*, it means that a malignancy gene(s) is able to over-ride the action of the normal genes responsible for

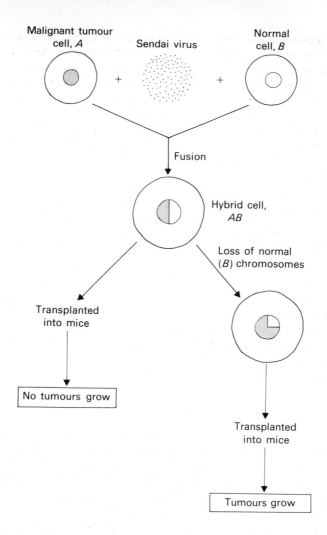

Figure 6.12 Analysis of malignancy by cell fusion (Harris-Klein experiment).

regulation of growth, differentiation, etc. On the other hand, if it is *recessive*, then the normal genes must exert a dominant controlling effect on the cell; neoplasia would then arise only when the normal genes had been lost, either by mutation or other damage to the gene or by physical chromosomal loss. In the case of a dominant malignancy gene, a hybrid formed between a tumour cell and a normal cell should be malignant; alternatively for a recessive malignancy gene, such 'tumour × normal' hybrids are expected to be normal, since the normal cell would contribute genes capable of suppressing the malignant state. Experiments to test these possibilities were carried out as shown in Figure 6.12. Malignant cells were used which were able to produce a high frequency of malignant tumours if transplanted into recipient animals; they were fused with another cell type which was either normal or very weakly tumourigenic (i.e. rarely produced tumours in recipient mice). The hybrids were tested for malignancy by transplantation into mice and counting the number of animals which developed cancers. At first such experiments seemed to show that the hybrids were as malignant as the cancer cell itself, i.e. that the cancer genes were dominant and were unaffected by the presence of the genes of the normal cell. However, at that time it was not known that hybrid cells lose chromosomes spontaneously; when this phenomenon was discovered, it was suggested that perhaps malignant hybrids had in fact lost some normal chromosomes and that this was a necessary condition for expression of malignancy. Harris and Klein in Oxford explored this possibility with various types of hybrids and found that malignancy in fact behaves as a *recessive* character. If a hybrid is formed by fusing a malignant cell with a normal cell, it will not be malignant if it retains a complete set of chromosomes of both cells. In those cases where hybrid cells were malignant, it was always found that they had lost chromosomes. Hence, genes from the normal or less malignant cell are able to suppress the deviant cancer genes, and the latter are only expressed when specific normal chromosomes have been shed. The conclusion that malignancy is recessive was reinforced by hybridisation of two malignant cell lines with each other. Here the hybrids were almost always malignant and did not require chromosome loss for the expression of malignancy. These results suggest that when a cell becomes neoplastic, certain normal genes, probably responsible for growth regulation, either become defective or are physically lost from the cell; fusion with a normal cell corrects this situation by supplying normal genes, thereby making good the defect or loss. In principle, it should be possible to discover which particular chromosomes carry the crucial genes, by correlating the loss of certain chromosomes from the hybrid with the appearance of malignant properties.

While the experiments described above have used mouse cancer cells produced in a variety of ways (e.g. spontaneously appearing, virus-transformed or chemically induced), some experiments with virus-transformed human cells have produced rather different conclusions. The human cells were transformed (i.e. caused to undergo a neoplastic change) by the tumour virus SV40 (see also p. 779). When SV40-transformed cells were fused with normal mouse cells, the hybrids produced were all malignant, even though they retained all the mouse chromosomes. Thus, in this case the malignant state appeared to be dominant. Moreover, it was possible to pinpoint the individual chromosome which was responsible for malignancy, because in some hybrids all human chromosomes except one, chromosome 7, had been lost and yet the hybrids were still malignant. When viruses transform cells, viral DNA is incorporated into the host genome; in this case it was also found that the SV40 virus DNA had been inserted specifically into chromosome 7 and had presumably dictated the change to a cancer cell. The dominant effect of SV40 virus contrasts with the recessive nature of the other malignancies tested by hybridisation.

More recently, the question of whether transformation involves dominant or recessive genetic changes has been studied by physical transfer of genes from neoplastic to normal cells by *transfection*. This is described more fully on page 805 (Figure 6.32). In brief, DNA prepared from neoplastic cells is incubated with a line of cultured normal mouse fibroblasts (NIH/3T3 cells);

some cells take up the DNA and integrate it stably into their own genomes, and after a few days the incidence of transformation in the recipient fibroblasts can be assessed. Transfection has shown that many neoplastic cells, whether spontaneously occurring or induced by chemical, physical or viral agents, possess active, *dominant* genes which can transform NIH/3T3 cells. Such genes are called *transforming genes* or *oncogenes* and at least some code for enzymes involved in growth regulation (p. 807). Evidently these genes have escaped from the repression normally exerted by cellular regulatory mechanisms. On the other hand, DNA from approximately 50% of chemically induced and spontaneous tumours does not induce efficient transformation in the transfection assay, confirming the possible occurrence of recessive genetic alterations as indicated in the Harris–Klein experiments. The divergence of results does serve to make the point that there is more than one pathway to the neoplastic phenotype and that one should not expect to find the same genetic explanation for all cancers.

For tumours in which the malignancy genes are recessive, and therefore suppressible by fusion with a normal cell, hybridisation can be used to answer the question of whether the same genes are responsible for malignancy in two unrelated cancer cells. The approach is to look for *gene complementation*, i.e. a situation in which fusion of two cancer cells produces a *non-malignant* hybrid. The implication of such complementation would be that the two parent cancer cells have different genetic defects and that each possesses the normal gene (or genes) missing in the other (Figure 6.13). However, in practice the hybrids formed by fusing two malignant cell types have nearly always been malignant. This lack of complementation suggests that the same genetic abnormality is present in the few cancer cells which have been studied in this way. One cannot say from this how many genes are abnormal in a malignant cell. In theory, a mutation at a single gene locus would produce the above result.

Figure 6.13 Principle of gene complementation.
(a) *A* and *B* are both neoplastic cells but have mutations in different genes (*x* and *y*). The hybrid therefore receives a normal *x* and *y* and behaves as a normal cell, in spite of having neoplastic parents.
(b) Cells *C* and *D* are neoplastic due to mutations in the same gene (*x*). The hybrid does not receive a normal *x* gene and is therefore neoplastic.

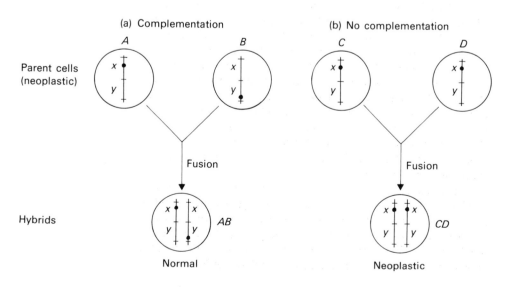

733

4. SPREAD OF MALIGNANT NEOPLASMS

The most important characteristic of malignant neoplasms, and
the one which contributes most to the death of the host, is the
ability to spread. This includes both local invasion of the surrounding tissue and spread to new near or distant sites via the
circulation. The latter is called *metastasis*, which is defined as the
colonisation by a tumour of a new site as a result of transportation
in the lymph or blood of malignant cells which break away from
the original tumour. The ability to invade locally and to metastasise varies from one tumour to another. Certain cancers, notably
the basal cell carcinoma of the skin ('rodent ulcer') are entirely
confined to local invasion, while others, including malignant
melanoma, and carcinoma of the breast and lung, metastasise
widely and set up secondary growths in different organs. Figure
6.14 shows diagrammatically the events involved in spread of
malignant melanoma. Some of the cellular properties of cancer
cells which allow them to spread are described below.

Local (primary) invasion

Cancers spread in the local tissue along lines of least resistance, notably the natural cleavage planes. Certain tissue components resist invasion, including the capsules of organs such as
kidney and liver, artery walls and the periosteum of bones. Dense
fibrous tissue and cartilage also act as barriers to invasion,
probably because they are resistant to breakdown by tumour cells
or their products. Three distinct components in tumour invasion
are recognised, namely mechanical pressure of the growing
tumour cell mass, the amoeboid motility of malignant cells, and
their release of enzymes which destroy host tissue matrix.

Pressure

It is likely that the increased pressure within a tumour, especially
one which is growing rapidly, will force cells out into the tissue
and into adjoining spaces. However, some tumours are highly
invasive yet relatively slow growing, such as carcinoma of the
breast. Moreover, if fragments of normal and cancer tissue are
placed together in culture, the neoplastic cells still infiltrate
the normal tissue under conditions where no pressure is
generated. Clearly other factors must also be involved.

Motility of cancer cells

The abnormal behaviour of cancer cells in tissue culture has been
described (p. 710), and includes the loss of normal contact inhibition of movement. For example, when normal fibroblasts are
placed in a culture dish, they migrate over the surface until they
make contact with neighbouring cells, whereupon motility is inhibited. Sarcoma cells, in contrast, continue to migrate over each
other and their movement is not inhibited by normal fibroblasts.
It seems very likely that the membrane changes seen in malignant

734

cells which are responsible for their decreased adhesiveness are also involved in loss of inhibition of motility. These changes, which include increased surface charge, lectin agglutinability and decreased formation of junctions, have been described on pages 710–719. Treating the surface of malignant cells with lectins such as concanavalin A, under non-agglutinating conditions, can cause them to revert to normal motility in culture, as well as restoring contact inhibition of division. Once again, cyclic nucleotides are probably the link between membrane contact and intracellular events, such as changes in the structures of microfilaments and microtubules responsible for cell movement. Thus normal growth characteristics, including motility inhibition, are restored when tumour cells are treated with cyclic AMP. In some cases, contact with normal cells also inhibits the movement of cancer cells in culture, suggesting that the latter could still receive, but not send out, inhibitory signals, though in other experiments the growth and movement of tumour cells was not affected by the presence of normal cells in the culture.

Release of enzymes by tumour cells

Invasive tumours have been found to release enzymes which both damage host cells and digest connective tissue and tissue matrix. The enzymes found associated with cancers include collagenase, hyaluronidase and lysosomal enzymes. The latter are often increased in tumour cells and could be released when the cells die or divide. The invasiveness of breast carcinoma has been correlated with the amount of collagenase produced by the tumour. We have noted previously that release of lysosomal enzymes is one way in which the membranes of the tumour cells themselves may be damaged, leading to loss of adhesiveness and contact inhibition of movement and mitosis (p. 718).

Metastasis

The local invasion of the tissue is the start of a process which for many cancers eventually leads to the establishment of new (*secondary*) growths at sites removed from the original (*primary*) tumour. Metastasis involves the *detachment* of cells from the primary tumour following their *invasion* of lymphatics and blood vessels; then follows their *transportation* as emboli in the lymphatics to regional lymph nodes and/or in the blood to more distant sites; and finally their *arrest, penetration* and *growth* as secondary deposits in the new tissue. These events are illustrated in Figure 6.14.

Detachment

Detachment of cells from the primary tumour is made possible by the reduced adhesive forces holding them together. Enzymes may also play a role in weakening cell junctions.

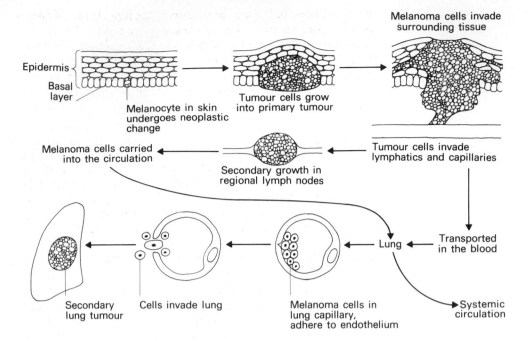

Epidermis

Basal layer

Melanocyte in skin undergoes neoplastic change

Tumour cells grow into primary tumour

Melanoma cells invade surrounding tissue

Melanoma cells carried into the circulation

Secondary growth in regional lymph nodes

Tumour cells invade lymphatics and capillaries

Transported in the blood

Lung

Systemic circulation

Secondary lung tumour

Cells invade lung

Melanoma cells in lung capillary, adhere to endothelium

Figure 6.14 Spread of malignant melanoma.

Lymphatic spread

Initial spread via lymphatics is particularly common for carcinomas, whereas sarcomas are dispersed in the blood rather than the lymph. (Carcinoma cells can, of course, also be transported by the blood, but generally at a later stage). It is not known how tumour cells enter lymphatics, but having done so they may sometimes grow in cords inside the vessel to the regional lymph node or more frequently form clumps or emboli which are transported in the lymph. They then reach the local nodes via the afferent lymphatics and if trapped in the node set up a secondary growth. Gradually the lymph node is entirely replaced by the metastatic tumour growth, and spread to the next group of nodes may then occur. Some cancers tend to invade local lymphatics and spread to the lymph nodes very early, including malignant melanoma and carcinoma of the tongue; others, such as squamous cell skin carcinoma, spread to the nodes rather late. Basal cell carcinomas do not colonise the nodes at all. It is not known why carcinomas are spread more frequently to lymph nodes than sarcomas; it may be due to differences in the cell surfaces of the two types of neoplasm. The lymph nodes are not perfect filters of tumour cells and it is quite possible for cancer cells to pass through them without being trapped; they then feed quickly into the circulation.

Blood spread

Cancer cells can be carried to the bloodstream in lymph via the thoracic duct, or alternatively may penetrate veins directly at the site of the primary tumour. Again, the details of such penetration are unknown. Sarcomas, as noted above, are commonly spread in the circulation, and so are carcinomas of the lung, breast, kidney, prostate and thyroid. The presence of tumour cells in the circulation is not in itself an indication of bad prognosis, since the overwhelming majority quickly die there and only a very small percentage survives to set up secondary tumours. In the circulation, tumour cells again form emboli by aggregating with each other or with lymphocytes or platelets.

Arrest of tumour cells

Tumour emboli eventually become trapped in the narrow lumen of capillaries and stick to the endothelium. Their adherence is encouraged by formation of fibrin and the development of a local thrombus around them, which may be initiated by release of thromboplastic agents from the tumour cells themselves. The administration of anticoagulants such as heparin or fibrinolytic agents such as plasmin (p. 636) reduces the incidence of metastasis by interfering with the development of these fibrin thrombi. While the formation of fibrin is probably not essential for metastasis, it does serve to protect the tumour cells from haemodynamic forces and circulating host lymphocytes. Somehow the tumour cells then penetrate the vessel wall into the tissue, though the details are not clear. Tumour cells seem to move between endothelial cell junctions rather like emigrating leucocytes in inflammation (Section 1), though much more slowly. The release of tumour enzymes probably aids invasion and destruction of the basement membrane.

Growth of metastases

If the tumour cells are to establish a successful secondary growth in the new tissue, they must soon acquire a fibrovascular stroma to provide them with sufficient blood supply. To this end, the cells may release factors which stimulate angiogenesis (proliferation of blood vessels). Some tumours secrete prostaglandins (PGE_2) which may also play a role in establishing the new growth. Once established with adequate blood supply, the tumour will usually grow relentlessly in its new site and eventually become clinically evident. Sometimes, however, metastases become apparent years after surgical removal of the primary growth. This phenomenon is known as *dormancy* and is seen with cancers of the breast and kidney. Apparently, tumour cells can remain in a viable, but resting, non-proliferative state for a very long time, to become reactivated years after seeding, perhaps as a result of a change in local conditions. The factors responsible for reactivating growth of these cells may include an enhanced blood supply to the tissue, or mechanical or chemical damage; a decrease in host immunological resistance could also be involved.

Distribution of metastases

The occurrence of metastases in lymph nodes is readily

understood as the result of invasion of the local lymphatics by tumour cells and their transportation, or growth, to the regional nodes. Cancer cells carried in the blood do not set up metastases in all tissues equally. The favoured sites for secondary growths are the liver, lungs, bone marrow, brain and adrenal glands, in that order. In contrast, tissues such as skin and spleen are rarely and skeletal muscle hardly ever involved. To some extent this pattern can be explained on the basis of mechanical trapping of tumour emboli by the narrow lumen of capillaries. Thus, emboli which enter the systemic veins, either directly from the primary tumour itself or from the thoracic duct lymph, will inevitably pass through the lung capillaries, which will act as a first filter, and indeed the lung is a very common site of secondary growths. The liver, however, is an even more frequent site, and although cells of tumours of the gastrointestinal tract may be drained there in the portal vein, the liver also attracts cells of other tumours, such as breast and kidney carcinomas, and melanomas. Likewise, the development of metastases in the brain and adrenals can only be explained by transportation of cancer cells in the arterial circulation. Tumour cells can enter the arteries either from secondary deposits in the lung, or can perhaps squeeze through pulmonary capillaries or even bypass them altogether by traversing shunts. Certainly systemic metastases can occur without evidence of lung deposits. Once in the arterial circulation, there is obvious selectivity of tumour cells for certain 'favourable' organs. This phenomenon can be studied experimentally by injecting tumour cells directly into the left side of the heart. When this is done, some organs such as the spleen or skeletal muscle generally resist metastatic growth while others, such as the liver and lung, apparently favour growth. Furthermore, cancer cells of different origins show distinctive patterns of organ involvement. The basis for the resistance of some sites and the favourable nature of others is not well understood, but probably involves the ease of access of the tumour to the tissue and the suitability of local conditions within the tissue, sometimes expressed in terms of a favourable 'soil' for the 'seeded' cancer cells.

Host factors

Host factors will play a role in the occurrence of metastases, perhaps the most important being the host immune system, as discussed in detail below. General immune depression enhances metastasis and may also affect the distribution of secondary growths in different tissues.

THE IMMUNE RESPONSE AGAINST NEOPLASTIC CELLS

The idea that the immune system prevents the development of tumours by recognising and eliminating neoplastic cells as they arise was first formulated at the turn of the century by Paul Ehrlich (1909) among others. The essential condition for immunological defence against tumours is that the tumour cells carry *specific antigens* which distinguish them from host cells, and for many tumours such antigens have been demonstrated. A variety of different mechanisms have recently been discovered whereby cell-mediated immunity can lead to killing of tumour cells; and moreover it has been found that individuals in whom such immune responses are depressed are more likely to develop certain malignant neoplasms than normal individuals. The term *immunological surveillance* is used to describe the concept that host immunity prevents the majority of neoplastic cells from developing into tumours, and the evidence in its favour is described below. A practical application of the surveillance concept is found in *immunotherapy* of tumours, in which attempts are made to treat cancer by improving the patient's own antitumour response. Recently, the optimistic view that all tumours are monitored by the immune system, and therefore potentially treatable by immunotherapy, has been called into question and it appears that the surveillance role of the immune system is probably more restricted than was originally supposed.

Antigenicity of tumours

The first suggestion that tumours may be recognised immunologically came from early attempts to transplant them from one animal to another. The fact that tumour transplants were regularly rejected by their recipients led to the conclusion that tumours are antigenic and should therefore be susceptible to rejection by their original host as well. However, since the donor and recipient in these early experiments were usually unrelated, rejection was caused by the reaction against transplantation (histocompatibility) antigens on the graft rather than antigens specific for the tumour. The demonstration that tumours have unique antigenic determinants of their own could only be achieved by transplantation between genetically identical (syngeneic) animals, which accept normal tissue grafts from each other. Immunological rejection of a tumour by a syngeneic animal must be due to recognition of tumour-specific antigens. Such experiments are often carried out in mice because of the availability of inbred strains, all mice within each strain being syngeneic. Before testing for tumour rejection, recipient animals are first immunised by injection of syngeneic tumour cells in a non-dividing state (e.g. after X-irradiation); such cells cannot grow but serve to stimulate specific antitumour immunity. Later, the same animals receive inoculations of living, dividing cells of the same tumour in numbers which would normally 'take', i.e. develop into tumours and kill the host. If the immunisation has been successful, the neoplastic cells are rejected and tumours fail to grow, and this has now been demonstrated for many tumours. The rejection by an animal of a syngeneic tumour graft proves that the tumour cells carry their own specific antigens, which are called *tumour-specific transplantation antigens* (TSTAs).

In the light of these findings, tumours would be expected to be antigenic in the animals in which they first arise and should stimulate an immune response. In fact a state of immunity often does exist even in animals which carry growing tumours. This can be demonstrated by taking some cells from an animal's own tumour and transplanting them to a different site on the same animal, whereupon it is found that the transplanted cells are indeed rejected, a phenomenon called *concomitant immunity*. Thus a seemingly paradoxical situation exists in which animals have developed immunity against their own tumour cells, yet the tumours continue to grow. Evidently the immune response can only deal efficiently with a small number of tumour cells and is inadequate to reject a large tumour load.

Types of tumour-associated antigens

The antigens which label the tumour cell as 'foreign' and which enable lymphocytes to kill it are present at the tumour cell surface. Membrane changes are a universal feature of neoplasia and some are intimately involved in the loss of growth control (p. 710). Some of these changes present themselves as TSTAs. There is an important difference between chemically-induced and virally-induced tumour cells in connection with their surface antigens. The TSTAs of each chemically-induced tumour are *unique* to that tumour and are not shared by other tumours, even those induced by the same agent, regardless of similarities in cell morphology. It follows that immunisation with one chemically-induced tumour, in the manner described above, is highly specific and will not protect the animal against the growth of any other tumour. In contrast, all cells transformed by the same oncogenic virus share *common* surface antigens regardless of differences in cell morphology. Thus any tumour produced by polyoma virus, for example, will be able to stimulate immunity against other polyoma-induced neoplasms, even if some are sarcomas and others are carcinomas; but a polyoma-induced tumour cell will not immunise against an SV40-induced tumour.

Virus-coded antigens on transformed cells are of two types. Some are evidently components of the virus particle itself and are found both on the virus envelope and the tumour cell membrane. This would be expected for RNA viruses which bud from the surface of tumour cells, since envelope glycoproteins enter the cell membrane as part of the budding process. There are also antigens on virus-transformed cells which, though coded by the virus, are not present on the virus particles. Virus transformation is also accompanied by the presence of antigens inside the transformed cell, particularly in the nucleus, e.g. the T antigen (p. 783). These intracellular antigens are not involved in the rejection of tumour cells.

In addition to the above antigens, many tumours also express proteins which are normally only present in *embryonic* cells and which are therefore antigenic in the adult. They are rather weak antigens and are probably not very important in tumour rejection. However, they are particularly significant in diagnosis since they are released into the blood where they can be detected by sensitive immunological assays. Some examples have been described on p. 726 and include the carcinoembryonic antigen of colonic cancer and alpha-fetoprotein associated with hepatomas.

740

We may note at this point that not all tumours are antigenic; in some, TSTAs are apparently absent.

Immunological surveillance

Since many neoplastic cells are antigenic, the immune system has the opportunity of recognising tumour cells as they arise and responding against them. According to the immunological surveillance hypothesis, tumour cells are continually arising in the body but the majority are eliminated by the immune response; only those cells which can 'escape' from surveillance can develop into tumours. One of the predictions of this theory is that neoplasms should be more frequent in individuals in whom the immune response is depressed, either by immunosuppression or immunodeficiency disease. This has been borne out by the high incidence of certain cancers in patients receiving immunosuppressive drugs following kidney transplantation and in children with various immunodeficiency syndromes. In both groups, the neoplasms most frequently seen are those of the lymphoid system itself (lymphomas, leukaemias, reticulum cell sarcomas), though others also arise. The increased cancer risk is a serious problem in transplant patients where, for the neoplasms mentioned, the incidence is at least 100 times that of the normal population. Skin cancers are also seen in transplant patients, especially in sunny climates. The use of cytotoxic drugs outside the transplantation field, for instance in rheumatoid arthritis, involves a similar hazard. (Note that immunosuppressants are often also mutagens; the increased incidence of neoplasms may owe as much to their carcinogenicity as to their immunosuppressive action.) Similarly, inherited deficiency of T lymphocyte function, as in severe combined immunodeficiency, the Wiskott–Aldrich syndrome and ataxia telangiectasia, is accompanied by a very high incidence of leukaemias and lymphoreticular neoplasms, which are again about 100 times more common than in children with normal immune systems.

Although this increase is very striking and confirms a role for surveillance by the immune system, it is clearly a selective increase; while other cancers do occur in these circumstances, they are far less frequent than the lymphoid neoplasms. It is possible that the lymphoid system is particularly prone to neoplasia, e.g. through viral infection, and that normally the surveillance process successfully destroys transformed cells as they appear (see EBV below). On the other hand, the relative infrequency of tumours of most other organs in immunosuppression or immunodeficiency argues against an important role for immune surveillance in limiting the appearance of neoplasms outside the lymphoid system. A similar conclusion comes from an animal model of T cell deficiency, namely the *nude mouse*. Besides being hairless, nude mice lack a thymus and consequently have no circulating T cells. They are very susceptible to fatal infection by pathogens which require cell-mediated immunity for their elimination, such as viruses. When the incidence of neoplasms is examined, there is again found to be an increase in frequency of lymphoreticular neoplasms, while most other organs have no more tumours than normal animals. Moreover, induction of neoplasms by chemical carcinogens such as methylcholanthrene is no more efficient in thymusless mice than normal mice, despite the strong antigens which such tumours can carry.

Some of the best examples of effective immunological surveillance are provided by the response against tumours induced by viruses. Polyoma in mice provides a good illustration. Despite the fact that polyoma virus infection is widespread both in wild and laboratory mice, polyoma-induced tumours hardly ever arise. To induce tumours in normal animals, it is necessary to inject polyoma virus at the neonatal stage. The reason adults do not succumb to polyoma tumours, even when injected with the virus, is that they are able to make an effective immune response against the virus-transformed cells. This can be proved by various immunosuppressive measures, such as neonatal thymectomy or treatment with antilymphocyte serum: immunosuppressed mice develop polyoma tumours even after infection as adults. The same is true of adult nude mice. Protection against the tumours in such animals can be provided by transfer of lymphocytes from syngeneic mice immunised with a polyoma tumour, but transfer of antibody is ineffective. Thus the main reason tumours do not develop in normal adult mice after infection with polyoma virus is that they mount an effective cell-mediated (T cell) response against the tumour cells. The oncogenicity of polyoma in newborns is a result of the relative slowness with which very young animals make an immune response, rather than the development of tolerance to polyoma antigens; by the time the response develops, the tumours are too large to be controlled. Neoplasms caused by other oncogenic viruses, such as murine and avian leukaemias, are evidently also controlled by immunological surveillance, as indicated by the need to inject the virus into very young animals for neoplasms to develop. In chicks, tolerance appears to be induced by early exposure to the virus and the birds have a permanent viraemia (Figure 6.30).

In man, infection with Epstein–Barr virus (EBV) provides an example of successful surveillance by the immune system. As described elsewhere (p. 794), outside certain tropical areas or particular racial groups, infection with EBV in childhood leads to immunity while infection as an adolescent can lead to infectious mononucleosis. The self-limiting character of this disease is due to the development of cytotoxic T cells which proliferate extensively and kill the EBV-transformed B lymphocytes. In contrast, in children infected with EBV in areas of hyperendemic malaria, Burkitt's lymphoma may develop. It has been suggested that malaria may exert an immunosuppressive effect which allows some transformed cells to grow into lymphomas (p. 795). Acute malarial infections in mice do suppress the immune response. A property of Burkitt's lymphoma which supports the hypothesis of 'escape from surveillance' is that although EBV transforms many B cells at the same time, the lymphomas are single clones (i.e. all the lymphoma cells are descended from a single transformed cell). An explanation for the monoclonality of Burkitt's lymphoma is that only the occasional cell is able to escape from surveillance and grow into a tumour. The significant rates of spontaneous regression and complete cure after chemotherapy indicate successes for the immune system in Burkitt's lymphoma. In the case of another EBV-associated neoplasm, nasopharyngeal carcinoma, an inherited defect in immune response associated with HLA-type may allow transformed cells to grow (p. 793). Finally, the appearance of lymphomas due to EBV in graft recipients undergoing immunosuppression is an excellent illustration of the importance of surveillance. Most normal adults carry a permanent latent infection by EBV in some B cells, and without the controlling action of cytotoxic T cells, transformed clones would grow out much more frequently than they do (see p. 173).

In summary, control of neoplastic cells by the immune system occurs in some, but by no means all cases. Certain neoplasms, notably those of the lymphoid system and those induced by viruses, are recognised and killed by T lymphocytes, while for other types of neoplasm immune surveillance does not play a significant role. One may reasonably ask why surveillance does not extend to all antigenic tumour cells. It is possible that lymphocytes cannot reach some peripheral sites and thus do not get the opportunity to react against certain tumours until they begin to spread, when the immune response is too late to be decisive. However, a beneficial effect of immunity even at this stage may be to reduce metastasis. It is often noted that secondary growths are relatively rare when compared with the frequency of tumour cells in the blood; in part, this may be because an immune reaction against tumour cells can occur in the circulation whereas the primary growth was inaccessible. In experimental animals, tumours which do not normally metastasise spontaneously will do so after immunosuppression.

Mechanisms of tumour cell destruction

Several mechanisms exist whereby the immune system can destroy neoplastic cells: in general they come under the category of cell-mediated immunity. Their study has depended largely on *in vitro* tests, two of which have been particularly useful. These are (a) the colony inhibition technique, which measures the ability of lymphocytes to inhibit the formation of tumour colonies from cells seeded onto small Petri dishes, and (b) the more generally applicable microcytotoxicity test, in which the release of isotope from tumour cells labelled with radioactive chromium ^{51}Cr is used as an index of cell destruction. At least four different modes of cell-mediated immunity against tumours can occur, in addition to the possible effects of antibody and complement, and are illustrated in Figure 6.15. In brief they are as follows.

Cytotoxic T lymphocytes

T cells can recognise surface antigens of tumour cells and develop into cytotoxic effector cells. Killing of the tumour cell requires direct contact with the T cell, but complement is not involved.

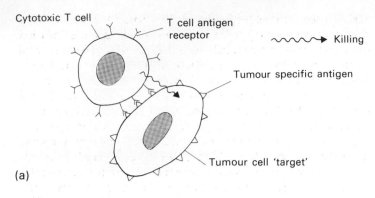

(a)

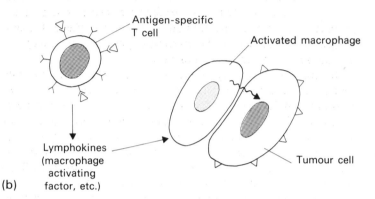

(b)

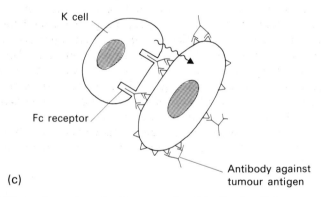

(c)

Figure 6.15 Mechanisms of cell-mediated killing of tumour cells.
(a) Cytotoxic T cell (role of MHC molecules is omitted).
(b) Activated macrophage.
(c) K cells (antibody-dependent cell-mediated cytotoxicity).

This has been described in some detail in Section 2, in connection with killing of virus-infected cells, and a similar mechanism probably applies to tumours. Thus the T cell needs to recognise both the tumour antigen and a histocompatibility molecule on the tumour cell for effective kill, as described on p. 177.

Natural killer (NK) cells

Recently it has been discovered that lymphocytes of *normal* human individuals can kill some tumour cells *in vitro*; a similar phenomenon has been found in mice, where it is correlated with the natural resistance of certain strains to transplantation of specific neoplasms. The term *natural killer*, abbreviated as

NK, is used for these cells, though like 'natural' antibodies they may have been stimulated by antigens to which the animal has been previously exposed. NK cells discovered to date react with tumour cells selectively, particularly with those carrying C-type RNA particles such as mouse leukaemias. NK cells are not T cells, since they are present in athymic (nude) mice, and indeed their origin is not well understood; they have some characteristics of macrophages, but may be an independent lymphocyte line. NK cells may play as important a role in immune surveillance as the better known cytotoxic T cells. We have previously noted the low incidence of spontaneous tumours among nude mice, and this has been used as a strong argument against an important role for cell-mediated immunity in the control of neoplasia. The discovery of the non-thymus-dependent NK cell provides an explanation for the resistance of nude mice to spontaneous tumour induction and emphasizes the diversity of possible immunological mechanisms involved in surveillance.

Because they lack cytotoxic T cells, nude mice are convenient animals in which to investigate the role of NK cells. Studies in nude mice have confirmed that NK cells can be a highly effective defence against certain tumours. For example, as few as 10–100 HeLa or BHK tumour cells will 'take' in all nude mice, but if these same cells are first infected with any of six C-type retroviruses, inocula of 10^6 or 10^7 cells fail to grow. The persistently infected tumour cells are eliminated by NK cells, whereas the uninfected parent cells are not. Another useful mouse strain is a mutant called *beige*, which is deficient in NK cells. The beige mouse seems to suffer the murine equivalent of the Chédiak–Higashi syndrome (p. 25), and people with the latter condition are also NK cell deficient. Tumour cells which can be killed by NK cells *in vitro*, such as a murine melanoma line, show enhanced growth and increased numbers of metastases in beige as compared with normal mice, suggesting that NK cells restrict metastasis. It is interesting that a high incidence of lymphomas is seen in Chédiak–Higashi patients, perhaps connected with their NK cell deficiency. Reports of diminished activity of NK cells in cancer patients lends similar support to the antitumour role of these cells.

Macrophages

These have also been found to kill tumour cells, killing being by contact between macrophage and tumour cell rather than by phagocytosis. The cytotoxic action of macrophages is generally non-specific and requires their activation by lymphokines released from specifically sensitised T cells (p. 147). This has been exploited as a means of cancer therapy, in which tumour cells are destroyed as a side-effect of a delayed hypersensitivity response against another antigen, such as tuberculin (p. 163). It seems that macrophages which are non-specifically activated by T cells responding to tuberculin can proceed to attack tumour cells in the same area. The clinical use of this antitumour action of inflammatory responses is described further on p. 749.

K cells

These cells are able to kill targets which have first been coated with specific antibody. The K cell possesses Fc receptors, rather than specific antigen receptors, and uses them to bind to antibody-coated tumour cells; hence the term 'antibody-dependent cell-mediated cytotoxicity' for K cell activity. Killing then follows membrane contact and does not require complement. K cells are not thymus-derived, nor are they B cells, but seem to be related to monocytes (see also p. 145).

Antibody and complement in killing of tumour cells

Other than in collaboration with K cells, antibody is believed to be much less significant as a means of killing tumour cells than cell-mediated mechanisms. Thus immunity against tumours in mice can be transferred with reactive cells, but usually not with specific antibody. Leukaemias may be an exception, however, and complement-mediated lysis by specific antibody may be important in immunity. In contrast, antibody often improves the growth of neoplastic cells *in vivo*, by protecting them from cell-mediated immunity, and this is described below.

Escape from surveillance

Given the existence of these immunological mechanisms for killing neoplastic cells, and assuming that at least in some cases tumours are accessible to lymphocytes, it is important to discover how successfully-growing tumours manage to avoid immunological destruction. A variety of possibilities can be envisaged. Perhaps the most obvious is that the successful tumour cell is one which has lost its antigenicity in the host and therefore does not stimulate an immune response. Not all tumours are strongly antigenic and those with poor antigenicity should be at a selective advantage when faced with the immune system. The weak antigenicity of many spontaneous tumours in animals may well reflect 'immunoselection'. Another possibility is that the host is unable for genetic reasons to recognise particular tumour antigens. Elsewhere (Sections 2 and 7) we have noted that immune response (Ir) genes in the major histocompatibility gene complex control the levels of immune responses to specific antigens, and that some individuals may be 'low responders' while others are 'high responders' to an antigen, depending on their genetic constitution. Such Ir genes may well determine the efficiency with which responses to specific tumour antigens develop. Inherited low responsiveness on the part of the host would allow specific neoplasms to grow even if carrying potentially strong antigens. We have noted a possible example of this in nasopharyngeal carcinoma, susceptibility to which seems to be associated with HLA type. An influence of HLA type on acute childhood lymphocytic leukaemia and Hodgkin's disease has sometimes been detected.

However in many cases, including human neoplasms, it is

possible to demonstrate clearly both that the tumour cells are antigenic in the host and that an immune response has been stimulated. The phenomenon of concomitant immunity has already been noted (p. 740). In man, it has been shown for carcinomas of the breast, colon, cervix and bladder, for neuroblastoma and for malignant melanoma that lymphocytes taken from the patient have the ability to kill the patient's own tumour cells *in vitro*. Despite this evidence of immunity in the patient, the tumour continues to grow. Escape from surveillance may be due to an inadequacy in the number of killer lymphocytes produced by the patient compared to the size of the tumour, i.e. the immune response cannot deal with a large number of tumour cells, although it can stop a small number from growing. If the development of the immune response is for any reason delayed while neoplastic cells are starting to grow, the tumour has a chance to develop to a size that cannot later be destroyed, an effect which has been called 'sneaking through'. It is therefore significant that many chemical carcinogens exert an immunosuppressive effect, which would help the neoplastic cells to get a 'head start' over the immune response.

The discovery which has received most attention as an escape pathway for tumours is the presence in the serum of cancer patients or tumour-bearing animals of factors which specifically interfere with cell-mediated immunity against tumour antigens. Such *blocking factors* were first demonstrated in the colony inhibition assay (p. 743), which measures the ability of lymphocytes to prevent the growth of tumour colonies *in vitro*. Appropriate sera taken from patients in which the tumour was growing could inhibit the action of antitumour lymphocytes, and allow tumour colonies to form despite the presence of killer cells. The serum blocking effect was tumour-specific. At first it was thought that blocking factors were *antibodies* against the tumour antigens, which by binding to the surface of tumour cells would inhibit contact by cytotoxic or other effector cells (Figure 6.16a). It could be demonstrated that antitumour antibodies were sometimes able to improve the growth of tumours *in vivo*, just as antibodies against histocompatibility antigens can increase the survival of foreign tissue grafts (*immunological enhancement*, p. 174). However, this explanation for the blocking activity of sera is now untenable, because it was found that blocking factors rapidly disappear from sera when tumours are surgically removed from the animal or patient. It seems more likely, therefore, that the blocking factor is the *tumour-specific antigen* itself, possibly in the form of a complex with antibody. It is known that cells shed their surface antigens as they grow. Free antigen in the fluid around a growing tumour could block cell-mediated immunity by combining with the specific receptors on cytotoxic T cells or NK cells, as shown in Figure 6.16b. Complexes of tumour antigen and antibody would provide even more effective blockade of T cell receptors (Figure 6.16c). Blocking factors could also account for the inverse relationship we have noted between the effectiveness of antitumour immunity and tumour size—the larger the number of

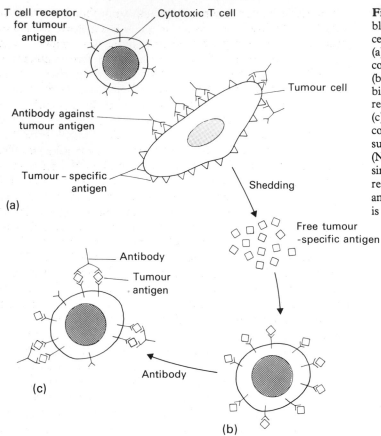

T cell receptor for tumour antigen

Cytotoxic T cell

Antibody against tumour antigen

Tumour cell

Tumour – specific antigen

Shedding

(a)

Antibody

Tumour antigen

Free tumour -specific antigen

Antibody

(c)

(b)

Figure 6.16 Mechanisms of blocking the cytotoxic action of T cells.
(a) Blocking by antibody covering tumour antigens.
(b) Blocking by free antigen binding to T cell or NK cell receptor.
(c) Blocking by antigen–antibody complexes at T cell or NK cell surface.
(Note that, for purposes of simplification, associated recognition of tumour antigen and an MHC molecule by T cells is ignored in b and c.)

tumour cells, the more tumour antigen would be shed to block cell-mediated immunity.

Thus there is a variety of possible methods by which tumours might avoid destruction by host immune defence. A combination of different escape mechanisms may be required to enable the tumour to establish itself, especially in the period when the tumour mass is small and therefore most vulnerable.

Immunotherapy of cancer

There has been considerable interest for many years in using the specific antitumour potential of the immune system in the treatment of cancer, though for the present this remains an area of promise rather than great achievement. It is unlikely that immunological methods alone will be successful as a treatment for widespread malignant disease. Rather, immunotherapy may have its place as an adjunct to surgery, radiotherapy and chemotherapy where these methods fail to eradicate cancer cells completely. For instance, chemotherapy in its present form, with a few exceptions, cannot completely eliminate disseminated tumour cells because the doses required would be toxic to normal tissues. Immune responses which, as we have noted, are successful in dealing with a small tumour load, may be useful in seeking out and killing remaining neoplastic cells. One approach in current use is active immunisation of patients using their own tumour cells, killed by irradiation, as the antigen. The method, as used in treatment of acute myeloblastic leukaemia, is to remove large numbers of leukaemic cells from the patient before commencing chemotherapy and to store them frozen. The patient then receives intensive chemotherapy until remission is secured; chemotherapy is then continued and at the same time the patient's own irradiated leukaemia cells are injected subcutaneously together with attenuated mycobacteria (BCG). The latter act as an adjuvant, improving the immune response to the inoculated cells. It seems that leukaemic patients maintained by a combination of chemotherapy and immunotherapy survive longer than control groups on chemotherapy alone. It was also reported by Mathé in 1970 that BCG alone was effective in controlling childhood leukaemia after chemotherapy. This generated a great deal of interest in the possible use of adjuvants such as BCG or *Corynebacterium parvum* as antitumour agents which would act by increasing the activity of the reticuloendothelial system (e.g. activation of macrophages). However, controlled clinical trials in Britain and America have failed to demonstrate a beneficial effect of administration of BCG alone in acute leukaemia after chemotherapy.

BCG has also been used in the local treatment of tumours, by virtue of the fact that delayed hypersensitivity reactions can lead to nonspecific killing of tumour cells by activated macrophages (p. 745). When injected directly into skin melanomas, BCG sometimes causes regression following an intense inflammatory response (the patient being sensitive to BCG as a result of previous exposure). It appears that macrophages which infiltrate the area of the delayed hypersensitivity response become endowed with antitumour properties after activation by lymphokines (p. 147). The activated macrophages do not kill normal cells in the area. The use of BCG in this way is not usually recommended if surgery could be used instead to remove a local tumour deposit. A similar approach is also successfully applied in treatment of skin carcinomas. Patients are first sensitised to dinitrochlorobenzene (DNCB) to produce a state of specific reactivity; DNCB is then later painted on the skin at the site of the tumour. In this way a delayed hypersensitivity response to DNCB is elicited at the tumour site, which can successfully eradicate basal cell carcinomas. Once again, macrophages are the agents of nonspecific tumour cell destruction following their activation by T cells reacting against the sensitising agent (DNCB). (Alternatively tuberculin can be used after BCG sensitisation.)

Uses of monoclonal antibodies against tumour cells

The diagnosis and therapy of cancer is already benefiting from the availability of monoclonal antibodies against tumour antigens. The characteristics of monoclonal antibodies have been described in Section 2 and it will be recalled that their particular advantages over antisera are their homogeneity, unique specificity and potentially unlimited supply. Monoclonal antibodies have been made against the antigens of several neoplasms, including leukaemias, melanoma, colorectal carcinoma, neuroblastoma, etc.; they do not all show an absolute specificity for tumour cells, however, as some tumour antigens are expressed at a low level on normal cells. Diagnostically, these antibodies can be used to identify neoplastic cells in tissue sections and blood samples and to discriminate between cell types which may be hard to distinguish morphologically (e.g. leukaemias due to different classes of lymphocyte). By conjugation with a radioactive label, monoclonal antibodies can be used to detect cancer cells in the body by imaging techniques (scintigrams).

Particular interest centres on the therapeutic potential of monoclonal antibodies. Those of the appropriate classes would be expected to kill tumour cells *in vivo* by the cytotoxic action of complement or K cells or, if the neoplastic cells are present in the circulation, by specific opsonisation. However, a more promising general application is in the *targeting* of drugs or other cytotoxic agents: the monoclonal antibody is conjugated to a drug, enzyme or toxin subunit and used as a carrier to specifically direct the agent onto the tumour cell. Thus, the antibody is given a 'warhead' to destroy tumour cells to which it binds. (Ehrlich originally coined the term 'magic bullet' for antibodies which he thought could be used to destroy specific cellular targets in the body responsible for a disease, but 'warhead' is more in line with modern developments in weaponry!) Because antibody targeting makes a drug specific for the tumour, many of the toxic side-effects of chemotherapy should be avoidable. As well as standard cytotoxic agents, the active moieties of toxins such as diphtheria toxin, ricin and abrin have been conjugated to monoclonal anti-tumour antibodies, creating 'immunotoxins'. The action of these conjugates depends on the ability of the active (A) fragment to enter the cell after binding and exert its lethal enzymatic action (p. 410). Antibody–toxin conjugates will indeed kill tumour cells selectively *in vitro* and their use *in vivo* is being explored. However, it seems unlikely in principle that targeting of drugs or toxins with antibodies could be wholly effective in eradicating tumours. One forseeable problem is that if just a few of the cells in the tumour failed to express the specific antigen, they would survive and the tumour would thus ultimately grow back.

Another application of monoclonal antibodies in therapy is in the removal of malignant cells from bone marrow. Doses of chemotherapeutic drugs are often limited by myelotoxicity, and one way to overcome this is to remove cells from the patient's bone marrow before starting the treatment and reinfuse them afterwards. Neoplastic cells which may have infiltrated the bone marrow must obviously be eliminated before reinfusion, and this can be achieved with cytotoxic monoclonal antibodies.

CAUSES OF NEOPLASIA

There is little doubt that major causative factors for most cancers are present in the environment. This emerges clearly from the epidemiological evidence described on pages 699–709, particularly from the associations between certain cancers and individual habits or occupations. The fact that international variations in the frequencies of various cancers disappear in the children of individuals who migrate from one country to another is good evidence that these cancers are environmentally rather than racially determined. Genetic factors play a major role in only a few rare forms of human cancer, such as skin cancer in *xeroderma pigmentosum* (p. 773), colonic cancer in *familial polyposis* and some rare tumours of the nervous system. In common cancers, such as lung, stomach, colon and breast, a certain inherited predisposition can be demonstrated in studies with identical twins or families, and it would indeed be anticipated that the effects of environmental agents would in some cases be influenced by host genotype. By and large, however, genetic susceptibility seems to play only a minor part in common cancers (see p. 875).

A *carcinogen* can be defined as a substance which increases the risk of development of a cancer, compared with the risk in its absence. (The general term for an agent which induces neoplasia is an *oncogen*, Gk. onkos = mass.) A distinction can be made between true carcinogens and agents which act as *co-carcinogens*; the latter increase the activity of carcinogens but cannot themselves give rise to cancer in the absence of a carcinogen (p. 766). Carcinogenic agents are of three main types, namely chemical, physical and viral. The different classes of carcinogens and their likely modes of action are described in the following pages.

1. CHEMICAL CARCINOGENESIS

The history of the induction of cancer by chemical agents goes back two hundred years to the observation by Percivall Pott in 1775 that chimney sweep boys were 'peculiarly liable' to cancer of the scrotum. From this first indication of the carcinogenic properties of the products of combustion of coal has come an intensive study of *polycyclic aromatic hydrocarbons* as causes of cancer. They very probably play a key role in the incidence of lung cancer, through their presence in tobacco smoke and polluted air. The development of the dye industry at the end of the nineteenth century brought to light the carcinogenic properties of *aromatic amines* and related compounds. Research into the production of cancer by chemical agents usually involves animal experiments in which the activities of chemically pure substances can be investigated, in the hope of finding reasonable models of human cancers. One problem with this approach is that the carcinogens to which humans are exposed often occur in complex mixtures. For example, the risk of lung cancer is strongly associated with tobacco smoking, yet the smoke contains a variety of substances, none of which seems to be present in sufficient concentration to cause cancer on its own. We should be aware, therefore, that in man, cancer may frequently result from the combined effects of several chemical carcinogens acting together.

Polycyclic hydrocarbons

These were the first carcinogenic chemicals to be recognised and isolated in pure form. Polycyclic aromatic hydrocarbons are widely distributed in our environment, in cigarette smoke, in polluted city air and in some cooked (especially smoked) foods. They are in fact products of the combustion of almost all carbon-containing materials. The first description of the carcinogenic effects of soot by Pott has already been noted; the apparent specificity for scrotum which he found is probably attributable to the lack of proper washing facilities, such as bathrooms, at that time. It was also the first of many examples of cancer as an occupational hazard. Soot consists of small coal dust particles held together by *coal tar* and, a hundred years later, the latter was shown to contain the active principle, when coal tar workers developed cancer of the hands and forearms. The turning point in research into the carcinogenic properties of coal tar was the achievement of the Japanese workers, Yamagiwa and Ichikawa who, in 1915, successfully induced skin tumours on the ears of rabbits by repeated painting with tar over several months. In the 1920's, Kennaway and his colleagues in London attempted to isolate the active principles from coal tar, using as a guide a characteristic fluorescence spectrum given by all tars tested at that time. This spectrum turned out to be that of a *benzanthracene* type of structure (Figure 6.17). In 1929, the group synthesized 1:2, 5:6-dibenzanthracene and showed it to be a potent carcinogen; this was the first pure carcinogen discovered, though dibenzanthracene itself is not present in coal tar. The isolation of a carcinogenic component from tar required extraction from two tons of pitch! The yield was 50 grams of a chemically pure carcinogen, *3:4-benzpyrene*. Figure 6.17 shows the structures of these and other polycyclic hydrocarbons widely studied experimentally. 3:4-Benzpyrene is a common component of our environment—in car exhaust, cigarette smoke, city air and smoked food. These molecules are able to induce a variety of tumours in different tissues, depending on the route of administration. When applied to the skin they lead to papillomas and carcinomas at the site of application, and when injected or fed produce tumours of internal organs. They are also toxic, in common with other carcinogens, and this may indeed be of importance to the cancer-inducing events (p. 767).

It will be apparent even from the small number of structures shown in Figure 6.17 that polycyclic hydrocarbons can be very closely related structurally, yet show marked differences in carcinogenic potency. Thus, while 3:4-benzpyrene and 1:2, 5:6-dibenzanthracene are strong carcinogens, the very similar molecules 1:2-benzpyrene and 1:2, 3:4-dibenzanthracene are not carcinogenic. The deciding factor seems to be the chemical reactivity of the molecules, in particular the ability of certain double bonds on the ring structure to undergo addition reactions. The critical bonds are located in a part of the molecule which has been termed the *K-region*, indicated on the next page for benzanthracene. It was also realised that the 7, 12 carbon atoms

Figure 6.17 Polycyclic
hydrocarbons in carcinogenesis.
N: non-carcinogenic
W: weakly carcinogenic
S: strongly carcinogenic

(N)

Anthracene

(W)

1:2-Benzanthracene

(S)

3-Methylcholanthrene

(S)

7,12-Dimethylbenzanthracene

(S)

1:2,5:6-Dibenzanthracene

(W)

1:2,3:4-Dibenzanthracene

(S)

3:4-Benzpyrene

(N)

1:2-Benzpyrene

should be inactive in a carcinogenic molecule and the term
L-region was applied to this part of the molecule:

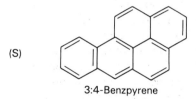

It was originally envisaged that the K-region would react directly
with target molecules in the cell (at first thought of as proteins,
but more likely to be DNA) and that this binding would lead in
some way to neoplastic change. It now seems probable that once
within the cell, polycyclic hydrocarbons are converted
enzymatically into compounds that are more water soluble and
reactive and which would be better able to bind to cell
constituents. The metabolic pathway of these molecules involves
addition of oxygen to the K-region double bond to form an
epoxide; this is believed to be the intermediate which reacts
with cell DNA, etc.:

O$_2$

microsomal enzyme
(*aryl hydrocarbon hydroxylase*)

epoxide

H

H   O

Reacts with
protein or
DNA

It has been found that some polycyclic hydrocarbons will induce the production in the cell of the microsomal enzyme *aryl hydrocarbon hydroxylase* which catalyses this reaction. From work with cultured cells, metabolism of the hydrocarbons appears to be an essential step if they are to react with cell DNA, RNA or protein.

As indicated above, the mechanism whereby polycyclic hydrocarbons produce a neoplastic change is believed to involve binding to cell macromolecules; although binding to protein certainly occurs, it seems unlikely that this is the crucial step in carcinogenesis. Rather, reaction of the carcinogen with DNA provides a better explanation for the irreversible genetic change which takes place in neoplastic transformation. One can readily envisage that binding to DNA could lead directly to mutational events, perhaps in critical growth-regulating genes (p. 769). It has been demonstrated that polycyclic hydrocarbons will bind to DNA and that the extent of this binding correlates with carcinogenic potency; no such correlation is found for binding either to protein or RNA.

ROLE IN HUMAN CANCER

We have already noted that skin cancers arose in workers exposed to coal products, such as pitch, tar or tar products. Mineral oils also contain carcinogenic hydrocarbons and the distillation products of shale-oil mined in Scotland caused shale-oil cancer of the hands and arms. In the Lancashire cotton-spinning industry, there was a high incidence of skin cancer among weavers and machinists who used equipment lubricated with mineral oils (mule-spinner's cancer). Today, the main exposure to aromatic hydrocarbons is through polluted air of industrial cities, from car exhaust fumes and, most importantly, the condensate or 'tar' of tobacco smoke. The lungs of most individuals are thereby frequently exposed to 3:4-benzpyrene and other hydrocarbons known to produce cancer in animals. There is no doubt that smoking is one of the principal causative factors in lung cancer (this association is discussed more fully on p. 707), and it is likely that carcinogenic hydrocarbons are partly responsible. At present it is not possible to attribute the carcinogenic properties of tobacco tar to a single substance; tar contains a mixture of known carcinogens, radioactive substances and co-carcinogens. While individual polycyclic hydrocarbons can produce cancer in the lungs of experimental animals, in man the combined effect of several agents is probably responsible. An example of such combination is seen in the increased incidence of lung cancer among workers in the *asbestos* industry. This is now one of the commonest occupational cancers (p. 700). It has been found that the risk of developing lung cancer is very much higher when inhalation of asbestos dust is combined with cigarette smoking. Whereas workers who do not smoke have only a moderately increased risk of asbestos-induced cancer, in smokers the risk is about 90 times that of the general population.

Genetic susceptibility probably plays some role in development of lung cancer. Since metabolism by microsomal enzymes is required for the carcinogenic action of polycyclic hydrocarbons it is possible that inheritable differences in the levels of such enzymes could influence the cancer process. Aryl hydrocarbon hydroxylase (AHH) is induced in tissue cells by the presence of the hydrocarbon substrate and it has been found that its inducibility is under genetic control. Two alleles at a single locus are indicated in man for the induction of this microsomal enzyme. It is therefore possible that individuals in whom the enzyme is more readily induced will be more susceptible than others to lung cancer caused by carcinogenic hydrocarbons. This is illustrated in mice, where mutations which block the induction of AHH make the animals less sensitive to the carcinogenic effects of certain polycyclic hydrocarbons.

Aromatic amines, azo-dyes and aminofluorenes

The carcinogenic properties of aromatic amines were first noticed in the dye factories of Europe at the end of the last century. Workers engaged in production of *aniline dyes* (magenta, mauve, etc.) suffered cancers which principally affected the urinary bladder. Aniline itself did not cause these tumours, but other amines involved in the dye-making process were carcinogenic, notably *β-naphthylamine* and *benzidine* (Figure 6.18). Industrial production of the aniline dyes was soon followed by that of the *azo-dyes*, produced by diazotisation of aromatic amines, and some of these such as 'scarlet red' and 'butter yellow' are also carcinogens. Butter yellow is the name given to dimethylamino-azobenzene (DAB) from the use of this dye to colour butter or margarine—needless to say, this practice has been abandoned. Azo-dyes such as DAB usually only induce liver tumours. The *aminofluorenes* are a third group of molecules with carcinogenic properties related to aromatic amines. A well-studied example is *2-acetylaminofluorene* (AAF), originally introduced as an insecticide, which was found to induce tumours in a variety of species. Here again, bladder and liver cancers predominate. Figure 6.18 shows the structures of some of the carcinogenic aromatic amines, azo-dyes and aminofluorenes. As in the case of polycyclic hydrocarbons, it is found that molecules with close structural similarities can have very different carcinogenic activity. α-Naphthylamine is only weakly carcinogenic, but β-naphthylamine is very active. Similarly in the azo-dyes, the 'parent' molecule 4-aminoazobenzene is only very weakly

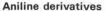

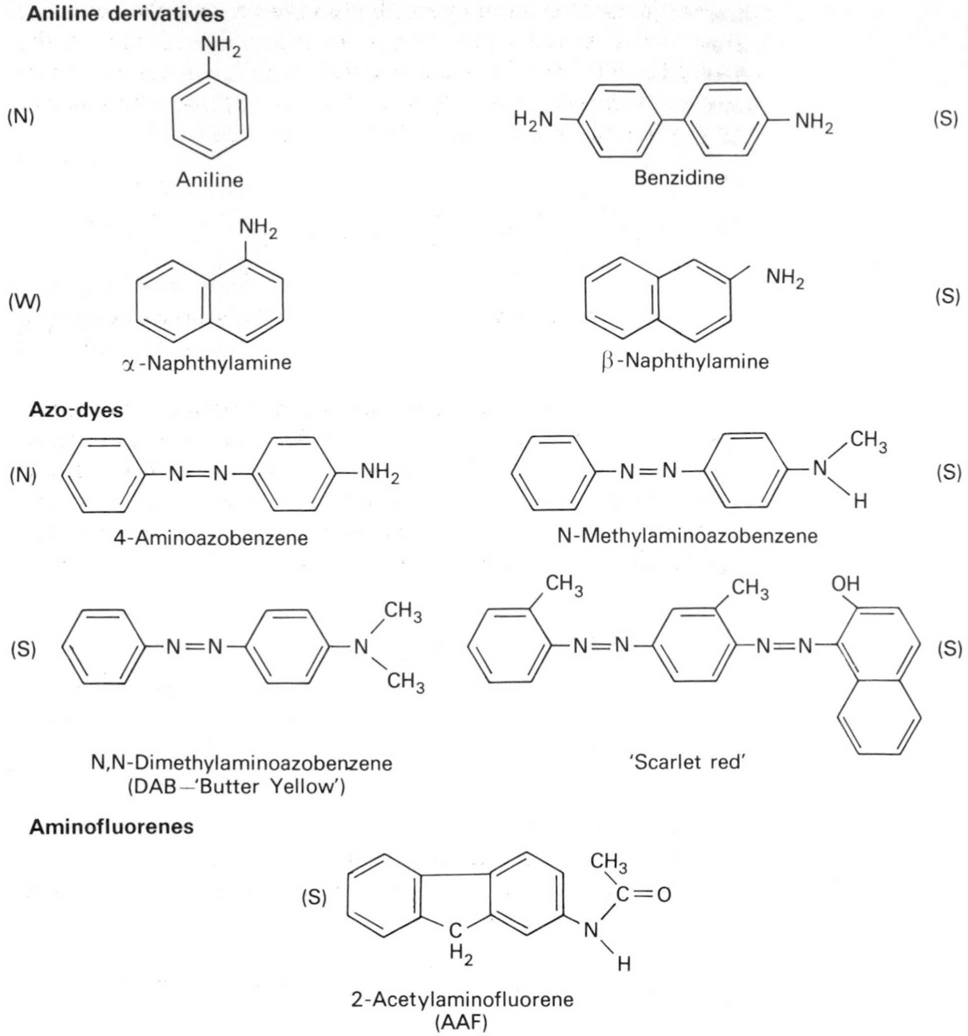
Aniline derivatives
NH2
(N)
Aniline
H2N
NH2
(S)
Benzidine
NH2
(W)
α-Naphthylamine
NH2
(S)
β-Naphthylamine
Azo-dyes
(N)
N=N
NH2
4-Aminoazobenzene
N=N
N
CH3
H
(S)
N-Methylaminoazobenzene
(S)
N=N
N
CH3
CH3
N,N-Dimethylaminoazobenzene
(DAB—'Butter Yellow')
CH3
CH3
OH
N=N
N=N
(S)
'Scarlet red'
Aminofluorenes
(S)
C
H2
CH3
C=O
N
H
2-Acetylaminofluorene
(AAF)

Figure 6.18 Carcinogenic aromatic amines and related molecules.
N: noncarcinogenic
W: weakly carcinogenic
S: strongly carcinogenic

carcinogenic, but the mono- and di-N-methyl derivatives are strong carcinogens (Figure 6.18).

An important feature of carcinogenesis by the aromatic amines and related molecules is that, unlike polycyclic hydrocarbons, they do not usually induce tumours at the site of their original contact or application; tumours develop instead at distant sites, principally the bladder and liver. The term *remote carcinogenesis* describes this phenomenon. The reason for this effect is that the native molecules are not themselves the carcinogens, but must be metabolised in order to exert a carcinogenic action. The tissues in which tumours arise are those in which the enzymes required to convert them to their carcinogenic derivatives are found; the active derivatives are called the *ultimate* carcinogens.

A good example of the production of ultimate carcinogens through metabolism is provided by *β-naphthylamine.* This produces bladder cancer if fed to animals, yet if introduced directly into the bladder in the form of small pellets is non-carcinogenic. It appears that β-naphthylamine is converted into

its ultimate carcinogen by metabolism elsewhere in the body, and the active product then exerts its effects specifically on the bladder (or liver in some species). The sequence of events involves the conversion, by *hydroxylation*, of β-naphthylamine to the aminophenol, 1-hydroxy-2-aminonaphthalene:

β-naphthylamine → 1-hydroxy-2-aminonaphthalene
ultimate carcinogen

The aminophenol is carcinogenic and will produce tumours if implanted into the bladder. The hydroxylation reaction takes place enzymatically in the liver, yet in most species, including the dog, hamster and man, tumours arise preferentially in the bladder. This is because the liver is able to *detoxify* the aminophenol by conjugation to glucuronic acid:

2-amino-1-naphthylglucuronic acid
(*aminophenol-glucuronic acid conjugate*)

Unfortunately the bladder reverses this detoxification by virtue of the enzyme glucuronidase, which acts on the glucuronic acid conjugate in the urine to release the aminophenol, the ultimate carcinogen in this case:

glucuronic acid-aminophenol conjugate $\xrightarrow{\text{glucuronidase}}$ aminophenol $\longrightarrow$ cancer

Bladder cancer only develops in species which possess bladder glucuronidase (dog, man); animals lacking this enzyme are not susceptible. Thus, the initiation of bladder cancer by exposure to β-naphthylamine involves a rather complex series of events—hydroxylation, detoxification and reactivation—which accounts for the high degree of tissue selectivity.

As we have seen, the activation of β-naphthylamine takes place by hydroxylation of the aromatic ring at the position adjacent to the amino group (ortho-hydroxylation). For the fluorenes and azo-dyes, however, the hydroxylation reaction takes place on the amino nitrogen itself (N-hydroxylation). In the case of the fluorene AAF, for example, the N-hydroxy derivative is excreted in the urine and is a more potent carcinogen than AAF itself:

AAF → N-hydroxy-AAF

This type of reaction is important in the activation into carcinogens of many aromatic amines and related molecules; almost invariably, the N-hydroxy form is more carcinogenic than the parent molecule. However, these derivatives are not the ultimate carcinogens themselves, but a step on the pathway towards them; they are therefore called *proximate carcinogens*, to indicate that they are more closely related to the final active form of the carcinogen than are the parent molecules. The N-hydroxy derivatives of the azo-dyes have been more difficult to detect in free form, probably because of their high reactivity. Before it can be hydroxylated, the azo-dye DAB is first demethylated:

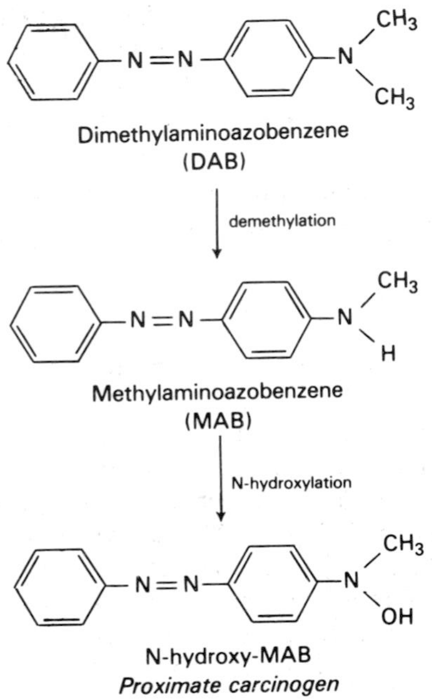

Dimethylaminoazobenzene
(DAB)

demethylation

Methylaminoazobenzene
(MAB)

N-hydroxylation

N-hydroxy-MAB
Proximate carcinogen

The ultimate carcinogen for AAF and DAB is an ester of their N-hydroxy derivatives formed with sulphuric acid:

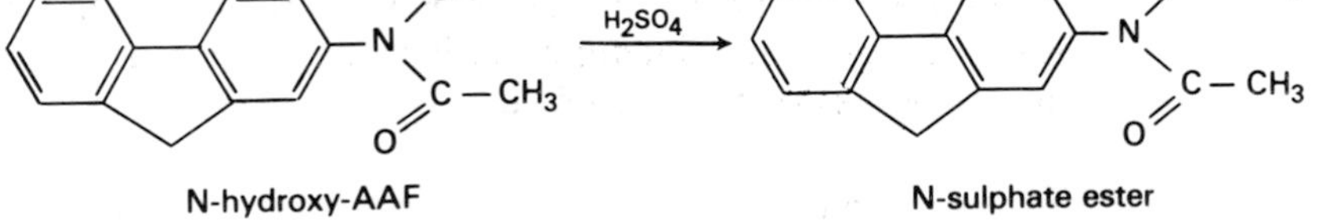

N-hydroxy-AAF

N-sulphate ester

These esters are reactive molecules and can interact with proteins and, of special significance, with nucleic acids. The preferred base of attack in the latter is guanine:

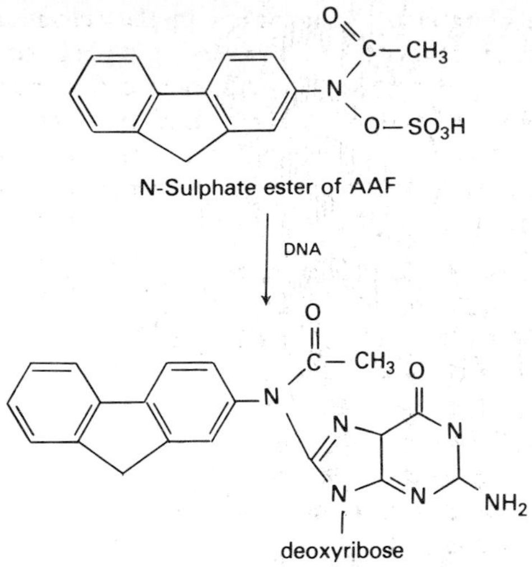

N-Sulphate ester of AAF

↓ DNA

deoxyribose

Guanine-bound AAF

This reaction probably forms the basis of the alteration of the genetic material by the carcinogen (p. 769).

ROLE IN HUMAN CANCER

Besides affecting workers in the dye industry itself, aromatic amines are causes of bladder cancer among workers in the rubber and cable manufacturing industries, textile dyers and printers, and gas workers. The major route of absorption is often through the lungs. The neoplasms appear in middle age and the disease has an induction period of 15–20 years. However, a few months' exposure to β-napthylamine may be sufficient to initiate the cancer process. Cancer of the bladder is also associated with heavy cigarette smoking, probably because β-naphthylamine is one of the products of tobacco combustion.

Nitrosamines

Considerable interest has developed in recent years in the cancer-inducing properties of these compounds for although they are not yet known to be responsible for any human cancers, many nitrosamines are carcinogenic and could be formed in the stomach by interaction of certain chemical components in food. The simplest member, dimethylnitrosamine, was to have been used as a solvent in the chemical industry until it was found to cause liver cancer when added to animal diets.

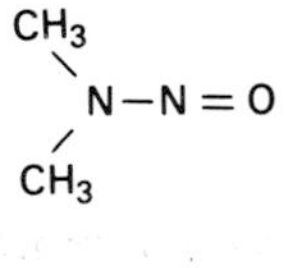

Dimethylnitrosamine

Nitrosamines are formed by a simple chemical reaction between a secondary amine with nitrous acid:

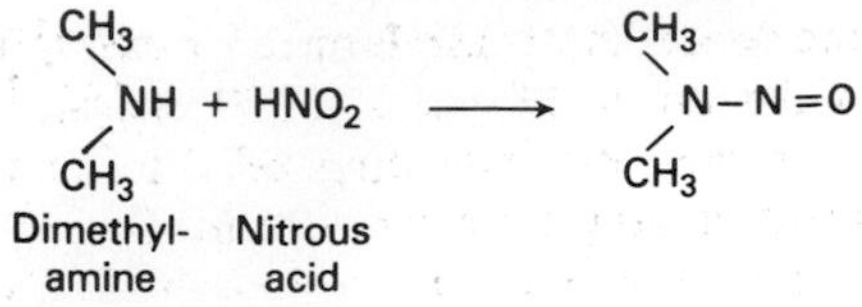

$$\begin{array}{ccc}
\text{CH}_3 & & \text{CH}_3 \\
\diagdown & & \diagdown \\
\text{NH} + \text{HNO}_2 \longrightarrow & & \text{N}-\text{N}=\text{O} \\
\diagup & & \diagup \\
\text{CH}_3 & & \text{CH}_3 \\
\text{Dimethyl-} \quad \text{Nitrous} & & \\
\text{amine} \qquad \text{acid} & &
\end{array}$$

Of particular concern is the possibility that this type of reaction might occur in the human stomach. Nitrites, which are abundant in sausages and certain preserved meats, will release nitrous acid if acted on by stomach hydrochloric acid; if secondary amines are also present in the food it is quite conceivable that potentially carcinogenic nitrosamines could be generated. Experimentally, it has been possible to induce tumours by feeding suitable mixtures of nitrites and amines. However, the extent to which nitrosamines are generated in man and are a human health hazard has still to be evaluated. A potent carcinogen, N-nitrosopiperidine, is present in tobacco smoke.

Alkylating agents

Unlike the preceding groups of chemical carcinogens which require conversion by metabolism to active ultimate carcinogens, some reactive molecules bind directly to DNA without the need for metabolic activation. They are alkylating agents and among those with carcinogenic properties are mustard gas, β-propiolactone, methylnitrosourea and alkyl sulphonates such as methyl methanesulphonate (Figure 6.19). Workers involved in the industrial manufacture of such agents may be at risk, as shown by the cases of respiratory cancer among men who had worked with mustard gas during World War II.

Aflatoxin

The toxic product of the fungus *Aspergillus flavus*, aflatoxin provides a good example of a naturally occurring carcinogen which is probably involved in a human cancer, namely liver carcinoma. Primary liver cancer is unusual in Europe and America, but has a high occurrence in parts of Africa, Hawaii and among the Chinese population of Singapore. In Africa there are pockets of

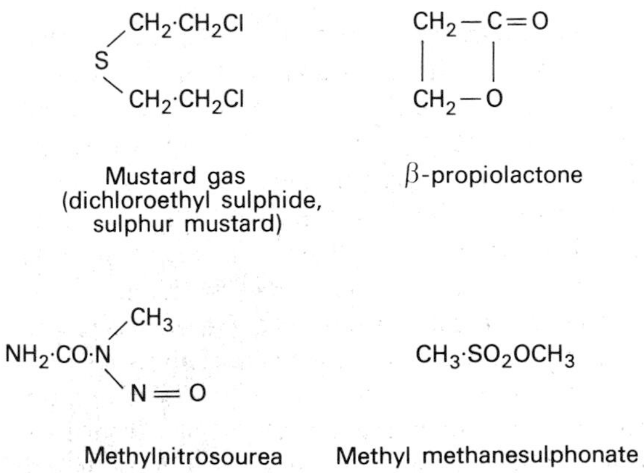

$$\begin{array}{cc}
\diagup \text{CH}_2\cdot\text{CH}_2\text{Cl} & \text{CH}_2-\text{C}=\text{O} \\
\text{S} & \qquad | \qquad | \\
\diagdown \text{CH}_2\cdot\text{CH}_2\text{Cl} & \text{CH}_2-\text{O}
\end{array}$$

Mustard gas $\qquad\qquad$ β-propiolactone
(dichloroethyl sulphide,
sulphur mustard)

$$\begin{array}{cc}
\diagup\text{CH}_3 & \\
\text{NH}_2\cdot\text{CO}\cdot\text{N} & \qquad \text{CH}_3\cdot\text{SO}_2\text{OCH}_3 \\
\diagdown\text{N}=\text{O} &
\end{array}$$

Methylnitrosourea $\qquad$ Methyl methanesulphonate

Figure 6.19 Carcinogenic alkylating agents.

760

especially high incidence: in Mozambique, for example, the rate is the highest in the world (98 per 100,000 males), fifty times greater than in Britain. An indication of the identity of an environmental agent causing liver cancer came in 1960 from an outbreak of fatal liver disease among turkeys in England, when 100,000 birds died of acute hepatic necrosis. The disease was traced to a dietary source, namely imported peanut meal contaminated with *Aspergillus flavus*. The products of the mould proved to be liver toxins and when tested in low doses in a number of species were also found to be potent liver carcinogens. Since *Aspergillus flavus* is a contaminant of certain staple foods (cereals, ground nuts) in many parts of the world, aflatoxin emerged as a candidate for a causative factor in liver cancer. Epidemiological evidence confirmed the association. In Kenya there was shown to be a significant association between aflatoxin and primary liver cancer among the Kikuyu; and in Mozambique, where aflatoxin levels in food were twenty times higher than in Kenya, a close correlation with liver cancer was also established. (Happily, the moulds used in certain soft cheeses, such as Camembert, Rocquefort and Gorgonzola, do not produce similar toxins and those used in the cheese-making process actively suppress infection by *Aspergillus*).

The structure of one of the four related aflatoxin molecules (B_1) is shown below. As with many of the other chemical carcinogens, aflatoxins probably undergo metabolism to ultimate carcinogens before binding to cellular macromolecules. The activation reaction is catalysed by microsomal aryl hydrocarbon hydroxylase, the enzyme also involved in metabolic activation of polycyclic hydrocarbons (p. 754). The hydroxy-derivative of aflatoxin binds to DNA, which as we have already noted is probably an essential part of chemical carcinogenesis.

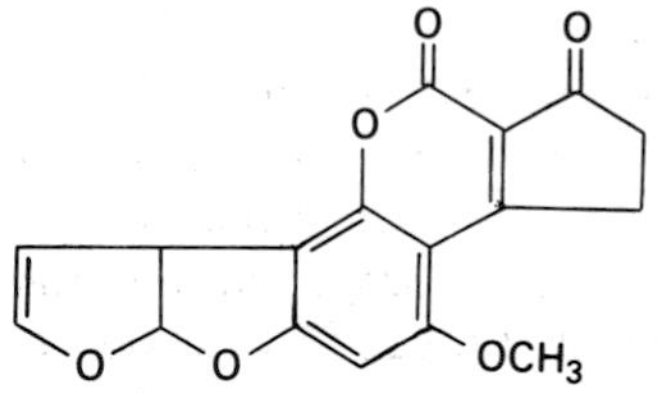

Aflatoxin B_1

However, the epidemiological studies on aflatoxin have been criticised on the grounds that the initiating events in liver cancer probably occur many years before the emergence of tumours, and the aflatoxin content in food at that time is not known. Moreover, the suggestion that aflatoxin is a primary agent of liver cancer in Africa has been been made less likely by the more recent universal finding of hepatitis B virus (HBV) in most liver cancer patients (p. 796). In some parts of the world over 90% of individuals with primary liver carcinoma are also chronic carriers of HBV, and this is the case both in areas where aflatoxin is present in the food and elsewhere. Thus, while it is undeniably one of the most potent carcinogens in some experimental animals, aflatoxin is evidently not present in high enough concentration in food even in Africa to produce many cancers in uninfected people. Perhaps its true role is to promote, through its hepatotoxic properties, the development of tumour cells initiated by HBV.

2. PHYSICAL AGENTS AS CARCINOGENS

The physical agents which can cause neoplasia are ionising radiations, such as X-rays and radioactivity, and solar radiation in the form of ultraviolet light. As with the chemical carcinogens, the cancer-inducing effects of these forms of radiation can be related to the damage which they produce in DNA.

Ionising radiations

The ionising radiations include X-rays and gamma rays, both of which are electromagnetic waves like visible light but of much greater energy, and radiations composed of subatomic particles, namely electrons (beta particles), protons, neutrons or alpha particles (two neutrons and two protons). All such radiations, as their name implies, produce ionisation, by removing electrons from the atoms of substances through which they pass. The resulting ionised molecules are extremely unstable and are rapidly (10^{-16} sec.) converted into highly reactive free radicals. The latter are responsible for the damaging effects of ionising radiation on biologically important molecules. Most of the biological damage is probably the result of the action on macromolecules of free radicals derived from ionised water molecules.

In sufficient dose, ionising radiation will kill cells as a result of chromosomal damage. The cells which are most sensitive to the lethal effects of radiation are those which are actively dividing, i.e. in the mitotic phase of the cell cycle; a higher dose is required to kill cells which are in the G_1, S or G_2 phases (p. 709). A high enough level of radiation damages DNA in all cells, including those which would not normally be capable of further division. However, the cell killing effect requires division as well as chromosomal damage. Thus differentiated, non-dividing cells are resistant to radiation killing not because their DNA is unharmed, but because DNA damage only becomes manifest on cell division (*mitotic death*). Bone marrow, intestinal epithelium, skin and germ cells are particularly sensitive to radiation death, being the most rapidly proliferating. Radiation induces breaks in DNA strands and this leads to various chromosomal aberrations. Fragmentation, deletion of parts of chromosomes, exchange of genetic material between chromosomes, and chromosome bridges can be seen in karyotypes of irradiated cells. It is the loss of genetic material in the form of chromosome fragments and the mechanical interference with mitosis by bridge formation which are responsible for mitotic death. Cells which survive irradiation may have sufficient alteration to their DNA to lead to neoplastic change.

In man, there are several examples of the production of neoplasms by ionising radiation, such as the many cases of skin cancer in the early radiologists and cancers in patients treated with radioactive materials and X-rays. The largest source of information on the effect of radioactivity on human health comes from the results of the atomic bomb explosions at Hiroshima and Nagasaki in August 1945. The main neoplasm found in survivors was *leukaemia* (acute and chronic granulocytic forms), after an average latent period of about 7 years; smaller increases in the incidence of cancer of the thyroid, breast and lung also occurred. Experimentally, irradiation of mice also gives rise to leukaemia, the most important feature of which is the presence of a transmissible virus in the leukaemic mouse cells (p. 798). Release of viral material is evidently triggered by irradiation. It is not known if a similar aetiology underlies human irradiation leukaemia. Some radioisotopes such as those of phosphorus (^{32}P), strontium (^{90}Sr), radium (^{226}Ra) and plutonium (^{239}Pu), cause bone neoplasms (*osteosarcomas*) if ingested (*bone-seeking isotopes*). The well-known 'dial painter's' cancer, caused by ingestion of radium by girls applying luminous paint to watch faces in the 1920's, has been noted previously (p. 700). For similar reasons, a certain apprehension attaches to the increased levels of radioactive strontium ^{90}Sr released into the atmosphere in H-bomb tests. ^{90}Sr is taken up by grass and can reach man via cow's milk, thereafter becoming deposited in bones. A radioisotope present in cigarette smoke is that of polonium (^{210}Po), the amount of which varies considerably with the soil in which the tobacco is grown. It has been suggested that the different mortalities from lung cancer seen in countries with similar smoking habits, e.g. the UK compared with South Africa or the USA (Figure 6.2a), are due to differences in the level of radioactivity inhaled, though this is not yet settled.

It should be noted that ionising radiations are less potent and specific as carcinogens than the chemical agents described above. Radiation is a more effective cytotoxic agent than oncogen. It is reasonable to assume that the carcinogenic effect of such radiation is due to chromosomal damage and consequent mutation. After irradiation, besides the physical breaks and rearrangements of the chromosomes described, changes in specific bases occur which can lead to miscoding (e.g. cytosine can be converted into uracil and guanine to hypoxanthine). The mutagenic effect of irradiation has been demonstrated in various test systems (p. 775). There is great interest in the cellular mechanisms for repairing damaged DNA, though these are better understood for u.v. damage than ionising radiation (see p. 769). The relation between DNA damage, mutation and carcinogenesis is discussed further on pp. 768–775.

Ultraviolet radiation

Exposure to u.v. radiation in sunlight is a major contributor to cancer of the skin. The distribution of squamous and basal cell carcinomas of the skin in the general population is directly related to the degree of exposure to sunlight, determined by geography, climate, altitude and personal occupation. Farmers, ranchers, sailors, sportsmen and others habitually exposed to the sun show high incidences of these cancers, which naturally occur on the most exposed parts of the body (hands, arms and face). Carcinomas are preceded by benign but precancerous lesions called *senile* or *actinic keratoses*. Skin pigmentation absorbs u.v. radiation and prevents neoplastic change in the proliferative layer of the skin; hence pigmented races have a lower incidence of skin cancer (7–8 times less frequent among Negroes than Whites).

Ultraviolet radiation is both toxic to cells and mutagenic, and its action spectrum follows closely that of its absorption by DNA, with a peak around 2600 Å. The basis of u.v. damage is the absorption of photons by DNA resulting in base alterations, of which the most important is dimerisation of pyrimidines, especially *thymine*. The formation of thymine dimers is shown in Figure 6.20. The presence of such dimers can prevent the normal replication of DNA and lead to the introduction of mutations, and it is assumed therefore to neoplasia (p. 768). As described in detail below, cells are able to prevent the harmful effects of u.v. irradiation from being 'fixed' in daughter cells on DNA replication by *repair mechanisms*, one of which involves the excision of thymine dimers and replacement of the damaged stretch of DNA by new synthesis. In a rare inherited disease, *xeroderma pigmentosum*, this excision repair mechanism is at fault and as a result patients with this disease are very sensitive to skin damage by sunlight and particularly prone to skin cancer (see p. 773). This emphasises the frequency of potential cell damage induced by u.v. in the normal skin and the importance of DNA repair in preventing its manifestation as neoplasia.

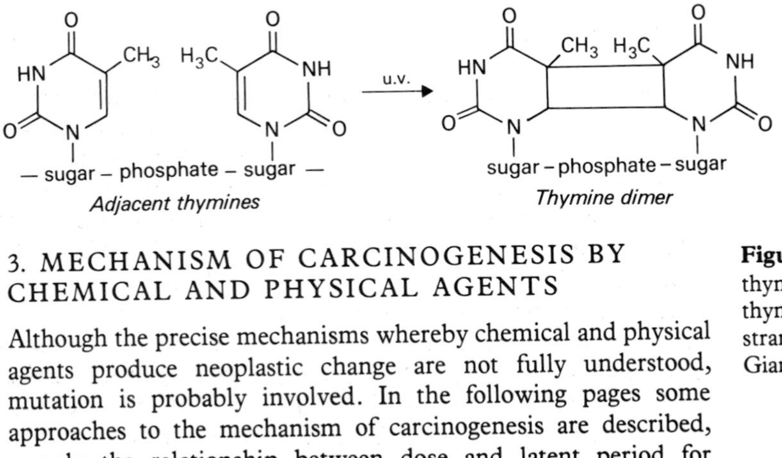

Adjacent thymines   *Thymine dimer*

3. MECHANISM OF CARCINOGENESIS BY CHEMICAL AND PHYSICAL AGENTS

Although the precise mechanisms whereby chemical and physical agents produce neoplastic change are not fully understood, mutation is probably involved. In the following pages some approaches to the mechanism of carcinogenesis are described, namely the relationship between dose and latent period for chemical carcinogens, the role of co-carcinogens (the *two-stage theory*) and the importance of the interaction of the carcinogen with cell genetic material (the *mutation theory*).

Figure 6.20 Formation of thymine dimer from two adjacent thymines on the same DNA strand by u.v. irradiation (from Giannelli, 1976).

Dose-response and latent period

The quantitative parameters used to assess the potency of a carcinogenic chemical *in vivo* are the dose of carcinogen, the yield of tumours in test animals and the time taken for tumours to arise (the *latent period*). A measure which has been used since 1939 in the comparison of carcinogens is the *Iball index* of carcinogenicity (*I*) which is the ratio of the percentage of animals with tumours (*A*) to the average latent period in days (*B*) at a standard dose of carcinogen:

$$I = A/B \times 100$$

For skin carcinogenesis, a standard amount of an 0·3% solution of the chemical in benzene or acetone is applied to the test animals twice weekly until tumours appear. The percentage tumour yield and latent period can then be measured. However, the Iball index is clearly an inadequate description of carcinogenic potency, because it does not take into account the way carcinogenic activity varies with dosage. A more accurate comparison of carcinogenic agents is provided by dose-response curves, in which tumour yield is determined over a range of different doses. Unless this is done, carcinogenic potency may be underestimated.

The latent period in tumour induction can be quite considerable depending on the carcinogen and its dose. In studying the relationship between dose and latent period experimentally, it is usual to apply a carcinogen repeatedly, e.g. daily, at different doses until tumours appear. A simple proportionality between daily dose and latent period is found for some carcinogens, such as DAB (dimethylaminoazobenzene, p. 755). For example, at a daily dose of DAB of 30 mg per animal, the latent period is about 30 days, while at 3 mg it is approximately 350 days. In such cases the relationship

$$d \times t = \text{constant} \tag{1}$$

applies where d = daily dose and t = latent period. Thus the total dose of DAB required to induce tumours is the same irrespective of the size of the daily dose administered. This leads to the important and somewhat surprising conclusion that the effects of individual doses, even when very small, can be summated and that therefore each dose must have an *irreversible* effect. This conclusion is confirmed by experiments designed to give the animal an opportunity to reverse the action of the carcinogen, by leaving longer time intervals between successive applications of the agent; it is found that this merely prolongs the induction time (by the sum of the increased intervals), but does not increase the dose of carcinogen required. Thus, once exposure to a carcinogen has occurred, the animal is unable to reverse its effect.

For other carcinogens, the simple linear relationship of dose to latent period does not hold. Instead, as the daily dose is reduced, so too is the total dose required; that is, the effect of an increased induction time is to decrease the amount of carcinogen needed to produce tumours. The dose–time relation is now expressed as

$$d \times t^n = \text{constant} \tag{2}$$

the value of the integer n varying from 1·1 to 6·5. The value of n is

765

useful as an indicator of carcinogenic potency. Where the above relationship (2) applies, a graph of log d against log t yields a straight line of slope n. It might be thought that at very low doses a point would be reached where the amount of carcinogen was below the threshold of effect, so that this equation would no longer hold. However, in practice the log plot of d vs. t is a straight line even down to the smallest doses. The implication is that *no threshold exists* below which cancer cannot be induced. Of course, at very low doses the latent period cannot be measured as it exceeds the normal lifespan of the animal, but within this limitation subthreshold doses have not been demonstrable.

In summary, measurements of latent period in relation to dose have demonstrated two related concepts for chemical carcinogens, namely that their effects are irreversible and that there is no measurable threshold dose below which exposure has no effect. Let us now consider the carcinogenic events themselves.

Initiation and promotion: the 2-stage theory of neoplasia

In important experiments in the 1940's, Berenblum demonstrated that the process of induction of tumours in mouse skin could be divided into two stages, which he called *initiation* and *promotion*. It was known that skin tumours could be produced by repeated skin-painting with carcinogens such as the polycyclic hydrocarbons dimethylbenzanthracene, benzpyrene or methylcholanthrene. A single low dose (e.g. 25 μg) of any of these compounds applied locally fails to produce skin tumours during the lifespan of the animal. Berenblum showed that if such a single painting with carcinogen was followed by repeated application of a solution of an irritant, but non-carcinogenic substance, namely *croton oil*, benign tumours appeared after a few weeks. Croton oil itself was incapable of producing such tumours on its own; pretreatment of the skin with carcinogen was essential. The effect of the croton oil was therefore to *promote* a process which had been *initiated* by a carcinogenic hydrocarbon. In accord with this explanation, the order of application of the two substances was very important: if croton oil was applied first, no tumours were produced. The carcinogenic process thus seemed to begin with a primary induction event produced in cells by the initiator, the result of which was a latent tumour cell (Figure 6.21). The croton oil then in some way encouraged growth of the potential neoplastic cell into a tumour and was therefore termed a *co-carcinogen* or *promoter* (Figure 6.21). Since the polycyclic hydrocarbons, aromatic amines and other carcinogens can give rise to tumours when administered alone, either in a sufficiently large single dose or in small doses over a long enough period, they can be termed *complete carcinogens*. In contrast, exposure of tissues to co-carcinogens leads to neoplasia only if the tissues have previously been in contact with a true carcinogen in a subcarcinogenic dose.

Croton oil is obtained from the seeds of the tropical plant *Croton tiglium* (*Euphorbiaceae*) and is highly irritating to the skin. When applied it causes notable cell multiplication and hence

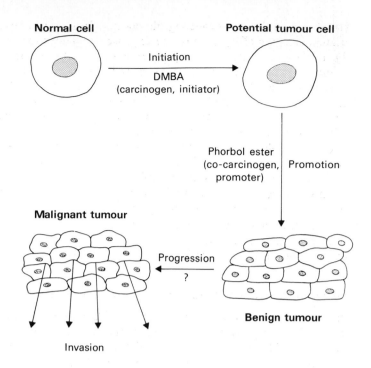

Figure 6.21 Initiation, promotion and progression as successive stages in the development of cancer (in the mouse skin model). (After Hecker, 1976)

hyperplasia and this is probably important in its co-carcinogenic properties. Other processes in which hyperplasia occurs, in particular wound healing and regeneration, also promote tumour growth, and it is noteworthy that complete carcinogens are all toxic for tissues and hence initiate proliferative and hyperplastic events. On the other hand, hyperplasia cannot be the whole basis of promotion, since many injurious substances produce regenerative hyperplasia but do not act as co-carcinogens. The active molecule in croton oil has been isolated and in structure is a di-ester of the diterpene *phorbol*. Other promoters include the detergent Tween 60, coal tar phenols and anthraline (trihydroxyanthracene). Substances acting as promoters are probably present in carcinogenic mixtures which affect man, such as coal tar and tobacco smoke.

An important difference between initiation and promotion is that initiation is an irreversible event, while promotion is reversible. Thus, after a single treatment with polycyclic hydrocarbon, the application of croton oil can be delayed for several months and still be successful (though after a year the effect of a single initiating dose may fade). After they have been acted on by carcinogen, potential tumour cells do not revert to normal but await a further promoting signal. In contrast, the reversible nature of promotion is seen if long time intervals are allowed between the required applications of croton oil, whereupon there is a considerable loss of promotional activity, i.e. a reduction in tumour yield. Furthermore, the promoter must be given in suitably large doses: if the amount of croton oil required for promotion is divided into small doses administered more frequently, promotion is again less effective. Thus, in addition to its reversibility, promotion has a demonstrable threshold and the effect of small doses cannot be summated; in these respects it can be distinguished from initiation or complete carcinogenesis.

While the experiments with mouse skin provided an important conceptual framework for understanding the carcinogenic process, they have some important shortcomings. Whereas complete carcinogens can give rise to carcinomas, the tumours produced in the skin as a result of independent initiation and promotion are always benign (papillomas). In some experiments, a two-stage process can be shown to be involved in induction of malignant neoplasms: for example, sesame seed oil injections promote the development of sarcomas in rats after feeding methylcholanthrene. However, the general applicability of a simple two-stage theory of carcinogenesis remains debatable. At least one extra stage is indicated, namely the *progression* from benign to malignant tumour (Figure 6.21). *In vivo*, hormones may function as co-carcinogens able to mediate both promotion and progression. The dependence of cancers of the breast and prostate on oestrogens and androgens respectively during part of their development probably reflects such a co-carcinogenic action of hormones. Ultimately such cancers achieve hormone independence.

Carcinogens and the mutation theory of neoplasia

We have noted that a tumour arises as a result of an irreversible, inheritable change which takes place originally in a single cell; the cell divides and gives rise to a *clone* of similar cells, all of which carry the same alteration. The involvement of the genetic material in the neoplastic change is also evident from the karyotypic abnormalities of tumour cells (p. 729) and, as expected from their clonal origin, cells from any single tumour show similar karyotypic changes, in contrast to the diversity of karyotypes found in different tumours. These observations led to the *mutation theory* of neoplasia, which can be summarised in the proposal that an alteration in the DNA is a necessary part of the neoplastic change. For chemical as well as physical carcinogens, there is little doubt that production of a tumour is related to the ability of these agents to react with DNA and produce mutations. By now, practically all chemical carcinogens have been shown to bind to DNA, either directly or following metabolism to reactive products. The damaging effect of ionising and u.v. irradiation on DNA has been noted above. Further, using a variety of sophisticated mutagenicity tests (p. 775), most chemical and physical carcinogens have been shown to be mutagens, though the reverse is not necessarily true, i.e. some mutagenic substances are non-carcinogenic. The reaction of carcinogenic agents with DNA may lead directly to mutational events as described below. However, cells possess complex mechanisms to counter the mutagenic effect of these agents by eliminating damaged segments of DNA and replacing them. A great deal of attention is now given to these DNA repair mechanisms and there is good evidence that defects in DNA repair increase the likelihood of mutation and hence the risk of at least some forms of cancer.

We have seen that while some chemicals, notably alkylating agents, can react with DNA directly, others require metabolism to ultimate carcinogens before interaction with DNA can take place. Despite the differences in their chemical structures, the reactive molecules are all essentially electrophiles (i.e. possess electron-deficient atoms) which react with nucleophilic centres (sites with atoms rich in electrons) present on DNA. Although there are several such sites, *guanine* is the preferred base of attack, usually at the N7 or C8 position. Some characteristic reaction products are shown in Figure 6.22. Bivalent reagents such as the sulphur mustards can cross-link guanines on adjacent DNA strands to produce guanine dimers. Other agents, such as acridines carrying a reactive group, intercalate in the DNA, i.e. slot between two bases, before binding covalently to one of them. Ultraviolet light causes the formation of dimers of adjacent thymines on the same DNA chain, while ionising radiations lead to physical breaks and other chromosomal changes.

The result of all these reactions is to damage DNA and if this is not repaired by the enzymatic processes described below, mutation can result in different ways. The simplest examples are *point mutations*, which can be *base-pair substitutions* or *frame-shift mutations* (Figure 6.23). The former can arise if an altered guanine pairs incorrectly with thymine or adenine instead of its correct partner cytosine (Figure 6.23a). This mispairing leads to a permanent single change in the sequence of nucleotides in the replicated DNA; when translated into protein, this causes a single amino acid substitution in the sequence. Intercalation, on the other hand, can cause the introduction of a new, additional base pair in the sequence of nucleotides (Figure 6.23b), and since this alters the reading of all subsequent triplets, such a 'frame-shift' can lead to a greatly altered protein product. More complex chromosomal changes can also occur. For example DNA may be replicated above and below the aberrant base leaving a small gap; unless this is repaired, chromosomal fragmentation and rearrangement can occur and, if the cell survives, mutation due to gene loss can ensue. Note that all these mutational events are 'fixed' permanently in the genome when the DNA replicates; they are then passed on to a daughter cell and become permanently inheritable.

MECHANISMS OF DNA REPAIR

The mutagenic and other damaging effects of chemical and physical carcinogens can be prevented by DNA repair processes of which at least two types are known. In one, called *excision repair*, the segment of altered DNA is enzymatically removed and resynthesized correctly before DNA replication; in the other, termed *post-replication repair*, the DNA is first replicated despite the damage to the parent molecule, but leaving gaps opposite lesions in the template which are later filled in. Some of the enzymes involved in these processes show genetic variation and certain individuals have an inherited deficiency in a repair enzyme

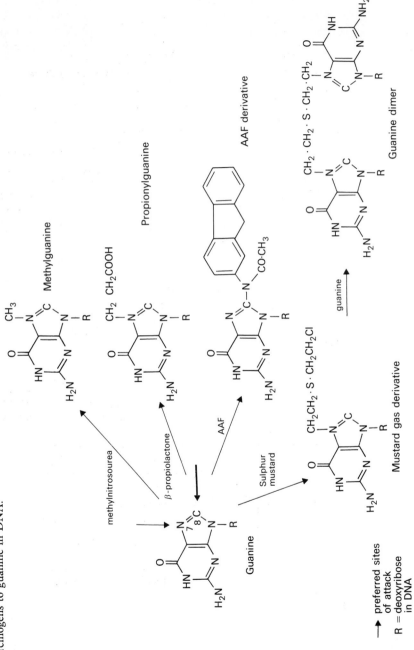

Figure 6.22 Binding of carcinogens to guanine in DNA.

Figure 6.23 Point mutations in DNA.
(a) Generation of a base-pair substitution in DNA by mispairing.
(b) Generation of a 'frame-shift' mutation by intercalation.
A: adenine
C: cytosine
G: guanine
Ⓖ: aberrant guanine
T: thymine

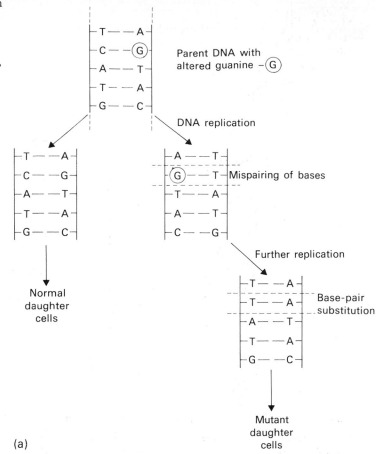

(a)

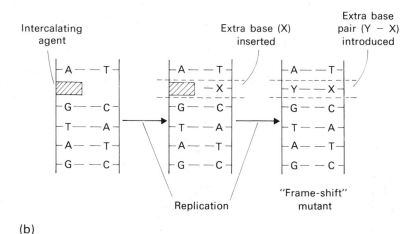

(b)

which leads to a special sensitivity to neoplasia. Hence DNA repair is believed to play an important role in preventing mutations which could lead to cancer.

771

Excision repair

This process has been studied mostly in bacterial cells exposed to u.v. irradiation to induce thymine dimers in the DNA, but the same repair events occur in mammalian cells treated with chemical carcinogens. Thymine dimers or bulky chemical groups bound to bases distort the DNA backbone locally and the distortion can be recognised by an endonuclease. This enzyme makes a 'nick' or incision near the damaged area and allows a second enzyme, an exonuclease, to remove the damaged piece of DNA, as shown in Figure 6.24. At the same time, DNA polymerase resynthesises the stretch of DNA chain which has been removed, using the opposite strand as template; finally the newly synthesised piece is joined to the free end of the old DNA strand by another enzyme, polynucleotide ligase. These events will successfully repair stretches of DNA damaged by u.v. or large chemical groups and since repair takes place outside the S phase of the cell cycle it is sometimes called *unscheduled* DNA synthesis. Excision repair may not function where only small alkyl groups are bound to DNA, as after methylation, because the DNA must be distorted by the agent to a sufficient degree for recognition by the endonuclease. Furthermore, even after binding of reasonably large molecules, such as AAF, excision repair does not work with

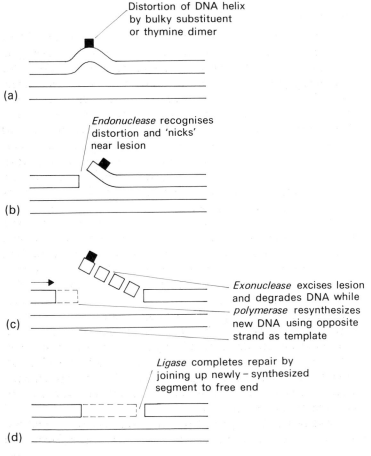

(a) Distortion of DNA helix by bulky substituent or thymine dimer

(b) Endonuclease recognises distortion and 'nicks' near lesion

(c) Exonuclease excises lesion and degrades DNA while polymerase resynthesizes new DNA using opposite strand as template

(d) Ligase completes repair by joining up newly–synthesized segment to free end

Figure 6.24 Excision repair of DNA after binding of carcinogen or u.v. irradiation (after Roberts, 1976).

100% efficiency, and a certain proportion of the carcinogenic moieties bound to DNA are not removed by this mechanism. About 50–75% of thymine dimers induced by u.v. light are excised by normal human cells, while the remainder persist in the DNA. For this reason, a second DNA repair mechanism is also available as a 'back-up' system, as follows.

Post-replication repair

This has also been studied using u.v.-induced dimerisation of thymine residues as a model system in bacterial and mammalian cells. If these dimers are not removed by excision repair, the DNA replicates up to the dimer, where it stops and then rein-itiates at a point beyond the damage. In this way gaps are produced in the replicated strand. Later these discontinuities are filled in with the correct nucleotide sequences by a complex mechanism involving recombination; hence the alternative name for this process, recombination repair. These events are blocked by caffeine and the fact that this inhibitor greatly increases the lethality of various alkylating agents in cultured cells and the frequency of chromosomal aberrations induced by such agents or u.v. light, indicates the importance of post-replication repair in cell survival after exposure to these substances.

Repair defects and human cancer

The importance of excision repair in preventing damage to DNA from being fixed as mutation and thus possibly leading to neoplasia is well illustrated by a rare inherited disease called *xerodema pigmentosum* (XP), characterised by extreme sensitivity to sunlight and a high incidence of u.v.-induced skin cancers. This was the first human condition in which a precise defect in DNA repair was defined. The disease is inherited as an autosomal recessive (p. 829) and is caused by a deficiency of the *endonuclease* required to commence excision repair. Children with this disease, which has its highest incidence in parts of North Africa, are very sensitive to sunlight and after repeated exposure the skin becomes dry, scaly and hypopigmented, and later atrophies; there are areas of hyperkeratosis (thickening of the stratum corneum) and tumours develop in the areas of the skin most exposed to the sun. Many of the neoplasms are malignant, and patients often die from disseminating carcinoma before the age of 20. Careful protection from sunlight is essential to prevent the appearance of skin cancers. Cells from XP patients fail to excise the thymine dimers formed in DNA after u.v. irradiation, but are able to repair the breaks in DNA caused by X-irradiation. Thus the enzymes other than endonuclease are apparently normal in XP cells. In addition, XP cells cannot repair damage to DNA caused by chemical car-cinogens which distort but do not break DNA strands, emphas-izing the role of the same enzyme in dealing both with u.v. and chemically induced changes.

A variant of XP is called the *De Sanctis-Cacchione syndrome* and there is evidence that the enzymatic defect is different from that of classical XP. This has been analysed by *somatic cell hybridisation* (p. 730) in which fibroblasts of XP and De Sanctis-Cacchione patients were fused together *in vitro* (Figure 6.25). While neither of the parent cells could repair u.v.-damaged DNA, hybrid cells were able to do so; in short, *complementation* of the defects in the two diseases had occurred (see also p. 733). This indicated that different enzymes were defective in the two parent cells, which could each therefore correct the deficiency of the other when fused to form a hybrid cell. The enzyme missing from De Sanctis-Cacchione cells is probably involved in post-replication rather than excision repair.

These discoveries with XP are clearly important in understanding how u.v. light produces tumours of the skin. As we have seen previously, the frequency of skin cancers in different parts of the world is dependent on the factors which govern the dose of u.v. absorbed by the proliferative layer of the skin. Ultraviolet light is known to be a powerful mutagen for both animal and bacterial cells. At a certain level of irradiation, skin cells may be unable to cope with the degree of DNA damage produced; alternatively, the repair processes themselves may be prone to error and may be a possible source of mutation (below). Ensuing mutations may well be the initiators of neoplastic change. It is interesting that XP patients do not show any obvious increase in the common fatal internal cancers of the lung, alimentary tract or breast. This may be because they do not survive long enough to experience them; alternatively, the other neoplasms may not be caused by the kind of DNA lesions which XP patients are specifically unable to repair. If correct, this second explanation would have important implications for the genetic mechanisms of carcinogenesis in common cancers.

Figure 6.25 Cell fusion showing complementation between cells of xeroderma pigmentosum and De Sanctis-Cacchione syndrome. Only the hybrid receiving the nuclei of both parents can repair DNA after u.v. exposure.

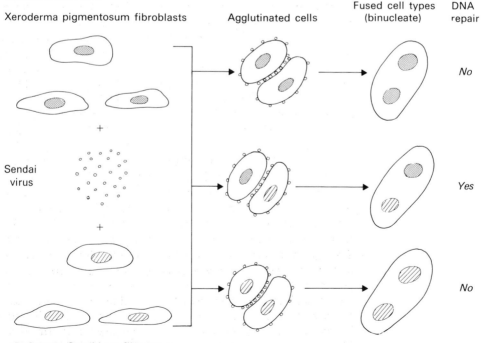

Xeroderma pigmentosum fibroblasts   Agglutinated cells   Fused cell types (binucleate)   DNA repair

+

Sendai virus

+

No

Yes

No

DeSanctis-Cacchione fibroblasts

There are two other diseases where defective DNA repair predisposes to cancer, namely *ataxia telangiectasia* (AT) and *Fanconi's anaemia*. In the former, the symptoms are cerebellar ataxia (muscular incoordination due to lesions in the cerebellum) and oculocutaneous telangiectases (small foci of abnormally prominent capillaries); there is a predisposition to leukaemias and other lymphoreticular neoplasms. AT cells are more sensitive to gamma radiation than to u.v. and are apparently unable to excise the gamma-ray modified bases. However, there is also a marked immunodeficiency in AT and this may be more important than the excision defect in development of neoplasia. In Fanconi's anaemia there is also a tendency to develop leukaemia, associated with an inability to excise thymine dimers after u.v. irradiation.

For the majority of human cancers, there is as yet no reason to believe that repair of DNA is abnormal. Sometimes the repair of DNA damage is liable to error and hence may be a possible source of mutation. A repair system induced in *E. coli* has been found to be 'error-prone' and if it exists in mammalian cells could be relevant in carcinogenesis.

TESTING FOR MUTAGENICITY

The correlation between carcinogenic and mutagenic properties of chemical and physical agents greatly strengthens the theory that the neoplastic state arises as a result of genetic mutation. Certain hormones such as oestradiol are exceptional in being carcinogenic but not mutagenic and there are some molecules, including base analogues, nitrous acid and some acridines, which are mutagens but not carcinogens. These exceptions are sufficiently rare to make it worthwhile screening various environmental substances for mutagenic, and by inference carcinogenic, properties with *mutagenicity test systems*. A simple and sensitive test for mutation has been devised which utilises bacteria, notably some special strains of *Salmonella typhimurium*. These are well-defined mutants which, unlike the wild-type organisms, have a specific requirement for histidine in their growth medium. The mutant strains can revert back to wild-type growth, i.e. growth on minimal medium, as a result of mutation and this tendency is accelerated by mutagenic agents. Different test strains of *S. typhimurium* have been developed to detect different types of mutation (base-pair substitution, frame-shift, chromosomal breaks, etc.). The test is simply to spot a small quantity of the suspected mutagen onto a lawn of tester strain, and then count the number of revertant colonies of the organism which subsequently grow out on medium not supplemented with histidine. This number is a measure of the mutagenicity of the test substance. The test has been refined by inclusion of a liver microsomal hydroxylase system to activate carcinogens requiring metabolism. So far some 85% of the carcinogens examined have proved to be mutagens, including many which are carcinogenic in man, such as cigarette smoke, coal tar, β-naphthylamine, aflatoxin, etc. Promoters such as phorbol are non-mutagenic in this test. Moreover, non-carcinogenic molecules closely related in structure to carcinogens are very rarely found to be mutagenic. The correlation between carcinogenicity and mutagenicity is thus very close indeed. Extensive screening with this test has revealed some disturbing activity in widely used substances of hitherto unknown mutagenicity—for example most common hair dyes are mutagens. Since there are literally millions of users of these dyes, investigations of their possible carcinogenic effect are now being actively pursued.

4. VIRUSES AND NEOPLASIA

It has long been established that viruses can cause cancer in animals and there is great interest in whether this is also true in man. Among malignancies with a viral aetiology in animals are sarcomas and leukaemias of chickens, mice and cats, murine mammary cancer and renal carcinoma in frogs. Scepticism about the notion of a viral role in human cancer existed for many years, partly because in the vast majority of cases the epidemiological characteristics of neoplasms do not suggest an infectious causation and also because the direct demonstration of tumour viruses in man has been very difficult. There are only a few instances in animals or man where neoplastic disease is clearly contagious under natural conditions. In chickens an infectious cancer of the lymphoid system called Marek's disease is definitely caused by a contagious herpesvirus and vaccination is used to prevent the disease; leukaemia in cats is spread by infection with the feline leukaemia virus. In mice, mammary cancer is caused by a virus passed from mother to offspring in milk. For human tumours, only the benign wart has been proven to be virally produced and transmitted (human papilloma virus), but evidence for a causal association between viruses and some human cancers has accumulated in recent years. Probably the strongest case can be made that a herpesvirus, Epstein-Barr virus, is the cause of two cancers, namely Burkitt's lymphoma and nasopharyngeal carcinoma, while another herpesvirus, herpes simplex type 2, may be responsible for carcinoma of the cervix. There is also good reason to link hepatitis B virus infection with primary liver cancer, while breast cancer and certain leukaemias also seem to be associated with viruses. In addition, experimental research has demonstrated mechanisms whereby viruses interacting with normal cells can cause neoplastic change and has led to stimulating theories of the relationship between viruses and cancer. In this section, some of the processes involved in viral production of tumours are described and the evidence that viruses are aetiological agents of cancer is discussed.

Classification of tumour viruses

Like other viruses, the tumour-causing or *oncogenic* viruses can be divided into DNA- and RNA-containing groups. The best known examples and the species in which they are oncogenic are shown in Table 6.6. The DNA tumour viruses include the *papovaviruses*, almost all members of which can cause tumours; some

Table 6.6 Oncogenic viruses.

Virus	Oncogenic in	Neoplasm
1. DNA VIRUSES		
Papovaviruses		
Papilloma	Man, rabbit, cattle	Wart, papilloma
Polyoma	Rodents	Various
SV40	Rodents	Sarcoma
Adenoviruses	Rodents	Sarcoma
Herpesviruses		
Marek's disease virus	Chicken	Lymphomatosis
Lucké virus	Frog	Adenocarcinoma
Epstein-Barr virus	Man?	Burkitt's lymphoma Nasopharyngeal carcinoma
Herpes simplex type 2	Man?	Cervical carcinoma
Herpesvirus saimiri	Monkey	Lymphoma
Poxviruses		
Shope fibroma virus	Rabbit	Fibroma
Yaba monkey virus	Monkey	Papilloma
Hepatitis viruses		
Hepatitis B virus	Man?	Liver cell carcinoma
Woodchuck hepatitis virus	Woodchuck	Liver cell carcinoma
2. RNA VIRUSES (ONCORNAVIRUSES)		
Sarcoma viruses		
Rous sarcoma virus	Chicken	Sarcoma
Murine sarcoma virus	Mouse, rat	Sarcoma
Feline sarcoma virus	Cat, dog, rabbit	Sarcoma
Bovine lymphosarcoma virus	Cattle	Sarcoma
Leukaemia viruses		
Avian leukaemia virus	Birds	Leukaemia
Murine leukaemia virus (Gross, Rauscher, Friend)	Mouse, rat	Leukaemia
Feline leukaemia virus	Cat, dog, rabbit	Leukaemia
Mammary tumour viruses		
Mouse mammary tumour viruses (Bittner, Mühlbock)	Mouse	Mammary carcinoma

adenoviruses, *herpesviruses* and *poxviruses* are also oncogenic. The RNA tumour viruses all belong to one group called *oncornaviruses* (i.e. *onco*genic-*rna-virus*). This is part of a larger family, the *Retroviridae*, which includes all viruses containing the enzyme *reverse transcriptase,* an essential element in the oncogenic properties of RNA viruses. They are broadly subdivided according to the types of tumour they produce into *sarcoma, leukaemia* and *mammary tumour* viruses, as well as to the species in which they are found (avian, murine, feline, etc.). Another description frequently used in reference to these viruses is based on their morphology in the electron microscope. Thus most RNA tumour viruses are *C-type* particles, an exception being the mammary tumour virus which is *B-type.* Each virus consists of a 'nucleoid', enclosed in a lipid-containing envelope; the nucleoid contains the RNA genome associated with structural (capsid) protein and reverse transcriptase. In C-type particles the nucleoid is centrally placed, while in B-type particles it is eccentric and surrounded by an inner membrane.

Interactions between tumour viruses and cells

TRANSFORMATION

The essential property of a tumour virus is its ability to alter permanently the characteristics of the cell it has infected, in particular to cause it to escape from normal restrictions of growth control. When this change is produced in culture it is known as *transformation.* Cells transformed *in vitro* lose contact inhibition of mitosis and movement; they are morphologically distinct from normal cells and show surface changes of the type characteristic of tumour cells (lectin agglutinability, altered intercellular junctions, etc.). They may also show some of the biochemical changes seen in tumour cells, such as increased anaerobic glycolysis and expression of foetal antigens, and exhibit karyotypic alterations. Moreover, in many cases cells transformed by viruses in culture will grow into tumours when inoculated into test animals. Because of these close parallels between virus-transformed cells and naturally occurring tumour cells, transformation *in vitro* is assumed to correspond to natural neoplastic change occurring *in vivo.* (See also Section 3, Figure 3.14.)

VIRUS REPLICATION

An important difference between DNA and RNA tumour viruses is that the DNA viruses do not replicate in the cells which they transform and intact virus is therefore not detectable intracellularly in transformed cells; in contrast, RNA tumour viruses are frequently produced by transformed cells. The reason for this difference lies in the effect of viral replication on the cell, for it is an obvious prerequisite that a tumour virus should not kill the cell destined for transformation. For a DNA tumour virus, there are two main possible outcomes of infection. In cells derived from its natural host, the virus will usually replicate to produce infectious progeny; ultimately the cell is lysed and progeny virus released. Such a cell is termed *permissive* and replication is called *productive* or *lytic.* On the other hand, when the infected cell is of a different species of origin, the virus often does not multiply and the cell is said to be *non-permissive*. Such cells lack certain factors required for viral replication. It is the non-permissive cells that are the main targets of transformation by DNA viruses, since it is clear that the normal replicative life-cycle of the virus is incompatible with cell survival. An alternative situation in which transformation rather than lytic replication can occur is where the virus itself lacks some of the genetic information required for replication. Transformation by such *defective* DNA viruses can occur in otherwise permissive cells.

In contrast to the DNA viruses, RNA tumour viruses do not lyse the cells in which they replicate; they are shed from the cell surface by *budding*, an event which leaves the cell intact (p. 238). Thus transformation and replication are perfectly compatible for RNA viruses and indeed often occur together. Hence, when virus particles are found inside transformed cells they are invariably of the RNA type. The phenomenon of defective replication is also seen for some RNA tumour viruses. Many sarcoma viruses, for example, will transform fibroblasts *in vitro*, but cannot replicate on their own. The fact that sarcoma virus replication frequently occurs in transformed cells is due to the simultaneous presence of a *helper* virus, which provides a product required for replication of the sarcoma virus, such as an envelope protein. The helper viruses are invariably leukaemia viruses; in the fibroblast they are capable of replication, but not transformation, though they will transform haematopoietic cells. This last point also shows that tumour viruses have specific target cells which they will transform, and that susceptibility to transformation is related to the differentiated nature of the cell.

PERSISTENCE OF VIRAL GENOME IN TRANSFORMED CELLS

Although it is frequently impossible to demonstrate viable virus particles in transformed cells, at least part of the genetic material of the virus is *always* permanently retained in the cell after transformation. For both DNA and RNA tumour viruses, the virus-specific genetic information is physically integrated into host DNA. This event is an essential step in the process of transformation, though it is not restricted to the oncogenic viruses. Whereas the genome of DNA tumour viruses can integrate directly into host chromosomes, that of RNA viruses is first transcribed into DNA by a process unique to this class of viruses and the DNA 'copy' is then integrated. The integrated form of the virus is called a *provirus*.

DNA viruses

Insertion of the DNA of these viruses directly into host chromosomes occurs by a process akin to recombination. We have already noted that complete DNA virus particles are not found in transformed cells. However, the persistence of the complete viral DNA has been demonstrated, at least in the case of SV40 virus, by fusion of transformed (non-permissive) cells with normal

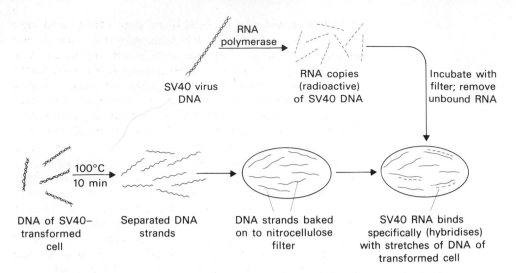

RNA polymerase

SV40 virus DNA

RNA copies (radioactive) of SV40 DNA

Incubate with filter; remove unbound RNA

DNA of SV40-transformed cell

100°C 10 min

Separated DNA strands

DNA strands baked on to nitrocellulose filter

SV40 RNA binds specifically (hybridises) with stretches of DNA of transformed cell

permissive cells. The reappearance of SV40 virus in the hybrid cells showed that all the genetic information required to produce virus had been carried by the transformed cells. (SV40 is unusual in that the *whole* of its genome is integrated into the host DNA. For most other DNA tumour viruses, only part of the genome becomes integrated). The existence of viral DNA in the host cell chromosomes can be revealed by the technique of *nucleic acid hybridisation* (not to be confused with cell hybridisation by fusion). In the DNA–RNA hybridisation technique illustrated in Figure 6.26, the DNA of SV40 virus has been used to prepare radioactive RNA *in vitro*, with DNA-dependent RNA polymerase; because the virus DNA is the template, the RNA produced is complementary to it. Since complementary sequences of nucleotides in nucleic acids associate with each other (as in the two strands of DNA), the labelled RNA can be used as a probe to detect viral DNA sequences in the host genome. Thus, if viral DNA has been incorporated into host cell chromosomes, the complementary RNA should adhere to individual strands of host DNA. In the experimental procedure, DNA of SV40-transformed cells is first heated to separate the strands ('melting') and then attached to a nitrocellulose filter. Radioactive RNA transcribed from SV40 DNA is then incubated with the same filter and the amount of radioactivity binding to the filter after washing is an indication of the complementarity of viral RNA and cell DNA. Using DNA of normal cells, binding is generally very low, but with DNA from SV40-transformed cells significant binding occurs and can be detected with high sensitivity. In this way it has been shown that human cells transformed in culture with SV40 virus carry at least one copy each of the SV40 genome; in some cases as many as ten copies have been found in a single cell.

Given that viral DNA integrates covalently into a host chromosome(s), it is important to know if this event occurs at random in the host DNA, or if insertion into a specific chromosome is necessary for transformation. This has been studied in SV40-transformed human cells using the cell fusion technique. It will be recalled from the earlier description of this method (p. 730)

Figure 6.26 Demonstration of SV40 DNA in the chromosomes of transformed cells by DNA–RNA hybridization.

that when diploid cells are fused by an agent such as inactivated Sendai virus, hybrid cells are produced which are initially tetraploid (at least). They are usually unstable in terms of chromosome number, however, and proceed to lose chromosomes seemingly at random. This phenomenon is of use in gene mapping, because it is possible to associate the expression of a cell property or product with the retention of a specific chromosome. Hence cell hybridisation can be used to identify the chromosomes into which a tumour virus has integrated. In the case of SV40, transformed human cells were fused with normal mouse cells; hybrids were obtained, some of which had lost human chromosomes but retained a full complement of mouse chromosomes. It was found that the expression of malignant properties by such cells was dependent on the retention of one particular human chromosome: only hybrids carrying human chromosome 7 continued to behave as transformed cells, to give rise to tumours in mice and to express certain definitive SV40 products (T antigen, p. 783). Hence the SV40 genome had become specifically incorporated into chromosome 7 in transformed human cells. The significance of this specific insertion locus for the mechanism of transformation by SV40 has yet to be elucidated. (It may also be recalled that the hybrids of SV40-transformed and normal cells were malignant *in vivo*, demonstrating the dominant effect of viral transformation, in so far as normal mouse cells did not contain genes able to suppress the malignant state. This contrasts with results obtained with other types of cancer cell, as described on page 732.)

RNA viruses

In order for the genetic information of RNA viruses to be incorporated into the cell genome, a DNA copy of the single-stranded viral RNA must first be made by a unique process called *reverse transcription* (RNA → DNA). As its name suggests, this is the reversal of the normal flow of genetic information in the cell (DNA → RNA); it is catalysed by an enzyme called *RNA-dependent DNA polymerase* or *reverse transcriptase*. The presence of this enzyme in a cell or associated with a particle is sufficiently unusual to be a very strong indication of the presence of an RNA tumour virus, although it is also found with a few non-oncogenic viruses. (The other viruses which carry reverse transcriptase are the unusual 'foamy agents' found in some cultured cells, and those causing 'slow', i.e. progressive, diseases of sheep, such as visna, p. 368.) The importance of reverse transcriptase is shown by the inability of mutant viruses which lack the enzyme either to replicate or to transform cells. Once the DNA copy of the viral genome has been made, it is inserted into a host chromosome as a provirus, and is carried permanently by the cell and its descendents. The provirus is required not only for transformation but also for viral replication and in this the RNA tumour viruses differ from the other RNA viruses. As shown in Figure 6.27, the latter replicate by using RNA as a template for RNA synthesis, whereas the tumour viruses are replicated by transcription from

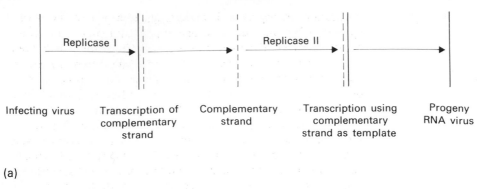

Infecting virus | Transcription of complementary strand | Complementary strand | Transcription using complementary strand as template | Progeny RNA virus

(a)

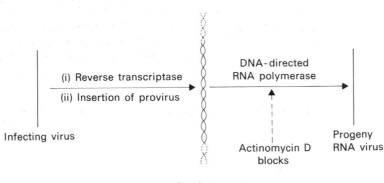

(b)

Provirus (⨉⨉⨉)
inserted into host DNA (⨉⨉⨉)

their DNA provirus. This reading of viral RNA from DNA is thus more akin to production of messenger RNA in the normal cell than it is to conventional replication of RNA viruses (see also Section 3, p. 235). These processes explain unexpected findings originally made with Rous sarcoma virus, that replication was prevented by inhibitors of DNA synthesis, such as bromodeoxyuridine, and by actinomycin D, an inhibitor of DNA-directed RNA synthesis, neither of which interferes with the cycle of most conventional RNA viruses (Figure 6.27).

A DNA provirus is always present in cells transformed by RNA viruses, even in cases where the virus does not produce infectious progeny (e.g. mammalian cells transformed by avian sarcoma virus). As with DNA viruses, the existence of the provirus can be demonstrated by nucleic acid hybridisation (Figure 6.26), in this case using DNA synthesized *in vitro* from viral RNA, by reverse transcriptase, as the radioactive 'probe'. This hybridises with the DNA of the transformed cell, proving the existence of the viral genome in cell chromosomes. Surprisingly, the DNA of *normal* cells also hybridises with that transcribed from RNA of some retroviruses indicating that normal cells can carry genes of RNA tumour viruses apparently without having been exposed to viral infection. This important discovery is discussed further on p. 787.

Significance of viral integration

Thus for both DNA and RNA tumour viruses the process of

Figure 6.27 Replication of RNA viruses.
(a) Replication of RNA viruses other than oncornaviruses.
(b) Replication of RNA tumour viruses.

transformation begins with the introduction of new, i.e. virus-specific, DNA into the host genome. In this way, viral information is fixed in the cell and inherited by the progeny of that cell when it divides. It is possible that viral integration is itself an oncogenic event. For example, since integration involves a form of recombination between host and viral DNA, it could be a source of mutations which, if they occurred in important regulatory genes, might have a transforming effect. Mutagenic effects of viral insertion are known for bacteria infected with certain bacteriophages, but have not been established in animal cells. Viral integration can also lead to chromosomal aberrations, another potential source of mutation. In general, however, the process of integration *per se* is not sufficient for transformation. Rather, its primary importance is in the permanent introduction into the host DNA of specific viral genes, the products of which then direct the process of transformation. The nature of such transforming genes and their products is discussed below.

Viral genes and products associated with transformation

DNA VIRUSES

T antigens

Transformation by DNA viruses such as the papovaviruses is associated with the appearance of a virus-specific protein in the nucleus, called the T (tumour) antigen; the term antigen is used because it can be detected immunologically, by means of antibodies present in the sera of tumour-bearing animals. The T antigens produced by different viruses do not cross-react. Although they are not part of the virus structure, they do appear in permissive as well as transformed cells and are produced early in the replicative cycle of the virus. The part of the viral DNA coding for the T antigen is therefore called the 'early' region. The presence of the T antigen is apparently essential both for integration of the viral DNA into the host genome and for transformation, since virus mutants which do not produce T antigen neither transform nor integrate. Very little is known of its exact role in transformation. Its importance may be in stimulating cell division, perhaps as a direct result of binding to DNA.

Transforming genes

The papovaviruses possess small genomes, with only enough DNA to code for between five and eight polypeptides depending on size. There is, therefore, a real possibility of identifying the products of specific viral genes in the hope of discovering one which is particularly crucial to transformation. One approach is the use of enzymes which cleave DNA at restricted sites, called *restriction endonucleases*. When viral DNA is digested by such enzymes, fragments are obtained which can be separated and tested for transforming ability. Some individual fragments do retain the ability both to integrate into cell DNA and to transform, while comprising only a fraction of the virus genome. Since a small fragment suffices to transform the cell, it may well carry a specific *transforming gene*. It is, therefore, very interesting that for papovaviruses, the transforming fragment corresponds to the early region of the genome which codes for the T antigens. Thus the T antigens are further implicated directly in the mechanism of transformation itself.

When *adenoviruses* transform cells, only part of their DNA becomes integrated and whole virus is not retrievable. The integrated viral DNA is always the 'left-hand' region of the adenovirus genome and as little as 6% of the adenovirus information is required for transformation.

TRANSFORMING GENES OF RNA VIRUSES
(ONCOGENES)

Among the oncornaviruses, a distinction can be made between those which cause rapid transformation (within hours or days), so-called 'acute' transforming viruses, and those which are slowly transforming. Among the former are sarcoma viruses, while the latter include several leukaemia viruses and mouse mammary tumour virus. The genome of acute transforming sarcoma viruses, such as the well-studied *Rous sarcoma virus* (RSV), includes one gene which is essential for transformation, but is not required for viral replication; in the case of RSV, this is called the *src* (for sarcoma) gene. Genes such as *src* which bring about neoplastic change are known as transforming genes or *oncogenes*; they are not present in the slowly transforming RNA viruses. Two lines of evidence indicate that the *src* gene is responsible for transformation by RSV. One is that cells transformed by RSV occasionally revert to the normal phenotype; such revertant cells produce RNA viruses which no longer transform target cells and in some cases have been shown to have deletions of the *src* gene. The other evidence comes from mutants of RSV which are *temperature sensitive* (*ts*): *ts* mutants will transform the cell only in a certain restricted (permissive) temperature range (35–37°C), while at 40–41°C (non-permissive temperatures) many such mutants replicate in the cell but cannot transform. Moreover, the continued expression of transformed characteristics by the infected cells is also temperature dependent, i.e. if cells transformed by a *ts* mutant at 35°C are shifted to 41°C, properties such as abnormal growth, lectin agglutinability, etc., are lost. These observations make the important point that both the process of transformation and the maintenance of the transformed state are dependent on the continued expression of viral genes. For some *ts* mutants, the

Figure 6.28 Proposed genetic map of Rous sarcoma virus. 'c' = common region, i.e. nucleotide sequences common to several viruses, not coding for protein.

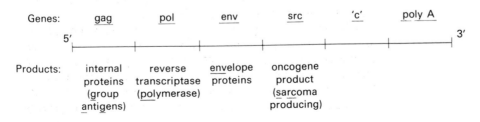

784

lesion has been mapped to the *src* region of the virus genome.

Oncornaviruses, like the papovaviruses, possess small genomes, making it possible to identify the functions of individual viral genes. A gene map for a 'complete' sarcoma virus, i.e. one which can both transform and replicate, is shown in Figure 6.28. In addition to the transforming gene *src*, there are three other genes. The gene called *gag* (from *g*roup-specific *a*nti*g*ens) codes for the internal or core proteins of the mature virus. The *pol* gene codes for reverse transcriptase, the *pol*ymerase enzyme which transcribes viral RNA into its DNA provirus. Another gene, *env*, codes for viral *env*elope proteins. These insert into the host cell membrane at the budding site, so that viral cores budding through are enveloped by host plasma membrane containing *env* gene products. Many strains of RSV and similar rapidly transforming sarcoma viruses are defective for the *env* gene and are therefore dependent on a helper virus to provide the envelope proteins required for replication.

The mechanism of action of the *src* gene is that it codes for a protein which can transform the cell. The *src* product has now been identified and is designated pp60^{src} to indicate that it is a phosphoprotein (phosphorylated protein, pp) of 60,000 mol.wt. pp60^{src} is a *protein kinase*, an enzyme which phosphorylates proteins by transferring phosphate from ATP to specific amino acid residues. It differs from the cellular protein kinases known hitherto in that it catalyses the phosphorylation of *tyrosine* in proteins, whereas other kinases phosphorylate serine or threonine. In normal cells, 90% of the phosphorylated residues in proteins are serines and 10% are threonines; phosphorylated tyrosines comprise less than 0.05%. In cells transformed by RSV, the amount of phosphorylated tyrosine increases approximately tenfold. The evidence that the *src* gene codes for this unusual kinase includes the following. (a) Deletion mutants of RSV which lack the *src* gene fail to produce kinase; (b) the kinase of *ts* mutants is only active at permissive temperatures; and (c) pp60^{src} has been synthesized *in vitro* by direct translation from fragments of viral RNA containing the *src* gene. That kinase activity correlates with the transformed state is shown by (a) the increase in phosphorylated tyrosine already noted and (b) the finding that in cells transformed by *ts* mutants, the level of phosphorylated tyrosine reverts to normal as cells are shifted from a permissive to a non-permissive temperature. Thus there is good reason to believe that this enzyme is responsible for transformation (Figure 6.29). Moreover, other retroviruses code for similar enzymes (Table 6.7). Protein kinase activity has also been found associated with transforming gene products of some DNA viruses, such as SV40, polyoma and adenoviruses, though the nature of this association is less clear-cut than with retroviruses.

Obviously the identity of the cellular protein(s) phosphorylated by pp60^{src} and related enzymes is of key interest; in fact several proteins, one or more of which are probably involved in growth control, have been found to be tyrosine-phosphorylated in RSV-transformed cells. One substrate for the enzyme is a cytoplasmic protein of 36,000 mol.wt present in cells in large quantity

Table 6.7 Transforming genes of acute transforming retroviruses.

Gene	Prototype virus	Protein kinase?	Isolation source
src	Rous sarcoma virus	+	Chicken
fps	Fujinami sarcoma virus	+	Chicken
fes	Snyder-Theilin feline sarcoma virus	+	Cat
yes	Y73 sarcoma virus	+	Chicken
fms	McDonough feline sarcoma virus	?	Cat
mos	Moloney sarcoma virus	?	Mouse
ras	Harvey sarcoma virus	+	Rat, mouse
sis	Simian sarcoma virus	?	Woolly monkey
myc	Myelocytomatosis virus MC29	?	Chicken
erb	Avian erythroblastosis virus	?	Chicken
myb	Avian myeloblastosis virus	?	Chicken
abl	Abelson leukaemia virus	+	Mouse
rel	Reticuloendotheliosis virus T	?	Turkey
ros	UR2 sarcoma virus	+	Chicken

After Cooper (1982) *Science*, **218**, 801.

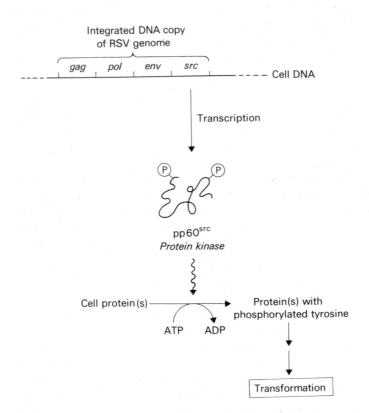

Figure 6.29 Mechanism of transformation by the *src* gene of Rous sarcoma virus.

(up to 0.5% of total cell protein) but of undetermined function. Another is *vinculin*, a protein which anchors actin filaments of the cytoskeleton to the inside of the cell membrane and assists in the adhesion of cells to basement membranes and solid surfaces via 'adhesion plaques'. Glycolytic enzymes also become phosphorylated by pp60^{src} and this may be related to the high rate of glycolysis of neoplastic cells (p. 723). Another significant finding is that pp60^{src} is itself localised on the inner surface of the cell membrane, from where it may direct the membrane alterations which are considered particularly important in the transformed cell. In any event, the fact that protein kinases do have a wide range of possible substrates may account for the large number of cellular changes associated with neoplasia and for the surprising discovery that a *single gene product* can lead to such complex disturbances of cell growth and function.

The technique of nucleic acid hybridisation (p. 780) has been used to demonstrate the presence of the *src* gene in the genome of RSV-transformed cells. A radioactive DNA copy of *src* was prepared by reverse transcriptase and used as a probe to detect cellular DNA of similar sequence. This led to a most important result, namely that the *src* gene can be detected not only in DNA from neoplastic cells, but also in that of normal, non-infected chickens and other birds, and is even found in fishes and in mammals, including man. In other words, it seems that the cells of all vertebrates possess a gene related or identical to *src*. Further investigation showed that the *src* gene of normal cells is structurally distinct from viral *src* and is therefore not a result of silent retroviral infection; rather, it is the *normal cellular gene* coding for one of the cell's own protein kinases, and is referred to as the c-*src* gene ('c' for cellular). A protein immunologically indistinguishable from pp60^{src} can be demonstrated at a low level in normal cells and is evidently the c-*src* product; the normal kinase is present at about 1–2% of the concentration of pp60^{src} in RSV-transformed cells. The findings with the *src* gene have now been extended to the oncogenes of about 20 other retroviruses and practically all have close relatives (homologues) in the genomes of normal cells.

Two major conclusions can be drawn from these discoveries. (i) The transforming genes of retroviruses are probably *copies of cellular genes*, acquired by the viruses at some point in their evolution. The viral proteins coded by these genes are thus closely related to normal cell constituents (e.g. protein kinases), and are involved in universal cellular functions such as control of cell division. Transformation by these retroviruses results from the relative overproduction in the cell of proteins such as pp60^{src} and the resulting uncontrolled increase in an otherwise normal cell reaction, in this case tyrosine-phosphorylation. (ii) Normal cells possess genes which, if activated, can transform them into neoplastic cells. The existence of such potential cellular oncogenes has profoundly influenced current views on the production of neoplasia. The 'oncogene hypothesis' suggests that the activation of oncogenes inherent in normal cells is a pathway common to many disparate carcinogenic agents, chemical and physical as well as viral. This hypothesis is discussed further on p. 805.

It should be noted that some oncogenic retroviruses do not contain specific transforming genes. In contrast with the acute transforming viruses, which cause rapid cell transformation in culture and have a short period of latency *in vivo*, these viruses are only weakly oncogenic, do not transform cells in culture and require long latent periods before neoplasms appear *in vivo*. They include mouse mammary tumour virus (MMTV, p. 801), some mouse leukaemia viruses and avian lymphoid leukosis virus. Oncogenesis by these retroviruses is thought to be more akin to the action of chemical carcinogens, e.g. via indirect activation of a cellular gene, rather than by introduction of an active viral transforming gene as in RSV infection.

Transmission of tumour viruses

There are two main ways in which oncogenic viruses can be transmitted. In *horizontal transmission* the virus is spread from one infected animal to another by contact or proximity and this is well illustrated by the contagious spread of certain cancers, notably Marek's disease of chickens and feline leukaemia. The alternative mode of spread is *vertical transmission* in which virus passes directly from parent to offspring. This can occur either because the parent is a carrier of live virus, in which case *congenital infection* occurs; or by *genetic transmission*, in which endogenous viral information is part of the genome of the parent and is therefore inherited in egg or sperm. Vertical transmission is illustrated by RNA tumour viruses. For example, the mouse mammary tumour virus (Bittner agent) is present in the milk of female mice of certain strains and is passed to neonatal offspring on suckling. On the other hand, murine leukaemia viruses are

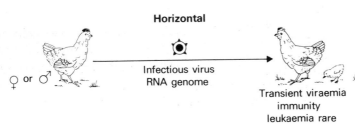

Horizontal

Infectious virus
RNA genome

♀ or ♂

Transient viraemia
immunity
leukaemia rare

Figure 6.30 Modes of transmission of avian leukaemia virus (from Tooze, *Molecular Biology of Tumour Viruses*, 1973).

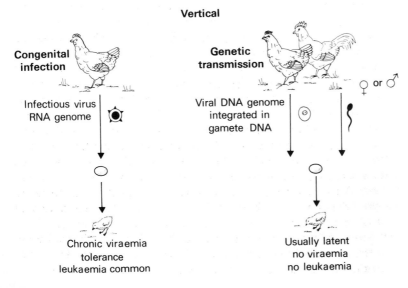

Vertical

Congenital infection

Infectious virus
RNA genome

Chronic viraemia
tolerance
leukaemia common

Genetic transmission

♀ or ♂

Viral DNA genome
integrated in
gamete DNA

Usually latent
no viraemia
no leukaemia

present as DNA proviruses in the genomes of certain mouse strains and are inherited as such rather than as free viable particles. Some RNA viruses, such as avian leukaemia virus, are transmitted by all three routes, horizontal, congenital and genetic, but the disease only develops as a result of congenital infection (Figure 6.30). Horizontal spread fails to induce leukaemia because the chicks or adult birds become immune to the virus; genetic transmission passes on latent provirus, but this is rarely activated. Only congenital infection, in which the virus is present as live particles in the egg, produces a successful infection during embryonic development and thereby avoids the immune response by inducing a state of specific tolerance. These tolerant birds are chronically viraemic and, because they are continually shedding virus, are the major sources of horizontal infection. Other RNA viruses share this inability to produce tumours unless introduced into very young, immunologically immature animals.

Some examples of tumour viruses

ONCOGENIC DNA VIRUSES

Papovaviruses

The name of this family of viruses derives from its three members, the *pa*pilloma viruses, *po*lyoma viruses and the simian '*va*cuolating' virus called SV40. Polyoma and SV40 are very similar in their physical and chemical properties and together form the polyomavirus group; they are among the most extensively studied of all tumour viruses and most of the events involved in transformation by DNA viruses described above have been discovered with them. In contrast, rather little is known about the molecular biology of papilloma viruses as they cannot be studied in cell culture.

Papilloma viruses have been known for many years to be the cause of *warts* of man and animals. Warts are benign growths, more akin to hyperplasia than true tumours. The common wart, *verruca vulgaris*, is a local outgrowth of the skin, most frequently on sites subject to trauma, such as the fingers and knees, though it may spread elsewhere. Another variety, the moist wart, *condyloma acuminatum*, is a pedunculated growth in the genital region which sometimes becomes malignant. An early wart virus discovered (1933) was the *Shope papilloma virus* of rabbits. (The human wart virus had been discovered by Ciuffo in 1907.) Shope made extracts of the large wart-like growths or 'horns' of wild cottontail rabbits and showed that they would cause papillomas to grow in domestic rabbits if rubbed into the scarified skin. There were interesting differences between the growths produced in this way in domestic rabbits and the natural tumours, both in the character of the warts, which grew faster and were less keratinised in domestic rabbits, but more importantly in the presence of free virus. Whereas the warts produced by infection in the wild could be transmitted with extracts, and therefore contained free virus, the tumours induced in domestic animals were apparently virus-free, i.e. extracts failed to transmit the tumour. From what has been described above, it will be realised that it is unusual to find quantities of free DNA viruses in tumours, as they do not replicate in transformed cells. The extraction of free virus from rabbit warts was only possible because the virus multiplies in the keratinised, non-dividing cells of the outer layer of the wart; virus is not detectable in the proliferating cells of the basal layer. In the latter cells, the virus is incorporated into the host genome, as described for other tumour viruses; it can evidently be 'released' and commence replication in dying cells. Apparently such release only occurs in cells of the natural rabbit host and not in the genetically distinct domestic rabbit. Unfortunately, these events have been difficult to study because papilloma viruses do not transform cells in culture, except with very low efficiency.

In man, papilloma virus is also extractable from warts and is presumably responsible for their infectious spread. Warts have been transmitted to volunteers by inoculation of human wart extracts. As in the cotton-tail rabbit, wart virus is absent from the dividing cells of the basal layer, but present in very large numbers in the outer keratinised tissue. Warts can be shown to be *clonal* growths, i.e. each originates from a single transformed cell, rather than a local collection of independently infected neoplastic cells. This can be proved in women heterozygous for a variant of an enzyme coded on the X-chromosome: since only one X-chromosome is active in any one female cell, a clonal growth should only express one form of the enzyme and this was indeed found to be the case for warts (see also p. 860 for similar applications of the inactive-X phenomenon).

In contrast with the papilloma viruses, neither polyoma nor SV40 viruses cause tumours in their natural hosts. *Polyoma virus* was discovered by Gross in 1953 in extracts of the organs of leukaemic mice. In order to demonstrate its oncogenic properties it was necessary to inject it into newborn mice, since it failed to produce tumours in adults. The name is derived from the great variety of different tumours which the virus will produce in the neonatal mouse — hence 'poly-oma'. (Note that Gross's leukaemia extracts contained two viruses—the leukaemia virus as well as polyoma.) Polyoma virus will also cause tumours in the newborn of other species, such as hamsters, rats and rabbits; monkeys and chickens are resistant. Polyoma virus transforms cells in culture, where it has been widely studied. It is a natural infection of wild and laboratory mice, but polyoma tumours are very rare in the natural state. This is attributable to the action of the immune system in producing neutralising anti-polyoma virus antibodies and in eliminating transformed cells by cell-mediated immunity. That this is so is shown by the susceptibility of nude (athymic) mice to polyoma tumours at any age. Since these mice lack T cells, they make neither antibody nor CMI against the virus or transformed cells (see also p. 742).

The *SV40 virus* was named after its discovery in monkey kidney cells which are used to grow polioviruses for vaccines (simian *v*irus number 40). Like polyoma virus, SV40 can produce tumours in newborn rodents and transform cells in culture. It

790

was, therefore, disturbing that many doses of polio vaccine had been contaminated with SV40 and administered, though happily no ill effects have been found in the recipients of contaminated vaccine. Indeed it is unlikely that SV40 ever produces tumours under natural conditions. SV40 is very similar to polyoma virus in size and structure and classified in the polyomavirus group. Both illustrate many of the properties described earlier, such as replication only in permissive and not in transformed cells, integration of viral DNA in one or more copies into host DNA, and production of T antigen.

Viruses closely resembling polyoma virus and SV40 are found in a rare, non-neoplastic human brain disease called *progressive multifocal leukoencephalopathy* (PML), which occurs in individuals whose immune response has been severely depressed by immunosuppressive therapy or malignant disease (see p. 368).

Adenoviruses (p. 272)

In the 1960's the startling discovery was made that a human adenovirus (type 12) caused tumours if injected into newborn hamsters and could transform cells *in vitro*. However, detailed investigation has failed to demonstrate any role for adenoviruses in human cancers.

Herpesviruses (p. 262)

These are of particular interest because at least one herpesvirus, *Marek's disease virus*, is the cause of a cancer which is highly contagious under natural conditions, namely avian neurolymphomatosis (Marek's disease), and another, the *Epstein-Barr virus*, is closely associated with two human malignancies, Burkitt's lymphoma and nasopharyngeal carcinoma. In addition, *herpes simplex virus type 2* has been implicated in cervical cancer of women.

Marek's disease is a lymphoid cancer of chickens which for many years was a major economic problem for the poultry industry—an outbreak would commonly kill 30% of a flock in a short time. By 1970, the financial losses due to the disease ran into millions of pounds, but since then vaccination has virtually eliminated Marek's disease as a serious problem. It differs from the other leukaemias of chickens in that the agent involved is a DNA rather than an RNA virus. The typical herpesvirus was recovered from cultures of infective cells and was shown to produce the disease when injected into young chicks. The virus is ubiquitous in poultry populations and eventually all chickens become infected, though only a minority develops lymphomas. Infection is by horizontal spread (contact with infected birds) rather than vertical (direct passage from mother to offspring). The origin of infectious virus particles is a permissive form of replication which takes place in the chicken, but in localised cells outside the lymphoid system, namely in the epithelium of feather follicles. When feathers are shed, the virus is released into the birds' environment and thereby spreads. Neoplastic change occurs in lymphocytes, apparently T cells. Like other DNA viruses, MDV cannot be found in tumour cells, though several copies of the virus genome are incorporated into the DNA of the transformed cell. The neoplastic cells then proceed to proliferate into lymphomas, especially in the peripheral nerves, leading to demyelination and paralysis. Fortunately it has been possible to develop an attenuated form of Marek's disease virus and its use as a vaccine has virtually eliminated the disease.

Epstein-Barr virus (EBV). Herpesviruses have come into prominence as possible agents of human cancer mainly through the association of EBV with *Burkitt's lymphoma* and *nasopharyngeal carcinoma*. A particularly interesting feature of both these malignant conditions is their restricted geographical distribution—Burkitt's lymphoma in parts of Africa and nasopharyngeal carcinoma in Southern China and S.E. Asia. In Europe and the U.S.A., on the other hand, the same virus is the cause of a common proliferative but self-limiting disorder of lymphoid tissue, *infectious mononucleosis (glandular fever)*. The reasons for the production of such different diseases by the same virus are of great interest. In many people, EBV is carried permanently as a latent infection in some B lymphocytes and can give rise to lymphomas in patients undergoing immunosuppressive therapy.

Burkitt's lymphoma is unusual both in its clinical features and its epidemiology. It is a childhood tumour, a lymphocytic lymphoma (a solid proliferation of malignant lymphocytes) with a unique predilection for the jaw, though tumours are also found in internal organs such as the ovaries, liver and adrenals. It is a rare tumour in most parts of the world, and has its principal occurrence in parts of Africa. Within Africa, the distribution is also geographically determined; thus it is not common in any region where the temperature falls below 60°F in any season or where the annual rainfall is less than 30 in. This restricted distribution strongly suggested an environmental agent and the most likely was thought to be an insect vector carrying an oncogenic virus. It has since become clear that the 'vectored virus' theory is incorrect, since EBV, with which the tumour is associated, is ubiquitous and no more frequent in areas with a high incidence of Burkitt's lymphoma than elsewhere. It was subsequently realised that Burkitt's lymphoma was only frequent in areas where *malarial incidence* was high; hyperendemic malaria and Burkitt's lymphoma seemed to be invariably associated. Particularly impressive was the complete absence of the tumour from the two areas in tropical Africa where malaria had been most successfully eradicated, namely Zanzibar and the area around Kinshasa in Zaire. Also in accord with a malarial association is the lower incidence of the tumour in carriers of the sickle-cell trait (p. 862) than in non-sickle controls.

Tumour cells from patients with Burkitt's lymphoma will grow indefinitely in culture as lymphoblastoid cell lines and it was in such cells that Epstein and Barr discovered, in 1964, the herpesvirus which bears their name. The virus was produced by a small proportion of such cells in culture; the majority do not release EBV, but it can be shown by nucleic acid hybridisation that they carry several copies of the EBV DNA integrated in proviral form into their chromosomes. They can also be induced to produce EBV particles by chemical treatment (e.g. with bromodeoxyuridine). EBV DNA is invariably associated with cells in biopsies of Burkitt's lymphoma. EBV will also transform human peripheral blood lymphocytes in culture into permanently growing cells which closely resemble those of Burkitt's lymphoma. Cells transformed *in vitro* and natural lymphoma cells both have a characteristic nuclear antigen (EBNA), analogous to the T antigen of other oncogenic DNA viruses, specific membrane antigens at the cell surface and proviral copies of the EBV genome. Further evidence for the aetiological role of EBV in Burkitt's lymphoma is the consistent presence in patients of antibody levels against EBV which are several times higher than in normal groups or in patients with unrelated tumours.

Thus there is good reason to believe that Burkitt's lymphoma is caused by EBV in areas of endemic malaria. One explanation for the malarial association is that malaria has a direct effect on lymphoid cells which allows EBV to produce malignant transformation *in vivo*. Alternatively, the immunosuppressive effect of malarial infection may reduce the 'surveillance' activity of the immune system (p. 741) and allow malignant cells to grow which would otherwise be immunologically killed. In agreement with this second hypothesis is the known immunosuppressive action of malaria in mice and the high antigenicity of the tumour, indicated by a significant rate of spontaneous regressions.

Nasopharyngeal carcinoma is a poorly differentiated cancer which arises from the lymphoepithelium of the nasopharynx. It is associated with a virus which is indistinguishable from EBV. The tumour is especially prevalent among natives of the southern provinces of China and emigrant Chinese in S.E. Asia and the Americas; it is rare in Caucasians. In the Kwangtung province of Southern China, for instance, it accounts for over 30% of all cancers (over 50% in Canton itself), and is the most frequent carcinoma throughout Southern China. It is far less prevalent in Northern China. It is particularly interesting that the high incidence among Chinese, and the difference between those from the north and south of China, persist in migrant Chinese populations who have settled in Hong Kong and Singapore and even in Australia, Hawaii and California. This is in contrast to the effect of migration on other cancers with geographical variation in incidence, in which the incidence in immigrants and their descendents comes to resemble that in the local population (see p. 701). There is thus a strong indication that genetic factors play a significant role in nasopharyngeal carcinoma, in addition to environmental agents such as EBV. Recently it has emerged that the genetic factor is associated with the histocompatibility (HLA) type of the individual, which is suggestive of a role for HLA genes in the aetiology of the disease. Chinese patients show a higher than average frequency of a particular HLA antigen, HLA-A2.

A causative role of EBV in nasopharyngeal carcinoma is suggested by observations similar to those made with Burkitt's lymphoma. Lymphoid cells obtained from biopsies grow permanently in culture and occasional cells produce EBV; the others contain EBV genetic information in proviral form and EBV nuclear antigens. The sera of patients likewise contain high levels of anti-EBV antibodies, which increase as the disease progresses. EBV DNA is also present in the malignant epithelial cells of the tumour as well as the lymphoblastoid cells, and is presumably responsible for the transformation of both.

Infectious mononucleosis (*glandular fever*) is a common disease of young adults (particularly college students) and is unequivocally caused by the Epstein-Barr virus. Its characteristic feature is a transient, but vigorous, hyperplasia of lymphoid tissue (lymphadenitis, splenomegaly) and an alarming leucocytosis in which atypical large lymphocytes (lymphoblasts) appear in the blood in large numbers, the white cell count reaching up to $50,000/mm^3$. Despite its similarity to malignant lymphoma, the disease is self-limiting and is over in 1–3 weeks. During the progress of the disease, diagnostic IgM antibodies called *heterophile agglutinins* appear in the patient's serum which can agglutinate red cells of sheep and other species. In the *Paul-Bunnell test*, these antibodies are detected by measuring the agglutination titre of the serum for sheep red cells (see p. 134 for details). Note that heterophile antibodies are not produced in Burkitt's lymphoma patients, despite infection with EBV.

The relationship between infectious mononucleosis and EBV was discovered fortuitously when a laboratory technician whose serum was negative for anti-EBV antibodies developed the disease and was subsequently found to have a positive serum. EBV is, as we have noted, widespread and most children are subclinically infected before school age and develop antibodies. Following the observations on the laboratory technician, a retrospective survey of sera of Yale University students sampled before and after they had infectious mononucleosis revealed that the disease only occurred in individuals whose sera had been anti-EBV negative; postrecovery sera were all positive for anti-EBV. It was also possible to understand why infectious mononucleosis has a particularly high incidence among college and university students: this is linked to socio-economic status. In the low socio-economic groups and in countries with a low standard of living, the large majority of children (70–80%) are infected with EBV, develop antibodies and are therefore protected against adult infection. In higher socio-economic groups, fewer children become infected with EBV and so a larger proportion of adolescents and young adults are anti-EBV negative. It seems that development of infectious mononucleosis only occurs when adolescents are infected for the first time (i.e. are anti-EBV negative). Since college and university populations contain a high proportion of young adults of the higher socio-economic groups, the prevalence of infectious mononucleosis is explained.

We have noted that abnormal lymphocytes appear in the blood in infectious mononucleosis. Some of these are the result of non-productive infection by EBV; *in vitro*, these cells will grow into lymphoblastoid lines which are indistinguishable from those from Burkitt's lymphoma or nasopharyngeal carcinoma. Although EBV is not expressed in these cells it can be 'rescued' by treatment with bromodeoxyuridine or by culture. It appears that these infected cells originate from B rather than T lymphocytes. The specificity of EBV for B cells arises from the presence of a receptor for the virus on the B cell surface, which is not expressed on T cells. Not surprisingly, this receptor binds EBV fortuitously rather than by design, and its true function is to bind a *complement fragment* called C3d. Having bound to the C3d receptor, essentially by cross-reaction, EBV gains access to the cell and ultimately transforms it. Antibody to EBV prevents the infection of B cells by binding to the virus and preventing cellular attachment. In infectious mononucleosis itself, however, only a small proportion ($\sim$ 10%) of the proliferating lymphocytes in lymphoid tissue or blood are transformed B cells; most are *T cells* responding to the presence of EBV-coded antigens on the membranes of infected B cells. These T cells constitute the cell-mediated immune response against the abnormal B cells, their function being to kill them (T cell cytotoxicity). T cells destroy their B cell targets in the same way as they kill cells during other virus infections, by engaging the cell directly via specific surface receptors and damaging the target cell membrane (see Section 2). It is probably due to the efficiency of the T cell response that lymphoproliferation is limited in duration to only one or two weeks.

If we accept that EBV is the aetiological agent of Burkitt's lymphoma and nasopharyngeal carcinoma, we must ask how the same virus can cause these neoplasms in some parts of the world, yet produce the benign infectious mononucleosis in others. The difference probably depends on environmental (e.g. malaria) or genetic (e.g. HLA) cofactors which determine the outcome of EBV infection. A current hypothesis is that the effectiveness of the immune response against the infected cells is the key factor. After EBV-induced transformation, proliferating cells reveal their presence to the immune system by the expression on their membrane of new antigens determined by the EB virus. In infectious mononucleosis, T cells respond effectively and kill the transformed cells. Malaria is known to have an immunosuppressive effect in experimental animals; if such suppression of cell-mediated immunity also occurs in man during malarial infection, it could permit neoplastic B cells to establish themselves permanently. This would account for the close association between Burkitt's lymphoma and endemic malaria. For nasopharyngeal carcinoma we have noted that genetic factors seem to be more important and that there is an apparent predisposition to the disease in individuals of a particular HLA type. As discussed in Section 2, the HLA complex contains genes which regulate the level of the immune response (*Ir genes*). It is thus possible that an inherited defect in the ability to respond to the membrane (or other) antigens of EBV-transformed cells depresses the T cell response sufficiently to allow a neoplasm to develop. This hypothesis assumes that in most individuals, T cells successfully carry out a role of surveillance against EBV-transformed cells. In strong support of this view is the fact that lymphomas which appear in patients undergoing immunosuppression (with cyclosporin A) after organ grafting are often caused by EBV (p. 173). EBV infection is life-long, but normally latent and clinically inapparent, the tendency of B cells to transform being checked by cytotoxic T cells; immunosuppression upsets this balance by removing T cells, whereupon neoplastic B cells are free to proliferate.

Herpes simplex virus type 2 and cervical carcinoma. Carcinoma of the uterine cervix has been shown by epidemiological studies to be associated with sexual activity (see also p. 699). It has its lowest frequency in virgins and highest in women with an active and promiscuous sexual life or in those who began intercourse during adolescence. Another observation suggesting venereal transmission is the occurrence of cervical carcinoma in two or more wives of the same man. Several such clusters have been found in the USA. An implication of the epidemiological findings is that an agent transmitted venereally by males to susceptible females is responsible for cervical cancer and a causative virus has been sought. Herpes simplex virus type 2 (HSV-2) is a likely candidate for several reasons. As described in Section 3, it produces genital infections (genital herpes) which are spread venereally and are therefore related in frequency to sexual activity, being rare among nuns and frequent in promiscuous women. Often, patients with cervical carcinoma have previously been infected with HSV-2, and sometimes have higher levels of antibodies to this virus than matched controls. More suggestive still are the finding of HSV-2 antigens in exfoliated cervical tumour cells and occasional isolation of active virus from cultures of these cells. However, as in the case of EBV, infection with HSV-2 is common in the general population and additional factors have to be invoked to explain the relative infrequency of cervical carcinoma. Such factors could include genetic susceptibility, depression of immune response or hormonal imbalance, so that only certain women are receptive to the oncogenic effect of viral infection.

Hepatitis B virus (HBV)

The properties of this virus, the agent of serum hepatitis, have been described in Section 3, and evidence associating it with primary liver cancer (liver cell or hepatocellular carcinoma) is summarised on p. 363. A sizeable proportion (10–20%) of individuals infected with HBV become chronic (life-long) carriers; viral multiplication continues in liver cells and viral particles and surface antigen (HBsAg) are present in the blood. With the development of sensitive assays for HBsAg, it emerged that in certain parts of the world, usually where socio-economic conditions are poor, 10–30% of the population may be HBV carriers; these are also the areas where liver cancer is most frequent. Studies in high incidence areas of Southern Africa, Senegal and parts of Asia showed that over 90% of patients with primary liver cancer carry the virus, probably having been infected years or decades before tumour development. (A similar correlation is found in other parts of the world.) Even in Mozambique, where a close association with dietary aflatoxin was discovered in the 1960's, liver cancer only develops in people chronically infected with HBV (p. 761). The risk for a chronic HBV carrier of developing primary liver cancer is estimated to be as high as 1%, and is about the same in New York as it is in Senegal. Since there are approximately 200 million carriers in the world, one can expect about 2 million new cases of liver cancer to appear in the next ten years, or about 500 cases per day.

Further evidence for the causal role of HBV comes from related animal viruses. The first to be found was the woodchuck hepatitis virus (WHV). Post-mortem examination of woodchucks maintained in American zoos revealed a high incidence of liver cancer; chronic WHV infection was present in many animals. Since the animals were reared in captivity under ideal nutritional conditions, with no likelihood of ingested hepatotoxins, the only predisposing factor seemed to be the chronic viral infection. Another virus resembling HBV exists in ducks. (The characteristics of HBV and related liver-tropic viruses are quite distinct from other DNA viruses (p. 358) and they seem to constitute a separate, as yet unclassified, viral family.)

Cellular studies also support a direct oncogenic role for HBV. A human cell line which grows continuously in culture (the Alexander cell line) was established in 1976 from the liver tumour of a Mozambiquan male and shown to produce hepatitis B surface antigen (HBsAg). Using cloned HBV DNA as a probe, it has been demonstrated that four complete and two partial copies of the hepatitis B genome are incorporated into the DNA of Alexander cells; HBV DNA was also found to be integrated into the genome of cells from a patient's tumour tissue (cf. Epstein–Barr virus DNA in cells of Burkitt's lymphoma). Cells of another line established from the liver tumour of an American patient also produce HBsAg and contain multiple integrated copies of the HBV genome. While integration of viral DNA does not prove that the virus is oncogenic (and it has not been shown to transform cells *in vitro*) it is very suggestive, for reasons already discussed (p. 782). Moreover, almost all woodchuck liver tumours examined to date (14/15) have WHV DNA integrated with the cell DNA.

ONCOGENIC RNA VIRUSES

As Table 6.6 shows, RNA tumour viruses are responsible for sarcomas, leukaemias and mammary tumours in animals. There is also some evidence for their involvement in human leukaemias and breast cancer.

Sarcoma viruses

The discovery by Rous in 1911 that a chicken sarcoma could be transmitted by cell-free sarcoma filtrates was the starting point for research on tumour viruses, and the *Rous sarcoma virus* (RSV) is the most extensively studied of the RNA tumour viruses. (The name 'Rous sarcoma virus' is now applied to several chicken viruses which cause sarcomas; they are also termed *avian sarcoma viruses*.) Rous found that the sarcoma extract induced tumours with greater efficiency in young chickens than in adult birds, and this principle has proved to be the case for many other tumour viruses; it probably reflects the immunological immaturity of the young animal which gives the tumour cells a chance to 'take' without immune attack. RSV is a *C-type particle*, in common with most oncornaviruses. It transforms chick fibroblasts in culture: if added to a fibroblast monolayer, it causes the development of foci of transformed cells which stand out and can easily be counted (Figure 3.14). The number of foci is directly proportional to the concentration of virus added, a result which makes the important point that infection by a single RSV particle can transform a normal cell into a cancer cell. The chief events involved in transformation by RSV are described in Figure 6.31, namely reverse transcription of RNA into DNA, incorporation of the DNA provirus into a host chromosome(s) and expression of the *src* gene leading to transformation. Some strains of RSV also carry the full complement of genes required for replicating infective virus particles, whereas others are *defective*—they transform but do not replicate. One such defective strain, the Bryan strain, lacks a surface component required for successful infection; this component can be provided by a co-infecting helper virus (an avian leukaemia virus). As described on p. 785, the *src* gene codes for a protein kinase (pp60^{src}) which phosphorylates tyrosines in a number of cell proteins, and this seems to be a key event in transformation (Figure 6.29). The details of how transformation occurs thereafter are, however, still speculative.

Leukaemia viruses

These viruses are associated with leukaemias and lymphomas of mice, chickens, cats and cattle. The *avian leukaemia virus* was one of the first viruses to be discovered, when Ellerman and Bang in 1908 successfully transmitted chicken leukaemia with an extract of leukaemic cells after passing it through filters that removed bacteria. The avian viruses cause a variety of tumours of haematopoietic cells, some of which are of economic importance in the poultry industry. They can spread both horizontally and vertically (Figure 6.30, p. 788), vertical transmission being the most important for induction of the disease. Avian leukaemia viruses are all C-type RNA viruses closely resembling RSV, with the notable exception of Marek's disease virus (p. 791). In common with other leukaemia viruses, they transmit disease most effectively to very young animals, probably because they can induce a state of immunological tolerance at the neonatal stage.

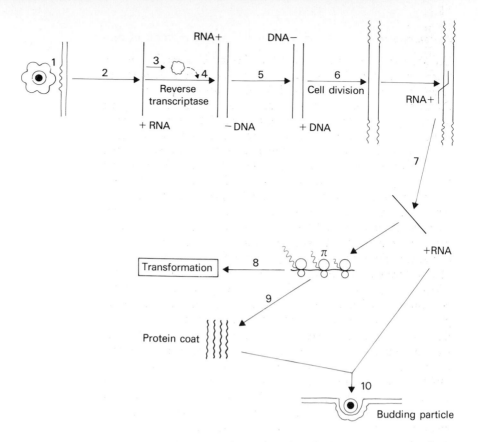

Figure 6.31 Life cycle of an
RNA tumour virus.
(1) Virus binds to cell surface
receptor, (2) enters cell and is
uncoated. (3) Reverse
transcriptase is translated from a
viral gene and (4) catalyses
synthesis of a DNA strand
($-$DNA) complementary to viral
RNA template ($+$RNA).
(5) DNA strand with same base
sequence as viral RNA ($+$DNA)
is synthesized and (6) after cell
division the double-stranded
DNA is integrated as a provirus
into host cell DNA. (7) The
proviral DNA is transcribed into
viral RNA ($+$RNA) which serves
as messenger for translation of
(8) protein causing transformation
(*src* gene product, pp60^{src}) and
(9) virus coat proteins. (10) The
coat proteins and virus RNA
form virus particles which bud
from the cell surface. (After
Tooze, *The Molecular Biology of
Tumour Viruses*, 1973)

However in contrast to sarcoma viruses, most leukaemia agents do
not transform cells in culture (though they may infect the cells
and replicate). This behaviour, which has greatly hindered their
detailed study, arises because, in general, they do not possess a
specific transforming gene as do the acute transforming sarcoma
viruses (Abelson leukaemia virus is an exception).

This discovery of the *mouse leukaemia viruses* sprang from the
observation that some inbred strains of mice were particularly
liable to develop a high frequency of spontaneous leukaemias in
middle and old age (e.g. the AKR strain); other strains (e.g. C3H)
showed a much lower incidence of leukaemia. In 1951, Gross
succeeded in transferring leukaemia from high incidence AKR
mice to low incidence C3H mice with cell-free extracts of
leukaemic cells. Once again, for successful neoplasm induction it
was essential to circumvent the immune system, by introducing
the extracts into neonatal C3H recipients; a state of tolerance
could thereby be established which enabled the virus to induce
neoplasms without a cell-mediated or antibody response developing. The targets of the virus are T cells within the
thymus; it does not induce leukaemia in thymectomised mice.
Specificity for T cells seems to be true of most RNA leukaemia
viruses; only the *Abelson virus* preferentially transforms B
lymphocytes. Most mouse leukaemia viruses have not been
shown to transform cells *in vitro*, though they replicate in
cultured cells and, as previously noted, act as helpers for
replication-defective sarcoma viruses.

The mouse leukaemia viruses provide a good example of vertical transmission. The viruses seem to be present endogenously in all mouse strains, including low incidence strains. This is indicated by the fact that leukaemia can be produced in the low incidence strains by large, sublethal doses of X-rays. A few days after irradiation, the virus appears in the tissues and eventually cells in the thymus are transformed. It is noteworthy that the viruses can arise in several tissues, but do not produce neoplasms in the absence of the thymus, i.e. the thymus cells are the target of action of the viruses, but not their only source. The implication is that many cells in the normal animal harbour virus in latent form and that this is released spontaneously with age in high incidence strains and on X-irradiation of low incidence strains of mice. Several chemical carcinogens, including methylcholanthrene and dimethylbenzanthracene, have the same effect as X-irradiation. These agents all produce other neoplasms besides leukaemias, and the possibility exists that release of latent viruses (i.e. from proviruses) is a common pathway for chemical carcinogens (see the oncogene theory, p. 805). The existence of a DNA provirus in uninfected cells has also been shown by nucleic acid hybridisation. Another indicator is the presence of group-specific viral antigens in normal, virus-negative mouse tissue. An even more intriguing finding is that leukaemia viruses can be found replicating in large numbers in the cells of mouse embryos and young mice of both high and low incidence strains without causing cancer; they disappear in adult animals and only re-emerge if leukaemia develops in the adult. The presence of replicating RNA tumour viruses seems to be a part of normal embryonic development and it is possible that they play an important role in differentiation. Subsequently their expression is suppressed, in most cases permanently. The induction of leukaemia would seem to involve a failure of a cellular control process which allows the proviral DNA to become reactivated inappropriately; such failures would be rare in wild-type animals and only revealed in high frequency in highly inbred laboratory strains.

Leukaemia in the cat is also associated with an RNA virus, *feline leukaemia virus* (FLV). The cat, like man, is a randomly outbred species and in many respects feline leukaemia is a better model for the human disease than that of highly inbred laboratory mice. There are some important differences between leukaemias of cats and mice. Although an endogenous form of FLV exists, it does not apparently have an important role in the disease; it is poorly infective for cat cells in culture, though highly infective for human cultured cells. Instead the disease spreads in a more conventional contagious manner, by transfer of FLV from infected to healthy animals (i.e. horizontal rather than vertical transmission). It is not uncommon to find clusters of unrelated leukaemic cats in households which keep many cats together. In most infected animals, immunity to the virus and to antigens on the surface membrane of virally transformed cells develops and prevents development of the neoplasm. However, the virus exerts a significant immunosuppressive effect and this may be crucial in allowing neoplasms to grow in the small proportion of animals which actually develop leukaemia. It is not always possible to recover FLV from leukaemic cats even though its causative role is well established. This fact is very relevant to consideration of the role of analogous viruses in human leukaemia, where they have only occasionally been demonstrated; the failure to demonstrate virus in tumour cells cannot be taken to mean that a virus is not causally involved.

If RNA leukaemia viruses are ubiquitous and present in the genome of all species—which has emerged as a real possibility—there is an obvious likelihood that they will be found in human leukaemic cells. This indeed seems to be the case. Viral genetic information similar to that of mouse leukaemia virus has been detected by DNA hybridisation techniques with human leukaemic cells; recently, budding virus particles carrying reverse transcriptase have also been detected under the electron microscope in some cultures of leukaemic leucocytes. A widespread incidence of leukaemia viruses in man is indicated by the demonstration of antibodies against them in most adults, and virus induction by chemical treatment of human cell lines in culture. Although for the time being the evidence is circumstantial, it seems likely that RNA viruses are causally associated with some leukaemias in man as in other animals. We should remember that the involvement of leukaemia viruses with the disease takes a different form in different species, from the transfer of latent provirus in the chromosomes of mice to the openly contagious transmission in cats. It remains to be seen whether man is 'cat-like' or 'mouse-like' in this respect.

Mouse mammary tumour viruses (MMTV)

These oncornaviruses cause mammary carcinoma in mice. They provide an example of a third mode of transmission, namely vertical by congenital infection of offspring by an infected mother. As in leukaemia, the occurrence of mammary tumours in mice is genetically determined—certain strains (e.g. C3H) have a high incidence of mammary tumours while other strains have a low incidence (e.g. C57). An important discovery was made when mice of these two strains were crossed. The female offspring (F1 hybrids) of such matings always had the same incidence of mammary cancer as the strain of their mothers. Thus, although the genetic constitution of the offspring of the mating (C3H♂ × C57♀) is the same as (C57♂ × C3H♀), only from the latter did daughters develop high levels of mammary cancer. This showed that the female parent type was more important than the genetic constitution of the hybrid and suggested the transmission of an agent from high incidence mothers to their offspring. In due course this was confirmed by Bittner, who showed that if newborn mice were removed from their high incidence mothers and subsequently nursed by mothers of a low incidence strain, they failed to develop the high incidence characteristic of their own strain. Likewise, low incidence offspring nursed by high incidence mothers showed a high incidence of mammary tumours in later life. The transmission of an infectious agent, now known as the *Bittner virus*, had taken place via the milk of the nursing high incidence mother mouse. The viruses were subsequently shown to be RNA particles, but of a different morphology (B-type) from leukaemia or sarcoma viruses (C-type). Like the mouse leukaemia viruses above, MMTV does not transform cells in culture, has a long latency *in vivo* and lacks a transforming gene.

In addition to the virus, genetic factors also proved to be important, since although the virus will induce tumours in low incidence strains, it ultimately disappears in successive generations of these strains. Another important discovery with the mouse mammary tumour was that, in the high incidence strains, tumours could be produced in male mice, which did not normally develop mammary cancer, if they were given large doses of *oestrogen*; conversely, ovariectomised females of the high incidence strain failed to develop mammary tumours. Hence for the first time hormones were demonstrably implicated in the development of a tumour. However, oestrogen alone was not a complete carcinogen, since in the low incidence strain it caused cystic hyperplasia of mammary tissue but not carcinoma. It is probably correct, therefore, to consider oestrogen as a promoter, through its ability to cause hyperplasia, of tumours initiated by virus. Breast cancer in humans is also hormone dependent.

Is there evidence for a Bittner-type virus in human breast cancer? This question has been explored in several ways, with some results that suggest a positive answer. There is electron microscope evidence for particles resembling the Bittner virus in human milk. Despite initial claims that the occurrence of such particles was related to a family history of breast cancer, careful studies show that this is apparently not the case. Similar particles have also been found in human breast cancer cells and shown to be RNA viruses containing reverse transcriptase. Moreover, the RNA of these human viruses is apparently similar in base sequence to the RNA of the murine Bittner virus. This has been demonstrated by nucleic acid hybridisation, in the following way. RNA of the Bittner virus is transcribed *in vitro* by reverse transcriptase to produce a complementary DNA strand; the latter is the probe used to detect Bittner-like RNA in human breast cancers. The 'Bittner DNA' probe does hybridise with RNA from this source, but not from normal breast tissue or benign tumours. Finally, human embryo cells have been treated in culture with human milk and found to produce RNA viruses carrying reverse transcriptase. However, all of these findings fall short of proof of viral causation of human breast cancer or of milk transmission. If the latter were important, we would expect a decline in breast cancer in parallel with a decline in breast feeding, but recent trends do not suggest this to be the case.

CELLULAR MECHANISMS OF NEOPLASIA

It is evident that neoplasia manifests itself as a diverse range of diseases in which the common denominator is a failure of cells to regulate their proliferation and, in malignant disease, their migration. The variety of neoplastic cells and of the agents which induce them creates a major difficulty in developing comprehensive explanations for the neoplastic process, namely, is there a single pathway to neoplasia which all cells follow or are there several different routes to the same phenotypic change? Although this cannot be answered with certainty, many theories have been put forward to explain the property common to all neoplastic cells —the permanent change in growth regulation. Some of these theories have already been discussed at some length and the following is intended as a comparative overview. Evidence for three principal mechanisms has been described, supporting the possibilities that neoplasia is (1) an abnormal pathway of differentiation, (2) a result of mutation in cell genetic material, or (3) determined by the acquisition of viral genes foreign to the cell.

(1) According to the *aberrant differentiation hypothesis*, a neoplastic cell arises as a result of an altered pattern of expression of normal genes which does not require a mutational change in the DNA. The difference between a normal and a neoplastic cell can be regarded as similar in kind to that between types of differentiated cells, which involves only the pattern of gene repression and derepression. The hypothesis argues that since, say, liver cells and kidney cells follow their distinct, stable pathways of differentiation without requiring gene loss or mutation, it is unnecessary to invoke mutation to explain inheritable change in neoplasia. The term *epigenetic* is used to describe inheritable changes such as those which occur in normal differentiation and do not involve alteration in the genetic material. The repression of genes normally expressed and the inappropriate derepression of others lends support to the concept of neoplasia as an abnormal differentiation pathway; moreover, the types of inappropriate products expressed by neoplastic cells (ectopic hormones, foetal proteins, etc.), are often characteristic of a particular type of tumour (p. 726).

Some evidence favouring an epigenetic rather than mutational basis for neoplasia is the apparent reversibility of neoplastic change which can be demonstrated under certain experimental conditions. Two recent approaches are particularly interesting. In the first, the nuclei of frog tumour cells were transplanted into frog egg cells from which the normal nuclei had been removed. It is known that nuclei of somatic, differentiated cells, introduced into such enucleated eggs, can direct the development of normal tadpoles, indicating that during differentiation no genetic information is lost or altered. The same result was obtained with nuclei of frog renal adenocarcinoma cells (Lucké carcinoma): *normal* tadpoles developed from eggs containing transplanted tumour cell nuclei. Neoplastic change had not apparently caused an irreversible alteration in the genome, nor any loss of nuclear potential. The other relevant experiments explored the ability of mouse malignant teratocarcinoma cells, which originate from germ cells, to participate in normal differentiation when introduced into embryos at the blastocyst stage. Mice which developed from such embryos were chimeras in which some normal tissues contained differentiated cells derived from the teratocarcinoma cells. Thus these neoplastic cells were apparently diverted into normal differentiation by their introduction into the early embryo. These experiments support the view that, at least in some cases, neoplasia results from alterations in gene expression similar to those involved in normal differentiation, rather than irreversible genetic change. To these examples may also be added the apparent suppression of malignancy in cell hybrids carrying the chromosomes of normal as well as neoplastic cells (p. 732).

(2) The *mutation hypothesis* presents the alternative and more widely accepted view that, in the majority of instances, alterations in DNA are involved in neoplasia. The best evidence in its favour is the frequent demonstration of chromosomal abnormalities in neoplastic cells and the fact that the vast majority of chemical and physical carcinogens react with DNA and are mutagenic. The predictive value of the hypothesis is borne out by mutagenicity testing in which several carcinogens have first come to light by their ability to produce mutations in bacteria (p. 775). Mutations affecting either regulatory or structural genes can be envisaged; the former could lead to inappropriate gene derepression and the latter to loss of function of specific proteins.

One difficulty is how a mutation in a single or small number of genes can lead to all the other cellular changes of neoplasia, such as the more extensive gene derepression, enzymatic and respiratory changes, etc. It is possible that mutation in a single regulatory gene could derepress a group of structural genes, leading to multiple effects. However, the discovery that transforming genes are often enzymes, potentially with many different substrates (p. 785), has made it easier to appreciate how a very limited genomic alteration can have complex and far-reaching cellular consequences. Mutation of itself apparently only initiates neoplasia; promotion is necessary for the expression of the mutant gene (p. 766). Some of the cellular abnormalities associated with neoplasia may be secondary changes which occur on promotion or progression. The strength of the mutation theory is its ready explanation of the carcinogenic action of chemical and physical agents. This is much less easy to explain as aberrant different- iation, though models have been proposed for epigenetic effects of such agents, by acting on histones or certain types of regulatory RNA and thereby leading to stable disruption of cellular control mechanisms without necessarily acting on DNA itself.

(3) *Acquisition of viral information.* Many viruses seem to cause neoplasia by a third type of mechanism, namely the introduction into the cell genome of new information which transforms the cells. In some cases, a single transforming gene is responsible, and the elucidation of the nature of the gene products has greatly advanced our understanding of the process of transformation (p. 785). Moreover, the discovery that viral transforming genes are closely related to and probably copies of normal cellular equivalents has indicated that the viral pathway is not radically different from the mechanisms discussed above. Infection by an

804

oncogenic virus such as a retrovirus is essentially an effective means of presenting to the cell an activated form of one of its own growth-controlling genes. This realisation has stimulated an intensive search for the potential transforming genes of normal cells and those active within neoplastic cells and has suggested a general theory of neoplasia which is described below.

Cellular oncogenes: A unifying theory of neoplasia

We have noted above and on p. 787 that the transforming genes of retroviruses, such as the *src* gene, are probably copies of normal cellular genes which at some time in the past became associated with retroviral genomes. Thus normal cells possess similar genes which must, therefore, have oncogenic potential; these are known as cellular oncogenes or transforming genes. Recent evidence suggests that neoplasia is often a consequence of an inappropriate activation or altered expression of these genes. The existence of cellular oncogenes has been established (a) by homology with retroviral transforming genes and (b) by the technique of *transfection*, in which fragments of purified DNA from neoplastic or normal cells are taken up by normal recipient cells in culture, integrated into their genomes and induce neoplastic transformation in them (Figure 6.32). A mouse fibroblast line called NIH/3T3 is often used as the recipient in transfection experiments. Purified cellular oncogenes from *normal* mouse cells (homologues of viral transforming genes) transform NIH/3T3 cells in the transfection assay, especially when first linked to a viral regulatory nucleotide sequence (promoter) to ensure efficient intracellular transcription. Furthermore, small fragments of

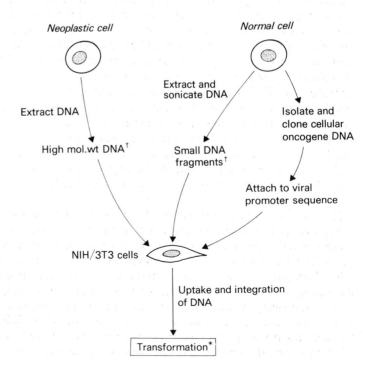

Figure 6.32 Demonstration of transforming genes of neoplastic and normal cells by transfection.

† High mol.wt DNA = 20×10^6; small DNA fragments = $0.3-3 \times 10^6$ mol.wt.
* Measured as number of colonies of transformed cells.

Neoplastic cell

Normal cell

Extract DNA

Extract and sonicate DNA

Isolate and clone cellular oncogene DNA

High mol.wt DNA†

Small DNA fragments†

Attach to viral promoter sequence

NIH/3T3 cells

Uptake and integration of DNA

Transformation*

DNA of normal chicken embryo fibroblasts and normal human embryo lung fibroblasts also induce transformation in NIH/3T3 cells. Evidently, fragmentation of normal DNA dissociates cellular oncogenes from normal regulatory sequences and leads to their expression in cells taking up and integrating the fragments. Larger pieces of DNA from a number of different types of neoplasm are highly efficient in transforming NIH/3T3 cells by transfection, producing 10–100 times more frequent transformation than the small fragments of normal cell DNA. These neoplasms include spontaneously occurring tumours, chemically-induced tumours and virus-induced tumours which do not contain specific viral transforming genes. Among human cancers in which transforming genes have been demonstrated by transfection are cells of bladder, lung, mammary and colon carcinomas, myelomas and T and B cell lymphomas. Thus, in all these cells an oncogene is active which behaves in a dominant fashion and can transform a normal recipient mouse cell.

The structure of transforming genes from different tumour cells has been analysed using restriction endonucleases (p. 472) and the important finding made that specific oncogenes exist for different cell types. Thus, the same oncogene is active, for example, in all mammary carcinomas (both human and mouse), while another oncogene appears to be common to all myelomas, and yet another in lymphomas, and so on. There must therefore be a considerable number of different potential oncogenes in the genome (50–100 seems likely), each apparently specific for a different cell type. Their normal function may be in tissue-specific control of cell proliferation. It is especially noteworthy that the particular gene activated in each case is apparently determined solely by the cell type and not by the nature of the carcinogen.

In some cases, the oncogenic activity of a cellular gene is a result of *mutation* of the normal gene rather than its activation. This was revealed recently when a transforming gene was isolated from human bladder carcinoma cells and its nucleotide sequence compared with its counterpart in normal bladder cells. It was found that the two genes were not completely identical, but differed in a single nucleotide, resulting in replacement of a glycine by valine in the protein coded by the gene. Evidently this point mutation has a crucial effect on the activity of the protein and can lead to neoplastic change. In this particular instance, the mutant product is not made in greater amount than the normal, in contrast with transformation which results from gene activation.

Figure 6.33 shows how these recent discoveries can be brought together into a general model to explain the genetic basis of neoplasia. The model takes as its starting point the normal cellular genes responsible for growth control. Some of these may code for protein kinases like pp60^{src}, while others may have different functions. Under normal circumstances in differentiated cells, the expression of growth-controlling genes is regulated to ensure that they are only activated in response to tissue requirements, growth factors, etc.; in a non-dividing cell, therefore, these genes will be expressed at a very low level or repressed altogether.

Figure 6.33 The cellular oncogene hypothesis.

Neoplasia is the result of activation of, or mutation in, a cellular gene responsible for normal growth control. When activated or altered, the cellular gene becomes an oncogene and directs neoplastic change.

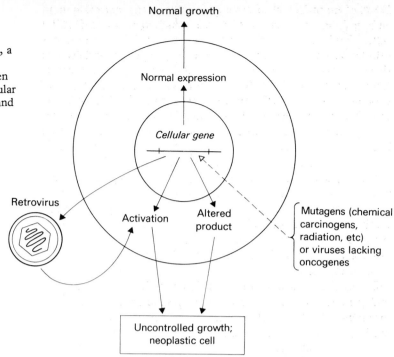

Their permanent activation or alteration leads to uncontrolled cell division; thus growth-controlling genes of normal cells are potential oncogenes. A pertinent illustration of the relationship between a gene's normal cellular function and its activation in neoplasia is provided by the tyrosine-phosphorylation reaction catalysed by the protein kinase product (pp60^{src}) of the *src* transforming gene of Rous sarcoma virus. Although it is an unusual enzymatic reaction, tyrosine-phosphorylation does occur in normal cells and in fact seems to be involved in stimulation of cell division. For example, a physiological stimulator molecule called *epidermal growth factor* (EGF) activates a cell membrane protein kinase which carries out this particular reaction. It has further been shown that some of the cell proteins phosphorylated as a result of stimulation by EGF are also phosphorylated by pp60^{src}. The fact that a stimulant of normal growth and an oncogene product share a common mode of action supports the view that neoplastic change can represent an abnormal over-activity of a physiological pathway of growth control.

A number of different routes may lead to activation of cellular transforming genes, including mutation at critical regulatory sites by chemical or physical carcinogens, the integration of non-oncogene viral DNA close to the cellular gene (e.g. leukaemia viruses), or the acquisition of the activated retroviral form of the gene (e.g. sarcoma viruses). Alternatively, mutation in a cellular gene may alter the function of its product sufficiently to cause uncontrolled growth (e.g. the bladder cancer gene cited above). Thus, in this scheme, cellular oncogenes are primarily genes essential to normal cell function, but lead to oncogenesis when expressed abnormally. Where their products are enzymes with several possible protein substrates, the diversity of the cellular abnormalities associated with neoplasia can be readily accounted for. In time, it may be possible to use the rapidly-growing knowledge of the function of these genes and their products to halt their action.

FURTHER READING

General

Becker F.F. (ed.) (1976) *Cancer: A Comprehensive Treatise*. 6 vols. Plenum Press.
Cairns J. (1978) *Cancer, Science and Society*. W.H. Freeman.
Committee on Professional Education of the U.I.C.C. (1978) *Clinical Oncology: A Manual for Students and Doctors*, 2nd edn. Springer Verlag.
Louis C.J. (1978) *Tumours. Basic Principles and Clinical Aspects*. Churchill Livingstone.
Pierce G.B., Shikes R. & Fink L.M. (1978) *Cancer: A Problem of Developmental Biology*. Prentice Hall.
Scott R.B. (1979) *Cancer: The Facts*. Oxford University Press.
Symington T. & Carter R.L. (eds.) (1976) *Scientific Foundations of Oncology* (with Supplement, 1980). Heinemann Medical.

Specific topics

Abercrombie M. (1979) Contact inhibition and malignancy. *Nature*, **281**, 259.
Alderson M. (ed.) (1982) *The Prevention of Cancer*. Edward Arnold.
Bishop J.M. (1982) Oncogenes. *Scientific American*, **246**, No.3, 68.
Bridges B.A. & Harnden D.G. (1981) Untangling ataxia telangiectasia. *Nature*, **289**, 222.
Cairns J. (1981) The origin of human cancers. *Nature*, **289**, 353.
Chemical Carcinogenesis. *British Medical Bulletin* (1980), **36**, no. 1.
Cooper G.M. (1982) Cellular transforming genes. *Science*, **218**, 801.
Cooper G.M., Okenquist S. & Silverman L. (1980) Transforming activity of DNA of chemically transformed and normal cells. *Nature*, **284**, 418.
Currie G.A. (1980) *Cancer and the Immune Response*, 2nd edn. Edward Arnold.
Doll R. & Peto R. (1981) *The Causes of Cancer*. Oxford University Press.
Fetal Antigens and Cancer. *Ciba Foundation Symposium* (1983), **96**. Pitman Books.
Hanafusa H. (1981) Cellular origin of transforming genes of RNA tumour viruses. *Harvey Lectures*, Series **75**, 255.
Herberman R. (ed.) (1980) *Natural Cell-Mediated Immunity against Tumours*. Academic Press.
Hynes R.O. (ed.) (1979) *Surfaces of Normal and Malignant Cells*. John Wiley.
Langan T. (1980) Malignant transformation and protein phosphorylation. *Nature*, **286**, 329.
Lennox E.S. & Sikora K. (1982) Definition of human tumour antigens. In McMichael A.J. & Fabre J.W. (eds.) *Monoclonal Antibodies in Clinical Medicine*, p. 111. Academic Press.
Loewenstein W.R. (1979) Junctional intercellular communication and the control of growth. *Biochim. Biophys. Acta*, **560**, 1.
Occupational Carcinogenesis. *Annals N.Y. Acad. Sci.* (1976), **271**.

Parkes W.R. (1982) *Occupational Lung Disorders*, 2nd edn. Butterworths.

Preger L. *et al.* (eds.) (1978) *Asbestos-related disease.* Grune and Stratton.

Ringertz N.P. & Savage R.E. (1976) *Cell Hybrids*. Academic Press.

Thorpe P.E. *et al.* (1982) Monoclonal antibody-toxin conjugates: aiming the magic bullet. In McMichael A.J. & Fabre J.W. (eds.) *Monoclonal Antibodies in Clinical Medicine*, p. 167. Academic Press.

Tooze J. (1981) *The Molecular Biology of Tumour Viruses: DNA Tumour viruses*, 2nd edn. Cold Spring Harbor Laboratory.

Weiss, R.A. (1982) *The Molecular Biology of Tumour Viruses: RNA Tumour Viruses*, 2nd edn. Cold Spring Harbor Laboratory.

Weissmann G. & Claiborne R. (1975) *Cell Membranes; Biochemistry, Cell Biology and Pathology*. H.P. Publishing Co.

Introduction

All human disease is the outcome of a combination of genetic and environmental factors, of 'nature and nurture'. The relative contributions of inheritance and environment, however, vary over a wide range. At one extreme are diseases which are the result of mutations in *single genes* and which follow simple Mendelian patterns of inheritance, including haemophilia, cystic fibrosis, muscular dystrophies and the 'inborn errors of metabolism'. Individually such conditions are generally rather rare, but collectively their contribution to disease is very considerable, affecting almost 1% of all births. Similarly, conditions resulting from *chromosomal aberrations*, such as Down's syndrome, are another category in which the individual's genetic material is the paramount cause of disease. On the other hand, there are many situations in which genetics plays a relatively small role, for example in infectious disease, though here too a genetic influence in susceptibility and speed of recovery may be present. Between these extremes, there is a long list of important common diseases in which there is an interaction between multiple genetic and environmental factors. Such *multifactorial diseases* include many congenital defects, diabetes, peptic ulcer, hypertension, atherosclerosis, schizophrenia, some neoplasms, and so on. In these conditions, the genetic contribution is usually polygenic and therefore does not follow simple Mendelian patterns, while the environmental factors may be equally complex. This section illustrates the genetic contribution to disease processes in some well-studied examples of each of these classes.

CHROMOSOMAL ABNORMALITIES

The genetic material of man, as of all other species, is DNA which is organised in the form of chromosomes. Figure 7.1 is a chromosome preparation or *karyotype* of a normal human male, prepared from a single cell. Most somatic cells are diploid* and contain, in man, 22 pairs of *autosomes* or non-sex chromosomes, and one pair of *sex chromosomes*, the latter comprising two X chromosomes in the female and a single X and a Y chromosome in the male. This number of 46 chromosomes is maintained at division in somatic cells by *mitosis*, but is halved to 23 in the gametes by *meiosis* (for detailed accounts of these processes see references at end of this section). Figure 7.1 shows the variation in size and form of the chromosomes, which enables them to be arranged into seven groups (A–G). Such an arrangement clearly does not make it possible to distinguish all the pairs definitively; however, new staining methods have revealed characteristic bands which enable each pair to be identified with far greater accuracy (Figure 7.2).

The chromosomes are the carriers of the genes, which in turn code for all the structural, enzymatic, developmental and regulatory proteins of the body. It is clear that each chromosome,

---

* Some exceptions are noted below under polyploidy.

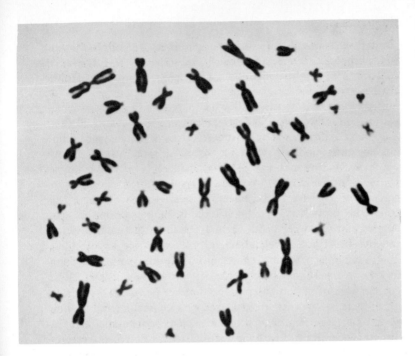

Figure 7.1 Human chromosomes: a normal male metaphase spread, traditional Giemsa staining. (Courtesy of Dr Maj Hulten.)

Figure 7.2 Human chromosomes showing banding patterns. In this normal male karyotype, chromosomes have been banded using hot saline Giemsa (one of several methods) to assist identification of homologous chromosome pairs. (Courtesy of Dr Maj Hulten.) Group A comprises chromosomes 1–3; B: chromosomes 4 and 5; C: chromosomes 6–12 and X; D: 13–15; E: 16–18; F: 19 and 20; G: 21, 22 and Y.

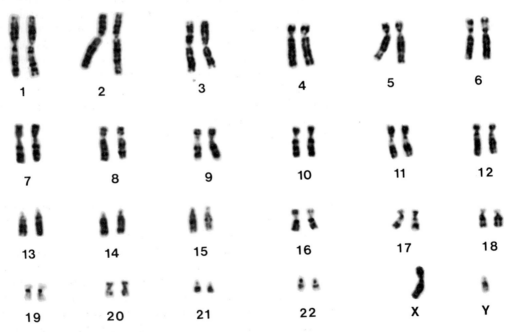

with the probable exception of Y, carries a large number of genes; it is therefore not very surprising that abnormalities of the chromosomes usually produce severe pathological conditions, which in many cases are not compatible with survival. Indeed, such abnormalities are a common cause of spontaneous abortion. For special reasons, aberrations of the sex chromosomes generally have less deleterious effects than corresponding changes in the autosomes.

Terminology

Chromosome abnormalities can be of two types, namely changes in the *number* of the chromosomes or alterations of their *structure*. A deviation in the normal total number of chromosomes, other than a multiple of the normal 46, is termed *aneuploidy*. For example, this may involve the presence of an extra chromosome, so that one set is represented three times in the cell rather than as the normal pair; this is called *trisomy*. Autosomal trisomy is the basis of *Down's syndrome* (*mongolism*). Alternatively, one member of a chromosome pair may be missing, a situation termed *monosomy*. Monosomy of an autosome is lethal; however monosomy can occur for the X-chromosome (*Turner's syndrome*, XO). Sexual abnormality syndromes involve a change in the number of sex chromosomes, e.g. XO (Turner's syndrome), XXY (*Klinefelter's syndrome*), XYY, XXY, and so on. *Polyploidy* is the term for a multiple of the normal diploid chromosome number, a phenomenon common in plants and insects, but very rare in mammals. Triploidy (69 chromosomes) and tetraploidy (92) are invariably lethal in man, but interestingly occur in a significant proportion of spontaneous abortions. (It may be noted that polyploidy is sometimes safely generated somatically—e.g. liver cells are frequently tetraploid—and some cell types are always polyploid, such as the tetraploid Purkinje cells and octaploid megakaryocytes.) Alterations of chromosomal structure which give rise to disease are usually the result of breakage and include *deletions*, i.e. loss of part of a chromosome, and *translocations*, in which a fragment of one chromosome is transferred (reciprocally) onto another. Chromosomal changes which are transmitted via the germ cells or occur in the early cleavage stages of the zygote result in disease syndromes which may be of considerable complexity, some of which are described below.

Down's syndrome

Also known as mongolism, this was first described by Langdon Down in 1866 and exemplifies some of these mechanisms of chromosomal abnormality. The most frequent cause is simple *trisomy* of chromosome 21, i.e. the presence of three copies of this chromosome rather than two. The condition is quite common, with an overall incidence of about 1 in 700 live births, and is the commonest single identifiable cause of severe mental deficiency. The characteristic facial appearance of affected individuals, notably the slanting eyes, gave rise to the term 'mongolism'. Patients are of retarded physical as well as mental development (mean IQ about 50), though normally placid and affectionate. An abnormal palm print is typical, often with a strong single midpalmar crease or 'simian line'. Congenital heart disease is quite frequent and may lead to an early death, but otherwise these individuals often survive to middle age (death is rare between 10 and 50). While trisomy 21 clearly has very severe effects, it is in fact the best tolerated of the autosomal trisomies. This is probably because chromosome 21 is the smallest chromosome, and therefore carries

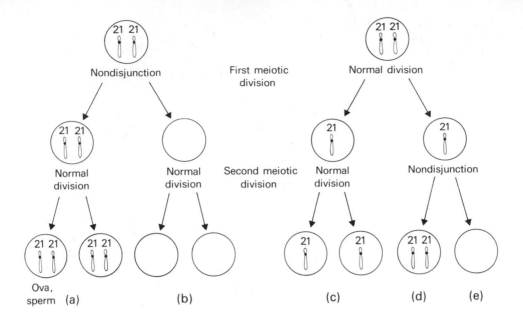

First meiotic division

Second meiotic division

Nondisjunction — Normal division — Normal division

Ova, sperm (a) (b) (c) (d) (e)

a correspondingly small amount of genetic material. Trisomy of larger chromosomes such as 13 or 18 is very much more severe and rare (1:3000 and 1:5000 respectively), and survival is for no more than a few months. On the other hand, monosomy for any autosomal chromosome is always lethal.

The incidence of Down's syndrome shows a marked dependence on maternal age, increasing from about 1:5000 live births in the 20–30 year age group of mothers, to 1:100 in mothers of 40 and 1:30 at 45. The cause of trisomy is a chromosomal 'accident', known as *non-disjunction*, in which a homologous pair fails to separate as it normally should at meiosis (Figure 7.3). The result of meiotic non-disjunction is the production of some gametes carrying the non-separated chromosome pair, and the fusion of such a gamete with a normal gamete at fertilisation leads to trisomy. The correlation with maternal age indicates that meiotic non-disjunction of chromosome 21 usually occurs in the ovum. Occasionally, non-disjunction of chromosome 21 is a *mitotic* event, occurring in an early cleavage stage of the zygote. In such cases, the mongoloid individual possesses two lines of cells, a normal 46 chromosome line and a trisomic 47 chromosome line (monosomic cells die); this mixture of cells with different karyotypes is termed *mosaicism* and the individual is a *mosaic* for these two cell types (Figure 7.4). Symptoms will then depend on the proportion of trisomic cells and will vary from case to case.

About 95% of all cases of Down's syndrome are due to non-disjunction. This is a relatively rare event, however, and is unlikely to occur twice in the same family. Therefore, the finding of some instances of a familial tendency to Down's syndrome (e.g. two or more cases in the same generation) strongly suggests that it may also be caused by direct inheritance from one of the parents. In such families, the mongoloid individuals possess the normal number of 46 chromosomes and so do not have simple trisomy 21.

Figure 7.3 Meiotic non-disjunction for chromosome 21.

The constitution of the gametes depends on whether non-disjunction occurs at the first or second meiotic division as shown. When fused with a normal gamete, (a) and (d) lead to trisomy for 21, i.e. Down's syndrome; (c) are normal ova or sperm; (b) and (e) lack 21 and their fusion with a normal gamete would result in monosomy (non-viable zygote). (After Bodmer & Cavalli-Sforza, 1976).

Figure 7.4 Production of a chromosome mosaic (two cell lines) by mitotic non-disjunction after formation of a normal zygote.

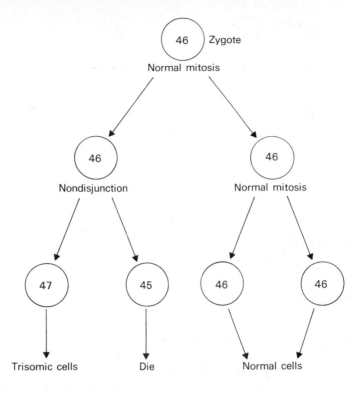

Nevertheless, the genetic material of chromosome 21 is again present in three copies in their genome, but this time through an aberrant *translocation* chromosome. This is formed by the fusion of parts of two chromosomes, namely the G-group chromosome 21 and a D-group chromosome (13, 14 or 15), most commonly 14; if such a translocation 14–21 chromosome is present in addition to the normal 21 pair, the 21 material is essentially represented three times, and Down's syndrome results. The 14–21 (or D/G) translocation is carried by one of the parents who is phenotypically normal but is found to possess only 45 rather than 46 chromosomes: instead of a chromosome pair 14/14 and a pair 21/21, this parent carries only one normal 14 chromosome, one normal 21 and the 14–21 translocation (Figure 7.5b). The genetic material of this individual is thus 'balanced' and there is no disease effect (a balanced carrier). However, this parent can produce some gametes carrying both 14–21 and 21, and fusion of such with a normal gamete will produce offspring of the type 14/14–21, 21/21, with the excess 21 material and hence Down's syndrome (Figure 7.5b). The figure also shows the way in which a 14–21 translocation occurs. It involves breakage of a 14 near the centromere and breakage of 21 on the long side; the long arms of 14 and 21 then join to form the translocation 14–21. The small fragment which is also formed is lost. This type of translocation is called *Robertsonian* after its discoverer, and is the most frequent obvious structural anomaly of autosomes. For unknown reasons, female carriers of 14–21 translocations have a higher proportion of offspring with Down's syndrome than male carriers.

Patients with Down's syndrome are more liable to develop

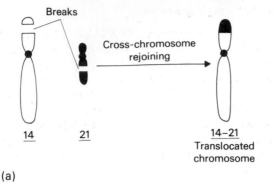

Breaks

Cross-chromosome
rejoining

14   21

Small fragment,
usually lost

14–21
Translocated
chromosome

(a)

Figure 7.5 Inheritance of Down's syndrome through chromosomal translocation. (After Bodmer & Cavalli-Sforza, 1976). (a) Origin of a 14–21 translocation.
(b) Possible offspring of mating between a normal individual and a 14–21 translocation carrier.
(Note that in (a) and (b) the relative length of the short chromosome arms has been exaggerated.)

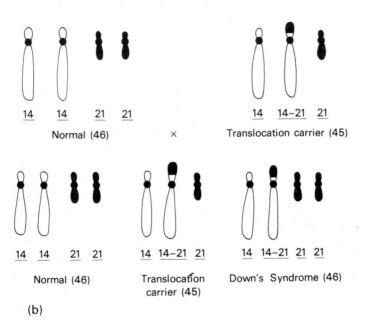

| 14 | 14 | 21 | 21 | | 14 | 14–21 | 21 |

Normal (46)   ×   Translocation carrier (45)

| 14 | 14 | 21 | 21 | 14 | 14–21 | 21 | 14 | 14–21 | 21 | 21 |

Normal (46)   Translocation carrier (45)   Down's Syndrome (46)

(b)

acute lymphocytic leukaemia than the normal population. For some time it appeared that an aberration of chromosome 21 was involved in leukaemia in another way as well—a large percentage of patients with chronic granulocytic leukaemia have a deletion of part of the long arm of a chromosome of the same group (G), the so-called *Philadelphia* chromosome (p. 729). However it is difficult to distinguish the G-chromosomes 21 and 22 by conventional microscopy, so until recently it was not clear whether the same chromosome was involved in leukaemia and Down's syndrome. Now, as a result of new staining techniques, it has been possible to identify the chromosome of Down's syndrome definitely as a 21 and the Philadelphia chromosome as a 22. Furthermore, the missing portion of the Philadelphia chromosome is now known to be translocated to chromosome 9. This particular aberration arises somatically in the bone marrow and is not present in other cells.

Cri du chat (cat's cry) syndrome

This is a rare condition (incidence 1:10,000 births) named after the unusual high-pitched cry of the affected infants which resembles a kitten in distress. There are various physical and cardiovascular anomalies in the syndrome, with mental retardation. It is caused by deletion of part of the short arm of chromosome 5. This is usually a sporadic event which is unlikely to recur in a family. However, it can also be inherited from a balanced carrier, an individual in which the missing part of chromosome 5 has been translocated to another chromosome and who is otherwise normal but can transmit the aberrant 5 to offspring. In contrast to Down's syndrome, the abnormalities of this syndrome result from a deficiency in the genes of chromosome 5 and the products they code for, the individuals being essentially monosomic for the deleted segment.

Sex chromosome abnormalities

Sex in man is determined by the sex chromosomes, X and Y, normal females having the constitution XX and males XY. X is one of the larger chromosomes and carries a large number of genes (more than 100 have been assigned), many of which are not related to its sex role. In contrast, Y is one of the smallest chromosomes and it is important to note that the X-linked genes have no equivalent on the Y chromosome. Thus males are effectively monosomic for X, while females have twice the dose of X-linked genes of males. The fact that this situation does not have serious consequences is in marked contrast to the autosomes, where we have already noted that monosomy is generally a lethal state and trisomy has very deleterious effects. Moreover, sex chromosomal aberrations include both true monosomy (XO) and trisomy (XXX, XXY, XYY) which, compared with similar autosomal anomalies, are relatively benign. Clearly the sex chromosomes are a special case and the reason for this is a unique mechanism of 'dosage compensation'. This involves the inactivation of either of the two X chromosomes in every somatic cell in the normal female, with the result that in terms of dose the somatic expression of genes on the X chromosome is the same in both females and males (the *Lyon hypothesis*, proposed by Mary Lyon in 1961). The decision of whether it is the paternal or maternal of the two X chromosomes that is inactivated in any particular female cell is apparently random, though in all the descendents of that cell the same chromosome is always 'switched off'. Thus, normal females who carry mutants or alleles of X chromosome genes are functional mosaics for those genes, since they will possess two somatic cell types depending on which X chromosome is inactivated. The inactive chromosome can in fact be seen under the microscope; the nucleus of a few somatic cells in the female carries a small darkly-staining mass known as the *sex chromatin* or *Barr body*, after its discoverer. The Barr body is absent from male cells and this fact enables the simple determination of sex from observation of the cell nucleus.

It was observations of Barr bodies which indicated the basis of the chromosomal aberrations involved in different sex abnormalities. For example, in the condition known as *Turner's syndrome* or gonadal dysgenesis, the individual is female but the Barr body is absent (sex chromatin negative), while in *Klinefelter's syndrome*, the patient is a male whose cells are nevertheless found to contain the Barr body (sex chromatin positive). These syndromes are caused by an abnormal number of sex chromosomes: in the former, one X chromosome is missing and the sex chromosome constitution is XO (i.e. monosomy for X), while in the latter, there is an extra X and the constitution is XXY, a trisomy. In general, the maximum number of Barr bodies in the nucleus is one less than the number of X chromosomes. Thus, where more than two X chromosomes are present, for example in the XXX syndrome, and even in the rare XXXX and XXXXX individuals, all but one may be visible as Barr bodies.

These observations and the Lyon hypothesis provide an explanation for why, compared with autosomal aberrations, an aberrant number of X chromosomes is reasonably well tolerated, since no matter how many X chromosomes are present in the cell only the genes of *one* will be actively expressed. On the other hand, the fact that well defined syndromes do result from the presence of an abnormal number of X chromosomes probably indicates that X inactivation is never really complete, and that the expression of some of the genes on the 'inactivated' X chromosome may in fact be necessary for normal female development.

The study of sex chromosome abnormalities made an important contribution to the understanding of how sex is determined in man. It became clear that, regardless of how many X chromosomes are present, an individual's sex phenotype is always determined solely by the presence or absence of the Y chromosome. In the absence of Y, the sex phenotype is always female, even if there is only one X chromosome as in Turner's syndrome (XO); and *vice versa*, the presence of a single Y establishes a male type, even if more than one X chromosome is present as in Klinefelter's syndrome (XXY). It is interesting that the male-determining role of the Y chromosome was only definitely established for man as recently as 1959. While the same effect is seen in other mammals, it is not the case in *Drosophila* and many non-mammals where sex is determined by the number of X chromosomes and Y plays no apparent role.

An abnormality in the number of sex chromosomes is the result of non-disjunction, which as in the case of the autosomes (p. 816), may occur at meiosis or mitosis. Meiotic non-disjunction leads to the production of abnormal sperm or ova, and since non-disjunction may occur at either of the two meiotic divisions, it can result in formation of four possible types of abnormal sperm (XY, XX, YY and O) and two types of abnormal ova (XX and O), as shown in Figure 7.6. The possible products of matings in which the abnormal gametes are involved are shown in Table 7.1. Note that any combination leading to the exclusion of both X chromosomes from the zygote, such as YO, is lethal. Mitotic non-disjunction of the sex chromosomes is also known, as for the auto-

Figure **7.6** Consequences of non-disjunction of sex chromosomes in male and female meiosis.
(a) Male meiosis.
(b) Female meiosis.
(After Bodmer & Cavalli-Sforza, 1976).

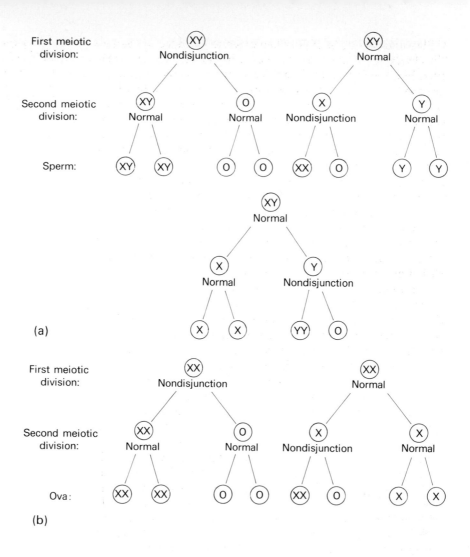

First meiotic division:
Second meiotic division:
Sperm:

(a)

First meiotic division:
Second meiotic division:
Ova:

(b)

somes, and its occurrence in the early cleavage division of the embryo gives rise to a mosaic with two (or more) cell lines, one of which is abnormal. The condition of the individual then depends on the proportion of abnormal cells present.

The following are some of the syndromes which are produced by sex chromosome abnormality.

Table 7.1 Non-disjunction of sex chromosomes: constitution of offspring after fertilisation involving (a) abnormal sperm and (b) abnormal ova.

Abnormal sperm	Normal ova X
	Offspring:
XY	XXY
XX	XXX
YY	XYY
O	XO

(a)

Normal sperm	Abnormal ova XX O
	Offspring:
X	XXX XO
Y	XXY YO

(b)

XO = Turner's syndrome; XXY = Klinefelter's syndrome;
XXX = Abnormal female; XYY = Abnormal male; YO = Inviable.

Turner's syndrome (gonadal dysgenesis, XO)

As mentioned above, Turner's syndrome results from the absence in the female of one X chromosome, so that the constitution is 45, XO and there is no Barr body. Reference to Table 7.1 shows that this may arise by meiotic non-disjunction in production either of a sperm or ovum; in the majority of cases the non-disjunction event seems to occur in the father. The affected individual is, as expected, female in outward appearance. However, some cases show characteristic physical abnormalities, including very short height, broad shield-like chest with widely spaced nipples, webbing of the neck, and occasionally coarctation of the aorta (Figure 7.7). Moreover, the ovaries are usually replaced by streaks of fibrous ovarian stroma and the individual is therefore infertile. It thus appears that, despite the normal inactivation of one of the X chromosomes in each somatic cell, the presence of both X chromosomes is essential for development of functioning ovaries and normal physical development in the female. Information on which parts of the X chromosome are responsible for these functions has been obtained from an interesting abnormality of the structure of the X chromosome known as an *isochromosome*. This is an X chromosome which,

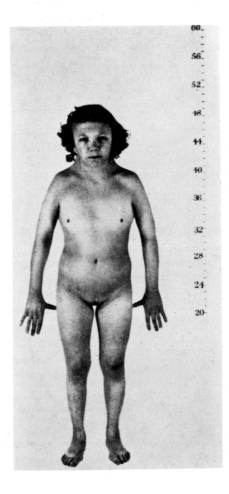

Figure 7.7 Turner's syndrome. Patient aged 21. Note short stature, webbing of the neck, broad shield-like chest, underdeveloped breasts and widely spaced nipples.
(From Gaisford & Lightfoot, *Paediatrics for the Practitioner*, courtesy of Butterworth & Co.)

instead of the normal long and short arms, is composed of either two identical long arms or two identical short arms; it is believed to be produced by a misdivision of the X chromosome during mitosis (Figure 7.8). An individual possessing a normal X and a long arm X isochromosome apparently has 46 chromosomes and possesses a Barr body, but is effectively monosomic for the short arm of X (i.e. carries the short arm genes in a single dose only). Such an individual has the typical clinical picture of Turner's syndrome, including the physical anomalies. On the other hand, when in rare cases the short arm X isochromosome is present, in addition to the normal X, the individual is infertile with streak gonads, but is outwardly normal in physical appearance. It thus appears that normal physical development is dependent on genes on the short arm of the X chromosome, whereas development of ovaries requires genes on both arms, and that to be a normal female a diploid (double) set of both X chromosome genes is essential. Clearly, therefore, the Lyon X-inactivation hypothesis must be modified to account for the Turner syndrome: either the functioning of both X chromosomes is required at certain stages in development, or alternatively perhaps some of the genes on the 'inactive X' are never really switched off at all.

Turner's syndrome is rather rare, with an incidence of 1 in 3500 female births and, as we have seen, is relatively well tolerated compared with the autosomal monosomies which are always lethal. However, the XO type occurs in the remarkably

Figure 7.8 Production of isochromosomes by misdivision of centromere at mitosis.
(a) Normal division of centromere.
(b) Misdivision of centromere.
(After Harnden, 1962).

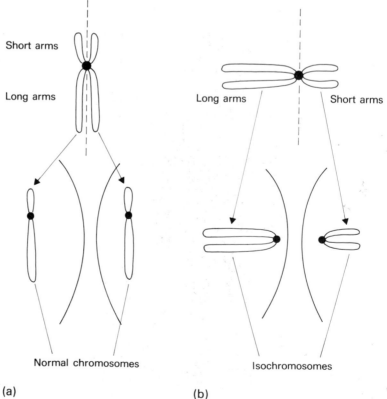

Short arms

Long arms

Long arms   Short arms

Normal chromosomes

Isochromosomes

(a)   (b)

high proportion of about 1 in 15 spontaneous abortions. Thus, not only is meiotic non-disjunction for X a very much more frequent genetic event than the number of live cases suggests, but also it seems that as few as 1 in 50 conceptions with the XO condition proceeds to a live birth.

Klinefelter's syndrome (XXY)

This has the rather frequent occurrence in male births of about 1 in 500. It is caused by the addition of an extra X chromosome to the normal male XY complement, so that there are 47 chromosomes and the abnormal (for a male) presence of a Barr body. The individuals appear as normal males until adolescence. Subsequently, the testes are characteristically very small and spermatogenesis rare; infertility is the commonest cause of detection. Sometimes there is development of female breast tissue (gynaecomastia), which may require surgical removal. The fact that Klinefelter patients (XXY) are males whereas Turner patients (XO) are females demonstrates the male-determining capacity of the Y chromosome.

The XYY syndrome

This attracted a great deal of interest when it was discovered in 1965 that a significant proportion of violent criminals in maximum security prison hospitals carry an extra Y chromosome. XYY males are usually taller and more aggressive than normal XY males. However, it is clear that only a small proportion ($\sim 5\%$) have criminal records, and many XYYs are indistinguishable from normal males. Nevertheless, the fact that an extra Y chromosome may be accompanied by a gross inability to adjust to contemporary society makes this an important discovery in behavioural genetics. The frequency is about 1 in 2000 male births.

Other possible outcomes of mating involving abnormal gametes are trisomy for X or *XXX syndrome*, tetra-X (XXXX) and penta-X (XXXXX). The XXX female may have mental retardation or be infertile, though most appear intellectually normal and fertile. The rare tetra-X patients are more retarded than the XXX individuals, while the patients with penta-X syndrome are severely retarded.

DISEASES CAUSED BY SINGLE-GENE (MENDELIAN) DEFECTS

It is difficult to analyse in detail the biochemical mechanisms underlying the syndromes produced by the chromosomal aberrations described above because they probably involve an imbalance in the function of the products of several genes. In contrast, there are many disease states which result from changes (mutations) in *single genes* where as a result it is possible to be precise about the processes involved. Although diseases caused by single-gene defects are individually rather rare, with frequencies ranging from 1:2000 to 1:100,000, taken together they may affect almost 1% of the newborn population. As expected, these diseases follow simple Mendelian patterns of inheritance, and the most important genetic information comes from studying their occurrence in families. With such information it is not only possible to draw meaningful inferences about the mechanisms of these diseases, but for individuals of affected families the risks of occurrence can be assessed and advice given (genetic counselling).

Terminology

A *mutation* is an inheritable change in a gene, often involving the replacement of a single base by another in the DNA sequence of the gene (*point mutation*; see also p. 769 and Figure 6.23). The original form of the gene and the mutant form are called *alleles*, meaning alternatives at that locus. As a result of mutation, the amino acid sequence of the protein coded by the gene is changed and consequently the tertiary structure and function of the protein may be altered. If the change in function is deleterious, as is often the case, and sufficiently profound, it may lead directly to a disease. Since proteins have a variety of roles in the body—structural, enzymatic, regulatory—it is apparent that a whole range of possible abnormalities can occur, depending on the gene in which the mutation occurred.

If an individual inherits a mutant allele, the outcome will depend on whether the effect of that allele, i.e. the trait it specifies, is *dominant* or *recessive*. To define these terms, we must bear in mind that each individual has a double chromosome set (paternal and maternal) and therefore possesses two copies of the gene at every locus (with the important exception of genes on the X chromosome in males). If both copies of a particular gene are identical, the individual is *homozygous* for that genetic locus, whereas if they are different the individual is *heterozygous* and carries two alleles at the locus. A *dominant* trait is one that is fully expressed in heterozygotes, i.e. even if only one copy of the allele determining it is present. A trait is *recessive* if it is only expressed in homozygotes, i.e. a double dose of the allele must be present for the trait to appear. Thus a dominant disease will, in principle, affect every individual possessing a single copy of a deleterious mutant allele, whereas a recessive disease only affects those having two copies of the mutant allele, i.e. homozygotes. Individuals who are heterozygous for a recessive allele will nevertheless be *carriers*, in the genetic sense, of the trait. An exception exists for mutant genes on the X chromosome: recessive X-linked genes will always be expressed in *males* even though only one copy is present, because the Y chromosome does not carry any genes homologous to those on X (p. 819). The male is said to be *hemizygous* for genes on the X chromosome. Because of this different pattern of expression of X-linked genes, it is usual to divide the single-gene diseases into autosomal (dominant and recessive) and X-linked (dominant and recessive).

Tables 7.2–7.4 give examples of single-gene diseases and indicate their frequencies. These are only a small fraction of the more than 2000 Mendelian conditions catalogued by McKusick in his *Mendelian Inheritance in Man* (1975). Also note that despite the apparent simplicity of the genetic event, these conditions may have a complex set of characteristic symptoms and in many cases are therefore termed 'syndromes'.

Dominant and recessive disorders

The mode of inheritance of a single-gene disorder as a dominant or recessive trait depends on the nature of the protein product of the gene and its normal level of activity. In particular, the crucial factor is often whether there is sufficient of the unaltered gene product in a heterozygote to ensure normal function; if there is, the disease will only be seen in homozygotes and is recessive, but if not, then the mutant trait or condition will be dominant. For example, if the gene product is an enzyme, the result of mutation may be a molecule which is enzymatically defective or inactive. Enzyme defects are common causes of genetic disease. In the heterozygote, however, the normal as well as the defective enzyme will be synthesized and there is usually sufficient of the former to enable the individual to function normally. Hence, enzyme defects will in general express themselves only in individuals who are homozygous for the mutant allele, and the resulting diseases are therefore recessives.

Many of the conditions in Tables 7.3 and 7.4 are caused by mutant enzymes and in more than 150 such disorders the enzymes have been identified. In contrast, diseases manifested as dominants are rarely caused by enzyme deficiencies. An unusual exception is found in *acute intermittent porphyria*, which involves deficiency of an enzyme in porphyrin metabolism, uroporphyrinogen I synthetase, yet is inherited as a dominant. Apparently the level of this enzyme is sufficiently limiting in the normal state to lead to overt deficiency in the heterozygote and hence a dominant pattern of inheritance. However, in general, dominant conditions involve alteration in proteins other than enzymes. Unfortunately, it is far more difficult at present to be precise about the molecular basis of most dominant diseases than it is for recessives.

Although dominant disorders are, by definition, expressed in heterozygotes, who carry only one copy of the defective or disease gene, they can of course also occur in homozygotes where they appear in a much more severe form. In practice, however, it is rare to observe homozygotes for dominant disorders, both because they are probably often lethal and because a homozygote could only be produced in the rare mating of two affected individuals. Dominant conditions are generally less severe than recessive disorders, which can only be expressed when two copies of a mutant gene are present.

Pedigree patterns

To establish that a disease is the result of a single-gene mutation it is, of course, essential to study its inheritance in families. Each of the possible categories defined above—autosomal dominant and recessive, X-linked dominant and recessive—has a characteristic pedigree pattern which follows Mendelian principles. The main features of the inheritance of each category are described below. In representing pedigrees, the following symbols are used:

Normal male, female	□ , ○
Male, female affected with the trait under study	■ , ●
Heterozygous carriers of recessive trait	◨ , ◖
Female carrier of X-linked trait	⊙
Mating	□─○
Consanguinous mating (i.e. mating between blood relatives)	□═○
Sibs (brothers & sisters)	□ ○ □

AUTOSOMAL DOMINANT INHERITANCE

Table 7.2 gives some examples of diseases inherited as dominant Mendelian traits. Well-studied examples are *Huntington's chorea*, a disease characterised by involuntary muscular movements and progressive mental deterioration; *brachydactyly*, or shortening of the fingers; and *Marfan's syndrome*, a connective tissue disorder (p. 866). These diseases are rare: Huntington's chorea, for example, has a frequency of 1:20,000 in the population in the UK. For dominant diseases, individuals inheriting the mutant gene will inherit the disease, regardless of the other allele present. Practically all cases will be heterozygotes; production of a homozygote would require a mating between two affected individuals, which is certain to be very rare, and moreover homozygosity for such dominant mutant genes may be lethal. A typical pedigree which might be found is shown in Figure 7.9. The important features are the following. (i) Every affected individual has one affected parent (unless the disease represents a new mutation). (ii) The disease trait appears in every generation. (iii) Males and females are equally affected. (iv) An affected person mating with a normal individual has, on the average, one half normal and one half affected offspring. (v) Offspring of normal relatives of affected persons are normal.

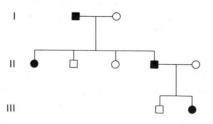

Figure 7.9 Pedigree of autosomal dominant inheritance. I, II, III: generations in family. ■ ● : heterozygous affected individuals. □ ○ : homozygous normal individuals.

827

Table 7.2 Autosomal dominant diseases.

Disease	Incidence at birth	Features
Achondroplasia	1:20,000	Form of dwarfism; 90% of cases are new mutations, implying very high mutation rate
Ankylosing spondylitis (p. 879)		Arthritic disease with fusion of sacroiliac and vertebral joints; spinal immobility. Generally males (sex-influenced). Close association with HLA-B27
Brachydactyly		Shortening of the fingers
Deafness, dominant forms		Includes many different forms of deafness
Elliptocytosis		Abnormal red cell morphology; may be associated with haemolytic anaemia
Epidermolysis bullosa		Superficial blistering, especially of ankles and feet
Huntington's chorea	1:20,000	Irregular, jerky (choreic) movements; dementia; onset around 30–40 years
Marfan syndrome (p. 866)	1:20,000	Disorder of connective tissue; long, thin limbs, disorders of the cardiovascular system and the eye. Probably abnormality of collagen or elastin structure
Methaemoglobinaemia (p. 864)	(About 10 cases in UK)	Cyanosis, hypoxia; abnormal haemoglobin M in which iron of haem is oxidised to ferric form
Myotonic dystrophy	1:20,000	Progressive, disabling muscular weakness and wasting
Neurofibromatosis (von Recklinghausen's disease)	1:20,000	Multiple tumours (neurofibromas) of peripheral nerves, cranial nerves and skin; café-au-lait pigmented spots in skin; 50% are new mutations
Polyposis of the colon		Malignant change to carcinoma of colon is common
Porphyria, hepatic (p. 826)		Enzymatic abnormality of porphyrin metabolism
Von Willebrand's disease (p. 639)		Bleeding disorder with prolonged bleeding time and factor VIII deficiency (cf. haemophilia). Impaired adhesion of platelets to collagen, but normal aggregation. Deficiency of von Willebrand factor required for both platelet adhesion and factor VIII activity

One of the problems encountered in establishing pedigrees, especially with dominant disorders, is that the severity of the disease can vary widely between individuals even within the same family; the term *expressivity* is used to indicate the degree to which symptoms appear in an individual. Sometimes, the expressivity may be so low that the disease cannot be detected at all, even though the pedigree shows the gene to be present in the individual. The disease is then said to be *non-penetrant* in that individual. Variation in expressivity is the result of the interaction of the effects of the disease gene with products of other genes and factors in the environment. Note that penetrance and expressivity are often functions of the sensitivity of the diagnostic methods used to detect the condition, since these set the threshold for defining the presence of disease.

AUTOSOMAL RECESSIVE INHERITANCE

As Table 7.3 shows, many of these diseases are caused by enzyme defects, which may lead to a disruption of events in intermediary metabolism (*inborn errors of metabolism*), storage of certain substrates at abnormally high levels (*storage diseases*), and so on. As already noted, enzyme aberrations are recessive because their effects can generally only be expressed in homozygotes. The deleterious genes must therefore have been present in both parents, who will usually be heterozygous and unaffected carriers of the disease gene. Figure 7.10 shows a possible pedigree. Note the following typical features. (i) Parents of affected individuals are not themselves affected. (ii) On the average, ¼ of the offspring of the mating of two heterozygotes will be homozygous recessives and therefore affected, ½ will be heterozygous carriers and ¼ homozygotes for the normal gene. (iii) The disease does not appear in all generations since it requires the rare mating between heterozygotes. (iv) Males and females are affected equally. (v) The disease is more likely to occur in the offspring of parents who are themselves related (consanguinous), since this will greatly increase the likelihood of both being heterozygous for a rare gene (Figure 7.10). The less common the disease, the more likely it is that the parents of an affected child are themselves blood relations.

Like the dominant disorders, the recessive conditions are rare. One recessive disease which is rather common, however, is *cystic fibrosis (mucoviscidosis)*, which has a frequency among Caucasians of about 1 per 2500 births and accounts for over 1% of admissions

Figure 7.10 A pedigree of autosomal recessive inheritance. I, II, III: generations in family □ ○ : homozygous normal individuals. ◨ ◑ : heterozygous carriers (normal). ■ : homozygous affected individual. ◨=◑ : first-cousin marriage. ◑ ◨ : sibs.

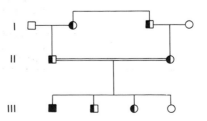

Table 7.3 Autosomal recessive diseases.

Disease	Approx. incidence at birth	Features
Adrenogenital syndrome (p. 848)	1:10,000	Premature virilisation in males, pseudohermaphroditism in females. Caused by excessive secretion of androgens by the adrenal cortex following defect in enzyme 21-hydroxylase
Albinism (p. 842)	Tyrosinase-negative form, 1:20,000 (Higher in N. Ireland, 1:15,000)	Absence of melanin from skin, hair and eyes; lack of an enzyme required for conversion of tyrosine into melanin (e.g. tryosinase). At least six genetically distinct types
Alkaptonuria (p. 843)	1:200,000	Excretion of homogentisic acid causes darkening of urine; black pigment deposited in cartilage (ochronosis). Lack of homogentisic acid oxidase in metabolism of tyrosine
Alpha-1-antitrypsin deficiency (p. 41)	1:1500	Lack of serum inhibitor of trypsin. Associated with lung disease in adults (emphysema) and liver disease in children (cirrhosis). Increased risk of lung disease in heterozygotes (frequency $\sim$ 1:20) which is exacerbated by smoking
Aminoacidurias and aminoacidaemias (see specific examples)	1:3500 (total)	Deficiencies in enzymes involved in metabolism or transport of amino acids
Ataxia telangiectasia (p. 775)	1:100,000	Cerebellar ataxia; oculo-cutaneous telangiectasis; immunodeficiency. Recurrent sinopulmonary infections due to deficient CMI and poor IgA production
Chédiak-Higashi syndrome (p. 25)		Recurrent infections due to defective killing of pyogenic organisms by neutrophils; partial albinism; CNS abnormalities; lymphoreticular neoplasms. Giant lysosomes in neutrophils. Death in childhood
Combined immunodeficiency (Swiss-type) (p. 78)		Severe deficiency of both cell-mediated and humoral immunity (T and B cells); life-threatening infections with viruses, fungi and bacteria
Cystic fibrosis (p. 829)	1:1000-1:4000 in Caucasians. Rare in Africans or Orientals	Disorder of exocrine glands affecting pancreas, respiratory system and sweat glands; chronic pulmonary disease and pneumonia; lack of pancreatic enzymes; excessive salt loss, especially in sweat

Table 7.3 *continued*

Disease	Approx. incidence at birth	Features
Cystinuria (p. 857)		Excessive excretion of cystine; cystine stones deposited in urinary tract; defect in cystine transport in renal tubule
Deafness	1:2000	75% of cases of congenital deafness are recessive; several forms
Ellis van Creveld syndrome	Very rare	Dwarfism; polydactyly (6 fingers); several cases in in-bred Amish community in Lancaster County, Pennsylvania
Fanconi syndrome (p. 859)		Generalised defect of renal tubular transport, with excess excretion of amino acids, glucose, phosphate
Galactosaemia (p. 844)	1:200,000	Vomiting, diarrhoea and jaundice following first milk feed, progressing to wasting and severe brain damage. Inability to metabolise galactose in milk; treated by milk-free diet
Gangliosidoses (p. 855)		Accumulation of gangliosides in brain, viscera. Several types, including Tay-Sachs disease (q.v.). Deficiencies of enzymes which degrade gangliosides
Gaucher's disease (p. 856)	Chiefly in Jewish families	Acute form in infancy (neurological deterioration, hepatosplenomegaly) ranging to childhood and adult chronic form (bone and joint involvement). Deficiency of glucocerebrosidase leads to excessive storage of ceramide glucoside
Glycogen storage diseases (glycogenoses) (p. 852)		Deficiencies of enzymes of glycogen metabolism cause excessive storage of glycogen; see von Gierke's and Pompe's diseases
Hartnup disease (p. 858)		Urinary excretion of tryptophan and inability to absorb tryptophan from intestinal tract due to deficient transport mechanism. Symptoms resemble pellagra
Histidinaemia		Delayed speech development, some mental retardation; raised plasma histidine, urinary histidine excretion. Defect in histidase

Table 7.3 *continued*

Disease	Approx. incidence at birth	Features
Homocystinuria (p. 844)		Syndrome involving circulation, connective tissue and CNS. Urinary excretion of homocystine; lack of cystathionine synthetase in metabolic pathway from methionine to cystine
Hurler syndrome (p. 851)	1:40,000	Mucopolysaccharide storage disease. Fatal by age 10; skeletal defects, corneal clouding, hepatospleno-megaly, 'gargoyle' facies, mental retardation. Lysosomal storage of dermatan sulphate and heparan sulphate due to absence of degradative enzyme. Corrected by enzyme from cells of Hunter syndrome patients (Table 5.4)
Maple syrup urine disease	1:300,000	Urinary excretion of branched-chain amino acids valine, leucine and isoleucine. Urine has characteristic maple syrup odour. Early death after neurological deterioration unless these amino acids are excluded from the diet. Lack of ketoacid decarboxylase
Mucopolysaccharide storage diseases (p. 850)	1:20,000	Six types, incl. Hurler, Scheie and Sanfilippo syndromes (Hunter syndrome is X-linked). Excessive storage and excretion of mucopoly-saccharides due to absence of lysosomal degradative enzymes
Niemann-Pick disease (p. 856)	Chiefly in Jewish families	Fatal disorder, extreme hepatosplenomegaly and CNS damage; excess storage of sphingomyelin in lysosomes due to absence of sphingomyelinase
Phenylketonuria (p. 843)	1:15,000 in Caucasians; 1:10,000 in Irish; very rare in Negroes and Finns	Mental retardation; seizures. Excretion of phenylketoacids, raised plasma phenylalanine; deficiency of phenylalanine hydroxylase. Clinical syndrome prevented by low phenylalanine diet; hence screening of newborns advisable
Pompe's disease (p. 852)		Most severe glycogen storage disease. Absence of lysosomal acid maltase leads to accumulation of glycogen. Cardiac enlargement, muscular hypotonia, early death

Table 7.3 *continued*

Disease	Approx. incidence at birth	Features
Sickle-cell disease (p. 862)	Up to 1:100 in West and Central Africa and among US Negroes; also common in Greece and N. India	Homozygosity for abnormal haemoglobin gene HbS. Chronic anaemia; sickling of red cells in lowered oxygen tension; often fatal. Malaria-associated
Tay–Sachs disease (p. 855)	1:2000 in Ashkenazi Jews; rare elsewhere	Developmental retardation, paralysis, blindness; fatal. Excess storage of ganglioside G_{M2} in CNS due to absence of lysosomal enzyme hexosaminidase A required for degradation of G_{M2}
Thalassaemia major (p. 865)	1:100 in some Mediterranean areas, also common in Africa and India	Severe anaemia due to defective production of haemoglobin α or β chains; often fatal. Especially prevalent in Mediterranean malarial areas. Partial compensation by production of foetal or unusual haemoglobins
Von Gierke's disease (p. 852)		Severe glycogenosis. Glycogen stored extralysosomally in cytoplasm due to lack of glucose-6-phosphatase required for release of glucose from liver. Liver enlargement, hypoglycaemia, convulsions, coma
Wilson's disease		Toxic deposits of copper in many organs, causing liver disease (jaundice, cirrhosis) and neurological disturbance (tremor, etc.). Defect in copper excretion. Kayser-Fleischer ring in cornea. Low copper diet

to children's hospitals. Interestingly, its frequency among Orientals and Africans is much lower. Sufferers frequently die in childhood, though as many as 70 percent may survive to adulthood under special care. Cystic fibrosis (CF) is a disease of exocrine glands (pancreas, salivary glands, sweat glands, bronchial glands). Its pathogenesis involves the production of very viscous mucous or eosinophilic material which blocks in particular the pancreatic ducts and leads to fibrosis (the islets are not affected); as a result there is a paucity of digestive enzymes in the intestine. In the lungs the mucus secretion causes obstruction which is followed by infection and chronic bronchitis. Many of the children die of pneumonia or other pulmonary complications caused especially by opportunistic infection with *Staphylococcus aureus* or *Pseudomonas aeruginosa* (p. 571). A characteristic feature is the high salinity of the sweat. Unfortunately, the biochemistry of the disease is poorly understood and as yet no specific enzyme defect has been shown to be responsible.

Although the frequency of cystic fibrosis itself is only 1:2500 it is important to realise that the frequency of heterozygous genetic carriers *is very much higher*. This is immediately obvious on consideration that only homozygotes for the mutant CF allele have the disease, and that to produce a homozygote requires a mating of two heterozygotes. Indeed the frequency of heterozygous carriers of the CF gene is about 1:25—i.e. one in every 25 individuals in the population carries the disease allele for cystic fibrosis. This figure, which may seem surprisingly high at first sight, is calculated from the frequencies of the normal gene and its disease allele in the population. The relationship between gene frequencies and affected or carrier individuals is given by the *Hardy–Weinberg law*, a rule of fundamental importance in population genetics. For a gene locus with a dominant and a recessive allele having frequencies of p and q respectively, the proportion of individuals homozygous for the dominant allele is p^2, while the proportion which is homozygous for the recessive allele is q^2; the frequency of heterozygotes, the carriers of the recessive allele, is $2pq$. Since these account for the whole population, i.e. $(p + q) = 1$, then

$$p^2 + 2pq + q^2 = 1, \text{ or } 100\%.$$

The Hardy–Weinberg principle states that these expected frequencies, p^2, $2pq$ and q^2, remain constant from one generation to the next (ignoring factors such as mutation and selection). Applying this to cystic fibrosis, the gene frequencies are calculated from the proportion of homozygotes, i.e. the incidence of the disease (q^2). If we assume this to be 1:2500 or 0.0004 for CF, the frequency q of the recessive (disease) gene is the square root of 0.0004, which is 0.02 or 2%. The frequency p of the dominant (normal) allele is therefore 0.98 or 98 per cent. Hence the proportion of heterozygotes $2pq = 0.04$ (4%). Thus one person in every 25 is a carrier of the CF disease gene.

Note that for a fully penetrant dominant disease, the frequency of the disease gene in the population is the same as that of the disease itself, whereas for a recessive disease it is the square root of the disease incidence—and therefore much higher. In other words, as the above example shows, deleterious recessive genes are much more widespread in the population than might be expected from the rarity of the diseases themselves. It follows that we are all likely to be heterozygous carriers of some recessive alleles which in the homozygous state could produce serious or lethal diseases. The term *genetic load* expresses this concept. It has been estimated that man carries about two 'lethal equivalents' of detrimental recessives, i.e. the equivalent of two genes which, if homozygous, would be lethal. This figure is the sum of several recessive genes, determining conditions of varying mortality, which remain hidden because of heterozygosity. Such conditions are commoner in the offspring of consanguinous marriages.

Clearly it would be advantageous to be able to detect hetero-zygotes for the more frequent recessive diseases. Unfortunately, this is not yet possible for cystic fibrosis.

X-LINKED INHERITANCE

Recessive

Haemophilia, colour blindness, Duchenne muscular dystrophy and *Bruton-type agammaglobulinaemia* are all recessive conditions for which the genes involved are located on the X chromosome (Table 7.4). They have a characteristic pattern of inheritance which readily distinguishes them from the autosomal recessives described above. Figure 7.11 shows a typical pedigree. The most obvious feature is that only males are affected by the disease. This results from the fact that the male has only one X chromosome, so that all X-linked genes will be expressed in males even if recessive. Females possessing an X-linked recessive gene, on the other hand, are almost all heterozygous unaffected carriers, just as for an autosomal recessive. Therefore, since homozygous recessive females are very infrequent, these diseases occur virtually exclusively in males. The other key features of the inheritance are as follows. (i) The affected male generally arises from a mating between a carrier female and a normal male. Since the affected male receives a Y chromosome from his father, the X-linked recessive gene can only come from his mother. (ii) In such a mating, half the sons are affected and half are normal; similarly, half the daughters are carriers and half normal. (iii) If an affected male is married to a normal female, *none* of his sons will be affected or be carriers since they cannot inherit his X-linked gene, but all his daughters will be carriers, since they must receive his X chromosome; hence father-to-son transmission is impossible. (iv) The disease occurs in sons of the normal sisters of affected males (Figure 7.11). The inheritance is 'oblique', 'like the knight's move in chess', in contrast with autosomal dominant 'vertical' inheritance, which occurs in each generation, and autosomal recessive 'horizontal' inheritance, which occurs in sibs of one generation.

The most famous example of such a pedigree is the family of Queen Victoria, the disease being haemophilia (Figure 7.12). Victoria herself was a carrier and through her carrier daughters Alice and Beatrice the disease gene was carried into the ruling families of Prussia, Russia and Spain. Haemophiliac males were born to all these families, with historic consequences. The gene is

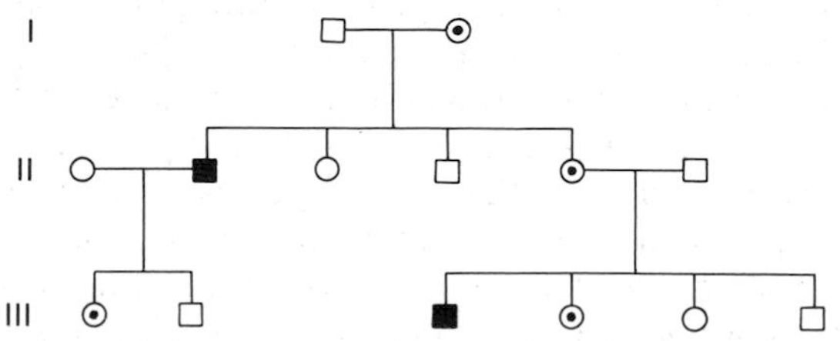

Figure 7.11 A pedigree of X-linked recessive inheritance.
■ : affected male.
⊙ : carrier female.

Table 7.4 X-linked recessive diseases.

Disease	Incidence at birth (males only)	Features
Agammaglobulinaemia (Bruton-type) (p. 78)		Absence of antibodies and immune defence mechanisms requiring antibody; normal cell-mediated immunity (i.e. B cell deficiency only). Severe recurrent infections by encapsulated bacteria, e.g. pneumococci, but normal resistance to viral and fungal infection
Angiokeratoma, diffuse (Fabry disease)		Nodular lesions on skin of lower trunk and mucous membranes; burning pain in extremities; death of adults from renal failure. Lipidosis, with excess storage of ceramide trihexoside (p. 842), due to deficiency of degradative enzyme ceramide trihexosidase
Chronic granulomatous disease (p. 24)		Susceptibility in childhood to pyogenic infections by catalase-positive bacteria (*Staph. aureus*, enterobacteria); granuloma formation. Eventually fatal despite antibiotics. Defect in phagocyte oxidative killing due to deficiency of super-oxide-forming enzyme
Diabetes insipidus (nephrogenic form)		Excessive urinary water loss (polyuria) due to unresponsiveness of renal tubules to ADH, antidiuretic hormone. (More commonly, diabetes insipidus is due to inadequate ADH production by the posterior pituitary and is not inherited.) Dehydration, pyrexia, vomiting, collapse
Glucose-6-phosphate dehydrogenase (G6PD) deficiency (p. 859)	1:10 in U.S. Negroes; 1:4 in parts of Africa, Sardinia	More than 80 G6PD variants are known. Deficiency leads to haemolytic anaemia after contact with agents such as drugs (primaquine) or fava beans (favism). Lysis related to intracellular level of reduced glutathione. Protection against malaria
Haemophilia A (classic form) (pp. 640, 835)	1:10,000 (A and B)	Deficiency of clotting factor VIII. Prolonged bleeding, life-threatening haemorrhage, bleeding into joints (haemarthrosis) leads to crippling. Replacement therapy with plasma or purified factor VIII

Table 7.4 *continued*

Disease	Incidence at birth (males only)	Features
Haemophilia B (Christmas disease) (p. 640)		Deficiency of clotting factor IX. Clinically similar to above
Hunter syndrome (p. 851)	1:200,000	Mucopolysaccharidosis; less severe than Hurler; no corneal clouding. Excess storage of dermatan sulphate and heparan sulphate due to absence of degradative enzyme in lysosomes. Corrected by enzyme from cells of Hurler syndrome patients
Ichthyosis		Skin disease; dry, scaly appearance of skin at birth ('fish-skin') due to hypertrophy of epidermis. Abnormality of keratinisation
Lesch–Nyhan syndrome (p. 845)	1:500,000	Gross neurological disturbance, including tendency to self-mutilation; very high uric acid levels in plasma and urine; renal uric acid stones. Lack of enzyme (HGPRT) in purine (uric acid) metabolism
Muscular dystrophy	1:5000	Three types including Duchenne, the commonest form of muscular dystrophy. Duchenne symptoms begin around 5 years with progressive muscular deterioration; death at around 20 years. Level of creatine phosphokinase is usually raised in female carriers, enabling detection in close relatives. However, a high proportion of cases have no family history (new mutations)
Testicular feminisation syndrome (p. 838)		Male, with testes, but female external genitalia (no uterus). Chromosomally 46, XY, no Barr body. Abnormality in pathway of androgen metabolism. Patients identify themselves as female
Wiskott–Aldrich syndrome		Thrombocytopenia with eczema and immunodeficiency. Severe bleeding episodes; recurrent infection with viruses, fungi and bacteria (especially pneumococci and enteric organisms). Defect in CMI and IgM production; poor IgM response to polysaccharide (thymus-independent) antigens of pneumococci and salmonellae

no longer present in the British Royal family, Queen Elizabeth II having descended from Victoria's normal *son* Edward VII.

Nearly 100 traits have been shown to be linked to the X chromosome in man, many of them pathological. Progress has been made in mapping the genes for these traits in relation to each other on the chromosome by observing recombinations between X-linked genes in families. A recent gene map is shown in Figure 7.13.

Some inherited conditions are expressed almost exclusively in males, but are determined by autosomal dominant rather than X-linked recessive genes. They are restricted to males for physiological rather than genetic reasons and are termed *sex limited* conditions. The distinction from true sex linkage is usually evident from the pedigree. Thus *pattern baldness*, in which the hair is thinned or lost altogether from the top of the head but grows at the sides, is far more common in males than females; however, the trait is transmitted from affected father to son, ruling out X-linked inheritance. The determining gene is an autosomal dominant, the effects of which are limited to males. Inherited disorders of sex organs themselves are naturally limited to one sex. If an affected male cannot reproduce, the distinction between autosomal dominant and X-linked recessive may not be possible from the pedigree. A good illustration is provided by *testicular feminisation*, in which individuals are genotypically male (XY) but phenotypically female. This is the result of interference with the action of testosterone on target organs; the affected individuals, who regard themselves as female, have undescended testes, a shortened vagina and no uterus. The condition requires the presence of testes to be expressed and therefore can only occur in males; as the individuals cannot reproduce, the criterion of father to son transmission is inapplicable. Thus the disorder may be X-linked or autosomal dominant.

Dominant

There are very few dominant X-linked diseases. One example is *vitamin D-resistant (hypophosphataemic) rickets*. The difference between this and autosomal dominant inheritance is that father to son inheritance cannot occur, for the same reason as in X-linked recessive traits. For X-linked dominants, an affected male transmits the disease to none of his sons but to all his daughters (there are no carriers). Affected females transmit the disease equally to half their male and half their female children.

MECHANISMS IN SINGLE-GENE DISEASES

In this section we describe some of the ways in which an inherited mutation at a single genetic locus can lead to disease. The result of mutation is production of a protein with an altered amino acid sequence; in consequence, the structure of the protein may be altered sufficiently to lead to defective function. Most of the examples in which it is possible to relate abnormal protein function to a pathological process are enzyme defects. The history

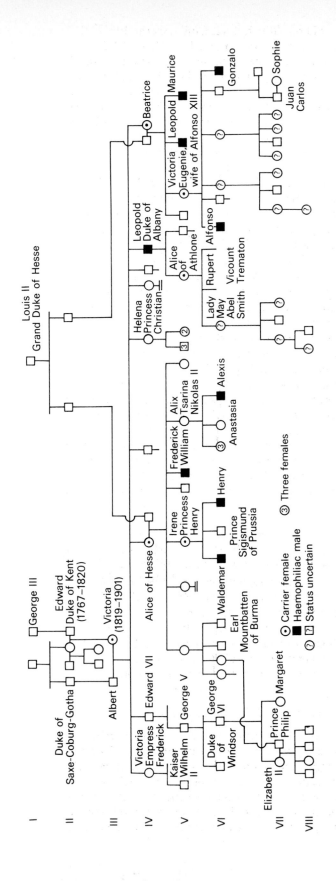

Figure 7.12 Pedigree of Queen Victoria and her descendents illustrating transmission of haemophilia, an X-linked recessive trait (from McKusick, 1969).

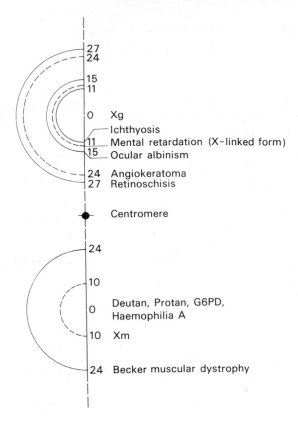

Figure 7.13 Genetic map of the human X chromosome.
Xg: a blood group
Xm: a plasma protein
G6PD: glucose-6-phosphate dehydrogenase
Deutan, protan: forms of colour blindness.

The map is based on family studies. Numbers are map distances (in centimorgans) based on recombination fractions. Semicircles are used to show that the relative positions of the loci in each cluster are unknown. There are at least 90 other loci, most unmapped. (After Race & Sanger, 1975 and McKusick, 1977).

Text labels in figure:
27
24
15
11
0 Xg
Ichthyosis
11 Mental retardation (X-linked form)
15 Ocular albinism
24 Angiokeratoma
27 Retinoschisis

Centromere

24

10

0 Deutan, Protan, G6PD, Haemophilia A

10 Xm

24 Becker muscular dystrophy

of the latter dates to the pioneering contribution of Sir Archibald Garrod who in 1909 defined the concept of the *inborn errors of metabolism*, conditions which result from blocks in specific metabolic pathways, caused by the inherited absence of a single enzyme. The four conditions he studied were alkaptonuria, albinism, pentosuria and cystinuria, and he noted the typical inheritance pattern of recessive characteristics, including a high incidence of parental consanguinity in the affected families (p. 829). As well as disrupting intermediary metabolism, enzyme defects may also cause excessive storage of the substrates of defective enzymes, leading to conditions known as *storage diseases*. Together, the inborn errors of metabolism and storage diseases include a long list of abnormalities involving amino acids, carbohydrates, mucopolysaccharides, lipids, steroids and purine and pyrimidine nucleotides (see Tables 7.3 and 7.4). Other enzyme abnormalities may only be revealed by adverse reactions to drugs or environmental agents. Another mechanism of single-gene disease is the inability to transport certain small molecules across cell membranes, causing so-called *transport diseases*; defects in receptor molecules or enzymes may be involved, though the molecular basis is generally not well understood. Finally, there remains a great diversity of other proteins which are not enzymes and whose functions may be altered by mutation. Here the relationship between genetics, biochemistry and pathology is well illustrated by the variants of haemoglobin and the anaemias they may produce.

Figure 7.14 Possible outcomes of inborn errors of metabolism.

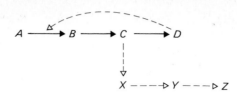

Normal Pathway

A = initial substrate; B,C = intermediates; D = final product;
X,Y,Z = minor products; ———▶ major pathway; − − − −▷ minor pathway;
feedback regulation.

Defect in enzyme catalysing C ———▶ D may lead to:

(i) Absence of end-product D

A ———▶ B ———▶ C —‖▶ D

(ii) Accumulation of intermediates, B and C.

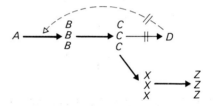

(iii) Increased use of minor pathway and overproduction of X,Y and Z

A ———▶ B ———▶ C —‖▶ D
X ———▶ Y ———▶ Z

(iv) Absence of feedback regulation by product

A ———▶ B ———▶ C —‖▶ D
    B C
    B C
X ———▶ Z
X Z
X Z

Inborn errors of metabolism

These diseases are the consequences of inherited deficiencies in enzymes involved in intermediary metabolism. In homozygotes, the enzyme may either not be produced at all or be produced in an aberrant form with reduced activity. Since a metabolic pathway involves a series of steps, each catalysed by a different enzyme, the absence of a particular enzyme will block the pathway and may lead to one of several situations as shown in Figure 7.14. A disease may result from (i) the absence of an important product; (ii) the excessive production of intermediates on the pathway just before the block; (iii) the diversion of intermediates into subsidiary pathways; or (iv) breakdown in the regulation of the pathway by end-products. The following illustrative examples are drawn from different areas of metabolism.

AMINO ACID METABOLISM

Examples of the first three of the above possibilities occur in the metabolism of the amino acids *phenylalanine* and *tyrosine*. The pathways involved are shown in Figure 7.15.

841

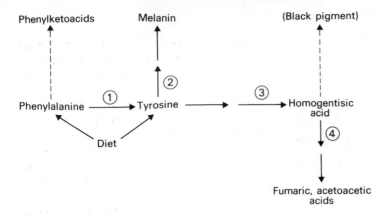

Figure 7.15 Pathways in the metabolism of tyrosine and phenylalanine, indicating the diseases produced by different enzyme deficiencies.
① : PKU (phenylalanine hydroxylase).
② : Albinism (tyrosinase).
③ : Tyrosinaemia (hydroxyphenylpyruvate oxidase).
④ : Alkaptonuria (homogentisic acid oxidase).

Albinism

Tyrosine is the precursor of melanin, the major pigment of the skin, hair and eyes: the pathway involves the conversion of tyrosine into DOPA (3,4-dihydroxyphenylalanine) and ultimately dihydroxyindole which is polymerised into melanin. Tyrosinase catalyses the first steps in this process:

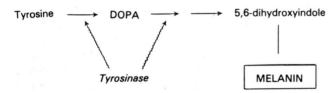

In albinism there is a failure to make melanin, so that albino individuals have white hair, very light skin and pink eyes. As a result, they are sensitive to sunlight and often have poor eyesight. One of the causes of albinism is lack of tyrosinase in the melanin-producing cells (melanocytes). However, more than one enzyme step is involved in melanin production, so it is perhaps not surprising that in some albinos tyrosinase is present in the melanocytes and another enzyme in the pathway, not yet identified, is lacking. It is usual to refer to the two forms of generalized albinism as *tyrosinase-positive* and *tyrosinase-negative* respectively. The two enzymes are controlled by two non-allelic autosomal loci. The fact that two distinct genes are involved has been demonstrated by *complementation* of the genetic loci involved, i.e. in some cases a marriage of two albinos has given offspring that have been normally pigmented. This can occur when the enzyme defect in each of the two parents is different, one being a tyrosinase-positive albino and the other a tyrosinase-negative. The children then receive a normal tyrosinase gene from one parent and a normal gene for the second enzyme from the other parent, and are therefore normal. This observation makes the basic point that diseases which appear to be the same, i.e. are phenotypically identical, can be caused by defects in different genes. This is conveyed by the term *genetic heterogeneity*.

Alkaptonuria

While albinism provides an example of a disease where an important end-product is missing, in alkaptonuria the absence of an enzyme causes the accumulation of an excess of a substrate proximal to the block (Figure 7.14 (ii)), in this case one of the oxidation products of tyrosine, homogentisic acid (Figure 7.15). The defective enzyme is homogentisic acid oxidase, and since homogentisic acid cannot be further metabolised it accumulates in the blood and is excreted in the urine. It is oxidised to a black pigment, which causes the urine to turn black on standing and darkens the napkins of affected babies. It is also polymerised in the body and deposited as a black pigment in cartilage, discolouring the ears and sclerae of the eyes, and causing arthritis through degeneration of cartilage in joints (ochronosis). It is a very rare autosomal recessive which, like albinism, was one of Garrod's original inborn errors.

Phenylketonuria (PKU)

This classic error in amino acid metabolism is caused by absence of the liver enzyme phenylalanine hydroxylase. As Figure 7.15 shows, this enzyme catalyses the main fate of phenylalanine, other than incorporation into protein, namely its conversion into tyrosine. When this cannot occur, phenylalanine accumulates in the blood and is metabolised by what are normally minor pathways to phenylketoacids and phenylacetic and phenyl-lactic acids. It is thus an example of the third type of 'error' in Figure 7.14. Phenylalanine and its products are very deleterious to early brain development, so that affected children are severely retarded (IQ $\sim$ 20). PKU is the most frequent single-gene cause of mental retardation. Fortunately, PKU can be detected at birth by screening blood phenylalanine levels in newborns and can then be prevented by immediately excluding phenylalanine from the diet. Such screening is now routinely carried out in many countries. Heterozygous carriers, though not affected, can be detected by the reduced rate at which they clear excess phenylalanine from the blood (phenylalanine tolerance test). The incidence of PKU shows ethnic variation, being highest among Caucasians (about 1:25,000 in UK) and lowest among American Negroes and Ashkenazi Jews. PKU also illustrates a phenomenon known as a *phenocopy*: if a child is born to a PKU-affected mother, it will develop mental retardation regardless of its own genotype. This is because the high phenylalanine level in the mother's blood crosses the placenta and affects the developing brain of her offspring. The child therefore appears to have PKU, even though it is only heterozygous for the gene. A phenocopy can be prevented by ensuring that the mother is kept on the special diet during her pregnancy. Since phenylalanine is a precursor of tyrosine, PKU individuals generally have very light skin pigmentation and fair hair.

Besides these examples, there are many other *aminoacidurias*, with 'overflow' excretion of the excess amino acid which accumulates proximal to the metabolic block. In some cases, syndromes of considerable complexity can result from defects in a single enzyme, as the following shows.

Homocystinuria

In this condition there is an absence of the enzyme cystathionine synthetase which occurs in the pathway from methionine to cysteine (Figure 7.16). Normally this enzyme converts homocysteine and serine into cystathionine, which in turn is an important precursor of cysteine. Deficiency of the enzyme leads to accumulation and excretion of homocysteine and lack of cystathionine. The resulting syndrome manifests a variety of clinical features, involving the circulation, connective tissue and nervous system. Among some unusual features are a very widespread tendency to thrombosis throughout the circulatory system, dislocation of the lens of the eye (ectopia lentis) and skeletal changes (osteoporosis). Apparently, excessive homocysteine increases the adhesiveness of platelets, leading to thrombosis, and inhibits the cross-linking of collagen fibres in connective tissue. In addition, the lack of cystathionine in the brain seems to be responsible for the mental retardation and psychiatric disturbances which frequently form part of the syndrome.

CARBOHYDRATE METABOLISM

Galactosaemia

Intermediate carbohydrate metabolism also provides examples of

Figure 7.16 Homocystinuria (from McKusick, 1972 *Heritable disorders of connective tissue*, 4th edn.).

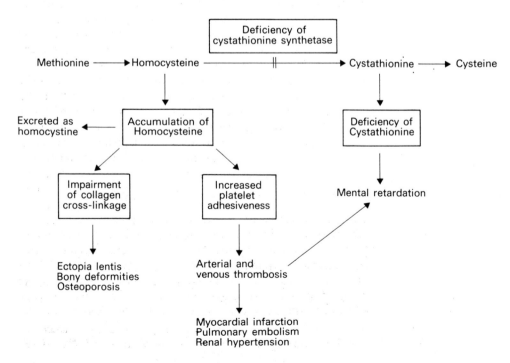

844

inborn errors. In galactosaemia the milk sugar galactose cannot be metabolised because the enzyme which converts galactose-1-phosphate into glucose-1-phosphate, before storage or utilisation, is missing (galactose-1-phosphate uridyl transferase), Figure 7.17. The presence of excess unmetabolised galactose-1-phosphate in the blood is detectable in newborns after feeding milk and can be prevented subsequently by a milk-free diet. Otherwise, vomiting, diarrhoea and jaundice ensue, with subsequent poor growth and liver damage, and either death from wasting and malnutrition or severe brain damage in survivors.

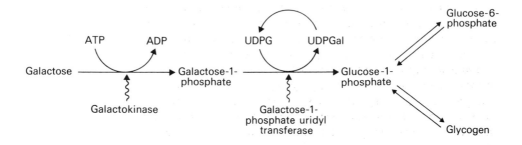

Figure 7.17 Pathway of galactose metabolism. UDPG: uridine diphospho-glucose. UDPGal: uridine diphospho-galactose

PURINE METABOLISM

Lesch–Nyhan syndrome

Metabolic pathways are frequently regulated in feedback manner, both negative and positive, by products of the pathway; this regulation normally acts on the first steps in the sequence. Another category of inborn error arises when this regulation is disturbed (Figure 7.14(iv)). For example, lack of the normal product may overactivate the initial steps in the sequence because feedback inhibition by the end-product is missing. An example of this occurs in the metabolism of the purine bases guanine and adenine, which are required as nucleotides for nucleic acids, energy metabolism, etc. The nucleotides GMP and AMP can be synthesized *de novo* in the cell from glutamine and PRPP (5-phosphoribosyl-1-pyrophosphate) by a pathway outlined in Figure 7.18. Dietary guanine and adenine can also be utilised by means of phosphoribosyl transferases; thus, in the case of GMP, the enzyme hypoxanthine guanine phosphoribosyl transferase, HGPRT, catalyses the reaction:

$$\text{Guanine} + \text{PRPP} \rightarrow \text{GMP}$$

This reaction is important in 'salvaging' guanine which would otherwise be catabolised to xanthine and uric acid. Accordingly, there is regulation of the *de novo* synthesis of the purine nucleotides by feedback inhibition by GMP, AMP and IMP (inosinic acid) on the first step of the synthetic reaction (Figure 7.18). If the level of GMP falls, for example, the synthetic pathway is stimulated until the requirement for GMP is satisfied. This happens in an unusual disease, the *Lesch-Nyhan syndrome*, which is caused by the inherited lack of HGPRT. In the absence

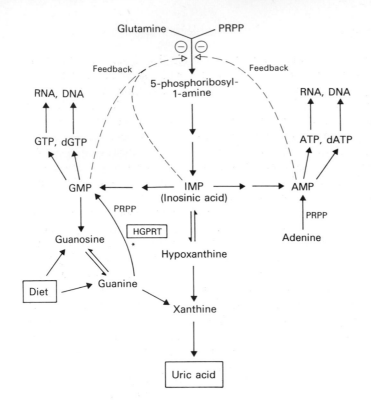

Figure 7.18 Regulation of purine metabolism.
PRPP: 5-phosphoribosyl-1-pyrophosphate
HGPRT: hypoxanthine guanine phosphoribosyl transferase
*: salvage pathway

of this enzyme the purine salvage mechanism cannot operate and preformed guanine is catabolised to xanthine and uric acid. The loss of guanine activates the synthetic pathway, but besides making up the cellular nucleotide requirement, this increases the formation of uric acid. The latter accumulates in the blood (*hyperuricaemia*) and urine; it is deposited as renal stones which often cause severe damage to the kidney. Uric acid deposited in the joints leads to gouty arthritis (below). However, the most striking feature of the Lesch–Nyhan syndrome is a progressive neurological and behavioural disturbance. There is an almost unique tendency to violent self-mutilation, in which an affected child—always a male because the condition is X-linked—will bite his own fingers and destroy his lips by chewing with his teeth, often requiring to be physically restrained. Most patients are mentally deficient as well. It is not really clear how HGPRT deficiency causes the neurological disorder, though the enzyme is normally very active in brain. It may be that, in the absence of purine salvage, the synthetic pathway cannot maintain GMP and IMP levels needed for normal brain function. It is clear that the nervous system involvement is not simply secondary to hyperuricaemia, since the two can occur independently. Hyperuricaemia is easily relieved with allopurinol, but there is as yet no effective therapy for the nervous dysfunction. Lesch-Nyhan syndrome can be detected in the foetus *in utero* and affected males aborted.

Gout is caused by hyperuricaemia, often resulting from aberrations in purine metabolism. It is a recurrent acute arthritis of peripheral joints which follows the deposition of monosodium urate in and around joints and tendons; in addition, deposition of free uric acid as calculi (stones) in the kidney leads to possibly life-threatening renal damage. Genetically and biochemically, gout is heterogeneous. Primary, familial gout may be caused by one of a number of genetic defects leading to increased production of uric acid (occasionally gout is secondary to administration of diuretics or chronic lead poisoning and is then not an inborn error). The mode of inheritance has been problematic: a case has been made for autosomal dominant inheritance, but polygenic inheritance has also been suggested and environmental factors can also influence the uric acid level. The hyperuricaemia of gout is usually the result of over-production of uric acid, though in some cases under-excretion is responsible. With rare exceptions, such as HGPRT deficiency (above), the specific enzyme aberration of primary gout has not been identified. Gout is predominantly a male disease; its scarcity in women in perhaps due to the lower circulating urate levels in females before the menopause (almost all female patients are post-menopausal).

Acute gout consists of excruciatingly painful attacks of arthritis, most frequently involving the great toe and also commonly the instep, ankle, heel, knee and wrist. Acute attacks are precipitated by minor trauma, such as a tightly-fitting shoe, or over-indulgence in food or alcohol. Each attack lasts for several days, during which the affected joints show all the signs of intense acute inflammation, with swelling, warmth, reddening and pain (Section 1). The attack eventually subsides and joint functions return to normal until the next one. As the disease progresses, attacks become more prolonged and the asymptomatic periods between them shorter; eventually there may be several attacks a year, each often lasting several weeks. Ultimately, chronic gout supervenes, with characteristic deposits of monosodium urate in large, bulbous lesions called *tophi* around the joints and with renal calculi of uric acid. The tophus consists of a mass of urate crystals surrounded by a chronic inflammatory reaction, with fibroblasts, lymphocytes, plasma cells and foreign body giant cells (Section 1). Tophi are responsible for progressive, permanent joint deformity.

The solubility of uric acid and its salts is low and even in normal individuals urate levels approach the limits of solubility. In gouty patients, the blood is often supersaturated, i.e. contains urate in excess of theoretical solubility, because of a stabilising effect of plasma proteins. Evidently in and around the joints this stability is lost, and urates crystallise out of solution, while in the lower pH of the kidney uric acid itself is precipitated. The cause of joint damage and inflammation is the release of lysosomal enzymes from neutrophils which engulf crystals of monosodium urate. After phagocytosis, the crystals are present in phagosomes with which lysosomes fuse and into which they discharge their enzymes, as described in Section 1 (p. 21). However, urate crystals disrupt phagosomes by forming hydrogen bonds with phospholipids in the phagosome membrane. Following rupture of a phagosome, the cell is soon killed by its own lysosomal enzymes released into the cytoplasm; the subsequent extracellular release of these enzymes leads to tissue damage and acute inflammation. A factor which may contribute to the low incidence of gout among women is the stabilisation of the phagosome membrane by female hormones. An acute gouty attack is rapidly terminated by colchicine, which seems to prevent the union of lysosomes with the phagosome. Long-term therapy of gout is by reduction of the circulating urate level, either by blocking uric acid production with allopurinol or by increasing uric acid excretion. In this way, tophaceous deposits may be resolved and erosive joint damage prevented.

STEROID METABOLISM

Adrenogenital syndrome

The biosynthesis of steroid hormones by the adrenal cortex provides an example of how inborn errors and regulation of metabolism combine to produce disease. In this case the condition is the *adrenogenital syndrome* associated with congenital adrenal hyperplasia. The characteristic symptom is *virilisation*—females possess male-like external genitalia, while males are masculinised prematurely. The adrenal cortex synthesizes several steroids from cholesterol, the two major types being glucocorticoids such as cortisol (hydrocortisone), and mineralocorticoids, notably aldosterone; in addition the cortex produces, normally in a minor way, androgenic sex hormones such as androstenedione and testosterone. This last pathway is the one which becomes excessively utilised in the adrenogenital syndrome. Figure 7.19 shows the pathway of synthesis and the enzymes involved; note that one enzyme may catalyse parallel steps in more than one pathway.

Figure 7.19 Biosynthesis of cortisol, sex hormones and aldosterone from cholesterol.
Dm: desmolase
A: 3β-hydroxysteroid dehydrogenase
B, B': 17-hydroxylase
C, C': 21-hydroxylase (commonest defect in cortisol and aldosterone production)
D, D': 11-hydroxylase
E, E': 17-hydroxycorticoid clearing enzyme
F: 17-hydroxysteroid dehydrogenase

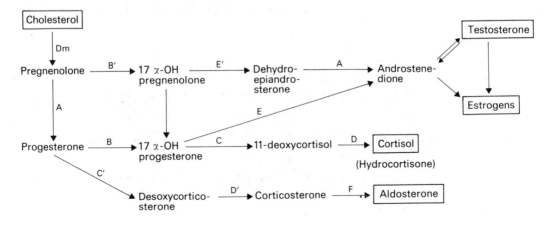

848

The rate of production of the adrenal steroids is itself under hormonal control, which involves a pituitary-adrenocortical homeostatic mechanism. The hypothalamus is sensitive to cortisol levels and when they fall it produces an ACTH-releasing factor which stimulates the release of ACTH from the anterior pituitary. ACTH promotes growth of the adrenal cortex and stimulates conversion of cholesterol into pregnenolone (Figure 7.20).

The commonest 'error' in steroid metabolism is the absence of 21-hydroxylase (enzyme C in Figure 7.19), which catalyses steps in the formation of the critically important hormones cortisol and aldosterone. The defect is an autosomal recessive. In response to the resulting deficiency of these hormones, the pituitary secretes ACTH, which causes adrenal cortex hyperplasia and stimulation of the adrenocortical pathways of Figure 7.19. However, these can only function up to the blocked reaction; intermediates therefore accumulate and are diverted into an alternative pathway, namely the production of androgens such as androstenedione and testosterone. The excess of adrenal androgens while the genitals are developing during early intrauterine life causes the adrenogenital syndrome. This is most marked in the female, where virilisation is apparent at birth; while the ovaries and ducts are normal, the external genitalia are unusual and resemble those of the male. The individual is a *pseudohermaphrodite*: her 'penis' is formed by hypertrophy of the clitoris, while the enlarged labial folds resemble a scrotum. In extreme cases it may be difficult to assign sex—other than by nuclear sexing—and some subjects are brought up as boys, though of course there are no testes and a buccal smear would reveal the Barr body (p. 819). In males, adrenal hyperplasia may cause premature masculinisation, though this would not be apparent until late infancy or childhood. Complications resemble those of Addison's disease (chronic adrenocortical insufficiency) and in many cases include excessive salt loss, vomiting, diarrhoea and dehydration. The salt loss is attributable to the very depressed aldosterone level (see p. 677). The condition can be arrested by administration of cortisol, which suppresses ACTH release and thereby diminishes the stimulation of the adrenal cortex. 21-Hydroxylase deficiency has a particularly high frequency in Switzerland, where an incidence of 1:5000 births has been found, and among

Figure 7.20 Feedback regulation of the adrenal cortex by cortisol and ACTH (adrenocorticotrophic hormone) and its breakdown in adrenogenital syndrome.

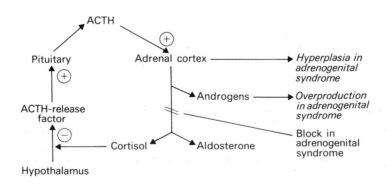

Eskimos—1:490 for the Yupik Eskimos of Alaska (cf. 1:67,000 in the USA.). Prenatal diagnosis is unsuccessful. Other enzyme defects in the steroid pathways do occur, but are very rare.

Storage diseases

We have already noted in Figure 7.14 that one consequence of the absence of an enzyme in a metabolic pathway is the accumulation of the substrate(s) proximal to the block. When these substrates are small, soluble molecules, they are distributed around the body by overflowing into the blood and are excreted in the urine, as described above. Substrates of limited solubility, on the other hand, are retained inside the cells which would normally be able to metabolise them, but which because of the inherited enzyme defect are unable to do so. The resultant excessive intracellular accumulation of such substances leads to disorders known collectively as storage diseases. The most important examples are *glycogen storage diseases, mucopolysaccharidoses* and *lipidoses*. Excessive storage occurs because of the absence of an important degradative enzyme rather than over-synthesis. Normally the intracellular degradation of mucopolysaccharides, glycogen, lipids, etc., frequently takes place inside lysosomes, the organelles which contain a variety of hydrolytic enzymes. Therefore, when a critical enzyme is missing, it is often inside lysosomes that the substrate accumulates and the cells become laden with vacuoles containing the unmetabolisable substrate. The term *lysosomal diseases* is used to refer to such conditions.

MUCOPOLYSACCHARIDOSES

In these diseases, the stored materials are the acid mucopolysaccharides which form a large part of the ground substance or matrix of connective tissue. These molecules are high molecular weight polymers, having subunits of a hexosamine (frequently *N*-acetyl-α-D-glucosamine or galactosamine) and a hexuronic acid (glucuronic or iduronic); some, such as hyaluronic acid and chrondroitin, are non-sulphated, while in the others the hexosamine residues carry sulphate groups (keratan sulphate, heparan sulphate, dermatan sulphate, etc.), Figure 7.21. In connective tissue itself, the polysaccharide chains are linked to a protein core. The mucopolysaccharides are synthesized in connective tissue by fibroblasts and this can be studied *in vitro* in fibroblast cultures. It appears that while most ($\sim$ 75%) of the mucopolysaccharide is secreted and leaves the cell, a certain proportion is always retained and degraded by lysosomal enzymes. At least four enzymes are essential in degradation of mucopolysaccharides in the lysosome, namely α-L-iduronidase, heparan sulphate sulphatase, β-glucuronidase and *N*-acetyl-α-D-glucosaminidase. It

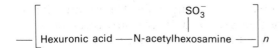

Figure 7.21 Repeating subunit structure of a sulphated acid mucopolysaccharide.

is the inherited lack of one of these enzyme activities which leads to the excess storage of mucopolysaccharides intracellularly and the pathological syndromes of mucopolysaccharidosis (MPS).

Although six distinct MPS types have been defined, the most important syndromes are the *Hurler syndrome* and the *Hunter syndrome*, of which the former is the more severe. In both, the excess storage products are dermatan sulphate and heparan sulphate, which are also excreted in the urine in considerable amount. The Hurler syndrome (frequency $\sim$ 1:100,000) is a fatal autosomal recessive condition which leads to death by about the age of ten. The chief clinical symptoms are skeletal defects, including dwarfism and stiff stubby fingers, clouding of the cornea which may lead to near-blindness, mental retardation, abdominal extension due to enlargement of the liver and spleen, and a facial appearance uncharitably termed 'gargoyle-like', which is shared by other MPS syndromes. Death is often due to cardiac complications caused by the deposition of mucopolysaccharide in the coronary arteries, which become thickened, and in the heart valves. Deposits of mucopolysaccharide are found in large amounts in fibroblasts in many sites ('gargoyle cells') and in nerve cells in the brain, accounting for the hepatosplenomegaly and mental retardation. The fundamental defect in the Hurler syndrome is a deficiency of α-L-iduronidase, the enzyme which degrades the iduronic acid-containing molecules dermatan sulphate and heparan sulphate. This accounts for the appearance of both these in the urine in this syndrome. In comparison, the Hunter syndrome is a less severe condition which is also inherited differently, namely as an X-linked recessive. Patients survive well into adulthood, do not show corneal clouding and suffer less from mental deterioration. Nevertheless, dwarfism, gargoylism and hepatosplenomegaly are features, as well as frequent progressive deafness. Once again, dermatan sulphate and heparan sulphate are stored in excess and excreted in the urine.

The fact that these two MPS syndromes differ in their mode of inheritance (autosomal vs. X-linked) immediately suggests a difference in the basic defect, despite the identity of the stored products. This has been proven by *in vitro* experiments with the fibroblasts of Hurler syndrome and Hunter syndrome patients. It was found that fibroblasts from either type of patient would, as expected, accumulate mucopolysaccharides excessively in culture, compared with normal fibroblasts. However, when fibroblasts from patients with the two syndromes were mixed together, mutual correction of the metabolic defects occurred, i.e. cultures containing the mixed Hunter and Hurler cells behaved exactly like cultures of normal fibroblasts. Furthermore, the culture medium in which cells of one MPS type had been growing could correct the defect in the other MPS type. It appeared that fibroblasts from a Hurler patient could release a soluble factor which corrected the defect in cells of a Hunter patient, and *vice versa*. It is now known that the corrective factors are themselves the fibroblast lysosome enzymes. Cross-correction is explained because there are *two* enzymes involved in the degradation of both dermatan sulphate and heparan sulphate;

defect of one of the enzymes causes the Hurler syndrome while lack of the other causes the Hunter syndrome. Hence each type of patient will still have one of the degradative enzymes and can therefore make good, or complement, the defect in the other patient. This is what is observed in the culture experiments, where fibroblasts release lysosomal enzymes which are taken up by and remain active in other fibroblasts, leading to cross-correction of defects. This result also has therapeutic potential, since administration of the missing enzyme might be expected to correct the defect in patients (replacement therapy). In fact normal human plasma contains these enzymes and normal plasma infusions are reported to have beneficial effects on Hurler and Hunter patients.

The cell culture approach has proved a very useful tool in analysing the underlying enzymatic defects in these apparently complex syndromes. For example, if the fibroblasts of two patients do not cross-correct each other in culture, it is very likely that they carry the same enzymatic deficiency. This turned out to be the case, surprisingly, for two MPS syndromes which are clinically quite distinct, namely the Hurler and the *Scheie* syndromes. Possibly the degree of enzyme deficiency is different in the two syndromes and determines the clinical features. Another unexpected finding was that in another MPS disease, the *Sanfilippo syndrome*, cross-correction between clinically identical patients could occur; in other words two distinct enzyme defects were demonstrable (keratan sulphate sulphatase and N-acetyl-α-D-glucosaminidase), but only one clinical syndrome was produced.

GLYCOGEN STORAGE DISEASES

Glycogen is the chief form in which carbohydrate is stored in animals. It is a multibranched polymer of glucose which is synthesized and stored in the liver and muscle. When glucose is required for energy metabolism, it is released from glycogen by the action of the enzyme phosphorylase. The pathways for the synthesis and degradation of glycogen are shown in Figure 7.22. Many enzyme defects in glycogen metabolism are known, some of which are indicated in the figure. Defect in an enzyme involved in glycogen breakdown causes a reduction in the level of circulating glucose (*hypoglycaemia*) and/or an excessive storage of glycogen (*glycogenosis*). The most severe forms are *von Gierke's disease* and *Pompe's disease*. The former disease is of historical interest as the first inherited deficiency of a known tissue enzyme to be demonstrated, by the Coris in 1952. In von Gierke's disease there is a lack of the enzyme glucose-6-phosphatase which is essential for the release of glucose from the liver. In the absence of this enzyme there is hypoglycaemia, which may be severe and lead to convulsions in children, and a tremendous enlargement of the liver due to storage of excess glycogen. Glucose-6-phosphatase is not a lysosomal enzyme and the glycogen is found in the cytoplasm of the liver cells rather than in vacuoles. Affected individuals may have a reasonably long life and survive to adulthood. Pompe's

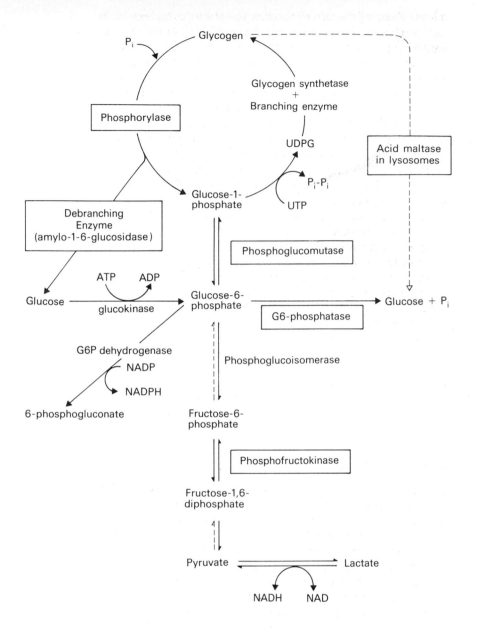

Figure 7.22 Pathways of
glycogen metabolism.

☐ : sites of enzyme defects
in different glycogen-storage
diseases.

disease differs in many respects. It is the most severe glycogenosis
and death is at five to six months of age. The striking clinical
manifestations are profound muscular hypotonia and gross enlargement of the heart, due to stored glycogen. In contrast with
von Gierke's disease, this is a lysosomal disorder caused by
absence of the enzyme α-1,4-glucosidase (acid maltase). As
opposed to phosphorylase and other enzymes involved in glycogen catabolism, which are found in the cytoplasm,
α-1,4-glucosidase is responsible for the breakdown to glucose
of glycogen fragments which enter lysosomes. When it is
missing, glycogen accumulates in lysosomes, eventually
forming large glycogen-filled vacuoles. This contrasts with

normal liver cells where glycogen is stored in the cytoplasm. In Pompe's disease, lysosomal accumulation takes place even though the cell contains the other glycogenolytic enzyme phosphorylase because the latter is extralysosomal. Thus it is the compartment- alisation of these enzymes within the cell that makes Pompe's disease possible. In other glycogen-storage diseases, the enzymes involved include muscle phosphorylase (*McArdle's disease*), liver phosphorylase (*Hers disease*) and phosphoglucomutase (*Thomson's disease*).

LIPIDOSES

The class of lipids with which we are concerned here are the *sphingolipids*. While they were originally discovered (by Thudichum) in brain, many are in fact widely distributed in cell membranes, though some termed gangliosides are predominantly found in brain and nervous tissue. The sphingolipids all share a basic structural unit called a *ceramide*, which consists of the long-chain base sphingosine linked by an amide bond to a long-chain fatty acid:

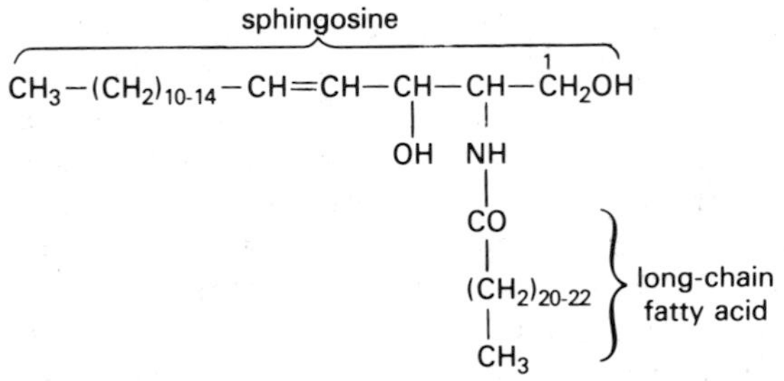

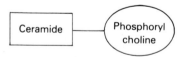

$$CH_3-(CH_2)_{10\text{-}14}-CH{=}CH-CH-CH-\overset{1}{CH_2}OH$$

with branches: OH, NH, CO, $(CH_2)_{20\text{-}22}$, CH_3 — long-chain fatty acid

Ceramide

The different classes of sphingolipids are distinguished by the moiety which is linked by ester bond to the carbon C-1 of the ceramide. For example, in *sphingomyelin* it is phosphorylcholine:

Ceramide — Phosphoryl choline

while in the *neutral sphingolipids* it is a sugar or oligosaccharide:

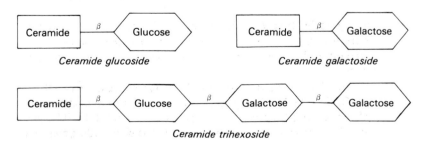

Ceramide —β— Glucose   Ceramide —β— Galactose
Ceramide glucoside   *Ceramide galactoside*

Ceramide —β— Glucose —β— Galactose —β— Galactose
Ceramide trihexoside

854

and in the *gangliosides* it is an oligosaccharide containing sialic acid and often an *N*-acetyl-hexosamine:

```
┌──────────┐  β  ╱─────────╲  β  ╱─────────╲  β  ╱───────────────╲
│ Ceramide ├────⟨  Glucose  ⟩────⟨ Galactose ⟩────⟨   N-acetyl     ⟩
└──────────┘    ╲─────────╱     ╲─────────╱      ╲ galactosamine  ╱
                                     │
ganglioside G_M2                   NANA
```

```
┌──────────┐  β  ╱─────────╲  β  ╱─────────╲  β  ╱───────────╲  β  ╱─────────╲
│ Ceramide ├────⟨  Glucose  ⟩────⟨ Galactose ⟩────⟨  N-acetyl  ⟩────⟨ Galactose ⟩
└──────────┘    ╲─────────╱     ╲─────────╱      ╲galactosamine╱    ╲─────────╱
                                     │
ganglioside G_M1                   NANA
```

(NANA = N-acetylneuraminic acid, sialic acid)

In the lipidoses, these molecules accumulate because of the inherited absence of specific enzymes which degrade these moieties or remove them from ceramide. The classic examples are Tay-Sachs disease, Gaucher's disease and Niemann-Pick disease.

Tay-Sachs disease (gangliosidosis G_{M2} or amaurotic family idiocy), a lethal autosomal recessive, is named after the British ophthalmologist Tay and the American neurologist Sachs who first described its symptoms in the 1880's. These are chiefly confined to the nervous system and include developmental retardation, paralysis, dementia and blindness. The blindness is characteristically associated with a cherry-red spot in the retina, first noted by Tay (amaurosis = blindness). The disease becomes apparent by 5–6 months and invariably leads to death by about 3–4 years. Biochemically, there is an accumulation in the brain of what is normally a minor sphingolipid component, the ganglioside G_{M2}. In the cerebral cortex, for example, ganglion cells become swollen and distorted by the enormous excess of ganglioside which is stored in vacuoles in their cytoplasm; the ganglion cells eventually disintegrate and are, of course, irreplaceable. Similar changes occur in the cerebellum and the rest of the central nervous system. They are accompanied by extensive demyelination of axons. The deficient enzyme is *hexosaminidase A*, a lysosomal enzyme normally involved in degrading ganglioside G_{M2}:

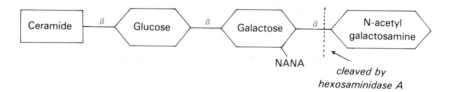

cleaved by
hexosaminidase A

In Tay-Sachs disease, undegraded ganglioside becomes stored in lysosomes, which then become the lipid-laden vacuoles of the ganglion cells; thus, this is another example of a lysosomal disease.

One of the striking features of Tay-Sachs disease is its ethnic distribution: 90% of all patients are Jews. Its frequency among Ashkenazi Jewish populations is as high as about 1:4000 births, while in Sephardic Jews or in non-Jews it is about 100 times less frequent. Ashkenazi Jews are those of Eastern European ancestry while Sephardic Jews are of Spanish descent. Approximately 1 in 30 Ashkenazi Jews will be a heterozygous carrier of the defective hexosaminidase gene, almost as high as the frequency of carriers of the defective gene for cystic fibrosis in Caucasians (p. 834). Fortunately, heterozygotes can be detected and it is advisable for Jewish couples to be tested for such heterozygosity before having children; if both are heterozygous carriers, the chances of an offspring having the disease are 1 in 4. Tay-Sachs disease can be detected in the foetus by amniocentesis and, if present, the pregnancy is terminated. The possible causes of ethnic variation in this and other diseases are discussed on p. 864.

Both *Gaucher's disease* and *Niemann–Pick disease* are also more commonly found among Ashkenazi Jews than other groups: in Israel, Gaucher's disease has a frequency of between 1:2000 and 1:20,000 in Ashkenazis. In contrast with the neurological manifestations of Tay-Sachs disease, the abnormalities of the commonest form of Gaucher's disease are found mainly in the viscera, with gross enlargement of the spleen and liver. A typical feature is the presence of Gaucher cells in these organs, as well as in the bone marrow and lymph nodes. These are reticulo-endothelial cells (macrophages) which have accumulated large quantities of the sphingolipid ceramide glucoside. The metabolic defect in these cells is the absence of the enzyme *glucocerebrosidase* (*β-glucosidase*) which splits off the glucose residue from the ceramide:

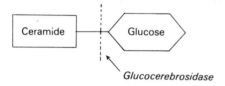

This form of Gaucher's disease can appear at any age and follows a chronic course. A much more severe form occurs in the first few months of life, with progressive neurological dysfunction in addition to hepatosplenomegaly. Death occurs in 1–2 years. Despite the disparity in their clinical symptoms, both forms of Gaucher's disease involve deficiency of the same enzyme, a situation akin to that of the Hurler and Scheie syndromes (p. 852). One can only assume that there is a difference in degree of deficiency and that the two forms of Gaucher's disease are caused by different mutations in the same enzyme.

Niemann–Pick disease is also a very severe disorder with extreme hepatosplenomegaly and irreparable damage to the nervous system. The commonest form leads to death by about the age of four years, though less severe types also occur. The cause is a deficiency of the enzyme *sphingomyelinase*, which breaks down sphinogmyelin, an important component of the membranes of all animal cells. The deficiency is again lysosomal, with excess sphingomyelin becoming stored in large "foam" cells—macrophages laden with vacuoles of sphingomyelin, which are found in the spleen, bone marrow and lymphoid tissue. The concentration of sphingomyelin in the liver may increase up to 30-fold and, for unknown reasons, cholesterol also accumulates. As for most of these diseases, there is no specific therapy.

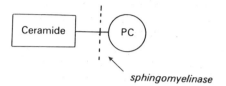

(PC = phosphorylcholine)

Transport diseases

In these diseases, the inherited deficiency does not lie in a step in intermediary metabolism, but in the transport of substrates across cell membranes, primarily in the epithelial cells of the kidney and intestine. The chief indications of such conditions are excessive excretion of the substrate in the urine and its impaired absorption from the gut. The disorders are relatively benign, but clinical effects may arise from deposition of the substrate in the kidney, from its deficiency in the body if it is an essential metabolite, or from the harmful effects of its metabolism by gut bacteria. However, such diseases have a significance which goes beyond their clinical interest, for the information they have provided on mechanisms of transport in cell membranes; in this respect they are valuable 'experiments of Nature'. In many cases, these inherited defects have been the first evidence for specific transport sites for different substances.

AMINO ACID TRANSPORT

Some *aminoacidurias* are the result of defects in the reabsorption of amino acids in the proximal renal tubule. An indication of a renal transport defect would be the excessive excretion of an amino acid without an increase in its concentration in the blood. The classic example is *cystinuria*, in which cystine is excreted in excess and precipitates in the urinary tract as cystine stones. This was originally thought by Garrod to be an inborn error of cystine catabolism, but some 40 years later it was shown that plasma cystine levels are not raised as they would be if cystine was merely being excreted by an 'overflow' effect. It was therefore suggested that there is a specific renal mechanism for the reabsorption of cystine in the renal tubule and that this is defective in cystinuria. In fact, other amino acids are also excreted in cystinuria, namely lysine, ornithine and arginine which, like cystine, are all dibasic; this implies a shared renal absorption system for the group of dibasic amino acids, acting through recognition of their common feature of two free amino residues (Figure 7.23). Investigation of other aminoacidurias has revealed two other group-specific renal transport mechanisms for amino acids, one for glycine, pro-line and hydroxyproline, and another for the monoamino-

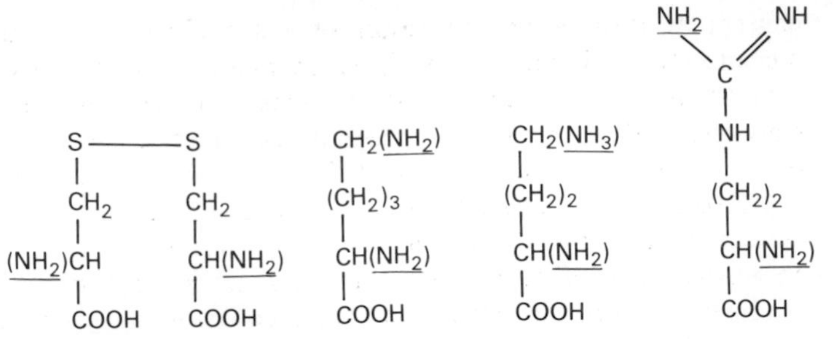

S——S		$CH_2(NH_2)$	$CH_2(NH_3)$	 NH$_2$ NH \ / C | NH
CH_2 CH_2		$(CH_2)_3$	$(CH_2)_2$	$(CH_2)_2$
$(NH_2)CH$ $CH(NH_2)$		$CH(NH_2)$	$CH(NH_2)$	$CH(NH_2)$
COOH COOH		COOH	COOH	COOH
Cystine		Lysine	Ornithine	Arginine

Figure 7.23 Dibasic amino acids which share a common transport mechanism. Amino groups are underlined.

monocarboxylic acids. *Iminoglycinuria* involves excess excretion of the former group, and *Hartnup disease* of the latter.

The same transport mechanisms appear to operate across the intestinal epithelium and this can lead to deficiency syndromes. For example, in Hartnup disease the symptoms resemble those of pellagra, the classical result of dietary deficiency of nicotinic acid (niacin). This is because tryptophan is among the group of amino acids which are poorly absorbed in Hartnup disease, and tryptophan is an important source of nicotinic acid in the body. Moreover, bacterial degradation of the excess tryptophan remaining unabsorbed in the intestine can lead to production of toxic metabolites, which can be absorbed and which may have damaging effects on the nervous system. Hence, in Hartnup disease the clinical symptoms have little to do with the urinary excretion of amino acids from which the diagnosis is made.

PHOSPHATE TRANSPORT

Specific transport defects are not restricted to amino acids. *Familial vitamin D-resistant (hypophosphataemic) rickets* is a disease caused ostensibly by failure of the normal mechanism of reabsorption of phosphate in the renal tubule. There is excessive excretion of phosphate (hyperphosphaturia) and low blood phosphate level. An adequate supply of calcium and phosphate is essential for the normal process of calcification of growing bones and the term *rickets* refers to the maldevelopment of the skeleton which results when this supply is diminished. Vitamin D is required for the intestinal absorption of calcium, its role being in the synthesis of a calcium-binding protein found in the cells of the small intestine, and the commonest cause of rickets is vitamin D deficiency. Rickets is therefore normally not inheritable and is easily remedied by providing adequate dietary vitamin D. However, the vitamin D-resistant form is a familial disorder which does not respond to physiological levels of the vitamin. The apparent cause of this condition is the excessive loss of phosphate in the urine which results from defective reabsorption in the kidney. The most obvious reason for this would be a defect in a specific transport mechanism for phosphate in the renal tubule. However, the pathogenesis is more complicated than it seems, for in addition to hyperexcretion of phosphate, there often occurs inadequate intestinal absorption of calcium, which may be the more immediate cause of rickets. Poor calcium absorption appears in turn to be the result of a specific defect in the metabolism of vitamin D itself, which must be converted enzymatically to an active product before calcium uptake is stimulated. Thus the root of vitamin D-resistant rickets could be an error of vitamin D metabolism, but how this causes impaired renal phosphate absorption has yet to be satisfactorily explained. Another unusual feature of this disease is its X-linked dominant mode of inheritance, of which it provides the best example. As with autosomal dominants, females as well as males can be affected, but father-to-son transmission is impossible (see p. 838). As would be expected, the heterozygous females are often less severely affected than the hemizygous males. Nevertheless, dominant inheritance is unusual where enzymatic defects are causative, unless the enzyme is normally present at or near rate-limiting concentrations.

Other transport defects include failure to reabsorb glucose (renal glucosuria), glucose-galactose malabsorptions and the *Fanconi syndrome*. The latter is less specific and involves a wider variety of substances, including amino acids.

Inherited reactions to drugs and environmental agents

Another category of single-gene disorder can be defined in which there is an inherited adverse reaction to administered agents such as drugs or to external environmental factors such as u.v. light.

PHARMACOGENETICS

Glucose-6-phosphate dehydrogenase deficiency

Pharmacogenetics concerns itself with altered responsiveness to pharmacological agents, usually resulting from specific enzyme defects. The classic disorder is sensitivity to the antimalarial drug *primaquine* in individuals with deficiency of *glucose-6-phosphate dehydrogenase* (*G6PD*). Under normal circumstances, G6PD deficiency has no clinical effects, but on administration of primaquine or a variety of other drugs a severe *haemolytic anaemia* occurs, with massive destruction of red blood cells, jaundice and excretion of a dark or black urine. The discovery of a deficiency of G6PD in the red blood cells in this condition opened the way to important biochemical and genetic studies with this enzyme. The basis of the red cell destruction provoked by the drug cannot be completely explained, although the key points are known. G6PD is important in glucose metabolism in red cells, oxidising glucose-6-phosphate (G6PD) to 6-phosphogluconate and producing the reduced coenzyme NADPH. The latter is required to maintain the substance *glutathione* in its reduced form (GSH), which is essential to the normal functioning of red cells and indeed to all other cells in the body. A major role of G6PD therefore is to ensure the conversion of oxidised glutathione (GSSG) to GSH (Figure 7.24). Drugs such as primaquine cause a fall in red cell GSH, the level of which can be rapidly re-established in normal, but not in G6PD-deficient, red cells. The

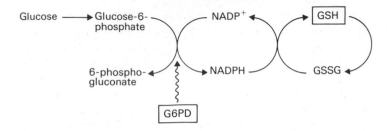

Figure 7.24 Reduction of glutathione requires G6PD (glucose-6-phosphate dehydrogenase). GSH, GSSG: reduced, oxidised forms of glutathione

fall in GSH leads, by means not yet clarified, to red cell destruction. Interestingly, the deficiency mainly affects old red cells, so that continued administration of the drug in fact leads to recovery and disappearance of symptoms as old red cells are replaced by young ones. Haemolytic anaemia is also seen in some G6PD-deficient individuals after eating fava beans (*Vicia fava*), a condition known as *favism* (Pythagoras may have been a famous sufferer). The active principle in the beans which induces haemolysis is DOPA-quinone.

There are several other important aspects to G6PD deficiency. It is an X-linked recessive, so that mainly males are affected. The gene has been a very useful marker for the X-chromosome in mapping studies, being closely linked to the genes for colour blindness and haemophilia (p. 828). The G6PD variants have been used to test the Lyon or 'inactive X' hypothesis (p. 807). For example, while nearly all Europeans possess the normal or B type of G6PD, a variant with near normal activity, called A+, is common in populations of African origin (including American Negroes). Females who are heterozygous for these two forms, i.e. G6PD-A+/B, possess two types of somatic cell: one type produces the normal B form while the other has the A+ variant. Similarly, there is a form of G6PD deficiency common among African populations and caused by a variant called A−. In females heterozygous for the A− gene, e.g. G6PD-A+/A−, there are again two populations of cells, one of which has normal G6PD activity (A+) while the other is G6PD-deficient (A−), a result of the random inactivation of one X chromosome in each somatic cell (p. 819). For this reason, some heterozygous females also show symptoms of G6PD deficiency. G6PD variants can thus be used to establish the *clonality*, or common origin, of a group of cells, and a recent application of this principle has been described in studies on atherosclerosis (Section 5, p. 670).

More than 60 variants of G6PD have been described, most of which have deficient activity. Some are found with high frequency in certain populations. For example, about 10% of American Negroes carry the common A− form of G6PD, as do their African counterparts; other forms are found in Mediterranean areas and among Asian populations. How is this high incidence of G6PD deficiency accounted for? Like other red cell abnormalities, it is connected with the prevalence of malaria in those areas. It is more difficult for the malaria parasite to multiply in G6PD-deficient red cells, so there is a considerable advantage for individuals with the deficiency in such an environment. Hence malaria exerts a selective pressure to maintain the deficient gene at a high level in the population; very similar considerations apply to the high incidence of the sickle-cell haemoglobin trait and thalassaemia in malarial areas (p. 863).

Other inherited enzyme defects which are revealed by drugs include *pseudocholinesterase deficiency*, which causes prolonged paralysis after anaesthesia with muscle-relaxant drugs such as succinylcholine and suxamethonium; and deficiency of a liver acetylase which inactivates isoniazid, the drug widely used in the treatment of tuberculosis. Individuals who inactivate the drug rapidly are less likely to suffer toxic side effects of isoniazid and other drugs detoxified by acetylation.

ENVIRONMENTAL FACTORS

In *xeroderma pigmentosum* an enzyme defect is revealed, not by the effect of a drug, but by an abnormal sensitivity of the skin to u.v. light. Patients with this condition suffer from disfiguring skin damage on exposure to sunlight, with a marked tendency for basal cell and squamous cell carcinomata to develop; so much so that the patients' exposed parts must all be covered to protect them from sunlight if an early death is to be avoided. It is valuable as an illustration of a rare clear-cut instance of hereditary predisposition to cancer. The basis of the disease lies in defective repair of DNA damaged by exposure to u.v. light and is described in detail in Section 6 (p. 773).

Defects in non-enzymatic proteins

HAEMOGLOBINOPATHIES

The inherited abnormalities in the structure of haemoglobin provide excellent examples of genetically determined variation in protein structure in man. The haemoglobin molecule consists of four polypeptide chains making up the protein globin, to which the four haem groups, which bind oxygen, are attached. The haemoglobin variants are the result of amino acid substitutions in the polypeptide chains. Normal adult haemoglobin is denoted HbA and contains two types of polypeptide chain known as α and β, two α and two β chains being non-covalently associated in the molecule; this is summarised in Figure 7.25. The foetus has a different form, HbF, in which two α chains are associated with two γ chains rather than β; HbF is the major form up to birth, but disappears by 4 months. While HbA comprises 98% of adult haemoglobin, there is also a minor component, HbA_2, consisting of two α and two δ chains. In short, each of the normal haemoglobins is made up of a pair of α chains associated with a pair of non-α chains, either β, δ or γ (and there is also an embryonic chain, ε). The β, δ, and γ genes are linked together, while the α gene is on a different chromosome (Figure 7.25). The α chain has 141 amino acids, the β chain 146. The variants of normal haemoglobin generally arise as a result of point mutations in the DNA coding for these chains; such mutation causes the

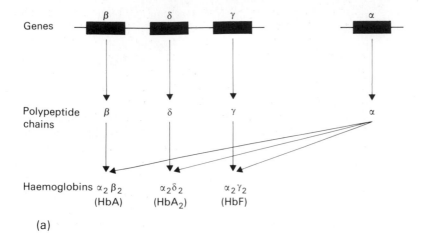

(a)

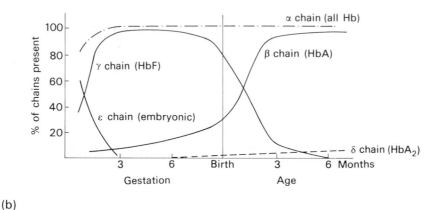

(b)

substitution of a normal amino acid in the sequence of the polypeptide chains. Since the 3-dimensional structure of the protein is determined by the amino acid sequence of its chains, such substitutions can lead to abnormalities in structure and properties of the haemoglobin molecule, and hence perhaps to pathological consequences.

Sickle-cell phenomenon

The best known abnormal haemoglobin is the haemoglobin HbS, which causes the sickle-cell phenomenon. In this molecule, a glutamic acid residue present at position 6 of the normal β chain is replaced by valine. This single change of a polar into a non-polar residue has a dramatic effect on the physical properties of haemoglobin, reducing the solubility of the deoxygenated form by about 15-fold. While oxygenated HbS and HbA have similar solubilities, HbS comes out of solution on deoxygenation to form a semi-solid gel. In the red cell, this causes an alteration of cell shape so that instead of the normal discs, curved sickle cells result. Heterozygotes for the abnormal sickle β gene produce both

Figure 7.25
(a) Haemoglobin genes and polypeptide chains.
The β and δ genes are closely linked; γ is linked to them and may be adjacent as shown. The α gene is not linked to β, δ or γ.
(b) Sequential appearance of haemoglobins during development.
The ϵ chain is embryonic and is present for the first few months only; it is replaced by the foetal γ chain of HbF. After birth, HbA, containing β chains, predominates.

the normal HbA and abnormal HbS (codominant expression); such individuals have the *sickle-cell trait*, in which sickling does not normally occur *in vivo* but can be demonstrated by deoxygenation of the blood *in vitro*. In contrast, homozygotes for the sickle gene have mainly HbS and cannot produce normal HbA; they suffer from *in vivo* sickling, which causes the severe disease *sickle-cell anaemia*. The high concentration of HbS in the red cells leads to sickling on deoxygenation and increases blood viscosity. The abnormal red cells are removed and destroyed by phagocytes, causing anaemia, while the vascular changes lead to thrombosis and infarction. The outlook is poor and homozygotes do not usually survive childhood. Note that while the expression of the sickle cell gene is codominant, only the sickle-cell *trait* shows dominant inheritance; sickle-cell anaemia behaves as an autosomal recessive, since it will occur only in homozygotes.

Haemoglobin polymorphism and malaria

A striking feature of the sickling abnormality is the very high frequency of the HbS gene in Negro populations in Africa and the United States—as many as 15% of Negroes may be heterozygous for the gene and hence carry the sickling trait, while deaths from sickle-cell anaemia number almost 100,000 annually in these populations. When an allele, such as the HbS gene, attains a gene frequency of more than 1% the locus is said to be *polymorphic*. There are many examples of polymorphism in man—the ABO blood group is perhaps the most familiar, with high frequencies of the A, B and O alleles in all populations. However, it is unusual for a deleterious or disease gene to reach the frequency of a polymorphism, because of the working of natural selection. A gene which reduces the ability to reproduce of the individuals carrying it can normally be maintained in the population only by new mutations; with mutation rates of the order of 1:10,000 or less, genes which are subject to this selection/mutation balance should not be able to reach the level of a polymorphism. The finding of a very high frequency for the S allele of haemoglobin therefore requires a special explanation, there being no evidence for an unusually high rate of mutation in the haemoglobin genes. The answer lies in a *selective advantage* conferred on heterozygous carriers of the S allele over normal individuals under special circumstances, namely in a malarial environment. That malaria was a selective force behind red cell anomalies was first suggested by J.B.S.Haldane and substantiated for HbS by A.C. Allison. The distribution of the S allele in Africa and Asia is quite well correlated with that of malaria, and malaria is rarely found in carriers of the sickle-cell trait. Moreover, if the malarial parasite is inoculated both into normal individuals and 'sicklers', it will grow only in the former. The likely mechanism for this protection from malaria is that red cells infected with *Plasmodium falciparum* tend to adhere to the walls of blood vessels, where they become deoxygenated. If they contain HbS, the red cells then sickle and are removed by phagocytes, thereby also eliminating the malarial parasite. A significant incidence of sickle-cell anaemia (i.e. homozygosity) will be the price paid by the population for this advantage.

A polymorphism which is maintained in this way by heterozygote advantage and selection is called a *balanced polymorphism*. Balanced polymorphism is also seen in relation to malaria for another haemoglobin allele, HbC, for thalassaemia genes (below) and for deficiency of the enzyme G6PD (p. 860). HbC, in which a glutamic acid at residue 6 of the β chain is replaced by lysine, produces less pronounced anaemia in the homozygous state than HbS, and also a lesser degree of protection against malaria; it is most common in West Africa, especially in Ghana where it must have originated.

The effect of heterozygote advantage may also explain the unusually high incidence of other disease genes in certain ethnic groups. For example, the genes causing phenylketonuria and cystic fibrosis have a much higher frequency among Caucasians than in Negro or Oriental populations, while Tay–Sachs disease is far more common in Ashkenazi Jews than other groups. The disease alleles for these genes are around 1% in frequency in the most affected groups. The selective pressures which might be involved are generally unknown; one which has been suggested is an advantageous resistance for carriers of the Tay–Sachs allele against tuberculosis in the ghetto conditions of Eastern Europe.

Other abnormal haemoglobins

A large number of haemoglobin variants besides HbS and HbC have been described. Identification of haemoglobin variants is usually accomplished by electrophoresis; this will pick out substitutions involving change of charge, as between HbA and HbS. Some of the variants lead to dominantly-inherited anaemias because of the instability of the mutant molecule and its tendency to precipitate and cause haemolysis. In another type of variant, the oxygen-carrying capacity of the molecule is impaired by substitution of important histidine residues, which lie adjacent to the haem groups in the molecule in both the α and β chains. The iron atom in the haem moiety in deoxyhaemoglobin is in the ferrous form (Fe^{2+}); it gives up an electron to become the ferric form (Fe^{3+}) when oxygen is bound, but reverts to ferrous when the oxygen is lost on deoxygenation. If the iron is permanently oxidised to Fe^{3+} it cannot bind or release oxygen, and the molecule is called *methaemoglobin*. This can be produced by substitution of a histidine in the α chain (position 58 or 87) or β chain position 63 or 92) by tyrosine. The tyrosine interacts with the iron atom of haem and stabilises the ferric state. Methaemoglobins produced in this way are called M haemoglobins, to distinguish them from oxidised (Fe^{3+}) haemoglobins produced by inherited absence of a reducing enzyme in the red cell (methaemoglobin reductase). The result of either condition is a disease called methaemoglobinaemia in which there is cyanosis (blueness of the skin and mucous membranes due to inadequate oxygenation of the circulating blood) and hypoxia. The condition is a dominant when produced by an M haemoglobin and a recessive when caused by the enzyme deficiency. Absence of the reducing enzyme can be reversed by administration of reducing agents such as ascorbic acid, but this is without effect on M haemoglobins.

THALASSAEMIAS

In contrast with these abnormalities of haemoglobin structure, thalassaemias are anaemias caused by a *reduced rate of synthesis* of haemoglobin chains. Thus in β-thalassaemia, for example, there is an insufficiency in β-chain production, but those β chains which are synthesized are functionally normal. Thalassaemia is particularly common in Mediterranean countries, such as Italy and Greece (Gk. *thalassa*, sea), where it may attain a very high incidence and where in some regions frequencies of thalassaemia genes can be as high as 10%. It is also found in Africa and India. Once again, a good correlation can be drawn between the incidence of thalassaemia and malaria; as with HbS, the thalassaemia gene confers protection against malaria, giving a selective advantage to carriers of the gene. As with the haemoglobinopathies, the effects of thalassaemia are much more severe in homozygotes than heterozygotes. Production of either α or β chains is commonly affected, leading to severe, life-threatening anaemia in homozygotes, but a much milder anaemia in heterozygotes. Partial or complete absence of β chains in β-thalassaemias leads to a corresponding lack of HbA and this is compensated to a certain extent by continued production of HbF, the foetal form of haemoglobin, in adult life. Deficiency in α chain production (α-thalassaemia) is potentially even more serious, since the α chain is required for all haemoglobins, foetal as well as adult; here a certain degree of compensation is provided by formation of tetramers of γ chains only (haemoglobin Barts) or β chains (haemoglobin H). In an interesting rare form of thalassaemia, a haemoglobin variant called the *Lepore haemoglobin* was discovered. Instead of the β chain of HbA or the δ chain of HbA_2, the Lepore molecule possesses a composite 'δ-β' chain, one end of which is like β and the other end like δ. The gene for this chain arises by an unusual genetic event known as unequal crossing-over, a recombination in which the homologous genes are misaligned, as shown in Figure 7.26. A gene is produced which is part-δ and part-β, and although the protein product of the gene is functional in haemoglobin, it is synthesized at a reduced rate, causing thalassaemia. Unequal crossing-over may be an important mechanism in evolution since it increases the number of adjacent genes, as Figure 7.26 illustrates.

The molecular basis of different forms of thalassaemia has been clarified recently by detailed studies of the α and β genes in patients, including sequence analysis of cloned genes. Contrary to the earlier assumption that a defect in genetic controlling elements (regulator genes, operators, etc.) was involved, it is now clear that in both α- and β-thalassaemias, there is either a deletion or a mutation in the *structural* genes themselves. Thus, in most cases of α-thalassaemia, the entire α gene is deleted. In β-thalassaemia, a variety of genetic alterations have been found

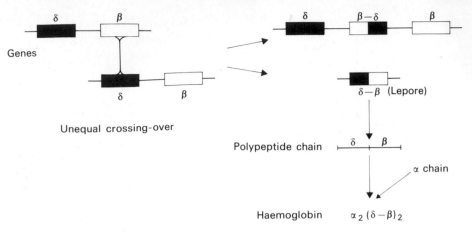

Genes

Unequal crossing-over

$\delta - \beta$ (Lepore)

Polypeptide chain

α chain

Haemoglobin $\alpha_2(\delta - \beta)_2$

Haemoglobin Lepore

among different patients, including deletions and point mutations. The latter are such as to reduce or totally prevent β-chain synthesis, rather than produce structurally abnormal β chains as in the haemoglobinopathies. For example, in β°-thalassaemia, a point mutation within the β gene makes it impossible for the RNA transcript of the gene to be 'spliced' into messenger (m) RNA; patients homozygous for this mutation therefore make no β-chain mRNA and hence no β chains. On the other hand, in β^+-thalassaemia, a different point mutation leads to a large reduction in the amount of mRNA, but patients are still able to make small amounts of normal β chains. (This is the form of thalassaemia most common in Cyprus and, therefore, in London.) Yet another type of mutation causes premature termination of the β chain during its translation. The fact that many independent types of mutation causing thalassaemia are seen is not surprising in view of the protection against malaria afforded to carriers.

Figure 7.26 Origin of haemoglobin Lepore by unequal crossing-over.

CONNECTIVE TISSUE PROTEINS:
THE MARFAN SYNDROME

The Marfan syndrome is a dominant disorder of connective tissue in which the most striking feature is the excessive length and loose-jointedness of the limbs and extremities (another term used is *arachnodactyly* or 'spider limbs'), Figure 7.27. The most famous sufferer may well have been Abraham Lincoln, whose unusual physical appearance, loose joints and enormous hands and feet, have led to the suggestion that he had this disease. Other abnormalities occur in the eye (*ectopia lentis*—dislocation of the lens) and the cardiovascular system. There is an inadequacy in the elastic tissue of the arterial wall, leading to *dissecting aneurysm* of the ascending aorta in which bleeding occurs into the media, generally through an intimal tear. In this condition the intima and upper third of the media become separated (dissected) from the lower two thirds of the media, creating a blood-filled space (the aneurysm) within the aorta wall. The wall may be dissected in this way along a considerable length. Death results from rupture of the aneurysm, which frequently occurs into the

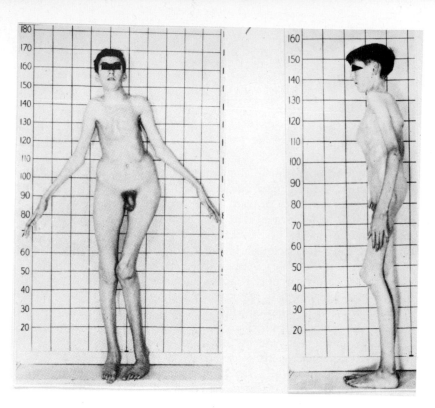

Figure 7.27 The Marfan syndrome.
(a) Patient, aged 13 years, is tall, very thin and shows arachnodactyly (note very elongated fingers).
(b) Same patient in profile, aged 11 years, showing chest deformity (pigeon breast, *pectus carinatum*).
(From McKusick, 1972, *Heritable Disorders of Connective Tissue*, 4th edn.)

pericardial sac. (Note the difference between the dissecting aneurysm of Marfan's syndrome and the more common aortic aneurysms associated with atherosclerosis, in which the aortic wall is stretched into a sac, but not dissected.) Since the Marfan syndrome shows dominant inheritance, an enzymatic defect is unlikely to be involved. Rather, it is probable that an inherited structural abnormality of collagen or elastin is the primary cause, though the details are obscure. The condition can be mimicked in animals by certain toxic agents (aminonitriles) which interfere with cross-linking of collagen.

MULTIFACTORIAL DISEASE

The diseases which result from single mutant genes are for the most part rare, generally with a frequency of less than one per thousand. Much more common are diseases which result from an interaction between genetic and environmental factors, i.e. are multifactorial in their causation. The genetic component involves more than one gene (polygenic), so that simple Mendelian patterns of inheritance are not apparent in family studies. The inherited contribution is often a predisposition in the individual to the adverse effects of environmental factors, such as infectious or chemical agents, diet, etc. The diseases responsible for the greatest human mortality, namely atherosclerosis and cancer, have significant genetic as well as environmental contributions, as do diabetes, peptic ulcer, schizophrenia, many birth defects, chronic infectious diseases, and so on. There is virtually no disease which is entirely free from genetic effects on its incidence

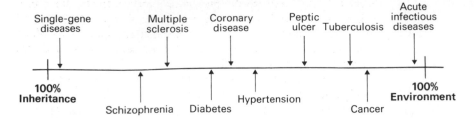

Figure 7.28 Spectrum of the relative importance of inheritance and environment in selected diseases.

or severity. An approximate comparison of the importance of inheritance in some common diseases is shown in Figure 7.28.

Several approaches have been used to estimate the role of inheritance in these diseases. The most obvious is evidence of a history of the disease in the families of affected individuals, care being taken to distinguish inherited effects from those of a shared environment. Valuable information can be obtained from studying the frequency of the disease in twins and comparing monozygotic and dizygotic twins. Since monozygotic twins are genetically identical, they should show greater similarity or 'concordance' than dizygotic twins for a disease with a significant inheritable component, and the degree of concordance should reflect the degree of genetic determination or *heritability*. From such studies, estimates of heritability in percentage terms have been derived for many diseases, e.g. about 20–30% for some cancers, 50–70% for hypertension, coronary disease and diabetes and 70–100% for schizophrenia, mental deficiency and manic-depressive psychosis. Differences in disease incidence between ethnic groups can also indicate genetic determination, especially if these cut across geographical barriers. Another approach is to look for an *association* between the disease and a genetic trait such as blood group or histocompatibility (tissue) type. Such associations can both confirm the genetic influence on the disease and also give an indication of possible aetiology. Examples include the increased risk of duodenal (peptic) ulcer in individuals of blood group O, and the associations between HLA type and a range of diseases, many involving autoimmunity. Some instances of multifactorial inheritance will now be discussed.

CONGENITAL MALFORMATIONS (BIRTH DEFECTS)

These are gross abnormalities of development which are evident at birth. It is important to be aware of the distinction between the terms 'congenital' and 'genetic' or 'inherited'. *Congenital* only refers to the presence at birth of a character or defect but does not mean that the defect has been inherited, since environmental factors can affect the developing foetus *in utero*. Conversely, disorders which are wholly genetically determined may not be apparent at all at birth and therefore not congenital. Indeed, congenital malformations cover a range from those which are wholly genetically determined to those which are almost wholly determined by non-genetic factors. In practice, those most commonly encountered, such as *cleft lip*, *cleft palate*, *club foot*, *spina bifida, anencephaly*, and *heart malformations*, are multi-factorial in causation, resulting from a combination of genetic and extrinsic factors. The latter include substances and agents which can influence the development of the foetus, such as drugs, viruses, chemicals and radiation.

Agents capable of inducing abnormal foetal development are called *teratogens* (lit. 'monster-producing'), and the study of abnormal development is *teratology*. The extreme examples of teratogens are agents which are capable of inducing abnormalities in most individuals exposed at the appropriate time in embryonic life; among those most clearly recognised in man are *rubella virus* (the agent of German measles), *cytomegalovirus* (CMV) and the sedative drug *thalidomide*. Both rubella virus and CMV can cross the placenta from the mother's bloodstream to infect the foetus *in utero* and produce congenital syndromes. Congenital rubella is described on p. 312; with the widespread practice of vaccination of girls, rubella is now a less frequent cause of abnormality than CMV infection (e.g. cytomegalic inclusion disease of the newborn, p. 270). The thalidomide tragedy is the extreme example in man of drug-induced teratogenesis. Following administration of this sedative/anti-emetic between the 3rd and 5th week of pregnancy, a range of malformations was produced of which the most severe were complete absence of all limbs (amelia) or gross limb underdevelopment (phocomelia—seal limbs).

Fortunately, teratogenic agents as potent as thalidomide are rarely encountered and it is more common for a teratogen to produce a malformation only where a genetic tendency exists for such a malformation to occur. Animal studies indicate that teratogens act to increase the frequency of malformations which already occur in the population at a low level of incidence, emphasizing the importance of an hereditary predisposition to the malformation in addition to the action of a teratogenic agent. Experience shows that this is also true in man. There are probably hundreds of agents with potentially teratogenic properties, given the appropriate genetic circumstances and timing of their action. This relationship has led to the desire wherever possible to avoid administration of, or exposure to, any conceivably damaging substances—drugs, chemicals, viruses—during early pregnancy.

DIABETES MELLITUS

This common disease provides a good example of multifactorial causation, though neither the genetic nor the environmental factors involved have been fully defined as yet. Diabetes mellitus results from a relative or absolute lack of the hormone insulin, produced by the β cells of the islets of Langerhans in the pancreas, though there is wide variation in degree of insulin deficiency among patients and hence in clinical severity of the disease. The estimate of the prevalence of diabetes is in the range of 1–8% depending on the criteria used for assessing the disease (overt clinical symptoms vs. glucose tolerance test) and the age groups considered (diabetes increases with age). Two major types of disease can be distinguished with regard to this latter point, namely *juvenile onset diabetes* in persons under 25 years (frequency $\sim$0.15%) and *adult onset diabetes*, the majority form. As will be further discussed below, there are sufficient differences between these two forms of diabetes, both in probable aetiology and pathogenesis, for them to be considered distinct disease entities. Insulin deficiency is greatest in juvenile diabetics, where there is usually a complete lack of insulin production and hence the most severe acute forms of the disease; insulin lack in adults is of variable degree.

The clinical effects of insulin lack stem from its central role in the metabolism of carbohydrate and fat, particularly in the storage and utilisation of these substrates of energy metabolism. Insulin is very much the hormone of the 'fed' state of the animal, facilitating the uptake of glucose by adipose tissue and muscle, and its storage as fat in adipose tissue and as glycogen in muscle and liver. Figure 7.29 indicates the effects of insulin on substrate metabolism in these tissues. Its main effects can be summarised as follows.

1   The efficient uptake of glucose by muscle and adipose tissue is insulin-dependent; the hormone accelerates membrane transport of glucose into these tissues by an unknown mechanism. The uptake of glucose by the brain and liver is not dependent on insulin.

2   In adipose tissue, insulin encourages lipogenesis (synthesis of fat), both through its facilitation of glucose entry and by enhancing phosphorylation of glucose to glucose-6-phosphate (G6P). This is the precursor both of α-glycerophosphate, required for the glycerol moiety of triglyceride, and of acetyl-CoA, from which fatty acids are synthesised. At the same time, insulin inhibits the breakdown of stored triglyceride (lipolysis) and thus prevents release of free fatty acids.

3   In muscle, the storage of glucose as glycogen after feeding is enhanced by insulin, ensuring that stored energy is present for immediate use on exercise (on prolonged exercise, muscle utilises fatty acids mobilised from adipose tissue).

4   In the liver, the central organ in the regulation of energy metabolism, insulin also acts to encourage storage of glucose as glycogen and inhibits glycogenolysis (glycogen breakdown). The hormone also inhibits gluconeogenesis, the conversion of non-carbohydrate substrates such as amino acids, glycerol and lactic acid into glucose.

It is clear that insulin deficiency will have major effects on the storage and utilisation of carbohydrate and fat. The key indicator of insulin deficiency is *hyperglycaemia* (abnormally raised blood glucose level) since removal of glucose from the blood into several tissues is insulin-dependent; in the absence of clinical signs, hyperglycaemia is detectable by a glucose tolerance test. In diabetes, the renal threshold for reabsorption of glucose is exceeded and glucose appears in the urine (glycosuria), leading to excessive urinary loss of water (polyuria), thirst and hunger. In adipose tissue, lipolysis now exceeds lipogenesis (Figure 7.29) and free fatty acids are mobilised; they are partially converted by the

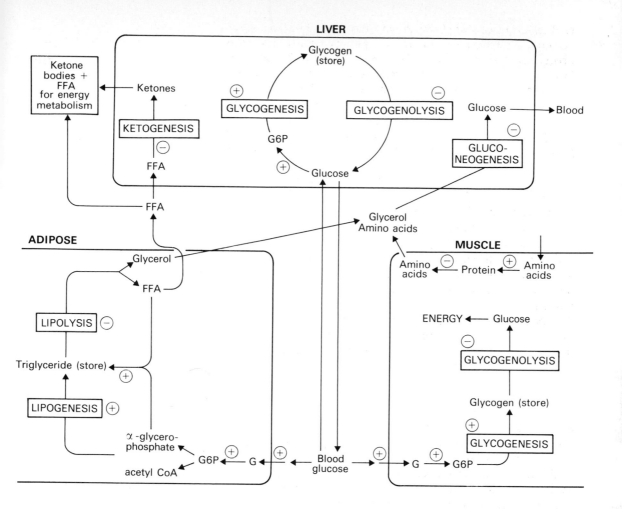

Figure 7.29 Effects of insulin on carbohydrate and fat metabolism. ⊕ : insulin-enhanced or -dependent (decreased in diabetes) ⊖ : insulin-inhibited (increased in diabetes)
FFA: free fatty acids
G: glucose
G6P: glucose-6-phosphate

liver into 'ketone bodies', i.e. the acids β-hydroxybutyric acid and acetoacetic acid, which together with free fatty acids serve as the energy source for muscle, heart, kidney and, in due course, brain (Figure 7.29). Body proteins are broken down to provide amino acids for gluconeogenesis, in an attempt to correct what appears to the tissues as a lack of blood glucose, but this leads to further hyperglycaemia and glucose excretion and contributes to the weight loss seen in diabetes. Eventually, fatal consequences can result from the excessive accumulation of ketone bodies (ketosis), including acetone, both in the blood with increased blood acidity and excreted in the urine with the loss of Na^+ and K^+ ions. Finally, diabetic coma and death ensue.

While these comprise the acute events of severe insulin deficiency, diabetes of chronic duration also has important effects on the vascular system. A major hazard is the accelerated atherosclerosis which occurs when part of the mobilised lipid is diverted into cholesterol, causing hypercholesterolaemia; diabetics are at significantly greater risk of coronary artery disease and myocardial infarction than the normal population. Another important consequence is thickening of capillaries, arterioles and venules by deposition of glycogen and mucopolysaccharides in basement membranes; major damage can result to the kidney (glomerulosclerosis) and the eye, where retinal damage leading to blindness is a relatively common complication of diabetes.

The causes of insulin deficiency are both genetic and environmental, with growing evidence for distinct aetiologies of juvenile and adult onset forms. That there is a strong inherited component in both is shown by the greater frequency of diabetes in the families of affected individuals than in the general population, and by the significant degree of concordance in monozygotic, compared with dizygotic, twins. However, it is equally clear that, while a recessive gene or genes may be involved, genetic expression depends on additional environmental factors. Thus, while concordance in monozygotic twins is about 50%, compared with about 8% for dizygotic twins, it is nevertheless well short of the expected 100% for a disease determined solely by genetic factors. It is also possible that inheritance is polygenic, the disease requiring the combined effects of two or more genes.

Recent family and population studies indicate that an important gene determining predisposition to juvenile diabetes is present in the major histocompatibility complex HLA. The significance of this and similar findings in other diseases is discussed at length on p. 877, and probably derives from the presence in the HLA complex of genes which regulate immune responses, *immune response* or *Ir genes* (see also Section 2). The Ir genes control the level and type of antibody or cell-mediated response, and since a range of these genes exist in the population (polymorphism) they are responsible for inherited differences in immune response between individuals. Thus some individuals respond better than others to pathogenic agents, while other individuals may have inherited an increased tendency to autoimmune reactions, and so on. These considerations are particularly relevant to the aetiology of juvenile diabetes, where evidence exists both for the involvement of a virus and for autoimmunity.

That a virus could be the environmental factor has been suggested by a temporal relationship between certain virus infections and onset of diabetes. Those possibly involved are rubella, mumps and coxsackievirus infections. A role in human diabetes is well established only for rubella virus, which produces diabetes in congenitally infected subjects. More than twenty cases of diabetes have been reported in association with mumps, and antibodies to islet cells have been found in mumps patients (but not in children infected with other viruses). Mumps virus may have an affinity for islet cells, in which it will grow in culture. The possible involvement of coxsackieviruses B3 and B4 has been discussed on p. 296. One could envisage that a genetically determined low or inappropriate antiviral immune response might allow a virus to damage the pancreas, and if sufficiently severe this could in itself produce diabetes. Alternatively, virus-induced damage to the pancreatic islets could trigger an autoimmune response, i.e. a response directed against 'self' body components which might be revealed to the immune system following pancreatic damage. The tendency to autoimmunity may itself be inherited as an effect of Ir genes. Evidence for an autoimmune basis for pancreatic damage in juvenile diabetes comes from lymphocytic infiltration of the pancreas ('insulitis') and the demonstration in patients of antibodies reacting with the insulin-producing β cells themselves, islet-cell antibodies. (It is unlikely that normal insulin is itself recognised as an antigen in diabetes, as spontaneous anti-insulin antibodies are rare). Such autoimmune reactions against the pancreatic islet cells mediated either by lymphocytes or antibodies could produce β cell destruction by the hypersensitivity mechanisms described in Section 2, notably types II, III and IV. Figure 7.30 indicates the postulated interactions between genetic and environmental factors in juvenile diabetes.

In contrast with the juvenile form, there is little evidence for involvement of immune response genes, viruses or autoimmunity in adult onset diabetes. However, other genetic factors are undoubtedly involved and environmental factors which are well recognised are *diet* and *physical exercise*. These are illustrated by the striking decline in diabetes during wartime, which correlates better with the period of food shortage than with the duration of the war itself, and its increase as food supplies became more available again. Also, an exceptionally high incidence of diabetes is seen in populations who have recently changed to the typical modern Caucasian diet rich in refined carbohydrate and fat, coupled with a reduction in their physical activity. This has been seen in Indian tribes in North America, such as the Pima Indians, where abnormal glucose tolerance has been found in over 50% of individuals over 50 years of age; similar observations have been made in New Zealand Maoris and South African populations newly moved to cities. A plentiful carbohydrate-rich diet and lack of physical activity lead to *obesity*, and the high proportion of adult diabetics who are obese is well recognised (about 80%); similarly, some 60% of obese individuals have abnormal glucose tolerance. The obese individual has an increased insulin requirement, which may either reveal latent insulin insufficiency or exhaust the insulin-producing capability of the β cells. Weight reduction frequently has an ameliorating effect. Note that obesity is characteristic of the adult form of diabetes, juvenile diabetics being of normal weight.

Figure 7.30 Possible aetiology of juvenile diabetes.

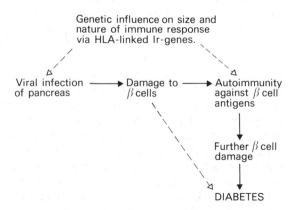

The degree of insulin deficiency in adult diabetes is quite variable, in contrast with the absolute lack of insulin common in the juvenile form. In both cases, however, deficiency lies in the production or release of insulin from the pancreas, rather than synthesis of an inactive mutant insulin molecule or an excess of an insulin antagonist, both of which possibilities have been suggested in the past. A particular phase of insulin release from the β cell has been shown to be defective in adult onset diabetes. In the normal response to glucose, there is a prompt release of insulin stored in the β cell, followed by a gradual further release of presumably newly synthesized insulin molecules. It seems that the adult diabetic with partial insulin insufficiency lacks the early, rapid insulin-release phase while retaining gradual secretion, leading to a delay in reaching appropriate insulin levels. The exact nature of the cellular defect in the β cells and the way this is genetically determined in adult diabetes are, however, yet to be elucidated.

The therapeutic control of diabetes depends on the degree of insulin lack. Where this is only partial, as in most obese adult diabetics, weight reduction and the use of oral hypoglycaemic drugs, such as sulphonylureas, to lower the blood sugar are often sufficient. In severe diabetics, including some obese adults and most cases in children and young people, insulin replacement therapy is required. In most instances, insulin treatment is completely effective. Rarely, however, resistance to insulin is encountered. An interesting immunological mechanism for this has been discovered. Insulin-resistant patients produce an antibody against the receptor for insulin on the surface of tissue cells, thereby blocking insulin action (a further example of autoimmunity in diabetes). A form of therapy for severe diabetes which will doubtless be seen in the future is pancreatic transplantation.

Table 7.5 summarises the major differences between the two forms of diabetes, emphasizing their distinct natures.

	Juvenile	Adult
Age of onset	< 25 years	> 25 years
Insulin deficiency	complete	variable
Genetics	HLA association; immune response genes	no HLA association
Environmental factors	virus	diet, exercise
Weight	normal	obese
Mechanism	autoimmunity, β cell damage	failure of rapid release by β cells (non-immunological)
Therapy	insulin-dependent	diet, hypoglycaemic drugs, insulin

Table 7.5 Comparison of juvenile and adult forms of diabetes

874

The commonest mental disorders are schizophrenia and manic-depressive psychosis and both have a major genetic component. The population incidence of schizophrenia is about 1%, with a strong familial tendency. Concordance between monozygotic twins ranges from 20% to 70% in different studies, depending on the criteria used in defining the disease; however, concordance is always considerably less than 100%, indicating an important role for environmental factors as well. The biochemical basis of schizophrenia is not yet understood. Manic-depressive psychosis often takes the 'bipolar' form of alternation of periods of excitement and elation with stuporous depression, though in some patients episodes are confined to depressions. There is evidence for an X-linked dominant mode of inheritance in the bipolar disease, from families which follow quite closely the pattern described on page 838. There is also tentative evidence from genetic linkage for a gene controlling manic-depressive psychosis located on the X-chromosome, between those for colour blindness and the Xg blood group (Figure 7.13, p. 840). Once again, the biochemical basis of the disorder is unknown.

NEOPLASIA

Environmental factors involved in neoplasia—chemical, viral, irradiation, etc.—have been discussed at length in Section 6. The inherited component in most common neoplasms is obscure; though several examples of familial incidence of neoplasms are known, their inheritance is non-Mendelian, most probably polygenic and multifactorial. However, in a few instances, mostly rare, simple Mendelian genetics do apply, showing that single mutant genes can be responsible for certain neoplasms. Mostly these are autosomal dominants, for example familial polyposis of the colon, neurofibromatosis (von Recklinghausen's disease) and some cases of bilateral retinoblastoma in children. Some enzyme deficiencies, autosomal recessives, predispose to neoplasia, e.g. albinism and xeroderma pigmentosum (p. 773) which predispose to carcinoma of the skin. Neoplasms are also frequently associated with the inherited immune deficiency diseases (p. 78), which has been taken to indicate that an important role of the immune system is to prevent the appearance of neoplasms (p. 741). Conditions involving chromosomal aberrations are also associated with increased incidence of neoplasms, often leukaemia, as in Down's syndrome (p. 818).

Some of the common neoplasms which recur in families in non-Mendelian fashion include carcinomas of the breast, uterus, stomach and lung; leukaemia and Hodgkin's disease; neuroblastoma and medulloblastoma. Twin studies indicate a significant, but limited, genetic component (average concordance for monozygotic twins is around 20%). Here the genetic component interacts with environmental factors in a multifactorial inheritance and a variety of possible mechanisms for such interactions can be envisaged (Section 6). The fact that information for oncogenic viruses can exist in the host genome and be inherited directly (vertical transmission) may provide the basis of one possible mechanism. Genetic determination of the level of the immune response may also be important, either against a virus or the neoplasm itself. In this regard, possible associations between the major histocompatibility complex HLA and acute lymphatic leukaemia and Hodgkin's disease may be noted (p. 878). Studies of the inheritance of carcinoma of the breast show that daughters of women with this neoplasm are 3–4 times more likely to develop the same carcinoma than the general population, and evidence from the mouse supports a significant genetic component in breast carcinoma (p. 801). The existence of high and low incidence strains of mice for a variety of spontaneous specific neoplasms—mammary, lymphoid, lung, etc.—is also good evidence of the important role genetic constitution must play in the incidence of neoplasia.

ATHEROSCLEROSIS

It will be recalled from Section 5 that several factors contribute to the development of atherosclerosis, including blood cholesterol levels, diet, hypertension, cigarette smoking and so on. The role of inheritance is a reflection of the degree to which these individual factors are genetically determined. Once again an interaction between genetic and environmental factors is indicated, with the genetic factors themselves being complex and often polygenic (Figure 7.31). The major inherited factors in atherosclerosis concern the determination of serum cholesterol levels and blood pressure. *Hyperlipoproteinaemias* (hyperlipidaemias), where they involve raised cholesterol levels, produce increased atherosclerosis. Six types of hyperlipoproteinaemia have been distinguished and the inheritance of most of these is itself complex. Type II hyperlipoproteinaemia (familial hypercholesterolaemia, p. 663.) seems to be inherited as an autosomal dominant, with cholesterol levels two or three times normal. In heterozygotes, this leads to considerably increased risk of coronary disease (over 50% at age of 50); homozygotes are very severely affected and many die in youth. *Blood pressure* is controlled by several genes and in many cases the basis of essential hypertension appears to be polygenic, though it is quite likely that in some instances a single mutant gene can lead to hypertension. *Diabetes* as a cause of atherosclerosis has been discussed on p. 871. Finally, the effects of inheritance on *personality* in relation to coronary disease should not be

Figure 7.31 Aetiological factors in atherosclerosis and coronary artery disease.

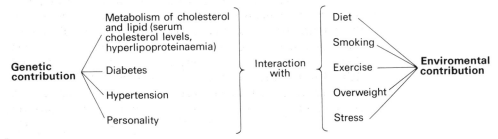

886

overlooked. Certain behaviour patterns predispose to heart disease—for example a characteristic combination would be ambition, aggressiveness, competitiveness and heavy cigarette smoking—and the genetic component in such behavioural traits is undoubtedly significant.

DISEASE ASSOCIATIONS

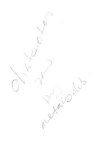

One means of providing information on the genetic basis of a multifactorial disease is to search for a relationship in individuals in the population between the occurrence of the disease and other genetic traits carried by the same individuals. When there is a concurrence of the disease and another trait in a frequency greater than that expected on a chance basis, an *association* is said to exist. This should not be confused with genetic linkage, which refers to the proximity of two genetic loci on a chromosome. Indeed, the fact that two polymorphic loci are linked would not be expected to lead to permanent association in the population of the traits they specify, since in time recombination should lead to random combinations of the traits (unless 'linkage disequilibrium' occurs, p. 878.) A classic example of disease association is that between duodenal ulcer and blood group O. The latter is found about 1.4 times more frequently in patients than in the normal population, indicating that group O individuals have a significantly higher risk of developing a duodenal ulcer than the rest of the population. This is not due to genetic linkage, but is an (undetermined) effect of blood group O on the physiology of the individual. Similarly, cancer of the stomach is slightly more common in individuals of blood group A. Associations of disease with blood group, however, are weak and generally unhelpful as regards the pathogenesis of the disorder; those between HLA and disease promise to be much more fruitful and are described below.

HLA and disease

An important insight has been provided into several diseases by the discovery of associations with the major histocompatibility complex of man, HLA. This is the genetic system which controls the antigens responsible for graft rejection, coding for antigenic molecules found on the surface of most tissue cells with the exception of red cells. The HLA system is highly polymorphic; the fact that tissue grafted between unrelated individuals is very unlikely to be accepted is a reflection of the great variety of HLA antigens in the population as a result of this genetic variation. It is now recognized that HLA plays a vital role as part of the immunological defence system and reference should be made to Section 2 for a fuller account of the structure and function of the HLA complex. In summary, there are four defined loci or regions, denoted HLA-A, B, C and D, each of which has several alleles which are detected as HLA antigens. In addition, the region contains genes which code for complement components, such as C2 and C4 as well as factor B of the alternative pathway. There are also genes which regulate the immune response, the immune response or Ir genes, which are linked to the HLA-D region. The complement and Ir genes are also polymorphic. Figure 2.46b is a map showing the positions of these genes as far as is known. The role of the products of these loci is described on pp. 176–180.

Many of the diseases which have been found to be HLA-associated share certain common features. They are all of unknown aetiology and lack a clearly identified causative agent. They are multifactorial and, while they run in families, the inherited component is probably due to more than one gene. In some there is evidence that the environmental agent is a virus. Many of these diseases involve autoimmune reactions and some have been discussed in Section 2 (pp. 187–212). Table 7.6 lists some of the diseases and shows the HLA antigens with which each is associated.

LINKAGE DISEQUILIBRIUM

This is a characteristic genetic feature of the HLA system which has an important bearing on the interpretation of the association between HLA and disease. We have noted that each of the HLA loci is highly polymorphic with many alleles in the population. The fact that recombination can occur between, for example, the HLA-A and HLA-B loci with a frequency of about 1% means that, given enough time (the half-life is about 2000 years), the alleles at each of these loci should not be found in any particular association in the population, other than that governed by chance. Thus, if particular alleles of HLA-A and HLA-B each have a frequency in the population of 0.1 (10%), the chance of finding

Disease	HLA antigen*	Relative risk†
Ankylosing spondylitis	B27	86
Reiter's disease	B27	38
Juvenile rheumatoid arthritis	B27	5
Yersinia arthritis	B27	
Multiple sclerosis	B7	1.6
	DW2	5
Myasthenia gravis	B8	4
Psoriasis vulgaris	BW37	6
Juvenile diabetes	B8	2
	BW15	3
Graves' disease	B8	4
Addison's disease	B8	6
Coeliac disease	B8	10
De Quervain's thyroiditis	BW35	27
Hodgkin's disease	B5	1.6
Acute lymphocytic leukaemia	A2,B12	‡

Table 7.6 Associations between HLA and disease

* The letters A, B and D refer to HLA loci, and the numbers following are serologically detected antigens coded by those loci; W, for Workshop, indicates an antigen which is not fully characterised.
† The number of times more frequently the disease occurs in individuals of the HLA type indicated than in the rest of the population.
‡ Small increase reported, but controversial at present.

them in combination on one chromosome is $(0.1)^2$ or 0.01 (1%). While this principle indeed holds in practice for most HLA alleles, some combinations are found more frequently than predicted from the gene frequencies (i.e. are in association in the population.). For example, the alleles of the A and B loci known as *A1* and *D8* occur together in Northern (Celtic) European populations about four times more frequently than expected. The tendency for certain alleles of linked loci to occur in combination is conveyed by the term *linkage disequilibrium*. Disequilibrium probably arises as a result of natural selection and indicates an advantage for certain combinations of HLA alleles over others. Quite likely the selective advantage lies in increased resistance to infectious disease conferred by certain combinations. The possible significance of linkage disequilibrium in some examples of HLA-associated diseases is discussed below.

ANKYLOSING SPONDYLITIS

One of the most striking associations discovered to date is that between the HLA antigen B27 and ankylosing spondylitis. This is a form of arthritis involving fusion (ankylosis) of the sacroiliac and vertebral joints and ossification of spinal ligaments, leading to rigidity of the spine ('bamboo spine'). The sacroiliac joints are usually affected first, with attendant lower back pain and stiffness, progressing to involvement of the whole of the spine and also the large peripheral joints. Changes in the vertebral joints resemble those of rheumatoid arthritis (p. 207), though the latter does not lead to ankylosis. Rheumatoid factor is not present in patients with ankylosing spondylitis and there is no evidence for autoimmunity. A further difference from rheumatoid arthritis is that males are affected about eight times more frequently than females. There is a strong familial tendency, with autosomal dominant inheritance (p. 827). The affected family members all carry the B27 antigen, though not all male siblings with B27 will develop ankylosing spondylitis. In many families, a healthy mother transmits the B27 antigen to sick male offspring, similar to an X-linked inheritance pattern, but note that this disease is *sex-influenced* and not sex-linked. In individuals homozygous for B27, females seem to be affected as often as males, indicating that the double gene dosage may overcome the sex influence. Within the population, B27 is found in 90% of all patients, compared with its frequency of only 9% among normal individuals. Individuals carrying B27 are about 100 times more likely to develop ankylosing spondylitis than non-B27 individuals and this is called the *relative risk*. Even in countries with a very low incidence of B27 in the population, e.g. 1% in Japan, the majority of patients again carry B27; and in African Negroes where B27 is very rare, ankylosing spondylitis does not occur at all. This very close association suggests that the B27 allele itself plays an important part in the aetiology of the disease, though the fact that 10% of patients lack B27 indicates a role for other genes too.

How might this high degree of association be explained? One possibility is that B27 resembles an antigen on a pathogenic micro-organism involved in the disease process. B27 carriers would be naturally tolerant of this antigen and might therefore have increased susceptibility to the organism. Such a situation is called 'molecular mimicry'. Alternatively, B27 might have an affinity for a pathogen and act as its receptor, causing the agent to be bound to B27-bearing cells and hence leading to pathogenic affects in B27-positive individuals. A third possibility is that there is a separate 'disease gene' linked to B27 and with a high degree of linkage disequilibrium between it and B27. In this case B27 is only a 'marker' for the presence of the disease gene and is not itself involved in the disease process. Unfortunately details of the causes of the disease are unknown. Environmental factors, such as bacterial infection with *Yersinia, Shigella* or *Salmonella* species, are probably involved as only 10% of males carrying B27 develop ankylosing spondylitis.

HLA AND AUTOIMMUNITY

Ankylosing spondylitis appears not to involve an autoimmune reaction. Many of the other HLA-associated diseases, on the other hand, are autoimmune disorders, including Addison's disease, myasthenia gravis, chronic active hepatitis and systemic lupus erythematosus (see Section 2). Others in which an autoimmune origin is suspected include coeliac disease (gluten enteropathy), multiple sclerosis and juvenile onset diabetes. In none of these is the association with HLA as strong as in ankylosing spondylitis, the relative risk ranging from 1·5 to 10. The association is almost always with an allele of the HLA-B locus rather than HLA-A, and is frequently even stronger with the HLA-D locus. The explanation for these associations most favoured at present is that the tendency towards organ-specific autoimmunity is governed by Ir genes in the HLA-D region. Some alleles of Ir genes are likely to be in linkage disequilibrium with alleles of the HLA-D or HLA-B loci. Thus the Ir gene responsible for juvenile onset diabetes would be linked to and in linkage disequilibrium with HLA-B15, while that for multiple sclerosis would be in disequilibrium with HLA-DW2 (Table 7.6). The association with HLA would therefore not be due to the HLA-B or D loci themselves. However, definitive explanations for these associations cannot be given at present because of the obscurity of the aetiology of many of these diseases. External agents are often involved and Ir genes may determine the immune response to them as well. The following examples indicate some of the complexities.

COELIAC DISEASE (GLUTEN ENTEROPATHY)

In this condition there is impaired absorption of nutrients from the small intestine due to atrophy of the intestinal villi, which leads to a typical *malabsorption* syndrome. In children, onset is usually between 6–18 months, with failure to thrive, muscular wasting, iron-deficiency anaemia, folate deficiency, diarrhoea and vomiting as characteristic symptoms. Symptoms of malabsorption may also appear or reappear in adults. The underlying cause of disease is a sensitivity to *gluten*, the protein component of wheat and rye, and the clinical effects and intestinal damage are alleviated by a gluten-free diet. The basis of gluten sensitivity is unknown. Patients often have serum antibody to gluten and delayed hypersensitivity is demonstrable by skin testing with gluten fractions. However, it is impossible to say whether these immunological findings are important to the aetiology of coeliac disease or whether they develop secondarily to direct gluten-induced intestinal damage. Consequently, the role of HLA genes in the disease is speculative, but could be an effect on the binding of gluten to the intestinal epithelium or on the level of immune response (hypersensitivity) developed to gluten. Coeliac disease is commonest in HLA-B8-positive individuals with a relative risk factor of about 10.

MULTIPLE SCLEROSIS (MS)

MS has also been found to be associated with certain HLA antigens. MS is a gradually progressive disease of the brain and spinal cord characterised by patches of demyelination of nerve fibres. It is the commonest neurological disease of young adults in temperate climates. The onset of symptoms occurs around the age of 30 and there may be long periods of remission followed by relapses at intervals of months or years. Early symptoms are mild, frequently affecting vision, but gradually there is involvement of the limbs, disturbances of speech, emotion, sensation and bladder control, and ultimately paralysis. The course of the disease is highly variable and the average duration is probably more than 25 years. At first, periods of remission lasting months or years often separate episodes, but these intervals grow shorter until disablement is permanent and progressive. However, the variety of clinical patterns in different patients is so great as to suggest that there may be more than a single aetiology.

MS is a multifactorial disease, caused by a combination of inherited and environmental factors; the former include tissue (HLA) type, and the latter may involve an infectious agent (a virus). The global distribution of MS shows some interesting features. It is principally a White man's disease, with a low incidence in Negroes and Orientals. In addition to racial distribution, geography has an intriguing influence, in that MS becomes more frequent the greater the distance from the equator, i.e. at increasing latitude. This applies particularly in the Northern hemisphere, and Northern and Central Europe are considered high risk areas. Some of the highest rates of MS are found in the northern areas of the UK, in Scotland and the Orkney and Shetland Islands (152 per 100,000 in the latter compared with 1–2 per 100,000 in Japan). However, South Australia and New Zealand are also high risk zones, while South Africa has a lower incidence. These differences suggest an environmental factor, possibly an infectious agent or diet, though the distribution of certain HLA antigens (below) among different populations may also be an important factor.

The main feature of the pathology of MS is the loss of myelin from nerve fibres in the brain and spinal cord. The effect of demyelination is an inability to transmit nerve impulses across the demyelinated zone (conduction block). Demyelination occurs in foci or plaques, which show signs of inflammation and accumulation of lymphocytes and monocytes around blood vessels (perivascular cuffing). The myelin of the nerve sheath is taken up by phagocytes. The presence of invading lymphocytes and macrophages is a strong indication of a cell-mediated response akin to delayed (Type IV) hypersensitivity, in which the target of response is myelin itself. This would put MS in the category of an autoimmune disease. Support for this concept has come from an experimental autoimmune reaction induced in animals by injection of whole brain homogenate in complete Freund's adjuvant. This disease—*experimental autoimmune encephalitis, EAE*—has the characteristic demyelination of MS and macrophages can be seen to attack the myelin sheath, which is taken up and digested by them. EAE can also be produced by immunisation with the characteristic *basic protein* which forms about 15% of the myelin sheath. EAE can be transferred with T cells, but not with antimyelin antibodies, and is a true cell-mediated autoimmune reaction to the basic protein in the brain. However, although these is a strong similarity between EAE and MS, the nature of the antigen in the latter is not yet known.

The geographical distribution of MS may be related to diet, in particular to the high consumption of saturated animal fat in countries where MS is common (e.g. Western Europe, North America) and a low consumption where MS is rare (e.g. Black Africa, Asia, Japan). Similarly, the feeding of babies on cow's milk rather than breast milk also correlates with the geographical prevalence of MS. One hypothesis is that a diet which is rich in dairy fat from birth may be deficient in essential polyunsaturated fatty acids which are necessary for the metabolism of myelin, and that in consequence the myelin laid down in infancy is somehow 'defective'. Such meylin might later be more susceptible to damage by the initiating agent of MS (as yet unidentified) and hence become a target of immunological attack more easily than 'normal' myelin. It was shown some time ago that rats are more susceptible to EAE if reared from birth on a diet deficient in certain essential fatty acids.

Recently, there has been considerable interest in a possible viral aetiology for MS. This is based partly on epidemiology, including the effect of migration of individuals from high risk areas, such as Northern Europe, to low risk areas, such as South Africa. It is found that if migration occurs after the age of 15 years, individuals take the high-incidence risk with them to the low risk zone; before 15 years, the tendency is to adopt the risk of the host country. Together with the age distribution of onset between 20 and 40 years, these observations have suggested that MS may be a late consequence of a virus infection occurring before the age of 15 years. Moreover, there are similarities between demyelination in MS and that in encephalitis following certain virus infections such as *measles*. If a virus is involved, it would have to be capable of very prolonged latency and duration of infection. Viruses with this as their major characteristic are known as *slow viruses* (p. 366) and have indeed been found in diseases of the CNS such as kuru and progressive multifocal leucoencephalopathy in man, and scrapie and visna in sheep, though the pathology of diseases produced by the slow viruses is quite unlike MS. Subacute sclerosing panencephalitis (SSPE) is a rare complication of measles infection in which the virus multiplies and spreads in the brain (p. 342). The measles virus has become a likely candidate for the initiating agent of MS, partly because it fulfils the criteria of a childhood infection capable of producing complications years later. A search for measles antibodies in MS patients has revealed a raised level compared with normal controls and has reinforced the suspicion that measles may be the slow virus involved in MS. Antimeasles antibody can also be found in the cerebrospinal fluid and is probably produced locally.

Deriving a likely train of events leading to MS from the above information must, of necessity, be very speculative at present. However, it is helpful to bring together the following key points of viral involvement, diet, hypersensitivity and HLA-association.

1 MS may be a late consequence of a childhood virus infection, the virus persisting in latent form in cells of the CNS for several years. The measles virus may be directly involved. The virus is likely to persist following infection in individuals who are slow to mount an efficient cell-mediated immune response against it. Although most of the virus is eventually successfully removed in the acute infection, some particles may lie dormant in nerve cells for many years. For unknown reasons, the virus may reactivate in adulthood, perhaps expressing viral antigen at the surface of its host cell or altering either a histocompatibility antigen (p. 177) or myelin itself. The myelin of individuals who were not breast fed and who have had a diet rich in animal fat may be particularly liable to alteration. For any of these reasons, the cell surface is now recognisable as antigenic by T lymphocytes (passing through the blood-brain barrier) and hence becomes the target of immune attack. Note that the virus itself does not demyelinate the nerve cell; this is a result of the host immune response (hypersensitivity).

2 There is good evidence that demyelination in MS does indeed have an immunological basis. The response is cell-mediated, with lymphocyte and macrophage involvement, as in a Type IV hypersensitivity reaction (p. 163). It is likely that sensitised T cells recognise an antigen on nerve fibres and release lymphokines to attract macrophages and other lymphocytes to the area (perivascular cuffing). Activated macrophages may then proceed to attack the myelin sheath. In addition, there may be a direct action of T cells on the target nerve cell. An unfortunate gap in our knowledge at present is the identity of the antigen recognised on the demyelinating cells. It may be a component of myelin itself, such as the basic protein, in which case MS is an autoimmune condition resembling EAE. Alternatively, it could be a viral antigen expressed on nerve cells, perhaps in association with a histocompatibility antigen (p. 177), or even an altered

histocompatibility molecule itself (Figure 2.48).

3 The HLA antigens showing association with MS in the population are HLA-A3, HLA-B7 and HLA-DW2, coded by the A, B and D loci respectively. The three alleles are themselves in linkage disequilibrium, i.e. in the population they occur more frequently together on the same chromosome than expected from their individual gene frequencies. The MS association is strongest with DW2 and progressively less with B7 and A3. Individuals carrying DW2 are about 5 times more likely to develop MS than the rest of the population. The fact that these associations are rather weak in comparison, for example, with those for B27 and ankylosing spondylitis, is an indication that DW2 itself is not involved in MS. The gene predisposing to the disease is very likely an immune response gene linked to DW2 and in disequilibrium with it, thus producing an association with DW2 in the population. If susceptibility to MS is governed by an HLA-linked immune response gene, several mechanisms could be envisaged. (a) An Ir gene could control the level of CMI response to the initial virus infection, perhaps increasing the antibody response to the detriment of cell-mediated immunity and hence causing inefficient clearance of virus. (b) The Ir gene could influence the

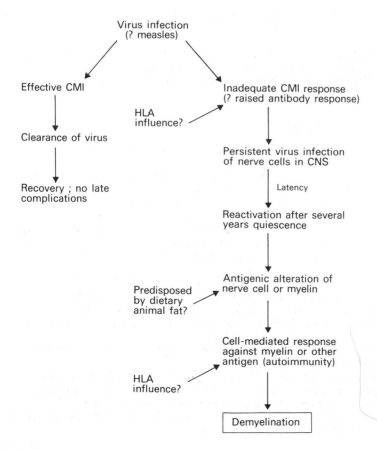

NORMAL INDIVIDUAL   **MS PATIENT**

Figure 7.32 Possible events in multiple sclerosis.

immune response to the antigens expressed much later, on nerve cells following virus reactivation. (c) It might predispose to the development of a harmful response against myelin, i.e. to autoimmunity. In these last two cases, the presence of the Ir gene in the individual would, in the right circumstances, allow a demyelinating immune response to occur. These possibilities are necessarily vague in the present state of ignorance concerning the details of the immune responses involved.

A summary of these possible mechanisms for MS is shown in Figure 7.32.

FURTHER READING

General

Bodmer W.F. & Cavalli-Sforza L.L. (1976) *Genetics, Evolution and Man.* W.H. Freeman.

Bondy P.K. & Rosenberg L.E. (1980) *Metabolic Control and Disease,* 8th edn. W.B. Saunders.

Clarke C.A. (1974) *Human Genetics and Medicine.* Institute of Biology's Studies in Biology No. 20. Edward Arnold.

McKusick V.A. (1969) *Human Genetics,* 2nd edn. Foundations of Modern Genetics Series. Prentice Hall.

McKusick V.A. (1975) *Mendelian Inheritance in Man: Catalogs of Autosomal Dominant, Autosomal Recessive and X-linked Phenotypes,* 4th edn. Johns Hopkins Press.

McMurray W.C. (1977) *Essentials of Human Metabolism.* Harper Row.

Nora J.J. & Fraser F.C. (1974) *Medical Genetics: Principles and Practice.* Lea and Febiger.

Stanbury J.B., Wyngaarden J.B. & Fredrickson D.S. (1978) *The Metabolic Basis of Inherited Disease,* 4th edn. McGraw-Hill.

Thompson J.S. & Thompson M.W. (1980) *Genetics in Medicine.* 3rd. edn. W.B. Saunders.

Specific topics

Barnhart M.I., Henry R.L. & Lusher J.M. (1976) *Sickle Cell.* A Scope Publication, The Upjohn Company.

Emerson P.M. & Grimes A.J. (1982) Red-cell metabolism: hereditary enzymopathies. In Hardisty R.M. & Weatherall D.J., *Blood and its Disorders,* 2nd edn., p. 265. Blackwell Scientific Publications.

HLA and Disease Susceptibility. *Immunological Reviews* (1983), **70**.

Huehns E.R. (1982) The structure and function of haemoglobin: clinical disorders due to abnormal haemoglobin. In Hardisty R.M. & Weatherall D.J., *Blood and its Disorders,* 2nd edn., p. 323. Blackwell Scientific Publications.

Human Malformations. *British Medical Bulletin* (1976), **32**, No. 1.

McVicar E.M. (1979) Hartnup disease. *J. Clin Invest.,* **69**, 999.

Multiple Sclerosis. *British Medical Bulletin* (1977), **33**, No. 1.

Neufeld E.F. (1981) Lessons from genetic disorders of lysosomes. *Harvey Lectures,* Series 75, 41.

Race R.R. & Sanger R. (1975) *Blood Groups in Man,* 6th edn. Blackwell Scientific Publications.

The Muscular Dystrophies. *British Medical Bulletin* (1980), 36, No. 2.

Weatherall D.J. & Clegg J.B. (1982) The molecular genetics of human haemoglobin: the thalassaemia syndromes. In Hardisty R.M. & Weatherall D.J. (eds.), *Blood and its Disorders,* 2nd edn., p. 401. Blackwell Scientific Publications.

INDEX

Abelson virus 799
ABO blood groups
  antibodies 88, 131
  detection by haemagglutination 131
  disease associations 877
  matching in transfusion 131
  polymorphism 863
Abortion, spontaneous 814, 824
Abrin 750
Abscess 26–27, 525
  chronic 57
  'cold' 63
  stitch 526
Acetylaminofluorene (AAF)
  as carcinogen 755–759
  mechanism of carcinogenesis 757–759
Acetylcholine receptor
  autoantibodies in myasthenia gravis 198–199
  isolation 199
N-Acetylglucosamine
  in mucopolysccharides 850
  on neoplastic cells 716–718
N-Acetylneuraminic acid 135, 716, 855
Achlorhydria 481
Achondroplasia 828(t)
Acid phosphatase
  in prostate cancer 724
Acquired immunity 165–168
Actinomycetes, thermophilic 163
Actinomycin C
  immunosuppression by 171
Actinomycin D
  immunosuppression by 171
  inhibition of viral replication 236, 321
Acute haemorrhagic conjunctivitis 289
Acute haemorrhagic cystitis 276
Acute pharyngoconjunctival fever 276
Acute respiratory disease (ARD) 272, 275
Acute phase
  protein 42, 67
  reaction 42
Acyclovir 268
Adamantanamine 332
Addison's disease 849, 878(t)
Adenine arabinoside 267
Adeno-associated virus (AAV) 240, 246, 274, 276, 283
Adenocarcinoma 692(t), 693, 721
Adenoma 692(t), 693
  endocrine glands 695, 725(t)
Adenoviridae 272–276
Adenoviruses 272–276
  as helper 240, 246
  cellular infection 274–275
  classification 274

common cold 298
diseases 275–276
hybrids with SV40 275
inclusion body 244, 274
latent infection 273, 275
oncogenic properties 272, 777, 784, 791
replication 233–234, 240, 274
structure 221, 223(a), 224(b), 272–273
transmission 275
vaccination 276
Adenylate cyclase 40, 56, 414, 421–423, 432–433, 629
  bacterial 426–427
  cholera toxin 414, 421–423
  components 422–423
  mast cells 153
  mechanism of activation 422–423
Adhesions 27, 48, 58
Adjuvant 80, 166, 399, 591, 593–594
  Freund's 80, 167, 193, 194, 400, 594, 882
ADP
  in haemostasis 637
  in platelet granules 626
  in platelet reactions 626–630
ADP-ribosylation 414
  adenylate cyclase 414, 421–423
  elongation factor 2 414, 416–417
ADP-ribosyltransferases 410–426
Adrenal gland
  aldosterone release 677
  autoimmunity 188, 201
  control of steroid production 849
  cortical hyperplasia 849
  tumours 677, 725(t)
Adrenaline (epinephrine)
  and blood pressure 676
  in pulmonary oedema 685
Adrenocorticotrophin (ACTH) 849
  produced by cancer cells 725(t), 726
Adrenogenital syndrome 830(t), 848–850
Adventitia 650, 651, 652
Aedes mosquito 302, 307, 308
  Aedes aegypti 307, 308, 309
Aerobacter aerogenes 24
Affinity chromatography 101, 102
Aflatoxin 706, 760–762, 797
Agammaglobulinaemia
  Bruton-type (X-linked) 78, 117, 571, 836(t)
  infections in 79, 150, 483, 571
Ageing
  autoimmunity 194
  decline in immune response 80
Agglutination tests 131–136
  antiglobulin 133, 159, 196
  bacterial 131, 135
  Coombs' 133, 159, 196
  direct 133

Hashimoto's thyroiditis 134
infectious mononucleosis 134
latex 134
passive 133, 134
Paul-Bunnell 134
procedure 133
prozone 133
red cell (haemagglutination) 133–135
rheumatoid arthritis 134
Rose-Waaler 134
typhoid fever 135
Widal 135
Agranulocytosis 196, 483
Alastrim 278, 280
Albinism 830(t), 842
  complementation 842
  skin carcinoma 875
  tyrosinase-negative 842
  tyrosinase-positive 842
Aldosterone 676–678, 680, 848–849
Aldosteronism 677, 678, 725(t)
Aleutian disease of mink 262, 367(t), 369
  glomerulonephritis 262, 369
Alexander cell line 797
Alkaline phosphatase
  deficiency in CML cells 723
Alkaptonuria 830(t), 842, 843
Alkylating agents
  carcinogens 760
  immunosuppression by 171
Allele 825
Allelic exclusion 96
Allergic asthma 156
Allergic encephalomyelitis 350
Allergy, *see* Hypersensitivity
Allograft 168
Allopurinol 846, 848
Alpha-fetoprotein (AFP) 727(t), 727–728
Alpha-1,4-glucosidase
  deficiency 853
Altered-self hypothesis 109, 178–179
Alum
  adjuvant 166
Alzheimer's senile dementia 367
Amantadine 332
Amaurotic family idiocy 855–856
Amelia 869
Aminoacidaemias 830 (t)
  see specific examples
Amino acid metabolism
  defects in 841–844
  see specific examples
Amino acid transport
  defects 857–858
Aminoacidurias 830 (t), 857
Aminofluorenes
  carcinogens 755–759
Aminoglycosides
  resistance to 463(t), 464–465

892

558–560, 561, 567, 579, 583–584)
Clostridium perfringens 579, 581, 583–584
Salmonella 552, 558–560
Vibrio parahaemolyticus 561, 567
Foot and mouth disease 284
vaccine 477
Foreign body
in chronic abscess 57
response 59, 63–64
Forssman antigen 134
Fowlpox 277
Frame-shift mutation 769, 771
Fungi 151
cell-mediated immunity 74, 78, 79, 151
hypersensitivity 164–165
immunological defence 74, 78, 79
infection in T cell deficiency 79, 151
skin tests 165

Gajdusek 371
Galactosaemia 831(t), 844–845
β-Galactosidase 541
Galen 3
Gamma radiation 762
Ganglion
dorsal root 257
sacral 258, 267
trigeminal 258, 267
Gangliosides, G_{M1}, G_{M2} 855
cholera toxin receptor 424
neurotoxin receptors 434, 435, 437
storage disease (gangliosidosis) 831(t), 855–856
Gangliosidoses 831(t), 855–856
Gangrene
gas 581–583
primary 581
secondary 581
Gap junctions 713(c), 714–715
Gargoyle cells 851
Garrod, Sir Archibald 840, 857
Gas gangrene 409, 429–430, 578, 579, 581–583
epidemiology 583
pathogenesis 581–582
septicaemia 582
toxins 409, 413(t), 429–430, 580, 582
treatment 583
Gastroenteritis 487, 545, 548–549, 558–560
acute infectious 284
coronaviruses 299
echoviruses 297
E. coli 456, 540, 545, 547, 548–549
non-bacterial 284, 364–366
Norwalk virus 283–284, 297, 365
rotaviruses 297, 364–366
Salmonella 545, 552, 554, 558–560
transmissible, of piglets 299
Gastrointestinal tract
opportunistic infections 481

Gaucher's disease 831(t), 856
osteomyelitis in 560
Gelatinous lesion 652
Gemfibrozil 671
Gene cloning 470
Gene complementation 733, 774
albinism 842
General paralysis of the insane 615
Genetic engineering 446, 470–477
practical applications 476–477
Genetic heterogeneity 842
Genetic load 834
Genital herpes 257, 258, 262, 263(t), 266–268
Gentamicin 465
German measles, *see* Rubella
Ghon, Anton 598
Ghon complex 598
Ghon focus 598
Giant cells 59–60, 64, 265, 266, 332, 335, 340, 598, 604
Aschoff 504
Langhans 60, 604
Warthin-Finkeldy 340, 341
Giant cell pneumonia 151, 341
Gingivitis 509, 510
Gingivostomatitis 263(t), 266
Glandular fever, *see* Infectious mononucleosis
Glomerular basement membrane, *see also* Glomerulonephritis, Goodpasture's syndrome
antibodies and renal damage 202–203
immunofluorescent staining 138–139, 162, 202
Glomerulonephritis 138–139, 162, 506, 508, 614
see also Goodpasture's syndrome
acute 506
Aleutian disease of mink 369
antigen–antibody complexes and 126, 139, 162, 202, 506, 614
hypertension 676
immunofluorescence 138–139, 162, 202
LCM virus 262
mechanisms 162, 202
post-streptococcal 162, 506
syphilis 614
Glucocerebrosidase 856
Glucocorticoids
in wound healing 48, 65
Glucose-6-phosphatase 852, 853
deficiency 852
Glucose-6-phosphate dehydrogenase
deficiency 24–25, 483, 836(t), 859–861
genetic studies 860
haemolytic anaemia 859–860
hexose monophosphate shunt 22
malaria 860–861
variants (A+, A−, B) 670, 860
X-linkage 840
Glucose tolerance test 870
Glutathione 22, 431, 859–860
Glutathione peroxidase 22

Gluten enteropathy 880–881
Glycogen
metabolism 852–853
storage diseases (glycogenoses) 831(t), 852–854
Glycosaminoglycans, *see* Mucopolysaccharides
Glycosyltransferases 628, 711–712
Gm types 190
Goldblatt, H. 676
Gonococci 26
see also Neisseria gonorrhoeae
infection in complement deficiency 125
pili 403, 531, 532, 533, 538
Gonorrhoea 530, 536–540
carriers 486, 538
control 540
females 538
immunity 539
males 538
ophthalmia neonatorum 538, 539
prevalence 537, 611
transmission 489, 537–538
treatment 461, 467, 539
Goodpasture's syndrome 138–139, 188(t), 203
Gout 26, 847–848
inheritance (primary familial) 847
joint damage 26, 847
tophi 847
Graft rejection 168–176
antibody-mediated 175
mechanisms 173–176
T-cell mediated 174–175
Graft-versus-host (GVH) reaction 176
Gram, Christian 386
Gram stain 386
Granulation tissue 44–46
Granulocytes, *see specific types*
Granulocytopenia 16
Granulomas 59–64, 591, 597, 601, 604, 614
Aschoff body 503
foreign body reaction 59, 63–64
Hodgkin's disease 61
leprosy 61, 601, 604
syphilis 614
tubercle 61–63, 597
Grass sickness 590
Graves's disease, *see* Thyrotoxicosis
Greenland
measles in 327, 340
Griffith, F. 450
transformation experiment 450–451
Growth hormone 470, 476
Guanine
reaction with carcinogens 758–759, 769–770
Guanylate cyclase 153, 433
Guarnieri body 244, 278, 280
Guatemala
dysentery in 461
Guillain-Barré syndrome 329, 331
Gumma 614, 616
Gut-associated lymphoid tissue 74, 75

896

898

natural killer cells in 745
neoplasms in 741–742

Obesity 873
Ochronosis 843
Ocular albinism 840
Oedema 681–686
  cardiac 684–685
  defined 681
  famine (nutritional) 683
  formation 682–683
  inflammatory 6, 682–683
  laryngeal 153
  pitting 682
  postural 683
  pulmonary 685–686
  renal 684
Oesophagus, cancer of
  incidence 699, 703(c), 706
Oncogen
  defined 751
Oncogene hypothesis 787, 805–808
Oncogenes 784–788, 805–808
Oncornaviruses 777–789, 797–802
  gene map 784
  transforming genes 784–788, 798,
    805, 807
O'nyong-nyong 301(t), 303
Oophoritis 338, 339
Ophthalmia neonatorum (528, 529)
Opportunistic infections, pathogens
    151, 173, 381, 478–485
  antimicrobial drug resistance 467,
    484
  clostridia 579
  conditions for 481–485
  cytomegalovirus 262, 270, 271
  fungi as 151
  hospital acquired 485
  neonates 485
  nosocomial 485
  transplant recipients 173
  viruses as 151
Opsonic adherence 146
Opsonin 16–19, 78, 402
  C-reactive protein 42
Opsonisation 16–19, 143(d), 145
Orbivirus 364
Orchitis 338, 339, 605
Orfvirus
  structure 223(e), 278
Organisation 46–47
  infarcts 649
  thrombi 646, 668–669
Original antigenic sin 325
Orthomyxoviridae 313–332
Orthomyxoviruses 218, 219, 313–332
  see also Influenza viruses
  budding 238, 239, 321
  replication 235–240
  structure 222, 223, 314–317
Orthopoxviruses 278
Osteitis 526
Osteomyelitis 57, 518, 526–527, 560
  chronic 527
    amyloidosis in 66
  pyaemia 490, 527

Osteoporosis 844
Osteosarcoma 692(t), 700, 763
  interferon treatment 252
Otitis media 502, 514
Ouchterlony double diffusion method
    127–130
  applications 129–130
Owl-eye cells 270
Oxidation-reduction potential 409,
    579, 582, 583, 586
Oxygen-dependent killing 21–23
  inherited defects 24–25

P, red cell antigen 196
Panama canal 308
Pancarditis 503
Pancreas
  autoimmunity 188, 872–873
Pannus 207–209
Panton–Valentine leucocidin 411(t),
    432–433, 524
Papanicolaou, G.N. 695
Papilloma 692(t), 693
Papillomaviruses 283, 777(t),
    789–790
  human 789–790
  Shope 789
Papovaviridae 283
Papovaviruses 368, 776, 777(t),
    789–791
  see also SV40 virus
  helper virus 246
  progressive multifocal
    leucoencephalopathy 368
  replication 233–234
Papule 269
Parabiosis 56
Paracortical areas 75–76
Parainfluenza viruses 332, 333(t),
    334(t), 336, 337–338
  common cold 298
  diseases due to 337
  structure 223
  transmission 253
  types 337
Paralysis
  flaccid 292, 434, 437, 589
  infantile, see Poliomyelitis
  spastic 434
Paramyxoviridae 332–345
  compared with Orthomyxoviridae
    333(t)
Paramyxoviruses 332–345
  cell fusion by 243, 332, 333(t),
    334, 335, 336–337
  cellular infection 334–336
  classification 332–334
  common cold 290
  haemadsorption 243
  haemagglutinin 331–335
  inclusion bodies 333(t), 335, 336
  measles virus 340–344
  mumps virus 338–339
  neuraminidase 331–335
  parainfluenzaviruses 337–338
  persistent infection 243, 332, 336
  properties 334(t)

replication 334–336
respiratory syncytial virus 344
structure 222, 223(b), 334–335
Parathyroid hormone (PTH) 725(t),
    726
Paratyphoid fever 554–558
  see also Typhoid fever
Parkinson's disease 367
Parotitis 338, 339
Paroxysmal cold haemoglobinuria
    196
Parvoviridae 283–284
Parvoviruses 283–284
  acute infectious gastroenteritis 283,
    284
  adeno-associated virus 240, 274,
    283
  Ditchling 284
  Hawaii 284
  Norwalk virus 283, 284
  size 217
Pasteur, Louis 346, 349–350, 502
Pasteurisation 592, 595
Patent ductus arteriosus 310
Pathogenicity
  bacterial structure and 383–409
  defined 381
  introduction to bacterial 381–382
  opportunistic 478–485
Pattern baldness 838
Paul–Bunnell test 134
Pavementing of leucocytes 4, 8–11
Pedigree patterns (Mendelian)
    826–838
  autosomal dominant 827
  autosomal recessive 829
  symbols 827
  X-linked dominant 838
  X-linked recessive 835
Pellagra 858
Penetrance 829
Penicillamine 162
Penicillin
  action 386, 390
  anaphylaxis 153
  as hapten 81, 160, 192
  haemolytic anaemia 160, 192
  resistance to 463–464, 467–468,
    530
  serum sickness-like syndrome 162
Penicillinase 463(t), 464, 467
Penis, carcinoma of 700
Penton 221
Peptic ulcer 27–28, 58
  and blood group O 877
  chronic 58
  multifactorial disease 868
  perforation 58, 172
Peptidoglycan 387–391
  action of lysozyme 390–391
  structure 388–390
Periarteritis 613
Pericarditis, fibrinous 6, 503
Periodontal disease 509–510
Periodontitis 509–510
Periosteitis 526
Peritonitis 27